A PEARSON AUSTRALIA CUSTOM BOOK

INDIVIDUAL DETERMINANTS OF HEALTH AND HUMAN BEHAVIOUR

This custom book has been compiled from:

SOCIAL PSYCHOLOGY
7TH EDITION
Vaughan & Hogg

PSYCHOLOGY AND LIFE
2ND EDITION
Gerrig, Zimbardo, Campbell, Cumming & Wilkes

INTRODUCTION TO HEALTH PSYCHOLOGY IN AUSTRALIA
2ND EDITION
Morrison, Bennet, Butow, Mullan & White

PSYCHOLOGY: FROM INQUIRY TO UNDERSTANDING
2ND EDITION
Lilienfeld, Lynn, Namy, Woolf, Jamieson, Marks, Slaughter

HEALTH: THE BASICS
11TH EDITION
Donatelle

PSYCHOSOCIAL ASPECTS OF HEALTHCARE
3RD EDITION
Drench, Noonan, Sharby, Ventura

PERSONALITY, INDIVIDUAL DIFFERENCES AND INTELLIGENCE
3RD EDITION
Maltby, Day, Macaskill

AN INTRODUCTION TO HEALTH PSYCHOLOGY
2ND EDITION
Morrison & Bennet

PSYCHOLOGY: CORE CONCEPTS
7TH EDITION
Zimbardo, Johnson, McCann

MANAGING STRESS AND ANXIETY IN VARIOUS CONTEXTS
Smith

OB THE ESSENTIALS
Robbins, Judge, Millet & Jones

LA TROBE UNIVERSITY

Pearson Australia
707 Collins Street
Melbourne VIC 3008
Australia
www.pearson.com.au

Project Management Team Leader: Jill Gillies
Production Manager: Aida Reyes Cruz
Copy Editor: Catherine du Peloux Menagé
Indexer: Mary Coe
Production Controller: Brad Smith
Custom Product Specialist: Lucie Bartonek

ISBN: 978 1 4886 1822 2

Printed and bound in Australia by The SOS Print + Media Group

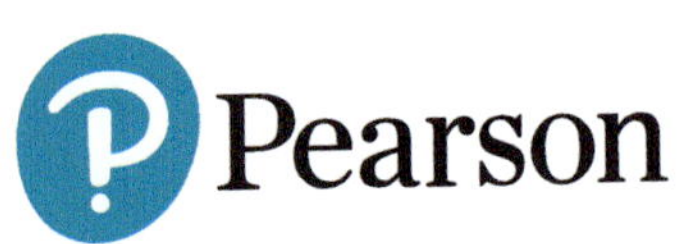

Acknowledgements

We would like to thank Kirsty Vondeling, Daphne Konas and Tammy Rendina for their help, suggestions and editing provided during the preparation of this book. We also appreciate the support received from the ever enthusiastic publishing team of Pearson, in particular, Lucie Bartonek and Victoria Rood.

Table of Contents

CHAPTER 1: LEARNING 1

The content in this section has been compiled from:

Lilienfeld, Lynn, Namy, Woolf, Jamieson, Marks & Slaughter, Chapter 6

Lilienfeld, S. O., Lynn, S. J., Namy, L. L., Woolf, N. J., Jamieson, G., Marks, A., & Slaughter, V. (2015). Learning: How nurture changes us. In S. O. Lilienfeld, S. J. Lynn, L. L. Namy, & N. J. Woolf (Eds.), *Psychology: From inquiry to understanding* (2nd ed., pp. 220–237, 239–249, 253–259). Melbourne, VIC: Pearson Australia.

CHAPTER 2: HUMAN DEVELOPMENT 37

The content in this section has been compiled from:

Gerrig, Zimbardo, Campbell, Cumming & Wilkes, Chapter 11

Gerrig, R. J., Zimbardo, P. G., Campbell, A. J., Cumming, S. R., & Wilkes, F. J. (Eds.). (2012). Human development across the lifespan. In *Psychology and life* (2nd ed., pp. 358–371, 373, 377–407). Frenchs Forest, NSW: Pearson Australia.

CHAPTER 3: MEMORY 87

The content in this section has been compiled from:

Gerrig et al., Chapter 8

Gerrig, R. J., Zimbardo, P. G., Campbell, A. J., Cumming, S. R., & Wilkes, F. J. (Eds.). (2012). Memory. In *Psychology and life* (2nd ed., pp. 239–278). Frenchs Forest, NSW: Pearson Australia.

CHAPTER 4: INTELLIGENCE 137

The content in this section has been compiled from:

Maltby, Day & Macaskill, Chapter 12

Maltby, J., Day, L., & Macaskill, A. (2013). Theories and measurement of intelligence. In J. Maltby, L. Day, & A. Macaskill (Eds.), *Personality, individual differences and intelligence* (3rd ed., pp. 279–297, 301). Harlow, Essex: Pearson Education.

Maltby, Day & Macaskill, Chapter 13
Maltby, J., Day, L., & Macaskill, A. (2013). The use of intelligence tests: What question emerge from the measurement of intelligence. In J. Maltby, L. Day, & A. Macaskill (Eds.), *Personality, individual differences and intelligence* (3rd ed., pp. 306–307, 313–321). Harlow, Essex: Pearson Education.

Gerrig et al., Chapter 10
Gerrig, R. J., Zimbardo, P. G., Campbell, A. J., Cumming, S. R., & Wilkes, F. J. (2012). Intelligence and intelligence assessment. In R. J. Gerrig, & P. G. Zimbardo, A. J. Campbell, S. R. Cumming, & F. J. Wilkes (Eds.), *Psychology and life* (2nd ed., pp. 331–333). Frenchs Forest, NSW: Pearson Australia.

Maltby, Day & Macaskill, Chapter 14
Maltby, J., Day, L., & Macaskill, A. (2013). The use of intelligence tests: What question emerge from the measurement of intelligence. In J. Maltby, L. Day, & A. Macaskill (Eds.), *Personality, individual differences and intelligence* (3rd ed., pp. 338–358, 370–371). Harlow, Essex: Pearson Education.

Maltby, Day & Macaskill, Chapter 15
Maltby, J., Day, L., & Macaskill, A. (2013). Further discussions and debates in intelligence: Sex differences in intelligence and emotional intelligence. In J. Maltby, L. Day, & A. Macaskill (Eds.), *Personality, individual differences and intelligence* (3rd ed., pp. 391–408). Harlow, Essex: Pearson Education.

Maltby, Day & Macaskill, Chapter 16
Maltby, J., Day, L., & Macaskill, A. (2013). The application of personality and intelligence in education and the workplace: The introduction of other intelligences. In J. Maltby, L. Day, & A. Macaskill (Eds.), *Personality, individual differences and intelligence* (3rd ed., pp. 410–422). Harlow, Essex: Pearson Education.

CHAPTER 5: PSYCHOLOGICAL DISORDERS **219**

The content in this section has been compiled from:
Lilienfeld, Lynn, Namy, Woolf, Jamieson, Marks & Slaughter, Chapter 16
Lilienfeld, S.O., Lynn, S. J., Namy, L. L., Woolf, N. J., Jamieson, G., Marks, A., & Slaughter, V. (2015). Psychological disorders: When adaptation breaks

down. In S. O. Lilienfeld, S. J. Lynn, L. L. Namy, N. J. Woolf, G. Jamieson, A. Marks, & V. Slaughter (Eds.), *Psychology: From inquiry to understanding* (2nd ed., pp. 449–460). Melbourne, VIC: Pearson Australia.

CHAPTER 6: HEALTH-RISK BEHAVIOURS **270**

The content in this section has been compiled from:

Morrison, Bennet, Butow, Mullan & White, Chapter 3

Morrison, V., Bennet, P., Butow, P., Mullan, B., & White, K. (2015). Health-risk behaviour. In V. Morrison, P. Bennet, P. Butow, B. Mullan, & K. White (Eds.), *Introduction to health psychology in Australia* (2nd ed., p. 63). Melbourne, VIC: Pearson Australia.

Donatelle, Chapter 10

Donatelle, R. J. (2015). Reaching and maintaining a healthy weight. In R. J. Donatelle (Ed.), *Health: The basics* (11th ed., pp. 293–294, 297–298). Upper Saddle River, NJ: Pearson Education.

Donatelle, Chapter 11

Donatelle, R. J. (2015). Improving your personal fitness. In R. J. Donatelle (Ed.), *Health: The basics* (11th ed., pp. 330–332). Upper Saddle River, NJ: Pearson Education.

Donatelle, Chapter 7

Donatelle, R. J. (2015). Recognizing and avoiding addiction and drug abuse. In R. J. Donatelle (Ed.), *Health: The basics* (11th ed., pp. 206–226). Upper Saddle River, NJ: Pearson Education.

Donatelle, Chapter 8

Donatelle, R. J.(2015). Drinking alcohol responsibly and ending tobacco use. In R. J. Donatelle (Ed.), *Health: The basics* (11th ed., pp. 228–258). Upper Saddle River, NJ: Pearson Education.

CHAPTER 7: MOTIVATION **340**

The content in this section has been compiled from:

Zimbardo, Johnson & McCann, Chapter 9

Zimbardo, P. G., Johnson, R. L., & McCann, V. (2014). Motivation and emotion. In P. G. Zimbardo, R. L. Johnson, & V. McCann (Eds.), *Psychology: Core concepts* (7th ed., pp. 363–387, 407-408). Upper Saddle River, NJ: Pearson Education

CHAPTER 8: BEHAVIOUR CHANGE **367**

The content in this section has been compiled from:

Drench, Noonan, Sharby & Ventura, Chapter 6

Drench, M. E., Noonan, A. C., Sharby, N., & Ventura, S. H. (2012). Motivation, adherence and collaborative treatment planning. In M. E. Drench, A. C. Noonan, N. Sharby, & S. H. Ventura (Eds.), *Pyschosocial aspects of health care (*3rd ed., pp. 114–141). Upper Saddle River, NJ: Pearson Education.

CHAPTER 9: SOCIAL PSYCHOLOGY **394**

The content in this section has been compiled from:

Vaughan & Hogg, Chapter 2

Vaughan, M. G., & Hogg, M. A. (2014). Social cognition and social thinking. In *Social psychology* (7th ed., pp. 38–43, 45–46, 56–72). Frenchs Forest, NSW: Pearson Australia.

Vaughan & Hogg, Chapter 3

Vaughan, M. G., & Hogg, M. A. (2014). Attribution and social explanation. In *Social psychology* (7th ed., pp. 74–78, 80–101). Frenchs Forest, NSW: Pearson Australia.

Vaughan & Hogg, Chapter 5

Vaughan, M. G., & Hogg, M. A. (2014). Attitudes. In *Social psychology* (7th ed., pp. 136–155, 159–162). Frenchs Forest, NSW: Pearson Australia.

Vaughan & Hogg, Chapter 6

Vaughan, M. G., & Hogg, M. A. (2014). Persuasion and attitude change. In *Social psychology* (7th ed., pp. 174–212). Frenchs Forest, NSW: Pearson Australia.

Vaughan & Hogg, Chapter 7

Vaughan, M. G., & Hogg, M. A. (2014). Social Influence. In *Social psychology* (7th ed., pp. 214–244). Frenchs Forest, NSW: Pearson Australia.

Vaughan & Hogg, Chapter 9

Vaughan, M. G., & Hogg, M. A. (2014). Leadership and decision making. In *Social psychology* (7th ed., pp. 312–313). Frenchs Forest, NSW: Pearson Australia.

CHAPTER 10: COMMUNICATION **529**

The content in this section has been compiled from:
Drench, Noonan, Sharby & Ventura, Chapter 5.
Drench, M.E., Noonan, A.C., Sharby, N., & Ventura, S.H. (2012). Motivation, adherence and collaborative treatment planning. In *Pyschosocial aspects of health care* (3rd ed., pp. 77-113). Upper Saddle River, NJ: Pearson Education.

CHAPTER 11: PERSONALITY **565**

The content in this section has been compiled from:
Maltby, Day & Macaskill, Chapter 4
Maltby, J., Day, L., & Macaskill, A. (2013). Theories and measurement of intelligence. In J. Maltby, L. Day, & A. Macaskill (Eds.), *Personality, individual differences and intelligence* (3rd ed., pp. 77–88). Harlow, Essex: Pearson Education.

Maltby, Day & Macaskill, Chapter 6
Maltby, J., Day, L., & Macaskill, A. (2013). Theories and measurement of intelligence. In J. Maltby, L. Day, & A. Macaskill (Eds.), *Personality, individual differences and intelligence* (3rd ed., pp. 124–150). Harlow, Essex: Pearson Education.

Maltby, Day & Macaskill, Chapter 7
Maltby, J., Day, L., & Macaskill, A. (2013). Theories and measurement of intelligence. In J. Maltby, L. Day, & A. Macaskill (Eds.), *Personality, individual differences and intelligence* (3rd ed., pp. 152–174). Harlow, Essex: Pearson Education.

CHAPTER 12: PAIN **635**

The content in this section has been compiled from:
Morrison, Chapter 16
Morrison, V., & Bennett, P. (2009). Pain. In V. Morrison & P. Bennett (Eds.), *An introduction to health psychology* (2nd ed., pp. 479–510). Harlow, Essex: Pearson Education.

CHAPTER 13: EMOTIONS 662

The content in this section has been compiled from:
Robbins, Judge, Millet & Jones, Chapter 6
Robbins, S. P., Judge. T. A., Millet, B., & Jones, M. (2010). Emotions and moods. In S. P. Robbins, T. A. Judge, B. Millet, & M. Jones (Eds.), *OB: The essentials* (pp. 154–160), Frenchs Forest, NSW: Pearson Australia.

Lilienfeld, Lynn, Namy, Woolf, Jamieson, Marks & Slaughter, Chapter 11
Lilienfeld, S. O., Lynn, S. J., Namy, L. L., Woolf, N. J., Jamieson, G., Marks, A., & Slaughter, V. (2015).Emotion and motivation. In S. O. Lilienfeld, S. J. Lynn, L. L. Namy, N. J. Woolf, G. Jamieson, A. Marks, & V. Slaughter (Eds.), *Psychology: From inquiry to understanding* (2nd ed., pp. 449–460). Melbourne, VIC: Pearson Australia.

CHAPTER 14: STRESS 686

The content in this section has been compiled from:
Lilienfeld, Lynn, Namy, Woolf, Jamieson, Marks & Slaughter, Chapter 12
Lilienfeld, S. O., Lynn, S. J., Namy, L. L., Woolf, N. J., Jamieson, G., Marks, A., & Slaughter, V. (2015). Stress, coping and health. In S. O. Lilienfeld, S. J. Lynn, L. L. Namy, N. J. Woolf, G. Jamieson, A. Marks, & V. Slaughter (Eds.), *Psychology: From inquiry to understanding* (2nd ed., pp. 503–510, 510–521). Melbourne, VIC: Pearson Australia.

Smith, Chapter 5
Smith, J. (1993). The transactional matrix. In J. Smith (Ed.), *Understanding stress and coping* (pp. 69–89). New York, NY: Macmillan.

Donatelle, Chapter 3
Donatelle, R. J. (2015). Managing stress and coping with life's challenges. In R. J. Donatelle (Ed.), *Health: The basics* (11th ed., pp. 75–83). Upper Saddle River, NJ: Pearson Education.

Smith, Chapter 8
Smith, J. (1993). The transactional matrix. In J. Smith (Ed.), *Understanding stress and coping* (pp. 133–146). New York, NY: Macmillan.

REVIEW ANSWERS 745

REFERENCES 756

INDEX 848

How To Use This Custom Book

Welcome to **Individual Determinants of Health and Human Behaviour.**

The chapters in this custom book have been chosen specifically to meet your course requirements by your lecturers.

In reading this book, please be aware that this custom edition includes content from 11 different source titles. When referencing please look at the superscript letters (A, B etc) added at the end of some paragraphs. These will take you to the footer of your book where you will find where the section starts and where it ends as well as the reference you need to use when working on your assignments.

We hope that you will find this text easy to follow and enjoyable.

surprisingly well. This principle can be called 'grandma's rule', because our grandmothers reminded us to finish our vegetables before moving on to dessert. If we give children the opportunity to choose between spinach and chocolate ice-cream, they will vote with their mouths and choose to eat chocolate ice-cream at a much higher frequency than they eat spinach. In this way, we can get children to eat spinach by reinforcing them with chocolate ice-cream if, but only if, they have finished their much-dreaded spinach.

If you find yourself putting off a reading or writing task, think of behaviours you would typically perform if given the chance—perhaps hanging out with a few close friends, watching a favourite TV programme or going for a swim. Then, reinforce yourself with these higher frequency behaviours *only* after you have completed your homework.[A]

Therapeutic applications of operant conditioning

We can apply operant conditioning to clinical settings as well. One of the most successful applications of operant conditioning has been the *token economy*.

Token economies are systems, often set up in psychiatric hospitals, for reinforcing appropriate behaviours and extinguishing inappropriate ones (Carr, Fraizer & Roland, 2005; Kazdin, 1982). Typically, psychologists who construct token economies begin by identifying *target behaviours*—that is, actions they hope to make more frequent. Staff members reinforce patients who exhibit these behaviours, using tokens, chips, points or other secondary reinforcers. Secondary reinforcers are neutral objects that become associated with primary reinforcers—things, like a favourite food or drink, that naturally increase the target behaviour.

Secondary reinforcers Neutral objects that people can trade in for reinforcers themselves.

Primary reinforcers Items or outcomes that are naturally pleasurable.

One psychiatric hospital unit in which one of the authors of your textbook worked consisted of children with serious behaviour problems, including yelling and swearing. In this unit, one target behaviour was being polite to staff members. So, whenever a child was especially polite to a staff member, he or she was rewarded with points, which could be traded in for something he or she wanted, like ice-cream or attending a movie with staff members. Whenever a child was rude to a staff member, he or she was punished with a loss of points.

Research suggests that token economies are often effective in improving behaviour in hospitals, group homes and juvenile detention units (Ayllon & Milan, 2002; Paul & Lentz, 1977). Nevertheless, token economies remain controversial, because the behaviours learned in institutions do not always transfer to the outside world (Wakefield, 2006). This is especially likely if the patients return to settings, like deviant peer groups, in which they are reinforced for socially inappropriate behaviours.

Operant conditioning has also been helpful in the treatment of individuals with autism, especially in improving their language deficits. *Applied behaviour analysis* (ABA) for autism makes extensive use of shaping techniques; mental health professionals offer food and other primary reinforcers to individuals with autism as they reach progressively closer approximations to certain words and, eventually, complete sentences.

Ivar Lovaas and his colleagues have pioneered the best-known ABA programme for autism (Lovaas, 1987; McEachin, Smith & Lovaas, 1993). The results of Lovaas's work have been promising. Children with autism who undergo ABA training emerge with better language and intellectual skills than do control groups of children with autism who do not undergo such training (Green, 1996; Matson et al., 1996; Romanczyk et al., 2003).

Nevertheless, because Lovaas didn't randomly assign children with autism to experimental and control groups, his findings are vulnerable: perhaps the children in the experimental group had higher levels of functioning to begin with. Indeed, there is

[A]Lilienfeld, S. O., Lynn, S. J., Namy, L. L., Woolf, N. J., Jamieson, G., Marks, A., & Slaughter, V. (2015). Learning: How nurture changes us. In S. O. Lilienfeld, S. J. Lynn, L. L. Namy, & N. J. Woolf (Eds.), *Psychology: From inquiry to understanding* (2nd ed., pp. 220–237) Melbourne, VIC:Pearson Australia.

References – This is the citation of the original source text. You need to quote these details, including the relevant page numbers, when referencing your assignments.

Preface

Individual Determinants of Health and Human Behaviour has been designed to incorporate substantial coverage of a variety of psychological topics not only to help students develop foundational knowledge, but also to help readers build clinical competence and professional excellence. Whether working in a hospital, or a community and residential setting such as a school or prison, understanding how psychological person-related factors influence individuals' behaviour and interactions can help optimise therapeutic outcomes.

This customised textbook addresses content that will not only foster learning and understanding on a number of topics central to understanding individual health behaviours (e.g., principles of learning, development, communication, personality, and memory processes), but in doing so will draw on theory, research and evidence-based practice. In addition to this, the final sections of the book address psychological features, or specific constructs (e.g. pain), that may be a response to injury or disease – all of which can influence an individual's behaviour and interpersonal interactions.

This book is structured so that chapters and/or groups of chapters can be read independently in almost any order. Further, you will notice that some of the theories will occur in more than one chapter. This is because theories often contain common assumptions that can be applied to multiple concepts in health and human behaviour.

Health care environments are often dynamic organisations which will inevitably require skills in communication, interpersonal relations and more generally, skills that come from a broad knowledge of psychology to work effectively in collaborative interdisciplinary health care teams, and with clients of diverse cultural, economic and intellectual backgrounds. We hope this book helps you develop knowledge and abilities that will contribute to the advancement of your immediate scholarly pursuits, as well as generate practical knowledge for life-long application.

CHAPTER 1

Learning

The content in this section has been compiled from:
Lilienfeld, Lynn, Namy, Woolf, Jamieson, Marks & Slaughter, Chapter 6

Lilienfeld, S. O., Lynn, S. J., Namy, L. L., Woolf, N. J., Jamieson, G., Marks, A., & Slaughter, V. (2015). Learning: How nurture changes us. In S. O. Lilienfeld, S. J. Lynn, L. L. Namy, & N. J. Woolf (Eds.), *Psychology: From inquiry to understanding* (2nd ed., pp. 220–237, 239–249). Melbourne, VIC: Pearson Australia.

CHAPTER 1

Learning

Learning is defined in this chapter as a relatively permanent change in behaviour as a result of experience. It is the lifelong, dynamic process by which individuals acquire new knowledge or skills and alter their thoughts, feelings, attitudes, and actions. Learning enables individuals to adapt to demands and changing circumstances and is crucial in health care—whether for clients and/or patients acquiring new information and learning necessary skills to manage a diagnosis and/or chronic health condition, or for healthcare staff understanding particular individual learnt health behaviours e.g., phobias and how this may influence interactions with clients and patients. This chapter will cover *learning theories* and apply principles that will describe, explain, or predict how people learn.

After studying this chapter you should be able to:

- Describe Pavlov's classical conditioning model
- Describe the principles of classical conditioning
- Apply principles of classical conditioning to everyday life
- Describe the principles of operant conditioning
- Distinguish between operant conditioning from classical conditioning
- Describe Thorndike's law of effect
- Distinguish reinforcement from punishment and its outcome on behaviour
- Describe the four schedules of reinforcement, and the response pattern associated with each
- Describe cognitive models of learning
- Describe biological influences on learning.

The three most famous figures in the psychology of learning were each colourful characters in their own way. The discoverer of classical conditioning, Ivan Pavlov, was a notoriously compulsive fellow. He ate lunch every day at precisely 12 noon, went to bed at exactly the same time every night and departed St Petersburg, Russia, for holiday the same day every year. Pavlov was also such a rapid walker that his wife frequently had to run frantically to keep up with him. The life of the founder of behaviourism, John B. Watson, was rocked with scandal. Despite becoming one of the world's most famous psychologists, he was unceremoniously booted out of Johns Hopkins University for having an affair with his graduate student, Rosalie Rayner. Watson also had rather unusual ideas about parenting; for example, he believed that all parents should shake hands with their children before bedtime. B. F. Skinner, the founder of radical behaviourism, was something of a prankster in his undergraduate years at Hamilton College in New York. He and a friend once spread a false rumour that comedian Charlie Chaplin was coming to campus. This rumour nearly provoked a riot when Chaplin did not materialise as expected.

By **learning**, we mean a change in an organism's behaviour or thought as a result of experience. When we learn our brain changes along with our behaviours. Remarkably, your brain is physically different now than it was just a few minutes ago, because it underwent chemical changes that allowed you to learn novel facts.

Learning
Change in an organism's behaviour or thought as a result of experience.

Habituation
Process of responding less strongly over time to repeated stimuli.

Learning lies at the heart of just about every domain of psychology. Virtually all behaviours are a complex stew of genetic predispositions and learning. Without learning, we would be unable to do much; we could not walk, talk or read an introductory psychology textbook chapter about learning.

Psychologists have long debated how many distinct types of learning there are. We are not going to try to settle this controversy here. Instead, we will review several types of learning that psychologists have studied in depth, starting with the most basic.

Before we do, place your brain on pause, put down your pen or highlighter, close your eyes and attend to several things that you almost never notice: the soft buzzing of the lights in the room, the feel of your clothing against your skin, the sensation of your tongue on your teeth or lips. Unless someone draws our attention to these stimuli, we do not even realise they are there, because we have learned to ignore them. **Habituation** is the process by which we respond less strongly over time to repeated stimuli. It helps to explain why loud snorers can sleep peacefully through the night while keeping their irritated roommates wide awake. Chronic snorers have become so accustomed to the sound of their own snoring that they no longer notice it.

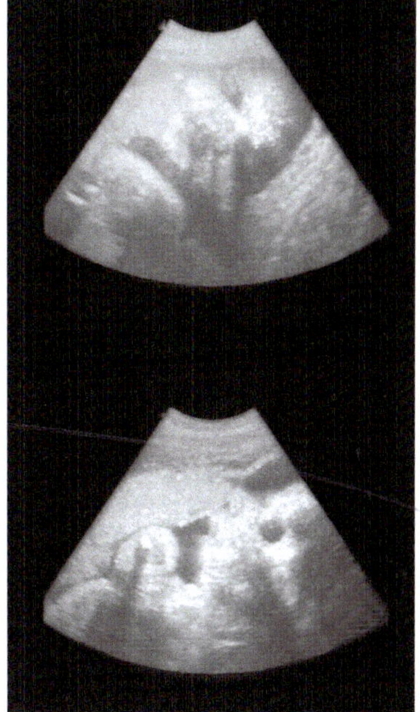

Even foetuses as young as 32 weeks have displayed habituation. While they first experience shock when a gentle vibrator is applied to the mother's stomach, the shock later becomes a mere annoyance.
(**Source:** Olga Makarova/Dreamstime.com.)

Habituation is the simplest and probably earliest form of learning to emerge in humans. Foetuses as young as 32 weeks display habituation when we apply a gentle vibrator to the mother's stomach. At first, the foetus jerks around in response to the stimulus, but after repeated vibrations it stops moving (Morokuma et al., 2004). What was first a shock to the foetus's system later became a mere annoyance that it could safely ignore.

In research that earned him the Nobel Prize in 2000, neurophysiologist Eric Kandel uncovered the biological mechanism of habituation of *Aplysia*, a 12-centimetre-long sea slug. Prick an *Aplysia* on a certain part of its body and it retracts its gill in a defensive manoeuvre. Touch *Aplysia* in the same spot repeatedly and it begins to ignore the stimulus. This habituation, Kandel found, is accompanied by a progressive decrease in the release of the neurotransmitter serotonin at *Aplysia*'s synapses (Siegelbaum, Camardo & Kandel, 1982). This discovery helped psychologists unravel the neural bases of learning (see Figure 1.1).

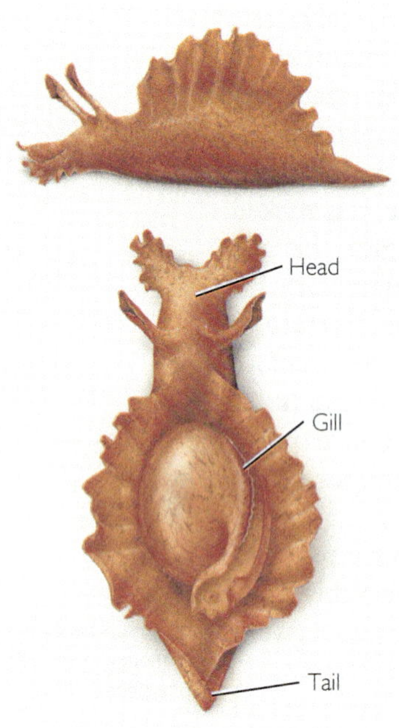

Figure 1.1 Habituation in a simple animal.

Aplysia californicus is a sea slug about 12 centimetres long that retracts its gill when pricked, but then habituates (stops retracting its gill) if pricked repeatedly.

Psychologists have studied habituation by measuring—of all things—sweat. Because perspiration on our fingertips is a good indicator of anxiety (Fowles, 1980), scientists measure it by using an electrical conductivity measure called the skin conductance response. Most research shows that our hands stop sweating sooner for weak stimuli than they do for strong stimuli, meaning that weak stimuli stop producing anxiety fairly quickly compared with strong stimuli. In the case of very strong stimuli, like painful electric shocks, we often see no habituation at all—people continue to sweat anxiously at the same high levels—even across many trials (Lykken et al., 1988).

This research suggests that habituation makes good sense from an evolutionary standpoint. We wouldn't want to attend to every tiny sensation that comes across our mental radar screens, because most pose no threat. Yet we wouldn't want to habituate to stimuli that could be dangerous. Fortunately, not all repeated stimuli lead to habituation, only those that we deem safe or worth ignoring do.

Some cases of repeated exposure to stimuli lead to *sensitisation*—that is, responding more strongly over time—rather than habituation. Sensitisation is most likely when a stimulus is dangerous, irritating, or both. *Aplysia* show sensitisation as well as habituation. Have you ever tried to study when the person next to you was whispering, and the whispering kept getting more annoying to the point that you could not concentrate? If so, you have experienced sensitisation.

Classical conditioning

The story of habituation could hardly be more straightforward. We experience a stimulus, respond to it and then stop responding after repeated exposure. We have learned something significant, but we have not learned to forge connections between two stimuli. Yet a great deal of learning depends on associating one thing with another. If we never learned to connect one stimulus, such as the appearance of an apple, with another stimulus, such as its taste, our everyday life would be a world of disconnected sensory experiences.

In the nineteenth century, a school of thinkers called the British Associationists believed that we acquire virtually all of our knowledge by *conditioning*—that is, by forming associations among stimuli. Once we form these links, like the connection between our mother's voice and her face, we need only recall one element of the pair to retrieve the other. The British Associationists believed that simple connections provided the mental building blocks for all of our more complex ideas. Their armchair conjectures were to be confirmed by a pioneering Russian physiologist who demonstrated these processes of association in the laboratory.

Pavlov's discovery of classical conditioning

That physiologist's name was Ivan Pavlov. Pavlov's primary research was on digestion in dogs—in fact, his discoveries concerning digestion, not classical conditioning, earned him the Nobel Prize in 1904. Pavlov placed dogs in a harness and inserted a collection tube into their salivary glands to study their digestive responses to meat powder. In doing so, he observed something unexpected: dogs began salivating (more informally, they started to drool), not only at the meat powder itself, but at previously neutral stimuli that had become associated with it, such as the research assistants who brought in the powder. Indeed, the dogs even salivated to the sound of these assistants' footsteps as they approached the laboratory. The dogs seemed to be anticipating the meat powder and responding to stimuli that signalled its arrival.

We call this process of association **classical conditioning** (or **Pavlovian or respondent conditioning**): a form of learning in which animals come to respond to a previously neutral stimulus that had been paired with another stimulus that elicits an automatic response. Pavlov's initial observations were merely anecdotal; so, like any good scientist, he put his informal observations to a more rigorous test.

Classical (Pavlovian or respondent) conditioning
Form of learning in which animals come to respond to a previously neutral stimulus that had been paired with another stimulus that elicits an automatic response.

The classical conditioning phenomenon

This is how Pavlov first demonstrated classical conditioning systematically (see also Figure 1.2).

1. He started with an initially neutral stimulus, one that didn't elicit any particular response. In this case, Pavlov used a metronome, a clicking pendulum that keeps time (in other studies, Pavlov used a tuning fork or whistle; contrary to urban legend, Pavlov did not use a bell).
2. He then paired the neutral stimulus again and again with an **unconditioned stimulus (UCS)**, a stimulus that elicits an automatic—that is, a reflexive—response. In the case of Pavlov's dogs, the UCS was the meat powder, and the automatic, reflexive response it elicits is the **unconditioned response (UCR)**. For the dogs, the UCR was salivation. The key point is that the animal does not need to learn to respond to the UCS with the UCR: dogs naturally drool in response to food. The animal generates the UCR without any training at all, because the response is a product of nature, not nurture.
3. As Pavlov repeatedly paired the CS and the UCS, he observed something remarkable. If he now presented the metronome alone, it elicited a response, namely salivation. This new response is the **conditioned response (CR)**: a response previously associated with a non-neutral stimulus that comes to be elicited by a neutral stimulus. Lo and behold, learning has occurred. The metronome had become a **conditioned stimulus (CS)**—a previously neutral stimulus that comes to elicit a conditioned response as a result of its association with an unconditioned stimulus. The dog, which previously did nothing when it heard the metronome except perhaps turn its head towards it, now salivates when

Factoid

Classical conditioning may occur not only in animals but in plants. One researcher found that a *Mimosa* plant that folds its leaves (UCR) when touched (UCS) can be conditioned to fold its leaves (CR) in response to a change in lighting condition (CS) that has been repeatedly paired with a touch (Haney, 1969). Nevertheless, this finding is scientifically controversial.

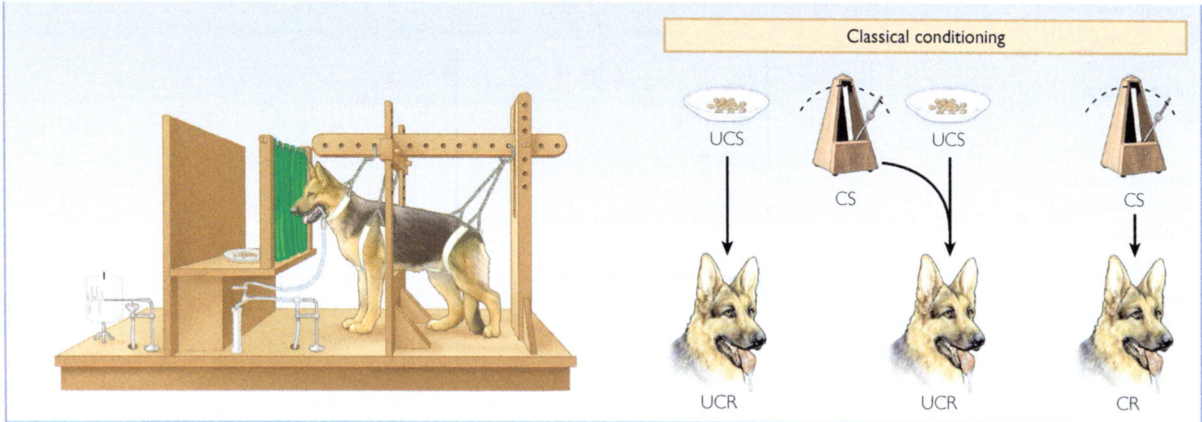

Figure 1.2 Pavlov's classical conditioning model.

The UCS (meat powder) is paired with the CS (metronome clicking) and produces the UCR (salivation). Then the CS is presented alone, and the CR (salivation) occurs.

Factoid

Backward conditioning—in which the UCS is presented *before* the CS—is extremely difficult to achieve. Because the CS fails to predict the UCS and the UCR often begins before the CS has even occurred, organisms have difficulty using the CS to anticipate the UCS.

it hears the metronome. The CR, in contrast to the UCR, is a product of nurture, not nature.

In most cases, the CR is similar to the UCR but it is rarely identical to it. For example, Pavlov found that dogs salivated less in response to the metronome (the CS) than to the meat powder (the UCS).

Few findings in psychology are as replicable as classical conditioning. We can apply the classical conditioning paradigm to just about any animal which has an intact nervous system, and demonstrate it repeatedly without fail. If only all psychological findings were so dependable!

Principles of classical conditioning

We will next explore the major principles underlying classical conditioning. Pavlov noted, and many others have since confirmed, that classical conditioning occurs in three phases—acquisition, extinction and spontaneous recovery. In addition, as we will see, once classical conditioning to a stimulus occurs, it often extends to a host of related stimuli, making its everyday life influence surprisingly powerful.

Acquisition

In **acquisition**, we gradually learn—or acquire—the CR. If you look at Figure 1.3(a), you will see that, as the CS and the UCS are paired over and over again, the CR increases progressively in strength. The steepness of this curve varies somewhat depending on how close together in time the CS and UCS are presented. In general, the closer in time the pairing of the CS and the UCS, the faster learning occurs, with about a half-second delay typically being the optimal pairing for learning. Longer delays usually decrease the speed and strength of the organism's response.

Unconditioned stimulus (UCS) Stimulus that elicits an automatic response.

Unconditioned response (UCR) Automatic response to a non-neutral stimulus that does not need to be learned.

Conditioned response (CR) Response previously associated with a non-neutral stimulus that is elicited by a neutral stimulus through conditioning.

Conditioned stimulus (CS) Initially neutral stimulus.

Acquisition Learning phase during which a conditioned response is established.

Extinction Gradual reduction and eventual elimination of the conditioned response after the conditioned stimulus is presented repeatedly without the unconditioned stimulus.

Extinction

In a process called **extinction**, the CR decreases in magnitude and eventually disappears when the CS is repeatedly presented alone—that is, without the UCS (see Figure 1.3[b]). After numerous presentations of the metronome without the meat power, Pavlov's dogs eventually stopped salivating. Most psychologists once believed that extinction was similar

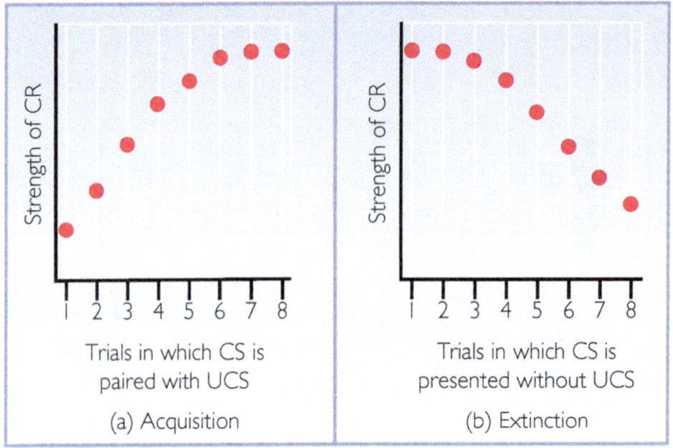

Figure 1.3 Acquisition and extinction.

Acquisition is the repeated pairing of the UCS and the CS, increasing the CR's strength (a). In extinction, the CS is presented again and again without the UCS, resulting in the gradual disappearance of the CR (b).

to forgetting: the CR fades away over repeated trials, just as many memories gradually decay. Yet the truth is more complicated and interesting than that. Extinction is an active, rather than passive, process. During extinction a new response, which in the case of Pavlov's dogs was the *absence* of salivation, gradually 'writes over' or inhibits the CR, namely salivation. The extinguished CR does not vanish completely; it is merely overshadowed by the new behaviour. This contrasts with most forms of traditional forgetting, in which the memory itself disappears. Interestingly, Pavlov had proposed this hypothesis in his writings, although few people believed him at the time. How do we know he was right? Read on.

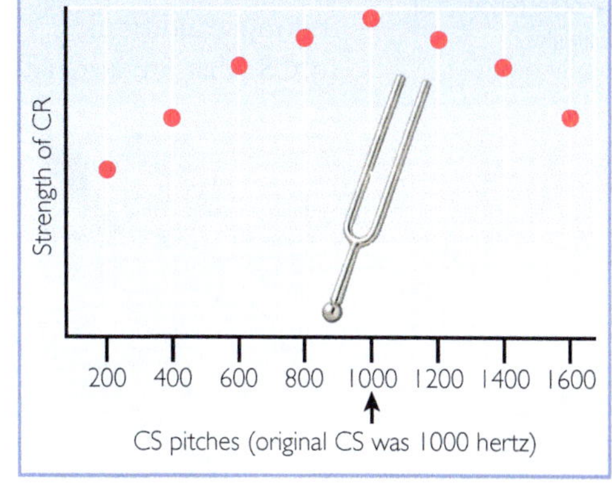

Figure 1.4 Generalisation gradient.

The more similar to the original CS the new CS is (for example, Pavlov using a tone pitched close to the original tone's pitch), the stronger the CR will be.

Spontaneous recovery

In a phenomenon called **spontaneous recovery**, a seemingly extinct CR reappears (often in a somewhat weaker form) if the CS is presented again. It is as though the CR were lurking in the background, waiting to appear following another presentation of the CS. In a classic study, Pavlov (1927) presented the CS (the tone from a metronome) alone again and again, and extinguished the CR (salivation) because there was no UCS (mouth-watering meat powder) following it. Two hours later, he presented the CS again and the CR returned. The animal had not really forgotten the CR, just suppressed it.

A related phenomenon is the **renewal effect**, which occurs when we extinguish a response in a setting different from the one in which the animal acquired it. When we restore the animal to the original setting, the extinguished response reappears (Bouton, 1994). The renewal effect may help to explain why people with *phobias*—intense, irrational fears—who have overcome their phobias often experience a reappearance of their symptoms when they return to the environment in which they acquired their fears (Denniston, Chang & Miller, 2003). Even though it may sometimes lead to a return of phobias, the renewal effect is often adaptive. If you have been bitten by a snake in one part of a forest, it makes sense to experience fear when you find yourself there again, even years later. That same snake or his slithery descendants may still be lying in wait in the same spot.

Spontaneous recovery
Sudden re-emergence of an extinct conditioned response after a delay in exposure to the conditioned stimulus.

Renewal effect
Sudden re-emergence of a conditioned response following extinction when an animal is returned to the environment in which the conditioned response was acquired.

Stimulus generalisation

Pavlov found that following classical conditioning his dogs salivated not merely to the original metronome sound, but to sounds similar to it. This phenomenon is **stimulus generalisation**: the process by which CSs that are similar, but not identical, to the original CS elicit a CR. Stimulus generalisation occurs along a *generalisation gradient*: the more similar to the original CS the new CS is, the stronger the CR will be (see Figure 1.4). Pavlov found that his dogs showed their largest amount of salivation to the original sound, with progressively less salivation to sounds that were less and less similar to it in pitch. Stimulus generalisation is typically adaptive, because it allows us to transfer what we have learned to new things. For example, once we have learned to drive our own car, we can borrow a friend's car without needing a full tutorial on how to drive it.

Stimulus generalisation
Process by which conditioned stimuli similar, but not identical, to the original conditioned stimulus elicit a conditioned response.

Stimulus discrimination

Stimulus discrimination is the flip side of the coin to stimulus generalisation; it occurs when we exhibit a less pronounced CR to CSs that differ from the original CS. Stimulus discrimination helps us understand why we can enjoy scary movies. Although we may hyperventilate a bit while watching sharks circle the capsized sailors in the movie *The Reef*,

Stimulus discrimination
Displaying a less pronounced conditioned response to conditioned stimuli that differ from the original conditioned stimulus.

Higher-order conditioning Developing a conditioned response to a conditioned stimulus by virtue of its association with another conditioned stimulus.

we would respond even more strongly if we went on a shark dive while on holiday. We have learned to discriminate between a motion picture stimulus and the real-world version of it, and to modify our response as a result.

Higher-order conditioning

Taking conditioning a step further, organisms learn to develop conditioned associations to CSs that are associated with the original CS. If after conditioning a dog to salivate to a tone, we pair a picture of a circle with that tone, a dog eventually salivates to the circle as well as to the tone. That is **higher-order conditioning**: the process by which organisms develop classically conditioned responses to CSs associated with the original CS (Gewirtz & Davis, 2000, pp. 257–266). There are several levels of higher-order conditioning, defined by the number of steps between the CS and the UCS. As we might expect, second-order conditioning—in which a new CS is paired with the original CS—tends to be weaker than garden-variety classical conditioning, and third-order conditioning—in which a third CS is paired with the second-order CS—is even weaker. Fourth-order conditioning and beyond are typically difficult or impossible to achieve.

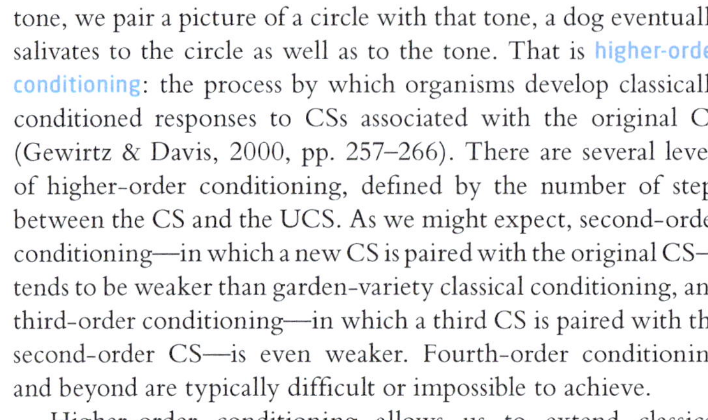

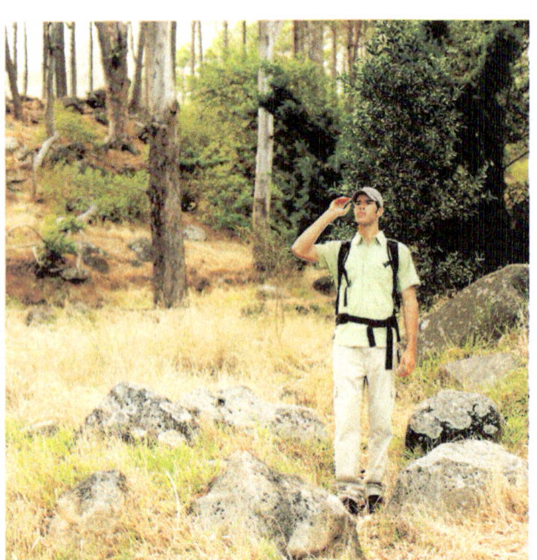

A person hiking through the forest may experience fear when he approaches an area if he has previously spotted a dangerous animal there.
(**Source:** Yuri Arcurs/Dreamstime.)

Higher-order conditioning allows us to extend classical conditioning to a host of new stimuli. It helps explain why we feel hungry after someone merely says 'kebab' after a late-night party. We have already come to associate the sight, sound and smell of a kebab with satisfying our hunger, and we eventually came to associate the word 'kebab' with these CSs.

Applications of classical conditioning to daily life

Classical conditioning applies to myriad domains of everyday life. We consider five here: advertising, the acquisition of fears and phobias, the acquisition of fetishes, and disgust reactions.

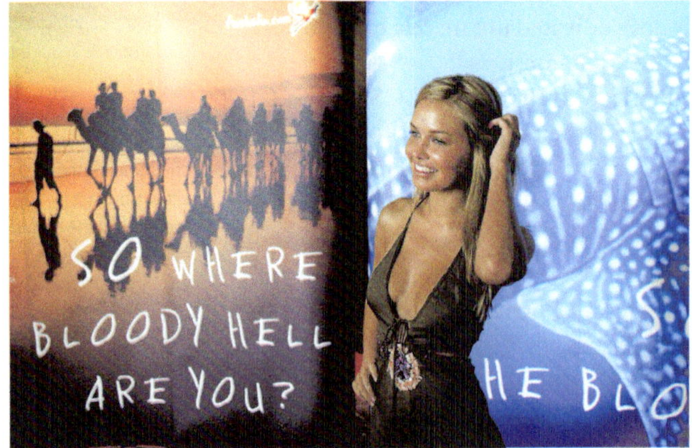

Advertisers use higher-order classical conditioning to get customers to associate their products with an inherently enjoyable stimulus.
(**Source:** Toby Zerna/Newspix/News Ltd.)

Classical conditioning and advertising

Few people grasp the principles of classical conditioning, especially higher-order conditioning, better than advertisers. By repeatedly pairing the sights and sounds of products with photographs of spunky football players and bikini-clad models, marketing whizzes try to establish classically conditioned connections between their brands and positive emotions. They do so for a good reason: it works.

Researcher Gerald Gorn (1982) paired slides of either blue or beige pens (the CSs) with music that participants had rated as either enjoyable or not enjoyable (the UCSs). Then he gave participants the opportunity to select a pen upon departing the lab. Whereas 79 percent of participants who heard music they liked picked the pen that had been paired with the music, only 30 percent of those who heard music they disliked picked the pen that had been paired with the music.

Nevertheless, not all researchers who have paired products with pleasurable stimuli have succeeded in demonstrating classical conditioning effects (Gresham & Shimp, 1985, pp. 10–49; Smith, 2001). But many of the negative findings are open to a rival explanation: latent inhibition. **Latent inhibition** refers to the fact that when we have experienced a CS alone many times, it is difficult to classically condition it to another stimulus (Vaitl & Lipp, 1997, pp. 85–93). Because some investigators who failed to obtain classical conditioning effects for products relied on brands with which participants were already familiar, their negative findings may be attributable to latent inhibition. Indeed, when researchers have used novel brands, they have generally been able to show classical conditioning effects (Stuart, Shimp & Engle, 1987, pp. 334–349).

Latent inhibition Difficulty in establishing classical conditioning to a conditioned stimulus we have repeatedly experienced alone; that is, without the unconditioned stimulus.

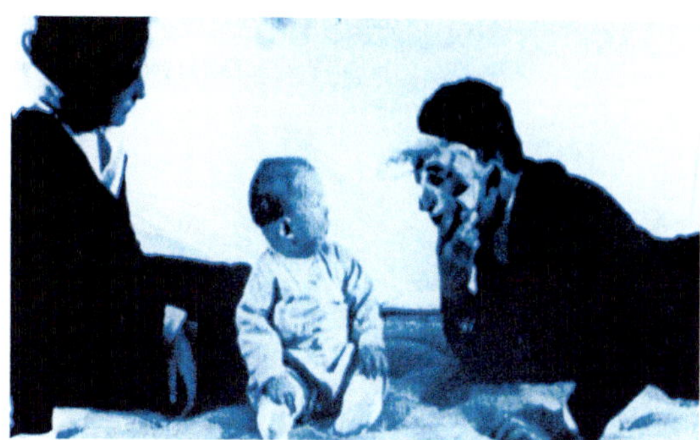

Classic study in which a nine-month-old boy was conditioned to fear white furry objects. Here, Little Albert, with John B. Watson and Rosalie Rayner, is crying in response to a Santa Claus mask.
(**Source:** Benjamin Harris, PhD.)

The acquisition of fears and phobias: the strange tale of Little Albert

Can classical conditioning help explain how we come to fear or avoid stimuli? John B. Watson, the founder of behaviourism, answered this question in 1920 when he and his graduate student, Rosalie Rayner, performed what must be regarded as one of the most ethically questionable studies in the history of psychology.

Watson and Rayner (1920) set out in part to show that the Freudian view of phobias, which proposed that phobias stem from deep-seated conflicts buried in the unconscious, was wrong. To do so, they recruited a nine-month-old infant who will be forever known in the psychological literature as Little Albert. Little Albert was fond of furry little creatures, like white rats. But Watson and Rayner were about to change that.

Watson and Rayner first allowed Little Albert to play with a rat. But only seconds afterward, Watson snuck up behind Little Albert and struck a gong with a steel hammer, creating an ear-splitting noise, which startled him out of his wits and made him cry. After seven such pairings of the rat and UCS (the loud sound from the gong), Little Albert displayed a CR (crying) to the rat alone, demonstrating that the rat had now become a CS. This conditioned response was still present when Watson and Rayner exposed Little Albert to the rat five days later. Moreover, Watson and Rayner observed that Little Albert had become a victim of stimulus generalisation, coming to fear not merely rats, but also a rabbit, a dog, a furry coat and, to a lesser extent, a Santa Claus mask and John B. Watson's hair. Fortunately, Little Albert also demonstrated at least some stimulus discrimination, as he did not display much fear towards cotton balls or the hair of Dr Watson's research assistants.

Incidentally, no one knows what became of poor Little Albert. His mother withdrew him from the study about a month after it began, never to be heard from again. Needless to say, because inducing a phobia-like condition in an infant raises a host of serious ethical questions, Watson and Rayner's Little Albert study would never get past a modern-day university ethical review board.

Stimulus generalisation, like that experienced by Little Albert, allows our learning to be remarkably flexible—which is often, although not always, a good thing. It allows us to develop fears of many stimuli. Certain phobias, like those of snakes, spiders, heights,

Table 1.1 Phobias galore. This sampling of phobias—some common, some exceedingly rare—illustrates just how enormously varied people's fears can be. Many of these phobias can be acquired at least partly by classical conditioning.

Alliumphobia: Fear of garlic	*Melissophobia:* Fear of bees
Arachibutyrophobia: Fear of peanut butter sticking to the roof of your mouth	*Ophidiophobia:* Fear of snakes
Brontophobia: Fear of thunderstorms	*Peladophobia:* Fear of bald people
Bufonophobia: Fear of toads	*Pentheraphobia:* Fear of one's mother-in-law
Catoptrophobia: Fear of mirrors	*Pogonophobia:* Fear of beards
Elurophobia: Fear of cats	*Rhytiphobia:* Fear of getting wrinkles
Epistaxiophobia: Fear of nose bleeds	*Samhainophobia:* Fear of Halloween
Latrophobia: Fear of doctors	*Taphephobia:* Fear of being buried alive
Lachanophobia: Fear of vegetables	*Xyrophobia:* Fear of razors

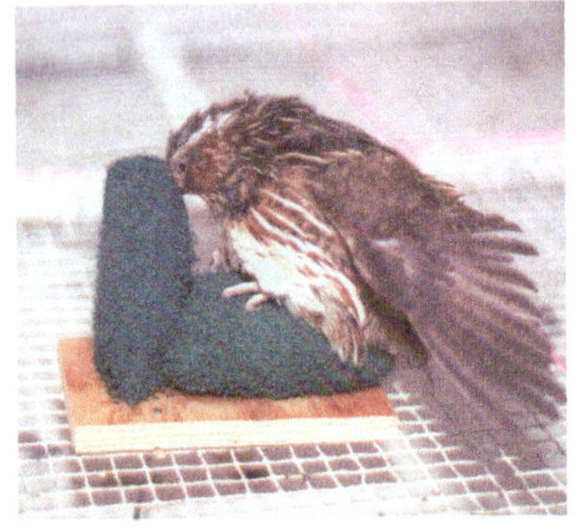

Michael Domjan and his colleagues used classical conditioning to instil a fetish in male quails.
(**Source:** Dr Michael Domjan.)

water and blood, are considerably more widespread than others (www.anxietyaustralia.com.au). And some are downright strange, as Table 1.1 illustrates.

The good news is that if classical conditioning can contribute to our acquiring phobias, it can also contribute to our conquering them. Mary Cover Jones, a student of Watson, treated a three-year-old named Little Peter, who had a phobia of rabbits. Jones (1924) treated Peter's fear successfully by gradually introducing him to a white rabbit while giving him a piece of his favourite lolly. As she moved the rabbit increasingly close to him, the sight of the rabbit eventually came to elicit a new CR: pleasure rather than fear. Modern-day psychotherapists, although rarely feeding their clients lollies, use similar practices to eliminate phobias. They may pair feared stimuli with relaxation or other pleasurable stimuli (Wolpe, 1990).

Fetishes

Fetishism
Sexual attraction to non-living things.

On the flip side of the coin from phobias, **fetishism**—sexual attraction to non-living things—may also arise in part from classical conditioning (Akins, 2004; Hoffmann, 2011). Like phobias, fetishes come in a bewildering variety of forms: shoes, stockings, dolls, stuffed animals, automobile engines (yes, that's right), and just about anything else (Lowenstein, 2002).

Although the origins of human fetishes are controversial, Michael Domjan and his colleagues were successful in classically conditioning fetishes in male Japanese quails. In one study, they presented male quails with a cylindrical object made of terrycloth, followed by a female quail with which they happily mated. After 30 such pairings, about half of the male quails attempted to mate with the cylindrical object when it appeared alone (Köksal et al., 2004). Although the generalisability of these findings to humans is unclear, there is good evidence that at least some people develop fetishes by the repeated pairing of neutral objects with sexual activity (Rachman & Hodgson, 1968; Weinberg, Williams & Calhan, 1995).

Disgust reactions

Imagine that a researcher asked you to eat a piece of fudge. No problem, right? Well, now imagine the fudge were shaped like dog faeces. If you are like most participants in the studies of Paul Rozin and his colleagues, you would hesitate (D'Amato, 1998; Rozin, Millman & Nemeroff, 1986).

Rozin and his colleagues have found that we acquire disgust reactions with surprising ease. In most cases, these reactions are probably the product of classical conditioning, because CSs associated with disgusting UCSs come to elicit disgust themselves. In many cases, disgust reactions are tied to stimuli that are biologically important to us, such as animals or objects that are dirty or potentially poisonous (Rozin & Fallon, 1987).

In another study, Rozin and his collaborators asked participants to drink from two glasses of water, both of which contained sugar (sucrose). In one case, the sucrose came from a bottle labelled 'Sucrose'; in another, it came from a bottle labelled 'Sodium Cyanide, Poison'. The investigators told participants that both bottles were completely safe. They even asked participants to select which label went with which glass, proving the labels were meaningless. Even so, participants were hesitant to drink from the glass that contained the sucrose labelled as poisonous (Rozin, Markwith & Ross, 1990, pp. 383–384). Participants' responses in this study were irrational, but perhaps understandable: they were probably relying on the heuristic 'better safe than sorry'. Classical conditioning helps keep us safe, even if it goes too far on occasion.

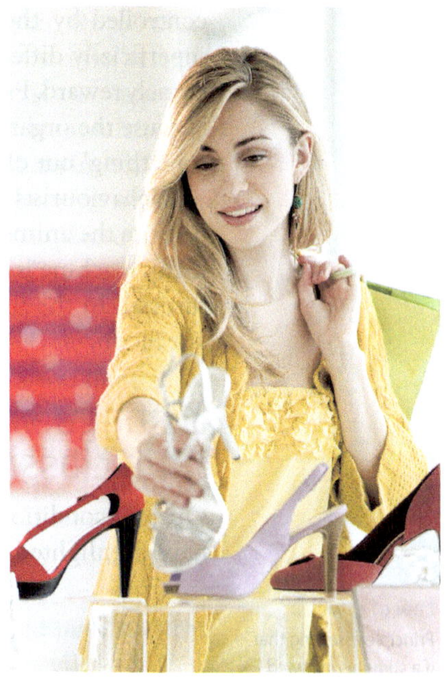

Some researchers have suggested that classical conditioning may similarly help to explain some human fetishes.
(**Source:** Photostogo/Photolibrary.)

Assess your knowledge — FACT or FICTION?

1. Habituation to meaningless stimuli is generally adaptive. **(True/False)**
2. In classical conditioning, the conditioned stimulus (CS) initially yields a reflexive, automatic response. **(True/False)**
3. Conditioning is most effective when the CS precedes the UCS by a short period of time. **(True/False)**
4. Extinction is produced by the gradual 'decay' of the CR over time. **(True/False)**

Answers: (1) T; (2) F; (3) T; (4) F

Operant conditioning

What do the following four examples have in common?

- Using bird feed as a reward, a behavioural psychologist teaches a pigeon to distinguish paintings by Monet from paintings by Picasso. By the end of the training, the pigeon is a veritable art aficionado.
- Using fish as a treat, a trainer teaches a dolphin to jump out of the water, spin three times, splash in the water and propel itself through a hoop.
- In his initial attempt at playing tennis, a frustrated 12-year-old hits his opponent's serve into the net the first 15 times. After two hours of practice, he returns his opponent's serve successfully more than half the time.
- A hospitalised patient with dissociative identity disorder (formerly known as multiple personality disorder) displays features of an 'alter' personality whenever staff members pay attention to him. When they ignore him, his alter personality seemingly vanishes.

The answer: all are examples of **operant conditioning**. The first, incidentally, comes from an actual study (Watanabe, Sakamoto & Wakita, 1995). Operant conditioning is learning

Operant conditioning
Learning controlled by the consequences of the organism's behaviour.

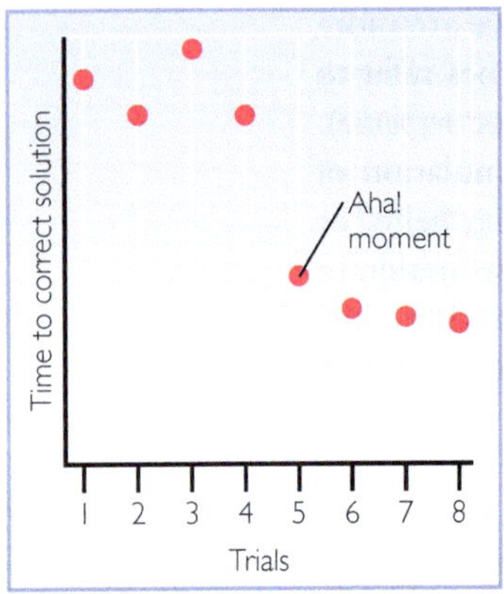

Figure 1.6 'Aha!' reaction. Insight learning: once the animal solves the problem, it gets the answer right almost every time after that.

Skinner found Thorndike's experimental set-up unwieldy, because the researcher had to stick around to place the unhappy cat back into the puzzle box following each trial. This limitation made it difficult to study the build-up of associations in ongoing operant behaviour over hours, days or weeks. So he developed what came to be known as a **Skinner box** (more formally, an operant chamber), which electronically records an animal's responses and prints out a *cumulative record*, or graph, of the animal's activity. A Skinner box typically contains a bar that delivers food when pressed, a food dispenser and often a light that signals when reward is forthcoming (see Figure 1.7). With this set-up, Skinner studied the operant behaviour of rats, pigeons and other animals, and mapped out their responses to reward. By allowing a device to record behaviour without any direct human observation, Skinner ran the risk of missing some important behaviours that the box was not designed to record. Nonetheless, his discoveries forever altered the landscape of psychology.

Terminology of operant conditioning

To understand Skinner's research, you need to learn some psychological jargon. There are three key concepts in Skinnerian psychology: reinforcement, punishment and discriminant stimulus.

Skinner box
Small animal chamber constructed by b. F. Skinner to allow sustained periods of conditioning to be administered and behaviours to be recorded unsupervised.

Reinforcement
Outcome or consequence of a behaviour that strengthens the probability of the behaviour.

Positive reinforcement
Positive outcome or consequence of a behaviour that strengthens the probability of the behaviour.

Negative reinforcement
Removal of a negative outcome or consequence of a behaviour that strengthens the probability of the behaviour.

Reinforcement

Up to this point, we have used the term *reward* to refer to any pleasant consequence that makes a behaviour more likely to occur. But Skinner found this term imprecise. He preferred the term **reinforcement**, meaning any outcome that strengthens the probability of a response (Skinner, 1953; 1971).

Skinner distinguished **positive reinforcement**, when we administer something pleasant, from **negative reinforcement**, when we take away something unpleasant. Positive reinforcement could be giving a child a sweet biscuit when he picks up his toys; negative reinforcement could be ending a child's time-out for bad behaviour once she has stopped whining. In both cases, the most frequent outcome is an increase or strengthening of the response. Note, though, that Skinner would call these actions 'reinforcements' *only* if they make the response more likely to occur in the future.

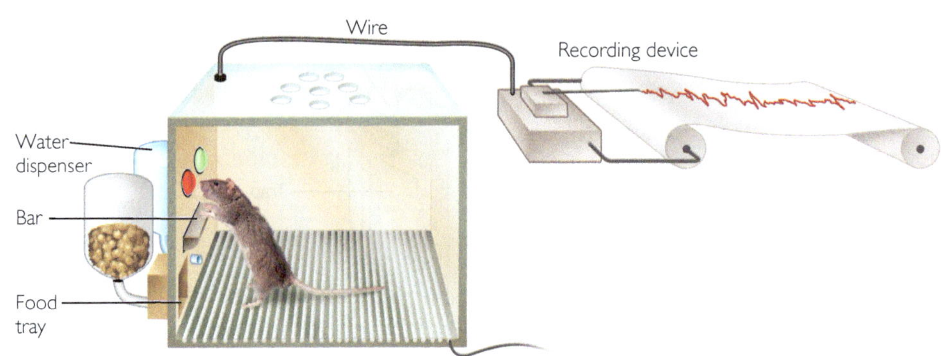

Figure 1.7 Rat in Skinner box and electronic device for recording the rat's behaviour.

B. F. Skinner devised a small chamber (the Skinner box) containing a bar that the rat presses to obtain food, a food dispenser, and often a light that signals when reward is forthcoming. An electronic device graphs the rat's responses in the researcher's absence.

Hundreds of psychology students over the years have demonstrated the power of reinforcement using an unconventional participant: their lecturer. In the game Condition Your Professor (Vyse, 1997), a class of introductory psychology students agrees to provide positive reinforcement—like smiling or nodding their heads—to their lecturer whenever he or she moves in a particular direction, such as to the far left side of the room. One famous introductory psychology teacher spent almost all of his time lecturing from behind a podium. During one class, his students smiled profusely and nodded their heads whenever he ventured out from behind the podium. Sure enough, by the end of class the lecturer was spending most of his time away from the podium. You and your classmates might want to attempt a similar stunt with your introductory psychology lecturer: just don't mention we suggested it.

Punishment

Negative reinforcement should not be confused with **punishment**, which is any *outcome* that weakens the probability of a response. Like reinforcements, punishment can be either positive or negative. If a punishment involves administering a stimulus, then it is positive; if it is taking away a stimulus, then it is negative.

Punishment Outcome or consequence of a behaviour that weakens the probability of the behaviour.

Positive punishment typically involves administering a stimulus that the organism wants to avoid, such as a physical shock or a smack, or an unpleasant social outcome, such as laughing at someone. Negative punishment involves the removal of a stimulus that the organism wishes to experience, such as a favourite toy or treat.

Punishment also should not be confused with the disciplinary practices often associated with it. Skinner, who insisted on precision in language, argued that certain actions that might superficially appear to be punishments are actually reinforcements. He defined reinforcements and punishments solely in terms of their consequences. Consider this scenario. A mother rushes into her three-year-old son's bedroom and yells 'Stop that!' each time she hears him kicking the wall. Is she punishing the child's demanding behaviour? There is no way to tell without knowing the consequences. If he kicks the wall more often following the scolding, then the mother is actually reinforcing his behaviour—strengthening the probability of a response. If his kicking decreases or stops altogether after he was scolded, then the mother's scolding is a punishment—weakening the probability of a response.

Try labelling each of the following examples as an instance of either negative reinforcement or punishment and explain why. (You can find the answers written upside-down in the margin at the bottom of the next page.)

1. A boy keeps making noise in the back of the classroom despite the teacher's repeated warnings. The teacher finally sends him to the principal's office. When he returns two hours later, he is much quieter.

Table 1.3 Distinguishing reinforcement from punishment

	Procedure	Effect on behaviour	Typical example
Positive reinforcement	Presenting a desirable stimulus	Increases target behaviour	Giving a gold star on homework, resulting in a student studying more
Negative reinforcement	Removing an undesirable stimulus	Increases target behaviour	Static on phone that subsides when you move to a different spot in your room, causing you to stand there more often
Positive punishment	Presenting a stimulus	Decreases target behaviour	Scolding by a pet owner, reducing a dog's habit of chewing on shoes
Negative punishment	Removing a stimulus	Decreases target behaviour	Taking away a favourite toy, stopping a child from throwing future tantrums

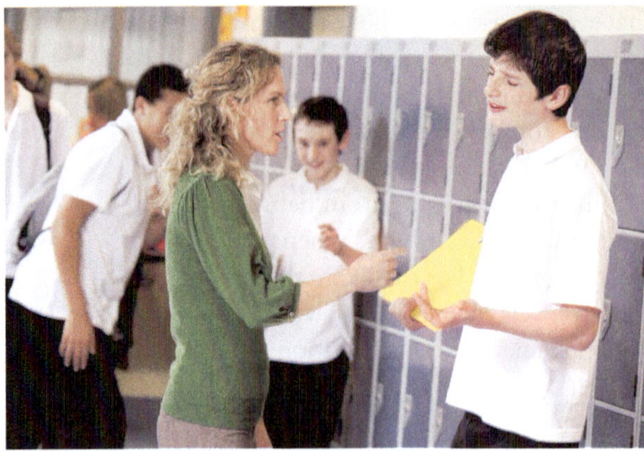

Forcing a student to see the principal is typically a form of punishment; nevertheless, it can instead serve as a negative reinforcement if it allows the student to escape from an unpleasant class.
(**Source:** Monkey Business Images/Dreamstime.)

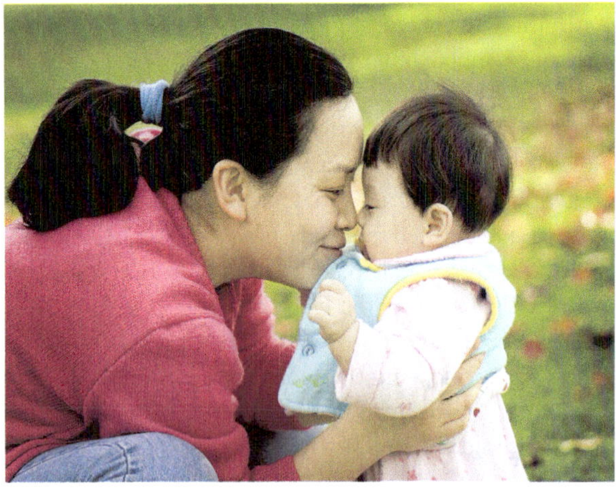

In some countries, such as China and Thailand, children are rarely punished.
(**Source:** Squall/Fotolia.)

2. A woman with diabetes works hard to control her blood sugar through diet and exercise. As a result, her doctor allows her to discontinue administering her unpleasant daily insulin shots, which increases her attempts to eat healthily and exercise.
3. A parole board releases a previously aggressive criminal from prison early for being a 'model citizen' within the institution over the past five years. On his release, he continues to behave in a law-abiding manner.
4. A woman yells at her roommate for leaving dirty clothing scattered all around her apartment. Her roommate apologises and never makes a mess again.

Does punishment work in the long run? Popular wisdom tells us that it usually does: 'Spare the rod, spoil the child.' Yet Skinner (1953) and most of his followers argued against the routine use of punishment to change behaviour. They believed that reinforcement alone could shape most human behaviours for the better.

According to Skinner and others (Azrin & Holz, 1966, pp. 380–447), punishment has several disadvantages:

1. Punishment tells the organism only what *not* to do, not *what* to do. A child who is punished for throwing a tantrum will not learn how to deal with frustration more constructively.
2. Punishment often creates anxiety, which in turn interferes with future learning.
3. Punishment may encourage subversive behaviour, prompting people to become sneakier about the situations in which they can and cannot display forbidden behaviour. A child who is punished for grabbing his brother's toys may learn to grab his brother's toys only when his parents are not looking.
4. Punishment from parents may provide a model for children's aggressive behaviour (Straus, Sugarman & Giles-Sims, 1997). A child whose parents slap him when he misbehaves may 'get the message' that slapping is acceptable.

Numerous researchers have reported that the use of physical punishment by parents is positively correlated with aggressive behaviour in children (Fang & Corso, 2007; Gershoff, 2002). Across many studies, Murray Straus and his colleagues (1998) found that physical punishment is associated with more behavioural problems in children.

Elizabeth Gershoff (2002) conducted a meta-analysis of 88 studies of corporal punishment based on a whopping 39,309 participants. Although she found some evidence that corporal punishment is associated with short-term improvements in children's behaviour, she also found that a history of such punishment in childhood is associated with an increased probability of becoming an abuser in adulthood.

Yet we must remember that these studies are correlational and do not demonstrate causality. Other interpretations are possible. For example, because children share half of their genes with each parent, and because aggression is partly heritable (Krueger, Hicks & McGue, 2001), the correlation between parents' physical aggression and their children's

Answers

1 Punishment because the boy's teacher reduced his rate of noise making.
2 Negative reinforcement because her doctor increased the woman's rates of eating well and exercising.
3 Negative reinforcement because the parole board increased the prisoner's rate of law-abiding behavior.
4 Punishment because the woman decreased her room-mate's rate of messy behaviour.

aggression may be due to the fact that parents who are physically aggressive pass on this genetic predisposition to their children (DiLalla & Gottesman, 1991, pp. 125–129). Or the correlation might be driven by environmental factors, such as family exposure to a lot of media violence, which could make the parents more likely to use harsh discipline and independently make their children more aggressive.

A recent study addressed this problem by investigating children of identical twins. Children of 887 twins participating in the Australian Twin Registry provided information about how they were disciplined by their parents; they also were interviewed about their lives, including their drug and alcohol use and their tendencies towards positive and negative behaviours. This experimental design is powerful because it untangles the effects of genes (shared by both twins and passed onto their children) from punishment styles (which sometimes differed from twin to twin). The results indicated higher levels of aggressive and delinquent behaviour and greater alcohol and drug use in children whose parents used harsh physical punishment compared with those whose parents used milder methods. The results ruled out a genetic explanation, because in pairs of twin parents who differed in their disciplinary styles, children of the harsh-punishing twin displayed more of these negative behaviours than children of the mild-punishing twin (Lynch et al., 2006).

That is not to say that we should never use any kind of punishment, only that we should use milder methods and use them sparingly. Most research suggests that punishment works best when it is delivered consistently and follows the undesired behaviour promptly (Brennan & Mednick, 1994). In particular, immediate punishment tends to be effective, whereas delayed punishment is often useless (Church, 1969; McCord, 2006; Moffitt, 1983). Punishment of an undesired behaviour also works best when we simultaneously reinforce a desired behaviour (Azrin & Holz, 1966).

Discriminative stimulus

The final critical term in operant conditioning lingo is **discriminative stimulus (S_d)**, which is any stimulus that signals the presence of reinforcement. When we snap our fingers at a dog in the hopes of having it come over to us, the dog may approach us to get a much-appreciated petting. For the dog, our finger snapping is a discriminative stimulus: it is a signal that if it comes near us, it will receive reinforcement. According to behaviourists, we are responding to discriminative stimuli virtually all the time, even if we are not consciously aware of it. A friend's waving at us from across campus is another common discriminative stimulus: it often signals to us that our friend wants to chat with us, thereby reinforcing us for responding to her wave.

Discriminative stimulus (S_d)
Stimulus associated with the presence of reinforcement.

Acquisition, extinction, spontaneous recovery, stimulus discrimination and stimulus generalisation

If you feel you are experiencing a case of déjà vu upon reading these bolded terms, do not be concerned, because you have indeed seen all of them before. Acquisition, extinction, spontaneous recovery, stimulus discrimination and stimulus generalisation apply just as much to operant conditioning as to classical conditioning. You can find the definitions in Table 1.4. Next, we examine how three of these concepts apply to operant conditioning.

Extinction

In operant conditioning, extinction occurs when we stop delivering reinforcement to a previously reinforced behaviour. Gradually, this behaviour declines in frequency and disappears. If parents give a screaming child a toy to quieten her, they may be inadvertently reinforcing her behaviour, because she is learning to scream to get something. If her parents

Table 1.4 Definition reminders of important concepts in both classical and operant conditioning

Term	Definition
Acquisition	Learning phase during which a response is established
Extinction	Gradual reduction and eventual elimination of the response after a stimulus is presented repeatedly
Spontaneous recovery	Sudden re-emergence of an extinguished response after a delay
Stimulus discrimination	Displaying a less pronounced response to stimuli that differ from the original stimulus
Stimulus generalisation	Eliciting a response to stimuli similar to, but not identical to, the original stimulus

buy earplugs and stop placating the child by giving her toys, the screaming behaviour will gradually extinguish. In such cases we often see an *extinction burst*. That is, shortly after withdrawing reinforcement the undesired behaviour initially increases in intensity, probably because the child is trying harder to get reinforcement. So there is some truth to the old saying that things sometimes need to get worse before they get better.

Schedule of reinforcement Pattern of reinforcing a behaviour.

Partial reinforcement Only occasional reinforcement of a behaviour, resulting in slower extinction than if the behaviour had been reinforced continually.

STIMULUS DISCRIMINATION. As we mentioned earlier, one group of investigators used food reinforcement to train pigeons to distinguish paintings by Monet from those by Picasso (Watanabe, Sakamoto & Wakita, 1995). That is stimulus discrimination, because the pigeons are learning to tell the difference between two different types of stimuli.

STIMULUS GENERALISATION. Interestingly, these investigators also found that their pigeons displayed stimulus generalisation. Following operant conditioning, they distinguished paintings by impressionist artists whose styles were similar to Monet's, such as Renoir, from paintings by cubist artists similar to Picasso, such as Braque.

Schedules of reinforcement

Skinner (1938) found that animals' behaviours differ depending on the **schedule of reinforcement**—that is, the pattern of delivering reinforcement. In the simplest pattern, *continuous reinforcement*, we reinforce a behaviour every time it occurs. **Partial reinforcement**, sometimes called *intermittent reinforcement*, occurs when we reinforce responses only some of the time.

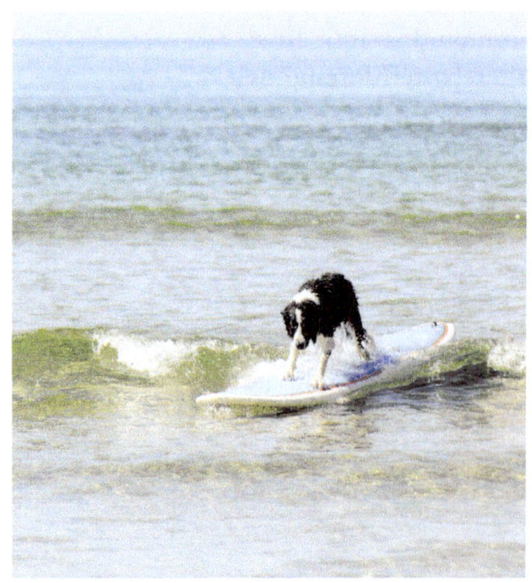

Behaviours that we reinforce only occasionally (partial reinforcement) are slowest to extinguish. So to train a dog to surf, we should reinforce it only intermittently.
(**Source:** Magnum/Fotolia.)

Try answering this question: If we want to train a dog to perform a trick, such as surfing, should we reinforce it for (a) each successful ride or (b) only some of its successful rides? If you are like most people, you will answer (a), which seems to match our commonsense notions regarding the effects of reinforcement. It seems logical to assume that the more consistent the reinforcement, the more consistent will be the resulting behaviour.

Nevertheless, Skinner's principle of partial reinforcement shows that our intuitions about reinforcement are inaccurate. According to the principle of partial reinforcement, behaviours we reinforce only occasionally are slower to extinguish than those we reinforce continuously—that is, every time. Does this idea seem counterintuitive? Think of it this way: if the dog has learned that he will be rewarded for staying on the board only sometimes, he is more likely to keep trying to stay on it in the hopes of getting reinforcement.

So, if we want an animal to maintain a trick for a long time, we should actually reinforce it for correct responses only occasionally. Skinner (1969) noted that continuous reinforcement allows animals to learn new behaviours more quickly, but that partial reinforcement leads to a greater resistance to extinction. This principle may help to explain why some people remain trapped for years in terribly dysfunctional, even abusive, relationships. Some relationship partners provide intermittent reinforcement to their significant others, treating them miserably most of the time but treating them well on rare occasions. This pattern of partial reinforcement may keep individuals 'hooked' in relationships that are not working.

Although there are numerous schedules of reinforcement, we will discuss the four major ones here. Remarkably, the effects of these reinforcement schedules are consistent across species as diverse as cockroaches, pigeons, rats and humans. That's impressive replicability. The principal reinforcement schedules vary along two dimensions:

1. *The consistency of administering reinforcement.* Some reinforcement contingencies are fixed, whereas others are variable. That is, in some cases experimenters provide reinforcement on a regular (fixed) basis, whereas in others they provide reinforcement on an irregular (variable) basis. Variable schedules tend to yield more consistent rates of responding than do fixed schedules. This finding makes intuitive sense. If we never know when our next treat is coming, it is in our best interests to keep emitting the response to ensure we have emitted it enough times to earn the reward.
2. *The basis of administering reinforcement.* Some reinforcement schedules operate on ratio schedules, whereas others operate on interval schedules. In ratio schedules, the experimenter reinforces the animal based on the number of responses it has emitted. In interval schedules, the experimenter reinforces the animal based on the amount of time elapsed since the last reinforcement. Ratio schedules tend to yield higher rates of responding than do interval schedules. This finding also makes intuitive sense. If a dog gets a treat every 5 times he rolls over, he is going to roll over more often than if he gets a treat every 5 minutes, regardless of whether he rolls over once or 20 times during that interval.

We can cross these two dimensions to arrive at four schedules of reinforcement (see Figure 1.8) each of which yields a distinctive pattern of responding:

1. In a **fixed ratio (FR) schedule**, we provide reinforcement after a regular number of responses. For example, we could give a rat a pellet after it presses the lever in a Skinner box 15 times.
2. In a **fixed interval (FI) schedule**, we provide reinforcement for producing the response at least once after a specified amount of time has passed. For example, a worker in a toy factory might get paid the same time every Friday afternoon for the work she has done, so long as she has generated at least one toy during that one-week interval.
   Fixed interval schedules are especially distinctive in the behaviours they yield; they are associated with a 'scalloped' pattern of responding (see Figure 1.9, overleaf). This pattern reflects the fact that the animal 'waits' for a time after it receives reinforcement, and then

Fixed ratio (FR) schedule
Pattern in which we provide reinforcement following a regular number of responses.

Fixed interval (FI) schedule
Pattern in which we provide reinforcement for producing the response at least once following a specified time interval.

Variable interval (VI) schedule
Pattern in which we provide reinforcement for producing the response following an average time interval, with the interval varying randomly.

Variable ratio (VR) schedule
Pattern in which we provide reinforcement after a specific number of responses on average, with the number varying randomly.

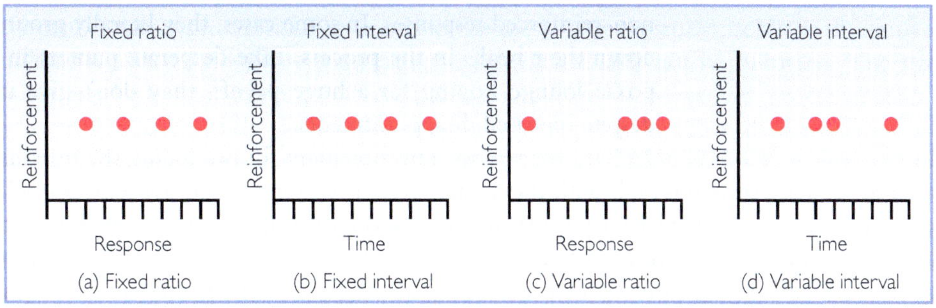

Figure 1.8 Four major reinforcement schedules.

The four major reinforcement schedules are (a) fixed ratio, (b) fixed interval, (c) variable ratio and (d) variable interval.

surprisingly well. This principle can be called 'grandma's rule', because our grandmothers reminded us to finish our vegetables before moving on to dessert. If we give children the opportunity to choose between spinach and chocolate ice-cream, they will vote with their mouths and choose to eat chocolate ice-cream at a much higher frequency than they eat spinach. In this way, we can get children to eat spinach by reinforcing them with chocolate ice-cream if, but only if, they have finished their much-dreaded spinach.

If you find yourself putting off a reading or writing task, think of behaviours you would typically perform if given the chance—perhaps hanging out with a few close friends, watching a favourite TV programme or going for a swim. Then, reinforce yourself with these higher frequency behaviours *only* after you have completed your homework.[A]

Therapeutic applications of operant conditioning

We can apply operant conditioning to clinical settings as well. One of the most successful applications of operant conditioning has been the *token economy*.

Token economies are systems, often set up in psychiatric hospitals, for reinforcing appropriate behaviours and extinguishing inappropriate ones (Carr, Fraizer & Roland, 2005; Kazdin, 1982). Typically, psychologists who construct token economies begin by identifying *target behaviours*—that is, actions they hope to make more frequent. Staff members reinforce patients who exhibit these behaviours, using tokens, chips, points or other **secondary reinforcers**. Secondary reinforcers are neutral objects that become associated with **primary reinforcers**—things, like a favourite food or drink, that naturally increase the target behaviour.

Secondary reinforcers Neutral objects that people can trade in for reinforcers themselves.

Primary reinforcers Items or outcomes that are naturally pleasurable.

One psychiatric hospital unit in which one of the authors of your textbook worked consisted of children with serious behaviour problems, including yelling and swearing. In this unit, one target behaviour was being polite to staff members. So, whenever a child was especially polite to a staff member, he or she was rewarded with points, which could be traded in for something he or she wanted, like ice-cream or attending a movie with staff members. Whenever a child was rude to a staff member, he or she was punished with a loss of points.

Research suggests that token economies are often effective in improving behaviour in hospitals, group homes and juvenile detention units (Ayllon & Milan, 2002; Paul & Lentz, 1977). Nevertheless, token economies remain controversial, because the behaviours learned in institutions do not always transfer to the outside world (Wakefield, 2006). This is especially likely if the patients return to settings, like deviant peer groups, in which they are reinforced for socially inappropriate behaviours.

Operant conditioning has also been helpful in the treatment of individuals with autism, especially in improving their language deficits. *Applied behaviour analysis* (ABA) for autism makes extensive use of shaping techniques; mental health professionals offer food and other primary reinforcers to individuals with autism as they reach progressively closer approximations to certain words and, eventually, complete sentences.

Ivar Lovaas and his colleagues have pioneered the best-known ABA programme for autism (Lovaas, 1987; McEachin, Smith & Lovaas, 1993). The results of Lovaas's work have been promising. Children with autism who undergo ABA training emerge with better language and intellectual skills than do control groups of children with autism who do not undergo such training (Green, 1996; Matson et al., 1996; Romanczyk et al., 2003).

Nevertheless, because Lovaas didn't randomly assign children with autism to experimental and control groups, his findings are vulnerable: perhaps the children in the experimental group had higher levels of functioning to begin with. Indeed, there is

---

[A]Lilienfeld, S. O., Lynn, S. J., Namy, L. L., Woolf, N. J., Jamieson, G., Marks, A., & Slaughter, V. (2015). Learning: How nurture changes us. In S. O. Lilienfeld, S. J. Lynn, L. L. Namy, & N. J. Woolf (Eds.), *Psychology: From inquiry to understanding* (2nd ed., pp. 220–237). Melbourne, VIC: Pearson Australia.

evidence that this was the case (Schopler, Short & Mesibov, 1989). The current consensus is that ABA isn't a miracle cure for the language deficits of autism, but that it can be extremely helpful in many cases (Herbert, Sharp & Gaudiano, 2002).

Putting classical and operant conditioning together

Up to this point, we have discussed classical and operant conditioning as though they were two entirely independent processes. Yet the truth is more complicated. The similarities between classical and operant conditioning, including the fact that we find acquisition, extinction, stimulus generalisation and so on, in both, have led some theorists to argue that these two forms of learning are not as different as some psychologists believe (Brown & Jenkins, 1968; Staddon, 2003).

Although there are certainly important similarities between classical and operant conditioning, brain-imaging studies demonstrate that these two forms of learning are associated with activations in different brain regions. Classically conditioned fear reactions are based largely in the amygdala (LeDoux, 1996; Veit et al., 2002), whereas operantly conditioned responses are based largely in the nucleus accumbens and related limbic systems linked to reward (Robbins et al., 1998).

These two types of conditioning often interact. To see how, let us revisit the question of how people develop phobias. We have seen that certain phobias arise in part by classical conditioning. A previously neutral stimulus (the CS)—say, a dog—is paired with an unpleasant stimulus (the UCS)—a dog bite—resulting in the CR of fear. So far, so good. But this tidy scheme does not answer an important question: why doesn't the CR of fear eventually extinguish? Given what we have learned about classical conditioning, we might expect the CR of fear to fade away over time with repeated exposure to the CS of dogs. Yet this often does not happen (Rachman, 1977). Many people with phobias remain deathly afraid of their feared stimulus for years, even decades. Indeed, only about 20 percent of untreated adults with phobias ever get over their fears (American Psychiatric Association, 2000). Why?

Enter *two-process theory* to the rescue as an explanation (Mowrer, 1947). According to two-process theory, we need both classical and operant conditioning to explain the persistence of anxiety disorders. People acquire phobias by means of classical conditioning. Then, once they are phobic, they start to avoid their feared stimulus whenever they see it. If they have a dog phobia, they may cross the street whenever they see someone walking towards them with a large German shepherd. When they do, they experience a reduction in anxiety—a surge of relief—which *negatively reinforces* their fear. Recall that negative reinforcement, which is one type of operant conditioning, is the removal of an unpleasant stimulus; in this case, anxiety. So, by avoiding dogs whenever they see them, dog phobics are negatively reinforcing their

Assess your knowledge — FACT or FICTION?

1. In classical conditioning, responses are emitted; in operant conditioning, they are elicited. **(True/False)**
2. Negative reinforcement and punishment are superficially different, but they produce the same short-term effects on behaviour. **(True/False)**
3. The principle of partial reinforcement states that behaviours reinforced only some of the time extinguish more rapidly than behaviours reinforced continuously. **(True/False)**
4. We can reinforce less frequent behaviours with more frequent behaviours. **(True/False)**

Answers: (1) F; (2) F; (3) F; (4) T

fear. Ironically, they are operantly conditioning themselves to make their fears more likely to persist. In essence, they are exchanging short-term gain for long-term pain.

Cognitive models of learning

Thus far, we have omitted one word when discussing how we learn: *thinking*. This is not accidental, because early behaviourists did not believe that thought played much of a causal role in learning. Skinner (1953) was an advocate of what he called *radical behaviourism*, so-called because he believed that observable behaviour, thinking and emotion are all governed by the same laws of learning; namely, classical and operant conditioning. For radical behaviourists, thinking and emotion *are* behaviours; they're just not observable.

Skinner believed that humans and other intelligent animals think (deBell & Harless, 1992; Wyatt, 2001). But he didn't believe that thinking is any different in principle from any other behaviour. For Skinner, this view is far more parsimonious than invoking different laws of learning for thinking than for other behaviours. Skinner (1990) even went so far to liken proponents of cognitive psychology, who believe that thinking plays a central role in causing behaviour, to pseudoscientists. Cognitive psychology, he argued, invokes unobservable and ultimately meaningless concepts—like 'mind'—to explain behaviour.

S-O-R psychology: throwing thinking back into the mix

Few psychologists today share Skinner's harsh assessment of cognitive psychology. In fact, the vast majority of psychologists now agree that the story of learning in humans is incomplete without at least some role for cognition—that is, thinking (Bolles, 1979; Kirsch et al., 2004, pp. 369–392; Pinker, 1997).

Over the past 30 or 40 years, psychology has moved increasingly away from a simple S-R (stimulus-response) psychology to a more complex S-O-R psychology, with 'O' being the *organism* that interprets the stimulus before producing a response (Mischel, 1973; Woodworth, 1929). For S-O-R psychologists, the link between S and R is not mindless or automatic. Instead, the organism's response to a stimulus depends on what this stimulus *means* to it. The S-O-R principle helps to explain a phenomenon we have probably all encountered.

You have probably had the experience of giving two friends the same mild criticism (like 'It bugs me when you show up late') and found that they reacted quite differently: one was apologetic, the other defensive. To explain these differing reactions, Skinner would have probably invoked your friends' differing *learning histories*; in essence, how each friend had been trained to react to criticism. In contrast, S-O-R theorists, who believe that cognition is central to explaining learning, would contend that the differences in your friends' reactions stem from how they *interpreted* your criticism. Your first friend may have viewed your criticism as constructive feedback; your second friend, as a personal attack.

S-O-R theorists do not deny that classical and operant conditioning occur, but they believe that these forms of learning usually depend on thinking. Take a person who has been classically conditioned by tones and shock to sweat in response to the tones. Her skin conductance response will extinguish suddenly if she is told that no more shocks are on the way (Grings, 1973). This phenomenon of *cognitive conditioning*, whereby our interpretation of the situation affects conditioning, suggests that conditioning is more than an automatic, mindless process (Brewer, 1974; Kirsch et al., 2004).

S-O-R theorists also emphasise the role of expectations in learning. They point out that classical conditioning occurs only if the CS regularly predicts the occurrence of the UCS (Rescorla, 1990; Rescorla & Wagner, 1972). If we repeatedly present the CS and UCS close together in time, that alone won't do the trick when it comes to producing classical conditioning. Organisms show classically conditioned reactions only when the CS reliably forecasts the UCS, suggesting that they are building up expectations about what comes next. So, according to S-O-R theorists, whenever Pavlov's dogs heard the ticking of the metronome, they thought—and the word 'thought' is crucial here—'Ah, I think some meat powder is on the way.'

To explain psychology's gradual transition from behaviourism to cognitivism, we need to tell the story of a pioneering psychologist and his rats.

Latent learning

One of the first serious challenges to the radical behaviourist account of learning was mounted by Edward Chace Tolman (1886–1959), whose contribution to the psychology of learning can't be overestimated. Tolman suspected that reinforcement wasn't the be-all and end-all of learning. To understand why, answer this question: 'Who was one of the first psychologists to challenge the radical behaviourist account of learning?' If you have been paying attention, you will have answered 'Tolman'. Yet immediately before we asked that question, you knew the answer, even though you had no opportunity to demonstrate it. According to Tolman (1932), you engaged in latent learning: learning that isn't directly observable (Blodgett, 1929, pp. 113–134). We learn many things without showing them. Putting it a bit differently, there is a crucial difference between *competence*—what we know—and *performance*—showing what we know (Bradbard et al., 1986).

Latent learning
Learning that is not directly observable.

Why is this distinction important? Because it implies that *reinforcement is not necessary for learning*. Tolman and C. H. Honzik (1930) demonstrated this point systematically by randomly assigning three groups of rats to go through a maze over a three-week period (see Figure 1.10). One group always received reinforcement in the form of cheese when it got to the end of the maze. A second group never received reinforcement when it got to the end of the maze. The first group made far fewer errors; that is no great surprise. The third group received no reinforcement for the first 10 days and then started receiving reinforcement on the eleventh day.

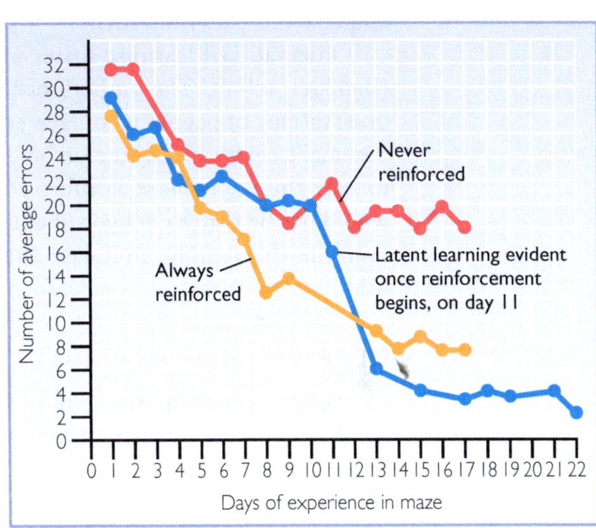

Figure 1.10 Tolman and Honzik's maze trials.

Graphs from Tolman and Honzik's classic study of latent learning in rats. Pay particular attention to the blue line. The rats in this group were not reinforced until day 11; note the sudden drop in the number of their errors on receiving reinforcement. The rats were learning all along, even though they were not showing it.
(**Source:** Tolman & Honzik, 1930.)

As can be seen in Figure 1.10, the rats in the third group showed a large and abrupt drop in their number of errors on receiving their very first reinforcement. In fact, within only a few days their number of errors did not differ significantly from the number of errors among the rats who were always reinforced.

Tolman argued that the rats in the third group had been learning all along. They just had not bothered to show it because they had nothing to gain. Once there was a payoff for learning, namely a tasty morsel of cheese, they promptly became miniature maze masters.

Cognitive maps
Mental representations of how a physical space is organised.

According to Tolman (1948), the rats had developed cognitive maps—that is, spatial representations—of the maze. If you are like most university students, you were hopelessly confused the first day you arrived on campus. Over time, however, you probably developed a mental sense of the layout of the campus, so that you now hardly ever become lost. That internal spatial blueprint is a cognitive map.

In a clever demonstration of cognitive maps, McNamara, Long and Wike (1956) had one set of rats run repeatedly through a maze to receive reinforcement. They put another set of rats in little moving 'trolley cars', in which the rats could observe the layout of the maze but not obtain the experience of running through it. When the researchers gave the second group of rats the chance to run through the maze, they did just as well as the rats in the first group. As rodent tourists in trolley cars, they had acquired cognitive maps of the maze.

The latent learning research of Tolman and others challenged strict behavioural models of learning, because their work suggested that learning could occur without reinforcement. To many psychologists, this research refuted the claim that reinforcement is necessary for all forms of learning.

Observational learning

Observational learning
Learning by watching others.

According to some psychologists, one important variant of latent learning is **observational learning**: learning by watching others (Bandura, 1965). In many cases, we learn by watching *models*: parents, teachers and others who are influential to us. Many psychologists regard observational learning as a form of latent learning, because it allows us to learn without reinforcement. We can merely watch someone else being reinforced for doing something and take our cues from them.

Observational learning spares us the expense of having to learn everything first-hand (Bandura, 1977). The authors of your book are not experts in skydiving, but from our observations of people who have gone skydiving we have the distinct impression that it is essential to have a parachute on before you jump out of the plane. Note that we did not need to learn this useful piece of information by trial and error—if we had made such an error, we would not be here to tell you about it. So, observational learning can spare us from serious, even life-threatening, mistakes. But it can also contribute to our learning of maladaptive habits.

Observational learning of aggression

In classic research in the 1960s, Albert Bandura and his colleagues demonstrated that children can learn to act aggressively by watching aggressive role models (Bandura, Ross & Ross, 1963). Bandura and his colleagues asked preschool boys and girls to watch an adult (the model) interact with a large Bobo doll, a doll that bounces back to its original upright position after being hit (Bandura, Ross & Ross, 1961). The experimenters randomly assigned some children to watch the adult model playing quietly and ignoring the Bobo doll, and others to watch the adult model punching the Bobo doll in the nose, hitting it with a mallet, sitting on it and kicking it around the room. As though that were not enough, the model in the latter condition shouted out insults and vivid descriptions of his actions while inflicting violence: 'Sock him in the nose', 'Kick him', 'Pow!'

Bandura and his colleagues then brought the children into a room with an array of appealing toys, including a miniature fire engine, a jet fighter and some dolls. Just as children began playing with these toys, the experimenter interrupted them, informing them that they needed to move to a different room. This interruption was intentional, as the investigators wanted to frustrate the children to make them more likely to behave aggressively. Then the experimenter brought them into a second room, which contained a Bobo doll identical to the one they had seen.

On a variety of dependent measures, Bandura and his colleagues found that previous exposure to the aggressive model triggered significantly more aggression against the Bobo doll than did exposure to the non-aggressive model. The children who had watched the aggressive model yelled at the doll as much as the model had done, and they even imitated many of his verbal insults. In a later study, Bandura and his colleagues (Bandura, Ross &

Ross, 1963, pp. 575–582) found essentially the same results when they displayed the aggressive models to children on film rather than in person.

Media violence and real-world aggression

The Bandura studies and scores of later studies of observational learning led psychologists to examine a theoretically and socially important question: does exposure to media violence, such as in films or movies, contribute to real-world violence—or what Bushman and Anderson (2001) called violence in the 'reel world'? The research literature addressing this question is as vast as it is confusing, and could easily occupy an entire book by itself. So, we will only briefly touch on some of the research highlights here.

Hundreds of investigators using correlational designs have reported that children who watch many violent television programmes are more aggressive than other children (Wilson & Herrnstein, 1985). These findings, though, do not demonstrate that media violence causes real-world violence (Freedman, 1984). They could simply indicate that highly aggressive children are more likely than other children to tune into aggressive television programmes. Alternatively, these findings could be due to a third variable, such as children's initial levels of aggressiveness. That is, highly aggressive children may be more likely than other children to both watch violent television programmes and to act aggressively.

Investigators have tried to get around this problem by using longitudinal designs, which track individuals' behaviour over time. Longitudinal studies show that children who watch many violent television shows commit more aggressive acts years later than do children who watch fewer violent television shows, even when researchers have equated children in their initial levels of aggression (Huesmann et al., 2003; see Figure 1.11). These studies offer somewhat more compelling evidence for a causal link between media violence and aggression than do correlational studies, but even they do not demonstrate the existence of this link. For example, an unmeasured personality variable, like impulsivity, or a social variable, like weak parental supervision, might account for these findings. Moreover, just because variable *A* precedes variable *B* does not mean that variable *A* *causes* variable *B*. For example, if we found that most common colds start with a scratchy throat and a runny nose, we should not conclude that scratchy throats and runny noses cause colds, only that they are early signs of a cold.

Still other investigators have examined whether the link between media models and later aggression holds up under strictly controlled conditions within the confines of the laboratory. In most of these studies, researchers have exposed participants to either violent or non-violent media presentations and seen whether participants in the former groups behaved more aggressively, for example by yelling at the experimenter or delivering electric shocks to another participant when provoked. In general, meta-analyses of these studies suggest a causal association between media violence and laboratory aggression (Wood, Wong & Chachere, 1991). The same conclusion may hold for the relation between violent video games and aggression (Anderson, Gentile & Buckley, 2007; Bushman & Anderson, 2001), although the causal link here is controversial and less well established

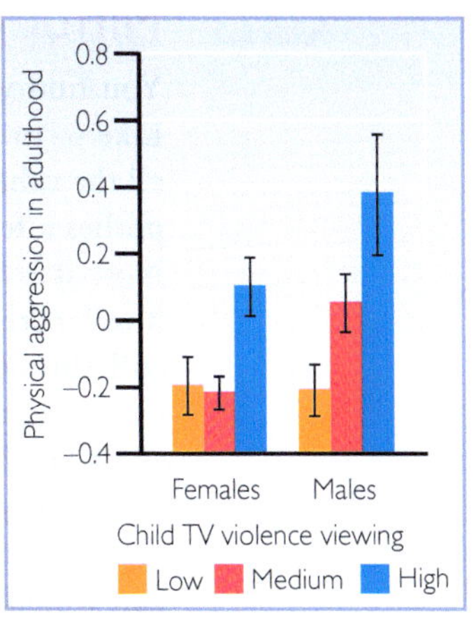

Figure 1.11 Longitudinal study of individuals who watched violent television programmes as children.

In both females and males, there is a positive correlation between viewing violent television in childhood and violent behaviour in adulthood. But this correlation does not demonstrate causality. Why?
(**Source:** Huesmann et al., 2003. Copyright © 2003 by the American Psychological Association. Reproduced with permission. The use of APA information does not imply endorsement by APA.)

Assess your knowledge — FACT or FICTION?

1. According to Skinner, animals do not think or experience emotions. **(True/False)**
2. Proponents of latent learning argue that reinforcement is not necessary for learning. **(True/False)**
3. Research on observational learning demonstrates that children can learn aggression by watching aggressive role models. **(True/False)**
4. There is no good evidence for insight learning. **(True/False)**

Answers: (1) F; (2) T; (3) T; (4) F

learn through insight rather than trial and error. There is good evidence that humans can, too (Dawes, 1994).

Biological influences on learning

For many decades, most behaviourists regarded learning as entirely distinct from biology. The animal's learning history and genetic make-up were like two ships passing in the night. Yet we now recognise this view as naïve, because our biology influences the speed and nature of our learning in complex and fascinating ways. Here are two powerful examples.

Conditioned taste aversions

One night in the 1970s, psychologist Martin Seligman went out to dinner with his wife. He ordered a filet mignon steak flavoured with sauce béarnaise, his favourite topping. Approximately six hours later, while at the opera, Seligman felt nauseated and became violently ill. He and his stomach recovered, but his love of sauce béarnaise did not. From then on, Seligman could not even think of, let alone taste, sauce béarnaise without feeling like vomiting (Seligman & Hager, 1972).

The *sauce béarnaise syndrome*, also known as *conditioned taste aversion*, refers to the fact that classical conditioning can lead us to develop avoidance reactions to the taste of food. Before reading on, ask yourself a question: does Seligman's story contradict the other examples of classical conditioning we have discussed, like that of Pavlov and his dogs?

In fact it does, in at least three ways (Garcia & Hankins, 1977):

1. In contrast to most classically conditioned reactions, which require repeated pairings between the CS and the UCS, conditioned taste aversions typically require *only one trial* to develop. This difference makes good sense. We would not want to have to experience horrific food poisoning again and again to learn a conditioned association between taste and illness. Not only would doing so be incredibly unpleasant, but in some cases, we would be dead after the first trial.
2. The delay between the CS and the UCS in conditioned taste aversions can be as long as six or even eight hours. Again, this fact makes good sense, because food poisoning often sets in many hours after eating toxic food, even though traditional conditioned learning works best when the CS and the UCS are presented close together in time.
3. Conditioned taste aversions tend to be remarkably specific and display little evidence of stimulus generalisation. For example, someone who becomes violently ill after eating lasagne may avoid lasagne at all costs but enjoy eating spaghetti, manicotti and veal parmigiana, despite their similarity to lasagne.

Conditioned taste aversions are a particular problem among cancer patients undergoing chemotherapy, which frequently induces nausea and vomiting. As a result, they frequently begin to avoid any food that preceded the chemotherapy, even though they realise it bears no logical connection to the treatment. Fortunately, health psychologists have developed a clever way around this problem. Capitalising on the specificity of conditioned taste aversions, the psychologists ask cancer patients to eat an unfamiliar *scapegoat food*—a novel food of which they are not fond—before they undergo chemotherapy. In general, the taste aversion becomes conditioned to the scapegoat food rather than to patients' preferred foods (Andresen, Birch & Johnson, 1990).

John Garcia and one of his colleagues helped to demonstrate biological influences on conditioned taste aversions. They found that rats exposed to X-rays, which make them nauseated, developed conditioned aversions to a specific taste but not to a specific visual or auditory stimulus presented after the X-rays (Garcia & Koelling, 1966). In other words, the rats more readily associated nausea with taste than with other sensory stimuli after a single exposure. Conditioned taste aversions are not much fun, but they are often adaptive. In the real world, poisoned drinks and foods, not sights and sounds, make animals feel sick. As a consequence, animals more easily develop conditioned aversions to stimuli that tend to trigger nausea in the real world (see Figure 1.12).

This finding contradicts the assumption of **equipotentiality**—the claim that we can pair all CSs equally well with all UCSs—a belief held by many traditional behaviourists (Plotkin, 2004). Garcia and others had found that certain CSs, such as those associated with taste, are easily conditioned to certain UCSs, such as those associated with nausea. Psychologists call this phenomenon *belongingness*, because certain stimuli are more likely than others to go together with certain responses (Rachman, 1977; Thorndike, 1911). Recall that following his night out with his wife, Martin Seligman felt nauseated at the thought of sauce béarnaise, but not at the thought of the opera or—thankfully, for his marriage—his wife.

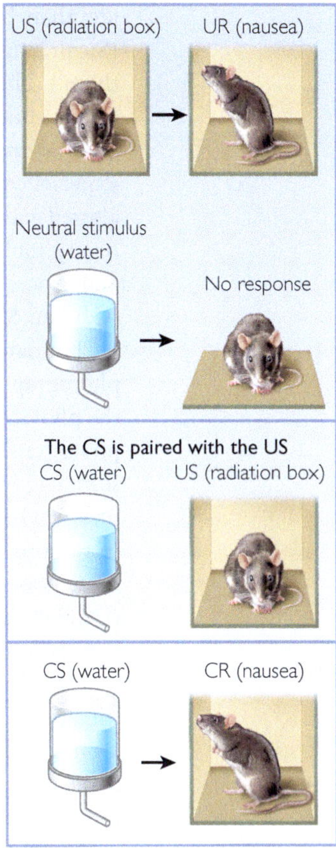

Figure 1.12 Conditioned taste aversion.

The work of John Garcia and his colleagues demonstrated that animals tend to develop conditioned taste aversions only to certain stimuli, namely those that trigger nausea in the real world.

Preparedness and phobias

A second challenge to the equipotentiality assumption comes from research on phobias. If we look at the distribution of phobias in the general population, we will find something curious: people are not always afraid of things with which they have had the most frequent unpleasant experiences. Phobias of the dark, heights, snakes, spiders, deep water and blood are commonplace, even though many people who fear these stimuli have never had a frightening encounter with them. In contrast, phobias of razors, knives, the edges of furniture, ovens and electrical outlets are extremely rare, although many of us have been cut, bruised, burned or otherwise hurt by them.

Seligman (1971) proposed that we can explain the distribution of phobias in the population by means of **preparedness**: we are evolutionarily predisposed to fear certain stimuli more than others. According to Seligman, that is because certain stimuli, like steep cliffs and poisonous animals, posed a threat to our early human ancestors (Ohman & Mineka, 2001). In contrast, household items and appliances did not, because they were not around back then. In the words of Susan Mineka and Michael Cook (1993), prepared fears are 'evolutionary memories': emotional legacies of natural selection.

Mineka and Cook (1993) showed lab-reared rhesus monkeys, who had no previous exposure to snakes, a videotape of fellow monkeys reacting in horror to snakes. Within

Equipotentiality
Assumption that any conditioned stimulus can be associated equally well with any unconditioned stimulus.

Preparedness
Evolutionary predisposition to learn some pairings of feared stimuli over others owing to their survival value.

less than half an hour, the monkeys acquired a fear of snakes by observational learning. (Surprisingly, rhesus monkeys who have never been exposed to snakes show no fear of them.) The researchers then edited the videotape to show the same monkeys reacting in horror, but this time in response to flowers, a toy rabbit, a toy snake and a toy crocodile. They then showed these doctored videotapes to different groups of monkeys who had no experience with flowers, rabbits, snakes or crocodiles. The monkeys who observed these altered videotapes acquired fears of the toy snake and toy crocodile, but not the flowers or toy rabbit. From the standpoint of preparedness, this finding is understandable. Snakes and crocodiles were dangerous to our primate ancestors, but flowers and rabbits were not (Ohman & Mineka, 2003).

Humans also show prepared learning. In fear-learning studies, participants look at photographs of various subjects, including spiders, snakes, flowers and mushrooms. Some of the photographs are always paired with a mild electric shock. Participants readily learn which photographs signal danger (the shock) and which ones do not, and they exhibit enhanced skin conductance (sweating) when those photographs are presented. In the extinction phase, when shocks are no longer administered, participants show resistance to extinction in response to the photographs of snakes and spiders—that is, they continue to sweat when these photographs are presented, but not so for the photographs of flowers and mushrooms (Ohman & Mineka, 2001). This suggests that people are prepared to associate danger with threats from our evolutionary history.

Visual search studies indicate that people may also be prepared to detect evolutionary threats. When presented with an array of photographs in which a snake is placed among a bunch of flowers, participants very quickly find the snake. However, when the task is reversed and participants have to look for a flower among snakes, they are slower to find the flower. This 'snake in the grass effect' (Ohman, Flykt & Esteves, 2001) may mean that evolution has put us on the lookout for stimuli that could threaten our safety and survival.

Preparedness may render us likely to develop *illusory correlations* between fear-provoking stimuli and negative consequences (Tomarken, Mineka & Cook, 1989). An illusory correlation is a statistical mirage; it is the perception of a non-existent association between two variables. One team of investigators administered intermittent mild electric shocks to participants—some of whom feared snakes and some of whom did not—while they watched slides of snakes and damaged electrical outlets. The pairings of the slide stimuli with the shocks were random, so that the actual correlation between them was zero. Yet participants with high levels of snake fear perceived a marked correlation between the occurrence of the snake slides, but not the electrical outlets, with the electric shocks. Participants with low levels of snake fear did not fall prey to this illusory correlation (Tomarken, Sutton & Mineka, 1995).

Snake-fearful participants were on the lookout for any threatening stimuli that might signal snakes, so they overestimated how often snake slides co-occurred with electric shock. Interestingly, they showed no such overestimation for electrical outlets, even though they are more closely linked in our minds than are snakes with electric shock. This finding suggests that preparedness may be at work, because snakes, but not electrical outlets, would have posed a threat to the safety of our distant ancestors.

Still, some of the laboratory evidence for preparedness points to explanations that are not evolutionary in nature. For instance, researchers at the University of Queensland have shown that participants sometimes respond to non-prepared stimuli, such as dogs and fish, in the same way that they respond to snakes and spiders, following a short training session in which the non-prepared stimuli were consistently associated with electric shock (Purkis & Lipp, 2008). These findings indicate that basic learning processes could account for common phobias, at least some of the time. Moreover, some authors have proposed that preparedness findings may be due to an alternative explanation: latent inhibition. As you will recall from earlier in the chapter, latent inhibition refers to the fact that CSs that have appeared alone (that is, without a UCS) many times are especially difficult to classically condition to a stimulus. Because we routinely encounter electrical sockets, stoves, knives and the like without experiencing any negative consequences, these stimuli may be resistant to classical conditioning. In contrast, because few of us have regular encounters with snakes and spiders, these stimuli may be more easily classically conditioned to aversive outcomes (Bond & Siddle, 1996).[2]

Aside from preparedness, genetic influences probably play a role in the acquisition of certain phobias. Dog phobics and non-dog phobics do not differ in their number of negative experiences with dogs, such as bites (DiNardo, Guzy & Bak, 1988). Moreover, only about half of dog phobics have ever had a scary encounter with a dog; the same holds for people with many other phobias. These results make it unlikely that classical conditioning alone can explain all cases of phobia. Instead, some people appear genetically predisposed to develop phobias given a history of certain classical conditioning experiences (Kendler et al., 1992).[B]

Assess your knowledge — FACT or FICTION?

1. Many conditioned taste aversions are acquired in only a single trial. **(True/False)**
2. Most research suggests that the assumption of equipotentiality is false. **(True/False)**
3. The phenomenon of preparedness helps explain why virtually all major phobias are equally common in the general population. **(True/False)**

Answers: (1) T; (2) T; (3) F

[B]Lilienfeld, S. O., Lynn, S. J., Namy, L. L., Woolf, N. J., Jamieson, G., Marks, A., & Slaughter, V. (2015). Learning: How nurture changes us. In S. O. Lilienfeld, S. J. Lynn, L. L. Namy, & N. J. Woolf (Eds.), *Psychology: From inquiry to understanding* (2nd ed., pp. 239–249). Melbourne, VIC: Pearson Australia.

Summary

Classical conditioning

- Classical conditioning is a form of learning discovered by physiologist, Ivan Pavlov.
- Classical conditioning occurs in three phases – acquisition, extinction and spontaneous recovery
- Classical conditioning can apply to many situations of daily life, e.g., acquisition of fears and phobias

Operant conditioning

- Operant conditioning is learning controlled by the consequences of the organism's behaviour
- Skinner's theory of operant conditioning was based on the work of Thorndike. Edward Thorndike studied learning in animals using a puzzle box to propose the theory known as the 'Law of Effect'
- There are three key concepts in Skinnerian psychology: reinforcement, punishment and discriminant stimulus

Cognitive models of learning

- S-O-R psychology is the abbreviation for stimulus-organism-response psychology. It deals with how an organism will respond to a stimulus
- S-O-R theorists emphasise the role of expectations in learning
- Edward C. Tolman first proposed the theory of latent learning in 1930, when his experiments with rats showed that learning was taking place even without the immediate presence of a reward
- Observational learning is learning that occurs through observing the behaviour of others

Biological influences on learning

- Taste aversion—learning to avoid a food that makes you sick—is a form of classical conditioning
- Seligman (1971) developed the preparedness theory of fear acquisition. Seligman noted that the common feature of stimuli that become the target of a phobic reaction is that they are biologically threatening

Review questions

A. Fill in the missing words to complete the following statements.

1. Classical conditioning is a form of learning whereby a ____________________ becomes associated with an unrelated ________________________ in order to produce a behavioural response known as a conditioned response (CR).
2. Acquisition is the _______________ phase during which a conditioned response is formed. In classical conditioning, repeated pairings of the _______________________________ and the ___________________________________ eventually leads to acquisition. After pairing the CS with the UCS repeatedly, the CS alone will come to elicit the response, which is now known as the ____________________________.
3. While classical conditioning depends on developing associations between events, the form of conditioning that involves learning from the consequences of our behaviour is called ____________________________.
4. Positive and negative punishment, ____________________ the likelihood of behaviour.
5. In operant conditioning, a ___________________________ is a schedule of reinforcement where a response is reinforced after an unpredictable number of responses. This schedule of reinforcement usually yields the highest rates of responding of all four schedules.

B. Read the following sentences and answer with the most correct definition.

6. In Pavlov's dog experiment, after numerous presentations of the metronome without the meat powder, the dogs eventually stopped salivating. This is an example of _____________.
7. Imagine a young child being introduced to different dog breeds for the first time. When the chid sees a Border Collie and responds "dog!", the parents reward the child with praise and they learn that the animal is indeed a dog. When the child sees a Terrier and responds "dog!", they are also rewarded with praise. The child responds the same way to both types of dog stimuli, and each response generates the same result. In this way the child learns to call all dog breeds "dogs," even though they are of different sizes and have different types of fur, and colour. This is an example of __________________________.
8. Edward Thorndike hypothesised that any behaviour that is followed by pleasant consequences is likely to be repeated, and any behaviour followed by unpleasant consequences is likely to be stopped. This is known as the ______________________.
9. You leave home at 8am to drive to work, and you always encounter heavy traffic. From now on you leave home at 7am, causing you to avoid the heavy traffic. This is an example of ____________________________.

C. Please select one statement that best answers each of the following questions.

10. Classical conditioning occurs when a(n)
a) neutral stimulus is paired with an unconditioned stimulus
b) conditioned stimulus is paired with an unconditioned stimulus
c) neutral stimulus is paired with a conditioned response
d) conditioned stimulus is paired with a conditioned response
e) unconditioned stimulus is paired with a conditioned response

11. A neutral stimulus is one that
a) does not elicit an unconditioned response
b) elicits an unconditioned response
c) elicits a conditioned response
d) elicits a controlled response
e) returns spontaneously during spontaneous recovery

12. A conditioned response will weaken and eventually disappear if the CS is presented in the absence of the US. This is referred to as
a) spontaneous recovery
b) generalisation
c) discrimination
d) reconditioning
e) extinction

13. Through classical conditioning, Marie has developed a fear of dogs. However, she fears only large, longhaired dogs and not small, longhaired dogs or large, shorthaired dogs. Marie is demonstrating
a) spontaneous recovery
b) stimulus discrimination
c) stimulus generalisation
d) latent learning
e) extinction

14. A man has a severe phobia involving spiders. He has this phobia because, as a child, he used to observe his mother scream every time a spider appeared. In this example, the spider is a(n)
a) conditioned stimulus
b) conditioned response
c) unconditioned stimulus
d) unconditioned response

15. The process of learning in which the consequences of a response determine the probability that the response will be repeated is called
a) classical conditioning
b) operant conditioning
c) insight learning
d) observational learning
e) latent learning

CHAPTER 2

Human Development

The content in this section has been compiled from:
Gerrig, Zimbardo, Campbell, Cumming & Wilkes, Chapter 11

Gerrig, R. J., Zimbardo, P. G., Campbell, A. J., Cumming, S. R., & Wilkes, F. J. (Eds.). (2012). Human development across the lifespan. In *Psychology and life* (2nd ed., pp. 358–373, 377–395). Frenchs Forest, NSW: Pearson Australia.

CHAPTER 2

Human Development

Health is often a consequence of multiple determinants from genetic, biological, behavioural and social contexts that change as a person develops across the lifespan. This chapter presents a number of theories that provide a framework for understanding how development occurs and how it affects behaviours, including health behaviours and the consequent health outcomes.

After studying this chapter you should be able to:

- Describe physical development across the lifespan
- Describe cognitive development across the lifespan
- Describe Piaget's stages of cognitive development
- Describe Erikson's stages of psychosocial development
- Describe Kohlberg's stages of moral reasoning.

Imagine you are holding a newborn baby. How might you predict what this child will be like as a 1-year-old? At 5 years? At 15? At 50? At 70? At 90? Your predictions would almost certainly consist of a mixture of the general and the specific—the child is extremely likely to learn a language but might or might not be a gifted author. Your predictions would also rely on considerations of heredity and of environment—if both of the child's parents were gifted authors, you might be willing to guess that the child would also show literary talent; if the child was educated in an enriched environment, you might predict that the child's accomplishments would exceed those of the parents. In this chapter, we describe the theories of developmental psychology that enable us to think systematically about the types of predictions we can make for the life course of a newborn child.

Developmental psychology is the area of psychology that is concerned with changes in physical and psychological functioning that occur from conception across the entire life span. The task of developmental psychologists is to find out how and why organisms change over time—to document and explain development. Investigators study the time periods in which different abilities and functions first appear and observe how those abilities are modified. The basic premise is that mental functioning, social relationships and other vital aspects of human nature develop and change throughout the entire life cycle. Table 2.1 presents a rough guide to the major periods of the life span.

Developmental psychology The branch of psychology concerned with interaction between physical and psychological processes and with stages of growth from conception throughout the entire life span.

In this chapter we will provide a general account of how researchers document development and the theories they use to explain patterns of change over time. We will then divide your life experiences into different domains and trace development in each domain. Early in the chapter, we focus on physical, cognitive and language development. We then shift our attention to the changing nature of social relationships over the life span as well as the specific tasks individuals face at different moments in their lives. Let's begin now with the question of what it means to study development.

Studying development

Suppose we ask you to make a list of all the ways in which you believe you have changed in the last year. What sorts of things would you put on the list? Have you undertaken a new physical fitness program? Or have you let an injury heal? Have you developed a range of new hobbies? Or have you decided to focus on just one interest? Have you developed a new circle of friends? Or have you become particularly close to one individual? When we describe development, we will conceptualise it in terms of *change*. We have asked you to perform this exercise of thinking about your own changes to make the point that change almost always involves trade-offs.

Often people conceptualise the life span as mostly *gains* (changes for the better) in childhood and mostly *losses* (changes for the worse) over the course of adulthood. However, the perspective on development we will take here emphasises that *options*, and therefore gains and losses, are features of all development (Dixon, 2003, pp. 151–167; Lachman, 2004). When, for example, people choose a lifetime companion, they give up variety but gain security. When people retire, they give up status but gain leisure time.

It is also important that you not think of development as a *passive* process. You will see that many developmental changes require an individual's *active* engagement with his or her environment (Bronfenbrenner, 2004).

Table 2.1 Stages in life span development

Stage	Age period
Prenatal	Conception to birth
Infancy	Birth at full term to about 18 months
Early childhood	About 18 months to about 6 years
Middle childhood	About 6 years to about 11 years
Adolescence	About 11 years to about 20 years
Early adulthood	About 20 years to about 40 years
Middle adulthood	About 40 years to about 65 years
Late adulthood	About 65 years and older

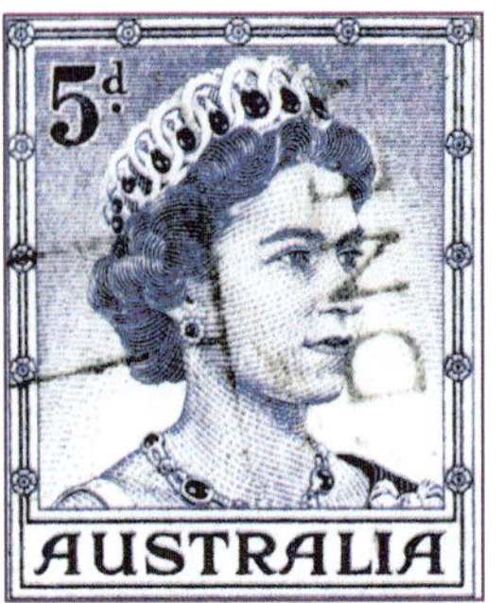

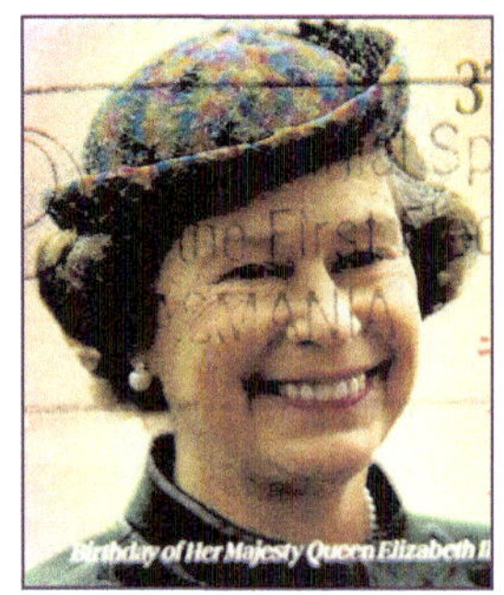

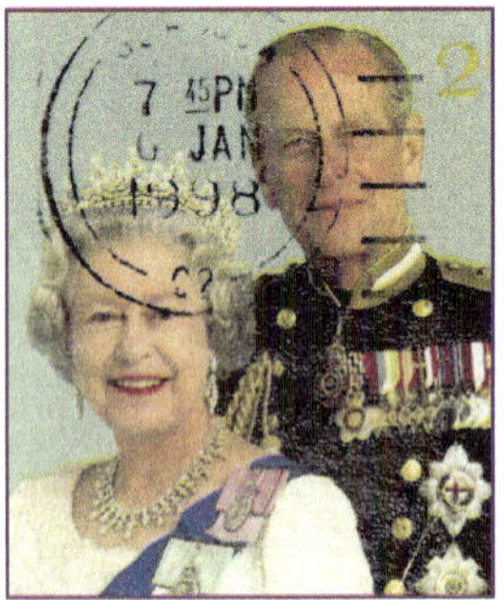

In a longitudinal design, observations are made of the same individual at different ages, often for many years. This well-known woman might be part of a longitudinal study of British children born in 1926. How might she be similar to and different from other children in that cohort? (**Source:** Sergey Ozerov/ Dreamstime.com, © Tiziano Casalta/ Dreamstime.com)

To document change, a good first step is to determine what an average person is like—in physical appearance, cognitive abilities, and so on—at a particular age. **Normative investigations** seek to describe a characteristic of a specific age or developmental stage. By systematically testing individuals of different ages, researchers can determine developmental landmarks. These data provide *norms*, standard patterns of development or achievement, based on observation of many people.

Normative standards allow psychologists to make a distinction between chronological age (the number of months or years since a person's birth) and **developmental age** (the chronological age at which most people show the particular level of physical or mental development demonstrated by that child). A 3-year-old child who has verbal skills typical of most 5-year-olds is said to have a developmental age of 5 for verbal skills. Norms provide a standard basis for comparison both between individuals and between groups.

Developmental psychologists use several types of research designs to understand possible mechanisms of change. In a **longitudinal design**, the same individuals are repeatedly observed and tested over time, often for many years (see Figure 2.1). In a study on the effectiveness of the High/Scope Perry preschool program researchers first collected data on a group of children when they were 3 and 4 years old (Schweinhart, 2004). To assess the long-term impact of the preschool program, the researchers studied the children every year until age 11, and then again at ages 14, 15, 19, 27 and 40. This

Normative investigation
A research effort designed to describe what is characteristic of a specific age or developmental stage.

Developmental age
The chronological age at which most children show a particular level of physical or mental development.

Longitudinal design
A research design in which the same participants are observed repeatedly, sometimes over many years.

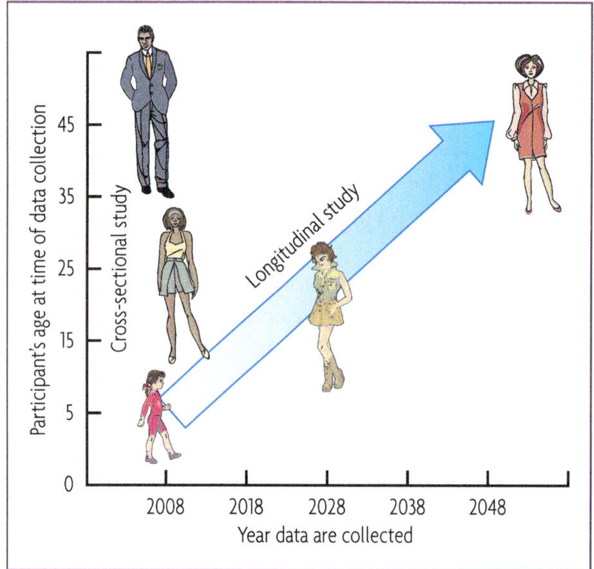

Figure 2.1 Longitudinal and cross-sectional research

In longitudinal studies, researchers follow the same group of individuals over days, months or years. In cross-sectional studies, researchers test individuals of different ages at the same moment in time.

longitudinal data collection allowed the researchers to draw strong conclusions about the program's lifelong benefits. Researchers also often use longitudinal designs to study *individual differences*. To understand the life outcomes of different people, researchers may assess a range of potential causal factors early in life and see how those factors influence each individual's life course.

A general advantage of longitudinal research is that because the participants have lived through the same socioeconomic period, age-related changes cannot be confused with variations in differing societal circumstances. A disadvantage, however, is that some types of generalisations can be made only to the same *cohort*, the group of individuals born in the same time period as the research participants. Suppose, for example, we discovered that current 50-year-olds showed a gain in happiness in the years after their children left home. That result might not apply to a future cohort of 50-year-olds who grew up with different expectations about how long children would remain in their parents' homes. Also, longitudinal studies are costly because it is difficult to keep track of the participants over extended time, and data are easily lost because participants quit or disappear.

Much research on development uses a **cross-sectional design**, in which groups of participants, of different chronological ages, are observed and compared at one and the same time. A researcher can then draw conclusions about behavioural differences that may be related to age changes. For example, researchers who wanted to determine how children learn to walk without falling down tested children of ages 15, 21, 27, 33 and 39 months on the same laboratory task (Joh & Adolph, 2006). A disadvantage of cross-sectional design comes from comparing individuals who differ by year of birth as well as by chronological age. Age-related changes are confounded by differences in the social or political conditions experienced by different birth cohorts. Thus a study comparing samples of 10- and 18-year-olds now might find that the participants differ from 10- and 18-year-olds who grew up in the 1970s, in ways related to their different eras as well as to their developmental stages.

Cross-sectional design
A research method in which groups of participants of different chronological ages are observed and compared at a given time.

Each methodology gives researchers the opportunity to document change from one age to another. Researchers use these methodologies to study development in each of several domains. As we now consider some of those domains—physical, cognitive and social development—you'll come to appreciate and understand some of the vast changes you've already experienced.

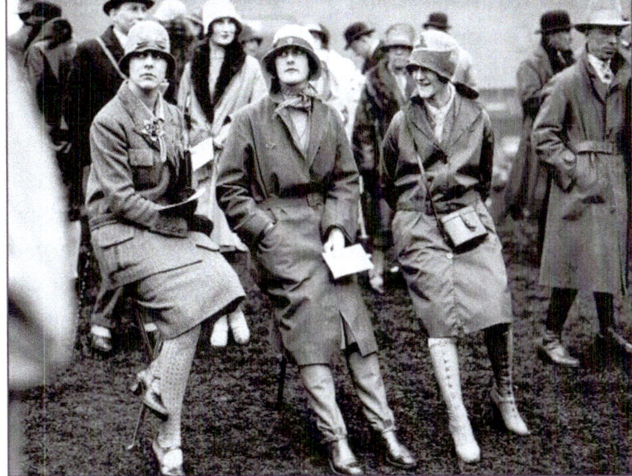

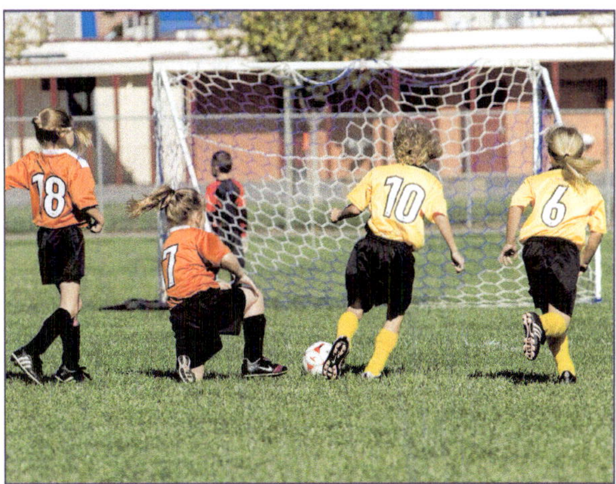

A drawback of cross-sectional research is the cohort effect. What differences might exist between these two groups of females as a result of the eras in which they lived?
(**Source:** Hulton Archive/Getty Images.)

Stop and review

1. What is developmental age?
2. Why are longitudinal designs often used to study individual differences?
3. What is the relevance of birth cohorts to cross-sectional designs?

Physical development The bodily changes, maturation and growth that occur in an organism, starting with conception and continuing across the life span.

Zygote The single cell that results when a sperm fertilises an egg.

Germinal stage The first two weeks of prenatal development following conception.

Embryonic stage The second stage of prenatal development, lasting from the third week through to 8 weeks after conception.

Foetal stage The third stage of prenatal development, lasting from the ninth week through to the birth of the child.

Physical development across the life span

Many of the types of development we describe in this chapter require some special knowledge to detect. For example, you might not notice landmarks in social development until you read about them here. We will begin, however, with a realm of development in which changes are often plainly visible to the untrained eye: **physical development**. There is no doubt that you have undergone enormous physical change since you were born. Such changes will continue until the end of your life. Because physical changes are so numerous, we will focus on the types that have an impact on psychological development.

Prenatal and childhood development

You began life with unique genetic potential: at the moment of conception a male's sperm cell fertilised a female's egg cell to form the single-cell **zygote**; you received half of the 46 chromosomes found in all normal human body cells from your mother and half from your father. In this section, we outline physical development in the *prenatal period*, from the moment of conception until the moment of birth. We also describe some of the sensory abilities children have obtained even before birth. Finally, we describe the important physical changes that you experienced during childhood.

Physical development in the womb

The first two weeks after formation of the zygote are known as the **germinal stage** of prenatal development. During this stage, cells begin to divide rapidly; after about 1 week a mass of microscopic cells attaches itself to the mother's uterine wall. The third through eighth week of prenatal development is called the **embryonic stage**. During this stage, rapid cell division continues, but the cells begin to become specialised to form different organs. As these organs develop, the first heartbeat occurs. Responses to stimulation have been observed as early as the sixth week, when the *embryo* is not yet an inch long; spontaneous movements are observed by the eighth week (Kisilevsky & Low, 1998).

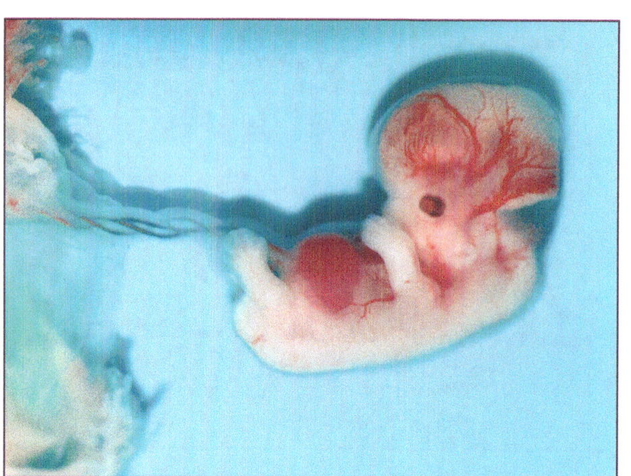

As the brain grows in the developing foetus, it generates 250,000 new neurons per minute. What must the brain be prepared to do, as soon as the child enters the world?
(**Source:** SMC Images/Getty Images.)

The **foetal stage** lasts from the end of the eighth week through to the birth of the child. The mother will feel the *foetus* move in about the sixteenth week after conception. At this point, the foetus is about 18 centimetres long (the average length at birth is 50 centimetres). As the brain grows in utero, it generates new neurons at the rate of 250,000 per minute, reaching a full complement of over 100 billion neurons by birth (Cowan, 1979). In humans and many other mammals, most of this cell proliferation and migration of neurons to their correct locations take place before birth; the development of the branching processes of axons and dendrites largely occurs after birth (Kolb, 1989). The sequence of brain development, from 30 days to 9 months, is shown in Figure 2.2.

Over the course of pregnancy, environmental factors such as infection, radiation or drugs can prevent the normal formation of organs and body structures. Any environmental factor that causes structural abnormalities in the foetus is called a **teratogen**. For example, when mothers are infected with rubella (German measles), their children often suffer negative consequences such as mental retardation, eye damage, deafness or heart defects. When the infection occurs in the first 6 weeks after conception, the probability of birth defects may be 100 percent (De Santis et al., 2006). If exposure occurs later in the pregnancy, the probability of adverse effects becomes lower (e.g., 50 percent in the fourth month; 6 percent in the fifth month). Mothers who consume alcohol during sensitive periods of pregnancy put their unborn children at risk for brain damage and other impairments (Bailey & Sokol, 2008). *Foetal alcohol syndrome* is the most serious consequence of a mother's alcohol

Teratogen
Environmental factors such as diseases and drugs that cause structural abnormalities in a developing foetus.

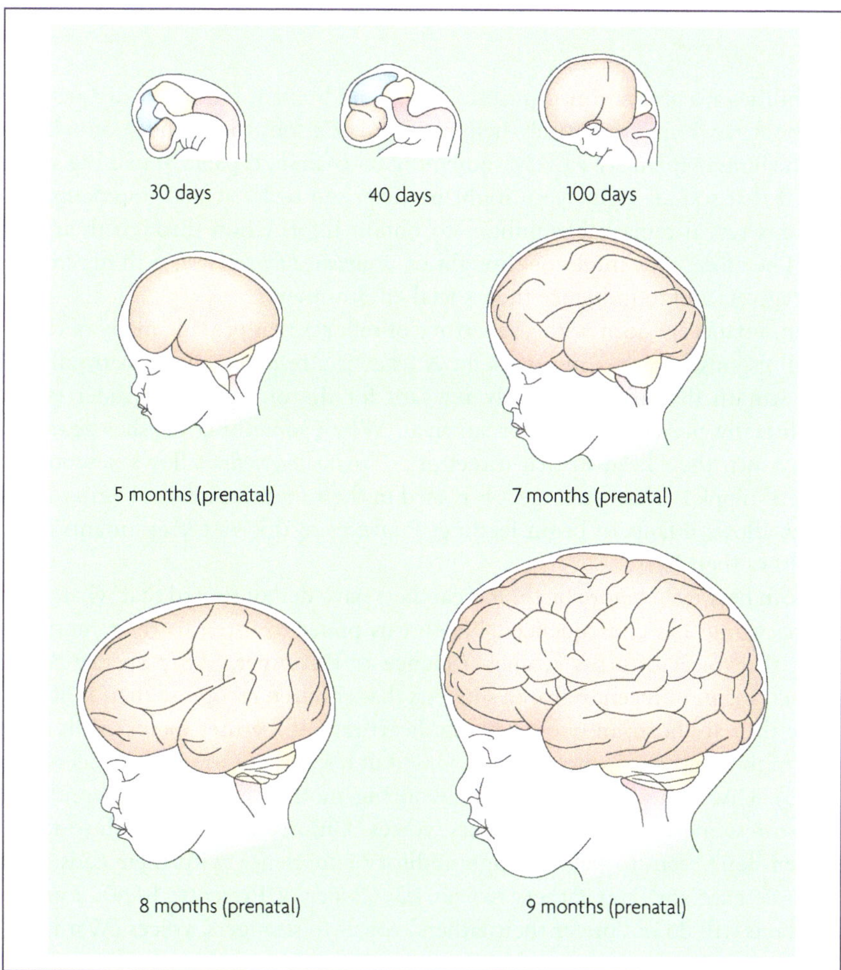

Figure 2.2 The development of the human brain

During the 9 months before birth, the brain reaches its complement of over 100 billion neurons.
Adapted from Cowan, W.M. (1979). *The Brain*. Copyright © 1979 W.M. Cowan.

consumption during pregnancy. Children with foetal alcohol syndrome often have small heads and bodies and facial abnormalities. Disruptions of the central nervous system cause cognitive and behavioural problems (Niccols, 2007).

Pregnant women who smoke also put their children at risk. Smoking during pregnancy increases the risk of miscarriage, premature births, and low birth-weight babies (Salihu & Wilson, 2007). In fact, women who are exposed to second-hand smoke during pregnancy are also more likely to have babies with low birth weights (Dejin-Karlsson et al., 1998). Finally, almost all illicit drugs cause damage to the foetus. Cocaine, for example, travels through the placenta and can affect foetal development directly. In adults, cocaine causes blood vessels to constrict; in pregnant women, cocaine restricts placental blood flow and oxygen supply to the foetus. If severe oxygen deprivation results, blood vessels in the foetus's brain may burst. Such prenatal strokes can lead to lifelong mental handicaps (Bennett et al., 2008; Singer et al., 2002). Research suggests that the brain systems most damaged by cocaine are those responsible for controlling attention: children exposed to cocaine in the womb may spend their lives overcome by the distractions of irrelevant sights and sounds (Savage et al., 2005). We use these examples to emphasise that nature and nurture interact to shape the body and brain even before a child is born.

Babies prewired for survival

What capabilities are programmed into this body and brain at birth? We are accustomed to thinking about newborns as entirely helpless. John Watson, the founder of behaviourism, described the human infant as 'a lively, squirming bit of flesh, capable of making a few simple responses'. If that sounds right, you might be surprised to learn that, moments out of the womb, infants reveal remarkable abilities to obtain information through their senses and react to it. Therefore, they might be thought of as *prewired for survival*, well suited to respond to adult caregivers and to influence their social environments.

To begin, infants are born with a repertory of reflexes that provide many of their earliest behavioural responses to the environment. A *reflex* is a response that is naturally triggered by specific stimuli that are biologically relevant for the organism. Consider two reflexes that quite literally prewire infants for survival. When something brushes against infants' cheeks, they turn their head in that direction. This *rooting reflex* allows newborns to find their mothers' nipples. When an object is placed in their mouths, infants begin to suck. This *sucking reflex* allows infants to begin feeding. Reflexes of this sort keep infants alive in the early months of their lives.

Infants can hear even before birth. Researchers have demonstrated that what infants hear while in the womb has consequences. Newborns prefer to listen to their mothers' voices rather than the voices of other women (Spence & DeCasper, 1987; Spence & Freeman, 1996). In fact, the most recent research suggests that children recognise their mothers' voices even before they are born: in one study, the heart rate of foetuses increased in response to recordings of their mothers' voices and decreased in response to strangers' voices (Kisilevsky et al., 2003). Given these strong results favouring mothers, you might wonder whether children also respond more to their fathers' voices. Unfortunately, research so far indicates that children don't seem to have enough auditory experience with their dads. Newborns show no preference for their fathers' voices (DeCasper & Prescott, 1984). Even at age 4 months, infants still do not prefer their fathers' voices to strangers' voices (Ward & Cooper, 1999).

Infants also put their visual systems to work almost immediately: a few minutes after birth, a newborn's eyes are alert, turning in the direction of a voice and searching inquisitively for the source of certain sounds. Even so, vision is less well developed than the other senses at birth. The visual acuity of adults is roughly 40 times better than the visual acuity of newborns (Sireteanu, 1999). Visual acuity improves rapidly over the first 6 months of a baby's life. Newborns are also ill equipped to experience the world in three dimensions. You use a great variety of cues to experience depth. Researchers have begun to document the time course with which infants are able to interpret each type of cue. For example, at 4 months, infants start being able to use cues such as relative motion and interposition to infer three-dimensional structures from two-dimensional images of objects (Shuwairi et al., 2007; Soska & Johnson, 2008).

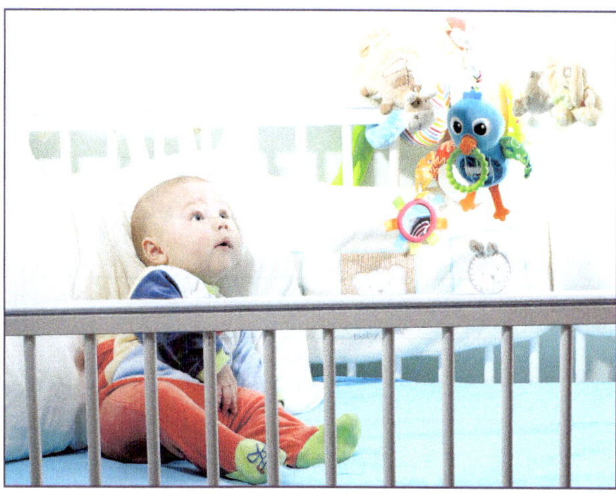

Early on, infants can perceive large objects that display a great deal of contrast. What visual experiences do newborns find particularly appealing?

Even without perfect vision, however, children have visual preferences. Pioneering researcher Robert Fantz (1963) observed that babies as young as 4 months old preferred looking at objects with contours rather than those that were plain, complex ones rather than simple ones, and whole faces rather than faces with features in disarray. More recent research suggests that—by the age of 3 days—infants have a preference for *top-heavy patterns* (Macchi Cassia et al., 2004). To experience a top-heavy pattern, take a look at your face in a mirror—your eyes, eyebrows, and so on, take up much more space than your lips. The fact that faces are top heavy might explain why infants prefer to look at human faces versus other types of visual displays.

Once children start to move around in their environment, they quickly acquire other perceptual capabilities. For example, classic research by Eleanor Gibson and Richard Walk (1960) examined how children respond to depth information. This research used an apparatus called a *visual cliff*. The visual cliff had a board running across the middle of a solid glass surface. As shown in Figure 2.3, checkerboard cloth was used to create a deep end and a shallow end. In their original research, Gibson and Walk demonstrated

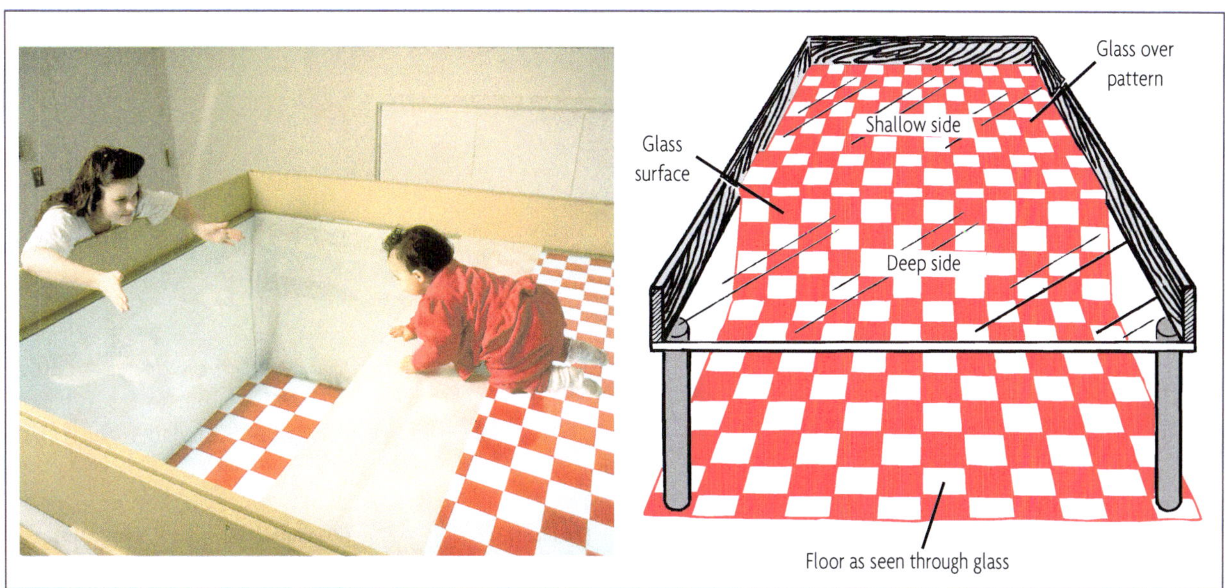

Figure 2.3 The visual cliff

Once children have gained experience crawling around their environment, they show fear of the deep side of the visual cliff.

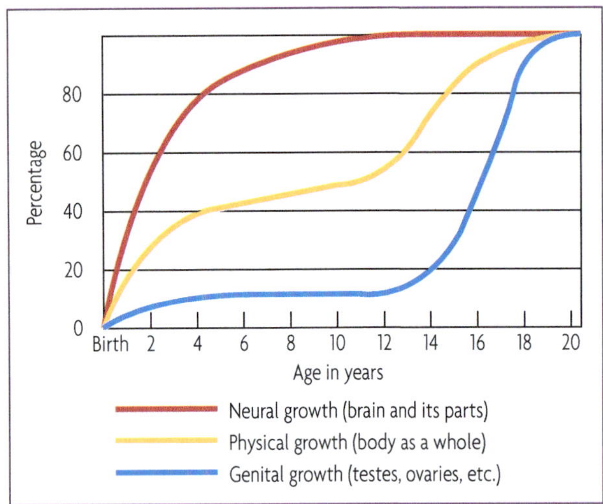

Figure 2.4 Growth patterns across the first two decades of life

Neural growth occurs very rapidly in the first year of life. It is much faster than overall physical growth. By contrast, genital maturation does not occur until adolescence.

that children would readily leave the centre board to crawl across the shallow end, but they were reluctant to crawl across the deep end. Subsequent research has demonstrated that fear of the deep end depends on crawling experience: children who have begun to crawl experience fear of the deep end, whereas their non-crawling same-age peers do not (Campos et al., 1992; Witherington et al., 2005). Thus wariness of heights is not quite 'prewired,' but it develops quickly as children begin to explore the world under their own power.

Growth and maturation in childhood

Newborn infants change at an astonishing rate but, as shown in Figure 2.4, physical growth is not equal across all physical structures. You've probably noticed that babies seem to be all head. At birth, a baby's head is already about 60 percent of its adult size and measures a quarter of the whole body length (Bayley, 1956). An infant's body weight doubles in the first 6 months and triples by the first birthday; by the age of 2, a child's trunk is about half of its adult length. Genital tissue shows little change until the teenage years and then develops rapidly to adult proportions.

Maturation The continuing influence of heredity throughout development; the age-related physical and behavioural changes characteristic of a species.

For most children, physical growth is accompanied by the maturation of motor ability. **Maturation** refers to the process of growth typical of all members of a species who are reared in the species' usual habitat. The characteristic maturational sequences newborns experience

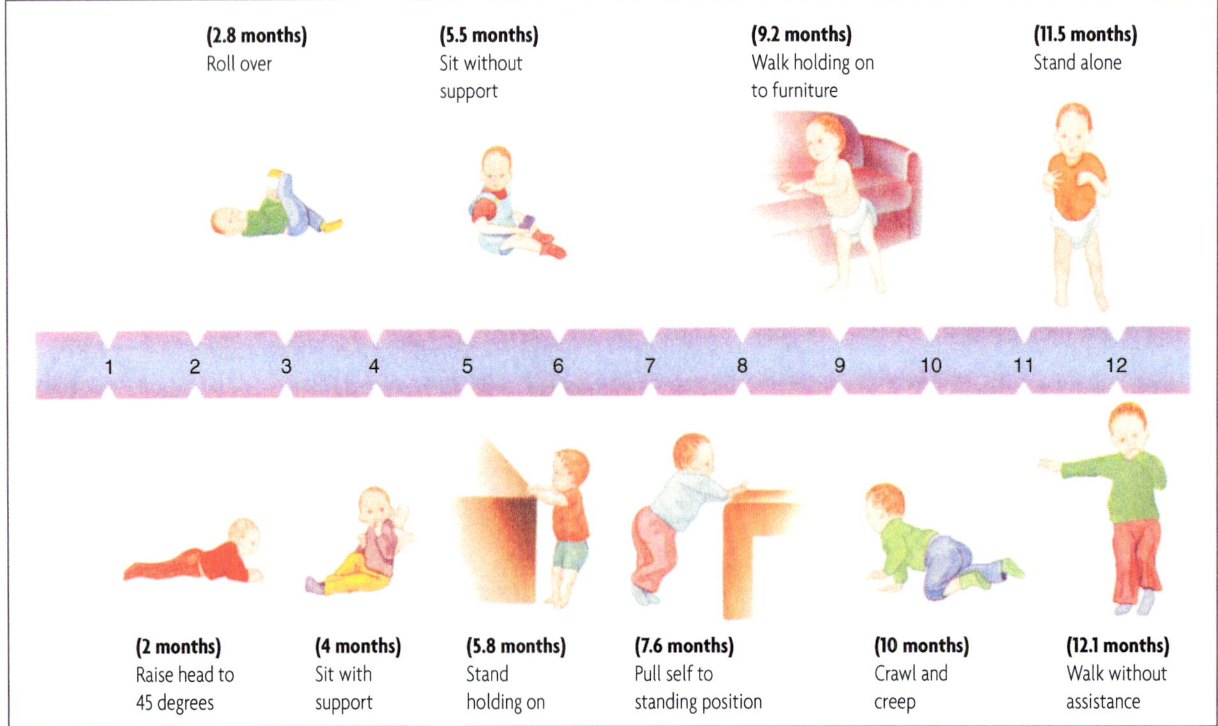

Figure 2.5 Maturational timetable for locomotion

The development of walking requires no special teaching. It follows a fixed, time-ordered sequence that is typical of all physically capable members of our species.

are determined by the interaction of inherited biological boundaries and environmental inputs. For example, in the sequence for locomotion, as shown in Figure 2.5, a child learns to sit up without special training. This sequence applies to the great majority of babies; a minority of children skip a step or develop their own original sequences. Even so, in cultures in which there is less physical stimulation, children begin to walk later. In typical non-Indigenous Australian society, most babies are pushed in strollers during their early infant years. This is not the case in Indigenous culture, where most babies are carried about on a relative's back or hip. The difference between these two cultural groups is that Indigenous children tend to develop faster motor skills due to their having exposure to more exercise in their environment than most non-Indigenous children. Although it is believed that Indigenous Australian children tend to develop faster in motor skill development, it is still important to note that infants across all cultural groups will develop their full potential of motor skills. Having said this, some infants are likely to excel in development over certain stages.

For more than a decade there has been an unheeded call for culturally relevant national legislation relating to Aboriginal and Torres Strait Islander child development. Such legislation would ensure that attention is given to Indigenous children's cultural and traditional needs in addition to the more obvious needs of food, clothing, health and safety. In the absence of this legislation, research has tended to learn more about specific health development, rather than psychological and motor development, in Indigenous children. This is perhaps due to there being a higher rate of immunity problems, asthma and nutritional problems in Indigenous communities than in non-Indigenous communities, and these issues more often than not lead to increased problems with normal physical and intellectual development (RHEF, 2005).

Physical development in adolescence

The first concrete indicator of the end of childhood is the *pubescent growth spurt*. At around age 10 for girls and age 12 for boys, growth hormones flow into the bloodstream. For several years, the adolescent may grow 8 to 15 centimetres a year and gain weight rapidly as well. The adolescent's body does not reach adult proportions all at once. Hands and feet grow to full adult size first. The arms and legs come next, with the torso developing most slowly. Thus an individual's overall shape changes several times over the teenage years.

Another important process that occurs during adolescence is **puberty**, which brings about sexual maturity. (The Latin word *pubertas* means 'covered with hair' and signifies the growth of hair on the arms and legs, under the arms and in the genital area.) Puberty for males brings about the production of live sperm; for girls it leads to **menarche**, the onset of menstruation. In Australia, the average time for menarche is between the ages of 12 and 13, although the normal range extends from 11 to 15. For boys, the production of live sperm first occurs, on average, between the ages of 12 and 14, but again there is considerable variation in this timing. These physical changes often bring about an awareness of sexual feelings.

Puberty
The process through which sexual maturity is attained.

Menarche
The onset of menstruation.

Some other important physical changes happen inside adolescents' brains. Researchers once thought that most brain growth was over within the first few years of life. However, recent studies using brain imaging techniques have demonstrated continuing development within the adolescent brain (Paus, 2005). Researchers have documented particularly important changes in the *limbic system*, which regulates emotional processes, and the *frontal lobes*, the areas responsible for planning and control of emotions. However, maturation of the limbic system precedes maturation of the frontal lobes. The relative timing of changes within those regions may explain one of most salient aspects of social development in adolescence (Casey et al., 2008; Steinberg, 2008): adolescents tend to engage in risky behaviour. Let's explore this insight.

We'll return to social aspects of risky behaviour when we review social development across the life span. For now, our focus is on physical development. Researchers speculate that maturation of the limbic system readies adolescents to go out into the world: 'Evolutionarily speaking, adolescence is the period in which independence skills are acquired to increase success upon separation from the protection of the family' (Casey et al., 2008, p. 70). In that evolutionary context, it makes sense that regions of the frontal cortex that inhibit and control the emotional drive toward independence would mature somewhat later in life. To survive apart from their families, adolescents would have to take some initial risks. The difficulty is that in contemporary times people no longer typically leave their families during adolescence. Thus, the evolutionary impulse toward novelty seeking and risk taking no longer has an adaptive function. Fortunately, as people develop from adolescence into adulthood, the frontal lobes achieve maturity (Steinberg, 2008). New connections form between the frontal lobes and limbic system. Those new connections enable individuals to exercise more cognitive control over their emotional impulses.

With the passing of adolescence, your body once again reaches a period of the life span in which biological change is comparatively minimal. You may affect your body in a variety of ways—by diet and exercise, for example—but the next striking set of changes that are consistent consequences of ageing occurs in middle and late adulthood.

Physical changes in adulthood

Some of the most obvious changes that occur with age concern your physical appearance and abilities. As you grow older, you can expect your skin to wrinkle, your hair to thin and grey, and your height to decrease by up to 5 centimetres. You can also expect some of your senses to become less acute. These changes do not appear suddenly at age 65. They occur gradually, beginning as soon as early adulthood. However, before we describe some common age-related changes, we want to make a more general point: many physical changes arise not from ageing but from *disuse*; research supports a general belief in the maxim, 'Use it or lose it'. Older adults who maintain (or renew) a program of physical fitness may experience fewer of the difficulties that are often thought to be inevitable consequences of ageing. (Note that we will reach exactly the same conclusion when we discuss cognitive and social aspects of middle and late adulthood.) Let's now look, however, at some changes that are largely unavoidable and frequently have an impact on the way adults think about their lives.

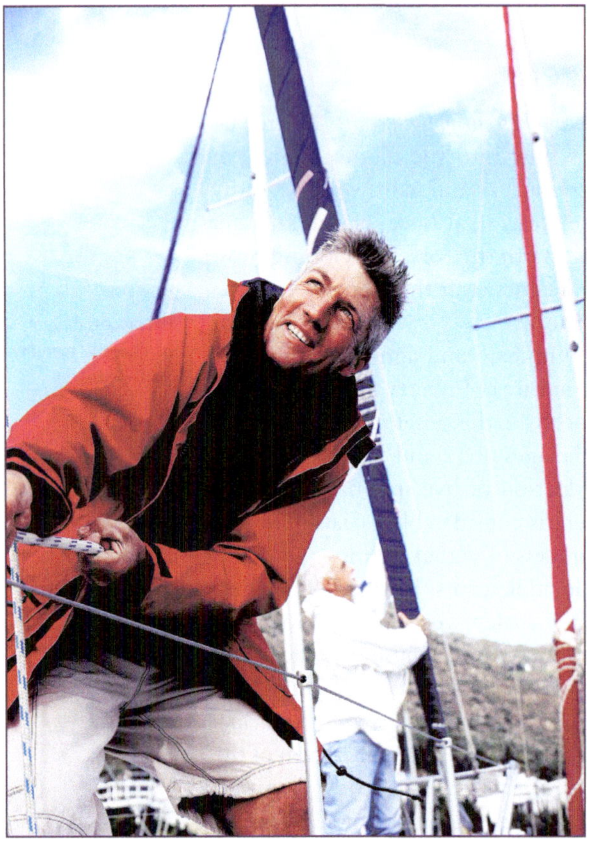

Why do researchers give the advice 'Use it or lose it'?
(**Source:** Stockbyte)

Vision

Beginning at ages 40 to 50, most people begin experiencing changes in the function of their visual system: the lenses of their eyes become less flexible and the muscles that change the thickness of the lens become less effective. These changes can make seeing objects at close range difficult. Lens rigidity also affects dark adaptation, making night vision a problem for older people. Many of these normal visual changes can be aided with corrective lenses. With age, the lenses of people's eyes also become yellowed. The yellowing of the lens is thought to be responsible for diminished colour vision experienced by some older people. Colours of lower wavelengths—violets, blues and greens—are particularly hard for some older adults to discriminate. By age 65, the vast majority of people experience some loss of visual function (Carter, 1982; Pitts, 1982).

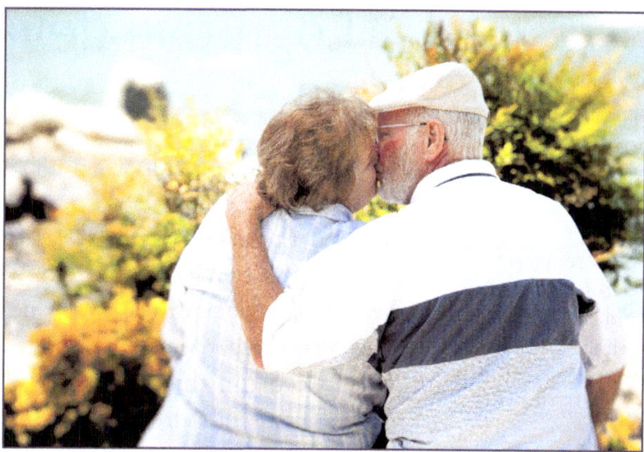

Older adults can and do enjoy the many benefits of intimacy and sexual relationships. Why does this image (Feverpitched/Dreamstime.com.) clash with stereotypes of late adulthood?
(**Source:** Feverpitched/Dreamstime.com.)

Hearing

Hearing loss is common among those 60 and older. The average older adult has difficulty hearing high-frequency sounds (Corso, 1977). This impairment is usually greater for men than for women. Older adults can have a hard time understanding speech—particularly that spoken by high-pitched voices. (Oddly enough, with age, people's speaking voices increase in pitch due to stiffening of the vocal cords.) Deficits in hearing can be gradual and hard for an individual to notice until they are extreme. In addition, even when individuals become aware of hearing loss, they may deny it because it is perceived as an undesirable sign of ageing. Some of the physiological aspects of hearing loss can be overcome with the help of hearing aids. You should also be aware, as you grow older or interact with older adults, that it helps to speak in low tones, enunciate clearly and reduce background noise.

Reproductive and sexual functioning

We saw that puberty marks the onset of reproductive functioning. In middle and late adulthood, reproductive capacity diminishes. Around age 50, most women experience *menopause*, the cessation of menstruation and ovulation. For men, changes are less abrupt, but the quantity of viable sperm falls off after age 40 and the volume of seminal fluid declines after age 60. Of course, these changes are relevant primarily to reproduction. Increasing age and physical change do not necessarily impair other aspects of sexual experience (DeLamater & Sill, 2005; Lindau et al., 2007). Indeed, sex is one of life's healthy pleasures that can enhance successful ageing because it is arousing, provides aerobic exercise, stimulates fantasy, and is a vital form of social interaction.

Let's now turn to the ways in which you developed an understanding of the world around you.

Stop and review

1. How does experience with crawling influence children's performance on the visual cliff?
2. What have recent studies demonstrated with respect to brain development in adolescence?
3. Why does increasing age often have an effect on colour vision?

Critical thinking

Consider the study on prenatal voice recognition. Why did the researchers have mothers tape-record the poems rather than having them read them 'live'?

Cognitive development across the life span

Cognitive development The development of processes of knowing, including imagining, perceiving, reasoning and problem solving.

How does an individual's understanding of physical and social reality change across the life span? **Cognitive development** is the study of the processes and products of the mind as they emerge and change over time. Because researchers have been particularly fascinated by the earliest emergence of cognitive capabilities, we will focus much of our attention on the earliest stages of cognitive development. However, we will also describe some of the discoveries researchers have made about cognitive development across the adult years.

As we begin this discussion of cognitive development, we want to remind you of the nature versus nurture distinction. The question is how best to account for the profound differences between a newborn and, for example, a 10-year-old: to what extent is such development determined by heredity (nature), and to what extent is it a product of learned experiences (nurture)? The debate concerning nature and nurture has a long history among philosophers, psychologists and educators. On one side of this debate are those who believe that the human infant is born without knowledge or skills and that experience, in the form of human learning, etches messages on the blank tablet (in Latin, the *tabula rasa*) of the infant's unformed mind. This view, originally proposed by British philosopher John Locke, is known as *empiricism*. It credits human development to experience. Empiricists believe that what directs human development is the stimulation people receive as they are *nurtured*. Among the scholars opposing empiricism was French philosopher Jean-Jacques Rousseau. He argued the *nativist* view that *nature*, or the evolutionary legacy that each child brings into the world, is the mould that shapes development. Our discussion of cognitive development should lead you to see that there is truth to both sides of the debate. Children have innate preparation to learn from their experiences in the world.

We begin our discussion of cognitive development with the pioneering work of the late Swiss psychologist Jean Piaget.

Piaget's insights into mental development

For nearly 50 years, Jean Piaget (1929, 1954, 1965, 1977) developed theories about the ways that children think, reason and solve problems. Perhaps Piaget's interest in cognitive development grew out of his own intellectually active youth: Piaget published his first article at age 10 and was offered a post as a museum curator at age 14 (Brainerd, 1996). Piaget used simple demonstrations and sensitive interviews with his own children and with other children to generate complex theories about early mental development. His interest was not in the amount of information children possessed but in the ways their thinking and inner representations of physical reality changed at different stages in their development.

Scheme Piaget's term for a cognitive structure that develops as infants and young children learn to interpret the world and adapt to their environment.

Assimilation According to Piaget, the process whereby new cognitive elements are fitted in with old elements or modified to fit more easily.

Accommodation Where existing schemes change to accommodate new information learnt by a child.

Building blocks of developmental change

Piaget gave the name **schemes** to the mental structures that enable individuals to interpret the world. Schemes are the building blocks of developmental change. Piaget characterised the infant's initial schemes as *sensorimotor intelligence*—mental structures or programs that guide sensorimotor sequences, such as sucking, looking, grasping and pushing. With practice, elementary schemes are combined, integrated and differentiated into ever more complex, diverse action patterns, as when a child pushes away undesired objects to seize a desired one behind him or her. According to Piaget, two basic processes work in tandem to achieve cognitive growth—assimilation and accommodation. **Assimilation** modifies new environmental information to fit into what is already known; the child accesses existing schemes to structure incoming sensory data. **Accommodation** restructures or modifies the

Table 2.2 Piaget's stages of cognitive development

Stage/Ages	Characteristics and major accomplishments
Sensorimotor (0–2)	Child begins life with small number of sensorimotor sequences.
	Child develops object permanence and the beginnings of symbolic thought.
Preoperational (2–7)	Child's thought is marked by egocentrism and centration.
	Child has improved ability to use symbolic thought.
Concrete operations (7–11)	Child achieves understanding of conservation.
	Child can reason with respect to concrete, physical objects.
Formal operations (11→)	Child develops capacity for abstract reasoning and hypothetical thinking.

child's existing schemes so that new information is accounted for more completely. The chapter on social cognitive and social thinking will examine this in more detail.

Consider the transitions a baby must make from sucking at a mother's breast, to sucking the nipple of a bottle, to sipping through a straw, and then to drinking from a cup. The initial sucking response is a reflex action present at birth, but it must be modified somewhat so that the child's mouth fits the shape and size of the mother's nipple. In adapting to a bottle, an infant still uses many parts of the sequence unchanged (assimilation) but must grasp and draw on the rubber nipple somewhat differently from before and learn to hold the bottle at an appropriate angle (accommodation). The steps from bottle to straw to cup require more accommodation but continue to rely on earlier skills. Piaget saw cognitive development as the result of exactly this sort of interweaving of assimilation and accommodation. The balanced application of assimilation and accommodation permits children's behaviour and knowledge to become less dependent on concrete external reality, relying more on abstract thought.

Stages in cognitive development

Piaget believed that children's cognitive development could be divided into a series of four ordered, discontinuous stages (see Table 2.2). All children are assumed to progress through these stages in the same sequence, although one child may take longer to pass through a given stage than another.

Sensorimotor stage
The period between birth and age 2 during which an infant's knowledge of the world is limited to their sensory perceptions and motor activities.

SENSORIMOTOR STAGE. The **sensorimotor stage** extends roughly from birth to age 2. In the early months, much of an infant's behaviour is based on a limited array of inborn

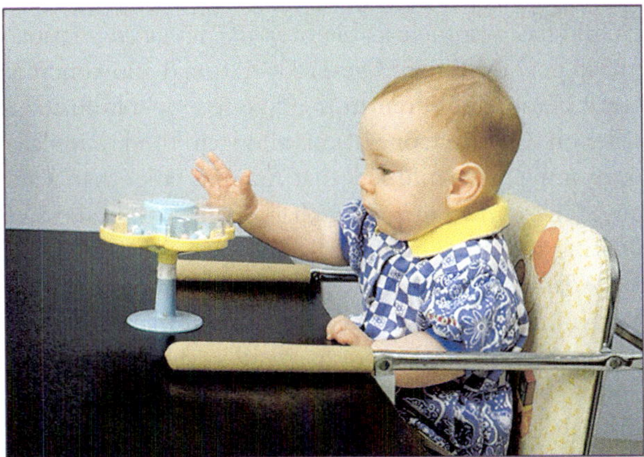

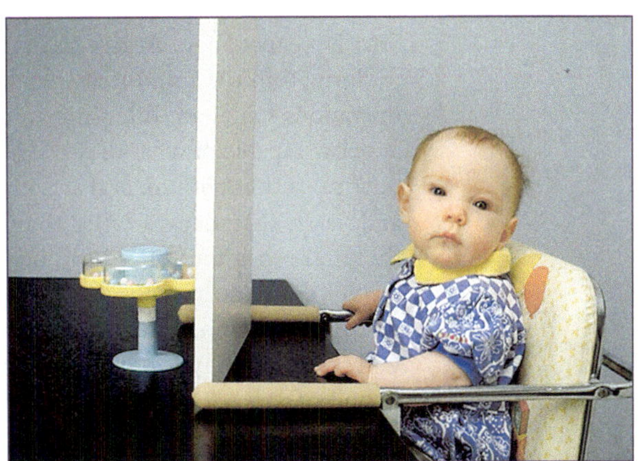

Piaget observed that the typical 6-month-old will attend to an attractive toy (left) but will quickly lose interest if a screen blocks the toy from view (right). What understanding about objects will the child achieve by age 2?
(**Source:** © Lew Merriam/Photoresearchers.Inc.)

schemes, like sucking, looking, grasping and pushing. During the first year, sensorimotor sequences are improved, combined, coordinated and integrated (sucking and grasping, looking and manipulating, for example). They become more varied as infants discover that their actions have an effect on external events.

The most important cognitive acquisition of the infancy period is the ability to form mental representations of absent objects—those with which the child is not in direct sensorimotor contact. **Object permanence** refers to children's understanding that objects exist and behave independently of their actions or awareness. In the first months of life, children follow objects with their eyes, but, when the objects disappear from view, they turn away as if the objects had also disappeared from their minds. At around 3 months of age, however, they keep looking at the place where the objects had disappeared. Between 8 and 12 months, children begin to search for those disappearing objects. By age 2 years, children have no remaining uncertainty that 'out of sight' objects continue to exist (Flavell, 1985).

Object permanence The recognition that objects exist independently of an individual's action or awareness; an important cognitive acquisition of infancy.

Preoperational stage The period between ages 2 and 7 during which a child learns to use language. During this stage, children do not yet understand concrete logic.

Egocentrism In cognitive development, the inability of a young child at the preoperational stage to take the perspective of another person.

Centration A thought pattern common during the beginning of the preoperational stage of cognitive development in a child.

PREOPERATIONAL STAGE.

The **preoperational stage** extends roughly from 2 to 7 years of age. The big cognitive advance in this developmental stage is an improved ability to represent mentally objects that are not physically present. Except for this development, Piaget characterises the preoperational stage according to what the child *cannot* do. For example, Piaget believed that young children's preoperational thought is marked by **egocentrism**, the child's inability to take the perspective of another person. You have probably noticed egocentrism if you've heard a 2-year-old's conversations with other children. Children at this age often seem to be talking to themselves rather than interacting.

Preoperational children also experience **centration**—the tendency to have their attention captured by the more perceptually striking features of objects. Centration is illustrated by Piaget's classic demonstration of a child's inability to understand that the amount of a liquid does not change as a function of the size or shape of its container.

> When an equal amount of lemonade is poured into two identical glasses, children of ages 5 and 7 report that the glasses contain the same amount. When, however, the lemonade from one glass is poured into a tall, thin glass, their opinions diverge. The 5-year-olds know that the lemonade in the tall glass is the same lemonade, but they report that it now is *more*. The 7-year-olds correctly assert that there is no difference between the amounts.

In Piaget's demonstration, the younger children centre on a single, perceptually salient dimension—the height of the lemonade in the glass. The older children take into account both height and width and correctly infer that appearance is not reality.

CONCRETE OPERATIONS STAGE.

The concrete operations stage goes roughly from 7 to 11 years of age. At this stage, the child has become capable of *mental operations*; actions performed in the mind that give rise to logical thinking. The preoperational and concrete operations stages are often put in contrast because children in the concrete operation stage are now capable of what they failed earlier on. Concrete operations allow children to replace physical action with mental action. For example, if a child sees that Adam is taller than Zara and, later, that Zara is taller than Tanya, the child can reason that Adam is the tallest of the three—without physically manipulating the three individuals. However, the child still cannot draw the appropriate inference ('Adam is tallest') if the problem is just stated with a verbal description. This inability to determine relative heights (and solve similar problems) without direct physical observation suggests that abstract thought is still in the offing in the period of concrete operations.

Conservation According to Piaget, the understanding that physical properties do not change when nothing is added or taken away, even though appearances may change.

The lemonade study illustrates another hallmark of the concrete operations period. The 7-year-olds have mastered what Piaget called **conservation**: they know that the physical properties of objects do not change when nothing is added or taken away, even though the objects' appearance changes. Figure 2.6 presents examples of Piaget's tests of conservation for

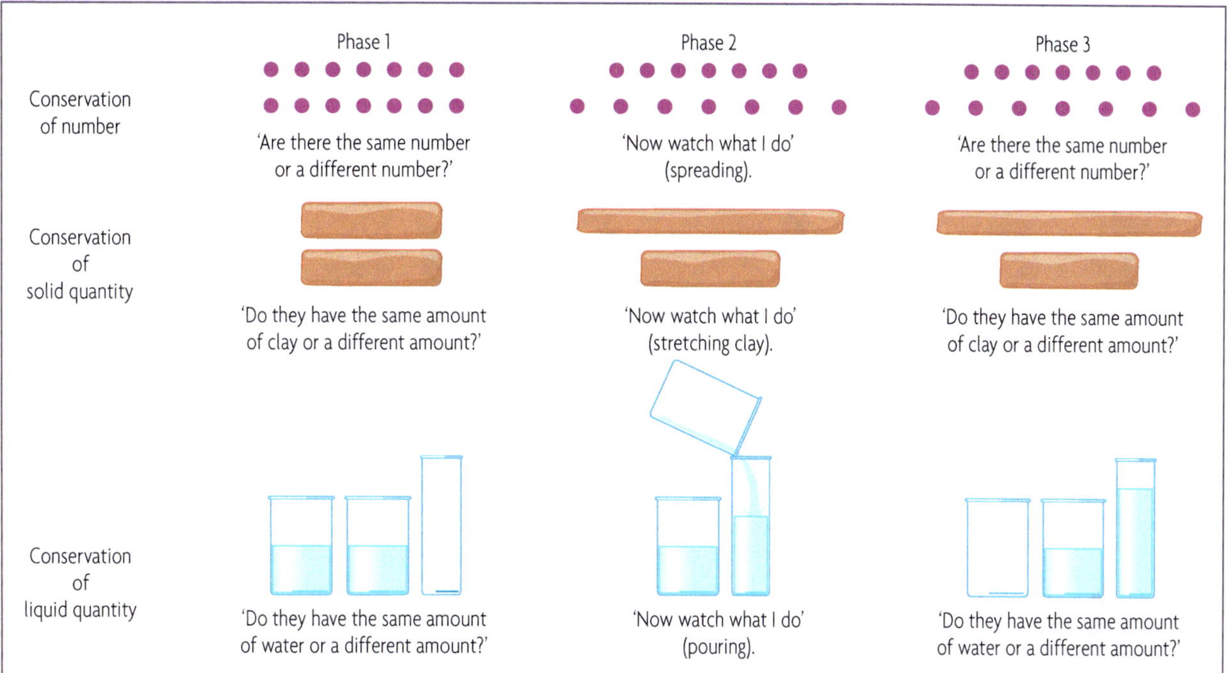

Figure 2.6 Tests of conservation

different dimensions. One of the newly acquired operations children can bring to bear on conservation tasks is reversibility. *Reversibility* is the child's understanding that both physical actions and mental operations can be reversed: the child can reason that the amount of lemonade *can't* have changed because when the physical action is reversed—when the lemonade is poured back into the original glass—the two volumes will once again look identical.

FORMAL OPERATIONS STAGE. The formal operations stage covers a span roughly from age 11 on. In this final stage of cognitive growth, thinking becomes abstract. Adolescents can see how their particular reality is only one of several imaginable realities, and they begin to ponder deep questions of truth, justice and existence. They seek answers to problems in a systematic fashion: once they achieve formal operations, children can start to play the role of scientist, trying each of a series of possibilities in careful order. Adolescents also begin to be able to use advanced deductive logic. Unlike their younger siblings, adolescents have the ability to reason from abstract premises ('If A, then B' and 'not B') to their logical conclusions ('not A').

Contemporary perspectives on early cognitive developments

Piaget's theory remains the classic reference point for the understanding of cognitive development (Feldman, 2004, pp. 175–231; Flavell, 1996, pp. 200–203; Lourenço & Machado, 1996; Scholnick et al., 1999). However, contemporary researchers have come up with more flexible ways of studying the development of the child's cognitive abilities.

Infant cognition

We've already detailed some of the tasks Piaget used to draw conclusions about cognitive development. However, contemporary researchers have developed innovative techniques

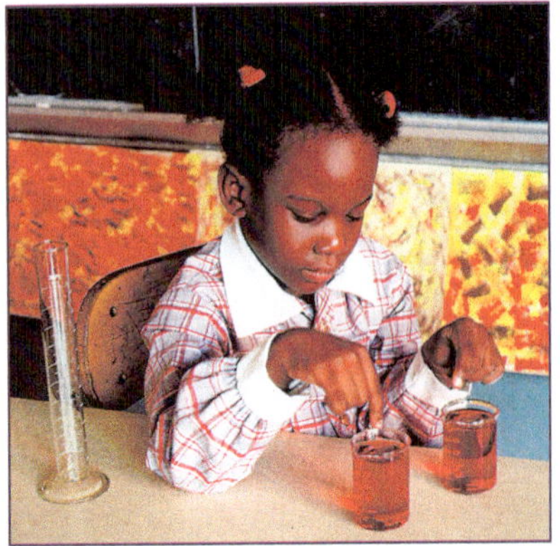
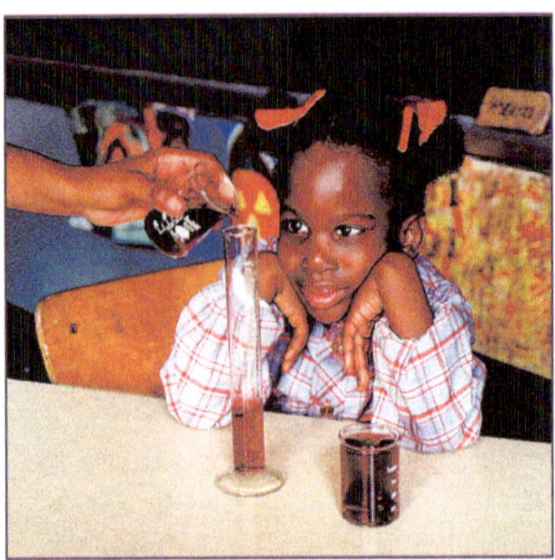
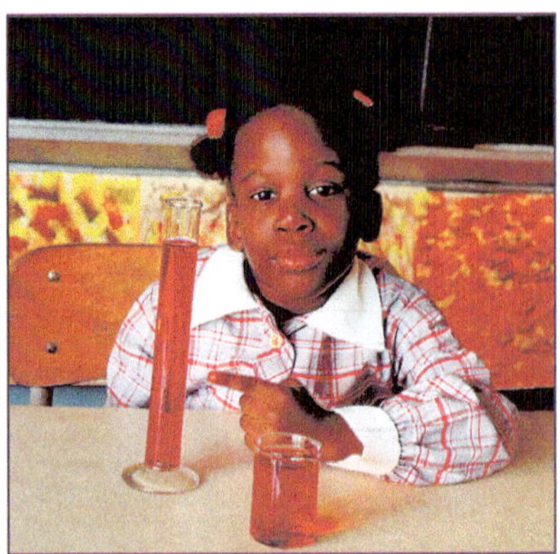

This 5-year-old girl is aware that the two containers have the same amount of coloured liquid. However, when the liquid from one is poured into a taller container, she indicates that there is more liquid in the taller one. She has not yet grasped the concept of conservation, which she will understand by age 6 or 7. Why wouldn't the 5-year-old child understand the concept, even if she were told the right answer?

that have allowed them to re-evaluate some of Piaget's conclusions. Consider object permanence, which Piaget suggested was the major accomplishment of the 2-year-old child. Contemporary research techniques suggest that infants as young as 3 months old have already developed aspects of this concept. This important finding has been shown with different tasks devised by researcher Renée Baillargeon and her colleagues.

In one study, 4-month-old infants watched while an experimenter lowered a wide rectangular object (see Figure 2.7) (Wang et al., 2004). In one condition, the path of the object would put it behind a *wide occluder*—a barrier wide enough to hide the rectangular object completely. In the other condition, the object was destined to pass behind a *narrow occluder*—a barrier too narrow to occlude the object fully. As this event unfolded, a screen appeared that hid the final moment in which the object was lowered. When the screen disappeared, the object was fully hidden. How did the infants respond in the two conditions? If they didn't have object permanence, we would expect them to be equally unbothered in both cases—once the rectangular object was gone, we would expect them to have no recollection that it had ever existed. Suppose they did have some recollection of the object. In that case, we would expect that they—like adults who watched the events—would be rather surprised that a wide object could be hidden by a narrow occluder. To assess the infants' degree of surprise, the researchers recorded how long infants looked at the displays after the screen disappeared. The infants who saw the narrow occluder event looked at the display for about 16 seconds longer than their peers who saw the wide occluder event.

We can't take the infants' surprise as evidence that they have acquired the full concept of object permanence—they may only know that something is wrong without knowing exactly what that something is (Lourenço & Machado, 1996). Even so, the research by Baillargeon and her colleagues suggests that even very young children have acquired important knowledge of the physical world.

The innovative methods researchers have developed to penetrate infants' minds continue to transform our understanding of what infants know and how they know it. Consider the relationship between actions and goals. As an adult, you are accustomed to inferring people's goals when you watch them perform actions. For example, if you see someone pull out a set of keys, you easily infer that he or she needs to unlock something. When did you start to understand how actions relate to goals? Research suggests that 7-month-olds have begun to divide the world up into actions that are goal-directed and those that are not (Hamlin et al., 2008). Consider an experiment in which infants sat in front of a display with a pair

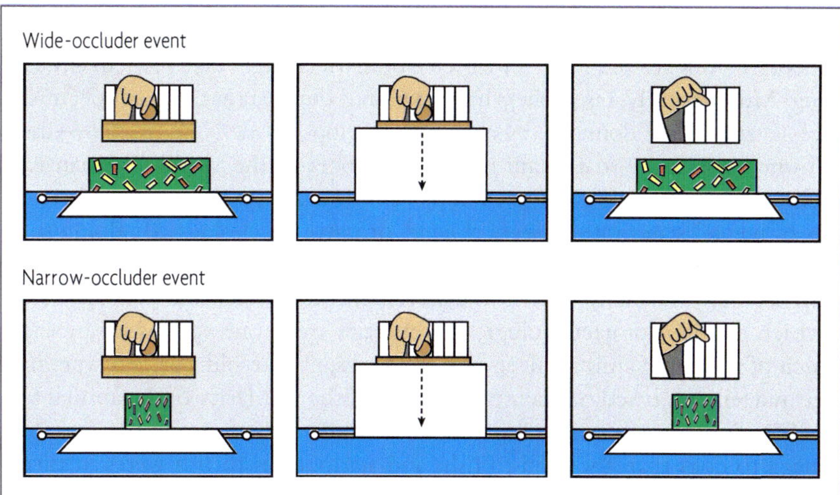

Figure 2.7 Four-month-olds and object permanence

Four-month-olds watched an experimenter lower a rectangular object (shown in brown) behind a wide occluder or a narrow occluder (each shown in patterned green). As the event unfolded, a screen appeared to mask the moment at which the object passed behind the occluder. When the screen disappeared, the experimenter's hand was empty. The infants who saw the narrow-occluder event spent more time looking at the display, suggesting they were surprised that a wide object could be hidden behind a narrow occluder. The infants' surprise suggests they have attained some aspects of object permanence: the rectangular object was out of sight but not out of mind.

From Su-hua Wang et al. (2004).

of toys. The infants watched an experimenter perform one of two actions with respect to the toys: some infants watched the researcher grasp a toy; other infants watched her touch a toy with the back of her hand. An adult watching the scene would find it relatively easy to interpret the grasp, but not the touch, as related to a specific goal (i.e., to acquire the toy). Infants' behaviours suggested that they also interpreted the actions differently. After the infants viewed the experimenter's actions, she told them 'Now it's your turn!' and put the toys within their reach. Infants who had viewed the grasping action were likely to touch the same toy the experimenter had grasped; infants who had viewed the back-of-the-hand contact didn't show a preference for touching one toy over the other. This pattern suggests that the infants interpreted only the grasping action as having goal-directed significance for just one of the two toys. This study illustrates how carefully infants attend to the world around them to understand the origins of other people's behaviours.

Further research suggests that 3-month-olds have begun to understand these relationships—but only when they have appropriate experience of their own (Sommerville et al., 2005). To support that claim, researchers outfitted one group of 3-month-olds with special Velcro mittens that allowed them to pick up toys. (Children of this age don't have the manual dexterity to grasp objects without this extra assistance.) A second group of children didn't have that novel experience of picking up toys. Both groups of children watched an experimenter perform a series of events that also involved grasping toys. An adult watching those events would infer that the experimenter had the particular goal, for example, of picking up a teddy bear. The group of children with grasping experience appeared to make that inference, but their inexperienced peers did not. This result brings us full circle to Piaget. Piaget suggested that children's knowledge is built up from active experience in the environment. This study confirms that active experience helps children learn how actions and goals fit together.

Children's foundational theories

Foundational theory
A framework for initial understanding formulated by children to explain their experiences of the world.

Piaget's theory is built around stages in which landmark changes take place in children's ways of thinking. More recently, researchers have explored the idea that changes occur separately, in each of several major domains, as children develop **foundational theories**—frameworks for initial understanding—to explain their experiences of the world (Gelman & Raman, 2002; Wellman & Inagaki, 1997). For example, children accumulate their experiences of the properties of mental states into a *theory of mind*, or naive psychology. By doing so, they are better able to understand the thought processes of themselves and others.

Researchers have formally studied the development of scientific concepts, such as the way in which children project biological properties from one species to another. When asked which of a series of animals sleep or have bones, 4-year-old children were inclined to make their judgements based on their perceptions of the similarity of the animal to humans (Carey, 1985). For example, more 4-year-olds attributed these properties (i.e., 'sleep' and 'have bones') to dogs than they did to fish, and attributions to fish were, in turn, greater than those to flies. Over time, children must replace a theory based on similarity to humans with one that acknowledges more structure in the animal kingdom—for example, they must acquire the formal distinction between *vertebrates* and *invertebrates* that defines which types of animals have bones. Similarly, 3- and 4-year-old children understand that what is inside objects affects their functions—although they have no clear idea what those insides are (Gelman, 2003; Gelman & Wellman, 1991). Thus, although 3- and 4-year-olds aren't entirely sure what kinds of things are inside dogs, they are quite certain that a dog would cease to be a dog if you removed whatever is inside. In each domain, you see that children begin to develop a general theory and then use a range of new experiences to provide successive refinements.

Social and cultural influences on cognitive development

Internalisation
According to Vygotsky, the process through which children absorb knowledge from the social context.

Another focus of contemporary research is on the role of social interactions in cognitive development. Much of this research has its origins in the theories of Russian psychologist Lev Vygotsky. Vygotsky argued that children develop through a process of **internalisation**: they absorb knowledge from their social context that has a major impact on how cognition unfolds over time.

The social theory that Vygotsky pioneered has found support in cross-cultural studies of development. As Piaget's theory initially seized the attention of developmental researchers, many of them sought to use his tasks to study the cognitive achievements of children in diverse cultures (Rogoff, 2003; Rogoff & Chavajay, 1995). These studies began to call into question the universality of Piaget's claims because, for example, people in many cultures failed to show evidence that they had acquired formal operations. Late in his life, Piaget himself began to speculate that the specific achievements he characterised as formal operations may rely more on the particular type of science education children obtain rather than on an unfolding of biologically predetermined stages of cognitive development (Lourenço & Machado, 1996).

Vygotsksy's concept of internalisation helps explain the effect culture has on cognitive development. Children's cognition develops to perform culturally valued functions (Serpell, 2000; Serpell & Boykin, 1994). Piaget, for example, invented tasks that reflected his own preconceptions about appropriate and valuable cognitive activities. Other cultures prefer their children to excel in other ways. If Piaget's children had been evaluated with respect to their understanding of the cognitive complexities of weaving, they probably would have appeared to be retarded in their development relative to Mayan children in Guatemala (Rogoff, 1990). Cross-cultural studies of cognitive development have quite often demonstrated that type of schooling plays a large role in determining children's achievement on Piagetian tasks (Rogoff & Chavajay, 1995). Psychologists must use these types of findings to sort out the nature and nurture of cognitive development.

The developmental changes we have documented so far are very dramatic. It's easy to tell that a 12-year-old has all sorts of cognitive capabilities unknown to a 1-year-old. We now shift to the more subtle changes that take place throughout adulthood.

Cognitive development in adulthood

As we have traced cognitive development across childhood into adolescence, 'change' has usually meant 'change for the better'. When we arrive at the period of late adulthood, though, cultural stereotypes suggest that 'change' means 'change for the worse' (Parr & Siegert, 1993). However, even when people believe that the course of adulthood brings with it general decline, they still anticipate certain types of gains very late into life (Dixon, 1999; Dixon & de Frias, 2004). We will look at intelligence and memory to see the interplay of losses and gains.

Intelligence

There is little evidence to support the notion that general cognitive abilities decline among the healthy elderly. Only about 5 percent of the population experiences major losses in cognitive functioning. When age-related decline in cognitive functioning occurs, it is usually limited to only some abilities. When intelligence is separated into the components that make up your verbal abilities (*crystallised intelligence*) and those that are part of your ability to learn quickly and thoroughly (*fluid intelligence*), fluid intelligence shows the greater decline with age (Baltes & Staudinger, 1993; Singer et al., 2003). Much of the decrease in fluidity has been attributed to a general slowing down of processing speed: older adults' performance on intellectual tasks that require many mental processes to occur in small amounts of time is greatly impaired (Salthouse, 1996; Sheppard & Vernon, 2008).

But all change is not in the direction of poorer functioning. For instance, psychologists are now exploring age-related gains in wisdom—expertise in the fundamental practices of life (Baltes & Kunzmann, 2003; Baltes & Staudinger, 2000). Table 2.3 presents some of the types of knowledge that define wisdom (Smith & Baltes, 1990). You can see that each type of knowledge is best acquired over a long and thoughtful life. Furthermore, individuals vary greatly in their later-life intellectual performance. Research indicates that older adults who pursue high levels of environmental stimulation tend to maintain high levels of cognitive abilities. One study, for example, focused on a group of older adults whose average age was 69 (Bielak et al., 2007). The adults whose everyday lives had the highest levels of social, physical and intellectual activities also showed the fastest processing speed on cognitive tasks. These results appear to support 'use it or lose it'. However, interpretation of results of this sort is muddied by the problem that correlation is not causation (Salthouse, 2006). The result *could* indicate that a high level of activity causes processing speed to remain relatively high. However, we must also consider the possibility that a smaller decline in processing speed allows some older adults to remain more active.

Table 2.3 Features of wisdom

- *Rich factual knowledge.* General and specific knowledge about the conditions of life and its variations
- *Rich procedural knowledge.* General and specific knowledge about strategies of judgement and advice concerning life matters
- *Life span contextualism.* Knowledge about the contexts of life and their temporal (developmental) relationships
- *Uncertainty.* Knowledge about the relative indeterminacy and unpredictability of life and ways to manage it

Even if it proves difficult to demonstrate that 'using it' prevents 'losing it', researchers have provided evidence that 'using it more' can bring about better intellectual functioning. They have devised training programs that are able to reverse older adults' decline in some cognitive abilities (Schaie, 2005). Let's consider an intervention that had a positive impact on measures of fluid intelligence.

Participants whose ages ranged from 60 to 75 were assigned either to an experimental or control group (Tranter & Koutstaal, 2008). Participants in the experimental group spent 10–12 weeks engaging in mentally stimulating tasks such as creative drawing activities and identification of mystery photographs; participants in the control group did not engage in special tasks. The researchers measured fluid intelligence both at the beginning of the experiment and again after the 10–12 week intervention. As the researchers predicted, participants in the experimental group showed greater gains in fluid intelligence compared to the control participants.

These results might encourage you to remain cognitively active across your life span. Meanwhile, if you're obtaining a university education you might already be giving yourself a long-term advantage. Research using fMRI scans has suggested that older adults with more education are better able to compensate for natural decline in their ageing brains than are their less educated peers (Springer et al., 2005). There's another good reason to continue your education!

The more general conclusion is that you should keep your mind at work. Warner Schaie and his colleagues have even been able to demonstrate that training programs can reverse older adults' decline in some cognitive abilities (Schaie, 2005). It appears that disuse, rather than decay, may be responsible for the deficits in intellectual performance that are not related to processing speed (Hultsch et al., 1998). With the massive uptake of video games for all ages, studies have now shown that video game playing that involves puzzle solving along with motor-skill exercises can actually impact health ageing for the brain by promoting new learning (Green & Bavelier, 2008). As promised, we have again arrived at the conclusion that 'use it or lose it (or seek training to get it back)' is an appropriate motto for the wise older adult.

Memory

A common complaint among the elderly is the feeling that their ability to remember things is not as good as it used to be. On a number of tests of memory, adults over 60 *do* perform worse than young adults in their 20s (Hess, 2005). People experience memory deficits with advancing age, even when they have been highly educated and otherwise have good intellectual skills (Zelinski et al., 1993). Ageing does *not* seem to diminish elderly individuals' ability to access their general knowledge store and personal information about events that occurred long ago. In a study of name and face recognition, middle-aged adults could identify 90 percent of their high school classmates in yearbooks 35 years after graduation; older adults were still able to recognise 70 to 80 percent of their classmates some 50 years later (Bahrick et al., 1975). However, ageing affects the processes that allow new information to be effectively organised, stored and retrieved (Buchler & Reder, 2007).

As yet, researchers have been unable to develop a wholly adequate description of the mechanisms that underlie memory impairment in older adults—perhaps because the impairment has multiple sources. (Hess, 2005). Some theories focus on differences between older and younger people in their efforts to organise and process information. Other theories point to elderly people's reduced ability to pay attention to information. Another type of theory looks to neurobiological changes in the brain systems that produce the physical memory traces. We explore those ideas in the 'Psychology in your life' box. Note that these brain changes are not the same as the abnormal tangles of neural tissue and plaques that cause the memory loss of Alzheimer's disease. Researchers also believe that older adults' performance may be impaired by their very belief that their memory will be poor (Hess & Hinson, 2006). Researchers continue to evaluate the relative contributions of each of these factors.

Let's now narrow our focus from general cognitive development to the more specific topic of the acquisition of language.[A]

Stop and review

1. In Piaget's theory, what is the relationship between assimilation and accommodation?
2. What does it mean when a child is able to overcome centration?
3. How has contemporary research modified conclusions about object permanence?
4. What was the major emphasis of Lev Vygotsky's theory?
5. What happens to processing speed across the life span?

Critical thinking

Recall the experiment that looked at object permanence in 4-month-olds. Why was looking time an appropriate measure to test the researchers' hypothesis?[1]

Social development across the life span

We have seen so far how radically you change as a physical and cognitive being from birth to older adulthood. In this section of the chapter we explore **social development**: how individuals' social interactions and expectations change across the life span. We will see that your social and cultural environment interacts with biological ageing to provide each period of the life span with its own special challenges and rewards.

Social development The ways in which individuals' social interactions and expectations change across the life span.

As we discuss social development, it is particularly important for you to consider the way in which culture and environment affect certain aspects of our lives. For example, people who live in circumstances of economic hardship undergo types of stresses that are absent from the 'normal' course of development (Kohen et al., 2008; Scaramella et al., 2008). Current trends in the United States and in other countries throughout the world make it imperative for developmental psychologists to consider the difficult circumstances in which many children, adolescents and adults are forced to live—circumstances that continually put their sanity, safety and survival at risk (Huston, 2005). American culture also enforces different outcomes for men and for women and for individuals who belong to minority groups. For example, in 2006 12 percent of women over 65 were living in poverty compared to 7 percent of men in this age range; 27 percent of African-American women over 65 were living in poverty compared to 9 percent of white women over 65 (Federal Interagency Forum on Aging-Related Statistics, 2008).

Australian cultural groups also have differing living standards, be they immigrants from another culture or Anglo-Australian. A recent study on the division of homelessness in Australian youth compared to those in the United States showed marked differences in culture. For example, more homeless youth were of school age or younger in America and

---

[A]Gerrig, R. J., Zimbardo, P. G., Campbell, A. J., Cumming, S. R., & Wilkes, F. J. (Eds.). (2012). Human development across the lifespan. In *Psychology and life* (2nd ed., pp. 358–373). Frenchs Forest, NSW: Pearson Australia.

had conviction records, whereas in Australia, the majority of homeless youth were older than school age with greater numbers from an Indigenous or immigrant background (Milburn et al., 2006). These differences are direct products of structural inequities in contemporary society.

When we draw conclusions about the 'average' life course, keep in mind that culture dictates that some individuals will depart from this average; as we describe the psychological challenges facing the 'ordinary' individual, bear in mind that many individuals face extraordinary challenges. It is the role of researchers to document the impact of contemporary problems—and to design interventions to alleviate their harshest consequences.

As you read the remainder of this chapter, keep in mind how the tasks of life are jointly determined by a biological accumulation of years and a social accumulation of cultural experiences. To begin our discussion of social development, we will describe Erik Erikson's life span theory, which makes explicit the challenges and rewards in each of life's major periods.

Erikson's psychosocial stages

Psychosocial stages Proposed by Erik Erikson, successive developmental stages that focus on an individual's orientation toward the self and others.

Erik Erikson (1963), who was trained by Sigmund Freud's daughter, Anna Freud, proposed that every individual must successfully navigate a series of **psychosocial stages**, each of which presented a particular conflict or crisis. Erikson identified eight stages in the life cycle. At each stage, a particular crisis comes into focus, as shown in Table 2.4. Although each conflict never completely disappears, it needs to be sufficiently resolved at a given stage if an individual is to cope successfully with the conflicts of later stages.

Trust versus mistrust

In Erikson's first stage, an infant needs to develop a basic sense of *trust* in the environment through interaction with caregivers. Trust is a natural accompaniment to a strong attachment relationship with a parent who provides food, warmth and the comfort of physical closeness. But a child whose basic needs are not met, who experiences inconsistent handling, lack of physical closeness and warmth, and the frequent absence of a caring adult, may develop a pervasive sense of mistrust, insecurity and anxiety.

Table 2.4 Erikson's psychosocial stages

Approximate age	Crisis	Adequate resolution	Inadequate resolution
0–1½	Trust vs. mistrust	Basic sense of safety	Insecurity, anxiety
1½–3	Autonomy vs. self-doubt	Perception of self as agent capable of controlling own body and making things happen	Feelings of inadequacy to control events
3–6	Initiative vs. guilt	Confidence in oneself as initiator, creator	Feelings of lack of self-worth
6–puberty	Competence vs. inferiority	Adequacy in basic social and intellectual skills	Lack of self-confidence, feelings of failure
Adolescent	Identity vs. role confusion	Comfortable sense of self as a person	Sense of self as fragmented; shifting, unclear sense of self
Early adult	Intimacy vs. isolation	Capacity for closeness and commitment to another	Feeling of aloneness, separation; denial of need for closeness
Middle adult	Generativity vs. stagnation	Focus of concern beyond oneself to family, society, future generations	Self-indulgent concerns; lack of future orientation
Later adult	Ego integrity vs. despair	Sense of wholeness, basic satisfaction with life	Feelings of futility, disappointment

Autonomy versus self-doubt

With the development of walking and the beginnings of language, there is an expansion of a child's exploration and manipulation of objects (and sometimes people). With these activities should come a comfortable sense of *autonomy* or independence, and of being a capable and worthy person. Excessive restriction or criticism at this second stage may lead instead to self-doubts, whereas demands beyond the child's ability, as in too-early or too-severe toilet training, can discourage the child's efforts to persevere in mastering new tasks.

Initiative versus guilt

Toward the end of the preschool period, a child who has developed a basic sense of trust, first in the immediate environment and then in himself or herself, can now *initiate* both intellectual and motor activities. The ways that parents respond to the child's self-initiated activities either encourages the sense of freedom and self-confidence needed for the next stage or produces guilt and feelings of being an inept intruder in an adult world.

Competence versus inferiority

During the elementary school years, the child who has successfully resolved the crises of the earlier stages is ready to go beyond random exploring and testing to the systematic development of *competencies*. School and sports offer arenas for learning intellectual and motor skills, and interaction with peers offers an arena for developing social skills. Successful efforts in these pursuits lead to feelings of competence. Some youngsters, however, become spectators rather than performers or experience enough failure to give them a sense of inferiority, leaving them unable to meet the demands of the next life stages.

Identity versus role confusion

Erikson believed that the essential crisis of adolescence is discovering one's true *identity* amid the confusion created by playing many different roles for the different audiences in an expanding social world. Resolving this crisis helps the individual develop a sense of a coherent self; failing to do so adequately may result in a self-image that lacks a central, stable core.

Intimacy versus isolation

The essential crisis for the young adult is to resolve the conflict between *intimacy* and *isolation*—to develop the capacity to make full emotional, moral and sexual commitments to other people. Making that kind of commitment requires that the individual compromise some personal preferences, accept some responsibilities, and yield some degree of privacy and independence. Failure to resolve this crisis adequately leads to isolation and the inability to connect to others in psychologically meaningful ways.

Generativity versus stagnation

The next major opportunity for growth, which occurs during adult midlife, is known as *generativity*. People in their 30s and 40s move beyond a focus on self and partner to broaden their commitments to family, work, society and future generations. Those people who haven't resolved earlier developmental tasks are still self-indulgent, question past decisions and goals, and pursue freedom at the expense of security.

Ego integrity versus despair

The crisis in later adulthood is the conflict between *ego integrity* and *despair*. Resolving the crises at each of the earlier stages prepares the older adult to look back without regrets and to enjoy a sense of wholeness. When previous crises are left unresolved, aspirations remain unfulfilled, and the individual experiences futility, despair and self-depreciation.

You will see that Erikson's framework is very useful for tracking individuals' progress across the life span. We will begin with childhood.

Social development in childhood

Socialisation The lifelong process whereby an individual's behavioural patterns, values, standards, skills, attitudes and motives are shaped to conform to those regarded as desirable in a particular society.

Children's basic survival depends on forming meaningful, effective relationships with other people. **Socialisation** is the lifelong process through which an individual's behaviour patterns, values, standards, skills, attitudes and motives are shaped to conform to those regarded as desirable in a particular society. This process involves many people (relatives, friends, teachers) and institutions (schools, houses of worship) that exert pressure on the individual to adopt socially approved values and standards of conduct. The family, however, is the most influential shaper and regulator of socialisation. The concept of family itself is being transformed to recognise that many children grow up in circumstances that include either less (a single parent) or more (an extended household) than a mother, father and siblings. Whatever the configuration, though, the family helps the individual form basic patterns of responsiveness to others—and these patterns, in turn, become the basis of the individual's lifelong style of relating to other people.

Temperament

Temperament A child's biologically based level of emotional and behavioural response to environmental events.

Even as infants begin the process of socialisation, they do not all start at the same place. Children begin life with differences in **temperament**—biologically based levels of emotional and behavioural response to the environment (Thomas & Chess, 1977). Researcher Jerome Kagan and his colleagues have demonstrated that some infants are 'born shy' and others are 'born bold' (Kagan & Snidman, 2004). These groups of children differ in sensitivity to physical and social stimulation: the shy or *inhibited* babies are consistently 'cautious and emotionally reserved when they confront unfamiliar persons or contexts'; the bold or *uninhibited* babies are consistently 'sociable, affectively spontaneous, and minimally fearful in the same unfamiliar situations' (Kagan & Snidman, 1991, p. 40). In one sample, about 10 percent of the infants were inhibited and about 25 percent were uninhibited; the rest of the infants fell in between those endpoints (Kagan & Snidman, 1991). Researchers have demonstrated that differences in temperament can be detected even while babies are still in the womb: high levels of foetal activity are associated with increased difficulty once the children are born (DiPietro et al., 1996). Further to this, studies have begun to explore the genetic variations that bring about these temperamental differences (Rothbart, 2007).

Longitudinal studies have demonstrated the long-term impact of early temperament. Children who, at age 4 months, displayed inhibited and uninhibited temperaments continue to behave differently as they get older (Kagan & Snidman, 2004). At age 2, the inhibited children generally showed the most fear—and the uninhibited children the least fear—when they were faced with unfamiliar events. At age 4, the uninhibited children were considerably more likely to be sociable when interacting with unfamiliar children. However, not all children who start out at the extreme ends of the dimension of inhibited versus uninhibited remain at those extremes—some children become less shy or less bold as they age (Pfeifer et al., 2002). However, even when children's responses become less extreme, they very rarely shift from one category to the other. For example, a child who started out life as inhibited might become less shy over time, but he or she would rarely switch over to being a bold child. In a large Australian longitudinal study conducted by Prior et al. (2000), in which children's temperament development was studied between 1983 and 2000, it was found that of all children in the study who were found to be extremely shy in their early childhood years (ages 3–7) only 20 percent of them continued with this level of shyness into their teenage years (ages 13–14). The other 80 percent of extremely shy children identified in the study were found to be less introverted as they grew older, but still preferred to be less social than outgoing children of their age group due to their shyness.

A study of children's temperament being influenced by parenting styles in both Australia and the United States (Russell et al, 2003) found that between these two Westernised countries the child's own temperament dictated as to whether they would be more social or aggressive regardless of their parent's temperament and parenting style. Only in the United States sample of parents was it found that an authoritarian father had some minor impact on aggressiveness or social skills in both boys' and girls' social relationships.

Temperament development sets the stage for later aspects of social development. Next, we consider the *attachment* bonds children form as their first social relationships.

Attachment

Social development begins with the establishment of a close emotional relationship between a child and a mother, father or other regular caregiver. This intense, enduring, social–emotional relationship is called **attachment**. Because children are incapable of feeding or protecting themselves, the earliest function of attachment is to ensure survival. In some species, the infant automatically becomes *imprinted* on the first moving object it sees or hears (Bolhuis & Honey, 1998). **Imprinting** occurs rapidly during a critical period of development and cannot easily be modified. The automaticity of imprinting can sometimes be problematic. Ethologist Konrad Lorenz demonstrated that young geese raised by a human imprint on the human instead of on one of their own kind. In nature, fortunately, young geese mostly see other geese first.

Attachment
Emotional relationship between a child and the regular caregiver.

Imprinting
A primitive form of learning in which some infant animals physically follow and form an attachment to the first moving object they see and/or hear.

You won't find human infants imprinting on their parents. Even so, John Bowlby (1973), an influential theorist on human attachment, suggested that infants and adults are biologically predisposed to form attachments. That attachment relationship has broad consequences. Beginning with Bowlby (1973), theorists have suggested that the experiences that give rise to an attachment relationship provide individuals with a lifelong schema for social relationships called an *internal working model* (Bretherton, 1996). An internal working model is a memory structure that gathers together a child's history of interactions with his or her caregivers, the interactions that yielded a particular pattern of attachment. The internal working model provides a template that an individual uses to generate expectations about future social interactions.

One of the most widely used research procedures for assessing attachment is the *Strange Situation Test*, developed by Mary Ainsworth and her colleagues (Ainsworth et al., 1978). In the first of several standard episodes, the child is brought into an unfamiliar room filled with toys. With the mother present, the child is encouraged to explore the room and to play. After several minutes, a stranger comes in, talks to the mother, and approaches the child. Next, the mother exits the room. After this brief separation, the mother returns, there is a reunion with her child, and the stranger leaves. The researchers record the child's behaviours at separation and reunion. Researchers have found that children's responses on this test fall into three general categories (Ainsworth et al., 1978):

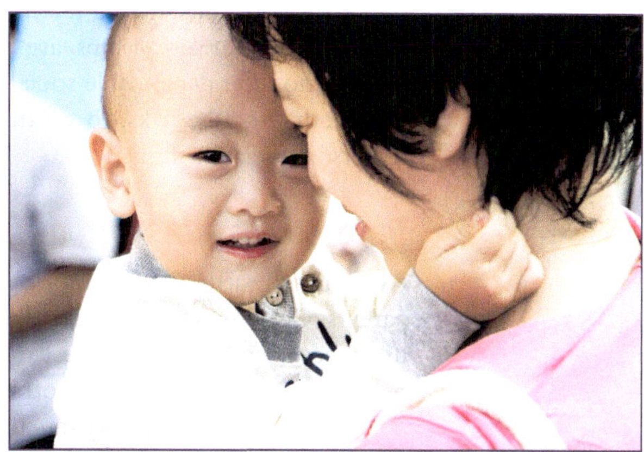

Why is it important for a child to develop a secure attachment to a parent or other caregiver?
(**Source:** © Mamahoohooba/Dreamstime.com.)

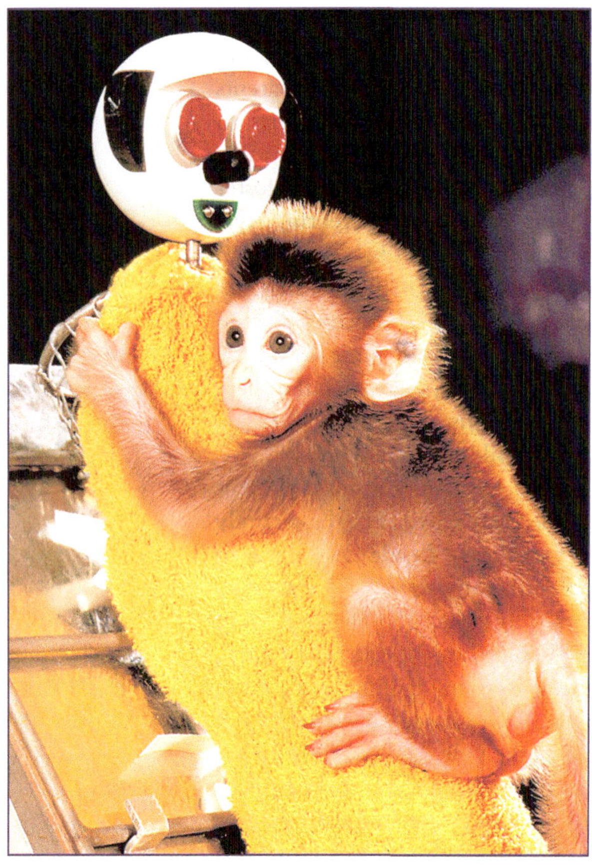

How did Harlow demonstrate the importance of contact comfort for normal social development?
(**Source:** © Martin Rogers/Stone/Getty Images)

interventions to improve parenting practices (Van Zeijl et al., 2006).

A close interactive relationship with loving adults is a child's first step toward healthy physical growth and normal socialisation. As the original attachment to the primary caregiver extends to other family members, they too become models for new ways of thinking and behaving. From these early attachments, children develop the ability to respond to their own needs and to the needs of others.

Contact comfort and social experience

What do children obtain from the attachment bond? Sigmund Freud and other psychologists argued that babies become attached to their parents because the parents provide them with food—their most basic physical need. This view is called the *cupboard theory* of attachment. If the cupboard theory were correct, children should thrive as long as they are adequately fed. Does this seem right?

Harry Harlow (1958) did not believe that the cupboard theory explained the importance of attachment. He set out to test the cupboard theory against his own hypothesis that infants might also attach to those who provide contact comfort (Harlow & Zimmerman, 1958). Harlow separated macaque monkeys from their mothers at birth and placed them in cages, where they had access to two artificial 'mothers': a wire one and a terry towelling one. Harlow found that the baby monkeys nestled close to the terry towelling mother and spent little time on the wire one. They did this even when only the wire mother gave milk! The baby monkeys also used the cloth mother as a source of comfort when frightened and as a base of operations when exploring new stimuli. When a fear stimulus (e.g., a toy bear beating a drum) was introduced, the baby monkeys would run to the cloth mother. When novel and intriguing stimuli were introduced, the baby monkeys would gradually venture out to explore and then return to the terry towelling mother before exploring further.

Parenting practices Specific parenting behaviours that arise in response to particular parental goals.

Contact comfort Comfort derived from an infant's physical contact with the mother or caregiver.

Further studies by Harlow and his colleagues found that the monkeys' formation of a strong attachment to the mother substitute was not sufficient for healthy social development. At first, the experimenters thought the young monkeys with terry towelling mothers were developing normally, but a very different picture emerged when it was time for the female monkeys who had been raised in this way to become mothers. Monkeys who had been deprived of chances to interact with other responsive monkeys in their early lives had trouble forming normal social and sexual relationships in adulthood.

Primate researcher Stephen Suomi (1999; Champoux et al., 1995) has shown that putting emotionally vulnerable infant monkeys in the foster care of supportive mothers virtually turns their lives around. Suomi notes that monkeys put in the care of mothers known to be particularly loving and attentive are transformed from marginal members of the monkey troop into bold, outgoing young males who are among the first to leave the troop at puberty to work their way into a new troop. This *cross-fostering* gives them coping skills and information essential for recruiting support from other monkeys and for maintaining a high social status in the group. Let's see now what lessons research with monkeys holds for human deprivation.

Human deprivation

Tragically, human societies have sometimes created circumstances in which children are deprived of contact comfort. Many studies have shown that a lack of close, loving relationships in infancy affects physical growth and even survival. In 1915, a doctor at Johns Hopkins Hospital reported that, despite adequate physical care, 90 percent of the infants admitted to orphanages in Baltimore died within the first year. Studies of hospitalised infants over the next 30 years found that, despite adequate nutrition, the children often developed respiratory infections and fevers of unknown origin, failed to gain weight, and showed general signs of physiological deterioration (Bowlby, 1969; Spitz & Wolf, 1946).

Contemporary studies continue to demonstrate patterns of disruption. For example, one study compared attachment outcomes for children raised at home to those for children largely (90 percent of their lives) raised in institutions (Zeanah et al., 2005). The researchers found that 74 percent of the home-reared children had secure attachments; for institution-reared children, only 20 percent had secure attachments. Moreover, a lack of normal social contact may have a long-lasting effect on children's brain development. One study compared a group of children who had spent about their first 1½ years in orphanages to those who had been raised by their biological parents (Wismer Fries et al., 2005). At age 4½, the two groups of children interacted with a stranger. The children who spent their earliest days in orphanages failed to show a normal pattern of brain response—as indicated by brain hormone levels—to the interaction with the stranger.

Unfortunately, no matter what the setting in which children live, there is a potential for abuse. In a recent analysis, the United States Government found that about 170,000 children experienced physical abuse in a single year, and roughly 90,000 experienced sexual abuse (United States Department of Health and Human Services, 2005a). In one sample of 375 young adults, nearly 11 percent reported having endured some type of physical or sexual abuse. Of that group, about 80 percent presented symptoms of one or more psychiatric disorders (Silverman et al., 1996). Instances of child abuse provide psychologists with a very important agenda: to determine what types of interventions are in the best interest of the child. In Australia, between the years 2005 and 2006, 266,745 cases of childhood neglect or abuse were reported (Australian Institute of Health and Welfare, 2007). Causes behind why child abuse occurs in Australia have strong correlations with community, culture, parenting styles and the levels of parent education across Anglo, multicultural and Indigenous communities. Child abuse in Australia ranges from physical injuries, sexual abuse, malnourishment, substance abuse, criminal behaviour and, of course, psychological abuse (Cicchetti & Carlson, 1989). In contrast to Australia, roughly 513,000 United States children and youths were removed from their homes and placed in some type of government-funded setting in 2005; for example, a foster home or group residence (United States Department of Health and Human Services, 2005b). Are these children always happy to be removed from their abusive homes? The answer is complex because even abused children have often formed an attachment to their caregivers: the children may remain loyal to their natural family and hope that everything could be put right if they were allowed to return. This is one reason that much research attention is focused on designing intervention programs to reunite families (Miller et al., 2006).

In this section, you have seen how experiences during childhood have an impact on later social development. We now shift our focus to later periods of life, beginning with adolescence.

Social development in adolescence

Earlier in the chapter, we defined adolescence by physical and cognitive changes. In this section, those changes will serve as background to social experiences. Because the individual has reached a certain level of physical and mental maturity, new social and personal challenges present themselves. We will first consider the general experience of adolescence and then turn to the individual's changing social world.

The experience of adolescence

The traditional view of adolescence predicts a uniquely tumultuous period of life, characterised by extreme mood swings and unpredictable, difficult behaviour: 'storm and stress'. This view can be traced back to romantic writers of the late 18th and early 19th centuries, such as Goethe. The storm-and-stress conception of adolescence was strongly propounded by G. Stanley Hall, the first psychologist of the modern era to write at length about adolescent development (1904). Following Hall, the major proponents of this view have been psychoanalytic theorists working within the Freudian tradition (e.g., Blos, 1965; Freud, 1946, 1958). Some of them have argued that not only is extreme turmoil a normal part of adolescence but that failure to exhibit such turmoil is a sign of arrested development. Anna Freud wrote that 'to be normal during the adolescent period is by itself abnormal' (1958, p. 275).

Two early pioneers in cultural anthropology, Margaret Mead (1928) and Ruth Benedict (1938), argued that the storm-and-stress theory is not applicable to many non-Western cultures. They described cultures in which children gradually take on more and more adult responsibilities without any sudden stressful transition or period of indecision and turmoil. Contemporary research has confirmed that the experience of adolescence differs across cultures (Arnett, 1999). Those cross-cultural differences argue against strictly biological theories of adolescent experience. Instead, researchers focus on the transitions children are expected to make in different cultures.

Recall that in Erikson's description of the life span, the essential task of adolescence is to discover one's true identity. For cultures such as the majority culture in Australia, one consequence is that children attempt to achieve *independence* from their parents. With approximately 1.2 million young people aged 12–24 in New South Wales, Australia (34,000 of these being Aboriginal or Torres Strait Islander), it is not unreasonable to suggest that a good portion of these adolescents are seeking to obtain independence and identity. Across the ages 10–17, part of the struggle teenagers and adolescents have to contend with are stages of puberty, which add angst to their battles for independence, as demonstrated in Table 2.5. Parents and their adolescent children must weather a transition in their relationship from one in which a parent has unquestioned authority, to one in which the adolescent is granted reasonable independence to make important decisions (Allen & Land, 1999; Holmbeck & O'Donnell, 1991). Consider the results of a study that followed 1330 adolescents from age 11 to age 14 (McGue et al., 2005). As 14-year-olds, these adolescents reported greater conflict with their parents than they had at age 11. At age 14, the adolescents' parents were less involved in their lives; the adolescents had less positive regard for their parents and they believed that their parents had less positive regard for them. This data illustrates some of the relationship costs that arise when children strive for independence. We don't want to paint an overly negative picture:

Table 2.5 Adolescent identity developmental stages

Identity development in early adolescence (age 10–14)
• Am I normal?
• Daydreaming
• Vocational goals change frequently
• Begin to develop own value system
• Emerging sexual feelings and sexual exploration
• Imaginary audience
• Desire for privacy
• Magnify own problems: no one understands
Identity develoment in middle adolescence (age 15–17)
• Experimentation with sex, drugs, friends, jobs and risk-taking behaviour
Identity development in late adolescence (age 18–21)
• Pursue realistic vocational goals with training or career employment
• Relate to family as an adult
• Realisations of own limitations and mortality
• Establishment of sexual identity; sexual activity is more common
• Establishment of ethical and moral value system
• More capable of intimate, complex relationships

most adolescents at most times are still able to use their parents as ready sources of practical and emotional support (Smetana et al., 2006). Most researchers reject 'storm and stress' as a biologically programmed aspect of development. Nonetheless, people typically do experience more extreme emotions and more conflict as they pass from childhood into adolescence. When we discussed physical development we noted that brain areas that control emotional responses show growth during adolescence. That brain maturation may explain why adolescents experience both extreme positive and extreme negative emotions (Casey et al., 2008; Steinberg, 2008).

Having stated this, adolescents' conflicts with their parents often do not lead to harmful outcomes. Many adolescents have conflicts with their parents that leave their basic relationship with them unharmed. When conflict occurs in the context of otherwise positive relationships, there may be few negative consequences. However, in the context of negative relationships, adolescent conflict can lead to other problems such as social withdrawal and delinquency (Adams & Laursen, 2007). Thus, family contexts may explain why some adolescents experience unusual levels of 'storm and stress'.

Now that we've considered the general adolescent experience, let's turn to the increasing importance of peers in adolescents' social experience.

Peer relationships

Much of the study of social development in adolescence focuses on the changing roles of family (or adult caregivers) and friends (Smetana et al., 2006). We have already seen that attachments to adults form soon after birth. Children also begin to have friends at very young ages. Adolescence, however, marks the first period in which peers appear to compete with parents to shape a person's attitudes and behaviours. Adolescents participate in peer relations at the three levels of friendships, cliques and crowds (Brown & Klute, 2003). Over the course of these years, adolescents come to count increasingly on their one-on-one *friendships* to provide them with help and support (Bauminger et al., 2008; Branje et al., 2007). *Cliques* are groups that most often consist of 6 to 12 individuals. Membership in these groups may change over time, but they tend to be drawn along lines of, for example, age and race (Smetana et al., 2006). Finally, *crowds* are the larger groups such as sport 'jocks' or 'nerds' that exist more loosely among individuals of this age. Through interaction with peers at these three levels, adolescents gradually define the social component of their developing identities, determining the kinds of people they choose to be and the kinds of relationships they choose to pursue (Smetana et al., 2006).

The peer relationships that adolescents form are quite important to social development. They give individuals opportunities to learn how to function in what can often be demanding social circumstances. In that sense, peer relationships play a positive role in preparing adolescents for their futures. At the same time, parents often worry—with reasonable cause—about negative aspects of peer influence. For example, research supports the conclusion that adolescents are more likely to engage in risky behaviours when they are under the influence of their peers.

To study developmental changes in peer influence, researchers recruited three groups of participants: adolescents (aged 13–16), young adults (aged 18–22) and adults (aged 24 and older) (Gardner & Steinberg, 2005). Participants in each age range played a video game called 'Chicken'. In this game, players act as drivers. They must decide how soon to stop their car when a light changes from green to orange. Their goal is to achieve as much distance as they can before the light turns red and a wall pops up. If they don't stop in time, they'll crash into the wall. About half of the participants played the game alone. The other half played in groups of three—each participant played in turn while the other two watched. Figure 2.9 presents the results of the experiment. As you can see, adolescents were

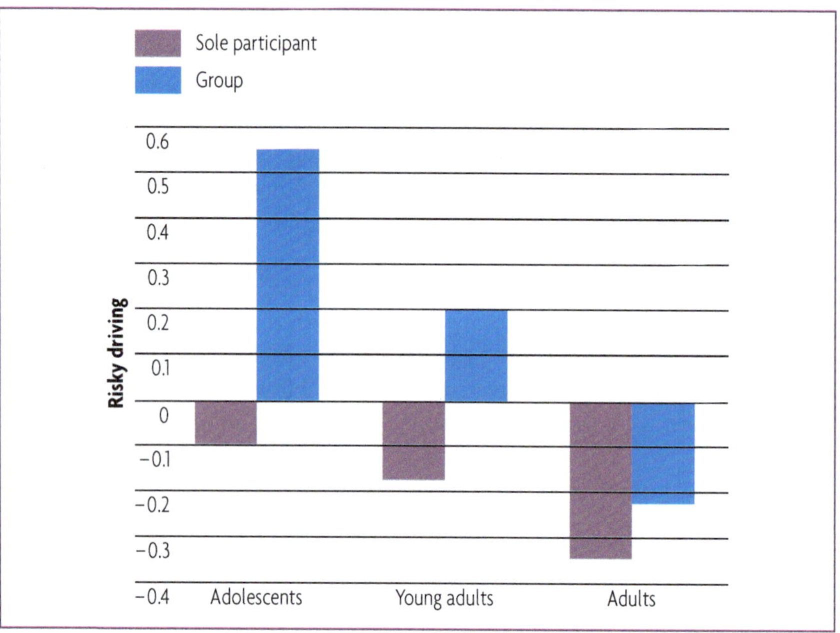

Figure 2.9 Peer influence on risky behaviour

Adolescents, young adults and adults played a video game called 'Chicken' by themselves or in a group setting. The video game allowed participants to take risks while driving. The y-axis plots a measure of risky driving: larger positive scores indicate higher risk. Adolescents showed the largest impact of the presence of peers.
From Gardner, M. and Steinberg, L. (2005). Copyright © 2005 by the American Psychological Association. Reprinted with permission.

far more likely to engage in risky driving (within the context of the video game) when in the presence of their peers.

This study confirms a general tendency for adolescents to demonstrate peer influence as a shift toward riskier behaviours. However, some adolescents are more susceptible to peer influence than others—and that susceptibility has consequences. In a longitudinal study, students who were more susceptible to their close friends' influence at the study's outset were more likely to have problems with drugs and alcohol 1 year later (Allen et al., 2006). We note, once again, that adolescence need not be a time of storm and stress. However, research of this type indicates the patterns of behaviour that indicate some adolescents are at risk.

Social development in adulthood

Erikson defined two tasks of adulthood as intimacy and generativity. Freud identified the needs of adulthood as *Lieben und Arbeiten*, or love and work. Abraham Maslow (1968, 1970) described the needs of this period of life as love and belonging, which, when satisfied, develop into the needs for success and esteem. Other theorists label these needs as affiliation or social acceptance and achievement or competence needs. The shared core of these theories is that adulthood is a time in which both social relationships and personal accomplishments take on special priority. In this section, we track these themes across the breadth of adulthood.

Intimacy

Intimacy
The capacity to make a full commitment—sexual, emotional and moral—to another person.

Erikson described **intimacy** as the capacity to make a full commitment—sexual, emotional and moral—to another person. Intimacy, which can occur in both friendships and romantic relationships, requires openness, courage, ethical strength and usually some compromise of one's personal preferences. Research has consistently confirmed Erikson's supposition that social intimacy is a prerequisite for a sense of psychological wellbeing across the adult life stages (Kesebir & Diener, 2008). Here, we focus on the role intimate relationships play in social development.

Figure 2.10 demonstrates that interactions with family and friends trade off over this long span of years to provide a fairly constant level in people's reports of their own wellbeing. The changes in these sources of support reflect, in part, the life events that are typically correlated with each age. Let's examine these correlations.

Young adulthood is the period in which many people enter into marriages or other stable relationships. The Australian Bureau of Statistics indicates that 19.7 percent of adolescents aged 20–24 were marrying in 2014, with the highest percentage of 45.2 percent in the 25–29 age demographic. The median age of marriage for males and females was 31.5 and 29.6 years respectively (Australian Bureau of Statistics, 2014). In comparison to the United States in 2010, 14 percent of 20- to 24-year-olds were married; with 25- to 29-year-olds that figure increased to 42 percent (Cohn, Passel, Wang & Livingston, 2011). This demonstrates that marriage rates between similar Western countries is very close, regardless of population size. It is also interesting to note that many other individuals live with partners to whom they are not married, or legally cannot marry. Statistics from the 2011 Census reveal that there were 33,714 same-sex couples in Australia with 16,100 same-sex female couples and 17,600 same-sex male couples (Australian Bureau of Statistics, 2013). While in recent years, a multitude of countries (e.g., New Zealand, France and parts of the United Kingdom) have legalised same-sex marriage, Australia is yet to follow suit (Neilsen, 2015). Researchers try to understand the consequences of all these types of relationships for social development in adulthood. For example, research attention has focused on differences and similarities between heterosexual and homosexual couples (Balsam et al., 2008; Roisman et al., 2008). Studies suggest that the strategies heterosexuals and homosexuals use to maintain relationships over time have much in common: both types of couples try to remain close by, for example, sharing tasks and activities together (Haas & Stafford, 2005). However, heterosexual couples obtain more societal support for their

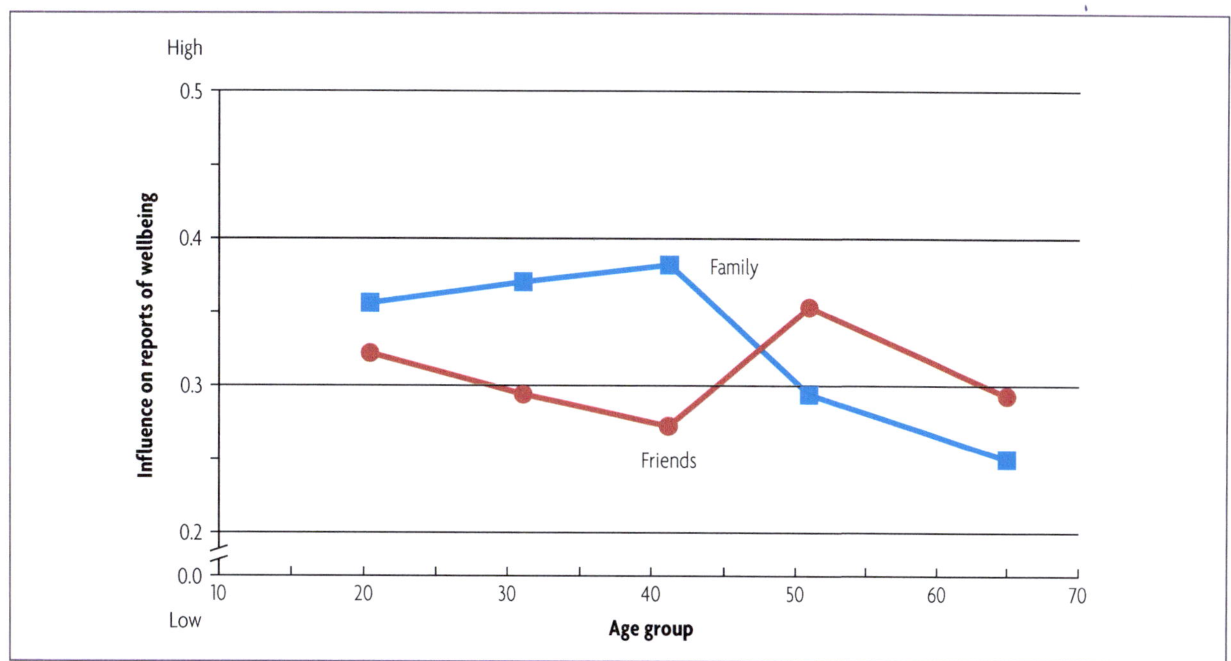

Figure 2.10 The effects of social interaction on wellbeing

Across the life span, social interactions with family and friends trade off to provide a fairly constant level of individuals' reports of wellbeing.

relationships (Herek, 2006). To combat a lack of social acceptance, homosexual couples often take special measures to maintain relationships, such as being publicly 'out' as a couple.

Each of these types of relationships increases the role of family in adults' social lives. Families also grow when individuals decide to include children in their lives. What may surprise you, however, is that the birth of children can often pose a threat to the overall happiness of a couple (Lawrence et al., 2007; Myrskylä & Margolis, 2014, pp. 1843-1866; Clark, Diener, Georgellis & Lucas, 2008, pp. 222–243). Why might that be? Researchers have focused on differences in the way that men and women make the transition to parenthood in heterosexual relationships (Cowan & Cowan, 2000) as well as sociodemographic factors (Myrskylä & Margolis, 2014, pp. 1843-1866). In contemporary Western society, marriages are more often founded on notions of equality between men and women than was true in the past. However, children's births can have the effect of pushing husbands and wives in the direction of more traditional gender roles. The wife may feel too much of the burden of child care; the husband may feel too much pressure to support a family. The net effect may be that, following the birth of a child, the marriage changes in ways that both spouses find to be negative (Cowan et al., 1985). As you might expect, homosexual relationships are less troubled by concerns about gender roles in the context of parenting (Goldberg & Perry-Jenkins, 2007; Patterson, 2002). Even so, in parallel to results for heterosexual couples, a study of lesbian couples found decreasing love and increasing conflict across the transition to parenthood (Goldberg & Sayer, 2006). In addition to research on the influence of gender roles and parental happiness, is research on the link between parental happiness and sociodemographic factors. Myrskylä and Margolis (2014, pp. 1843-1866) surmised that the trajectory of happiness following child birth is influenced by a range of sociodemographic factors including parental age at time of birth, parental educational attainment, marital status and number of pregnancies. In particular, Myrskylä and Margolis (2014, pp. 1843-1866) found that younger, resource-poor and less educated parents are more likely to experience a downward well-being trajectory.

For many couples, satisfaction with the marriage continues to decline because of conflicts as the child or children pass through their adolescent years. Contrary to the cultural stereotype, many parents look forward to the time when their youngest child leaves home and leaves them with an 'empty nest' (Dennerstein et al., 2003; Fingerman, 2000, pp. 95-106). Research suggests that empty nest parents enjoy improved relationships with their children and a greater opportunity to pursue their own goals and aspirations once their children leave the family home (Fingerman, 2000, pp. 95-106).

Have we discouraged you from having children? We certainly hope not! Our goal, as always, is to make you aware of research that can help you anticipate and interpret the patterns in your own life. Consider the following: if marriages are, on the whole, happier when the spouses reach late adulthood, should everyone try to stay married late into life? In Australia, approximately 40 percent of marriages end in divorce. ABS researchers would like to be able to determine which couples are fundamentally mismatched—with respect, for example, to their patterns of interactions—and which couples could avoid divorce (Orbuch et al., 2002; Story & Bradbury, 2004).

Researchers obtained information from 4460 couples in 1987–1988 and then again in 1992–1994 (Amato & Hohmann-Marriott, 2007). In that period of time, 509 of the couples had divorced or separated. To understand why relationships had ended, the researchers examined data from the study's outset. Participants had reported on their marital quality (such as their happiness with the relationship and the amount of conflict in the relationship). They also reported on their commitment to the marriage (e.g., their barriers to leaving the marriage or their alternatives to the marriage). The researchers' analyses revealed two clusters of people who ended relationships. One cluster had been in *high-distress* relationships in 1987–1988. They had reported low-quality relationships, which they brought to an end.

Couples in the other cluster had been *low-distress* relationships. Their marriage quality was about average. So why did they divorce? These couples had low barriers to ending the marriage and attractive alternatives beyond it.

These results suggest why you cannot always predict which couples are headed for divorce based on surface aspects of the relationships such as open conflict. When people have other alternatives, they may end relationships in which they are at least moderately happy.

When individuals stay together late into life, one member of the couple most often must cope with the death of a spouse. When we contemplate the death of a spouse or partner, we come back to one reason that the balance of social interactions shifts somewhat from family to friends late in life (see Figure 2.10). A stereotype about late adulthood is that individuals become more socially isolated. Although it is true that older individuals may interact socially with fewer people, the nature of those interactions changes so that intimacy needs continue to be met. This trade-off is captured by the **selective social interaction theory**. This view suggests that, as people age, they become more selective in choosing social partners who satisfy their emotional needs. According to Laura Carstensen (1991, 1998), selective interaction may be a practical means by which people can regulate their emotional experiences and conserve their physical energy. Older adults remain vitally involved with some people—particularly family members and long-time friends.

Selective social interaction theory
The view that suggests that as people age they become more selective in choosing social partners who satisfy their emotional needs.

Let's conclude this section where we began, with the idea that social intimacy is a prerequisite for psychological wellbeing. What matters most is not the quantity of social interaction but the quality (particularly, in Australian culture, for women). As you grow into older adulthood, you will begin to protect your need for intimacy by selecting those individuals who provide the most direct emotional support.

Let's turn now to a second aspect of adult development, generativity.

Generativity
A commitment beyond one's self and one's partner to family, work, society and future generations.

Generativity

Those people who have established an appropriate foundation of intimate relationships are most often able to turn their focus to issues of **generativity**. This is a commitment beyond oneself to family, work, society or future generations—typically a crucial step in development in one's 30s and 40s (McAdams & de St. Aubin, 1998). An orientation toward the greater good allows adults to establish a sense of psychological wellbeing that offsets any longing for youth.

George Vaillant studied the personality development of 95 highly intelligent men through interviews and observations over a 30-year period following their graduation from college in the mid-1930s. Many of the men showed great changes over time, and their later

Table 2.6 Differences between best- and worst-outcome subjects on factors related to psychosocial maturity

	Best outcomes (30 Men)	Worst outcomes (30 Men)
Personality integration rated in bottom fifth percentile during college	0%	33%
Dominated by mother in adult life	0%	40%
Bleak friendship patterns at 50	0%	57%
Failure to marry by 30	3%	37%
Pessimism, self-doubt, passivity and fear of sex at 50	3%	50%
Childhood environment poor	17%	47%
Current job has little supervisory responsibility	20%	93%
Subjects whose career choice reflected identification with father	60%	27%
Children's outcome described as good or excellent	66%	23%

behaviour was often quite different from their behaviour in college. The interviews covered the topics of physical health, social relationships and career achievement. At the end of the 30-year period, the 30 men with the best outcomes and the 30 with the worst outcomes were identified and compared (see Table 2.6). By middle life, the best-outcome men were carrying out generativity tasks, assuming responsibility for others, and contributing in some way to the world. Their maturity even seemed to be associated with the adjustment of their children—the more mature fathers were better able to give children the help they needed in adjusting to the world (Vaillant, 1977).

This study illustrates the prerequisites for generativity: for the best-outcome men, other aspects of their lives were sufficiently stable to allow them to direct their resources outwards, toward generations to come. When asked what it means to be well adjusted, middle-aged adults (average age 52) and older adults (average age 74) gave the same response as their most frequent answer. Both groups suggested that adjustment relies on being 'others oriented'—on being a caring, compassionate person and having good relationships (Ryff, 1989). This is the essence of generativity.

Let us also note that older adults looking back on their lives do so with a degree of wellbeing that is unchanged from earlier years of adulthood (Carstensen & Freund, 1994). As we have seen with respect to social relationships, late adulthood is a time when goals are shifted; priorities change when the future does not apparently flow as freely. Across that change in priorities, however, older adults preserve their sense of the value of their lives. Erikson defined the last crisis of adulthood to be the conflict between ego integrity and despair. The data suggest that few adults look back over their lives with despair. Most older adults review their lives—and look to the future—with a sense of wholeness and satisfaction.

We have worked our way through the life span by considering social and personal aspects of childhood, adolescence and adulthood. To finish the chapter, we will trace two particular domains in which experience changes over time, the domains of sex and gender differences and moral development.

Stop and review

1. At what life stage did Erik Erikson suggest people navigate the crisis of intimacy versus isolation?
2. What long-term consequences have been demonstrated for children's early attachment quality?
3. What dimensions define parenting styles?
4. In what levels of peer relationships do adolescents engage?
5. What impact does the birth of a child often have on marital satisfaction?

Critical thinking

Recall the study that examined risk taking in a video game. Why was it important that all three group members had a turn at the game?

Sex and gender differences

One type of information most children begin to acquire in the first few months in life is that there are two categories of people in their social world: males and females. Over time, children learn that there are many respects in which the psychological experiences of males and females are quite similar. However, when differences do in fact occur, children acquire an understanding that some of those differences arise from biology and others arise from cultural expectations. Biologically based characteristics that distinguish males and females are referred to as **sex differences**. These characteristics include different reproductive functions and differences in hormones and anatomy. However, the first differences children perceive are entirely social: they begin to sense differences between males and females well before they understand anything about anatomy. In contrast to biological sex, **gender** is a psychological phenomenon referring to learned sex-related behaviours and attitudes. Cultures vary in how strongly gender is linked to daily activities and in the amount of tolerance for what is perceived as cross-gender behaviour. In this section, we consider both sex differences and gender development: the nature and nurture of children's sense of maleness or femaleness.

Sex difference
A biologically based characteristic that distinguishes males from females.

Gender
A psychological phenomenon that refers to learned sex-related behaviours and attitudes of males and females.

Sex differences

Starting at about 6 weeks after conception, male foetuses begin to diverge from female foetuses, when the male testes develop and begin to produce the hormone *testosterone*. The presence or absence of testosterone plays a critical role in determining whether a child will be born with male or female anatomy. Testosterone also has an impact on brain development: experiments with nonhuman animals have demonstrated that sex differences in neural structure are largely brought about by this hormone (Morris et al., 2004).

The exact role of testosterone is less clear for the development of the human brain. However, brain scans have revealed consistent structural differences between men's and women's brains (Goldstein et al., 2001). Men typically have bigger brains than women—appropriate comparisons across the sexes adjust for that overall variation. The differences that remain after those adjustments are intriguing with respect to behavioural dissimilarities between men and women. For example, MRI scans reveal that the regions of the frontal lobe that play an important role in regulating social behaviour and emotional functioning are relatively bigger in women than in men (Gur et al., 2002).

Another interesting difference has been found with the levels of testosterone before and after birth and its relation to language development in British infants. At age 18–24 months, girls were found to have a significantly larger vocabulary than boys at their equivalent age. This suggested that foetal testosterone levels may have some impact on neural mechanisms underlying communication development. To confirm that sex differences of this type are biological—rather than the product of a lifetime of experience as men or women in particular cultural roles—researchers have undertaken similar studies with children and adolescents (Lenroot et al., 2007). Those studies confirm that sex differences emerge in the brain as a part of ordinary biological development.

Other analyses of sex differences focus on the distinct ways in which men's and women's brains accomplish cognitive and emotional tasks (Kimura, 1999). Consider the brain processes engaged when the two sexes view emotionally charged pictures.

Twelve men and 12 women underwent fMRI scans while viewing 96 pictures that ranged from neutral (e.g., a book or a fork) to negative (e.g., an autopsy or a gravestone) (Canli et al., 2002). As the participants viewed the pictures, they provided ratings of the intensity of their emotional experience on a scale ranging from 0 ('not emotionally intense at all') to 3 ('extremely emotionally intense'). Three weeks after this initial experience, the participants completed a test of recognition memory for the pictures—they had not been warned when they first viewed the pictures that this test was forthcoming. The researchers assessed the relationship between brain activity at the time of encoding and subsequent memory performance. They found distinct patterns of activity for men and for women. For example, greater activity in the left amygdala preceded recognition success for women; greater activity in the right amygdala preceded success for men.

Further studies of the brain at work confirm sex differences in the encoding and recognition of emotionally arousing stimuli (Cahill et al., 2004). These studies suggest that some of the behavioural differences that set men and women apart can be traced to biological differences rather than to cultural roles.

Most research on the biology of sex differences with human subjects focuses on global differences between men and women. However, researchers have recently begun to look at the biological origins of more fine-grained differences among individuals. These studies turn once again to the impact of the hormone testosterone on later development. In this case, the researchers determined the level of testosterone in the amniotic fluid of each individual participant. The researchers correlated those foetal testosterone levels with, for example, the quality of each boy's or girl's social relationships when they were 4-years-old (Knickmeyer et al., 2005). In general, boys had higher levels of foetal testosterone than girls. Against that background, individuals' higher levels of foetal testosterone were associated with poorer social relationships for both boys and girls. These results suggest that the extent to which individuals conform to expectations for male and female behaviour may depend, in part, on their prenatal hormonal environment (Morris et al., 2004).

Gender identity and gender roles

Gender identity One's sense of maleness or femaleness; usually includes awareness and acceptance of one's biological sex.

Gender stereotype Belief about attributes and behaviours regarded as appropriate for males and females in a particular culture.

You have just seen that important aspects of men's and women's behaviour are shaped by biological differences. However, cultural expectations also have an important impact on **gender identity**—an individual's sense of maleness or femaleness. Very early in life, children start to understand that the world is divided into two genders (Martin & Ruble, 2004; Martin et al., 2002). For example, 10- to 14-month-old children already demonstrate a preference for a video showing the abstract movements of a child of the same sex (Kujawski & Bower, 1993). In their earliest years, children begin to understand that they are either boys or girls—they settle into their gender identity. At the same time, they acquire knowledge of **gender stereotypes**, which are beliefs about attributes and behaviours regarded as appropriate for males and females in a particular culture.

Researchers have documented the time course with which most children acquire those gender stereotypes (Mulvey & Killen, 2015; LoBue & DeLoache, 2011). Through the preschool years, children's experience in the world provides them with knowledge about cultural expectations for men and women. Between ages 3 and 4, children consolidate their knowledge into gender stereotypes. However, by the ages of 5 and 6, children's rigidity with with respect to those stereotypes reduces. For example, one study assessed children's gender stereotypes by presenting participants with a pair of identical coloured items: one item was always pink and the other was either yellow, blue, green or orange (LoBue & DeLoache, 2011). Children were presented with the pairs of objects and asked 'Which one do you like better?' The results revealed that girls demonstrated a significant preference for the colour pink at the ages 3 and 4, while boys demonstrated a significant avoidance of pink at the same age. Further highlighted by this research was the finding that boys and girls develop more flexibility about gender roles by the ages of 5 and 6. Boys' avoidance of pink diminished, while girls' choice of other colours increased.

How do children acquire the information that leads to gender identity and gender stereotypes? Parents provide one ready source. In fact, this process more often than not starts while the child is in the womb with parents choosing to decorate the nursery and purchase toys and clothing consistent with traditional gender stereotypes (Zosuls, Miller, Ruble, Martin, & Fabes, 2011). Parents dress their sons and daughters differently, give them different kinds of toys to play with, and communicate with them differently (LoBue & DeLoache, 2011). When parents play with their children, they consider some toys to be 'masculine' and some to be 'feminine'. When they play with their children, they are more likely to choose gender-appropriate toys—though that preference may be stronger for play with boys than for play with girls (Wood et al., 2002). In general, children receive encouragement from their parents to engage in sex-typed activities (Boekee & Brown, 2015; McHale et al., 2003).

As children begin to spend more time socialising with other children, their peers provide an important source of gender socialisation by encouraging or discouraging certain behaviours. This may occur indirectly. For example, young children often engage in gender segregation, resulting in similar behaviours and interests (Martin et al., 2013; Mulvey & Killen, 2015). Alternatively, gender socialisation can also occur directly. For example, a preschool aged boy might say to his male peer "Barbie dolls are only for girls", while a young girl might reiterate to her female peer that "boys are not allowed to play with us". In fact, boys and girls show consistent differences in their patterns of social interaction. Some differences relate to the structure of those interactions. For example, at least by the age of 6, boys prefer to interact in groups outside, whereas girls prefer to play indoors in twos or threes (Benenson & Heath, 2006; Golombok, Rust, Zervoulis, Golding & Hines, 2012). Other differences between boys and girls relate to the content of their play (Rose & Rudolph, 2006). Girls are more likely than boys to engage in social conversations and disclose information about themselves. Boys are more likely than girls to engage in rough-and-tumble play. These differences become more prominent as children grow older.

We have been describing factors that affect gender development across all children. However, as with other domains of development, it's important to acknowledge individual differences among children. Consider a study that examined children's gender-typed behaviours over a 6-year period. The mothers of 5501 children provided information about their gender-typed behaviours when the children were aged 2½ (Golombok et al., 2008). The mothers completed the *Preschool Activities Inventory* (PSAI), which asked them to indicate, for example, how often their children had played with jewellery or engaged in fighting in the last month. The mothers provided PSAI ratings again when their children were 3½ and 5 years old. When the children were 8, they reported their own behaviour by completing the *Children's Activities Inventory* (CAI). For this inventory, children listened to pairs of statements that described different types of children: 'Some children play with jewellery … but other children don't play with jewellery' (p. 1586). The children indicated

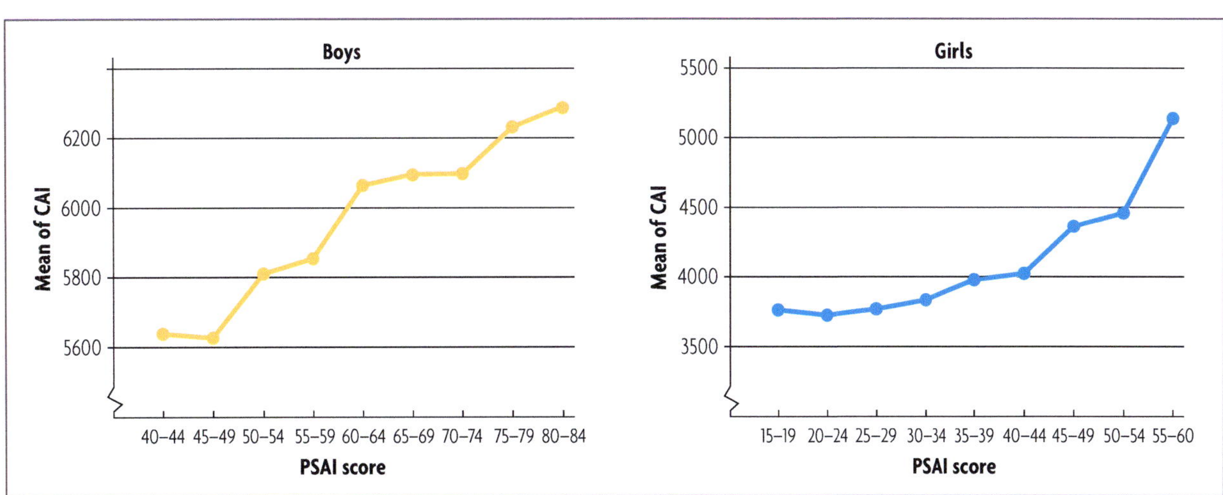

Figure 2.11 The stability of gender-typed behaviour over time

Mothers indicated children's gender-typed behaviour on the PSAI at age 3½, and children indicated their own behaviours at age 8. For each group of children who scored in a particular PSAI range at age 3½ (with lower scores indicating more stereotypically feminine behaviour), the researchers calculated their mean CAI value at age 8. The plot shows that children's levels of gender-typed behaviour were quite similar at the two points in time.

Stop and review

1. What is the distinction between sex differences and gender differences?
2. What does research suggest about differences between men and women for the processing of emotional stimuli?
3. In what ways are young children 'segregationists'?

how similar they felt to the two types of children. Based on these longitudinal assessments, the researchers concluded that the likelihood that individual children will engage in gender-typed behaviour remains very stable over time. For example, Figure 2.11 plots children's PSAI scores at age 3½ against their CAI scores at age 8. You can see a strong match between children's scores at the two ages.

Why is the children's behaviour so stable? The researchers pointed to both nature and nurture. With respect to nature, the researchers suggested that children may experience prenatal environments that cause their brains to be relatively more masculine or feminine. With respect to nurture, the researchers considered differences among the behaviours of both parents and peers. Parents who have less flexible gender stereotypes may also have children who produce more gender-typed behaviour. In addition, children may seek friends who are similar to them with respect to their levels of gender-typed behaviour—creating a context for those behaviours to be stable over time.

We have briefly considered how and why it is that boys and girls experience social development in different fashions. Let's now consider moral development.

Moral development

So far we have seen, across the life span, how important it is to develop close social relationships. Let's now consider another aspect of what it means to live as part of a social group: on many occasions you must judge your behaviour according to the needs of society, rather than just according to your own needs. This is the basis of *moral behaviour*. **Morality** is a system of beliefs, values and underlying judgement about the rightness or wrongness of human acts.

Morality
A system of beliefs and values that ensures that individuals will keep their obligations to others in society and will behave in ways that do not interfere with the rights and interests of others.

Before we consider how moral development unfolds for each individual, we want to consider the question for the whole human species: How did morality evolve? To answer that question, contemporary researchers have built on Charles Darwin's foundational observations about how humans function as a social species (Krebs, 2008). From an evolutionary perspective, moral behaviours are consequences of adaptive solutions to situations that have recurred across human history. For example, many early human endeavours (such as killing large game or defending territory) required cooperation among large groups of people. Thus, it was adaptive for humans to evolve a disposition 'to resolve fundamental social dilemmas in cooperative ways' (Krebs, 2008, p. 154). In contemporary times, moral questions often have a dimension of self-interested versus cooperative behaviour: Should a person drive his or her car less so that everyone can breathe cleaner air? The evolutionary perspective suggests that our reflexive responses to such questions is part of our genetic inheritance (Haidt, 2007).

However, even if people share some evolved moral responses, what constitutes moral and immoral behaviour in particular situations can become a matter of heated public debate. Perhaps it is no coincidence, therefore, that the study of moral development has also proved to be controversial. The controversy begins with the foundational research of Lawrence Kohlberg.

Kohlberg's stages of moral reasoning

Lawrence Kohlberg (1964, 1981) founded his theory of moral development by studying *moral reasoning*—the judgements people make about what courses of action are correct or incorrect in particular situations. Kohlberg's theory was shaped by the earlier insights of Jean Piaget (1965), who sought to tie the development of moral judgement to a child's general cognitive development. In Piaget's view, as the child progresses through the stages of cognitive growth, he or she assigns differing relative weights to the *consequences* of an act and to the actor's *intentions*. For example, to the preoperational child, someone who breaks 10 cups accidentally is 'naughtier' than someone who breaks one cup intentionally. As the child gets older, the actor's intentions weigh more heavily in the judgement of morality.

Children aged 3, 4 and 5 years old were asked to make moral judgements about people's behaviour that varied along three dimensions: actions, outcomes and intentions. The *actions* were defined as either positive or negative within a particular scenario (e.g., petting versus hitting an animal) as were the *outcomes* (e.g., the animal either cried or smiled). To vary *intentions*, the experimenters described some behaviour as intentional and others as accidental (e.g., the actor hit the pet either on purpose or by mistake). The children were asked to rate the *acceptability* of the behaviour by choosing one of a series of five faces that represented values from 'really, really bad' to 'really, really good'. The younger children based their acceptability ratings almost entirely on the outcome; only the 5-year-olds took intention into account. However, when children were asked whether the actor should be *punished*, more younger children took the actor's intention into account (Zelazo et al., 1996).

These results suggest that as children become more sophisticated cognitively, they are able to shift their focus from just outcomes to consideration of both outcomes and intentions together. However, the difference between acceptability judgements and punishment judgements suggests that some types of moral judgements allow children to consider more factors at an earlier age. As we saw earlier in the chapter, what children are specifically asked to do determines, in part, how 'mature' they seem.

Kohlberg expanded Piaget's view to define stages of moral development. Each stage is characterised by a different basis for making moral judgements (see Table 2.7). The lowest level of moral reasoning is based on self-interest; higher levels centre on social good, regardless of personal gain. To document these stages, Kohlberg used a series of dilemmas that pit different moral principles against one another:

> *In one dilemma, a man named Heinz is trying to help his wife obtain a certain drug needed to treat her cancer. An unscrupulous druggist will only sell it to Heinz for 10 times more than what the druggist paid. This is much more money than Heinz has and more than he can raise.*

Table 2.7 Kohlberg's stages of moral reasoning

Levels and stages	Reasons for moral behaviour
I Preconventional morality	
Stage 1 Pleasure/pain orientation	To avoid pain or not to get caught
Stage 2 Cost–benefit orientation; reciprocity—an eye for an eye	To get rewards
II Conventional morality	
Stage 3 Good-child orientation	To gain acceptance and avoid disapproval
Stage 4 Law and order orientation	To follow rules, avoid censure by authorities
III Principled morality	
Stage 5 Social contract orientation	To promote the society's welfare
Stage 6 Ethical principle orientation	To achieve justice and avoid self-condemnation
Stage 7 Cosmic orientation	To be true to universal principles and feel oneself part of a cosmic direction that transcends social norms

Heinz becomes desperate, breaks into the druggist's store, and steals the drug for his wife. Should Heinz have done that? Why? An interviewer probes the participant for the reasons for the decision and then scores the answers.

The scoring is based on the *reasons* the person gives for the decision, not on the decision itself. For example, someone who says that the man should steal the drug because of his obligation to his dying wife or that he should not steal the drug because of his obligation to uphold the law (despite his personal feelings) is expressing concern about meeting established obligations and is scored at stage 4.

Four principles govern Kohlberg's stage model: (1) an individual can be at only one stage at a given time; (2) everyone goes through the stages in a fixed order; (3) each stage is more comprehensive and complex than the preceding; and (4) the same stages occur in every culture. Kohlberg inherited much of this stage philosophy from Piaget, and, in fact, the progression from stages 1 to 3 appears to match the course of normal cognitive development. The stages proceed in order, and each can be seen to be more cognitively sophisticated than the preceding. Almost all children reach stage 3 by the age of 13.

Much of the controversy with Kohlberg's theory occurs beyond stage 3. In Kohlberg's original view, people would continue their moral development in a steady progression beyond stage 3. However, not all people attain stages 4 to 7. In fact, many adults never reach stage 5, and only a few go beyond it. The content of Kohlberg's later stages appears to be subjective, and it is hard to understand each successive stage as more comprehensive and sophisticated than the preceding. For example, 'avoiding self-condemnation', the basis for moral judgements at stage 6, does not seem obviously more sophisticated than 'promoting society's welfare', the basis for stage 5. Furthermore, the higher stages are not found in all cultures (Gibbs et al., 2007). We turn now to extended contemporary critiques of Kohlberg's theory that arise from considerations of gender and culture.

Gender and cultural perspectives on moral reasoning

Most critiques of Kohlberg's theory take issue with his claims of universality: Kohlberg's later stages have been criticised because they fail to recognise that adult moral judgements may reflect different, but equally moral, principles. In a well-known critique, Carol Gilligan (1982) pointed out that Kohlberg's original work was developed from observations only of boys. She argued that this research approach overlooked potential differences between the habitual moral judgements of men and women. Gilligan proposed that women's moral development is based on a standard of *caring for others* and progresses to a stage of self-realisation, whereas men base their reasoning on a standard of *justice*. Thus Gilligan's theory broadens Kohlberg's ideas about the range of considerations that may be relevant to moral judgements beyond childhood. Although we can value this contribution, research has suggested that she is incorrect to identify unique styles of moral reasoning for men and women. Let's examine the evidence.

Some studies have indicated that women mould their moral decisions to maintain harmony in their social relationships, whereas men refer more to fairness (Lyons, 1983). Even so, researchers continue to dispute whether gender differences in moral reasoning really exist at all (Donleavy, 2008; Friesdorf, Conway & Gawronski, 2015). Although men and women may arrive at their adult levels of moral development through different processes, the actual judgements they make as adults are highly similar (Boldizar et al., 1989). One possibility is that the gender differences are really consequences of the different types of social situations that arise in the lives of men and women. When asked to reason about the same moral dilemmas, men and women gave highly similar patterns of care and justice responses (Clopton & Sorell, 1993).

Cross-cultural research has also expanded researchers' understanding about the range of concerns that contribute to moral reasoning (Gibbs et al., 2007). One analysis has identified three types of concerns (Jensen, 2008). The first set of concerns relates to *autonomy:* 'A focus on people who have needs, desires, and preferences'; 'the moral goal is to recognise' people's right 'to the fulfilment of these needs and desires' (Jensen, 2008, p. 296). The second set of concerns relates to *community*: a focus on people 'as members of social groups such as family, school, and nation'; the moral goal is 'the fulfilment of role-based duties to others, and the protections and positive functioning of social groups'. The third set of concerns relates to *divinity:* a focus 'on people as spiritual or religious entities'; 'the moral goal is for the self to become increasingly connected to ... [the] pure or divine'.

If you think through these three types of concerns you can see how their importance might vary cross-culturally. Consider this situation: you see a stranger at the side of the road with a flat tyre. Should you stop to help? Suppose you decide not to stop. Is that immoral? If you have grown up in Australia, you probably think helping, under these circumstances, is a matter of personal choice, so it isn't immoral. But if you had grown up in India, in a culture that puts considerably more emphasis on interdependence and mutual assistance, you probably *would* view a failure to help as immoral (Miller et al., 1990).

It's also important to recognise that people's life experiences will have an impact on their judgements. Consider individuals who have grown up in circumstances of great violence.

The researchers recruited a group of children and adolescents from a highly impoverished area in Bogotá, Columbia (Posada & Wainryb, 2008). A large majority of the participants (88 percent) had witnessed or experienced some severe type of violence: they had, for example, seen people shot at, shot or killed. The researchers first asked the participants to share their moral judgements in the abstract. The participants answered questions like, 'Is it okay or not okay to take other people's things?' On such abstract questions, all the participants presented responses based on norms of justice. They indicated, for example, that it would not be okay to steal. However, the pattern changed when the participants made similar judgements in concrete contexts. For example, the participants read a scenario in which 15-year-old Julio had the opportunity to steal a bicycle from one of 'the people who hurt his father and his brother and forced his family to move' (p. 886). After hearing that scenario, participants often indicated their belief that Julio would steal the bicycle. In addition, despite their general aversion to stealing, many participants approved of that behaviour in this concrete instance.

The researchers note that the participants' violent life experiences have not completely overwhelmed ordinary moral development: 'Even the impoverished environments of war and displacement present youths with opportunities for reflecting on the intrinsic features of actions that harm others' (p. 896). Still, the researchers speculate that, because of their impact on moral judgements, 'contexts underscoring revenge might give rise to cycles of violence' (p. 896). The same behaviour that seems very wrong framed against one set of moral concerns may look very right framed against another.

Stop and review

1. What are the three major levels of moral reasoning in Kohlberg's theory?
2. What distinction did Carol Gilligan believe separates the moral reasoning of men and women?
3. What are three types of concerns people may bring to circumstances of moral reasoning?

Critical thinking

Consider the study that looked at moral judgements by children and adolescents in Columbia. Why might the researchers have chosen scenarios that involved revenge?

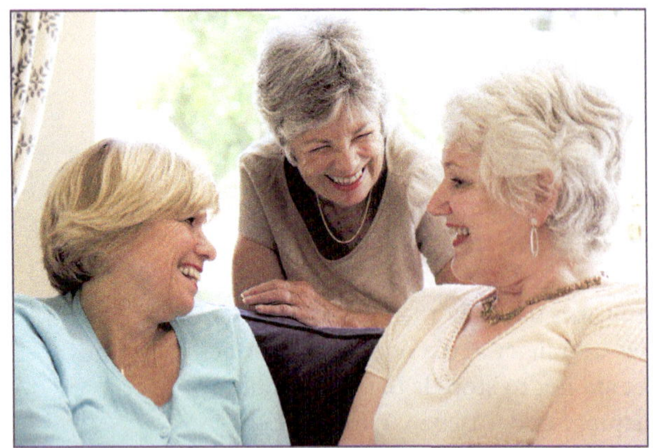

How do friends contribute to successful ageing?
(**Source:** 2100 (c) www.photostogo.com.au/all rights reserved.)

Learning to age successfully

Early in the chapter, we encouraged you to think of development as a type of change that always brings with it gains and losses. In this light, the trick to prospering across the life span is to solidify one's gains and minimise one's losses. Many of the changes that are stereotypically associated with ageing are functions of disuse rather than decay. Our first line of advice is straightforward: keep at it!

How can older adults cope successfully with whatever changes inevitably accompany increasing age? Successful ageing might consist of making the most of gains while minimising the impact of the normal losses that accompany ageing. This strategy for successful ageing, proposed by psychologists Paul Baltes and Margaret Baltes, is called **selective optimisation with compensation** (Baltes et al., 1992; Freund & Baltes, 1998). *Selective* means that people scale down the number and extent of their goals for themselves. *Optimisation* refers to people exercising or training themselves in areas that are of highest priority to them. *Compensation* means that people use alternative ways to deal with losses; for example, choosing age-friendly environments. Let's consider an example:

> *When the concert pianist [Arthur] Rubinstein was asked, in a television interview, how he managed to remain such a successful pianist in his old age, he mentioned three strategies: (1) In old age he performed fewer pieces, (2) he now practised each piece more frequently, and (3) he produced more ritardandos [slowings of the tempo] in his playing before fast segments, so that the playing speed sounded faster than it was in reality. These are examples of selection (fewer pieces), optimisation (more practice), and compensation (increased use of contrast in speed). (Baltes, 1993, p. 590)*

Although the selective optimisation perspective originated in research on the ageing process, it is a good way to characterise the choices you must make throughout your life span. You should always try to select the goals most important to you, optimise your performance with respect to those goals, and compensate when progress toward those goals is blocked. That's our final bit of advice about life span development. We hope you will age wisely and well.

[B]Gerrig, R. J., Zimbardo, P. G., Campbell, A. J., Cumming, S. R., & Wilkes, F. J. (2012). Intelligence and intelligence assessment. In *Psychology and life* (2nd ed., pp. 377–395). Frenchs Forest, NSW: Pearson Australia.

Summary

Studying development

- Researchers collect normative, longitudinal and cross-sectional data to document change.

Physical development across the life span

- Environmental factors can affect physical development while a child is still in the womb.
- Newborns and infants possess a remarkable range of capabilities: they are prewired for survival.
- Through puberty, adolescents achieve sexual maturity.
- Some physical changes in late adulthood are consequences of disuse, not inevitable deterioration.

Cognitive development across the life span

- Piaget's key ideas about cognitive development include development of schemes, assimilation, accommodation and the four-stage theory of discontinuous development. The four stages are sensorimotor, preoperational, concrete operational and formal operational.
- Many of Piaget's theories are now being altered by ingenious research paradigms that reveal infants and young children to be more competent than Piaget had thought.
- Researchers suggest that children develop foundational theories that change over time.
- Cross-cultural research has questioned the universality of cognitive developmental theories.
- Age-related declines in cognitive functioning are typically evident in only some abilities.

Social development across the life span

- Social development takes place in a particular cultural context.
- Erik Erikson conceptualised the life span as a series of crises with which individuals must cope.
- Children begin the process of social development with different temperaments.
- Socialisation begins with an infant's attachment to a caregiver.
- Failure to make this attachment leads to numerous physical and psychological problems.
- Adolescents must develop a personal identity by forming comfortable social relationships with parents and peers.
- The central concerns of adulthood are organised around the needs of intimacy and generativity.
- People become less socially active as they grow older because they selectively maintain only those relationships that matter most to them emotionally.
- People assess their lives, in part, by their ability to contribute positively to the lives of others.

Moral development

- Kohlberg defined stages of moral development.
- Subsequent research has evaluated gender and cultural differences in moral reasoning.

Learning to age successfully

- Selective optimisation with compensation is a strategy for improving health and wellbeing in older adults.
- The model proposed by Baltes & Baltes (1992, 1998) recommends that older adults select and optimise their best abilities and most intact functions, while compensating for declines and losses.[B]

Review questions

A. Fill in the missing words and/or key concepts to complete the following tables.

1. Stages of lifespan development

Stage	Age period
Prenatal	Conception to birth
	Birth at full term to about 18 months
Early childhood	
Adolescence	About 11 years to about 20 years
Early adulthood	
	About 40 years to about 65 years
Late adulthood	

2. Piaget's stages of cognitive development

Stages	Age	Characteristics and major accomplishments
Sensorimotor	0 – 2	
Preoperational	2 – 7	
Concrete Operational	7 – 11	
Formal Operations	11+	

3. Erikson's psychosocial stages

Approximate age	Crisis
0 – 1.5	Trust vs. mistrust
	Autonomy vs. self-doubt
3 – 6	
6 – puberty	
	Identity vs. role confusion
Early adult	Intimacy vs. isolation
Later adult	

B. Fill in the missing words to complete the following statements.

4. There are various research methods in developmental psychology. ____________ research involves studying the same group of individuals over an extended period of time. In contrast, ________________ research involves collecting data at a single point in time.
5. An important physical developmental process that occurs during adolescences is ________, which brings about sexual maturity.
6. In cognitive development, ________________ is considered to be the inability of a young child (at the preoperational stage) to take the perspectives of another person.
7. In Erik Erikson's theory of psychosocial stages, a commitment beyond one's self and one's partner to family, work, society and future generations is termed as ________________.
8. Four principles govern Kohlberg's stages of moral reasoning. These are:
   I.
   II.
   III.
   IV.

C. Read the following statements and answer with the most correct definition.

9. Any environmental factor (e.g., diseases, radiation and/or drugs) that causes structural abnormalities in a developing foetus is called a ________________.
10. When discussing physical development in the womb, the final stage which lasts from the end of the eighth week through to the birth of the child is called the __________ stage.
11. According to Piaget's stages of development, incorporating new information into your existing ideas is a process known as ____________________.
12. In regards to social and cultural influences on cognitive development, according to Vygotsky, the process through which children absorb knowledge from the social context is known as ________________________.

D. Please select one statement that best answers each of the following questions.

13. What is the correct order for the stages in Piaget's theory of cognitive development?
    a) sensorimotor, preoperational, concrete operational, formal operational
    b) sensorimotor, preoperational, formal operational, concrete operational
    c) preoperational, sensorimotor, formal operational, concrete operational
    d) preoperational, sensorimotor, concrete operational, formal operational
14. Which of the following is the first stage in Erikson's theory of development?
    a) initiative vs. guilt
    b) industry (competence) vs. inferiority
    c) trust vs. mistrust
    d) anatomy vs. self-doubt

15. The psychological conflict "industry (competence) vs. inferiority" takes place in which of Erickson's Psychosocial stages development?
a) adolescence
b) young adulthood
c) preschool
d) school age

16. According to Piaget's theory, if John is able to use skills of deductive reasoning and think about abstract concepts in his mathematics class, this indicates that he is in which stage of development?
a) postconceptional
b) formal operational
c) concrete operational
d) preoperational

17. If you have successfully resolved Erikson's conflict during the time you are 20-40 (early adulthood), what will the result be?
a) You feel a sense of wholeness vs. bitterness and regret for what could have been
b) You feel safe in your environment vs. insecure around the people in your life
c) You feel confident in your ability to create and initiate vs. feeling a low self-worth
d) You feel capable of developing closeness and commitment to another vs. feeling isolated and alone

18. Baby Ethan is drawn to looking at the blue ball on the floor. When his dad accidently covered the blue ball with a towel, baby Ethan began to cry because he thought the ball disappeared. He didn't know that all he had to do was lift the towel to find his blue ball again. According to this illustration, which specific aspect of cognitive development is baby Ethan still working on?
a) object permanence
b) conservation
c) centration
d) egocentrism

19. Children in the preoperational stage have difficulty taking the perspective of another person. This is known as
a) constructivism
b) reversibility
c) egocentrism
d) competence

20. During which of Erikson's stages do children begin to identify their strengths and take pleasure in their accomplishments?
a) autonomy vs. self-doubt
b) industry (competence) vs. inferiority
c) trust vs. mistrust
d) initiative vs. guilt

Chapter 3

Memory

The content in this section has been compiled from:
Gerrig et al., Chapter 8

Gerrig, R. J., Zimbardo, P. G., Campbell, A. J., Cumming, S. R., & Wilkes, F. J. (Eds.). (2012). Memory. In *Psychology and life* (2nd ed., pp. 239–278). Frenchs Forest, NSW: Pearson Australia.

CHAPTER 3

Memory

Memory can be defined as the retention of information over time. Memory processing is an important concept in health, and more specifically should be considered when consulting with clients and/or patients. Using the illustration of a patient being connected to various devices (i.e. experiencing unsettling noises, smells, lighting, and uncomfortable temperatures) demonstrates how both physical and mental stress, can influence memory retention – or working memory capacity. A patient overloaded with multiple stimuli is unlikely to be able to recall as accurately as when he/she is unencumbered by such stimuli overload. Consequently it is important to consider why people forget by recognising the effects of stress and anxiety on memory performance. While underpinned by the processes of memory, this chapter will further invoke consideration of techniques to expand individuals' ability to remember.

After studying this chapter you should be able to:

- Identify and describe types of memory
- Describe the process and capacity of the short term memory
- Describe the process and structures associated with long term memory, including encoding and retrieval
- Describe why people forget
- Identify techniques to improve memory
- Describe biological aspects of memory.

As you begin this chapter on memory processes, we'd like you to take a moment to retrieve your own earliest memory. How long ago did the memory originate? How vivid a scene do you recall? Has your memory been influenced by other people's recollections of the same event?

Now, a slightly different exercise. We'd like you to imagine what it would be like if you suddenly had no memory of your past—of the people you have known or of events that have happened to you. You wouldn't remember your mother's face, or your 10th birthday, or your Year 12 formal. Without such time anchors, how would you maintain a sense of who you are—of your identity? Or suppose you lost the ability to form any new memories. What would happen to your most recent experiences? Could you follow a conversation or untangle the plot of a television show? Everything would vanish, as if events had never existed, as if you had never had any thoughts in mind. Is there any activity you can think of that is not influenced by memory?

If you have never given much thought to your memory, it's probably because it tends to do its job reasonably well—you take it for granted, alongside other bodily processes, like digestion or breathing. But as with stomach aches or allergies, the times you notice your memory are likely to be the times when something goes wrong: you forget your car keys, an important date, lines in a play, or the answer to an examination question that you know you 'really knew'. These occasions are irritating, but keep in mind that the average human brain can store an estimated 100 trillion bits of information. The task of managing such a vast array of information is a formidable one. Perhaps you shouldn't be too surprised when an answer is sometimes not available when you need it!

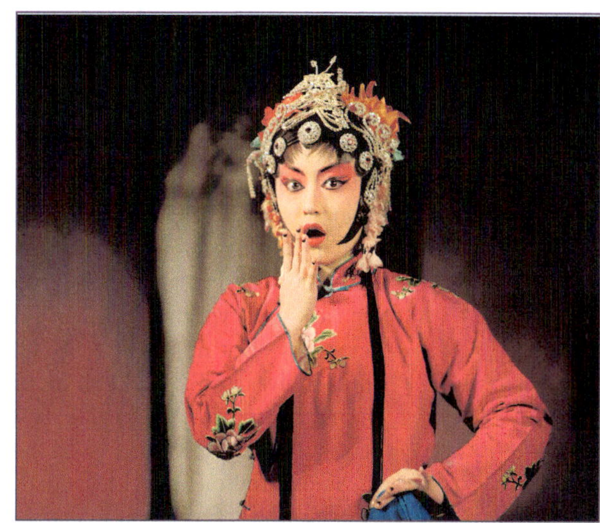

How are actors and actresses able to remember all the different aspects—movements, expressions and words—of their performances?

Our goal in this chapter is to explain how you usually remember so much and why you forget some of what you have known. We will explore how you get your everyday experiences into and out of memory. You will learn what psychology has discovered about different types of memories and about how those memories work. We hope that in the course of learning the many facts of memory, you will gain an appreciation for how wonderful memory is.

One last thing: because this is a chapter on memory, we're going to put your memory immediately to work. We'd like you to remember the number 46. Do whatever you need to do to remember 46. And yes, there will be a test!

What is memory?

To begin, we will define **memory** as the capacity to store and retrieve information. In this chapter, we will describe memory as a type of *information processing*. We will therefore focus on the flow of information in and out of your memory systems. Our examination of the processes that guide the acquisition and retrieval of information will enable you to refine your sense of what *memory* means.

Memory
The mental capacity to encode, store and retrieve information.

Types of memory

When you think about memory, what is most likely to come to mind at first are situations in which you use your memory to recall (or try to recall) specific events or information: your favourite movie, the dates of World War II, or your student ID number. In fact, one of the important functions of memory is to allow you to have conscious access to the personal and collective past. But memory does much more for you than that. It also enables you to have effortless continuity of experience from one day to the next. When you drive in a car, for example, it is this second function of memory that makes the landmarks along the roadside seem familiar. In defining types of memories, we will make plain to you how hard your memory works to fulfil these functions, often outside of conscious awareness.

Implicit and explicit memory

Imagine you are travelling on a bus. As soon as you sit down you realise that you know the person sitting next to you, but you have no idea *how* you know her. Is she the newsagent from around the corner? Your Introductory Psychology lecturer? The neighbour from three doors down who you rarely see? You know that the face is familiar, but no amount of searching through your memories of people helps you place her. Hours later, it pops into your head—she's the florist from the shopping centre, and you probably saw her yesterday when you were catching up with friends for a muffin and a coffee at the café near her shop.

Explicit use of memory
A conscious effort to encode or recover information through memory processes.

Implicit use of memory
The availability of information through memory processes without conscious effort to encode or recover information.

This simple example allows you to understand the difference between **explicit** and **implicit uses of memory**. Implicit memory is associated with a sense of familiarity: something about the face of the woman on the bus automatically triggers a sense that you know you have seen her before. But no amount of conscious thought can bring to mind who she is, or where you last saw her. Explicit memory refers to the conscious, deliberate retrieval of information from memory. In the example from the bus, you had a strong implicit memory of who she was, but you were unable to retrieve the explicit memory to go with that.

Thus, when it comes to using knowledge stored in memory, sometimes the use will be implicit (the information becomes available without any conscious effort) and sometimes it will be explicit (you make a conscious effort to recover the information).

We can make a similar distinction when it comes to the initial acquisition of memories. What shape is a 'give way' sign? If you think about it, you probably know that they are triangular. Did you ever memorise a list of road sign shapes? Probably not. Rather, it's likely that you acquired this knowledge incidentally, without conscious effort. By contrast, you probably learned the rules of the road intentionally; that is, at some point you practised the rules, or wrote them down, or otherwise used some conscious effort to learn them. To learn the association between words and experiences, your younger self needed to engage in explicit memory processes. You learned the word *refrigerator* because someone called your attention to the name of that object.

The distinction between implicit and explicit memory greatly expands the range of questions researchers must address about memory processes (Bowers & Marsolek, 2003; Buchner & Wippich, 2000). Most early memory research concerned explicit memory for intentionally acquired information. Experimenters most frequently provided participants with new information to retain, and theories of memory were directed to explaining what participants could and could not remember under those circumstances. However, as you will see in this chapter, researchers have now devised methods for studying implicit memory as well. Thus we can give you a more complete account of the variety of uses to which you put your memory. We can acknowledge that most circumstances in which you encode or retrieve information represent a mix of implicit and explicit uses of memory. Let's turn now to a second dimension along which memories are distributed.

Declarative and procedural memory

Can you whistle, or ride a bicycle, or use chopsticks? What kind of memory allows you to do these sorts of things? You probably remember having to learn these skills, but now they seem effortless. The examples we gave before of both implicit and explicit memories all involved the recollection of *facts* and *events*, which is called **declarative memory**. Now we see that you also have memories for *how to do things*, which is called **procedural memory**. Because the bulk of this chapter will be focused on how you acquire and use facts, let's take a moment now to consider how you acquire the ability to do things.

Declarative memory Memory for information such as facts and events.

Procedural memory Memory for how things get done; the way perceptual, cognitive and motor skills are acquired, retained and used.

PROCEDURAL MEMORY. refers to the way you remember how things get done. It is used to acquire, retain and employ perceptual, cognitive and motor skills. Theories of procedural memory most often concern themselves with the time course of learning (Anderson, 1996; Anderson et al., 1999). How do you go from a conscious list of declarative facts about some activity to an unconscious, automatic performance of that same activity? And why is it that after learning a skill, you often find it difficult to go back and talk about the component declarative facts?

We can see these phenomena at work in even the very simple activity of dialling a telephone number that, over time, has become highly familiar. At first, you probably had to think your way through each digit, one at a time. You had to work through a list of declarative facts:

First, I must dial 2,
next, I must dial 0,
then I dial 7,
and so on.

However, when you began to dial the number often enough, you could start to produce it as one unit—a swift sequence of actions on the touch-tone pad. The process at work is called *knowledge compilation* (Anderson, 1987). As a consequence of practice, you are able to carry out longer sequences of the activity without conscious intervention. But you also don't have conscious access to the content of these compiled units. Back at the telephone, it's not uncommon to find someone who can't actually remember the telephone number without pretending to dial it. In general, knowledge compilation makes it hard to share your procedural knowledge with others. You may have noticed this if your parents tried to teach you to drive. Although they may be good drivers themselves, they may not have been very good at communicating the content of compiled good-driving procedures.

You may also have noticed that knowledge compilation can lead to errors. If you are a skilled typist, you've probably suffered from the *the* problem: as soon as you hit the *t* and the *h* keys, your finger may fly to the *e*, even if you're really trying to type *throne* or *thistle.* Once you have sufficiently committed the execution of *the* to procedural memory, you can do little else but finish the sequence. Without procedural memory, life would be extremely laborious—you would be doomed to go step by step through every activity. However, each time you mistakenly type *the*, you can reflect on the trade-off between efficiency and potential error. Let's continue now to an overview of the basic processes that apply to all these different types of memory.

An overview of the memory processes

For any memory system to work, it must do at least three things: information has to get into it; it has to be kept somewhere; and it has to be able to be extracted from it. **Encoding** is the initial processing of information that leads to a representation in memory. **Storage** is the retention over time of encoded material. **Retrieval** is the recovery at a later time of the stored

Encoding The process by which a mental representation is formed in memory.

Storage The retention of encoded material over time.

Retrieval The recovery of stored information from memory.

information. Simply put, encoding gets information in, storage holds it until you need it, and retrieval gets it out. Let's now expand on these ideas.

Encoding requires that you form *mental representations* of information from the external world. You can understand the idea of mental representations if we draw an analogy to representations outside your head. Imagine we wanted to know something about the best gift you got at your last birthday party. (Let's suppose it's not something you have with you.) What could you do to inform us about the gift? You might describe the properties of the object. Or you might draw us a picture. Or you might pretend that you're using the object. These are all different representations of the original object. Although none of the representations is likely to be quite as good as having the real thing present, they should allow us to acquire knowledge of the most important aspects of the gift. Mental representations work much the same way. They preserve important features of past experiences in a way that enables you to *re-present* those experiences to yourself. There are no absolute rules about how 'best' to encode information. You may have friends who can only remember things if they've drawn a diagram of them, or who need to write things out in dot points, or who can only play their piano pieces if they are sitting at their own piano. All these are examples of the individuality of encoding.

Similarly, cultural and historical factors also serve to define the 'best' encoding strategy. Australians of English and European backgrounds tend to encode things verbally—their sense of 'self' is a narrative. For many Indigenous Australian groups, identity is defined by place. In a study of Aboriginal and non-Aboriginal children of different age groups, Kearins (1976, 1981) determined that the Aboriginal children had superior visual recall. As they encode information using predominantly visual strategies, they tend to show superior skill in spatial and visual recall, and are more likely to process information simultaneously rather than successively (Klich & Davidson, 1983). It has been suggested that the differences in visual memory in Aboriginal people are a result of living conditions in the bush and desert regions of Australia (Klekamp et al., 1989). Later in the chapter we will explore the relationship between how you encode information and how it is eventually retrieved.

If information is properly encoded, it will be retained in *storage* over some period of time. Storage requires both short- and long-term changes in the structures of your brain. At the end of the chapter, we will see how researchers are attempting to locate the brain regions responsible for these complex processes.

Retrieval is the payoff for all your earlier effort. When it works, it enables you to gain access—often in a split second—to information you stored earlier. Can you remember what comes before storage: decoding or encoding? The answer is simple to retrieve now, but will you still be able to retrieve the concept of encoding as swiftly and with as much confidence when you are tested on this chapter's contents days or weeks from now? Discovering how you are able to retrieve one specific bit of information from the vast quantity of information in your memory storehouse is a challenge facing psychologists who want to know how memory works and how it can be improved.

Although it is easy to define encoding, storage and retrieval as separate memory processes, the interaction among the three processes is quite complex. For example, to be able to encode the information that you have seen a tiger, you must first retrieve from memory information about the concept *tiger*. Similarly, to commit to memory the meaning of a sentence such as 'He's got the heart of Phar Lap', you must retrieve the meanings of each individual word, retrieve the rules of grammar that specify how word meanings should be combined in English, and retrieve cultural information that specifies exactly how brave and strong Phar Lap was.

We are now ready to look in more detail at the encoding, storage and retrieval of information. Our discussion will start with short-lived types of memories, beginning with sensory memory, and then we will move to the more permanent forms of long-term

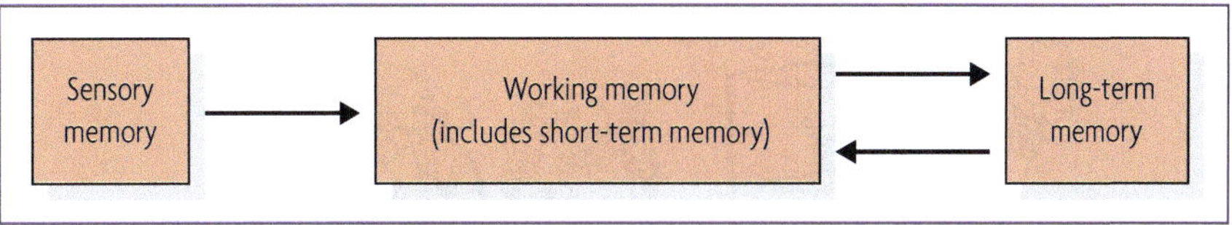

Figure 3.1 The flow of information in and out of long-term memory

Memory theories describe the flow of information to and from long-term memory. The theories address initial encodings of information in sensory and working memory, the transfer of information into long-term memory for storage and the transfer of information from long-term memory to working memory for retrieval.

memory (see Figure 3.1). We will give you an account of how you remember and why you forget. Our plan is to make you forever self-conscious about all the ways in which you use your capacity for memory. We hope this will even allow you to improve some aspects of your memory skills.

Stop and review

1. What is the difference between explicit and implicit uses of memory?
2. Suppose you are a skilled juggler. Does your skill rely more on declarative or procedural memory?
3. You suddenly can't remember the password for your email account. Which memory process is most likely to be causing the difficulty?

Memory use for the short term

Let's begin with a demonstration of the impermanence of some memories. In Figure 3.2 we have provided you with a reasonably busy visual scene. We'd like you to take a quick look at it—about 10 seconds—and then cover it up. Suppose we now ask you a series of questions about the scene:

1. What tool is the little boy at the bottom holding?
2. What is the middle man at the top doing?
3. In the lower right-hand corner, does the woman's umbrella handle hook to the left or to the right?

To answer these questions, wouldn't you be more comfortable if you could go back and have an extra peek at the picture?

This quick demonstration reminds you that much of the information you experience never lodges itself securely in your memory. Instead, you possess and use the information only for the short term. In this section, we examine properties of three less permanent uses of memory: *iconic memory*, *short-term memory* and *working memory*.

Iconic memory

When you first covered up Figure 3.2, did you have the impression that you could briefly still 'see' the whole picture? This extra peek at the picture is provided by your **iconic memory**—a memory system in the visual domain that allows large amounts of information to be stored for very brief durations (Neisser, 1967). Iconic memory is an example of a *sensory memory*. Researchers have speculated that each sensory system has a memory store that preserves representations of physical features of environmental stimuli for, at most, a few seconds (Radvansky, 2006). For example, people retain brief sensory representations of stimuli that

Iconic memory
Memory system in the visual domain that allows large amounts of information to be stored for very brief durations.

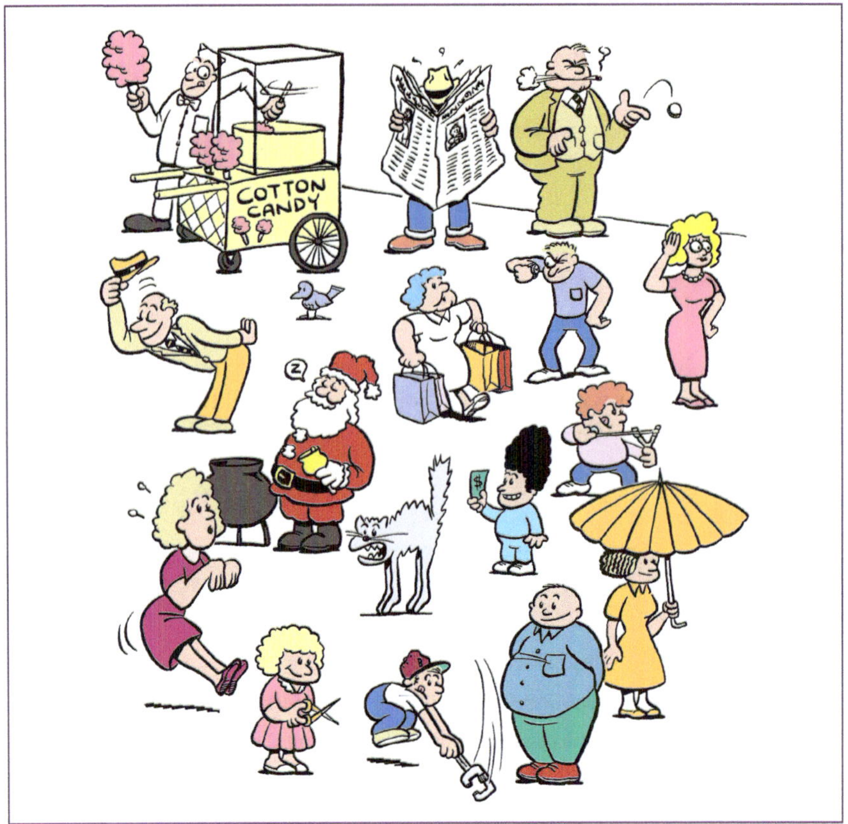

Figure 3.2 How much can you remember from this scene?

After viewing this scene for about 10 seconds, cover it up and try to answer the questions in the text. Under ordinary circumstances, iconic memory preserves a glimpse of the visual world for a brief time after the scene has been removed.

have touched their bodies (Gallace et al., 2008). We focus on iconic memory because it has received the most research attention.

A visual memory, or icon, lasts about half a second. Iconic memory was first revealed in experiments that required participants to retrieve information from visual displays that were exposed for only one-twentieth of a second.

George Sperling (1960, 1963) presented participants with arrays of three rows of letters and numbers.

7	1	V	F
X	L	5	3
B	4	W	7

Participants were asked to perform two different tasks. In a *whole-report procedure*, they tried to recall as many of the items in the display as possible. Typically, they could report only about 4 of 12, or one-third of the available items. Other participants underwent a *partial-report procedure*, which required them to report only one row rather than the whole pattern. The trick was that they didn't know *which* row they had to report until after the display was presented. A signal of a high, medium or low tone was sounded immediately after the presentation to indicate which row the participants were to report. Sperling found that regardless of which row he asked for, the participants' recall was well above the roughly 33 percent accuracy of the whole report condition.

Because participants could accurately report any of the three rows in response to a tone, Sperling concluded that all of the information in the display must have been stored, albeit briefly, in iconic memory. The difference between whole- and partial-report is that the image is fading so quickly that there isn't time to 'read out' all 12 items in whole report, but the fact that people can remember any three suggests that they are all available for a short period of time. That is evidence for the large capacity of iconic memory. At the same time, the difference between the whole- and partial-report procedures suggests that the information fades rapidly: the participants in the whole-report procedure were unable to recall all the information present in the icon. This second point was reinforced by experiments in which the identification signal was slightly delayed. Figure 3.3 shows that as the delay interval increases from 0 seconds to 1 second, the number of items accurately reported declines steadily. Researchers have measured quite accurately the time course with which information must be transferred from the fading icon (Becker et al., 2000; Tijus & Reeves, 2004). To take advantage of the 'extra peek' at the visual world, your memory processes must very quickly transfer information to more durable stores.

Note that iconic memory is not the same as the 'photographic memory' that some people claim to have. The technical term for 'photographic memory' is *eidetic imagery*: people who experience eidetic imagery are able to recall the details of a picture, for periods of time considerably longer than iconic memory, as if they were still looking at a photograph. 'People' in this case really means children: researchers have estimated that roughly 8 percent of pre-adolescent children are eidetickers, but virtually no adults (Neath & Surprenant, 2003). No satisfactory theory has been proposed for why eidetic imagery fades over time (Crowder, 1992). However, if you are reading this book as a high school or university student, you almost certainly have iconic memory but not eidetic images.

Short-term memory

Before you began to read this chapter, you may not have been aware that you had iconic memory. It is very likely, however, that you were aware that there are some memories

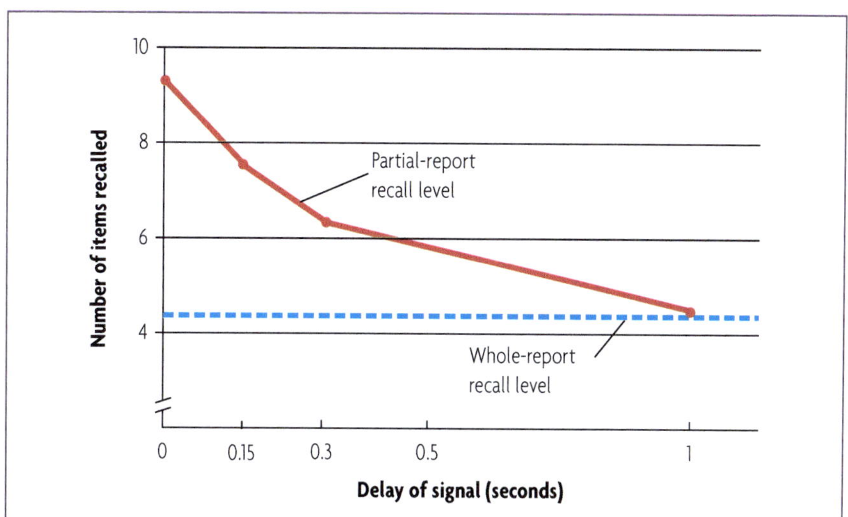

Figure 3.3 Recall by the partial-report method

The solid line shows the average number of items recalled using the partial-report method, both immediately after presentation and at four later times. For comparison, the dotted line shows the number of items recalled by the whole-report method.

Adapted from Sperling, G. (1960). The information available in brief visual presentations. *Psychological Monographs*, 74, 1–29. Copyright © 1960 by the American Psychological Association. Adapted with permission.

that you possess only for the short term. Consider the common occurrence of consulting a telephone book to find the number of a plumber or a shop and then remembering the number just long enough to dial it. If the number is engaged, you often have to go back to the telephone book and look it up again. When you consider this experience, it's easy to understand why researchers have hypothesised a special type of memory called **short-term memory (STM)**.

Short-term memory (STM) A memory process associated with preservation of recent experiences and with retrieval of information from long-term memory.

You shouldn't think of short-term memory as a particular place that memories go to, but rather as a built-in mechanism for focusing cognitive resources on some small set of mental representations (Shiffrin, 2003). But the resources of STM are fickle. As even your experience with telephone numbers shows, you have to take some special care to ensure that memories become encoded into more permanent forms.

The capacity limitations of STM

We know that your attentional resources are devoted to selecting the objects and events in the external world on which you will expend your mental resources. Just as there are limits on your capacity to attend to more than a small sample of the available information, there are limits on your ability to keep more than a small sample of information active in STM. The limited capacity of STM enforces a sharp focus of mental attention.

To estimate the capacity of STM, researchers at first turned to tests of *memory span*. At some point in your life, you have probably been asked to carry out a task like this one:

Read the following list of random numbers once, cover them, and write down as many as you can in the order they appear.

8 1 7 3 4 9 4 2 8 5

How many did you get correct?

Now read the next list of random letters and perform the same memory test.

J M R S O F L P T Z B

How many did you get correct?

If you are like most individuals, you probably could recall somewhere in the range of five to nine items. George Miller (1956) suggested that seven (plus or minus two) was the 'magic number' that characterised people's memory performance on random lists of letters, words, numbers, or almost any kind of meaningful, familiar item.

Tests of memory span, however, overestimate the true capacity of STM because participants are able to use other sources of information to carry out the task. When other sources of memory are factored out, researchers have estimated the pure contribution of STM to your seven (or so) item memory span to be only between three and five items (Cowan, 2001). But if that's all the capacity you have to commence the acquisition of new memories, why don't you notice your limitations more often? Despite the capacity limitations of STM, you function efficiently for at least two reasons. As we will see in the next two sections, the encoding of information in STM can be enhanced through rehearsal and chunking.

Rehearsal

You probably know that a good way to keep the plumber's telephone number in mind is to keep repeating the digits in a cycle in your head. This memorisation technique is called *maintenance rehearsal.* The fate of unrehearsed information was demonstrated in an ingenious experiment.

Participants heard three consonants, such as F, C and V. They had to recall those consonants when given a signal after a variable interval of time, ranging from 3 to 18 seconds.

To prevent rehearsal, a *distractor task* was put between the stimulus input and the recall signal—the participants were given a three-digit number and told to count backward from it by 3s until the recall signal was presented. Many different consonant sets were given, and several short delays were used over a series of trials with a number of participants.

As shown in Figure 3.4, recall became increasingly poorer as the time required to retain the information became longer. After even 3 seconds, there was considerable memory loss, and by 18 seconds, loss was nearly total. In the absence of an opportunity to rehearse the information, short-term recall was impaired with the passage of time (Peterson & Peterson, 1959).

Chunking
The process of taking single items of information and recoding them on the basis of similarity or another organising principle.

Performance suffered because information could not be rehearsed. It also suffered because of interference from the competing information of the distractor task. (We will discuss interference as a cause of forgetting later in this chapter.) You may have noticed that often a new acquaintance says his or her name—and then you immediately forget it. One of the most common reasons for this is that you are distracted from performing the type of rehearsal you need to carry out to acquire a new memory. As a remedy, try to encode and rehearse a new name carefully before you continue with a conversation.

Our conclusion so far is that rehearsal will help you to keep information from fading out of STM. But suppose the information you wish to acquire is, at least at first, too cumbersome to be rehearsed? You might turn to the strategy of chunking.

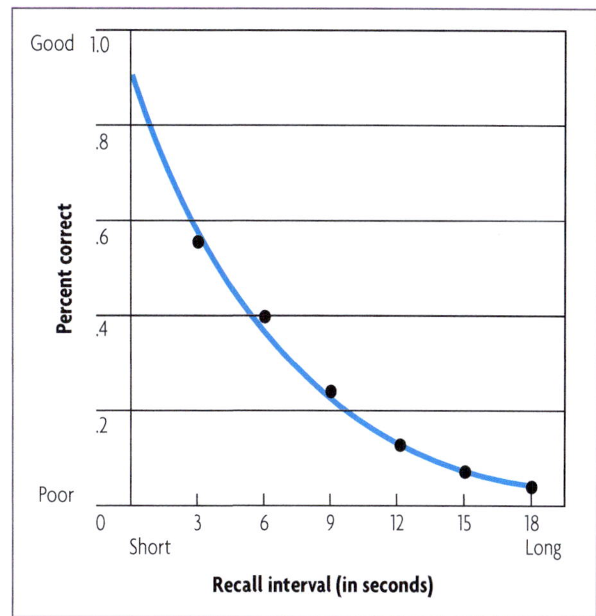

Figure 3.4 Short-term memory recall without rehearsal

When the interval between stimulus presentation and recall was filled with a distracting task, recall became poorer as the interval grew longer.

Chunking

A *chunk* is a meaningful unit of information (Anderson, 1996). A chunk can be a single letter or number, a group of letters or other items, or even a group of words or an entire sentence. For example, the letter sequence B-D-O-P-G consists of five letters that could exhaust your STM capacity. However, another five-letter sequence, A-N-Z-A-C is probably easier to remember, as it is the acronym for the Australian and New Zealand Army Corps, which is associated with the ANZAC Day public holiday and other events. While both are five-letter sequences, ANZAC constitutes only one chunk, leaving you much more capacity for other chunks of information. **Chunking** is the process of reconfiguring items by grouping them on the basis of similarity or some other organising principle, or by combining them into larger patterns based on information stored in long-term memory (Baddeley, 1994).

See how many chunks you find in this sequence of 12 letters: FBIABCUNICEF. You can answer '12' if you see the sequence as a list of unrelated letters,

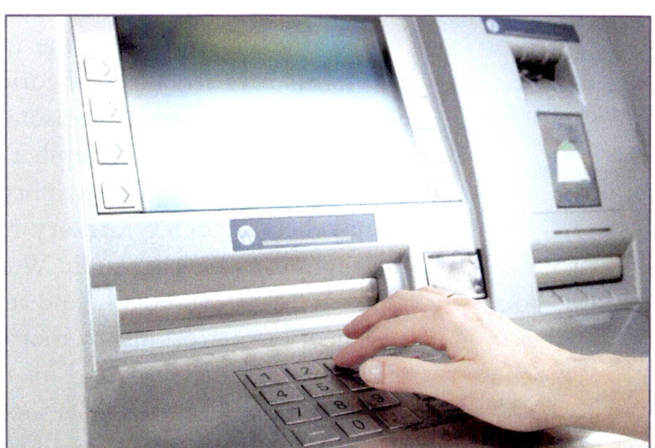

What role does short-term memory play when you punch in your ATM password?
(**Source:** © Roman Milert/Fotolia 2004–2010, all rights reserved)

or '3' if you break down the sequence into the well-known acronyms—FBI, ABC and UNICEF. If you do the latter, it's easy for you to recall all the letters in proper sequence after one quick glance. It would be impossible for you to remember them all from a short exposure if you saw them as 12 unrelated items.

Your memory span can always be greatly increased if you can discover ways to organise an available body of information into smaller chunks. A famous subject, S.F., was able to memorise 84 digits by grouping them as racing times (S.F. was an avid runner):

S.F.'s memory protocols provided the key to his mental wizardry. Because he was a long-distance runner, S.F. noticed that many of the random numbers could be grouped into running times for different distances. For instance, he would recode the sequence 3, 4, 9, 2, 5, 6, 1, 4, 9, 3, 5 as 3:49.2, near record mile; 56:14, 10-mile time; 9:35, slow 2 miles. Later, S.F. also used ages, years of memorable events, and special numerical patterns to chunk the random digits. In this way, he was able to use his long-term memory to convert long strings of random input into manageable and meaningful chunks. S.F.'s memory for letters was still about average, however, because he had not developed any chunking strategies to recall alphabet strings (Chase & Ericsson, 1981; Ericsson & Chase, 1982).

Like S.F., you can structure incoming information according to its personal meaning to you (linking it to the ages of friends and relatives, for example); or you can match new stimuli with various codes that have been stored in your long-term memory. Even if you can't link new stimuli to rules, meanings or codes in your long-term memory, you can still use chunking. You can simply group the items in a rhythmical pattern or temporal group (181379256460 could become 181, pause, 379, pause, 256, pause, 460). You know from everyday experience that this grouping principle works well for remembering telephone numbers.

Working memory

Our focus so far has been on short-term memory, and specifically the role that STM plays in the explicit acquisition of new memories. However, you need more memory resources on a moment-by-moment basis than those that allow you to acquire facts. For example, you also need to be able to retrieve pre-existing memories. At the start of this chapter, we asked you to commit a number to memory. Can you remember now what it was? If you can remember (if not, peek), you have made your mental representation of that memory active once more—that's another memory function. If we ask you to do something more complicated—suppose we ask you to toss a ball from hand to hand while you count backward by 3s from 132—you'll put even more demands on your memory resources.

Working memory A memory resource that is used to accomplish tasks such as reasoning and language comprehension.

Based on an analysis of the memory functions you require to navigate through life, researchers have articulated theories of **working memory**—the memory resource that you use to accomplish tasks such as reasoning and language comprehension. Suppose you are trying to remember a telephone number while you search for a pencil and pad to write it down. Whereas your short-term memory processes allow you to keep the number in mind, your more general working memory resource allows you to execute the mental operations to accomplish an efficient search. Working memory provides a foundation for the moment-by-moment fluidity of thought and action.

Theories of working memory often have as one component the 'classic' short-term memory. Alan Baddeley and his colleagues (Baddeley, 1986, 1992; Baddeley & Andrade, 2000) have provided evidence for three components of working memory:

- A *phonological loop*. This resource holds and manipulates speech-based information. The phonological loop overlaps most with short-term memory, as we have described it in the earlier sections. When you rehearse a telephone number by 'listening' to it as you run it through your head, you are making use of the phonological loop.

- A *visuospatial sketchpad*. This resource performs the same types of functions as the phonological loop for visual and spatial information. If, for example, someone asked you how many desks there are in your psychology classroom, you might use the resources of the visuospatial sketchpad to form a mental picture of the classroom and then estimate the number of desks from that picture.
- The *central executive*. This resource is responsible for controlling attention and coordinating information from the phonological loop and the visuospatial sketchpad. Any time you carry out a task that requires a combination of mental processes—imagine, for example, you are asked to describe a picture from memory—you rely on the central executive function to apportion your mental resources to different aspects of the task.

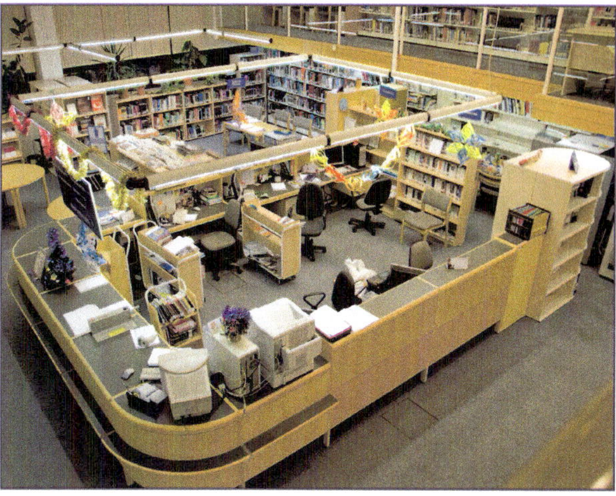
For a storage system to work efficiently, information has to be encoded, stored and retrieved. There also needs to be an 'executive' system that supervises and integrates all the other processes.
(**Source:** © Toxawww | Dreamstime.com)

The incorporation of short-term memory into the broader context of working memory should help reinforce the idea that STM is not a place but a process. To do the work of cognition—to carry out cognitive activities like language processing or problem solving—you must bring a lot of different elements together in quick succession. You can think of working memory as short-term special focus on the necessary elements. If you wish to get a better look at a physical object, you can shine a brighter light on it; working memory shines a brighter mental light on your mental objects—your memory representations. Working memory also coordinates the activities required to take action with respect to those objects.

Researchers have demonstrated that working memory capacity differs among individuals. They have devised several procedures to measure those differences (Conway et al., 2005). We will give you an example of one of those measures, which is called *working memory span*. Unlike standard short-term memory tasks, your working memory span is measured by asking you to remember something while doing something else with your cognitive processes. For example, researchers may ask participants to read aloud a series of sentences and then recall the final words. We've given you some sentences to try in Table 3.1. It's really not so easy! People are usually considered to be *high span* if they can recall 4 or more words and *low span* if they recall 2.5 or fewer—notice this is much smaller than the usual estimate of short-term memory capacity, as the task is much harder. These are averages across several trials and sets of sentences, so you shouldn't take too seriously your results from one attempt at Table 3.1.

Because working memory span is a measure of the resources individuals have available to carry out short-term cognitive processes, researchers can use it to predict performance

Table 3.1 A test for working memory span

Read these sentences aloud and then (without looking back) try to recall the final words of each sentence.
He had patronised her when she was a schoolgirl and teased her when she was a student.
He had an elongated skull which sat on his shoulders like a pear on a dish.
The products of digital electronics will play an important role in your future.
The taxi turned up Michigan Avenue where they had a clear view of the lake.
When at last his eyes opened, there was no gleam of triumph, no shade of anger.

From Daneman & Carpenter (1980).

on a variety of tasks. For example, working memory allows individuals to keep their attention focused on the tasks they need to accomplish. In general, the greater the working memory capacity, the more information individuals should be able to keep their minds from wandering.

To demonstrate the relationship between working memory capacity and mind wandering, a team of researchers recruited 124 university undergraduates for a study using experience sampling (Kane et al., 2007). At the start of the experiment, all participants completed measures of working memory capacity similar to the operations span task. In the experiment's next phase, participants carried handheld computers for a week. The computers signalled them eight times each day, between noon and midnight, to fill out a questionnaire. The questionnaires gathered information about the tasks on which the participants had been engaged when the beeps sounded. Participants indicated, for example, how challenging they had found the task at hand. The questionnaires also asked participants to report the extent to which their minds had wandered from each task. For nonchallenging tasks, participants' working memory capacity had no impact on the amount of mind wandering. However, when participants were engaged with challenging tasks, people with higher working memory capacity reported much less mind wandering than people with lower working memory capacity.

Recall that one component of working memory is the central executive. This experiment suggests that people with higher working memory capacity are better able to use that central executive resource: they can keep their attention tightly focused on the challenging tasks for which they need it most.

A final note on working memory: working memory helps maintain your psychological present. It is what sets a context for new events and links separate episodes together into a continuing story. It enables you to maintain and continually update your representation of a changing situation and to keep track of topics during a conversation. All of this is true because working memory serves as a conduit for information coming and going to long-term memory. Let's turn our attention now to the types of memories that can last a lifetime.

Long-term memory: encoding and retrieval

How long can memories last? At the chapter's outset, we asked you to recall your own earliest memory. How old is that memory? Fifteen years? Twenty years? Longer? When

Stop and review

1. Why do researchers believe that the capacity of iconic memory is large?
2. What is the contemporary estimate of the capacity of short-term memory?
3. What does it mean to *chunk* some group of items?
4. What are the components of working memory?

Critical thinking

Recall the study that demonstrated the importance of rehearsal to maintain information in short-term memory. In that study, why were participants asked to count backward by 3s (e.g., 167, 164, 161 . . .) rather than by 1s (167, 166, 165 . . .)?

psychologists speak of *long-term memory*, it is with the knowledge that memories often last a lifetime. Therefore, whatever theory explains how memories are acquired for the long term must also explain how they can remain accessible over the life course. **Long-term memory (LTM)** is the storehouse of all the experiences, events, information, emotions, skills, words, categories, rules and judgements that have been acquired from sensory and short-term memories. LTM constitutes each person's total knowledge of the world and of the self.

You may have noticed that it is easier to understand a class if the teacher tells you in advance what the main objectives are for the session. This is because you have a framework for understanding the incoming information. In this section of the book, our objective is to explain that your ability to remember will be greatest when there is a good match between the circumstances in which you encoded information and the circumstances in which you attempt to retrieve it. We will see over the next several sections what it means to have a 'good match'.

Retrieval cues

To begin our exploration between encoding and retrieval, let's consider this general question: How do you 'find' a memory? The basic answer is that you use retrieval cues. **Retrieval cues** are the stimuli available as you search for a particular memory. These cues may be provided externally, such as questions on a quiz ('What memory principles do you associate with the research of Sternberg and Sperling?'), or generated internally ('Where have I met her before?'). Each time you attempt to retrieve an explicit memory, you do so for some purpose, and that purpose often supplies the retrieval cue. It won't surprise you that memories can be easier or harder to retrieve depending on the quality of the retrieval cue. If a friend asks you, 'Who's the one Roman emperor I can't remember?', you're likely to be involved in a guessing game. If she asks instead, 'Who was the emperor after Claudius?', you can immediately respond 'Nero'.

To give you a full sense of the importance of retrieval cues, we will attempt to replicate classic memory experiments by asking you to learn some word pairs. Keep working at it until you can go through the six pairs three times in a row without an error.

Apple–Boat

Hat–Bone

Bicycle–Clock

Mouse–Tree

Ball–House

Ear–Blanket

Now that you've committed the pairs to memory, we want to make the test more interesting. We need to do something to give you a *retention interval*—a period of time over which you must keep the information in memory. Let's spend a moment, therefore, discussing some of the procedures we might use to test your memory. You might assume that you either know something or you don't and that any method of testing what you know will give the same results. Not so. Let's consider two tests for explicit memory, recall and recognition.

Recall and recognition

When you **recall**, you reproduce the information to which you were previously exposed. 'What are the components of working memory?' is a recall question. **Recognition** refers to

Long-term memory (LTM)
Memory processes associated with the preservation of information for retrieval at any later time.

Retrieval cue
An internal or external generated stimuli available to help with the retrieval of a memory.

Recall
A method of retrieval in which an individual is required to reproduce the information previously presented.

Recognition
A method of retrieval in which an individual is required to identify stimuli as having been experienced before.

the realisation that a certain stimulus event is one you have seen or heard before. 'Which is the term for a visual sensory memory: (1) echo; (2) engram; (3) icon; or (4) abstract code?' is a recognition question, as the correct answer is available to you, you only have to choose it. You can relate recall and recognition to your day-to-day experiences of explicit memory. When trying to identify a criminal, the police would be using a recall method if they asked the victim to describe, from memory, some of the perpetrator's distinguishing features: 'Did you notice anything unusual about the attacker?' They would be using the recognition method if they showed the victim photos, one at a time, from a file of criminal suspects or if they asked the victim to identify the perpetrator in a police line-up.

Let's now use these two procedures to test you on the word pairs you learned a few moments ago. What words finished the pairs?

Hat–? Bicycle–? Ear–?

Can you select the correct pair from these possibilities?

Apple–Baby	Mouse–Tree	Ball–House
Apple–Boat	Mouse–Tongue	Ball–Hill
Apple–Bottle	Mouse–Tent	Ball–Horn

Was the recognition test easier than the recall test? It should be. Let's try to explain this result with respect to retrieval cues.

Both recall and recognition require a search using cues. The cues for recognition, however, are much more useful. For recall, you have to hope that the cue alone will help you locate the information. For recognition, part of the work has been done for you. When you look at the pair *Mouse–Tree*, you only have to answer 'yes' or 'no' to 'Did I have this experience?' rather than, in response to *Mouse*—?, 'What was the experience I had?' In this light, you can see that we made the recognition test reasonably easy for you. Suppose we had given you, instead, recombinations of the original pairs. Which of these are correct?

Hat–Clock	Ear–Boat
Hat–Bone	Ear–Blanket

Now you must recognise not just that you saw the word before, but that you saw it in a particular context. (We will return to the idea of context shortly.) If you are a veteran of difficult multiple-choice exams, you have come to learn how tough even recognition situations can be. However, in most cases, your recognition performance will be better than your recall because retrieval cues are more straightforward for recognition. Let's look at some other aspects of retrieval cues.

Episodic and semantic memories

We have already made a pair of distinctions about types of memories. You have implicit and explicit memories and declarative and procedural memories. We can define another dimension along which declarative memories differ with respect to the cues that are necessary to retrieve them from memory. Canadian psychologist Endel Tulving (1972) first proposed the distinction between *episodic* and *semantic* types of declarative memories (see Figure 3.5).

Episodic memory
A long-term memory for autobiographical events and the contexts in which they occurred.

Episodic memories preserve, individually, the specific events or episodes that you have experienced. For example, memories of your happiest birthday or of your first kiss are stored in episodic memory. To recover such memories, you need retrieval cues that specify something about the time at which the event occurred and something about the content of the events. If you were asked what you had for breakfast yesterday, you would probably retrieve the answer by thinking about what you were doing: whether you ate at the table or on the train, whether

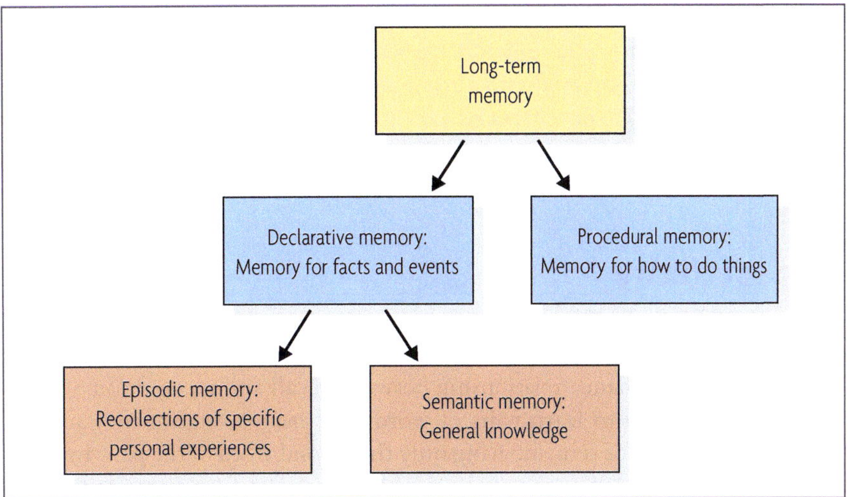

Figure 3.5 Dimensions of long-term memory

Researchers have suggested that people store different types of memories.

you had to be at uni early or not, and any number of other things that are not about breakfast itself, but about the events and experiences surrounding yesterday's breakfast. Depending on how the information has been encoded, you may or may not be able to produce a specific memory representation for an event. For example, do you have any specific memories to differentiate the tenth time ago you brushed your teeth from the eleventh time ago?

Semantic memory A generic, categorical memory, such as the meanings of words and concepts.

Everything you know, you began to acquire in some particular context. However, there are large classes of information that, over time, you encounter in many different contexts. These classes of information come to be available for retrieval without reference to their multiple times and places of experience. These **semantic memories** are generic, categorical memories, such as the meanings of words and concepts. For most people, facts like the formula $E = MC^2$ and the capital of France don't require retrieval cues that make reference to the episodes, the original learning contexts, in which the memory was acquired.

Events of personal importance, like seeing a relative or good friend for the first time after a year's separation, are retained in episodic memory. What types of information from semantic memory might contribute to a reunion?
(**Source:** © Galina Barskaya/Fotolia 2004–2010, all rights reserved

Of course, this doesn't mean that your recall of semantic memories is foolproof. You know perfectly well that you can forget many facts that have become dissociated from the contexts in which you learned them. A good strategy when you can't recover a semantic memory is to treat it like an episodic memory again. You will have been in examinations when an item of semantic knowledge has been hard to retrieve, and you might have gone back to episodic cues to attempt to retrieve it, thinking things like 'I studied it last week—after band practice and before Rob came over. It's in my yellow study notebook, near the bottom of the page...'

Context and encoding

To continue our exploration of encoding and retrieval, we want you to consider a phenomenon that you might call 'context shock'. You see someone across a crowded room,

Encoding specificity The principle that subsequent retrieval of information is enhanced if cues received at the time of recall are consistent with those present at the time of encoding.

and you know that you know the person but you just can't place her. Finally, after staring for longer than is entirely polite, you remember who it is—and you realise that the difficulty is that the person is in the wrong context. What is the woman who delivers your mail doing at your best friend's party? Whenever you have this type of experience, you have rediscovered the principle of **encoding specificity**: memories emerge most efficiently when the context of retrieval matches the context of encoding. Let's see how researchers have demonstrated that principle.

Encoding specificity

What are the consequences of learning information in a particular context? Endel Tulving and Donald Thomson (1973) first demonstrated the power of encoding specificity by reversing the usual performance relationship between recall and recognition.

Participants were asked to learn pairs of words like *train–black*, but they were told that they would be responsible for remembering only the second word of the pair. In a subsequent phase of the experiment, participants were asked to generate four free associates to words like *white*. Those words were chosen so that it was likely that the original to-be-remembered words (like *black*) would be among the associates. The participants were then asked to check off any words on their associates lists that they recognised as to-be-remembered words from the first phase of the experiment. They were able to do so 54 percent of the time. However, when the participants were later given the first words of the pair, like *train*, and asked to recall the associate, they were 61 percent accurate. In other words, directly contrary to what we have said above, this experiment seemed to produce conditions where participants were more able to recall the words than to recognise them.

Why was recall better than recognition? Tulving and Thomson suggested that what mattered was the change in context. After the participants had studied the word *black* in the context of *train*, it was hard to recover the memory representation when the context was changed to *white*. Given the significant effect of even these minimal contexts, you can anticipate that richly organised real-life contexts would have an even greater effect on your memory.

Researchers have provided several remarkable demonstrations of *context-dependent* memory. In one experiment, scuba divers learned lists of words either on a beach or under water. They were then tested for retention of those words, again in one of those two contexts. Performance was nearly 50 percent better when the context at encoding and recall matched—even though the material had nothing at all to do with water or diving (Gooden & Baddeley, 1975). Similarly, piano students performed a brief composition more accurately when they played it on the same piano on which they had first learned it (Mishra & Backlin, 2007). In another study, the use of consistent odour—either rosemary or lemon— at encoding and testing was associated with better word recall than switched odour conditions (i.e., lemon at encoding, rosemary at testing and vice versa) (Ball, Shoker & Miles, 2010).

In each of the examples we have provided so far, memories are encoded with respect to a context in the external environment—for example, the type of piano or an odour in the air. However, encoding specificity also occurs based on people's internal states. For example, in one study, participants drank a sweetened beverage containing either caffeine or a placebo before studying 40 pairs of words (Kelemen & Creeley, 2003). On the following day, participants drank either caffeine or a placebo before being tested on their recall ability. Participants who drank the same beverage (either caffeine or a placebo) at both study and test were able to recall more word pairs than those who drank different beverages on both days. When internal states provide the basis for encoding specificity, those effects are called *state-dependent memory*. Researchers have demonstrated that state-dependent memory occurs for other drugs such as marijuana, alcohol and amphetamines.

As a final example of encoding specificity, we want you to consider the experience of individuals who are bilingual and, thus, acquire information in more than one language.

Research suggests that memory performance can be strongly *language-dependent:* people find it easier to recall information when the language at encoding matches the language at retrieval.

Twenty Mandarin–English bilinguals agreed to participate in a study that tested their general world knowledge (Marian & Kaushanskaya, 2007). For one task, the experimenter asked each participant to name four examples from categories such as 'tourist attractions' and 'famous actors'. The questions were posed in either Mandarin or English. Participants' responses demonstrated language dependence: although they could name, for example, tourist attractions in both China and the United States, they were more likely to provide answers that matched the language in which the experimenter had posed the question. In a second task, participants received questions that each had two possible answers. Consider the question, 'In a famous love story, what were the names of two lovers who died because of family disapproval?' The answer can be either *Romeo and Juliet* or *Liang Shanbo and Zhu Yingtai*. Again, the participants' responses showed the impact of the language in which the question was posed: they provided more answers that matched the language of the question.

Your secret weapons for success at university

It is because we know that recall is better when there is a match of conditions between study and test, that most school and university student counsellors advise students to study under conditions that come close to matching the conditions of testing—that is, you should study, if possible, in a quiet, well-lit room, sitting at an uncluttered desk on a firm upright chair. This maximises the potential overlap between study conditions and examination conditions, and therefore allows you to use encoding specificity to your advantage.

The serial position effect

We can also use changes in context to explain one of the classic effects in memory research: the **serial position effect**. Suppose we required you to learn a list of unrelated words. If we asked you to recall those words in order, your data would almost certainly conform to the pattern shown in Figure 3.6: you would do very well on the first few words (the **primacy effect**) and very well on the last few words (the **recency effect**) but rather poorly on the middle part of the list. Figure 3.6 shows the generality of this pattern when students are asked to try to remember word lists of varying lengths (6, 10 and 15 words) using either *serial recall* ('Recite the words in the order you heard them') or *free recall* ('Recite as many words as you can') (Jahnke, 1965). Researchers have found primacy and recency in a wide variety of test situations (Neath & Surprenant, 2003). What day is it today? Do you believe that you would be almost a second faster to answer this question at the beginning or end of the week than in the middle (Koriat & Fischoff, 1974)?

The role context plays in producing the shape of the serial position curve has to do with the **contextual distinctiveness** of different items on a list, different experiences in your life, and so on (Neath et al., 2006). To understand contextual distinctiveness, you can ask the question, 'How different were the contexts in which I learned this information from the context in which I will try to recall it?' Let's focus on recency. Figure 3.7 is a visual representation of distinctiveness. Imagine, in part A, that you are looking at train tracks. What you can see is that they look as if they clump together at the horizon—even though they are equally spaced apart. We could say that the nearest tracks stand out most—are most distinctive—from your context. Imagine now that you are trying to remember the last 10

Serial position effect
A characteristic of memory retrieval in which the recall of beginning and end items on a list is often better than recall of items appearing in the middle.

Primacy effect
Improved memory for items at the start of a list.

Recency effect
Improved memory for items at the end of a list.

Contextual distinctiveness
The assumption that the serial position effect can be altered by the context and the distinctiveness of the experience being recalled.

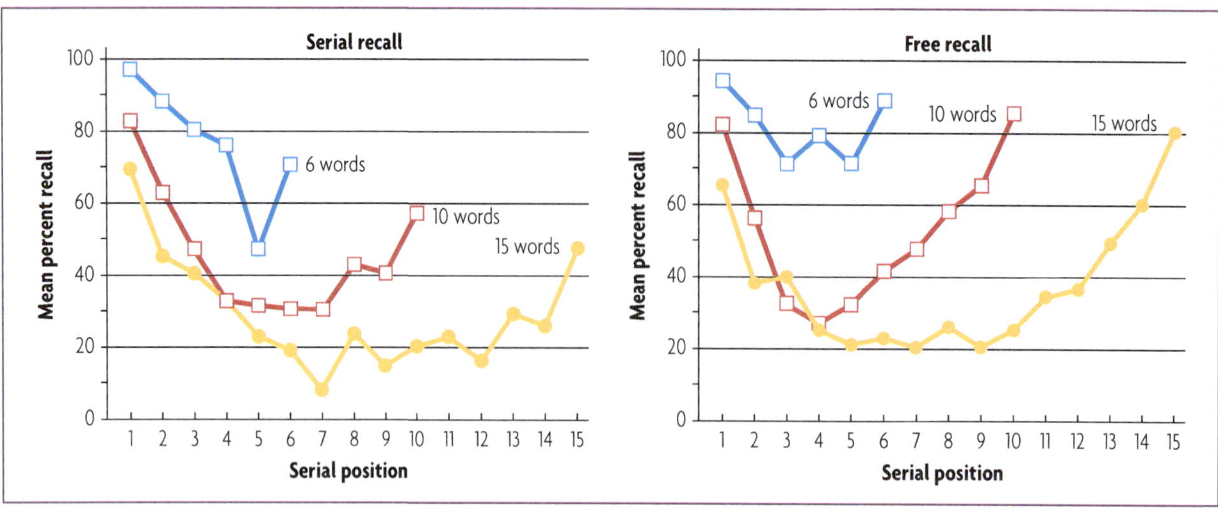

Figure 3.6 The serial position effect

This figure shows the generality of the serial position effect. Students were asked to try to remember word lists of varying lengths (6, 10 and 15 words) using either *serial recall* ('Recite the words in the order you heard them') or *free recall* ('Recite as many words as you can'). Each curve shows better memory for both the beginning (the *primacy* effect) and end (the *recency* effect) of the list.

movies you've seen. The movies are like the train tracks. Under most circumstances, you should remember the last movie best because you share the most overlapping context with the experience—it is 'closest' to the context of your current experiences. This logic suggests that 'middle' information will become more memorable if it is made more distinctive. The idea with respect to our analogy, as shown in part B of Figure 3.7, is to make the train tracks seem equally far apart.

To make the train tracks seem evenly spaced, engineers would have to make the more distant ones actually be farther apart. Researchers have used the same logic for a memory test, by exploiting the analogy between space and time. They had participants try to learn lists of letters, but they manipulated how far apart in time the letters were made to seem. This manipulation was accomplished by asking participants to read out some number of random digits that appeared on a computer screen between the letters. In the *conventional* condition (like part A of Figure 3.7), each pair of letters was separated by two digits. In the *proportional* condition (like part B), the first pair had four digits and the last pair had zero digits; this should have the effect of making the early digits more distinctive, just like moving distant train tracks farther apart. Participants, in fact, showed better memory for early items on the list when those items had been made more separate (Neath & Crowder, 1990).

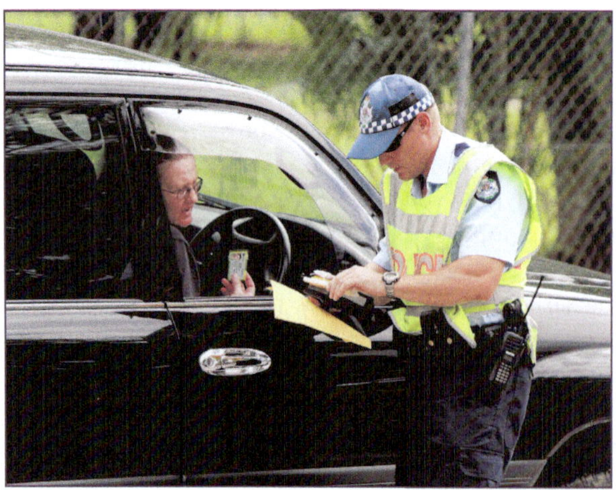

After receiving a traffic infringement warning from this officer, why might you not recognise him if you ran into him at a party?
(**Source:** © Newspix/News Ltd/3rd Party Managed Reproduction & Supply Rights)

This experiment suggests that the standard recency effect arises because the last few items are almost automatically distinctive. The same principle may explain primacy—each time you begin something new, your activity establishes a new context. In that new context, the first few experiences are particularly distinctive. Thus you can think of primacy and recency as two views of the same set of train tracks—one from each end!

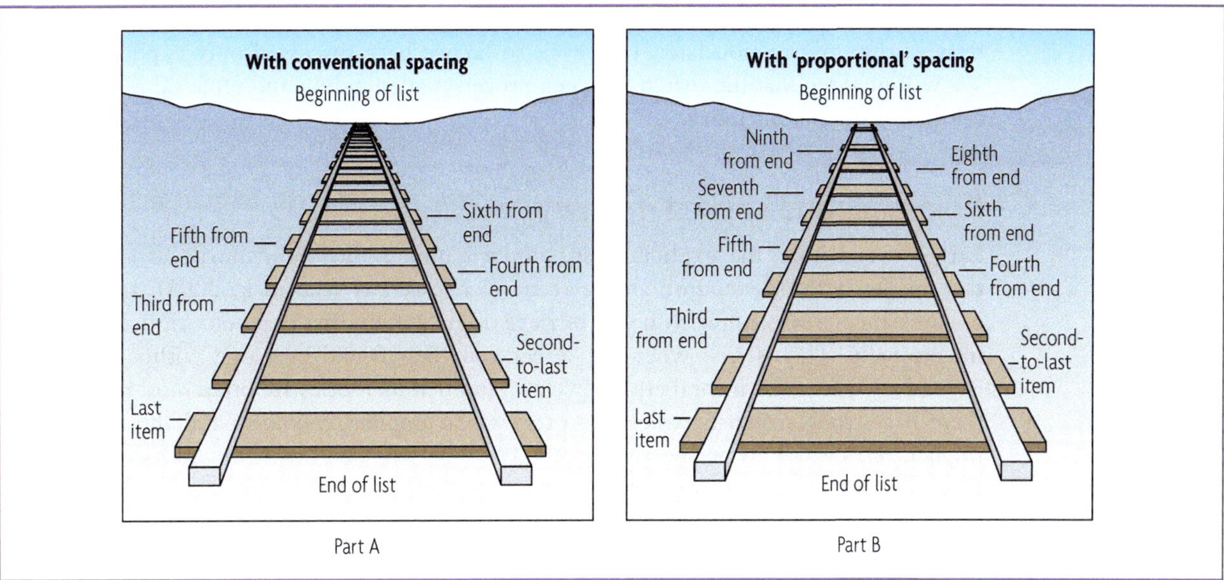

Figure 3.7 Contextual distinctiveness

You can think of items you put into memory as train tracks. In part A, you can imagine that memories farther back in time become blurred together, just like train tracks in the distance. In part B, you see that one way to combat this effect is to make the earlier tracks physically farther apart, so the distances look proportional. Similarly, you can make early memories more distinctive by moving them apart psychologically.

The processes of encoding and retrieval

We have seen so far that a match between the context of encoding and of retrieval is beneficial to good memory performance. We will now refine this conclusion somewhat by considering the actual processes that are used to get information to and from long-term memory. We will see that memory functions best when encoding and retrieval processes make a good match as well.

Levels of processing

Let's begin with the idea that the type of processing you perform on information—the type of attention you pay to information at the time of encoding—will have an influence on your memory for the information. **Levels-of-processing theory** suggests that the deeper the level at which information was processed, the more likely it is to be committed to memory (Craik & Lockhart, 1972; Lockhart & Craik, 1990). If processing involves more analysis, interpretation, comparison and elaboration, it should result in better memory. This is advice that we often give to students—they should read for meaning and understanding, rather than just skimming the words on the page.

Levels-of-processing theory A theory that suggests that the deeper the level at which information was processed the more likely it is to be retained in memory.

The depth of processing is often defined by the judgements participants are required to make when they first process material to be remembered. Consider the word *GRAPE*. We could ask you to make a physical judgement—is the word in capital letters? Or a rhyme judgement—does the word rhyme with *tape?* Or a meaning judgement—does the word represent a type of fruit? Do you see how each of these questions requires you to think a little bit more deeply about *GRAPE?* In fact, the deeper the original processing participants carry out, the more words they remember (Lockhart & Craik, 1990).

A difficulty of the levels-of-processing theory, however, is that researchers have not always been able to specify exactly what makes certain processes 'shallow' or 'deep'. Even so, results of this sort confirm that the way in which information is committed to memory—the mental processes that you use to encode information—has an effect on whether you can retrieve that information later. However, so far we have discussed only explicit memory. We will now see that the match between processes at encoding and retrieval is particularly critical for implicit memory.

Processes and implicit memory

Earlier, we defined the explicit versus implicit dimension for memories as a distinction that applies both at encoding and at retrieval (Bowers & Marsolek, 2003). Under many circumstances, for example, you will retrieve implicit memories that you originally encoded intentionally. This is true when you greet your best friend by name without having to expend any particular mental effort. Even so, implicit memories are often most robust when there is a strong match between the processes at implicit encoding and the processes at implicit retrieval. This perspective is called **transfer-appropriate processing**: memory is best when the type of processing carried out at encoding *transfers* to the processes required at retrieval (Roediger et al., 2002). To support this perspective, we will first describe some of the methodologies that are used to demonstrate implicit memories. Then we will show how the match between encoding and retrieval processes matters.

Transfer-appropriate processing The perspective that suggests that memory is best when the type of processing carried out at encoding matches the processes carried out at retrieval.

Let's consider a typical experiment in which implicit memory is assessed. The researchers presented students with lists of concrete nouns and asked them to judge the pleasantness of each word on a 1 (least pleasant) to 5 (most pleasant) scale (Rajaram & Roediger, 1993). The pleasantness ratings required participants to think about the meaning of a word without explicitly committing it to memory. After this study phase, participants' memories were assessed using one of four implicit memory tasks (suppose that a word on one list was *unicorn*):

- *Word fragment completion.* The participant is given fragments of a word, like ___*ni*___ *or*___, and asked to complete the fragments with the first word that comes to mind.
- *Word stem completion.* The participant is asked to complete a stem, like *uni*________, with the first word that comes to mind.
- *Word identification.* Words are flashed on a computer screen in such a fashion that participants cannot see them clearly. They must try to guess each word that is flashed. In this case, one of the words would be *unicorn*.
- *Anagrams.* Participants are given a scrambled word, like *corunni*, and asked to give the first unscrambled word that comes to mind.

Just like our example with *unicorn*, correct responses to each of the tasks can be provided by words from the earlier lists. What is critical, however, is that the experimenters have not called attention to the relationship between the words on the earlier list and appropriate responses on these new tasks—that's why the use of memory is implicit.

To assess the degree of implicit memory, the researchers compared the performance of participants who had seen a particular word, like *unicorn*, on the pleasantness lists with those who had not. Figure 3.8 plots the improvement brought about by implicit memory for a word—percentage correct when the word had appeared on the participant's list minus percentage correct when it had not. (Different participants experienced different word lists.) You can see that for each task there was an advantage to having seen a word before, even though participants had been asked only to say whether the word had a pleasant meaning. This advantage is known as **priming** because the first experience of the word *primes* memory for later experiences. For some memory tasks, like word fragment completion, researchers have found priming effects lasting a week and beyond (Sloman et al., 1988).

Priming In the assessment of implicit memory, the advantage conferred by prior exposure to a word or situation.

Let's turn now to the nature of the match between encoding and retrieval. The four implicit memory tests we've mentioned so far all rely on a *physical* match between the original stimulus and the information given at test. In a sense, whatever processes allow

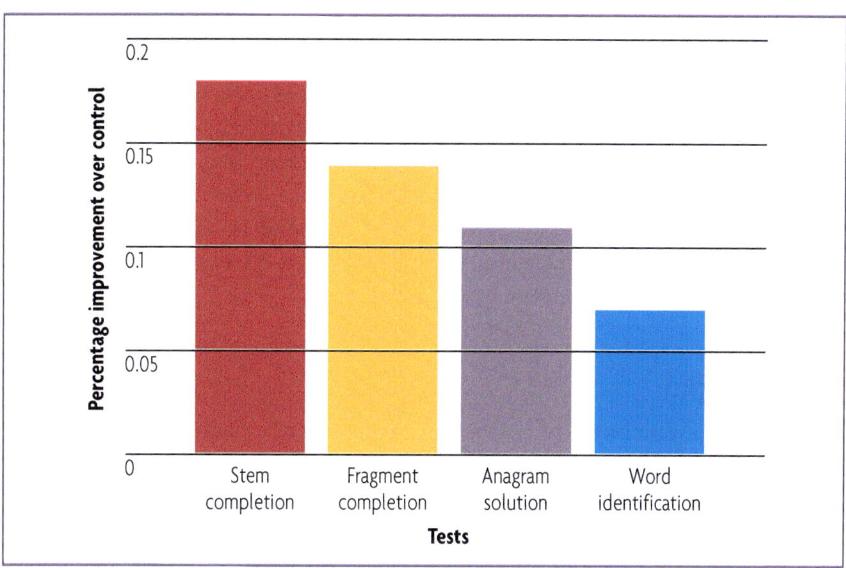

Figure 3.8 Priming on implicit memory tests

Priming indicates improvement on the various tasks over performance on control words. Some implicit memory tests demonstrate that priming can last a week or more.
Adapted with permission from Table 1 in Rajaram, S. & Roediger III, H.L. (1993).

you to encode *unicorn* also make that word available when you are asked to complete the stem *uni*_______, and so on. We can, however, introduce another test, *general knowledge*, which relies on *meaning* or *concepts* instead of on a physical match. Imagine we gave you the question, 'What mythological creature had a single horn?' You might very well say 'unicorn'. However, if you became more likely to say unicorn because you had seen the word on an earlier list, in a different context, that would be evidence of implicit memory.

Using two different types of implicit memory tests based on priming—by physical features or by meaning—we can look for a relationship between encoding and retrieval.

Memory researchers designed a levels-of-processing experiment to demonstrate that different implicit memories rely on different types of processes. Participants were asked to respond to each word on a list. For *deep* judgements, they responded to the words' meaning; for example, 'Can you buy this?' For *shallow* judgements, they responded to the words' physical features; for example, 'Does this word contain a *c*?' The researchers assessed implicit memory by using general knowledge questions and word fragment completion. Let's examine the tasks with an eye to transfer-appropriate processing. The deep judgements engage conceptual processes at encoding, but the shallow judgements do not. The general knowledge questions engage conceptual processes at retrieval, but word fragment completion does not. Accordingly, the researchers predicted that they should find a greater priming advantage for deep judgements when processes at encoding and retrieval matched (deep judgements with general knowledge questions) than when they mismatched (deep judgements with fragment completion). The results confirmed the prediction (Hamilton & Rajaram, 2001).

This type of research supports the idea of transfer-appropriate processing: if you use a certain type of processing—for example, physical or meaning analysis—to encode information, you will retrieve that information most efficiently when the processing uses the same type of analysis.

Earlier we made this assertion: your ability to remember will be greatest when there is a good match between the circumstances in which you encode information and the circumstances in which you attempt to retrieve it. This section provided the research evidence for this assertion. Note that this analysis defines both when your memory processes will function relatively well (i.e., when circumstances of encoding and retrieval match) and when those processes will function relatively less well (i.e., when there is a mismatch). In that sense, we've already provided you with some initial ideas about why you might not be capable of retrieving memories when you need them. Let's now look more generally at circumstances in which your memory processes fall short.

Why we forget

Much of the time, your memory works just fine. You see a new acquaintance walking toward you, and you retrieve her name from memory without hesitation. Unfortunately, every once in a while, you end up greeting her in awkward silence—with that awful realisation that you can't remember her name. How does that happen? Sometimes the answer can be provided by the processes we've already discussed. It could be the case, for example, that you're trying to recall the name in a context that's very different from the one in which you learned it. However, researchers have studied other explanations for forgetting. In fact, the earliest formal body of research on memory, published in 1885, focused directly on that topic. Let's begin with that work.

Ebbinghaus quantifies forgetting

See if this statement rings true: 'Facts crammed at examination time soon vanish, if they were not sufficiently grounded by other study and later subjected to a sufficient review.' In other words, if you cram for a test, you're not likely to remember very much a few days later. This astute, and very contemporary, observation was made in 1885 by the German psychologist Hermann Ebbinghaus, who outlined a series of such phenomena to motivate his new science of memory. (Ebbinghaus published his groundbreaking *Über das Gedächtnis*—'On Memory', later translated to English as *Memory: A Contribution to Experimental Psychology*—in 1885.) Ebbinghaus's observations added up to a convincing argument in favour of an empirical investigation of memory. What was needed was a methodology, and Ebbinghaus invented a brilliant one. Ebbinghaus used nonsense syllables—meaningless three-letter units consisting of a vowel between two consonants, such as CEG or DAX. He used nonsense syllables, rather than meaningful words, like DOG, because he hoped to obtain a 'pure' measure of memory—one uncontaminated by previous learning or associations that a person might bring to the experimental memory task. Not only was Ebbinghaus the researcher, he was also his own subject. He performed the research tasks himself and measured his own performance. The task he assigned himself was memorisation of lists of varying length. Ebbinghaus chose to use rote learning, memorisation by mechanical repetition, to perform the task.

Ebbinghaus started his studies by reading through the items one at a time until he finished the list. Then he read through the list again in the same order, and again, until he could recite all the items in the correct order—the *criterion performance.* Then he distracted himself from rehearsing the original list by forcing himself to learn many other lists. After this interval, Ebbinghaus measured his memory by seeing how many trials it took him to *relearn* the original list. If he needed fewer trials to relearn it than he had needed to learn it initially, information had been *saved* from his original study. (This concept should be familiar. Recall that there is often a savings when animals relearn a conditioned response.)

For example, if Ebbinghaus took 12 trials to learn a list and 9 trials to relearn it several days later, his savings score for that elapsed time would be 25 percent (12 trials – 9 trials = 3 trials; 3 trials ÷ 12 trials = 0.25, or 25 percent). Using savings as his measure, Ebbinghaus recorded the degree of memory retained after different time intervals. The curve he obtained is shown in Figure 3.9. As you can see, he found a rapid initial loss of memory, followed by a gradually declining rate of loss.

You have experienced the pattern revealed in Ebbinghaus's forgetting curve countless times in your life. Consider, for example, how you'd feel about taking an exam a week, or a fortnight, or a month after you studied for it. You know from experience that much of what you learned will no longer be accessible. Similarly, you might find it easy to recall a name right after you've learned it, but if a week goes by when you don't use it, you might find yourself thinking, 'I know I knew her name!'

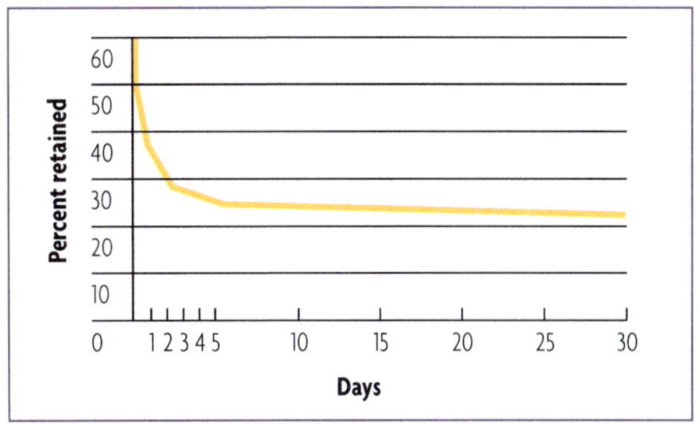

Figure 3.9 Ebbinghaus's forgetting curve

The curve shows how many nonsense syllables are remembered by individuals using the savings method when tested over a 30-day period. The curve decreases rapidly and then reaches a plateau of little change.

Interference

Why else might you forget a name that you knew a week ago? One important answer is that you didn't learn that name in isolation. Before you learned it, you had lots of other names in your head; after you learned it, you probably acquired a few more new ones. All those other names can have a negative impact on your ability to retrieve the one name you need in the moment. To make this point more formally, we want you to try to learn some new word pairs. Once again, keep working on these word pairs until you can repeat them three times in a row without an error.

Apple–Robe
Hat–Circle
Bicycle–Roof
Mouse–Magazine
Ball–Baby
Ear–coin

How did it go? Examine the list. You can see what we've done—we've paired the first word from the pairs we gave you earlier in the chapter with a new second word. Was it harder for you to learn these new pairs? Do you think it would now be harder for you to recall the old ones? (Go ahead and try.) The answer in both cases is typically 'yes'. This brief exercise should give you a sense of how memories can compete—or provide *interference*—with each other.

We have already given you a real-life example of the problem of interference when we asked you to try to differentiate your recollections of your episodes of toothbrushing. All of the specific memories interfere with each other. **Proactive interference** (*proactive* means 'forward acting') occurs when information you have acquired in the past makes it more difficult to acquire new information (see Figure 3.10). **Retroactive interference** (*retroactive* means 'backward acting') occurs when the acquisition of new information makes it harder for you to remember older information. The word lists we've provided demonstrate both of these types of interference. You've also experienced both proactive and retroactive interference if you've ever changed your telephone number. At first, you probably found

Proactive interference Circumstances in which past memories make it more difficult to encode and retrieve new information.

Retroactive interference Circumstances in which the formation of new memories makes it more difficult to recover older memories.

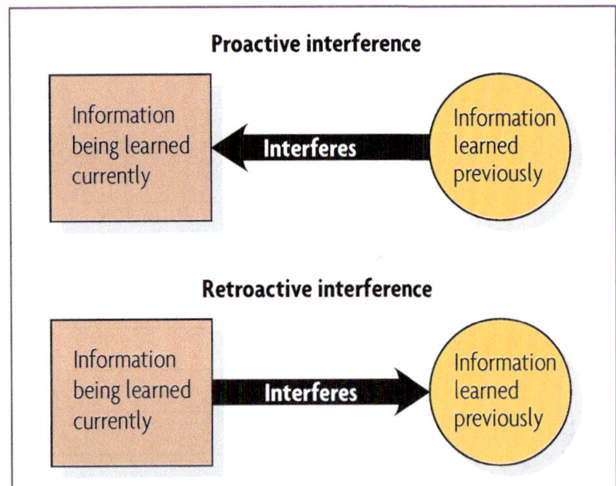

Figure 3.10 Proactive and retroactive interference

Proactive and retroactive interference help explain why it can be difficult to encode and retrieve memories. What you have learned in the past can make it more difficult for you to encode new information (proactive interference). What you are learning now can make it more difficult for you to retrieve old information (retroactive interference).

From Baron R.A., *Psychology* (5th edn, p. 225). Boston, MA: Allyn & Bacon. Copyright © 2002 by Pearson Education. Reprinted by permission of the publisher.

it hard to remember the new number—the old one kept popping out (proactive interference). However, after finally being able to reliably reproduce the new one, you may have found yourself unable to remember the old number—even if you had used it for years (retroactive interference).

As with many other memory phenomena, Hermann Ebbinghaus was the first researcher to document interference rigorously through experiments. Ebbinghaus, after learning dozens of lists of nonsense syllables, found himself forgetting about 65 percent of the new ones he was learning. Fifty years later, students at Northwestern University who studied Ebbinghaus's lists had the same experience—after many trials with many lists, what the students had learned earlier interferred proactively with their recall of current lists (Underwood, 1948, 1949).

In this section, we've suggested some reasons why you might forget information. It seems fitting that we move now to research that gives advice on how to make memory function better.

Improving memory for unstructured information

After reading this whole section, you should have some concrete ideas about how you could improve your everyday memory performance—how you can remember more and forget less. (The 'Critical thinking in your life' box, later in the chapter, will help you solidify those ideas with respect to your studies.) You know, especially, that you're best off trying to recover a piece of information in the same context, or by performing the same types of mental tasks, as when you first acquired it. But there's a slightly different problem with which we still must give you some help. It has to do with encoding unstructured or arbitrary collections of information.

For example, imagine that you are working as a sales assistant in a store. You must try to commit to memory the several items that each customer wants: 'The woman in the green blouse wants hedge clippers and a garden hose. The man in the blue shirt wants a pair of pliers, six 3 millimetre screws and a paint scraper.' This scenario, in fact, comes very close to the types of experiments in which researchers ask you to memorise paired associates. How did you go about learning the word pairs we presented earlier? The task probably was somewhat of a chore because the pairs were not particularly meaningful for you—and information that isn't meaningful is hard to remember. To find a way to get the right items to the right customer, you need to make associations seem less arbitrary. Let's explore *elaborative rehearsal* and *mnemonics*.

Elaborative rehearsal

Elaborative rehearsal
A technique for improving memory by enriching the encoding of information.

A general strategy for improving encoding is called **elaborative rehearsal**. The basic idea of this technique is that while you are rehearsing information—while you are first committing it to memory—you elaborate on the material to enrich the encoding. One way to do this is to invent a relationship that makes an association seem less arbitrary. For example, if you wanted to remember the pair *Mouse–Tree*, you might conjure up an image of a mouse scurrying up a tree to look for cheese. Recall is enhanced when you encode separate bits of information into this type of miniature story line. Can you imagine, in the sales assistant situation, swiftly making up a story to link each customer with the appropriate items? (It will work with practice.) You may have already guessed that it is also often helpful to supplement your story line with a mental picture—a visual image—of the scene you are trying to remember. Visual imagery can enhance your recall because it gives you codes for both verbal and visual memories simultaneously (Paivio, 1995).

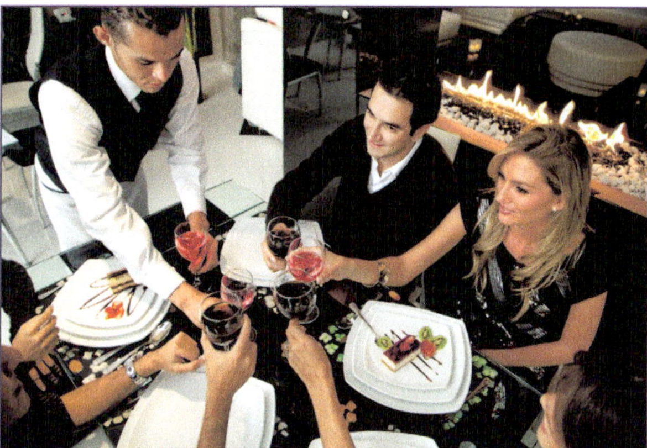

How might a waiter or waitress use elaborative rehearsal or mnemonics to get the right meals to the right customers?
(**Source:** © Andres Rodriguez/Fotolia 2004–2010, all rights reserved.)

Elaborative rehearsal can also help save you from what has been called the *next-in-line effect:* when, for example, people are next in line to speak, they often can't remember what the person directly before them said. If you've ever had a circle of people each give his or her name, you're probably well acquainted with this effect. What was the name of the person directly in front of you? The origin of this effect appears to be a shift in attention toward preparing to make your own remarks or to say your own name (Bond et al., 1991). To counter this shift, you should use elaborative rehearsal. Keep your attention focused on the person in front of you and enrich your encoding of his or her name: '*Deb—I'm caught in her web!*'

Mnemonics

Another memory-enhancing option is to draw on special mental strategies called *mnemonics* (from the Greek word meaning 'to remember'). **Mnemonics** are devices that encode a long series of facts by associating them with familiar and previously encoded information. Many mnemonics work by giving you ready-made retrieval cues that help organise otherwise arbitrary information.

Mnemonic
A strategy or device that uses familiar information during the encoding of new information to enhance subsequent access to the information in memory.

Consider the *method of loci*, first practised by ancient Greek orators. The singular of *loci* is *locus*, and it means 'place'. The method of loci is a means of remembering the order of a list of names or objects—or, for the orators, the individual sections of a long speech—by associating them with some sequence of places with which you are familiar. To remember a grocery list, you might mentally put each item sequentially along the route you take to get from home to school. To remember the list later, you mentally go through your route and find the item associated with each spot (see Figure 3.11).

The *peg-word method* is similar to the method of loci, except that you associate the items on a list with a series of cues rather than with familiar locations. Typically, the cues for the peg-word method are a series of rhymes that associate numbers with words. For example, you might memorise 'one is a *bun*', 'two is a *shoe*', 'three is a *tree*' and so on. Then you would associate each item on your list interacting with the appropriate cue. Suppose a history lecturer asked you to memorise, in order, the rulers of the Roman Empire. You might have Augustus eating a platter of buns, Tiberius wearing oversized shoes, Caligula sitting in a tree and so on. You can see that the key to learning arbitrary information is to encode the information in such a fashion that you provide yourself with efficient retrieval cues.

Metamemory

Suppose you're in a situation in which you'd really like to remember something. You're doing your best to use retrieval cues that reflect the circumstances of encoding, but you just

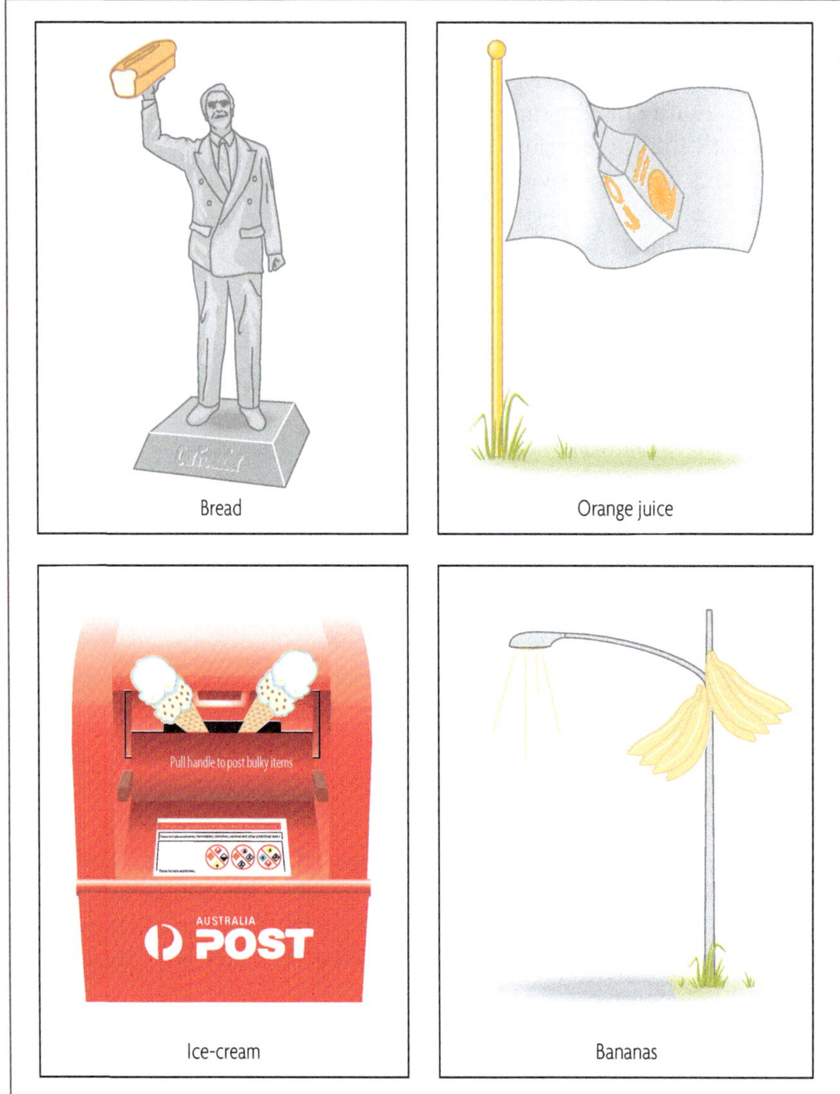

Figure 3.11 The method of loci

In the method of loci, you associate the items you wish to remember (such as the items on a grocery list) with locations along a familiar path (such as your route to and from school).

Metamemory Implicit or explicit knowledge about memory abilities and effective memory strategies; cognition about memory.

can't get the bit of information to emerge. Part of the reason you're expending so much effort is that you're sure that you are in possession of the information. But are you correct to be so confident about the contents of your memory? Questions like this one—about how your memory works or how you know what information you possess—are questions of **metamemory**. One major question on metamemory has been when and why *feelings-of-knowing*—the subjective sensations that you do have information stored in memory—are accurate.

Research on feelings-of-knowing was pioneered by J.T. Hart (1965), who began his studies by asking students a series of general knowledge questions. Suppose, for example, we asked you, 'What planet is the largest in our solar system?' Do you know the answer? If you don't, how would you respond to this question: 'Even though I don't remember the answer now, do I know the answer to the extent that I could pick the correct answer from among several wrong answers?' This was the question Hart put to his participants. He allowed them to give ratings from 1, to say they were quite sure they wouldn't choose correctly on the multiple choice, to 6, to say they were quite sure they would choose correctly. What would your rating be? Now here are your alternatives:

a. Mars
b. Venus
c. Earth
d. Jupiter

If you made an accurate feeling-of-knowing judgement, you should have been less likely to get the correct answer, d, if you gave a 1 rating than if you gave a 6. (Of course, to have a fair test, we'd want to give you a long series of questions.) Hart found that when participants gave 1 ratings, they answered the questions correctly only 30 percent of the time, whereas 6 ratings predicted 75 percent success. That's pretty impressive evidence that feelings-of-knowing can be accurate.

Research on metamemory focuses on both the processes that give rise to feelings-of-knowing and on how their accuracy is ensured (Benjamin, 2005; Koriat & Levy-Sadot, 2001; Metcalfe, 2000):

- The *cue familiarity hypothesis* suggests that people base their feelings-of-knowing on their familiarity with the retrieval cue. Suppose you were asked, 'What is the last name of the poet who wrote "I love a sunburnt country..."?' If you have prior familiarity with the poem *My Country* you might think that you probably would be able to recognise the correct alternative when given the multiple choice.
- The *accessibility hypothesis* suggests that people base their judgements on the accessibility, or availability, of partial information from memory. Thus, if the question 'poet who wrote, "I love a sunburnt country..."?' calls quite easily to mind information you believe to be related to the correct answer, you are likely to think that you will be able to recognise the correct answer as well.

Both of these theories have obtained empirical support—and both suggest that you can generally trust your instincts when you believe that you know something. (Later in the chapter, we will describe research on eyewitness testimony, which provides some exceptions to this general rule.)

You have now learned quite a bit about how you get information in and out of memory. You know what we mean by a 'good match' between the circumstances of encoding and of retrieval. In the next section, we will shift our focus from your memory processes to the content of your memories.

Stop and review

1. Do circumstances of recall or recognition generally provide more retrieval cues?
2. At a party, why might you have the best recall of the first person to whom you spoke?
3. What does the perspective known as transfer-appropriate processing suggest?
4. For your English class, you memorise *The Raven*. When you're done, you can no longer recite last week's assignment. Is this an example of proactive or retroactive interference?
5. How could you use the method of loci to remember the order of elements in the periodic table?
6. What two types of information contribute to feelings of knowing?

Critical thinking

Recall the experiment that tested Mandarin–English bilinguals. What would you expect to find if you tested the participants' episodic memories?

Structures in long-term memory

We have focused so far on how you encode and later retrieve information from memory. In this section we focus on an important aspect of memory storage: the way in which the information you acquire over time becomes represented in large bodies of *organised knowledge*. Recall, for example, that we asked you to consider whether *grape* is a fruit. You could say 'yes' very quickly. How about *porcupine?* Is it a fruit? How about *tomato?* In this section, we will examine how the difficulty of these types of judgements relates to the way information is structured in memory. We will also discuss how memory organisation allows you to make a best guess at the content of experiences you can't remember exactly.

Memory structures

An essential function of memory is to draw together similar experiences, to enable you to discover patterns in your interactions with the environment. You live in a world filled with countless individual events, from which you must continually extract information to combine them into a smaller, simpler set that you can manage mentally. But apparently you don't need to expend any particular conscious effort to find structure in the world. Just as we suggested when we defined the incidental acquisition of memories, it's unlikely that you ever formally thought to yourself something like, 'Here's the shape of a Give Way sign'. It is through ordinary experience in the world that you have acquired mental structures to mirror environmental structures. Let's look at the types of memory structures you have formed in your moment-by-moment experience of the world.

Categories and concepts

We will begin by previewing one of the topics we have covered in Chapter 1—the mental effort a child must go through to acquire the meaning of a word, such as *doggie*. For this word to have meaning, the child must be able to store each instance in which the word *doggie* is used, as well as information about the context. In this way, the child finds out what common core experience—a furry creature with four legs—is meant by *doggie*. The child must acquire the knowledge that *doggie* applies not just to one particular animal, but to a *whole category* of creatures. This ability to categorise individual experiences—to take the same action toward them or give them the same label—is one of the most basic abilities of thinking organisms (Murphy, 2002).

Concept
A mental representation of kinds or categories of items and ideas.

The mental representations of the categories you form are called **concepts**. The concept *doggie*, for example, names the set of mental representations of experiences of dogs that a young child has gathered together in memory. (As we saw in Chapter 1, if the child hasn't yet refined his or her meaning for *doggie*, the concept might also include features that adults wouldn't consider to be appropriate.) You have acquired a vast array of concepts. You have categories for *objects* and *activities*, such as *sheds* and *cricket*. Concepts may also represent *properties*, such as *red* or *large; abstract ideas*, such as *truth* or *love*; and *relations*, such as *smarter than* or *sister of*. Each concept represents a summary unit for your experience of the world.

As you consider the many categories you experience in the world, you will recognise that some category members are more or less typical. You can develop this intuition if you think about a category like *bird*. You would probably agree that a robin is a typical bird, whereas an emu or a penguin is atypical. The degree of typicality of a category member has real-life consequences. Classic research has shown, for example, that people respond more quickly to typical members of a category than to its more unusual ones. Your reaction time to determine that a robin is a bird would be quicker than your reaction time to determine that a penguin is a bird (Rosch et al., 1976). But what makes people consider a robin to be a typical bird, rather than an emu? Answers to this question have often focused on *family resemblance*—typical category members have attributes that overlap with many other members of the category (Rosch & Mervis, 1975). Robins have most of the attributes you associate with birds—they are about the right size, they fly, and so on. Emus, by contrast, are unusually large and they do not fly. These examples suggest that family resemblance plays a role in judgements of typicality. However, recent research suggests that the most typical category members are also the *ideal* category members.

A team of researchers recruited individuals from two communities who had several decades of fishing experience. One group was Native American Menominee Indians from northern central Wisconsin; the second group was European Americans from roughly the same geographical location (Burnett et al., 2005). The experiment used these two groups because they differ with respect to the species of fish they consider to be most desirable or ideal. For example, the Menominee people consider sturgeon to be sacred. The researchers presented the participants with a group of 44 cards printed with the names of local fish. Participants sorted these cards into groups—the researchers used the participants' verbal justifications (e.g., 'good eating') for which fish they grouped together as an index of desirability. Also, the participants rated the extent to which each species was a good example of the 'fish' category. The researchers found a 0.80 correlation between desirability and typicality. (Correlations range from –1.0 to +1.0.) That's impressive evidence that the participants' notions of the 'ideal' fish played a role in their judgements of typicality. In addition, the ratings were influenced by cultural differences in desirability. For example, the Menominee group rated sturgeon as even more typical than did the European–American group.

If you don't have a lot of fishing experience, you might have less of a sense than these participants did about which fish are desirable. However, you can think about categories with which you have a lot of experience to see how your notions of what is ideal inform your judgements about what is typical.

Basic levels and hierarchies

Concepts, and their prototypes, do not exist in isolation. As shown in Figure 3.12, concepts can often be arranged into meaningful organisations. A broad category like *animal* has several subcategories, such as *bird* and *fish*, which in turn contain exemplars such as *canary*, *ostrich*, *shark* and *salmon*. The animal category is itself a subcategory of the still larger category of *living beings*. Concepts are also linked to other types of information: you store the knowledge that some birds are *edible*, some are *endangered*, some are *birds of prey*.

There seems to be a level in such hierarchies at which people best categorise and think about objects. This has been called the **basic level** (Rosch, 1973, 1978). For example, when you buy an apple at the supermarket, you could think of it as a *piece of fruit*—but that seems imprecise—or a *Golden Delicious*—but that seems too specific or narrow. The basic level is just *apple*. If you were shown a picture of such an object, that's what you'd be likely to call it. You would also be faster to say that it was an apple than that it was a piece of fruit (Rosch, 1978). The basic level emerges through your experience of the world. You are more likely to encounter the term *apple* than its more or less specific alternatives. If you became an apple grower, however, you might find yourself having daily conversations about *Pink Ladies* or *Granny Smiths*. With those experiences, your basic level would probably shift lower in the hierarchy.

Basic level
The level of categorisation that can be retrieved from memory most quickly and used most efficiently.

Schemas

We have seen that concepts are the building blocks of memory hierarchies. They also serve as building blocks for more complex mental structures. Imagine that you are staying in a

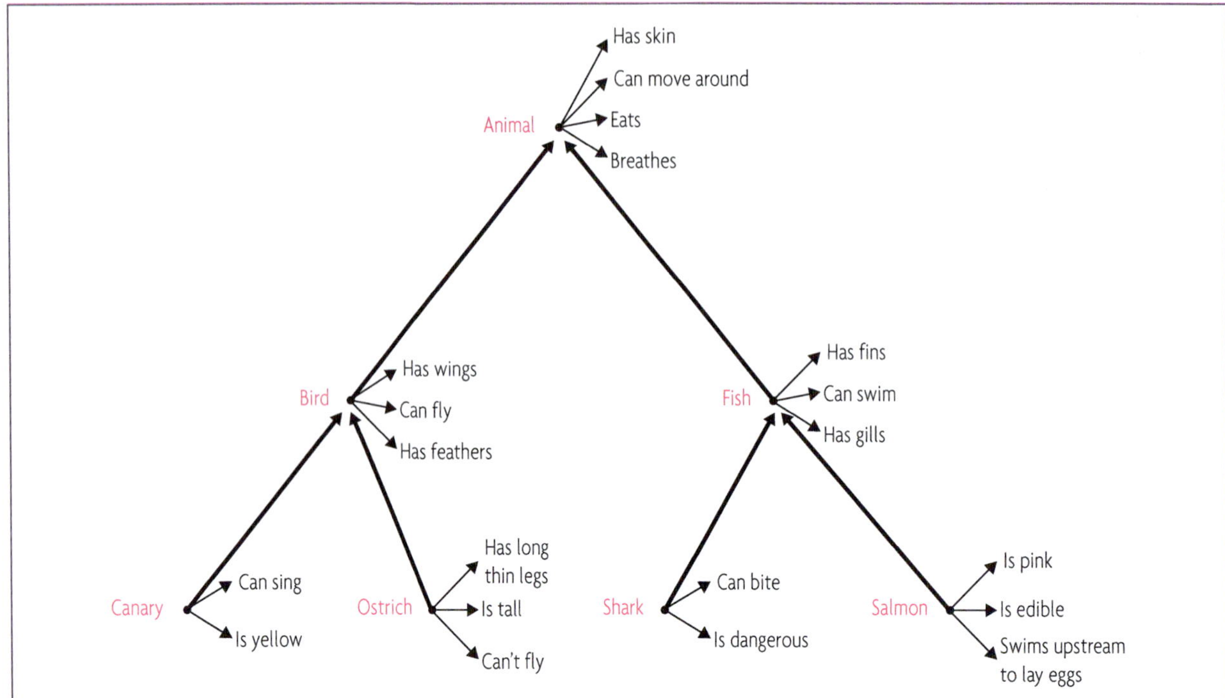

Figure 3.12 Hierarchically organised structure of concepts

The category *animal* can be divided into subcategories such as *bird* and *fish*; similarly, each subcategory can be further divided. Some information (such as *has skin*) applies to all concepts in the hierarchy; other information (such as *can sing*) applies only to concepts at lower levels (e.g., a *canary*).

holiday house that you have never been in before. You want to make a sandwich and you need to look for bread, margarine, jam and the like. You probably wouldn't start looking in the laundry—you'd go straight to the kitchen. Then, when you were in the kitchen, you'd look for the margarine in the fridge, not the microwave. This is because, even though this house is new to you, you have been in enough houses to have in mind a general idea of a house. Nested within that general idea of a house, you have a general idea of a kitchen. An important task of our memory system is to generalise from millions of isolated examples into a single organising concept that 'makes sense' of particular experiences or events. In this example, you have developed a single representation that combines the individual concepts of a kitchen—your knowledge about ovens, sinks and refrigerators—into a larger unit. We call that larger unit a schema. **Schemas** (sometimes called *Schemata*) are conceptual frameworks, or clusters of knowledge, regarding objects, people and situations. Schemas are knowledge packages that encode complex generalisations about your experience of the structure of the environment. You have schemas for kitchens and bedrooms, race car drivers and teachers, surprise parties and formals. There are many other types of schemas that shape your day-to-day experiences. For example, the attachment relationships children form with their

Schema
A general conceptual framework or cluster of knowledge regarding objects, people and situations.

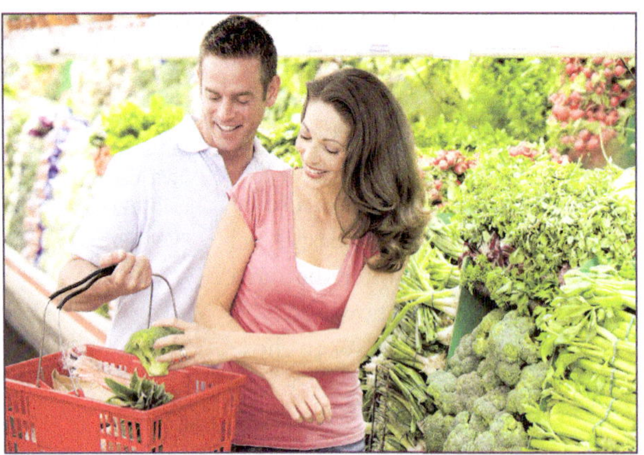

How does the formation of categories—such as what constitutes a healthy head of lettuce, a sweet strawberry, or a tasty tomato—help you make daily decisions such as what to buy for dinner?
(**Source:** ©Monkey Business Images Ltd/Photolibrary.)

parents provide schemas for later social interactions. The *self-schema* is a memory structure that allows you to organise information about yourself.

One thing you may have guessed is that your schemas do not include all the individual details of all your varied experiences. A schema represents your average experience of situations in the environment. Thus your schemas are not permanent but shift with your changing life events. Your schemas also include only those details in the world to which you have devoted sufficient attention. For example, what appears on the *tails* side of a 5-cent coin? You may have thought 'an echidna', but is there anything else? You probably didn't think to mention the number 5, because that has not been the focus of your attention since you were very young and had no other way of knowing the value of coins. Similarly, American students appeared to 'forget' the word *Liberty*, which appears on every coin (Rubin & Kontis, 1983). Thus your schemas provide an accurate reflection of what you've *noticed* about the world. Let's now look at all the ways in which you use your concepts and schemas.

Using memory structures

Let's consider some instances of memory structures in action. To begin, consider the picture in part A of Figure 3.13. What is it? Although we purposely chose an unusual member of the category, you probably reached the conclusion 'It's a chair' with reasonable ease. However, to do so, you needed to draw on your memory representations of members of that category. You can say 'It's a chair' because the object in the figure calls to mind your past experiences of chairs.

Researchers have provided two theories of how people use concepts in memory to categorise the objects they encounter in the world. One theory suggests that, for each concept in memory, you encode a **prototype**—a representation of the most central or average member of a category (Rosch, 1978). You recognise objects by comparing them to prototypes in memory. Because the picture in part A of Figure 3.13 matches many of the important attributes of the prototype in part B, you can recognise the picture as a chair.

Prototype
The most representative example of a category.

Exemplar
A member of a category that people have encountered.

An alternative theory suggests that people retain memories of the many different **exemplars** they experience for each category. In part C of Figure 3.13, we give you a subset of the exemplars of chairs you might have seen. You recognise an object by comparing it to the exemplars you have stored in memory. You recognise the picture as a chair because it is similar to several of those exemplars. Researchers have conducted a large number of studies to test between prototype and exemplar accounts of categorisation. The data largely support the exemplar view: people appear to categorise the objects they encounter by comparing them to multiple representations in memory (Nosofsky & Stanton, 2005; Voorspoels et al, 2008).

We intended the picture in Figure 3.13 to be an unusual chair but clearly a chair nonetheless. However, sometimes the world provides ambiguous stimuli—and you use prior knowledge to help interpret those stimuli. Look at Figure 3.14. Do you see a duck or a rabbit? Let's suppose we give you the expectation that you're going to see a duck. If you match the features of the picture against the features of a duck present in exemplars in memory, you're likely to be reasonably content. The same thing would happen if we told you to expect a rabbit. You use information from memory to generate—and confirm—expectations.

As we've previously noted, memory representations also allow you to understand when something is unusual in the world. Suppose that in the holiday house example from earlier the fridge did happen to be in the laundry. You would have to learn to override your 'house' schema and look in the laundry for margarine. You would probably also remember the house as 'the house with the fridge in the laundry' and that unusual fact would make this house memorable even after many holidays at more 'schema-consistent' houses. In one study, researchers illustrated that schema-inconsistent information is more memorable by filling a

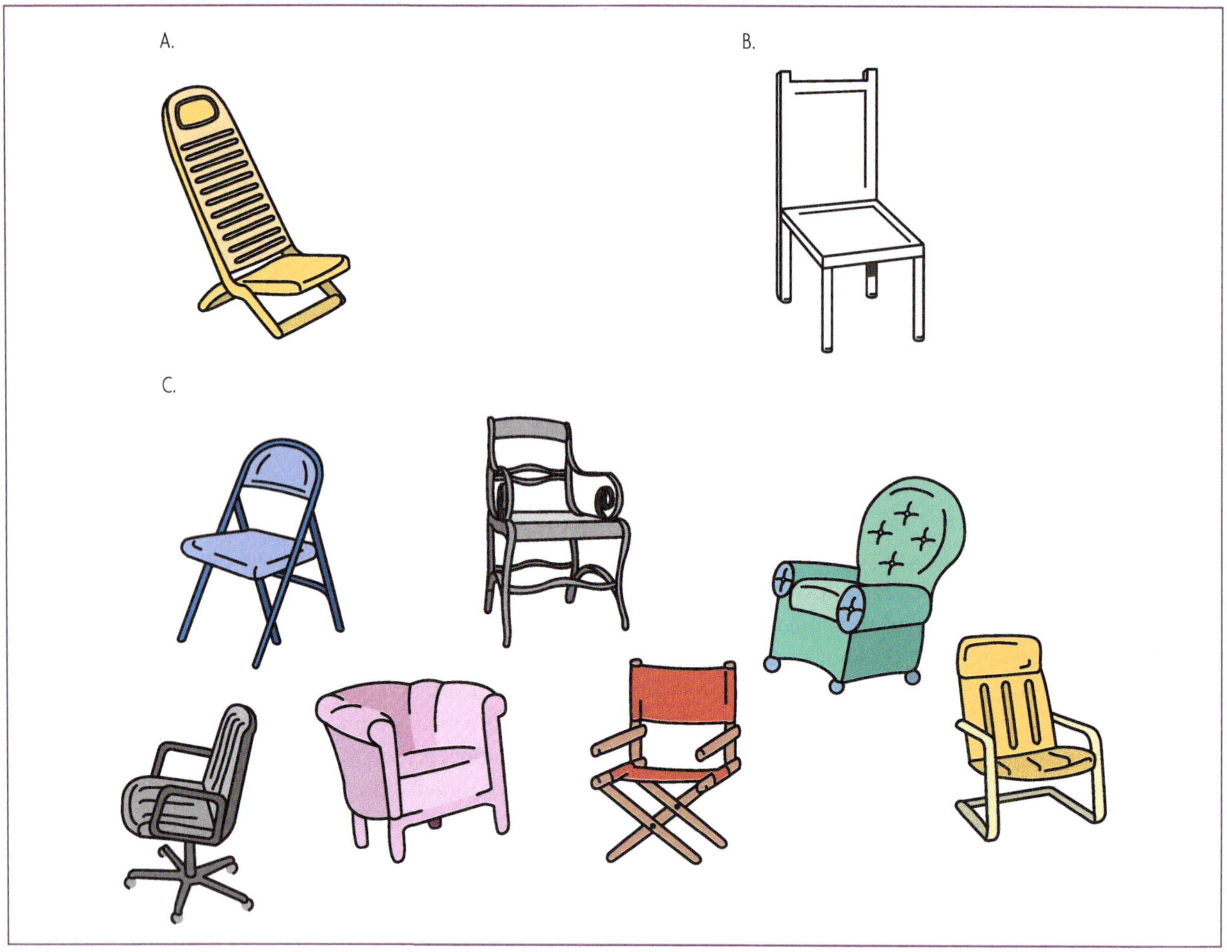

Figure 3.13 Theories of categorisation

A. What is this unusual object? B. One theory suggests that you categorise this object as a chair by comparing it to a single prototype stored in memory. C. An alternative theory suggests that you categorise this object by comparing it to the many exemplars you have in memory.

graduate student office with both typical objects (e.g., notebook, pencil) and atypical objects (e.g., harmonica, toothbrush) (Lampinen et al., 2001). Participants spent 1 minute in the room. In a later phase of the experiment, participants indicated which items on a list had been present in the room. Their memory was consistently more accurate for the atypical items than for the typical items. In addition, the participants were likely to have more specific memories of having seen the atypical items, whereas their memories for the typical items were based more on a general sense of familiarity. This study illustrates how memory structures direct your attention to unusual aspects of a scene.

Taken together, these examples demonstrate that the availability of memory structures can influence the way you think about the world. Your past experiences colour your present experiences and provide expectations for the future. You will see shortly that, for much the same reasons, concepts and schemas can sometimes work against accurate memory.

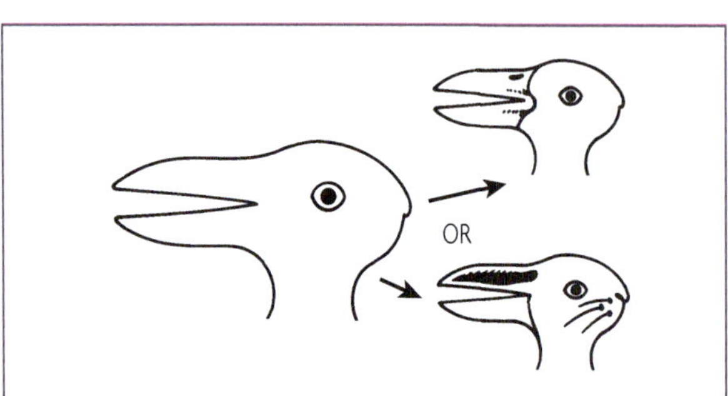

Figure 3.14 Recognition illusion

Duck or rabbit?

Remembering as a reconstructive process

Let's turn now to another important way in which you use memory structures. In many cases, when you are asked to remember a piece of information, you can't remember the information directly. Instead, you *reconstruct* the information based on more general types of stored knowledge. To experience **reconstructive memory**, consider this trio of questions:

Reconstructive memory The process of putting information together based on general types of stored knowledge in the absence of a specific memory representation.

- Did Chapter 1 have the word *the* in it?
- Did 1991 contain the day 7 July?
- Did you breathe yesterday between 2:05 and 2:10 p.m.?

You probably were willing to answer 'Yes!' to each of these questions without much hesitation, but you almost certainly don't have specific, episodic memories to help you (unless, of course, something happened to fix these events in memory—perhaps 7 July is your birthday or you crossed out all the *the*'s in Chapter 1 to curb your boredom). To answer these questions, you must use more general memories to reconstruct what is likely to have happened. Let's examine this process of reconstruction in a bit more detail.

The accuracy of reconstructive memory

If people reconstruct some memories, rather than recovering a specific memory representation for what happened, then you might expect distortions—or occasions on which the reconstructed memory differed from the real occurrence. One of the most impressive demonstrations of memory distortions is also the oldest. In his classic book *Remembering: A Study in Experimental and Social Psychology* (1932), Sir Frederic Bartlett undertook a program of research to demonstrate how individuals' prior knowledge influenced the way they remembered new information. Bartlett studied the way British undergraduates remembered stories whose themes and wording were taken from another culture. His most famous story was 'The War of the Ghosts', an American Indian tale.

Bartlett found that his readers' reproductions of the story were often greatly altered from the original. The distortions Bartlett found involved three kinds of reconstructive processes:

- *Levelling*—simplifying the story.
- *Sharpening*—highlighting and overemphasising certain details.
- *Assimilating*—changing the details to better fit the participant's own background or knowledge.

Thus readers reproduced the story with words familiar in their culture taking the place of those that were unfamiliar: *boat* might replace *canoe* and *go fishing* might replace *hunt seals*. Bartlett's participants also often changed the story's plot to eliminate references to supernatural forces that were unfamiliar in their culture.

Following Bartlett's lead, contemporary researchers have demonstrated a variety of memory distortions that occur when people use constructive processes to reproduce memories (Bergman & Roediger, 1999). How, for example, do you remember what you did as a child? Participants in one experiment were asked to indicate whether, before the age of 10, they had 'Met and shook hands with a favourite TV character at a theme resort' (Braun et al., 2002, p. 7). After answering that question—as part of a larger life-experiences inventory—some of the participants read an advertisement for Disneyland that evoked the idea of a family visit: 'Go back to your childhood . . . and remember the characters of your youth, Mickey, Goofy, and Daffy Duck'. Later the ad described circumstances in which the visitor was able to shake hands with a childhood hero: 'Bugs Bunny, the character you've idolised on TV, is only several feet away . . . You [reach up] to grab his hand' (p. 6). After reading this type of ad, participants were now more likely to indicate—though they hadn't before—that they shook a character's hand. Moreover, they were more likely to report a specific memory that they had shaken Bugs Bunny's hand at Disneyland: 16 percent of the participants in this advertisement group remembered having done so versus 7 percent of the participants in a group that hadn't read the autobiographical ad. Of course, none of these memories can be accurate: Bugs Bunny isn't a Disney character!

This study suggests how even memories for your own life events are reconstructed from various sources. The study also illustrates the fact that people with no reason to consciously distort or misrepresent their recollection are not always accurate at recalling the original sources for various components of their memories (Mitchell & Johnson, 2000). In fact, researchers have demonstrated that individuals will sometimes come to believe that they actually carried out actions that they, in fact, only accomplished in their imaginations.

A group of 40 students participated in an experiment that had three sessions. In session 1, the students joined an experimenter for a 1-hour walk around campus. The pair stopped 48 times during the walk. At each stop, the experimenter read an action statement such as: 'Check the Pepsi machine for change.' After hearing each statement, the students did one of four things: they performed the actions themselves, they watched the experimenter perform the actions, they imagined that they were performing the actions, or they imagined that the experimenter was performing them. In addition, half the actions were bizarre. For example, rather than 'Check the Pepsi machine for change', half the students were instructed to 'get down on one knee and propose marriage to the machine'. The experimenter and the participants took a second walk during session 2, which took place 24 hours later. On the second walk, the students imagined themselves or the experimenter performing some new and some old actions (both ordinary and bizarre) at locations that were also divided between new and old. In session 3, which took place two weeks after session 2, the students were asked to think back to the first session. They tried to recall whether each action had been performed or imagined. For both ordinary and bizarre actions, the same finding held true: students often recalled that the actions they had only been asked to imagine had actually been performed by them or the experimenter. Thus, some participants agreed that they had actually proposed marriage to a Pepsi machine or patted a dictionary to ask how it was doing when they had only imagined doing so (Seamon et al., 2006).

Can you find applications of this result in your own life? Suppose you keep reminding yourself to set your alarm clock before you go to bed. Each time you remind yourself, you form a picture in your head of the steps you must go through. If you imagine setting the clock often enough, you might mistakenly come to believe that you actually did so! Of course, the opposite can also happen: have you ever been away from the house and suddenly wondered if you *really* turned off the iron, or just *thought* about doing it before you left? Sometimes that worry can be so strong that you might have gone all the way home, only to find that you really had turned it off.

In this case, you have incorrectly 'forgotten' something that you have actually very recently done. It is important to keep in mind, however, that psychologists often infer the normal operation of processes by demonstrating circumstances in which the processes lead to errors. You can think of these memory distortions as the consequences of processes that usually work pretty well. In fact, a lot of the time, you don't need to remember the exact details of a particular episode. Reconstructing the gist of events will serve just fine.

Flashbulb memories

Flashbulb memory A person's vivid and richly detailed memory in response to personal or public events that have great emotional significance.

For most of your past life experiences, you would probably agree that you need to reconstruct the memories. For example, if we asked you to tell us how you celebrated your birthday 3 years ago, you'd likely count backwards and try to reconstruct the context. However, there are some circumstances in which people believe that their memories remain completely faithful to the original events. These types of memories—which are called **flashbulb memories**—arise when people experience emotionally charged events: people's memories are so vivid that they seem almost to be photographs of the original incident. The first research on flashbulb memories focused on people's recollections of public events (Brown & Kulik, 1977). For example, the researchers asked participants if they had specific memories of how they first learned about the assassination of President John F. Kennedy. All but one of the 80 participants reported vivid recollections.

The concept of flashbulb memory applies to both private and public events. People might have vivid memories, for example, of an accident they experienced or how they learned about the September 11 attacks. However, research on flashbulb memories has largely focused on public events. To conduct these studies, researchers recruit participants and ask them to share their memories of emotionally resonant events. For different age groups, such events might be the *Challenger* explosion, the death of Princess Diana, or the attack on Pearl Harbor. The content of flashbulb memories reflects how people learned about the events. For example, people who acquired their information from the media tend to include more event facts in their memory reports than do people who acquired information from another individual (Bohannon et al., 2007). United States citizens had more specific recollections of the September 11 attacks than did citizens of other countries such as Italy, the Netherlands and Japan (Curci & Luminet, 2006).

Research on these public events confirms that people acquire flashbulb memories. The question remains, however, whether these memories are as accurate as people believe them to be. To address the question of accuracy, researchers recruit participants directly after the events and then assess their memories at one or more points later in time. One such study began on 12 September 2001.

The researchers extended their project by inviting the original participants for another memory test after a full year had passed (Talarico & Rubin, 2007). The conclusions remained the same: in a pattern that was quite similar for both types of memories, the participants' ability to provide correct details decreased, whereas their tendency to introduce incorrect details increased. There was, however, one feature that set flashbulb memories apart from everyday memories: for their flashbulb memories, participants were considerably more confident that they were providing accurate memories.

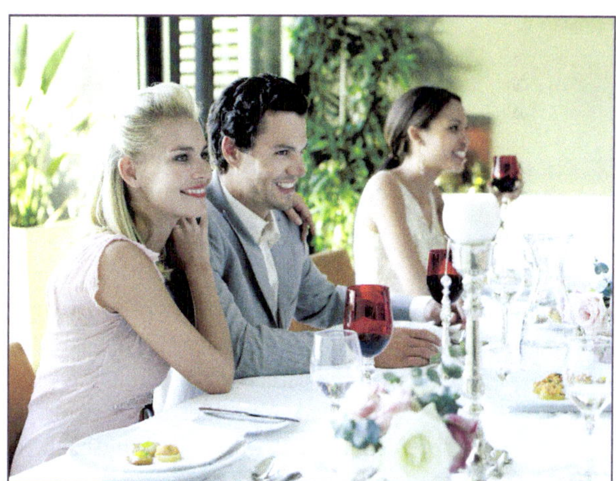

Suppose, while you were at this dinner party, someone told you the man in the middle was a millionaire. How would this affect your memories of his actions at the party? What if you had been told he only had delusions of being a millionaire?

(**Source:** © moodboard/Fotolia 2004–2010, all rights reserved.)

That final result indicates why it is often difficult for people to accept the results of research on flashbulb memories. How could memories that feel so vivid and true actually be inaccurate (or, at least, be no more accurate than other less vivid memories)? The same processes of reconstruction we discussed earlier apply to flashbulb memories. However, people's desire to hold tight to their memories for particularly emotional events makes it quite difficult for them to consider the possibility that those memories might not be accurate.

We turn now to a domain in which people's over-confidence in their memories can have negative real-world consequences. In the domain of eyewitness testimony, people are always held responsible for reporting *exactly* what happened.

The day after the September 11 attacks, students provided answers to a series of questions, including 'Where were you when you first heard the news?' and 'Were there others with you and, if so, who?' (Talarico & Rubin, 2003). For purposes of comparison, the students also reported memories for an everyday event (such as a party or sporting event) that occurred in the few days before the attack. The students answered the same types of questions for

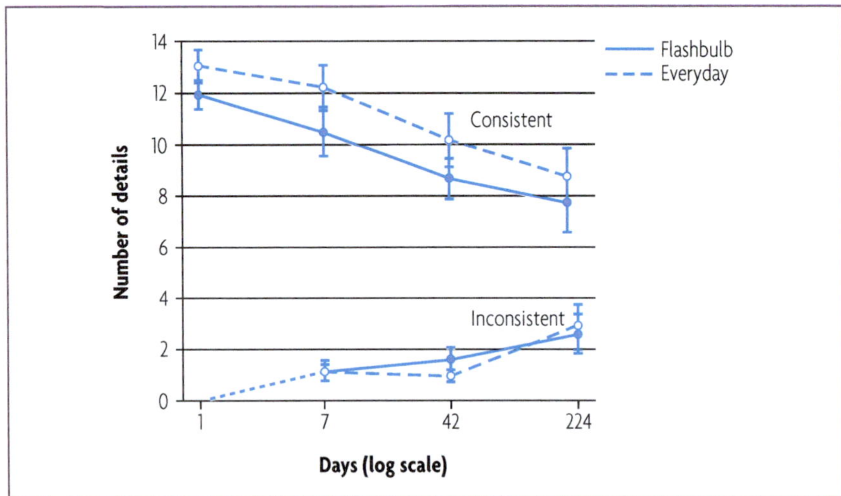

Figure 3.15 Students' recall of flashbulb and everyday memories

On 12 September 2001, students reported details of their memories of the September 11 attack as well as an everyday memory that occurred in the few days preceding that event. When they were tested for the memories 1, 6 or 32 weeks later, the students' performance was highly similar for both types of memories. Over time, they reported fewer details consistent with their first reports and more details that were inconsistent.
From Talarico, J.M. & Rubin, D.C. (2003). Confidence, not consistency, characterises flashbulb memories. *Psychological Science, 14*, 445–461. © Association for Psychological Science. Reprinted with permission of SAGE Publications.

those everyday memories (e.g., 'Where were you physically?' and 'Were there others present and, if so, who?'). The researchers called the students back to the laboratory 1, 6 or 32 weeks after the initial memory test. At each delay, the students answered the same series of memory questions they had answered on 12 September. The researchers determined which details were consistent with the original reports and which were inconsistent. As you can see in Figure 3.15, there were no differences between September 11 memories and everyday memories. The students recalled consistent details and introduced inconsistent details at nearly the same rate for both types of memories.

Eyewitness memory

A witness in a courtroom swears 'to tell the truth and nothing but the truth'. Throughout this chapter, however, we have seen that whether a memory is accurate or inaccurate depends on the care with which it was encoded and the match of the circumstances of encoding and retrieval. Consider the cartoon of a crowd scene we asked you to examine earlier in the chapter. Without looking back, try to write down or think through as much as you can about the scene. Now turn back to the cartoon. How did you do? Was everything you recalled accurate? Because researchers understand that people may not be able to report 'the truth', even when they genuinely wish to do so, they have focused a good deal of attention on the topic of *eyewitness memory*. The goal is to help the legal system discover the best methods for ensuring the accuracy of witnesses' memories.

Influential studies on eyewitness memory were carried out by Elizabeth Loftus (1979; Wells & Loftus, 2003) and her colleagues. The general conclusion from their research was that eyewitnesses' memories for what they had seen were quite vulnerable to distortion from *post-event information*. For example, participants in one study were shown a film of an automobile accident and were asked to estimate the speeds of the cars involved (Loftus & Palmer, 1974). However, some participants were asked, 'How fast were the cars going when they smashed into each other?' while others were asked, 'How fast were the cars going when they contacted each other?' *Smash* participants estimated the cars' speed to have been over 40 miles [60 kilometres] per hour; *contact* participants estimated the speed at 30 miles [almost 50 kilometres] per hour. About a week later, all the eyewitnesses were asked, 'Did you see any broken glass?' In fact, no broken glass had appeared in the film. However, about a third of the *smash* participants reported that there had been glass, whereas only 14 percent of the *contact* eyewitnesses did so. Thus post-event information had a substantial effect on what eyewitnesses reported they had experienced.

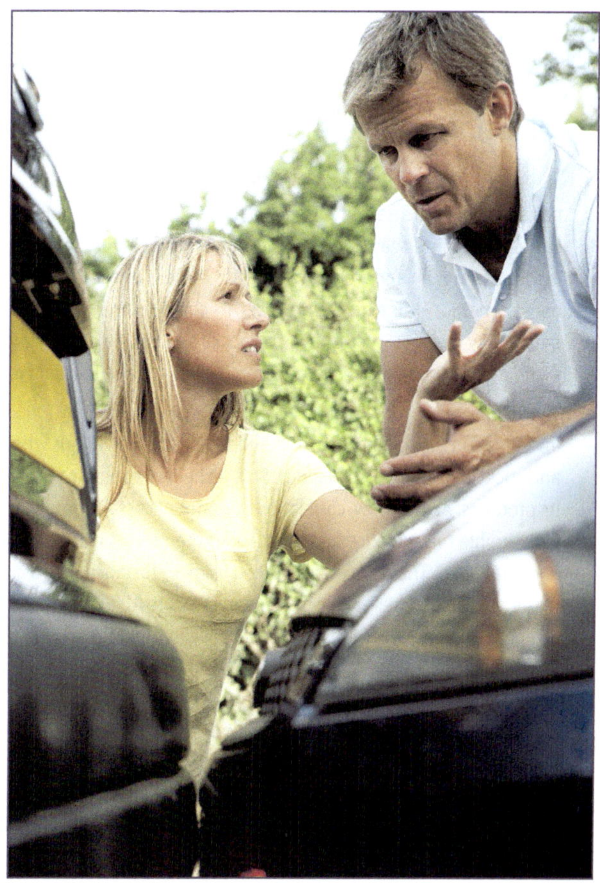

Why might the different words eyewitnesses use to describe an accident affect their later recall?
(**Source:** © 2011 www.photostogo.com.au/www.photolibrary.com.au/all rights reserved.)

This experiment represents what is probably the real-life experience of most eyewitnesses: after the events, they have a lot of opportunities to acquire new information that can interact with their original memories. In fact, Loftus and her colleagues demonstrated that participants often succumb to a *misinformation effect* (Loftus, 2005). For example, in one study participants watched a slide show of a traffic accident. They were then asked a series of questions. For half of the participants, one question was 'Did another car pass the red Datsun while it was stopped at the stop sign?' For the other half, the question read, 'Did another car pass the red Datsun while it was stopped at the yield sign?' The original slide show displayed a stop sign. Still, when participants were asked to recognise the original slide between options with a stop sign or a yield (give way) sign, those who had been asked about the stop sign were 75 percent correct, whereas those who had been asked about a yield sign were only 41 percent correct (Loftus et al., 1978). That's a large impact of misinformation.

A team of researchers sought to demonstrate that people's memory performance can be harmed if they discuss events with co-witnesses (Hope et al., 2008). The researchers also wished to assess the impact of the relationship between the co-witnesses by using pairs that were strangers, friends or romantic partners. The participants watched a video of a girl entering an office at a university. The events were filmed from two different angles so that some actions (such as the girl's theft of money) were visible from one angle but not the other. The members of each pair watched one or the other versions of the events. They then worked their way through a questionnaire that asked them to recall the events as if 'they were real witnesses waiting for the police to arrive' (p. 478). Finally, the participants completed separate memory questionnaires that instructed them to report only information that they themselves had witnessed. Even so, when participants interacted with strangers, 29 percent reported information they had obtained from their co-witness. When participants interacted with friends or romantic partners, 58 percent reported such information.

This experiment suggests that, after discussing events with co-witnesses, people may find it difficult to isolate their own eyewitness memories from what they have learned from others. This may be particularly the case if they have a prior relationship with the co-witnesses. Such results are important because, when people testify in court, they swear to report only information they obtained from their own experience of the events.

Psychology in your life

Why does Alzheimer's disease affect memory?

In the past 15-20 years, researchers have acquired a deeper understanding of how memories are formed in the brain. This knowledge has allowed for focused attention on *Alzheimer's disease*—a biological condition in which memory function gradually breaks down. In Australia, this disease afflicts approximately one in ten people over the age of 65 and three in ten people over the age of 85 (Australian Institute of Health and Welfare, 2012). Alzheimer's disease onset is deceptively mild—in early stages the only observable symptom may be memory impairment. However, its course is one of steady deterioration. Individuals with Alzheimer's disease may show gradual personality changes, such as apathy, lack of spontaneity, and withdrawal from social interactions. In advanced stages, people with Alzheimer's disease may become completely mute and inattentive, even forgetting the names of their spouse and children.

The symptoms of Alzheimer's disease were first described in 1906 by the German psychiatrist Alois Alzheimer. In those earliest investigations, Alzheimer noted that the brains of individuals who had died from the disease contained unusual tangles of neural tissue and sticky deposits called plaques. Still, Alzheimer could not determine whether those brain changes were the cause of the disease or its products. As we know, correlation does not necessarily imply causation.) Only in the past 15 to 20 years have researchers been able to assemble the evidence that the plaques themselves cause the brain to deteriorate (Esler & Wolfe, 2001; Hardy & Selkoe, 2002; Ono & Yamada, 2011). The plaques are formed from a substance called *amyloid* b-*peptide* (Ab). Ordinary processes in the human brain that aid in the growth and maintenance of neurons create Ab as a by-product. Normally, Ab dissolves in the fluid surrounding neurons, without any consequences. However, in Alzheimer's disease, Ab becomes deadly to neurons: Ab forms plaques and causes brain cells to self-destruct (Marx, 2001).

This understanding of the role of Ab in the progress of Alzheimer's disease has led to important recent breakthroughs. For example, researchers are beginning to improve their ability to diagnose the disease. As we know, human ageing is accompanied by some ordinary changes in memory function. To make a timely diagnosis of Alzheimer's disease, doctors need a way to determine whether older adults' memory impairments are something more than ordinary change. For most of the past 100 years that was a difficult task. Alzheimer's disease could be definitively diagnosed only when doctors could see the patients' brains—something that was not possible while the patients were living. However, researchers have begun to develop applications of PET scans that enable them to detect the presence of Ab in the living brain (Helmuth, 2002). The key advance was the manufacture of a radioactive marker that attaches itself to the Ab plaques. This radioactive marker becomes visible through PET scans—providing a mechanism for early diagnosis of ominous patterns of Ab in the brain.

Early diagnosis would allow early treatment, with the goal of minimising the negative impact of the disease. Although scientists are pursuing a number of preventive measures and treatments, several lines of research once again focus on Ab (Travis, 2005; Ono & Yamada, 2011). For example, researchers are seeking methods to interrupt the biochemical processes that produce Ab in the first place. They are also exploring techniques to destroy the Ab plaques once they have begun to form. Taken together, these approaches hold out great hope that Alzheimer's disease will be less devastating for future generations.

We have now considered several important features of the encoding, storage and retrieval of information. In the final section of the chapter, we discuss the brain bases of these memory functions.

Stop and review

1. What is the relationship between categories and concepts?
2. What claim is made by the exemplar theory of categorisation?
3. On Frederic Bartlett's account, what three processes create distortions in reconstructive memory?
4. How did Elizabeth Loftus and her colleagues demonstrate misinformation effects?

Critical thinking

Recall the study that investigated the typicality of fish. Why might the researchers have used two groups from the same geographical region?

Biological aspects of memory

The time has come, once again, for us to ask you to recall the number you committed to memory at the beginning of the chapter. Can you still remember it? What was the point of this exercise? Think for a minute about biological aspects of your ability to look at an arbitrary piece of information and commit it instantly to memory. How can you do that? To encode a memory requires that you instantly change something inside your brain. If you wish to retain that memory for at least the length of a chapter, the change must have the potential to become permanent. Have you ever wondered how this is possible? Our excuse for having you recall an arbitrary number was so that we could ask you to reflect on how remarkable the biology of memory really is. Let's take a closer look inside the brain.

Searching for the engram

Let's consider your memory for the number 46 or, more specifically, your memory that the number 46 was the number we asked you to remember. How could we determine where in your brain that memory resides? Karl Lashley (1929, 1950), who performed pioneering work on the anatomy of memory, referred to this question as the search for the **engram**, the physical memory representation. Lashley trained rats to learn mazes, removed varying-size portions of their cortexes, and then retested their memories for the mazes. Lashley found that memory impairment from brain lesioning was proportional to the amount of tissue removed. The impairment grew worse as more of the cortex was damaged. However, memory was not affected by *where* in the cortex the tissue was removed. Lashley concluded that the elusive engram did not exist in any localised regions but was widely distributed throughout the entire cortex.

Engram The physical memory trace for information in the brain.

Perhaps Lashley could not localise the engram partly because of the variety of types of memories that are called into play even in an apparently simple situation. Remember that rats are trained to run mazes for a food reward, so maze learning, in fact, involves complex interactions of spatial, visual and olfactory signals. Neuroscientists believe that memory for complex sets of information is distributed across many neural systems, even though discrete types of knowledge are separately processed and localised in limited regions of the brain (Fuster, 2009; Roth, Serences & Courtney, 2006).

Five major brain structures are involved in memory:

- the *cerebellum*, which is essential for procedural memory, memories acquired by repetition, and classically conditioned responses
- the *striatum*, which is a complex of structures in the forebrain and the likely basis for habit formation and for stimulus-response connections
- the *cerebral cortex*, responsible for sensory memories and associations between sensations
- the *hippocampus*, which is largely responsible for declarative memory of facts, dates and names, and the consolidation of spatial memories
- the *amygdala*, which plays a critical role in the formation and retrieval of memories of emotional significance.

Other parts of the brain, such as the thalamus, the basal forebrain and the prefrontal cortex, are involved also as way stations for the formation of particular types of memories (see Figure 3.16).

Let us take a look at the methods that neuroscientists use to draw conclusions about the role of specific brain structures for memory. We will examine two types of research. First, we consider the insights generated by 'experiments of nature'—circumstances in which individuals who have suffered brain damage volunteer to further memory research. Second, we describe the ways in which researchers are applying new brain-imaging techniques to improve their understanding of memory processes in the brain.

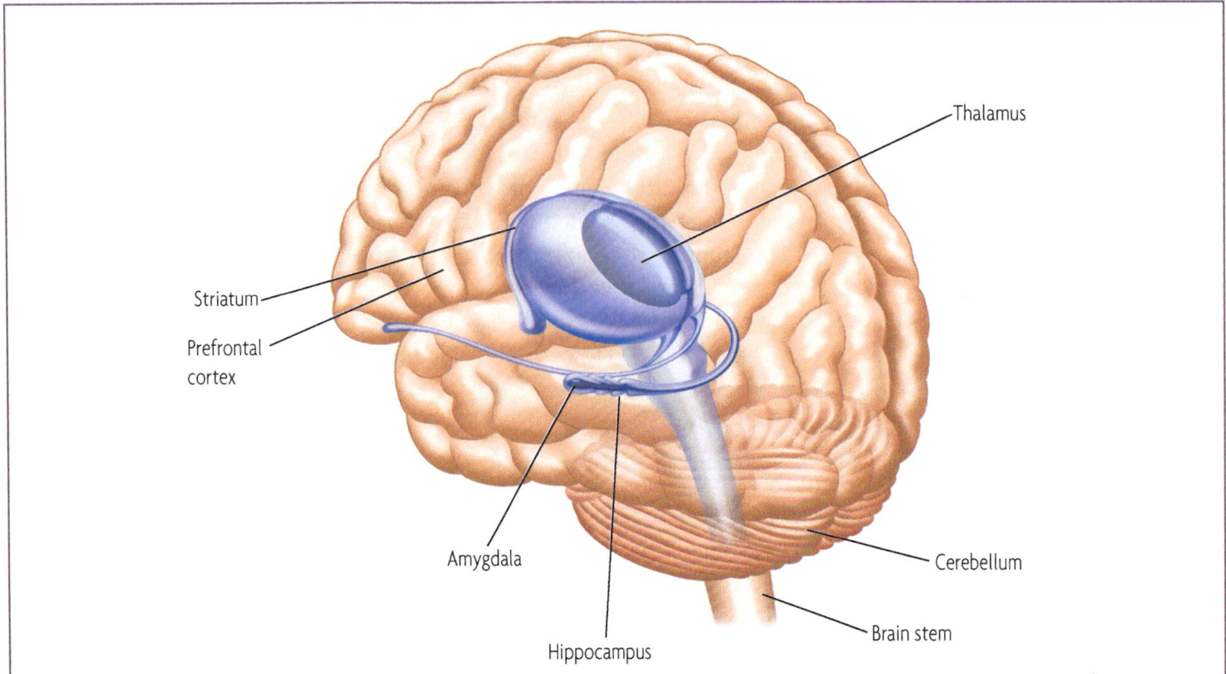

Figure 3.16 Brain structures involved in memory

This simplified diagram shows some of the main structures of the brain that are involved in the formation, storage and retrieval of memories.

Amnesia

In 1960, Nick A., a young air force radar technician, experienced a freak injury that permanently changed his life. Nick had been sitting at his desk while his roommate played with a miniature fencing foil. Then, suddenly, Nick stood up and turned around—just as his buddy happened to lunge with the miniature sword. The foil pierced Nick's right nostril and continued to cut upwards and backwards into the left side of his brain. The accident left Nick seriously disoriented. His worst problem was **amnesia,** the failure of memory over a prolonged period. Because of Nick's amnesia, he forgets many events immediately after they happen. After he reads a few paragraphs of writing, the first sentences slip from his memory. He cannot remember the plot of a television show unless, during commercials, he actively thinks about and rehearses what he was just watching. However, Nick has perfectly normal recall of events up to, and including, his brain injury. His memory problem is marked by an almost total inability to learn any *new* information—existing memories, acquired before the injury, are still well preserved.

Amnesia
A failure of memory caused by physical injury, disease, drug use or psychological trauma.

Anterograde amnesia
An inability to form explicit memories for events that occur after the time of physical damage to the brain.

Retrograde amnesia
An inability to retrieve memories from the time before physical damage to the brain.

The particular type of amnesia from which Nick suffers is called **anterograde amnesia**. This means that Nick can no longer form explicit memories for events that occur after the time at which he suffered physical damage. Other patients suffer from *retrograde* amnesia. In those cases, brain damage prevents access to memories that preceded the moment of injury. If you've ever had the misfortune of receiving a sharp blow to the head (during, for example, a car crash), you're likely to have experienced **retrograde amnesia** for the events leading up to the accident.

Researchers are grateful to patients like Nick for allowing themselves to be studied as 'experiments of nature'. By relating the locus of brain injuries like Nick's to patterns of performance deficit, researchers have begun to understand the mapping between the types of memories we have introduced you to in this chapter and regions of the brain (O'Connor

& Lafleche, 2005). Nick still remembers how to do things—his procedural knowledge appears to be intact even in the absence of declarative knowledge. So, for example, he remembers how to mix, stir and bake the ingredients in a recipe, but he forgets what the ingredients are.

The selective impairment of explicit memory of the sort demonstrated by Nick strongly suggests that different regions of the brain are involved for different types of encoding and retrieval. For that reason, damage to a single brain region may impair one memory process but not another. Researchers have demonstrated this type of dissociation by contrasting explicit and implicit uses of memory.

Twenty people with amnesia and 21 control individuals participated in a study that assessed their explicit and implicit memory ability (Verfaelli et al., 2006). In the experiment, participants read aloud word pairs such as *moss–newspaper* and also read statements that provided a relation between the words, such as: 'Adding moss to compost helps decompose newspaper.' Later, the participants performed explicit and implicit memory tasks. For the explicit task, participants were presented with the first word in each pair and asked to recall the second. By comparison to the control individuals, the people with amnesia performed quite poorly on this explicit task. For the implicit memory task, participants were given the first word from a pair (e.g., *moss* or *banana*) and then asked to generate four words from a category (such as 'reading material'). Both the control individuals and the people with amnesia were more likely to generate words as examples of categories if they had seen the word earlier in the experiment. This result illustrates that the people with amnesia were able to acquire new information. However, the responses of the people with amnesia didn't show evidence that they learned any new associations. For example, if participants had encoded a new association between *moss* and *newspaper*, we would expect that they would be even more likely to generate *newspaper* among their four examples of 'reading material' than they would have been without that association. In fact, the control individuals generated *newspaper* more often in the context of *moss*—but the people with amnesia did not.

This experiment demonstrates some of the subtle differences between the implicit memory processes that are spared and disrupted when people experience anterograde amnesia. People with amnesia are able to learn information about single items (so that, for example, *newspaper* is more accessible when they provide examples of 'reading material'). However, implicit memory processes do not generally allow people with amnesia to learn new associations.

The cases in which people lose the ability to recall past information or acquire new information are the most dramatic forms of memory disorders. However, people experience less extensive memory disruptions as a result of injury or disease. For example, the 'Psychology in your life' box describes the progressive course of Alzheimer's disease. Researchers study individuals who are at high risk for Alzheimer's disease to understand the biological basis for successive changes in memory function (Murphy et al., 2008). Researchers often seek out people who have damage in particular brain regions to test specific theories about the biology of memory processes. Recall, for example, our discussion of metamemory, which revealed that people's feeling-of-knowing judgements are often reasonably accurate. Researchers suggested that regions of the prefrontal cortex (PFC) (see Figure 3.16) provide the brain basis for those judgements (Modirrousta & Fellows, 2008). To test that claim, the researchers identified five individuals who had damage in those PFC regions. These individuals with PFC damage and matched controls all tried to learn new associations between faces and names. Even when the two participant groups performed equally well on a recognition test, the individuals with PFC damage were consistently less accurate on their feeling-of-knowing judgements. This experiment supports the claim that the prefrontal cortex plays a role in metamemory. It also provides an example of the value of research that examines more subtle forms of memory disorder.

Brain imaging

Psychologists have gained a great deal of knowledge about the relationship between anatomy and memory from the amnesic patients who generously serve as participants in these experiments. However, the advent of brain-imaging techniques has enabled researchers to study memory processes in individuals without brain damage (Nyberg & Cabeza, 2000). For example, using positron emission tomography (PET), Endel Tulving and his colleagues (Habib et al., 2003) have identified a difference in activation between the two brain hemispheres in the encoding and retrieval of episodic information. Their studies parallel standard memory studies, except that the participants' cerebral blood flow is monitored through PET scans during encoding or retrieval. As you can see in Figure 3.17, these researchers discovered disproportionately high brain activity in the left prefrontal cortex for encoding of episodic information and in the right prefrontal cortex for retrieval of episodic information. Thus the processes show some anatomical distinctions in addition to the conceptual distinctions made by cognitive psychologists.

Research with functional magnetic resonance imaging (fMRI) has also provided remarkable detail about the way that memory operations are distributed in the brain. For example, studies with fMRI have begun to identify the specific brain regions that are activated when new memories are formed. Consider a study in which participants underwent fMRI scans while watching an episode of the sitcom 'Curb Your Enthusiasm' that was new to them (Hasson et al., 2008). Over the course of 27 minutes, the main character engaged in a series of events such as attending a dinner party and arguing with friends. Three weeks later, the participants returned to the laboratory to take a 77-question memory test on the episode. Each participant remembered some details but not others. The researchers analysed the fMRI data to identify those brain regions that were particularly active when information was successfully encoded. As shown in Figure 3.18, several brain regions emerged from that analysis. Unless you pursue studies in cognitive neuroscience, you needn't worry why it is

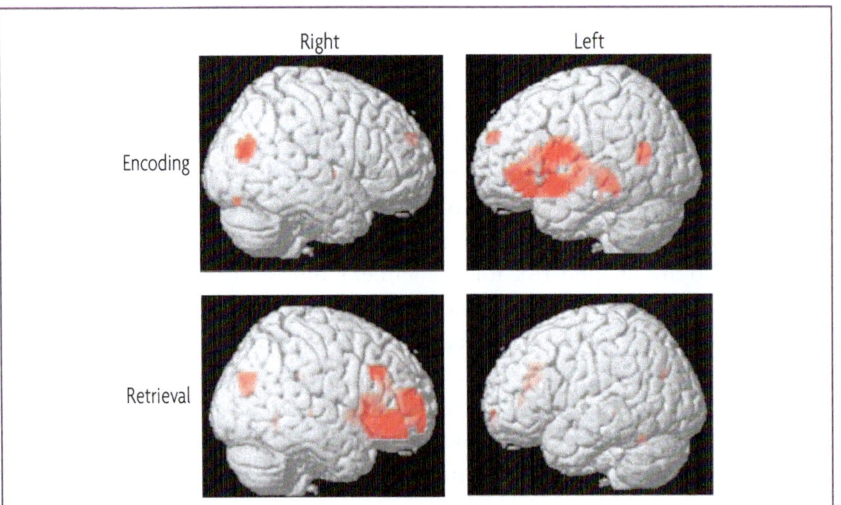

Figure 3.17 Brain activity for encoding and retrieval

The figure displays the regions of the brain that were most highly activated for encoding versus retrieval. The PET scans display disproportionately high brain activity in the left prefrontal cortex for the encoding of episodic information and in the right prefrontal cortex for the retrieval of episodic information.

Reprinted from Habib, R., Nyberg, L. & Tulving, E. (2003). Brain activity for encoding versus retrieval. *Trends in Cognitive Sciences*, *7*(6), 241. Copyright © 2003 with permission from Elsevier.

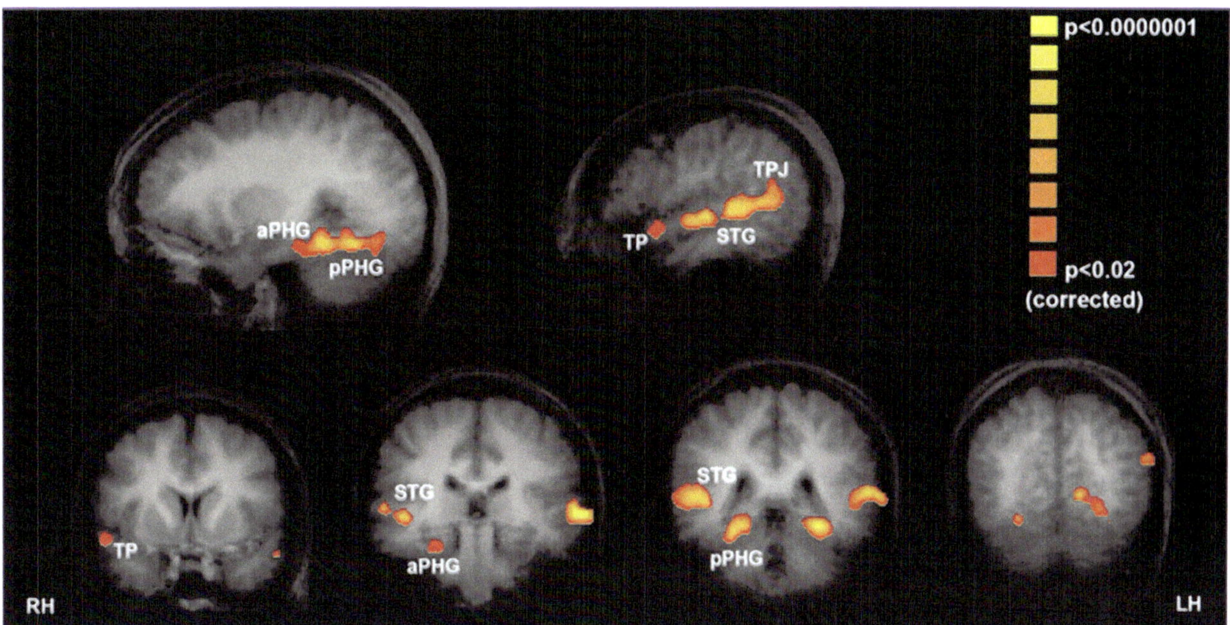

Figure 3.18 Brain regions that predict successful memory

When this set of brain regions was particularly active at time of encoding, people were more likely to remember details from their viewing of a sitcom. The areas are the right temporal pole (TP), superior temporal gyrus (STG), anterior parahippocampal cortex (aPHG), posterior parahippocampal gyrus (pPHG), and temporal parietal junction (TPJ). RH and LH refer to the right and left hemispheres.

Reprinted from Hasson, U. et al. (2008). Enhanced intersubject correlations during movie viewing correlate with successful episodic encoding. *Neuron, 57*(3), 11. Copyright © 2008 with permission from Elsevier.

activity in exactly this set of structures that predicts later recall. Figure 3.18 should suggest to you that researchers are making progress toward the goal of witnessing the birth and consolidation of new memories.

Brain scans also provide information about how memory processes unfold in time. If you try to recall the capital of New Zealand, the answer might present itself to you (or not) rather quickly. However, if you try to recall what happened the first time you met someone from New Zealand, you'll likely need more time to retrieve and elaborate that memory. For those sorts of rich autobiographical memories, the role of different regions of the brain changes over time.

A team of researchers asked participants to retrieve autobiographical memories while undergoing fMRI scans (Daselaar et al., 2008). Participants heard a cue word, such as *tree*, and attempted to bring a specific event to mind that was associated with the word. Participants pushed a button on a response box to indicate when they had retrieved a memory. Because this process unfolded over several seconds, the researchers were able to determine how different brain areas became involved in different aspects of autobiographical memory. For example, early on, structures like the hippocampus were active as participants searched their episodic memories. As participants elaborated their memories, activity in other areas became more prominent. For example, participants' visual cortex became more active as they enriched their memories with visual images. When the visual cortex was particularly active, participants reported the strongest sense that they were actually reliving the memory.

Take a moment to retrieve your own memory in response to *tree*. Do you feel your recollection of the event become more elaborate over time? The fMRI scans provide a moment-by-moment account of where and how that elaboration occurs in your brain.

The results from imaging studies illustrate why researchers from different disciplines must work closely together in the quest for a full understanding of memory processes. Psychologists provide the data on human performance that become fuel for neurophysiologists' detection of specialised brain structures. At the same time, the realities of physiology constrain psychologists' theories of the mechanisms of encoding, storage and retrieval. Through shared effort, scientists in these fields of research provide great insight into the operation of memory processes

Stop and review

1. What did Karl Lashley conclude about the location of the engram?
2. What has been learned about the impairment of implicit memory for individuals with amnesia?
3. What have PET studies indicated about the brain bases of encoding and retrieval of episodic information?

Critical thinking

Recall the study that looked at memory for sitcom details. Why was it important that participants hadn't seen the episode before?

[A]Gerrig, R. J., Zimbardo, P. G., Campbell, A. J., Cumming, S. R., & Wilkes, F. J. (Eds.). (2012). Memory. In *Psychology and life* (2nd ed., pp. 239–278). Frenchs Forest, NSW: Pearson Australia.

Summary

What is memory?

- Cognitive psychologists study memory as a type of information processing.
- Memories involving conscious effort are explicit. Unconscious memories are implicit.
- Declarative memory is memory for facts; procedural memory is memory for how to perform skills.
- Memory is often viewed as a three-stage process of encoding, storage and retrieval.

Memory use for the short term

- Iconic memory has large capacity but very short duration.
- Short-term memory (STM) has a limited capacity and lasts only briefly without rehearsal.
- Maintenance rehearsal can extend the presence of material in STM indefinitely.
- STM capacity can be increased by chunking unrelated items into meaningful groups.
- The broader concept of working memory includes STM.
- The four components of working memory provide the resources for moment-by-moment experiences of the world.

Long-term memory: encoding and retrieval

- Long-term memory (LTM) constitutes your total knowledge of the world and of yourself. It is nearly unlimited in capacity.
- Your ability to remember information relies on the match between circumstances of encoding and retrieval.
- Retrieval cues allow you to access information in LTM.
- Episodic memory is concerned with memory for events that have been personally experienced. Semantic memory is memory for the basic meaning of words and concepts.
- Similarity in context between learning and retrieval aids retrieval.
- The serial position curve is explained by distinctiveness in context.
- Information processed more deeply is typically remembered better.
- For implicit memories, it is important that the processes of encoding and retrieval be similar.
- Ebbinghaus studied the time course of forgetting.
- Interference occurs when retrieval cues do not lead uniquely to specific memories.
- Memory performance can be improved through elaborative rehearsal and mnemonics.
- In general, feelings-of-knowing accurately predict the availability of information in memory.

Structures in long-term memory

- Concepts are the memory building blocks of thinking. They are formed when memory processes gather together classes of objects or ideas with common properties.
- Concepts are often organised in hierarchies, ranging from general, to basic level, to specific.
- Schemas are more complex cognitive clusters.
- All these memory structures are used to provide expectations and a context for interpreting new information.
- Remembering is not simply recording but is a constructive process.
- People encode flashbulb memories in response to events with great emotional significance, but those memories may not be more accurate than everyday memories.
- New information can bias recall, making eyewitness memory unreliable when contaminated by post-event input.

Biological aspects of memory

- Different brain structures (including the hippocampus, the amygdala, the cerebellum, the striatum and the cerebral cortex) have been shown to be involved in different types of memories.
- Experiments with individuals with memory disorders have helped investigators understand how different types of memories are acquired and represented in the brain.
- Brain-imaging techniques have extended knowledge about the brain bases of memory encoding and retrieval.[A]

Review questions

A. Fill in the missing words to complete the following statements.

1. In reviewing the memory process, encoding gets information in, ____________ holds it until you need it, and ____________ gets it out
2. ____________ refers to the creation of more associations between a new memory and existing memories. When you are studying, and you tie in the concepts you are reading about in your textbook to events in your own life, you are ____________.

B. Read the following statements and answer with the most correct definition.

3. One technique to help overcome the limited capacity of STM is called ____________.
4. The process by which a mental representation is formed in memory is known as ____________.
5. The memory system in the visual domain that allows large amounts of information to be stored for very brief durations is known as ____________ memory.

C. Please select one statement that best answers each of the following questions.

6. Working memory is a special function of
   a) the sensory register
   b) short-term memory
   c) long term memory
   d) episodic memories
7. When you get to the grocery store, you realise you left your shopping list at home. According to the serial position effect, what items on the list are you most likely to recall?
   a) at the beginning of the list
   b) in the middle of the list
   c) at the end of the list
   d) a and c
8. An inability to store and/or retrieve new information in long-term memory is characteristic of
   a) anterograde amnesia
   b) retroactive amnesia
   c) schemas
   d) retrograde amnesia
9. A key brain structure that is often damaged in patients with anterograde amnesia is the
   a) cerebral cortex
   b) striatum
   c) hippocampus
   d) hypothalamus

D. Fill in the missing words and/or key concepts to complete the following diagram.

10.

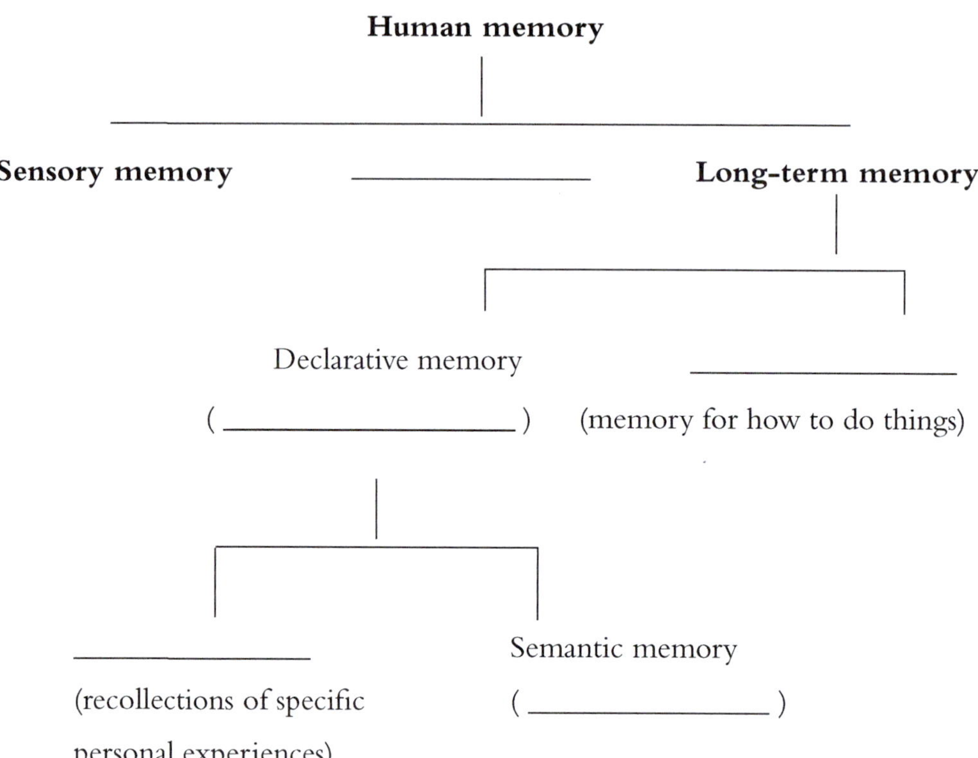

Chapter 4

Intelligence

The content in this section has been compiled from:

Maltby, Day, & Macaskill, Chapter 12

Maltby, J., Day, L., & Macaskill, A. (2013). Theories and measurement of intelligence. In J. Maltby, L. Day, & A. Macaskill (Eds.), *Personality, individual differences and intelligence* (3rd ed., pp. 279–297, 301). Harlow, Essex: Pearson Education.

Maltby, Day, & Macaskill, Chapter 13

Maltby, J., Day, L., & Macaskill, A. (2013). The use of intelligence tests: What question emerge from the measurement of intelligence. In J. Maltby, L. Day, & A. Macaskill (Eds.), *Personality, individual differences and intelligence* (3rd ed., pp. 306–307, 313–321). Harlow, Essex: Pearson Education.

Gerrig et al., Chapter 10

Gerrig, R. J., Zimbardo, P. G., Campbell, A. J., Cumming, S. R., & Wilkes, F. J. (2012). Intelligence and intelligence assessment. In R. J. Gerrig, & P. G. Zimbardo, A. J. Campbell, S. R. Cumming, & F. J. Wilkes (Eds.), *Psychology and life* (2nd ed., pp. 331–333). Frenchs Forest, NSW: Pearson Australia.

Maltby, Day, & Macaskill, Chapter 14

Maltby, J., Day, L., & Macaskill, A. (2013). The use of intelligence tests: What question emerge from the measurement of intelligence. In J. Maltby, L. Day, & A. Macaskill (Eds.), *Personality, individual differences and intelligence* (3rd ed., pp. 338–358, 370–371). Harlow, Essex: Pearson Education.

Maltby, Day, & Macaskill, Chapter 15

Maltby, J., Day, L., & Macaskill, A. (2013). Further discussions and debates in intelligence: Sex differences in intelligence and emotional intelligence. In J. Maltby, L. Day, & A. Macaskill (Eds.), *Personality, individual differences and intelligence* (3rd ed., pp. 391–408). Harlow, Essex: Pearson Education.

Maltby, Day, & Macaskill, Chapter 16

Maltby, J., Day, L., & Macaskill, A. (2013). The application of personality and intelligence in education and the workplace: The introduction of other intelligences. In J. Maltby, L. Day, & A. Macaskill (Eds.), *Personality, individual differences and intelligence* (3rd ed., pp. 410–422). Harlow, Essex: Pearson Education.

Chapter 4

Intelligence

Intelligence is derived from the Latin verb *intelligere*, meaning to comprehend or perceive. Put simply, it refers to an individual's ability to acquire and apply knowledge and skills. This chapter explores cognitive intelligence, and examines the history of intelligence testing, including the introduction and sometimes controversial use of intelligence tests. Later in this chapter, the importance of emotional intelligence and its application to work settings is presented. In health care, strong emotional intelligence can positively contribute to patient-health professional interactions, and substantially contribute to constructive consultations e.g., increased empathy and ability to identify patient emotions, can contribute to a greater repour and thus effective therapeutic outcomes.

After studying this chapter you should be able to:

- Describe early theorists in intelligence:
  - Galton
  - Binet
  - Terman
  - Yerkes
- Describe the theory of 'g' and alternative models
- Identify typical features and the application of intelligence tests
- Identify extremes of intelligence, including intellectual disability and learning disorders
- Describe genetic heritability and environmental influences of intelligence
- Describe models of emotional intelligence:
  - Salovey and Mayer
  - Goleman
  - Bar-On
- Understand the role and value that commonly known personality and intelligence tests have in predicting education and workplace achievements.

The birth of the psychology of intelligence: Galton and Binet

The modern foundations of intelligence theory and tests were formed just before the end of the nineteenth century through the work of two men: an Englishman, Francis Galton, and a Frenchman, Alfred Binet.

Galton

In 1865 Sir Francis Galton began to study heredity, after reading his cousin's (Charles Darwin) publication, *The Origin of Species*. Charles Darwin was the British naturalist (someone who studies natural history) who became famous for his theories of evolution and natural selection, which emphasised variations across species in nature. Following this work, Galton became interested in studying variations in human ability, and particularly intelligence. In particular, in his book *Hereditary Genius* (1869), Galton was convinced that higher intelligence was caused by superior qualities passed down to children by heredity. Much of this work was concerned with the hereditary nature of intelligence. What is important to theories and measurement of intelligence is that Galton was the first to be interested in showing that human beings did differ in intelligence.

Galton is the forefather of intelligence tests. His central hypothesis was that there were differences in intelligence, and he set out to explore this hypothesis. Galton maintained that it is possible to measure intelligence directly, and he used a variety of methods to provide such measures. His choices of measurements are based clearly on a biological background and on the thoughts of some of the early philosophers mentioned previously. Galton felt that intelligent people show the ability to respond to the large range of information experienced through the senses. However, he said that 'idiotic' people demonstrate problems dealing with information gained through the senses. Galton felt that people of low intelligence will show less response to sensory information, such as being unable to distinguish between heat and cold and being unable to recognise pain. Galton suggested several methods, such as reaction time, keenness of sight and hearing, the ability to distinguish between colours, eye judgement and strength, as a way to determine intelligence through responsiveness to stimuli. Therefore, he claimed that someone who has a slow reaction time, has poor sight and hearing, is unable to distinguish between colours and shows poor eye judgement can be considered unintelligent. Galton tested people at his Anthropometric Laboratory that was set up in the International Health Exhibition in 1884, where visitors to the exhibition could take the tests.

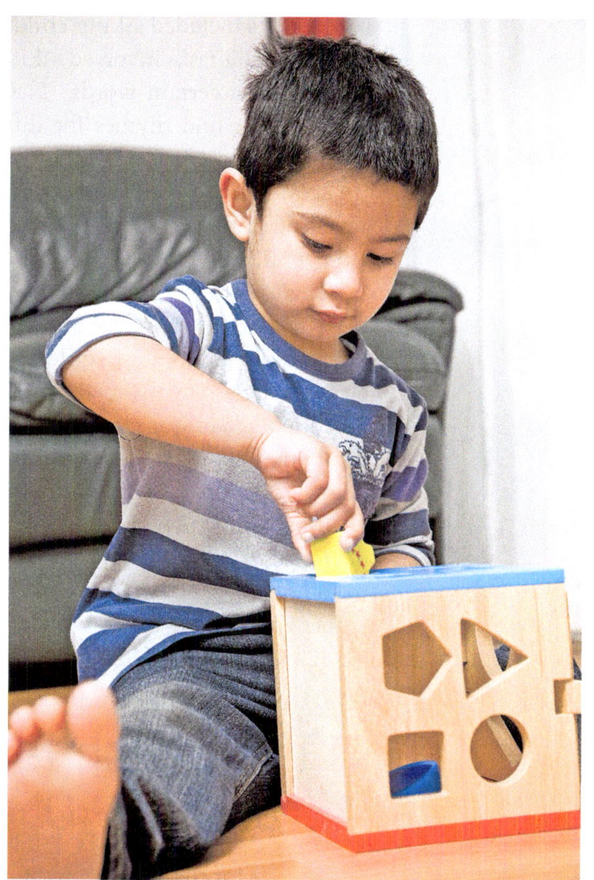

Early IQ tests involved elementary tasks.
(**Source:** Pearson Education Ltd. Lisa Payne Photography)

Perhaps it is easy to scoff at the reliability and validity of some of these measures. Clearly, poor eyesight does not determine poor intelligence, but is the result of a problem with the eyes. However, some of the measures that Galton developed, such as reaction time, are still used today. Galton's work presented the first attempt to measure intelligence directly.

Binet

Alfred Binet created the first intelligence test. In 1904, the French Ministry of Public Instruction commissioned him to provide techniques for identifying children at a primary age whose lack of success or ability might lead them to require special education. In 1905, with Theodore Simon, Binet produced the Binet–Simon scale, the first intelligence test, which Simon later described as 'practical, convenient, and rapid', that went on to be used with around 50 children.

To develop their test, Binet and Simon chose a series of 30 short tasks related to everyday life. This intelligence test included these tasks:

- following a lighted match with your eyes;
- shaking hands;
- naming parts of the body;
- counting coins;
- naming objects in a picture;
- recalling a number of digits after being shown a long list;
- word definitions;
- filling in missing words in a sentence.

The test questions were arranged in an increasing degree of difficulty to indicate levels of intelligence. The easiest of the tasks were tasks such as whether a child could follow a lighted match with their eyes; these tasks were expected to be completed by all children. Slightly harder tasks included asking children to name certain body parts or repeat simple sentences. More difficult tasks involved asking children to reproduce a drawing or construct a sentence that included certain words. The hardest tasks required children to repeat seven random digits and to find rhymes for difficult words. Each level of test was designed to match a specific developmental level for children based on ages ranging from 3 to 10 years old. The Binet–Simon test could be used to determine a child's 'mental age' and whether a child was advanced or backward for their age. A child of 7 who passed the tests designed for a 7-year-old but failed the tests for an 8-year-old would be assigned a mental age of 7.

This use of age in psychological testing is one of Binet's lasting contributions to psychology. Within Binet's system, age among children could be used as a criterion of intelligence. That is, the Binet–Simon test could determine what level in an intelligence test children should be attaining at any given age. You will certainly have come across this idea at school with the idea of reading age, in which children are judged on their ability in reading in relation to where they should be at a certain age (this is applied to the sales of books; for example, the Harry Potter series is determined as having a reading age of 9–11 years).

Binet and Simon's intelligence test was a turning point in psychology. Not only did they devise a test, but they devised a test in which the performance of the child was compared to the performance of children of the same age. The final publication of tests was in 1911 (Binet and Simon, 1911), with not only tests for 3- to 10-year-olds, but some further tests for 12- and 15-year-olds and adults.

The search for measurement continues: the birth of 'IQ' and standardised testing

The search for the measurement of intelligence then shifted to the United States. It is here that we see the growth of the measurement of intelligence, the birth of the intelligence quotient (IQ), standardised testing, cultural considerations and time limits on taking an intelligence test.

Terman

The first notable development was made when Lewis Terman of Stanford University in the United States decided to use the Binet–Simon test among California schoolchildren. He found that the age norms that Binet and Simon had devised for children in France didn't work very well for schoolchildren in California. So Terman revised the test, adapting some of the items and writing 40 new items. In 1916 Terman introduced the Stanford–Binet test, which was applicable for use with children aged from 4 to 14 years.

Items on the test were similar to Binet and Simon's test. At 4 years, children would be asked to do things such as: (1) compare two horizontal lines and say which is longer; (2) copy a square; and (3) find a shape that matches a target shape. At 9 years, a child would be asked to do things such as: (1) show awareness of dates, including what day of the week it is and what year; (2) arrange weights from highest to lowest; and (3) be able to do some mental arithmetic.

Terman went on to use the test with over 1,000 children aged from 4 to 14, which was a much larger group than the 50 children used by Binet. Terman was able to gain far more accurate information on how children typically scored on intelligence tasks because he had a much more representative sample of children. This issue of researchers using representative samples to determine accurate and representative scores was the beginning of recognising the need for 'standardised testing'. That is, to assess one child by comparing them with other children, researchers need to ensure that data they have on other children is representative so the assessment of the one child is fair.

One of the main advances towards standardised testing was made at this time. In 1912 a German psychologist, William Stern, developed the idea of the intelligence quotient, or, as it is more popularly known today, IQ. Stern had been using Binet's intelligence test in Germany. While studying scores on Binet's test, Stern noticed that 'mental' age varied among children proportionally to their real age. So, for example, if a child who at the age of 6 years scores 1 year below their age on the test and has a mental age of 5, then when they are 10 years of age, they will have a mental age of 8 – two years below their real age. Stern discovered that if the mental age were divided by the chronological age, the ratio was fairly constant (as shown in the following example). He named the ratio of the mental age divided by the chronological age the intelligence quotient (IQ).

In its fullest sense, the definition of IQ is (mental age ÷ chronological age) × 100.

This calculation set an IQ of 100 as an average intelligence. That is, if a child of 8 takes an intelligence test and receives a score that indicates a mental age of 8, they would have an IQ of 100 (8 divided by 8 = 1, and 1 multiplied by 100 = 100). An IQ score of 100 indicates that a child is performing at the expected age, and 100 sets the standard by which children are then compared. This allows children to be compared not only across a particular age group but also across ages. A child who is 8 and has the mental age of a child of 10 will have an IQ of 125 (10 divided by 8 = 1.25; 1.25 multiplied by 100 = 125). A child who is 10 years old and has a mental age of 6 will have an IQ of 60 (6 divided by 10 = 0.60; 0.60 multiplied by 100 = 60).

Let us use the imaginary scores given in Table 4.1 to show how IQ is calculated. As we can see from our example table, the child who scored the mental age scores at the following ages based on Stern's findings (mental age of 5 at 6 years, mental age of 8 at 10 years and mental age of 11 at 14 years) would score an IQ of around 80 over their childhood (between 79 and 83).

Table 4.1 Example of Stern's ratio of real age to mental age, used to develop his concept of intelligence quotient (IQ)

Mental age	Chronological age	Ratio (mental age ÷ chronological age)
5	6	0.83
8	10	0.80
11	14	0.79

Terman adopted this procedure for calculating IQ based on his test. Using this procedure, together with the items of the Stanford–Binet test and the need to obtain large and representative samples to develop age 'norms' for the test, the Stanford–Binet had developed into an intelligence test against which all other tests were compared.

Yerkes

The demand for intelligence tests quickly increased. In 1917 the United States entered the First World War, and a committee was appointed by the American Psychological Association to consider ways in which psychology could help the war effort. Head of this committee was Robert Yerkes, then President of the American Psychological Association (although the committee included Terman) and also a US Army major. The committee was quick to realise that psychology could help the Army because assessing the intelligence of recruits would enable the Army to classify and assign soldiers to suitable tasks. However, it was also realised that such an exercise would involve a huge number of people and that the sorts of tests developed by Binet and Terman were not suitable as they were time-intensive. That is, an experimenter had to sit down with the subject and take them through five or six tasks. The committee decided that what was needed was a test that could be completed simultaneously by a number of people, administered by one examiner. Yerkes' aim was to develop group intelligence testing.

Yerkes, alongside a staff of 40 psychologists (including Terman), developed two group intelligence tests, known as the Army Alpha and Army Beta tests. The Army Alpha was designed for literate groups and the Army Beta was designed for illiterates, low literates or non-English-speaking groups.

The army alpha test

The Alpha test battery for literates included the testing of a variety of cognitive abilities by examining the person's knowledge base in both oral language and written language. The Alpha test included eight tests of an individual's ability to:

- follow oral directions, involving the comprehension of simple and complex oral language directions;
- solve arithmetical problems, showing knowledge of arithmetic and the ability to perform simple computations;
- show practical judgement, involving the ability to make the 'correct' choice on a scenario presented to the individual;
- use synonyms and antonyms, knowledge of the 'same' and 'opposite' of words;
- rearrange disarranged sentences, such as 'I back it and door ran to the opened';
- complete an uncompleted series of numbers (1, 2, 4, 8, 16, . . .);
- see analogies, which requires the ability to see a similarity between two things that are otherwise dissimilar;
- demonstrate information, an examination of the person's everyday knowledge base.

The administration of each of the eight subtests was designed to be completed within a certain time.

The army beta test

The Beta test was an intelligence test comparable to the Alpha but freed of the influences of literacy and the English language. People who were non-English speakers or poor at speaking English, or those who typically had less than 6 years of experience in speaking the English language, were sent to Beta testing. Furthermore, those who had tried the Alpha test but were later judged to be poor readers, were retested using the Beta test.

The Beta test instructions were given by the tester and their aides by making hand signals. The examiners recorded responses. The Beta test included seven tests of ability in which the participants had to:

- complete a maze task, by finding the best route to be taken on a picture of a maze;
- complete a cube analysis, by counting cubes in a graphic representation;
- read an X–O series of graphic displays in left-to-right sequences;
- complete a test using digit symbols, requiring scanning and matching of numbers to symbols;
- complete a test using number symbols, requiring scanning and matching of symbols to numbers;
- complete a picture by looking at an uncompleted picture and using given objects to complete the picture (a little like a jigsaw);
- undertake geometrical construction, which involved working with graphics information and mentally rearranging it to construct a figure.

Again, like the Alpha test, the administration of each Beta subtest was completed within a certain time.

For each test, to determine each person's intelligence level, scores for all subtests were combined into one total score. Based on the total score, each individual was assigned a category based on a letter grade. A letter grade of A suggested superior intelligence; B, C+, C meant average intelligence, and C–, D, D– were considered as signifying inferior intelligence. The letter grade indicated the person's mental intelligence and was taken as a general indicator of the person's native intelligence.

In the end, Yerkes and his colleagues tested over 1.75 million people. This work was not completed until late in the war, and the work actually had little effect on the war effort; however, it did a lot to raise the status of psychology and the profile and potential usefulness of intelligence testing. For example, after the war, Yerkes received requests from the general public, business, industry and education for the intelligence test. In 1919 the National Intelligence Test was published and sold over half a million copies in its first year.

You can see that a growth in intelligence tests occurred from the work of Terman and Yerkes. Growth occurred not only in terms of what is measured and who can be measured but also: (1) in the number of people who can be measured at one time; (2) in developing an official way of scoring intelligence through IQ; and (3) in the consideration of culture and time limits on taking an intelligence test. These elements remain central to modern intelligence tests.

General intelligence (g): the theory and the measurement

Up to this point in the history of intelligence testing, approaches to intelligence had been very practical. Tests were developed for particular needs; that is, in response to French or American government demands. However, between 1904 and 1927, an English psychologist, Charles Spearman, introduced another way of conceptualising intelligence. He based his approach on the factor analysis of data (a technique for simplifying the relationships between a number of variables) that had already been collected. We will outline Spearman's research and theory of general intelligence and then introduce you to two measures of intelligence: the Wechsler and Raven's intelligence tests, which are designed to measure 'g'.

'g'

Charles Spearman (1904a; 1927), over the course of two publications – a journal article '"General Intelligence": Objectively determined and measured' and *The Abilities of Man*, introduced one of the most influential ideas in psychology, **general intelligence** or '**g**'.

General intelligence or 'g' A common factor measured by different intelligence tests.

In 1904 Spearman set out to estimate the intelligence of 24 children in the village school. Initially, Spearman used intelligence tests of memory, light, weight and sound in which participants were asked to identify changes in the illumination, weight and pitch of Spearman's instruments and perform memory tasks.

Spearman's first 24 participants were the oldest pupils of a village school in Berkshire. Spearman claimed that this sample was most favourable as it was within 100 yards of his own house, and all the families of the children resided in the immediate neighbourhood (perhaps the most convenient sample of what is known these days as 'convenience' sampling). Like other intelligence tests, the test was done on a one-to-one basis.

After this first experiment Spearman moved on to the next 36 oldest children in the school, and then to a local school which sent a lot of its pupils to Harrow (a well-known public school in the United Kingdom). Over a period of time, further data collections were taken among individuals who lived further from Spearman's home. Between 1904 and 1921, Spearman analysed the relationships between the data collected using a variety of intelligence tests and subjected them to factor analysis.

He found that his data indicated a trend towards positive correlations between intelligence tests. That is, a person who does well on one intelligence test will perform equally well on a variety of *intellectual* tests, be they tests concerned with vocabulary, mathematical or spatial (awareness of space and movement around oneself) abilities. Equally, if a person did poorly on one intelligence test, then they will also tend to perform poorly on other intellectual tasks. He called this positive correlation between tests the 'positive manifold'. Spearman used this idea of a positive manifold between intelligence tests to propose a two-factor theory of intelligence.

Specific abilities (s) Single aspects of intelligence.

The first factor of intelligence was **specific abilities**, or '**s**'. This was the name given to each type of intelligence needed for performing well on each different intelligence task that Spearman had observed. Therefore, vocabulary intelligence is a specific ability, mathematical intelligence is a specific ability and spatial intelligence is a specific ability.

The second factor was what Spearman thought was underlying all the positive correlations, and this was perhaps his most important and notable contribution to psychology: general intelligence, or 'g'. He argued that 'g' was underlying all the positive correlations: 'g' was the intelligence required for performance of intelligence tests of all types. Spearman envisaged 'g' as a kind of mental energy that underlies specific factors of intelligence. He saw it as a deeper fundamental mechanism which informed a number of intelligence abilities but was an intelligence also able to see relationships between objects, events and information and draw inferences from those relationships.

Spearman saw a person's ability in one specific ability test – for example, mathematical ability – as not only affected by one's specific ability to perform mathematical tasks but also as largely determined by that person's general intelligence. The main point of Spearman's findings was the idea of 'g', and this became a major theory that informs many subsequent approaches to intelligence. Proponents of general intelligence, or 'g', still exist amongst prominent psychologists.

Measuring 'g': the Wechsler and Raven's matrices

After Charles Spearman's introduction of his theory of intelligence, a central interest to intelligence developers was to develop a good measure of general intelligence, particularly among adults. Spearman's theory and research, together with the work of Terman and Yerkes, led to the development of more rigorous intelligence tests that could be used across the population to assess intelligence. However, there was some further work to be done. Both the Binet tests were primarily concerned with testing among children, and any testing done with adult samples involved relatively small samples. The Yerkes test was subject to a similar criticism. Although this test had been used with nearly one and a half million adults, they were all people who had applied to join the US Army. It was left for psychologists to devise intelligence tests that could be used to determine intelligence among the general population, and be used to assess a person's intelligence accurately in comparison to other people.

Two intelligence tests stand out in present psychology that show a historical move to standardised intelligence testing: the Wechsler test of intelligence and the Raven Matrices.

The Wechsler tests

David Wechsler was a US psychologist at Columbia University. In 1917 he had originally worked under the American Psychological Association/Yerkes' Army initiative and administered and interpreted intelligence tests that were used to assign army recruits to military jobs. During that time, the Army sent Wechsler to England and the University of London to work with Charles Spearman and Karl Pearson.

The history of what have now become known as the Wechsler tests spans the period from 1939 to the present day. Although Wechsler did not always agree with Spearman's view of intelligence, Wechsler's first tests were modelled on Spearman's two-factor model and Spearman's central position that intelligence covers a huge range of specific abilities that correlate within one another to form an overall measure of general intelligence (or 'g').

In 1939 Wechsler published the first of the Wechsler tests, the Wechsler–Bellevue Scale. The Wechsler–Bellevue Scale, unlike some former intelligence tests, was designed and standardised among a sample of 1,500 adults. However, in 1955 Wechsler introduced two tests:

- the Wechsler Adult Intelligence Scale (WAIS) that had been standardised among 2,000 adults aged between 16 and 75;
- the Wechsler Scale for Children (WISC) for children aged between 5 and 16 years.

As with the Binet tests, the Wechsler tests were administered on a one-to-one basis. Both Wechsler scales contained a number of subtests to measure several different aspects of intelligence, including verbal and performance tests such as:

- **Arithmetic (verbal)** – This subtest involves solving problems using mental arithmetic.
- **Block design (performance)** – In this subtest, the participant is presented with nine coloured blocks, each with two red, two white and two diagonally red and white sides. In this task the participant is asked to arrange the blocks to form certain patterns.
- **Comprehension (verbal)** – This subtest involves the participant demonstrating an understanding of the meaning of words and sayings, and the appropriate response to a number of scenarios (e.g. two trains are travelling in opposite directions 100 miles apart; one train is travelling at 40 miles an hour while the other is travelling at 60 miles an hour. How long before the two trains meet?).
- **Digit span (verbal)** – In this subtest the participant is asked to repeat a series of digits in exact or reverse order.
- **Digit symbol (performance)** – This subtest requires the participant to change symbols to numbers.
- **Information (verbal)** – This subtest requires the participant to show general knowledge of areas such as science, politics, geography, literature and history.
- **Object assembly (performance)** – This subtest requires a number of simple jigsaws to be completed within a particular time limit.

- **Picture arrangement (performance)** – In this subtest, participants are presented with a series of cards with a number of pictures. They must arrange the cards to tell a simple story.
- **Picture completion (performance)** – In this subtest, the participant has to complete line drawings of objects or scenes in which one or two lines are missing.
- **Similarities (verbal)** – This subtest involves the participant comparing two things that are alike.
- **Vocabulary (verbal)** – This subtest involves asking the participant for definitions of words.

Some examples from the Wechsler Adult Intelligence Scale are given in Figure 4.1.

(a)

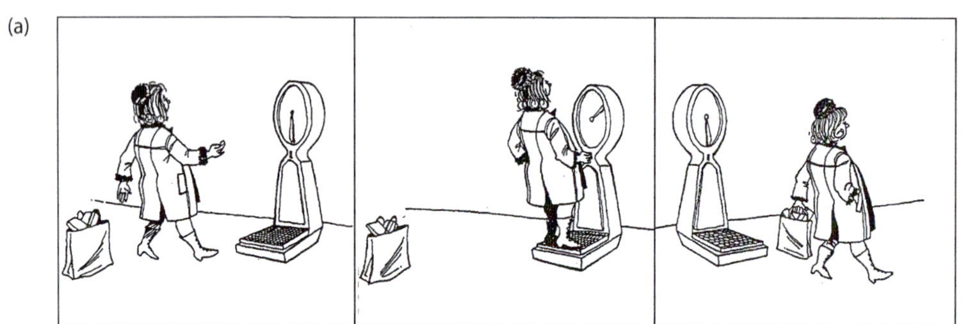

(b)

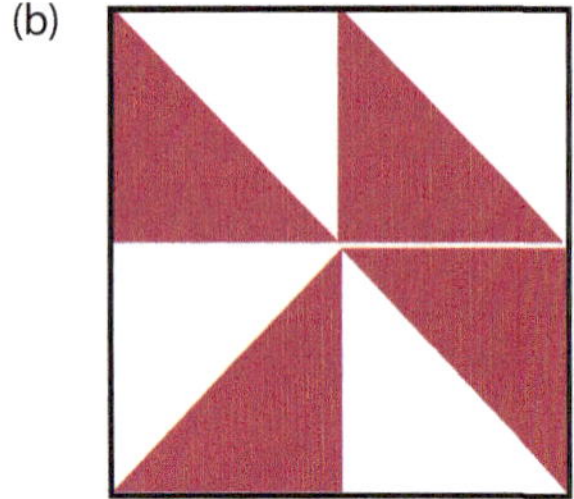

(c)

Item	Response
Q-3	3-Q
T-9-1	1-9-T
M-3-P-6	3-6-M-P
F-7-K-2-8	2-7-8-F-K
5-J-4-A-1-S	1-4-5-A-J-S
C-6-4-W-O-7-D	4-6-7-C-D-O-W

(d)

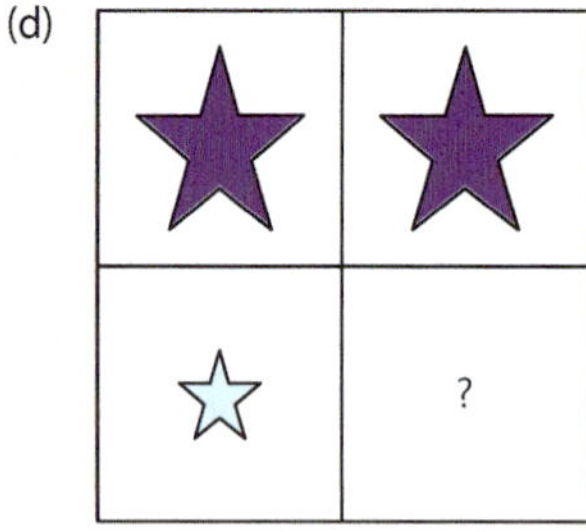

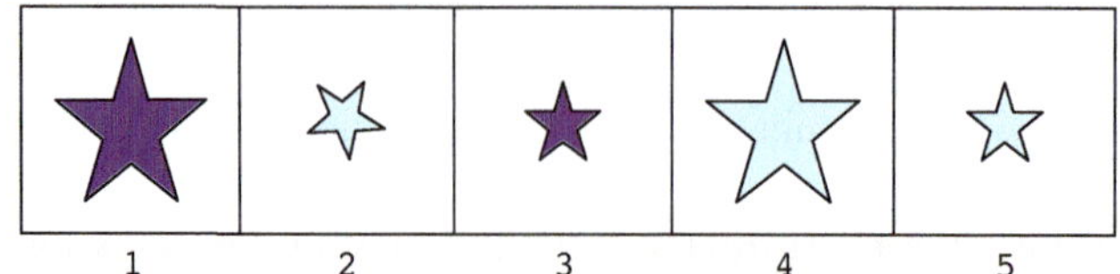

Figure 4.1 *(continues)*

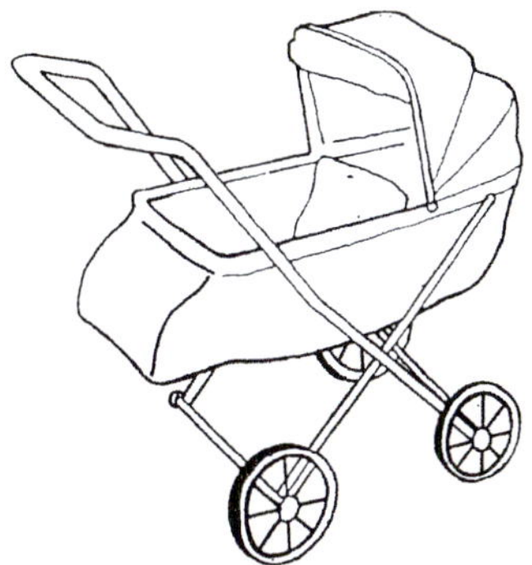

Paraphrased Wechsler-like Questions

Information

1 How many wings does a bird have?
2 How many nickels make a dime?
3 What is steam made of?
4 Who wrote *Tom Sawyer*?
5 What is pepper?

Comprehension

1 What should you do if you see someone forget his book when he leaves a restaurant?
2 What is the advantage of keeping money in a bank?
3 Why is copper often used in electrical wires?

Arithmetic

1 Sam had three pieces of candy and Joe gave him four more. How many pieces of candy did Sam have altogether?
2 Three women divided eighteen golf balls equally among themselves. How many golf balls did each person receive?
3 If two buttons cost $.15, what will be the cost of a dozen buttons?

Similarities

1 In what way are a lion and a tiger alike?
2 In what way are a saw and a hammer alike?
3 In what way are an hour and a week alike?
4 In what way are a circle and a triangle alike?

Vocabulary

This test consists simply of asking, 'What is a ____________?' or 'What does ____________ mean?' The words cover a wide range of difficulty.

Figure 4.1 (continued) Simulated items similar to those in the *Wechsler Adult Intelligence Scale*: picture arrangement (a), block design (b), letter-number sequencing (c), matrix reasoning (d), picture completion (e) and object assembly and Wechsler-like questions (f).
Source: *Wechsler Adult Intelligence Scale*, Third Edition (WAIS-III), Copyright © 1997 NCS Pearson, Inc. Reproduced with permission. All rights reserved. 'Wechsler Adult Intelligence Scale', 'WAIS' and 'Raven's Progressive Matrices and Vocabulary Scales' are trademarks, in the US and/or other countries, of Pearson Education, Inc. or its affiliate(s).

These scales are well-known tests that are still used today, although they have been revised. The Wechsler tests departed from previous intelligence tests in two important ways. First, the Wechsler scales were different from previous tests in that they were designed so that all people of all ages could take them. This was unlike Binet's test, which primarily required a 7-year-old to take tests designed for 7-year-olds, and 10-year-olds to take tests designed for 10-year-olds. Clearly, it would not have been useful or productive to design intelligence tests for all the years from early childhood to late adulthood. The Wechsler intelligence test includes a number of subtests for different aspects of intelligence, and within each subtest there are a variety of items with a wide range of difficulty. However, all participants are tested on the same items.

The second way in which the Wechsler tests differed from previous tests was the introduction of the concept of 'deviation IQ'. You will remember that Terman used the concept of IQ based on the mental age and the real age of the participant [(mental age ÷ chronological age) × 100]. However, Wechsler was primarily concerned with applying intelligence testing to adults, and the calculation that Terman used was not wholly applicable to adults. For example, let us apply Terman's method for calculating an average intelligence test score to adults. A 20-year-old and a 40-year-old take the same intelligence test and score in a way that indicates they are of the same mental age, thus the 40-year-old would appear to be half as intelligent as the 20-year-old (solely based on age). This problem stems from the fact that there is a huge range of years in adulthood as compared to childhood and that intelligence increases rapidly in childhood yet starts to level out in adulthood. Therefore, the challenge faced by Wechsler was to arrive at a fairer system of assessing IQ.

Wechsler's solution was not to define and score IQ based on mental and chronological age, but in terms of an individual's actual score on the intelligence test relative to the average scores obtained by others of the same age on the same intelligence test. The new formula for interpreting test scores in terms of deviation IQ was (actual test score ÷ expected score for that age) × 100.

However, this calculation involved two further steps to allow the standardisation in using the Wechsler IQ test: (1) determining the expected score for any particular age so all people could be compared; and (2) transforming the wide range of scores and variations among the population to a standardised form.

1. **Determining the expected score for a particular age.** Wechsler had to determine the average score on the intelligence test for all possible ages, so that it could be used effectively as a basis of comparison. To ensure that he had a reliable comparison, Wechsler collected data through stratified sampling, whereby sampling is based on randomly sampling individuals from mutually exclusive subgroups or strata of population (e.g. a certain number of 20-year-olds, 30-year-olds and so on). Wechsler ensured that he sampled people from various demographics, including social class, sex and region of the country. From this sampling Wechsler was able to establish intelligence norms for all ages.
2. **Transforming the wide range of scores and variations among the population to a standardised form.** You will remember that the original calculation of IQ was based on an observation by German intelligence tester William Stern that 'mental' age varies among children proportionally with their real age. It was this growth of mental age against chronological age that allowed Stern to make certain assumptions in calculating IQ. However, Wechsler could not make these assumptions. First, Wechsler was not surprised to find that mental age and chronological age do not grow or change proportionally. Rather, he found that mental age fluctuates (goes up, goes down, stays stable) compared with chronological age. He could not assume the proportional growth that Stern used in calculations.

Stop and think

IQ scores and the normal distribution

The introduction of mean scores to calculating IQ led to a complication of how IQ was calculated. Overall, researchers found that they were dealing with much more information by introducing numerous mean scores across a huge age range on an intelligence test (for example, 103.2 average IQ test score for 32-year-olds, 102.2 average IQ test scores for 33-year-olds and so on), rather than equally increasing absolute age over a limited time period (5–16 years). This result led to issues for allowing comparisons.

For example, if a company was interested in obtaining IQ scores in recruiting for jobs, then the present scoring system would be complicated. Suppose, for example, a recruiter has two candidates:

- Person A, aged 20 years, who scored 105 on the intelligence test; this was 10 points below the average for 20-year-olds (115 being the average intelligence test score among 20-year-olds).
- Person B, aged 25 years, who scored 100 on the intelligence test; this was 5 points below the average for 25-year-olds (105 being the average intelligence test score among 25-year-olds).

Who should the recruiter hire – the person with the highest IQ (Person A) or the person who scores nearest to the average for their age (Person B)?

Wechsler realised that he had to standardise the scoring of IQ. He had to find a way of comparing all these different scores and still provide a standardised scoring system. To do this, Wechsler used the normal distribution curve. You may remember from your statistics classes that a normal distribution curve (see Figure 4.2) is the symmetrical distribution of scores in a curve, with most of the scores situated in the centre and then spreading out, showing progressively lower frequency of scores for the higher and lower values.

What is particularly notable about this approach is that researchers have found that many of the variables measuring human attitudes and behaviour follow a normal distribution curve. This finding is one of statistics' more interesting elements. Statisticians and researchers are often not certain why many variables fall into a normal distribution; they have just found that many attitudes and behaviours do, including intelligence.

However, statisticians have noted that, if scores on a variable show a normal distribution, this is potentially a powerful statistical tool because we can then begin to be certain about how scores will be distributed in a variable (i.e. that many people's scores will be concentrated in the middle and few will be concentrated at either end). This certainty has given statisticians the impetus to develop ideas about statistical testing, including most notably probability and significance testing, but also intelligence.

Normal distribution and the certainty that surrounds the ability to calculate where people fall under different points of the curve allow the calculation of how much people deviate from the IQ score. Because of what we know about a normal distribution, and because Wechsler decided to use 100 as an average IQ (based on the original IQ calculations), we know that:

- 68 percent of scores lie within 1 standard deviation of the mean (plus/minus), so 68 percent of the population will score between 85 and 115.
- 95 percent of scores will fall within 2 standard deviations of the mean, therefore 95 percent of the population will score between 70 and 130. The average IQ score is 100. The standard deviation of IQ scores is 15.

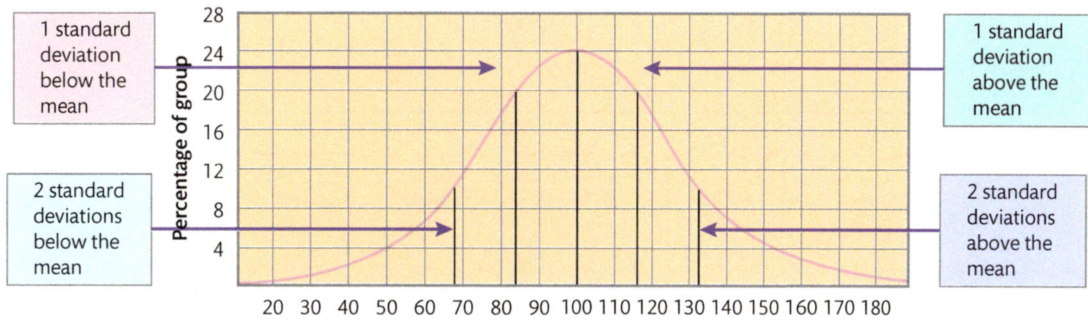

Figure 4.2 A normal distribution curve of intelligence scores.

It is then within these aspects that these scores are interpreted and classified. A score that is no more than 1 standard deviation (85–115) away from 100 can be interpreted as a normal score. A score that is between 1 and 2 standard deviations away from 100 can be interpreted as low (70–85) or high (115–130). A score that is more than 2 standard deviations away from 100 (lower than 70 or higher than 130) can be interpreted as very low (lower than 70) or very high (higher than 130). Therefore, Wechsler had provided a benchmark by which all people of all ages could be compared in IQ by using standard deviations.

Wechsler developed a measure that used a comparison of the person scores to means, rather than age. To do this, he still used the idea of average IQ as being 100. The choice of 100 was fairly arbitrary, but was based on the original IQ calculations suggested by Stern and used by Terman. Therefore, all ranges of intelligence tests score for all ages were transformed so they had a middle score of 100. If 35-year-olds had a mean score of 80.1 IQ points on the intelligence test, then their average would be transformed to 100, and all scores would be shifted around this average. Final IQ scores for each individual were based on how much they deviated from the average. Deviation IQ was calculated as how much someone deviated from the average IQ of 100.

If you want to read more on how IQ scores are calculated, go to Stop and think: IQ scores and the normal distribution.

IQ scores have been traditionally categorised to provide some understanding of level of general intelligence. Some labels that have been used to describe low, high and average scores are provided in Figure 4.3.

Raven's progressive matrices

Scottish psychologist John Carlyle Raven first published his Progressive Matrices in 1938. In comparison to the Wechsler tests, the Raven Progressive Matrices seem dramatically different. However, like the Wechsler test, their rationale is based on the theory of Spearman.

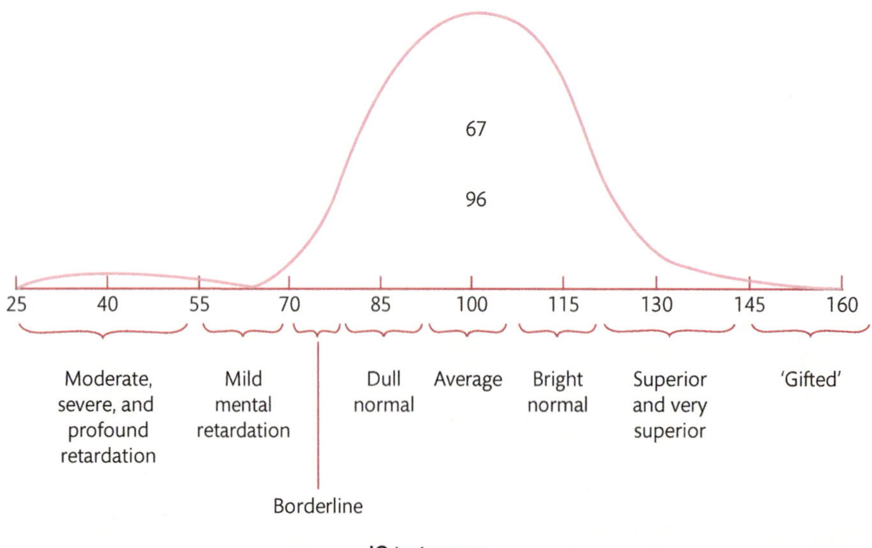

Figure 4.3 Labels traditionally given to IQ scores.

In his writing, Spearman had emphasised 'g' as the abstract ability (theoretical thought, not applied or practical) to see relationships between objects, events and information and draw inferences from those relationships. Raven thought the best way to test this abstract ability was to develop a test that was free of cultural influences, particularly language. As you have seen with the Wechsler tests, there was some reliance on culture and language (e.g. tests of general knowledge and vocabulary). Although this reliance on language is not always true of the Wechsler tests (e.g. block design, object assembly), Raven's Progressive Matrices were designed to minimise the influence of culture and language by relying on non-verbal problems that require abstract reasoning and do not require knowledge of a particular culture.

Examples of the items in Raven's Progressive Matrices are given in Figure 4.4. The participant is shown a matrix of patterns in which one pattern is missing. The aim of each item is to test a person's ability to form perceptual relations and to reason by analogy (seeing similarity between two subjects, and transferring information about one subject to another) independent of language. Put simply, the patterns within the matrix form certain rules, and the participant shows higher intelligence by being able to work out the rules that govern the patterns and then use these rules to select an item that best fits the missing pattern.

Raven's Progressive Matrices can be used with persons ranging from 6 years to adult. The overall test comprises 60 items, arranged into five sets of items, with each set of items arranged in increasing order of difficulty. Typically, like Wechsler's test and Spearman's theory of 'g', for the Progressive Matrices respondents are given an overall score. As in the Wechsler test, the overall IQ score is based on an individual's deviation from standardised norms. With the Matrices' emphasis on abstract (theoretical thought, not applied or practical) ability to see relationships among objects, events and information and draw inferences from those relationships and its non-dependence on language, the Matrices are often favoured as a good measure of 'g'. Arthur Jensen, a prominent IQ researcher, wrote that, when compared to other measures of general intelligence, Raven's Progressive Matrices are probably the best measure of a general intelligence factor (Jensen, 1998).

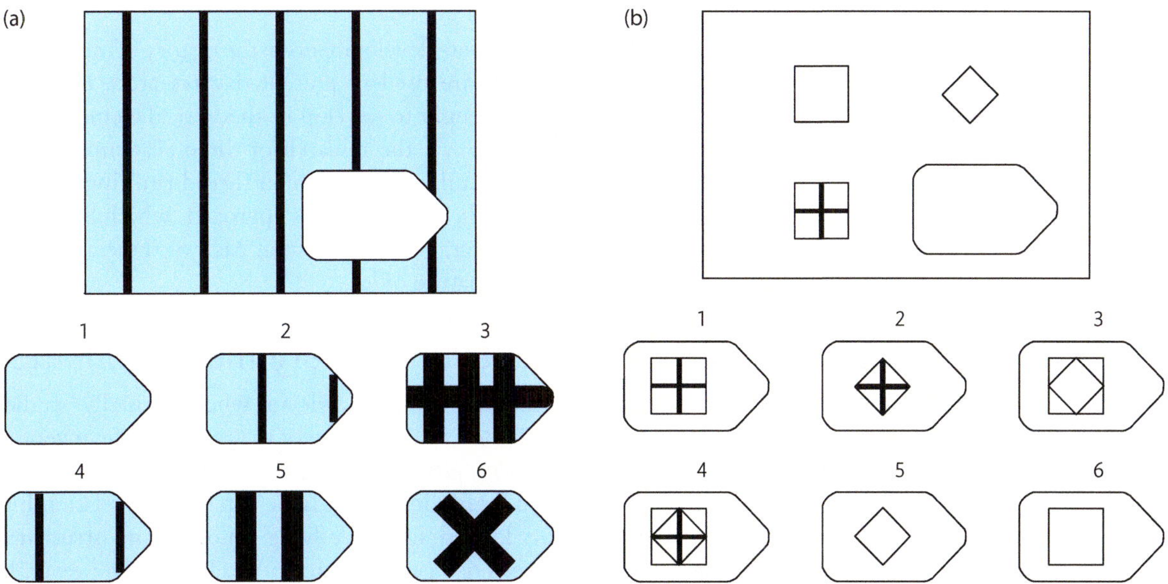

Figure 4.4 *(Continues)*

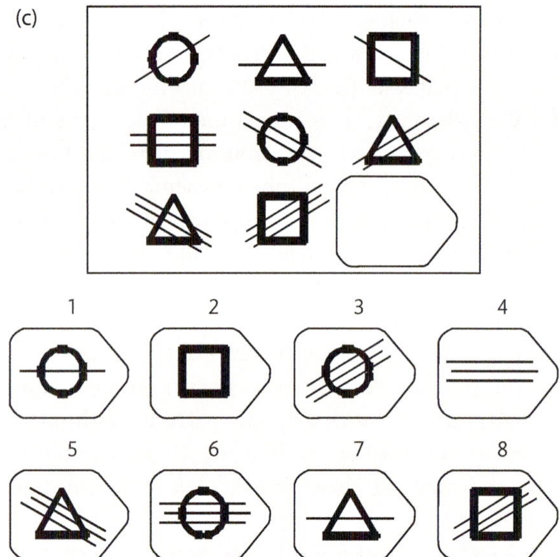

Figure 4.4 Simulated items similar to those in the Raven's Progressive Matrices: Raven's Colored Progressive Matrices (CPM) (a), Raven's Standard Progressive Matrices (b) and Raven's Advanced Progressive Matrices (APM) (c).

Multifactor theorists: Thurstone, Cattell and Guilford

Both Wechsler's and Raven's intelligence tests were developments in the history of intelligence based on Spearman's theory, and these tests are used in present-day research. However, other developments from Spearman's theory sought to develop its theoretical elements. The next section outlines three such developments via the research of three academics: Louis L. Thurstone, Raymond B. Cattell and J. P. Guilford. A common thread running through all these academics' work was that they used the factor analysis approach, which Spearman developed, to understand intelligence. However, you will see that each of these academics produced rather different perspectives on the nature of 'g'.

Thurstone: 'g' results from seven primary mental abilities

L. L. Thurstone was a US psychologist and psychometrician who originally studied engineering at Cornell University under Thomas Edison (one of the most prolific inventors of the late nineteenth century). Thurstone completed a PhD at the University of Chicago.

Thurstone used factor analysis to inform his findings. That is, he explored the relationships between a number of intelligences and looked for underlying patterns and structures. Thurstone agreed with Spearman's hypothesis of a general factor of intelligence; however, he viewed 'g' differently from Spearman. Spearman defined 'g' as a central factor of intelligence, underlying and informing all aspects of intelligence, including specific abilities. Thurstone disagreed. He couldn't see how, from Spearman's studies, he had shown that a general factor of intelligence was influencing all single aspects of intelligence. Thurstone argued that all Spearman had shown was that intelligence tests correlate positively, and he maintained that there was no evidence for Spearman's description of 'g'. Thurstone agued that 'g' results from, rather than lies behind, these seven primary mental abilities:

- **associative memory** – ability for rote (learning through routine or repetition) memory;
- **number** – ability to carry out mathematical operations accurately;
- **perceptual speed** – ability to perceive details, anomalies, similarities in visual stimuli;
- **reasoning** – ability in inductive and deductive reasoning;
- **space (spatial visualisations)** – ability to transform spatial figures mentally;
- **verbal comprehension** – ability in reading, comprehension, verbal analogies;
- **word fluency** – ability to generate and use effectively a large number of words or letters (i.e. in anagrams).

Within Thurstone's theory of intelligence, general intelligence was the result of these seven different aspects of intelligence, which formed parts of 'g'. Thurstone's approach to intelligence was the first real *multi*factor approach to intelligence. That is, he suggested there were a number of factors to intelligence, rather than just one or two.

Cattell: fluid and crystallised intelligence

Raymond B. Cattell was born, studied and lectured in the United Kingdom. He later moved to the United States, where he become a Research Associate of E. L. Thorndike at Columbia University in New York.

Cattell also used factor analysis in his studies of intelligence. He acknowledged Spearman's work in accepting that there was general intelligence, but he suggested that 'g' comprises two related but distinct components: crystallised intelligence and fluid intelligence.

Cattell described **crystallised intelligence** as acquired knowledge and skills, such as factual knowledge. It is generally related to a person's stored information and to their cultural influences. Knowledge of vocabulary, comprehension and general knowledge would all be tests of an individual's crystallised intelligence. Following Spearman's lead (who termed general intelligence 'g'), Cattell abbreviated this component as 'Gc' (the *c* standing for crystallised).

Crystallised intelligence
Acquired knowledge and skills, such as factual knowledge (abbreviated as Gc).

Fluid intelligence
Primary reasoning ability; the ability to solve abstract relational problems; free of cultural influences (abbreviated as Gf).

Cattell described **fluid intelligence** as a primary reasoning ability; the ability to solve abstract relational problems, free of cultural influences. This component is defined by intelligence abilities such as acquisition of new information, understanding new relationships, patterns and analogies in stimuli. Cattell abbreviated this component as 'Gf' (the *f* standing for fluid).

Cattell saw a dynamic relationship between these two intelligence components. Crystallised intelligence (for example, knowledge) is intelligence that increases throughout life and is a reflection of one's cumulative learning experience. Fluid intelligence is thought to be present from birth and then is meant to stabilise in adulthood. An example of how crystallised and fluid intelligence may work in society is seen in the way these different components inform certain types of thinking. It is often found that the great mathematicians do some of their best work when they are in younger adulthood. This is because mathematics is based on abstract thinking, and achievement in this area reflects fluid intelligence. However, in other disciplines, such as history and literature, some of the best work is produced by academics in later adulthood as they have accumulated more knowledge; achievement in this area reflects crystallised intelligence.

One interesting aspect of Cattell's work is the distinction between fluid and crystallised intelligence in relation to developments in IQ testing. The Wechsler tests are, to some extent, measuring crystallised intelligence, containing measures such as comprehension, knowledge and vocabulary. Raven's Progressive Matrices, which reflect abstract thinking, are often used as a measure of general fluid intelligence.

Guilford: many different intelligences and many different combinations

J. P. Guilford was a US psychologist who studied at the University of Nebraska and Cornell University. He also conducted research at the University of Southern California and Santa Ana Army Air Base.

Guilford disagreed with the stance of Spearman and, to some extent, with Thurstone and Cattell. He didn't acknowledge the existence of 'g'; instead, Guilford (1977) eventually proposed that intelligence was the result of 150 independent abilities (though originally he suggested 120 independent abilities [Guilford, 1959]). His theory was named the Structure of Intellect (SI) theory.

Guilford argued that these elementary abilities fall into three groups: operations, contents and products.

Operations
Within Guilford's theory of intelligence, operations are types of mental processing.

Contents
A term used in Guilford's Structure of Intellect (SI) theory that describes mental material that individuals possess.

Products
A term used in Guilford's Structure of Intellect (SI) theory that describes how information is stored, processed and used by the person to make associations or connections.

Operations are types of mental processing, for example, what a person does. There are five types of operations:

- **evaluation** – ability to examine and judge carefully and appraise;
- **convergent production** – ability to bring together information into a single theme (e.g. a list comprising 'cats, dogs, mice' would be converged into 'type of animals');
- **divergent production** – ability to produce ideas from a common point (e.g. if a person was asked to list animals, divergent production would be to list 'cats', 'dogs', 'mice', etc.);
- **memory** – mental faculty of retaining and recalling past experience and information;
- **cognition** – mental process of knowing, including aspects such as awareness, perception, reasoning and judgement.

Contents comprise the mental material we possess *on* which operations are performed. There are five types of contents:

- **visual** – material relating to or gained by the sense of sight;
- **auditory** – material relating to or gained by the sense of hearing;
- **symbolic** – material relating to or expressed by means of symbols or a symbol;
- **semantic** – material relating to meaning, especially meaning in language;
- **behavioural** – material relating to our own behaviour.

Products consist of the form in which the information is stored, processed and used by the person to make associations or connections. There are six types of products:

- **units** – comprises the ability to use information relating to something being classed as a unit. It may be an individual, group, structure or other entity regarded as part of a whole (e.g. a 1-euro note ["1] is a *unit* of money);
- **classes** – comprises the ability to use information relating to a set, collection, group or configuration containing members regarded as having certain attributes or traits in common (e.g. the monetary units of euros – (", "1, 50 cent, 20 cent, 10 cent, 5 cent, 2 cent and 1 cent – are a *class* of money);
- **relations** – comprises the ability to use information relating to seeing a logical or natural association between two or more things (e.g. there are 100 cents to (1; the association between these two units is a *relation*);
- **systems** – comprises the ability to use information relating to seeing a group of interacting, interrelated or interdependent elements forming a complex whole (e.g. the euro, sterling, US dollars, Chinese yen and all the other currencies in the world form a *system*);
- **transformation** – comprises the ability to understand the changing nature, function or condition of any information (e.g. exchange rates between currencies);
- **implication** – comprises the ability to use a variety of information and apply logic to it or further understand suggestions, meaning and significance relating to that information (e.g. If I had all the money in the world, that would mean I would be rich).

A popular way of illustrating Guilford's Structure of Intellect (SI) theory is given in Figure 4.5.

Guilford argued that, theoretically, 150 different components of intelligence emerge from the combinations of these different skills. So, for example, the ability to remember seeing a dog would use all of the following components:

- visual (content; the act of visualising the dog – remember *seeing* the dog);
- unit (product; the object itself – the dog – remember seeing the *dog*);
- memory (operation; the remembering part – *remember* seeing the dog).

Guilford suggested that the model could be simplified and that further groups of intelligence could be recognised by taking each of the five intelligence operations and applying them to the products and contents aspects (see Figure 4.5). Guilford recognised a further set of abilities:

- Reasoning and problem-solving intelligence could be fully understood by taking convergent and divergent operations and subdividing them into the 30 distinct abilities for the six products and five contents.
- Memory intelligence could be fully understood by subdividing the memory into the 30 distinct abilities for the six products and five contents.
- Decision-making skills could be fully understood by subdividing evaluation into the 30 distinct abilities for the six products and five contents.
- Language-related skills could be fully understood by subdividing cognition into the 30 distinct abilities for the six products and five contents.

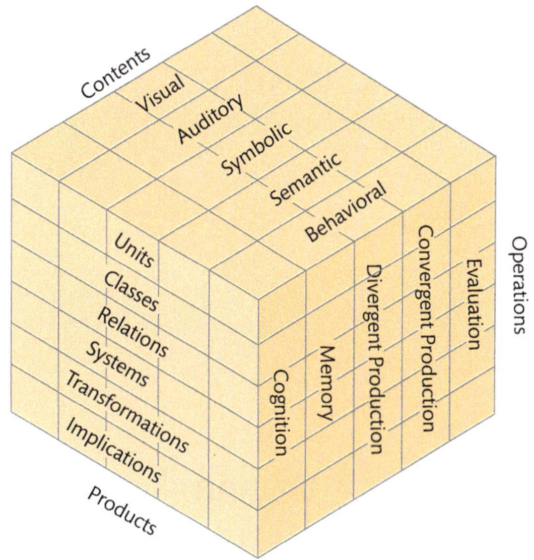

Figure 4.5 Guilford's Structure of Intellect (SI) theory.
Source: *The Analysis of Intelligence*, New York: McGraw-Hill (Guilford, J.P. and Hoepfner, R. 1971), copyright © 1971. Reproduced with permission of The McGraw-Hill Companies.

Guilford's model of intelligence really opens up the possibilities of intelligence. It clearly broadens the view of intelligence, while detailing how different aspects of intelligence intertwine to form specific abilities. However, it may be too complex to provide a definitive theory. Guilford researched and developed a wide variety of psychometric tests to measure the specific abilities predicted by SI theory. He largely based this work on groups of intelligence that could be found among the 150 different components. Although these tests may be useful on their own, when research has conducted factor analysis to examine whether these intelligences gather together in the way that Guilford suggests, there has been little support for his overall theory (Guilford and Hoepfner, 1971).

Intelligence and factor analysis – a third way: the hierarchical approach

So far we have considered theories of intelligence where 'g' is central (Spearman), apparent but not the most important (Thurstone and Cattell) or rejected (Guilford). Figure 4.6a shows how the theorists tend to be split between general theories of intelligence and specific abilities. However, there is a set of factor analysis theorists whose work fills the gap between the work of Spearman and Thurstone (see Figure 4.6b). These theorists developed hierarchical theories of intelligence, and we will now outline the work of Philip E. Vernon, John B. Carroll and John Horn.

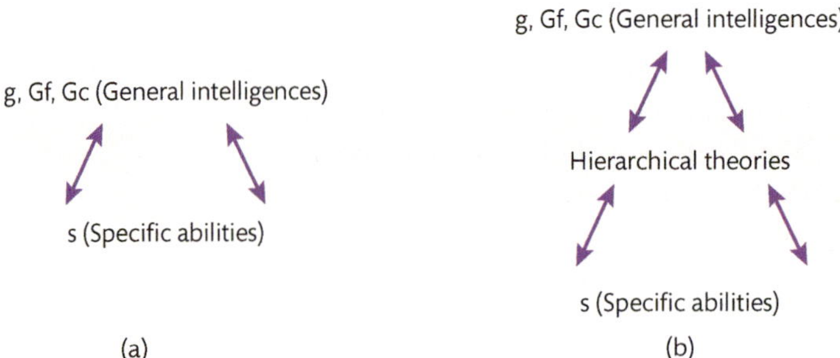

Figure 4.6 (a) Overview of theories by general intelligences and specific abilities. (b) How the hierarchical theories fit into this overview.

Vernon

Philip E. Vernon was an English psychologist educated at Cambridge University. He was a Professor of Psychology and Educational Psychology at the Institute of Education, University of London.

Vernon (1950) described several different levels of intelligence. He proposed that neither Spearman nor Thurstone had considered the existence of group factors that linked 'g' to specific intelligence abilities. Vernon argued that intelligence comprises various sets of abilities that can be described at various levels (i.e. from specific to grouped to general). Vernon's theory was the elaboration of 'g' to a series of group factors *in between* 'g' and 's' factors (see Figure 4.7).

Within Vernon's hierarchical theory, the highest intelligence level is 'g'. Like Spearman, Vernon thought 'g' was the most important factor underlying intelligence in human beings. The next level in Vernon's hierarchy comprises two *major group factors*, verbal/educational (v:ed) and spatial/mechanical abilities (k:m).

- The 'v:ed' factor represents largely verbal/educational intelligence, including verbal–numerical–educational abilities.
- The 'k:m' factor comprises spatial/mechanical intelligence, including practical–mechanical–spatial–physical abilities.

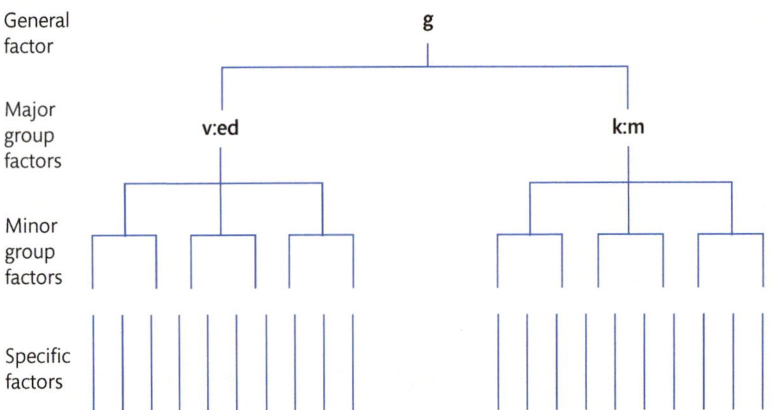

Figure 4.7 Vernon's hierarchical theory of intelligence.

The next level of Vernon's hierarchy contains *minor group factors*, divided from the major group factors. That is, from the major group factor, 'v:ed', verbal, numerical and educational abilities are minor group factors. Similarly, from the major group factor, 'k:m', practical, mechanical, spatial and physical abilities are minor group factors.

At the bottom of the hierarchy are the specific intelligence factors. These are divided from the minor group factors. That is, from the 'v:ed' major group factor family, and the educational abilities minor group factors, there would be specific abilities such as reading, spelling, use of grammar and punctuation. Similarly, from the 'k:m' major group factor family, and the spatial abilities minor group factors, there would be specific spatial abilities such as recognising an object when it is seen from different locations, the ability to imagine movement of an object and ability to think about spatial relations when the body of the observer is central.

Carroll: from the three-stratum model of human cognitive abilities to CHC

John B. Carroll, an American educational psychologist, proposed a hierarchical model of intelligence officially named the Three-Stratum Model of Human Cognitive Abilities.

Carroll (1993) proposed this hierarchical model of intelligence based on the factor analysis of 461 data sets obtained between 1927 and 1987. These data sets were important because they included a number of intelligence data sets from class intelligence studies reported during the past 50–60 years. Based on this analysis, Carroll proposed three hierarchical levels to intelligence, which he termed stratums:

- Stratum I comprises specific levels of intelligence. Overall, Carroll identified 69 different cognitive abilities/intelligences.
- Stratum II is made up of eight broad factors arising from these specific abilities:
  - fluid intelligence, abbreviated to (in a similar way to Cattell) Gf;
  - crystallised intelligence, abbreviated to Gc;
  - general memory and learning, abbreviated to Gy;
  - broad visual perception, abbreviated to Gv;
  - broad auditory perception, abbreviated to Gu;
  - broad retrieval ability, abbreviated to Gr;
  - broad cognitive speediness, abbreviated to Gs;
  - processing speed, abbreviated to Gt.
- Stratum III is the general level of intelligence representing general intellectual ability, similar to 'g'.

Carroll's work perhaps provided a much-needed systematic organisation and integration of over 50 years of research on the structure of human cognitive abilities. As you can see, it brings together a number of themes, including Spearman's 'g' and specific factors, Cattell's 'Gc' and 'Gf', Thurstone's specific factors and Vernon's hierarchical approach.

Cattell, Horn and Carroll (CHC): theory, research and practice together

Our story of factor-analytic studies and theories would be expected to stop with Carroll's 1993 work. However, it continues with recent convergence between Cattell's original work and Carroll's factor-analytic work.

US psychologist John Leonard Horn (Department of Psychology at the University of South Carolina), along with his advisor, Raymond B. Cattell, had been developing

Cattell's original theory of intelligence that specifies two broad factors, fluid and crystallised intelligence. The main thrust of Horn's work had been to look for numerous specific factors that support the general ones. However, by the middle 1980s, John Horn had begun to conclude that the available research supported the presence of seven additional broad 'g' abilities beyond that of Gf and Gc and had abandoned the notion of a general 'g' factor. Although Horn retained the title 'Gf–Gc' (known as Cattell–Horn 'Gf–Gc') to describe the theory, there were actually nine dimensions to the intelligence theory, with an abbreviation accompanying each intelligence:

- fluid reasoning (Gf);
- acculturation knowledge intelligence (Gc);
- short-term apprehension and retrieval abilities (SAR);
- visual processing (Gv);
- auditory processing (Ga);
- tertiary storage and retrieval (TSR/Glm);
- processing speed (Gs);
- correct decision speed (CDS);
- quantitative knowledge (Gq).

Together, Carroll's and Cattell and Horn's work had dramatically informed people who were developing and using psychometric tests. One such person was Richard W. Woodcock (a US psychologist who has a wide background in education and psychology). With his colleague, M. B. Johnson, Woodcock developed a series of intelligence tests called the Woodcock–Johnson Psychoeducational Battery, of which the latest, Woodcock–Johnson Psychoeducational Battery – Revised: Tests of Cognitive Ability, is used for measuring cognitive ability for people aged 2 years and older. The test battery contains 21 different subtests and measures seven broad intellectual abilities, including auditory processing, comprehension knowledge, processing speed, visual process, short-term memory, long-term retrieval and fluid reasoning.

Woodcock had noticed that researchers and testers in the educational and applied psychometric testing field have struggled with the subtle differences between Horn's and Carroll's theories. Woodcock felt, as you may have noticed, that some amalgamation could be made between the two theories.

For example, although Cattell–Horn's model of intelligence didn't acknowledge a general 'g' factor, Carroll's did. Cattell–Horn's model emphasised a factor of quantitative knowledge that was not matched by Carroll, and both recognised similar factors such as:

- fluid intelligence (be it reasoning [Cattell–Horn, CH] or intelligence [Cattell, C]);
- crystallised intelligence (be it acculturation knowledge [CH] or crystallised intelligence [C]);
- general memory and learning abilities (be it short-term apprehension and retrieval abilities [CH] or general memory and learning [C]);
- visual perception (be it visual processing [CH] or broad visual perception [C]);
- auditory perception (be it auditory processing [CH] or broad auditory perception [C]).

So, in 1999, Woodcock met with Horn and Carroll at Chapel Hill, North Carolina, to seek a more comprehensive model that would incorporate the similarities between their respective theoretical models, yet also acknowledge and incorporate their differences. Woodcock engaged Horn and Carroll in a sequence of conversations and private communications, and, as a result of those meetings, the Cattell–Horn–Carroll (CHC) theory of cognitive abilities was developed.

The CHC theory represents both the Cattell–Horn and Carroll models of intelligence and was first described in the psychological literature by Flanagan *et al.* (2000) and Lohman (2001).

There are two main strata in the CHC theory of cognitive abilities: a broad stratum (stratum II) and a narrow stratum (stratum I), with the abandonment of a general intelligence factor. Overall there are 16 intelligences in the broad stratum, with each of these being divided into a number of abilities that make up the narrow stratum (see Table 4.2).

The CHC model of intelligence shows an attempt to build a synthesis of several intelligence theories and measurements. However, we might here see some of the difficulties in combining the theoretical approach to intelligence with the practical use of intelligence tests. Clearly, the expectations of individual factor analysis academics working in a research setting and of those working in the applied setting might differ slightly. While individual factor analysis

Table 4.2 Cattell–Horn–Carroll (CHC) theory of cognitive abilities: a broad stratum (stratum II) and narrow stratum (stratum I)

Broad stratum (stratum II)	Narrow stratum (stratum I)
Fluid intelligence/Reasoning (Gf) – The use of mental operations to solve novel and abstract problems	General sequential (deductive) reasoning, inductive reasoning, quantitative reasoning, logical thinking and speed of reasoning
Crystallised intelligence/Knowledge (Gc) – Intelligence that is incorporated by individuals through a process of culture	Language development, lexical knowledge, listening ability, general (verbal) information, information about culture, communication ability, oral production and fluency, grammatical sensitivity, foreign language proficiency and foreign language aptitude
General (domain-specific) knowledge (Gkn) – Breadth and depth of acquired knowledge in specialised (not general) domains	Knowledge of English as a second language, knowledge of singing, skill in lip-reading, geography achievement, general science information, mechanical knowledge and knowledge of behavioural content
Visual-spatial abilities (Gv) – The ability to invent, remember, retrieve and transform visual images	Visualisation, spatial relations, closure speed, flexibility of closure, visual memory, spatial scanning, serial perceptual integration, length estimation, perceptual illusions, perceptual alternations and imagery
Auditory processing (Ga) – Abilities around hearing	Phonetic coding, speech sound discrimination, resistance to auditory stimulus, distortion memory for sound patterns, general sound discrimination, temporal tracking, musical discrimination and judgement, maintaining and judging rhythm, sound-intensity/duration discrimination, sound-frequency discrimination, hearing and speech threshold factors, absolute pitch and sound localisation
Short-term memory (Gsm) – The ability to encode, be aware of information in the short-term memory	Memory span and working memory
Long-term storage and retrieval (Glr) – The ability to store information in long-term memory	Associative memory, meaningful memory, free recall memory, ideational fluency, associational fluency, expressional fluency, naming facility, word fluency, figural fluency, figural flexibility, sensitivity to problems, originality/creativity and learning abilities
Cognitive processing speed (Gs) – The ability to perform cognitive tasks automatically and fluently	Perceptual speed, rate of test-taking, number facility, speed of reasoning, reading speed and writing speed
Decision/Reaction time or speed (Gt) – The ability to react and make decisions quickly in response to simple stimuli	Simple reaction time, choice reaction time, semantic processing speed, mental comparison speed and inspection time
Psychomotor speed (Gps) – The ability to perform body motor movements rapidly and fluently	Speed of limb movement, writing speed, speed of articulation and movement time
Quantitative knowledge (Gq) – A personal breadth and depth of other abilities gained primarily during formal educational experiences of mathematics	Mathematical knowledge and mathematical achievement
Reading/Writing (Grw) – Abilities relating to reading and writing skills and knowledge	Reading decoding, reading comprehension, printed language comprehension, cloze ability, spelling ability, writing ability, English usage knowledge, reading speed and writing speed
Psychomotor abilities (Gp) – Ability to perform body motor movements with precision and coordination	Static strength, multilimb coordination, finger dexterity, manual dexterity, arm–hand steadiness, control precision, aiming and gross body equilibrium
Olfactory abilities (Go) – Abilities relating to the sense of smell	Olfactory memory and olfactory sensitivity
Tactile abilities (Gh) – Abilities that depend on the sense of touch	Tactile sensitivity
Kinaesthetic abilities (Gk) – Abilities that depend on the sense that detects bodily position, weight or movement of the muscles, tendons and joints	Kinaesthetic sensitivity

academic researchers might ultimately be looking for a definitive model of intelligence, those individuals working in the psychometric test area might be looking not only for a definitive model of intelligence but also to develop an intelligence test that measures many aspects of intelligence (even those that are less popular) so they can produce a strong product that is of most use.

We can see that with the transfer of Carroll's work into applied test situations, his model of intelligence does not come through as strongly as it once seemed. Carroll's work seems to have led intelligence testing to a pinnacle by providing all sorts of definitive answers, with over 460 data sets on intelligence. However, following the meeting with educational test publishers, there seems to be a deviation from Carroll's concise eight-factor model to a more convoluted fifteen-factor model, which seems to satisfy the need of covering a number of possible dimensions in applied testing, but leaves us with the finding that some aspects of intelligence in this model (e.g. fluid intelligence and crystallised intelligence) are valid, comprehensive and more developed and understood than are other aspects (e.g. olfactory and tactile abilities).[A]

Overall, in this discussion we have taken you from the earliest conceptions of intelligence in psychology (Galton, Binet), through many of the major theorists (Spearman, Cattell, Carroll), major measures of intelligence and its estimation (the Wechsler and Raven's Matrices IQ tests, IQ and deviation IQ), multifactoral and hierarchical model (Guilford and Carroll). Taken together, you should now have an understanding of how intelligence, both the concept and its measurement, has developed for over a century. In the next three discussions we aim to develop some of the ideas and look at many of the debates and controversies that surround intelligence.[B]

Types of intelligence tests

Earlier in this chapter, we outlined the theory and gave you examples of the types of intelligence tests used to measure intelligence. We discussed earlier intelligence researchers such as Galton and Binet, who suggested that we could measure intelligence. Galton suggested that we could measure variability in intelligence, and he began to show that this was true through tests of sensory discrimination and motor coordination. Binet, meanwhile, was developing intelligence tests among children. His test, the Binet–Simon scale, used many of the techniques that we see in modern-day intelligence tests – items presented in an order of difficulty, varying techniques to assess intelligence and standardised scorings to determine IQ. Later we see work by Terman and Yerkes among US adults; this research introduced the idea of mass testing, deviation IQ and consideration of culture and culture-free specific tests. Later, Spearman's introduction of the notion of general intelligence ('g') led to the introduction of the Wechsler tests and Raven's Progressive Matrices. With the theoretical work of Cattell, Horn and Carroll we see the development of the Woodcock–Johnson Psychoeducational Battery–Revised: Tests of Cognitive Ability.

There are many intelligence tests in use today that reflect this theoretical and empirical growth in the understanding of intelligence and IQ. The Stanford–Binet test is now in its fifth edition (Roid, 2003), and is used among people aged from 2 to 90+ years. It can still be used not only to compute an overall measure of IQ but also to assess fluid reasoning, knowledge, quantitative reasoning, visual-spatial processing and working memory as well as

---

[A]Maltby, J., Day, L., & Macaskill, A. (2013). Theories and measurement of intelligence. In *Personality, individual differences and intelligence* (3rd ed., pp. 279–297). Harlow, Essex: Pearson Education Limited.

[B]Maltby, J., Day, L., & Macaskill, A. (2013). Theories and measurement of intelligence. In *Personality, individual differences and intelligence* (3rd ed., pp. 301). Harlow, Essex: Pearson Education Limited.

the ability to compare verbal and non-verbal performance. The Wechsler tests are still in use today, and comprise the Wechsler Preschool and Primary Scale of Intelligence (WPPSI) for use among 3- to 7-year-olds, the Wechsler Intelligence Scale for Children (WISC) for use among 7- to 16-year-olds and the Wechsler Adult Intelligence Scale (WAIS) for use among people who are 16 years and over. The scale contains measures of verbal and performance intelligence. The Woodcock–Johnson III Tests of Cognitive Abilities are used among people aged from 2 to 90+ years and also give an overall score of general intelligence (IQ score), as well as looking at working memory and executive function skills.[C]

Features, uses and problems surrounding intelligence tests

In the following sections we are going to consider the features, uses and problems found in intelligence tests.

Typical features of intelligence tests

Let us establish some of the important aspects that are essential to good intelligence tests. Sattler (2002) establishes three main aspects that tend to be typical in all good intelligence tests.

A variety of tasks are involved in intelligence tests

To assess a full range of abilities, a good intelligence test needs to contain a number of tasks. For example, tests such as the Wechsler Adult Intelligence Scale will contain various measures, including ability tests of general knowledge, digit span, vocabulary, arithmetic, comprehension, similarities, picture completion, picture arrangement, block design, digit symbol and object assembly. Such 'subtests' used together provide a fuller understanding of the overall intelligence of the person as well as their particular strengths.

Standardisation of administration

The aim of standardising administration is to provide a controlled environment in which the test is taken to allow comparisons among children (although note that different test authors differ in the emphasis they place on the importance of making comparisons *among* children). For example, if conditions differed during the test administration, such as the wording of questions or the exact time given for the test, then differences in intelligence between children might be (at least partly) attributed to the differences in administration conditions rather than to differences in their intelligence. The administration of any intelligence test is standardised, from instructions for completing the test, to the location of the test, to which and how many people should be present. Two further important aspects to this standardisation are the length of administration of the test and the conditions under which it is taken.

- As typically intelligence tests are administered to schoolchildren, the length of time children can take on a task will vary with the age of the child. For example, younger children will tend to be able to concentrate less over longer periods of time than older children will, and they will want to spend less time on more complicated tasks.

[C]Maltby, J., Day, L., & Macaskill, A. (2013). The use of intelligence tests: What question emerge from the measurement of intelligence. In *Personality, individual differences and intelligence* (3rd ed., pp. 306–307). Harlow, Essex: Pearson Education Limited.

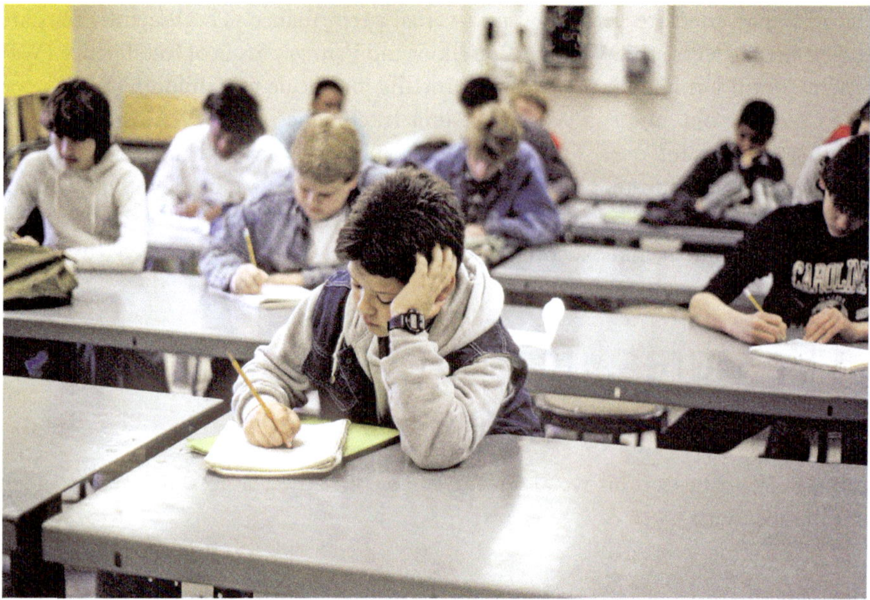

How do you think IQ tests have changed since the First World War?
Source: Alamy Images/Tina Manley

Researchers will seek to standardise the length of time of the test depending on the age of the child.

- There is a need for the actual test to be done in comfortable conditions and to be administered by a qualified test administrator. If you have ever taken an intelligence test at school, you will probably recall that it was administered by a trained staff member. This qualified person ensures the quality of administration of the test. This person ensures that test-takers are comfortable, and, particularly where children are concerned, the administrator might seek to develop a rapport with the students, responding to needs as they arise (i.e. when a student is in distress, making sure respondents aren't rushed into starting the test). You can see that without being provided with this type of approach, individuals might feel that their performance on the test wasn't only due to their intelligence, but to the conditions in which it was taken.

Norm referencing

This is another form of standardisation. The aim of making an intelligence test norm-referenced is to allow comparisons to be made with other children. There is no point in determining the IQ score of a person as being 140, unless you have something with which to compare it. All tests will have to be administered to a large group of people of around the same age (or at the same age among children) and of similar demographics (sex, race, area of residence, occupational status) to allow accurate comparisons to be made. The standard example is to use 100 to describe an average score and then compare all scores around that number. Some authors of intelligence tests play down the need to make comparisons on this basis among children because the tests are designed for individual assessment. However, even these intelligence tests will provide some norm-referenced material, so that the person using the intelligence test may have a context for understanding individual scores.

The uses of intelligence tests

Intelligence tests are used for all sorts of purposes, but mainly for the following three: selection, diagnosis and evaluation.

You may first come across intelligence tests in schools. Here, intelligence tests might be used for selection purposes, streaming children into high-ability and low-ability classes, or conceivably might be used by school selectors to ensure they only take on high-ability children. Intelligence tests might be used for diagnostic purposes, to help teachers determine whether there are problems in children with low ability and specifically where these problems might exist so children might be helped. They would also be used for evaluating the child's ability and could help teachers to decide which students might be capable of performing better in national examinations.

Similar ideas apply to intelligence tests when they are used in higher education and the workplace, with universities, universities and employers using them to select candidates. You can easily see how an applicant who scores well in general knowledge, vocabulary, arithmetic and comprehension (all specific intelligence abilities) might be more likely to get a vacancy over someone who does not achieve a high score in these abilities.

This application of tests is not without good reason. People who suggest and support the use of intelligence tests would argue that IQ tests are valid and useful as they show a positive correlation with school achievement and job performance.

As regards school achievement, research has looked at various indices, including examination ability, specific abilities in a particular topic (for example, mathematics, English) and whether students stay on in school. There are a number of reviews by psychologists. Jencks (1979) reported correlations between generally intelligence and academic achievement ranging from $r = 0.40$ to $r = 0.63$ for six longitudinal studies in the USA. US psychologists Alan Kaufman and Elizabeth Lichtenberger (Kaufman, 1990; Kaufman and Lichtenberger, 2005) provide a review of key papers that have looked at the correlation between general intelligence and school attainment and achievement. The authors conclude that the average correlation between IQ scores and a number of school indicators is around $r = 0.50$. Mackintosh (1998) estimates the correlation between general intelligence and achievement at school to be between $r = 0.4$ and $r = 0.7$.

A study in 2007 by Ian Deary, Steve Strand, Pauline Smith and Cres Fernandes (Deary *et al.*, 2007) reported on a 5-year prospective longitudinal study of 70,000 + English children and examined the association between psychometric intelligence at age 11 years (as measured by the cognitive ability test which gives an overall assessment of general intelligence, 'g') and educational achievement in national examinations in 25 academic subjects at age 16. In this study the authors used General Certificate of Secondary Education (GCSE) scores to measure educational attainment, which is the academic qualification awarded in a number of subjects (e.g. mathematics, English, history, etc.) by students in secondary education in the United Kingdom. Table 4.3 shows some of the correlations between general intelligence and GCSE scores across a number of subject areas.

Table 4.3 Correlations between general intelligence and GCSE scores (based on Deary *et al.*, 2007)

Subject	Correlation with general intelligence ($r =$)
GCSE total points	0.69
GCSE best 8	0.72
Mathematics	0.77
Biology	0.51
Chemistry	0.46
Physics	0.50
English	0.67
English literature	0.59
History	0.63
Geography	0.65
French	0.64
German	0.61
Spanish	0.62
Drama	0.47
Art and design	0.43
Music	0.54

Clearly, all these studies considered together suggest that intelligence does unambiguously predict academic achievement.

Two strong examples of this predictive power of intelligence tests can also be found in the workplace. In 1984 two US psychologists, John E. Hunter and R. F. Hunter (Hunter and Hunter, 1984), did a meta-analysis (a **meta-analysis** is a technique that combines the results of several studies) and put together the results of studies that examined various predictors at the start of a job with eventual job performance. In all, the authors looked at results for over 32,000 workers. They found that the correlation between general intelligence (IQ) and job performance was $r = 0.54$ (a medium-sized correlation) and had a much larger association with job performance than with the curriculum vitae of the candidate ($r = 0.37$), previous experience of the candidate ($r = 0.18$), job interviews ($r = 0.14$) and education of the candidate ($r = 0.10$).

The first ever meta-analysis of this type was repeated in the United Kingdom by UK psychologist Cristina Bertua, Dutch psychologist Neil Anderson and Spanish psychologist Jesús F. Salgado, who looked at over 280 samples, comparing 13,262 people's scores on different intelligence tests and their later job performance (Bertua *et al.*, 2005). In this study the researchers examined several different types of jobs, including clerical, engineering, professional, management and sales and ranging from low-skilled jobs to higher-skilled professional jobs. Bertua and her colleagues found that both general intelligence and specific ability tests were good predictors of job performance, with correlations being similar to those reported by Hunter and Hunter (1984) of between $r = 0.5$ and $r = 0.6$.

However, the potential usefulness of intelligence tests does not stop there. Some psychologists have shown that general intelligence in childhood can predict variables across the lifespan. In 1931 the Mental Survey Committee in Scotland met and decided (because there was no reliable way of getting a representative sample) to measure general intelligence and obtain IQ scores for everyone in Scotland. So on Wednesday, 1 June 1932, nearly every child attending school in Scotland who was born in 1921 took the same intelligence test ($n = 89{,}498$). This exercise was repeated in 1947, testing almost all people born in 1936 ($n = 70{,}805$).

A group of psychologists from Scotland – Ian Deary, Martha Whiteman, John Starr, Lawrence Whalley and Helen Fox (2004) – have pointed out that, in intelligence testing history, this sample is very unusual. Scotland remains the only nation with mental test data for an entire birth cohort, never mind two. In their study, the authors look at a number of factors in old age and their relationship to the test-takers' IQ scores from the 1932 and 1947 cohorts. Some of their main findings are summarised in Table 4.4. In this table we have taken some of the information from Deary *et al.*'s paper regarding the 1947 cohort in terms of those who were found to have died, those who had been diagnosed with cancer and those who had been diagnosed with a cardiovascular (involving the heart and the blood vessels) disease by the time of Deary *et al.*'s study.

What you can see from Table 4.4 is that people who were reported to have died and those having been diagnosed with cardiovascular disease had scored significantly lower on IQ in 1947 than those who had neither died nor been diagnosed with cardiovascular disease. However, note that no significant difference was found in the IQs of people who were later diagnosed with cancer. This finding suggests, at the very least, that IQ has some level of predictive strength very much later in life.

Table 4.4 The relationship between general intelligence (IQ) scores and a number of health outcomes in later life

Outcome	Number of people suffering from the outcome	Number of people not suffering from the outcome	Mean IQ of people suffering from the outcome	Mean IQ of people not suffering from the outcome	Significance
People dying	125	783	97.7	104.6	$P < 0.001$
People being diagnosed with cancer	78	830	101.3	103.9	$P > 0.05$
People being diagnosed with cardiovascular disease	98	810	100.1	104.1	$P < 0.05$

Source: Statistics from Deary *et al.* (2004).

Stop and think

What are the mechanisms that underpin the relationship between IQ and mortality?

In the section on intelligence and health we saw that researchers like Batty *et al.* examined possible mediating factors (such as blood pressure, body mass index or cigarette smoking) that explain the relationship between intelligence and health. Batty *et al.* (2007) and Calvin *et al.* (2011) have tried to summarise, in terms of areas, the possible mechanisms that might explain this relationship between IQ and mortality. Remember that these studies are looking at the measurement of IQ, usually at a relatively early age in people's lives (and that IQ tests are taken a long time before the person dies), and linking it to mortality rates.

Batty *et al.* (2007) have argued that it is important to realise that aspects such as parental intelligence, socioeconomic environment, nutrition and somatic and psychiatric illness all influence IQ. However, from this point on, Batty and his colleagues have suggested four possible domains that help us to understand the relationship between IQ before death (premorbid IQ) and mortality (see Figure 4.8). These are:

- disease and injury prevention: the extent to which one seeks to avoid developing disease or injuries;
- disease and injury management: the extent to which one seeks to manage and handle disease or injuries when they happen or emerge;
- high socioeconomic position: the extent to which individuals are living and working in healthier environments;
- psychiatric illness: many psychiatric illnesses (depression, schizophrenia) are lasting and permanent and are related to a number of factors or health behaviours related to mortality; for example, sucicide, smoking or drinking alcohol.

It is better to see these relationships as a chain in this part of the lifespan, with IQ leading to one of these four domains, which in turn leads to different levels of mortality. For example, Calvin *et al.* describe how higher IQ leads to better education and work successes. People will therefore have better jobs and be able to access not only safer living areas, but also better health services. Therefore those with a high socioeconomic position will spend their time in safer and healthier environments and therefore be less at risk of death.

Of course some of these relationships are complicated, because, as noted earlier, social and economic status might not only influence the relationship between IQ and mortality, but the socioeconomic environment also predicts IQ from an early age and therefore it may be a constant variable to account for. However, in this instance, look at the four domains and speculate for each domain how someone with a high IQ and someone with a low IQ might differ in terms of how they approach disease and injury prevention, disease and injury management, high socioeconomic position and psychiatric illness, and how this approach might eventually have an effect on mortality.

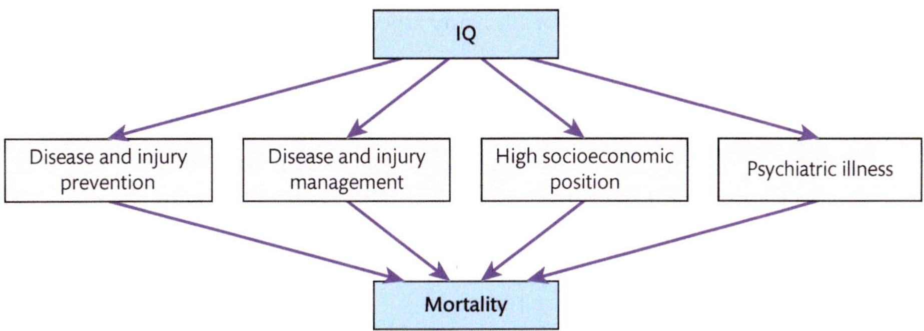

Figure 4.8 Possible mechanisms that explain the relationship between IQ at an early age and mortality (Batty *et al.*, 2007).

This type of study, exploring the relationship between intelligence at a young age and health in later life, is named cognitive epidemiology, a term introduced by Deary and Der (2005). One of the largest studies ever to explore the relationship between intelligence at an early age and health in later life was carried out by David Batty, who is at University College London, UK with several colleagues (Batty *et al.*, 2009). Up to 2010, in Sweden for the past 100 years all men in early adulthood have had to undertake conscription into either the military or the civil service. For many decades, on entering conscription individuals have been given intelligence tests and been given a particular unique identifier code (like a national insurance number or passport number) that can be revisited at a later date to match up each person with information (such as health outcomes) that are collected later or as part of public databases or surveys. Therefore, in Sweden, there is a database linking intelligence at an early age (at the time of conscription) to health outcomes at a number of stages in later life across a number of decades. Batty *et al.* studied mortality rate, a measure of the number of deaths. They found that, among nearly 1 million men (994,242) studied across an average of 20 years, there were nearly 15,000 deaths (14,498). When age, year of birth and where they were tested were controlled for, lower IQ score was associated with an increased risk of *all-cause mortality* (that is, total mortality rate for the population across all causes of death). Furthermore, this association was not mediated (mediation being a mechanism that explains the association) by blood pressure, body mass index or cigarette smoking, these being variables associated with both intelligence and health. However, when the authors controlled for education level (which, as we've noticed above, is clearly closely correlated with intelligence), they found that the association between IQ and mortality diminished markedly. When it came to the relationship between intelligence and specific causes of mortality, IQ was associated with deaths from accidents, coronary heart disease and suicide, but not cancer.

This high level approach to understanding the relationship between intelligence and health has also been carried out in other studies. Catherine Calvin and colleagues (Calvin *et al.*, 2011) carried out a meta-analysis of the 16 studies (encompassing longitudinal studies ranging from 17 to 69 years) that examined the relationship between intelligence in young people and all-cause mortality. In summarising these findings an increase of one standard deviation in the distribution of IQ scores led to a 24 percent lower risk of death.

The relationship between general intelligence and other factors is the focus of debate in the next two discussion. However, it is worth noting that, like the health variables just discussed, it is proposed that general intelligence predicts poverty, the likelihood of being in prison, being divorced or unemployed (Gottfredson, 1997). All in all, the evidence suggests that general intelligence – particularly IQ test scores – is not only related to, but may be a relatively important predictor of, many aspects of our lives.

Problems and issues with intelligence tests

However, intelligence tests are not without their criticisms. There are three main considerations of IQ tests that you will commonly find in the intelligence literature. These considerations are based on:

- the reliability of intelligence tests;
- the validity of intelligence tests;
- whether the usefulness of intelligence tests is over-emphasised.

Reliability of intelligence tests

The reliability of any test refers to two aspects:

- **Internal reliability** – any measure of intelligence with good internal reliability will have a number of items that correlate positively with one another; this suggests they are measuring the same construct.

- **Test–retest reliability (reliability of the test over time)** – a good intelligence test will show a good level of reliability over time. Your general intelligence is thought to be relatively stable over time. Therefore you would expect that if you took an intelligence test on one occasion (and got an IQ score) and you took the same intelligence test 3 months later (and got an IQ score), you would expect your IQ scores to be very similar.

The internal reliability of intelligence scales is often well established in the research programmes that accompany the development of intelligence tests. Tests such as the Stanford–Binet Intelligence Scales and the Wechsler Intelligence Scales will provide information in their test manuals that shows the items that make up the different subscales, and the subscales that are used to compute an overall IQ score are positively related to one another. However, as established intelligence items and intelligence scales have largely been developed on the basis that they should be correlated with one another (i.e. if one item or subscale is not correlated, then test developers omit it from the test), the concern surrounding the internal reliability of established intelligence tests is not a major issue in intelligence. The issues surrounding the stability of intelligence test scores over time present a much more important consideration.

People who question whether intelligence tests are reliable over time point to the fact that general intelligence (IQ) scores fluctuate. That is, if you took an intelligence test today and took the same one a week later, your IQ score computed from taking that test would probably be different. Some researchers have estimated that this fluctuation may be as much as 15 IQ points (Benson, 2003). Furthermore, individual performances on intelligence tests may fluctuate between administrations because the individual may perform differently while taking the test (they may be having a particularly good day or a particularly bad day). This fluctuation is further compounded because test-takers are not meant to take the same intelligence test twice, as they will have learnt some of the answers or the techniques involved in the test and consequently would be expected to perform better. The point is that, once you have taken one general intelligence test, you will be assigned an IQ score. It is not possible to take the test again, because your later scores will be influenced by having taken the test before. Furthermore, given that IQ test scores fluctuate between administrations, how can you be sure that your first (and only) IQ score is not just a fluctuation from your real intelligence? You can see that if we are to assign people IQ scores and compare people's IQ scores based on their performance on a single administration of an intelligence test, these fluctuations of IQ scores may present a concern about the accuracy of IQ tests.

This concern of IQ scores fluctuating has been a long-term consideration of intelligence researchers, and it has spawned a whole area of research to consider these fluctuations over time. Findings suggest that, although intelligence test scores do fluctuate, they do remain relatively stable over time. We will now outline some of this research.

US developmental psychologists Harold E. Jones and Nancy Bayley (1941) set up what is now known as the Berkeley Growth Study. This study was started in the late 1920s and represents data from people born in Berkeley, California, between 1928 and 1929. These researchers tested a sample of children annually throughout childhood and adolescence on a number of measures, including intelligence, and calculated their IQ scores. Jones and Bayley found that IQ scores of children at 18 years were positively correlated with their IQ scores at 12 years ($r = 0.89$) and 6 years ($r = 0.77$).

It is important to remember here what is meant by stable IQ in childhood (Neisser *et al.*, 1996). You will remember that IQ scores are based around a mean of 100 and are calculated by comparing the individual's score with other individuals at that age. An average IQ score for a typical 7-year-old would be stable if the same person, at age 18, showed the same average IQ score. A lack of variation in IQ score between age 7 and age 18 does not mean that their IQ has stayed the same, because individual knowledge, critical thinking, vocabulary and ability to reason will increase with age. Rather, it means that their score stays the same to relative to other people. A 7-year-old with an IQ score of 100 is at the mean IQ of 7-year-olds, while an 18-year-old with an IQ score of 100 is at the mean of 18-year-olds.

The findings of Jones and Bayley are supported by more recent studies. The longest follow-up study of intelligence and relationship between IQ scores used the Mental Survey Committee in Scotland that had measured intelligence in Scottish children born in 1921 and attending school on 1 June, 1932 (n = 87,498). Scottish psychologists Ian Deary, Lawrence Whalley, Helen Lemmon, J. R. Crawford and John Starr (2000) followed up 101 people at the age of 77 years. They found that the correlation between the two occasions was r = 0.63 (which was adjusted to r = 0.73 when corrected for fine details regarding ability range within the 77-year-olds). In a follow-up study (Gow *et al.*, 2011) reported correlations of r = 0.67 between the ages of 11 and 70 years, r = 0.66 for between the ages of 11 and 77 years, and r = 0.51 between the ages of 11 and 87 years. These findings show substantial stability from childhood to late life of IQ scores on tests.

The correlations between intelligence scores across these age ranges are impressive. However, they are not perfect; and, although we would not expect them to show perfect correlations, if there are fluctuations between IQ scores on administrations, you can see why people might be concerned or cautious when assigning a child a particular IQ score.

Validity of intelligence tests

Validity of tests refers to the question of whether the test measures what it claims to measure. In the context of intelligence tests we can ask, do intelligence tests measure intelligence?

Well, within one context they do; if we answer the question, 'Do intelligence tests measure what they *claim* to measure?' If you consider an intelligence test, like the Wechsler Adult Intelligence Scale, for example, then there is little doubt that the subtests of this intelligence test are measuring the different specific intelligence abilities that they have been designed to measure. Again, intelligence test developers set about establishing validity for all aspects of their intelligence test when developing them. If an intelligence test, or a particular intelligence subtest, did not show validity in development, then test developers would seek to improve that measure of intelligence. You can also see that, on the face of it (sometimes called **face validity**), an intelligence test that involves solving problems using mental arithmetic probably measures, to a greater degree, mental arithmetic intelligence. Similarly, a subtest that requires a number of simple jigsaws to be completed probably measures intelligence in object assembly.

Face validity
An aspect of validity that is concerned with what the measure appears to measure.

Concurrent validity
A type of validity that assesses a test's acceptable correlations with known and accepted standard measures of that construct.

Predictive validity
A type of validity that assesses whether a measure can accurately predict something in the future.

Furthermore, intelligence tests show **concurrent validity** due to their relationship with other measures of intelligence. Neisser and the rest of the Intelligence Task Force (Neisser *et al.*, 1996) argue that it is generally accepted that individuals perform equally as well or poorly on different intelligence tests, suggesting that intelligence tests tend to correlate with other intelligence tests – although there is evidence to suggest that, when IQ is calculated from different intelligence tests, scores can also fluctuate by up to 15 IQ points (Benson, 2003). Also, as we have just seen, intelligence tests have been used to predict 'real-world' measures of intelligence or achievement; for example, school achievement and job performance (this is known as **predictive validity**). All these findings suggest evidence for the general validity of intelligence tests measuring what they claim to measure – general intelligence (as defined by an IQ score) that is worked out by adding together the performance on several subtests of specific abilities (e.g. arithmetic, object assembly, comprehension).

However, the discussion takes a turn when we consider the general question of validity in a slightly different way: 'Do intelligence tests measure *intelligence*?'

Some critics argue that the main problem with intelligence tests is that they assume, particularly when they produce an overall IQ score, that there is an idea of general intelligence when in fact there is no agreement on whether such a global mental capacity exists (Benson, 2003). Although some theorists and researchers suggest there is a general factor of intelligence (e.g. Spearman), other theorists and researchers have questioned the idea of general intelligence. For example, psychologists such as Howard Gardner identified nine intelligences that comprise his multiple intelligence theory (Gardner, 1993; 1995), and Robert Sternberg devised the triarchic theory of intelligence (Sternberg, 1985b; 1988) that comprises three aspects of intelligence (componential, contextual and experiential). In the current discussion we saw that cognitive intelligence tests (such as the Kaufmans') emphasise sequential and simultaneous cognitive processes as well as more traditional achievement abilities.

What is crucial about these different approaches is that some critics of intelligence tests emphasise that intelligence is probably much more than what can be measured by intelligence tests; rather, intelligence is the result of the individual engaging in a variety of skills and information within their cultural context. For example, everyday theories that surround intelligence differ between eastern and western cultures, and those theories change within cultures owing to changing perceptions of intelligence with age or across different disciplines (for example, business and philosophy).

Consequently, the concern is that many intelligence tests cannot be valid, as no single intelligence test covers the many different theoretical interpretations and cultural considerations that need to be made when accurately measuring intelligence.

Modern-day intelligence researchers continually wrestle with these types of considerations and distinctions. However, it is timely to remember that early intelligence researchers strived to develop intelligence tests that allowed and considered cultural differences. Both Yerkes' Army Beta test and Raven's Progressive Matrices were developed around theories of intelligence that emphasised general intelligence and IQ scores but sought to make their tests free of influences of literacy and the English language. The Wechsler Intelligence Scale for Children (WISC) and the Stanford–Binet Intelligence Scale have recently been changed so they better reflect the abilities of test-takers from diverse cultural and linguistic backgrounds.

None the less, one of the big distinctions regarding the validity of intelligence tests is the exact question we ask when questioning their validity. If we ask whether intelligence tests measure what they claim to measure, then they probably do. If we ask whether intelligence tests measure intelligence, then the answer is much less certain; it depends on what your definition of intelligence is.

Is the usefulness of intelligence tests over-emphasised?

Another criticism of intelligence tests is that their capacity to predict intellectual performance in different walks of life is overplayed, overstated or over-emphasised (Benson, 2003). We have seen how intelligence tests have been known to predict, quite strongly, both academic achievement and job performance. In the latter case of job performance, the predictive strength of intelligence tests is greater than that of interviews, curriculum vitae and previous experience. You can see why people would put emphasis on intelligence testing as it is such a strong predictor of job performance.

However, critics of intelligence testing note that there are fluctuations in the predictive strength of intelligence tests. For instance, time has a great effect on the ability of the intelligence test to predict performance. That is, the longer the time between the administration of the test and the measurement of the performance, the weaker the relationship. Furthermore, the predictive strength of intelligence tests fluctuates when other variables are considered; for example, when different demographics are considered (such as age, race, sex) or situations or tasks change.

Benson (2003) notes that one area where these concerns are apparent is that of special education, which is concerned with people with learning disabilities. This concern arises from the use of IQ tests to classify learning disabilities using the 'IQ-achievement discrepancy

Stop and think

Alternatives to intelligence testing

Former APA President Dr Diane F. Halpern of Claremont McKenna College once said, 'Critics of intelligence testing often fail to consider that most of the alternatives are even more prone to problems of fairness and validity than the measures that are currently used.'

- What argument do you think Dr Halpern is trying to put forward?
- What alternatives do you think there are to intelligence testing?

model'. The IQ-achievement discrepancy model was based on comparing children's achievement to their IQ score. Where children's achievement scores are a standard deviation or more below their IQ scores, they are identified as learning disabled. Benson (2003) suggests that identifying students using the IQ-achievement discrepancy model does little to help teachers understand what they need to do practically to help the student to learn, and it holds no clue to the educational programme that that child may need to undertake to improve. Therefore, other assessments of children's needs (for example, the child's behaviour at school and home) might be a better indicator. Indeed, problems with the use of intelligence tests in this area have been recognised by the US government. On 3 October 2001, the then President George Bush established a Commission on Excellence in Special Education to collect evidence on federal, state and local special education programmes. The reason for this was to develop policies for improving the education performance of students with disabilities. The President's Commission on Excellence in Special Education (PCESE) delivered its report to President Bush on 1 July 2002. One recommendation of this report was to suggest that the use of intelligence tests to diagnose learning disabilities should be discontinued.

Benson suggests that supporters of intelligence tests would readily accept the possible flaws in this application of intelligence testing within an IQ-achievement discrepancy model. Researchers in the area of intelligence have been thinking about such problems for a long time. For example, Kaufman and Kaufman (2001) were suggesting, before the President's Commission on Excellence in Special Education, that intelligence tests should not be administered by anonymous research scientists in schools, but by specially trained educational practitioners or teachers with an expertise in child learning. These administrators wouldn't just total an IQ score, but look at the child, work with the child more and make special recommendations. Kaufman and Kaufman (2001) suggest that in this context there is no reason to dispense with intelligence tests altogether. Rather, intelligence testing should be used with a number of educational tools to arrive at as good an assessment as possible of the child.[D]

Extremes of intelligence

IQ scores are no longer derived by dividing mental age by chronological age. If you took the test today, your score would be added up and directly compared with the scores of other people your age. An IQ of 100 is 'average' and would indicate that 50 percent of those your age had earned lower scores. As you can see in Figure 4.9, scores between 90 and 110 are labelled 'normal'. In this section, we consider the individuals whose IQ scores fall on either side of this range.

Intellectual disability and learning disorders

When individuals below the age of 18 obtain valid IQ scores that are approximately two standard deviations below the mean on an intelligence test, they meet one criterion for a classification of **intellectual disability**. For the WAIS, that criterion would represent an IQ score of 70. However, as shown in Table 4.5, to be considered intellectually disabled, individuals must also demonstrate limitations 'in adaptive behaviour as expressed in conceptual, social, and adaptive skills' (American Association on Mental Retardation, 2002, p. 73). In earlier times, the term *mental retardation* was used to refer to people with IQs of 70 to 75 and below. However, because of the expanded definition that includes consideration of adaptive behaviour, intellectual disability has become the more appropriate term (Schalock et al., 2007). When clinicians diagnose individuals with intellectual disability, they attempt to understand as much as possible what limitations each individual has with adaptive skills. Rather than categorising people just on IQ, the contemporary goal is to provide environmental and social supports that are closely matched to each individual's needs.

Intellectual disability Condition in which individuals have IQ scores of 70 to 75 or below and also demonstrate limitations in the ability to bring adaptive skills to bear on life tasks.

Intellectual disability can be brought about by a number of genetic and environmental factors. For example, individuals with *Down syndrome*—a disorder caused by extra genetic material on the 21st chromosome—often have low IQs. Another genetic disorder, known as *phenylketonuria* (PKU), also has a potential negative impact on IQ (Gassió et al., 2005). However, through strict adherence to a special diet, people can control the negative effects of PKU if it is diagnosed in infancy. Family studies suggest that genetic inheritance likely plays a role only in the range of what historically would have been called mild retardation (see Figure 4.9) (Plomin & Spinath, 2004). The more severe forms of retardation appear to be caused by the occurrence of spontaneous genetic abnormalities in an individual's development that are not heritable. The environment that is most often critical for intellectual disability is the prenatal environment. Pregnant women who suffer diseases such as rubella and syphilis are at risk for having children with intellectual disabilities. In addition, pregnant women

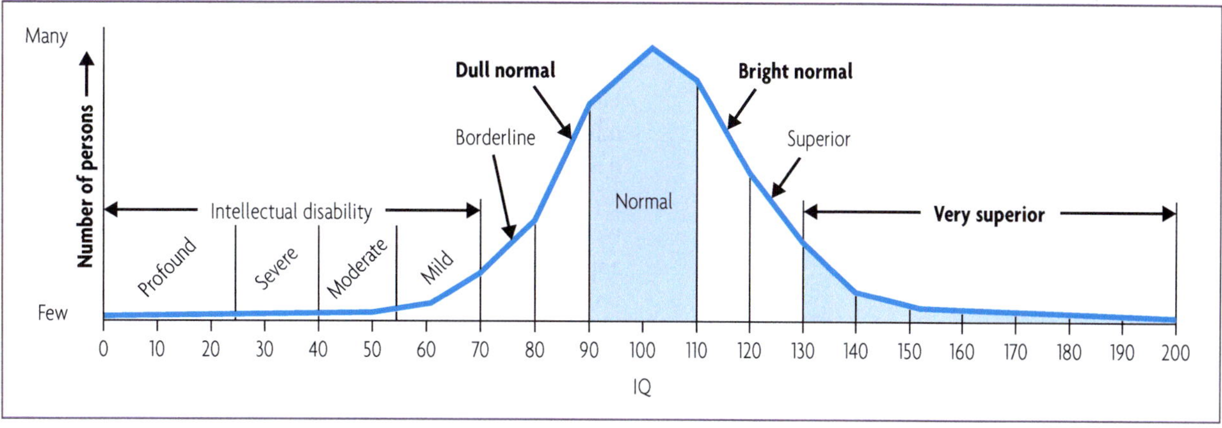

Figure 4.9 Distribution of IQ scores among a large sample

IQ scores are normed so that a score of 100 is the population average (as many people score below 100 as score above 100). Scores between 90 and 110 are labelled normal. Scores above 120 are considered to be superior or very superior; scores below 70 represent increasing levels of mental disability.

Adapted from Matarazzo, J.D. (1972). *Wechsler's Measurement and Appraisal of Adult Intelligence*, 5th edn. Copyright © 1972 by Oxford University Press, Inc. Used by permission of Oxford University Press, Inc.

[D]Maltby, J., Day, L., & Macaskill, A. (2013). The use of intelligence tests: What question emerge from the measurement of intelligence. In *Personality, individual differences and intelligence* (3rd ed., pp. 313-321). Harlow, Essex: Pearson Education Limited.

Table 4.5 Questions and problems similar to those on the WAIS-III

Verbal subtests	
Information	Who wrote *The Great Gatsby?*
Comprehension	What does it mean when people say 'Birds of a feather flock together'?
Arithmetic	If you paid $8.50 for a movie ticket and $2.75 for a bucket of popcorn, how much change would you have left from a $20 note?
Similarities	In what ways are aeroplanes and submarines alike?
Digit span	Repeat the following numbers: 3 2 7 5 9.
Vocabulary	What does *emulate* mean?
Performance subtests	
Digit symbol-coding	The examiner presents a key that matches digits (e.g., 1, 2, 3) with symbols (e.g., Φ, Θ, ∀). The test taker uses the key to complete a chart that gives just digits or symbols.
Picture completion	The test taker examines a picture and says what is missing (e.g., a horse without a mane).
Block design	The test taker uses patterned blocks to reproduce designs provided by the examiner.
Picture arrangement	The test taker puts a series of cartoon-like pictures into order so that they tell a story.
Object assembly	The examiner gives the test taker a set of cardboard puzzle pieces. The test taker arranges the pieces to form a picture of a common object.

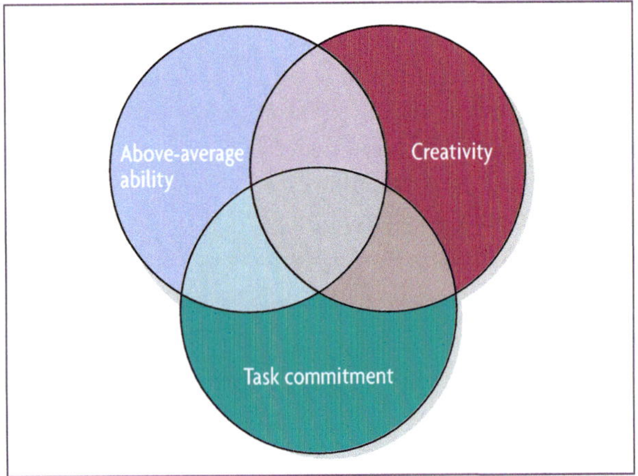

Figure 4.10 The three-ring conception of giftedness

According to the three-ring conception, gifted individuals are found at the intersection of above-average ability, high levels of creativity and high levels of task commitment.

From Renzulli, J.S. (1978). What makes giftedness? Re-examining a definition. *Phi Delta Kappan, 60*, 180–184. Copyright © Joseph S. Renzulli. Reprinted with permission.

who consume alcohol or other drugs, particularly during the early weeks of pregnancy, also increase the likelihood of having children with cognitive deficits (Bennett et al., 2008; Huizink & Mulder, 2006).

Historically, individuals with intellectual disabilities were educated—to the extent that they were educated—almost entirely in separate facilities. However, because evidence accumulated that these separate programs were not effective, the United States Government passed legislation requiring that students with disabilities be educated to the greatest extent possible in general classrooms (Williamson et al., 2006). The law recognises that some levels of impairment skill require students to receive separate instruction. However, about 45 percent of students diagnosed with an intellectual disability spend some or much of each school day in classrooms with their peers.

IQ scores give general information about how well people are able to perform—with respect to age-appropriate norms—on a variety of verbal and nonverbal tasks. In some instances, there is cause for concern when IQ scores and performance fail to match up. People who present a sufficiently large discrepancy between their achievement and their measured IQ might be diagnosed with a learning disorder. Before clinicians diagnose a **learning disorder**, they need to rule out other factors that can lead to poor performance such as low motivation, mediocre teaching or physical problems (such as visual deficits). Many schools provide special assistance to students who have been diagnosed with learning disorders.

Learning disorder A disorder defined by a large discrepancy between individuals' measured IQ and their actual performance.

Giftedness

Individuals are most likely to be labelled as *gifted* if they have an IQ score above 130. However, as with the definition of intellectual disability, researchers have suggested that the conception of giftedness is not adequately captured just by IQ. For example, Joseph Renzulli (2005) has argued in favour of a 'three-ring' conception of giftedness that characterises giftedness along the dimensions of ability, creativity and task commitment (see Figure 4.10). Individuals can be considered gifted with IQs that are above average but not necessarily superior. In addition, they need to show high levels of creativity and exert high levels of commitment to particular problems or domains of performance. This expanded definition of giftedness explains why people often are not gifted across the academic spectrum (Winner, 2000). Abilities, creativity, and task commitment may all differ, for example, between verbal and mathematical domains.

What qualities do gifted children generally possess? The formal study of gifted children began in 1921 when Lewis Terman (1925) began a long-term study of a group of over 1500 boys and girls who tested in the top 1 percent of their school populations. This group of individuals was followed all the way into their 80s (Holahan & Sears, 1995). Terman and his successors wanted to see how these children fared as they made their way through life. The questions Terman asked continue to shape the research agenda. For example, Terman explored the myth that gifted children have problems with social and emotional adjustment. Terman concluded just the opposite: he found his sample to be better adjusted than their less gifted peers. However, more contemporary studies support the conclusion that gifted children are more introverted—more internally oriented—than their peers (Sak, 2004). That orientation toward their own inner lives supports, in part, the task commitment that helps define giftedness. Still, gifted students report a reasonable level of participation in school activities. For example, a sample of 230 students attending a summer gifted program reported sports as their most frequent extracurricular or out-of-school activity (Olszewski-Kubilius & Lee, 2004). They were also involved in many academic clubs and competitions, with particular emphasis on mathematics.

Terman also documented that the children were largely successful in life. This is not surprising because IQ is a good predictor of occupational status and income. Thus the concern about gifted individuals is not that they aren't doing well. The concern, instead, is that they don't receive sufficient educational support to allow them to develop their gifts fully (Sternberg & Grigorenko, 2003; Winner, 2000). When giftedness is recognised as a multidimensional construct, gifted education must also have the flexibility to address individual students' particular talents.[E]

The heritability of intelligence

Intelligence: the nature versus nurture debate

Here we will outline what has become known as the nature versus nurture debate. We will compare and consider genetic versus environmental effects on intelligence.

Galton

As we saw earlier, in 1865 Sir Francis Galton began to study the heritability of intelligence, following his reading of his cousin Charles Darwin's publication *The Origin of Species*, which dealt with the idea that all species gradually evolve through the process of natural selection. In following this work, Galton soon became interested in studying the variations in human ability, and particularly intelligence. In his book *Hereditary Genius* (Galton, 1869), he began investigating why higher intelligence seemed to run in families. He suggested that man's

[E]Gerrig, R. J., Zimbardo, P. G., Campbell, A. J., Cumming, S. R., & Wilkes, F. J. (2012). Intelligence and intelligence assessment. In *Psychology and life* (2nd ed., pp. 331–333). Frenchs Forest, NSW: Pearson Australia.

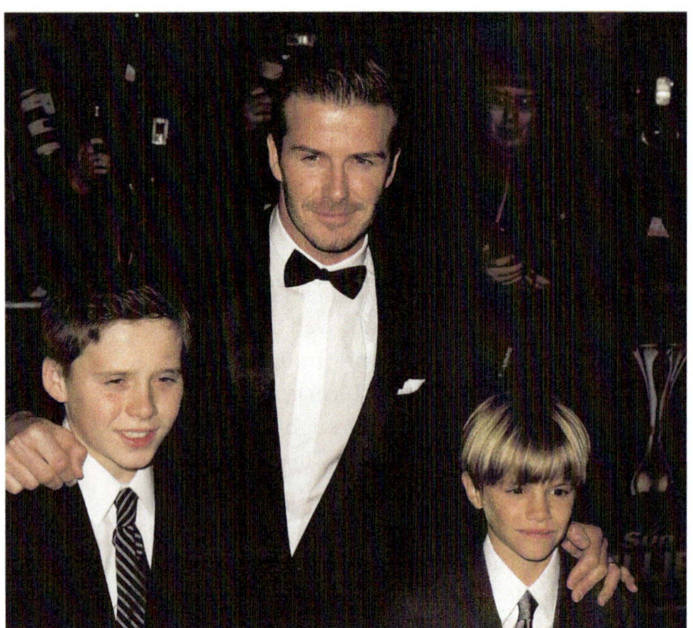

Galton felt that there was some value in studying eminent families as an indicator of the heritability of intelligence. How well would such an approach work today?
Source: Shutterstock.com/Featureflash/Simon Burchell

natural abilities are inherited under the same conditions as physical features of the animal world described by Darwin. Galton suggested that children inherit their intelligence from their parents.

To support such an assertion, Galton started analysing the obituaries of *The Times* newspaper so that he could identify the ancestry of eminent men. What Galton did was to compare different degrees of relationship between individuals in terms of being biological relatives (i.e. parents, siblings, cousins) and the eminence of each of these individuals. First-degree relatives are relatives with whom an individual shares an estimated average of 50 percent (half) of their genes (though note this is an estimated average percentage; you will learn more about why this is an estimated average later in this discussion). First-degree relatives include your parents, brothers and sisters and children. A second-degree relative is a relative with whom an individual shares an estimated average of 25 percent (a quarter) of their genes; that is, grandparents, grandchildren, aunts, uncles, nephews, nieces. A third-degree relative is a relative with whom an individual shares an estimated average of 12.5 percent (one-eighth) of their genes. Third-degree relatives include your great-grandparents, great-aunts, great-uncles and first cousins. Galton found that the number of eminent relatives of an eminent person was greater for first-degree relatives than for second-degree relatives; and again, the number was greater for second-degree relatives than for third-degree relatives. This result suggested to Galton that there is evidence for the heritability of intelligence.

However, Galton quickly became concerned with whether intelligence was simply heritable or whether it was also influenced by the environment. It was here that Galton was the first psychologist to make the distinction between 'nature' and 'nurture' (and he was the first to use this now-common phrase). To examine this idea, he surveyed 190 Fellows of the Royal Society, of which Galton was a member (Galton, 1874). The Royal Society is a highly prestigious scientific society dedicated to establishing the truth of scientific matters through experiment. It has had several famous scientists as members, including Robert Boyle, Sir Christopher Wren and Isaac Newton. Galton asked his fellow members of the Society several questions regarding their birth order and the occupation and race of their parents. He wanted to find out whether members of the Society's achievements and interest in science were caused by their natural makeup (nature) or their environment; for example, the encouragement of their talents by others (nurture).

You have to remember that many of Galton's speculations arose before we knew as much about genetics as we do today. That is why many recognise him as a truly great scientist. Galton himself recognised the inherent problems of such studies (Galton, 1875). For example, he speculated about the confounding effects of the environment and realised that eminent people might not have arisen to their current status alone, but with the help of relatives. Galton believed that the question of whether nature or nurture influences intelligence could be examined more carefully by comparing twins. He suggested that comparisons of twins who were similar at birth but had grown up in different environments, and comparisons of dissimilar twins who had grown up in similar environments, might hold the key to examining the nature–nurture debate surrounding intelligence. He also proposed that adoption studies might be useful to analyse the different effects of heredity and environment. His speculations about twins and adoption studies laid the groundwork for modern attempts to examine the nature–nurture debate in intelligence.

Heritability of intelligence

Within the nature versus nurture consideration of intelligence, we find ourselves concentrating on behavioural genetic principles. One area of behavioural genetics concentrates on the relationships between genes and environment, to compare the similarities and differences between individuals within a particular population and assess the relative influence of genes and the environment on any behaviour. In this case, the behaviour we are looking at is intelligence.

What do we mean by heritability of intelligence?

Behavioural geneticists such as Robert Plomin have written extensively about behavioural genetics (Plomin 2004; Plomin *et al.*, 2000). Heritability of intelligence begins with the fact that genes are biologically transmitted from biological parents to the child. Children inherit 50 percent of their father's genes and 50 percent of their mother's genes. We can use this information as a starting point to explore how genes influence intelligence.

The assessment of the extent to which any phenotype (any outward manifestation of the individual – physical attractiveness, behaviour, intelligence) is passed on from parents to children, from the results of their genes, is termed **genetic heritability**. The genetic heritability of any phenotype is assessed in terms of variability (i.e. how much they differ) between the parents and the child. This variability is often assessed within the *proportion of shared variance* of that behaviour between the parent and child. Proportion of shared variance is presented as a percentage (i.e. out of 100 percent). When a parent and child are very similar in a particular characteristic, there is thought to be a low variability between parent and child, and the proportion of shared variance of that behaviour is high (nearer 100 percent). In other words, the parent and child are not very different in this characteristic. Conversely, when a parent and child are quite different in a particular characteristic, there is thought to be a high variability between parent and child, and the proportion of shared variance of that behaviour is low (nearer 0 percent).

Genetic heritability
The extent to which genetic differences in individuals contribute to individual differences in a behaviour (e.g. personality or intelligence).

The heritability of a human physical characteristic, such as having a nose, is entirely genetic and not in any way influenced by factors such as the environment. In fact, the environment is seen as having zero variability, or a proportion of shared variance of 100 percent. However, some aspects of human behaviour (including intelligence), in which the environment is thought to have an influence, have greater amounts of heritable variability and lower shared variance. For example, choosing which football team to support would be heavily determined by environmental factors such as where you are born, your parents' football team, your friends and the first football team you see. Choosing a favourite football team has high variability between parent and child, but the proportion of shared variance of favourite football team caused by genetic heritability would be zero (0 percent).

In behavioural genetics of intelligence, researchers are primarily interested in *estimating* the extent of genetic heritability of intelligence across a population, and stating the genetic heritability of that behaviour in terms of shared variance. This estimated average of genetic heritability is known as h^2. Therefore, h^2 is the *average estimate* of the proportion of variance for intelligence thought to be accounted for by genetic factors across a population.

You may have noticed that we emphasised *estimating*, *estimate* ('estimate' meaning to calculate approximately) and *average*. This is because, for a long time in psychology, for any phenotype (characteristic or behaviour) the estimates of the strength of genetics factors were done and interpreted within a process called *additive assumption*. Additive assumption suggests that there are only two dimensions that determine heritability of any behaviour (in our case, intelligence): (1) the genetic part, which we've just outlined; and (2) the environment. Consequently, overall, heritability of intelligence is estimated in terms of the relative strength of both (e.g. nature versus nurture). Therefore, the influence of genetic (G) and environmental (E) components, in this theory, will always add together to account for 100 percent of the variance of intelligence. On the basis of this assumption, the heritability coefficient (h^2) can be subtracted from 100 percent to calculate the environmental contribution to intelligence. If researchers computed, for example, that genetics accounted for an average of 25 percent of the variance for intelligence, we would estimate that the environmental factors account for an average of 75 percent of the variance of intelligence. However, it is important to note that the additive assumption is now considered a starting point for calculating heritability of intelligence and for estimating the number of genes that people are expected to share (e.g. brothers and sisters are expected to share 50 percent). We will see later in this discussion that this view of assessing heritability has changed a lot. The idea of determining the relative strength of genetics and environmental factors by simply adding together genetic and environmental factors is more complicated than once thought, and psychologists really do emphasise the words 'estimate' and 'average' when referring to heritability.

Methods for assessing genetic heritability of intelligence

So, how might we assess genetic influences on intelligence? Well, as Galton himself mentioned, the relationship between genes and intelligence has traditionally been studied by concentrating on the similarities and differences between populations of individuals to assess the relative influence of their shared genes in intelligence.

Plomin (2004) identifies three main types of studies that use this technique: family studies, twin studies and adoption studies. As children share an estimated average of 50 percent of their genes with each of their parents, and they also share genes with their brothers and sisters, it is of interest to behavioural genetics researchers to examine possible associations between parents' and children's behaviours within a family. This leads to the first type of study, family studies. However, these studies on their own potentially tell us very little because all children share an estimated average of 50 percent of their genes with each of their parents and with their brothers and sisters. As well as this, using observation, interview or questionnaire measures also presents a problem because similarities between personalities might be caused by environmental influence (i.e. an intelligent daughter might be like her extraverted mother because she copies her behaviour). These are real concerns until we consider the occasions when families don't typically share genes in this way. There are two main examples: twin studies and adoption studies.

Twin studies provide an interesting area of research, as there is a possibility of comparing different types of genetic makeup to compare genetic influences. The term 'twin' refers to two individuals who have shared the same uterus (the uterus or womb is the major female reproductive organ). Identical (or monozygotic, MZ) twins occur when a single egg is fertilised to form one zygote, but the zygote then divides into two separate embryos. The two embryos develop into fetuses sharing the same womb. Identical twins are always of the same sex and have the same arrangement of genes and chromosomes (which contain the hereditary information necessary for cell life). These twins share 100 percent of genes with each other. Fraternal twins (non-identical, or dizygotic, DZ, twins) usually occur when two fertilised eggs are implanted in the uterine wall at the same time. The two eggs form two zygotes (hence they are dizygotic). These twins share an estimated average of 50 percent of their genetic makeup. Consequently, some researchers compare behaviours across non-twins, identical and fraternal twins to examine the relative influence of genetics.

The influence of the environment and genetics is often compared in adoption studies. Intelligence can be compared between parents and adopted children, as there is no genetic heritability. Variables are often compared between siblings, or twins, reared apart to examine the extent of genetic and environmental effects. For example, if two twins show similar behaviours, despite being raised in different environments, this suggests that genes may be important in that behaviour.

Once you consider all these types of studies together, in which intelligence is compared between parents and children, and siblings that share 0–100 percent genetic similarity, you can begin to make assessments of the extent of genetic heritability across a population.

It is important to remember that there is no physiological procedure in these sorts of studies. Behaviour geneticists do not have the ability to assess the genetic heritability of intelligence using advanced biological measures or a complex scientific genetic analysis (well, not yet). Rather, researchers look for similarities and differences in intelligence among individual people by using observation, interview or questionnaire measures. They look for similarities between parents' and children's intelligence (using intelligence measures) to determine the extent of genetic influence on intelligence. It is also important to remember that, when we deal with heritability estimates, we don't talk about heritability estimates for particular individuals; rather, researchers estimate the average heritability among certain populations of people – MZ (identical) twins, DZ (fraternal) twins, family members, parents and children. So, heritability estimate of 50 percent for intelligence does not mean that we all inherit 50 percent of that intelligence trait from our genes; it means that, across the population, the genetic heritability of intelligence has been estimated at an average of 50 percent.

Heritability estimates of intelligence

What is the heritability of intelligence from these types of studies? Well, some studies have estimated the heritability of intelligence based on family, twin and adoption studies.

For example, there have been a number of findings from Bouchard's Minnesota Study of Twins Reared Apart (overseen by US behavioural geneticist Thomas Bouchard). This research involves not only the medical and psychological assessment of identical (MZ) and fraternal (DZ) twins separated early in life and reared apart, on which figures are given, but also their intelligence. A well-cited documentation of these studies was recently provided by behavioural geneticist journalist Matt Ridley (Ridley, 1999). Ridley put together all the modern family, twin and adoption studies, which mainly included the findings of Bouchard and McGue's meta-analysis of 111 studies (Bouchard and McGue, 1981). The following analysis by Ridley is the concordance rate of IQ (the presence of the same intelligence level between two individuals) from all these studies (in parentheses are concordance rates given by Bouchard and McGue's meta-analysis; see also Figure 4.11):

- 100%: Perfect concordance rate;
- 87%: Same person tested twice;
- 86%: Identical twins reared together (86%);
- 76%: Identical twins reared apart (72%);
- 55%: Fraternal twins reared together (60%);
- 47%: Biological siblings reared together (47%);
- 40%: Parents and children living together (42%);
- 31%: Parents and children living apart (22%);

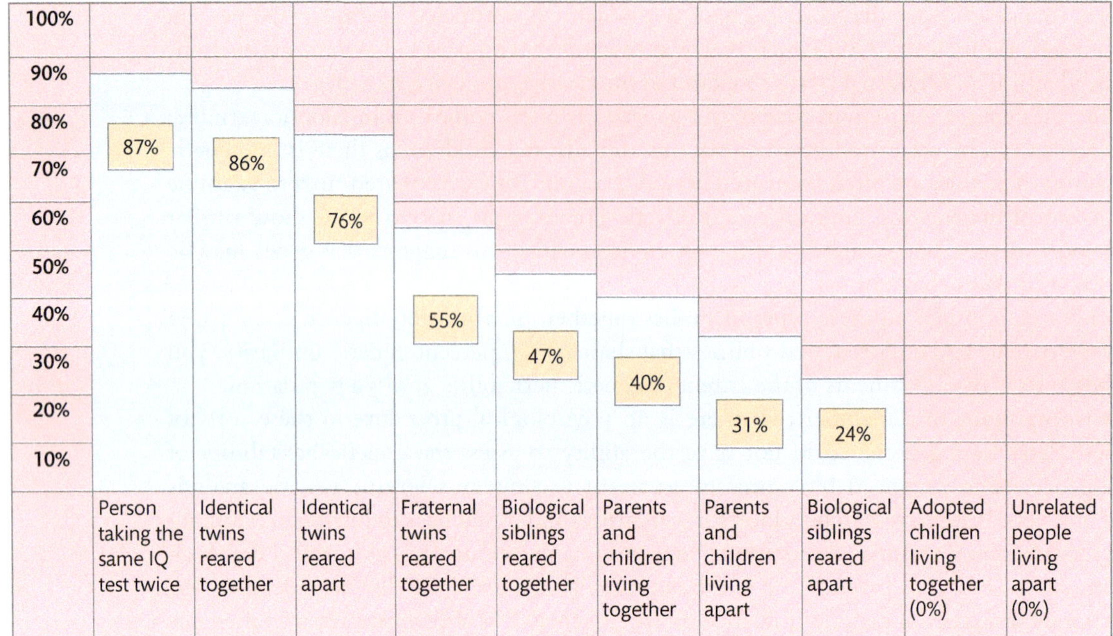

Figure 4.11 Concordance rates of intelligence.
Source: From Ridley, M. (1999). *Genome: the autobiography of a species in 23 chapters*. London: Fourth Estate. HarperCollins Publishers Ltd. © M. Ridley 1999.

- 24%: Biological siblings reared apart (24%);
- 15%: Cousins (Bouchard and McGue only);
- 0%: Adopted children living together;
- 0%: Unrelated people living apart.

Evidence such as this, coming from studies throughout the century, was consistent, and researchers were able to make estimates on the level of genetic heritability of intelligence. You can see from evidence like this how people would tend to estimate the influence of genetics on intelligence as in some instances relatively high, because the evidence for heritability, in some instances, is over 80 percent. For example, Professor Hans Eysenck (Eysenck, 1979) used this sort of evidence to suggest that the estimation of heritability of intelligence was around 69 percent in the general population. Later, Herrnstein and Murray (1994), whose work we will discuss at greater length later, estimated heritability in the general population at 74 percent.

Recent research suggests that previous figures quoted by Eysenck and Herrnstein and Murray may be a little high, but the view that genetics accounts for a weighty part of intelligence should not be ignored. In 2012 Ian Deary and a number of colleagues (Deary *et al.*, 2012) provided an estimate of the genetic contribution to stability of intelligence across most of the human lifetime. Deary compared the results of just under 2,000 unrelated individuals (n = 1,940) whose intelligence was measured first in childhood (age 11 years) and then again in old age (at age 65, 70 or 79 years). What was unique about this study was that the authors combined DNA analysis, a new statistical analysis, with data from the people in the study. They examined more than half a million genetic markers in this cohort to work out how genetically similar they were even though they were not related. What is important about this is that this method uses the same type of approach as that used in twin studies, looking for genetic similarity, and that the researchers are able to make, through the use of DNA analysis, more concise comparisons in terms of genetic similarity. Deary *et al.* found that the stability of cognitive ability from childhood to old age has a genetic contribution estimated at 38% of the variance.

However, in 2011, Deary (Deary, 2012) carried out a review on studies looking at the genetic contribution to stability of intelligence. An important point made by Deary is that the heritability of intelligence varies at different ages or across culture. In terms of age, Oliver Davis and colleagues (Davis *et al.*, 2009), using data in the Twins Early Development Study in the United Kingdom, found (from measures of verbal and non-verbal intelligence tests administered at ages 2, 3 and 4 years) that, for general intelligence, the heritability estimates were 23% in early childhood, and that this increased to 62% by middle childhood (from measuring intelligence from four mental ability tests at ages 7, 9 and 10 years). In terms of culture, studies among twin family studies in the Netherlands suggest the percentage of variance accounted for by genetic effects rises to over 80% for verbal IQ and just below 70% for performance IQ (Posthuma *et al.*, 2001). However, in Vietnam, findings suggest that genetic factors account for 49% of the variation in young adults and 57% in middle age (Lyons *et al.*, 2009).

Deary's research and reviews show that we are able to consider a lot more about the influences of genetics on intelligence today than previous work, and can provide a better consideration, though never perfect, of the relative influence of genetics and environment on intelligence. Some of these influences will now be outlined in detail so that you can see their relevance to the literature on intelligence as well as how estimates of the genetic influence on intelligence might be lower than previously estimated.

Considerations within behavioural genetics and intelligence

The idea of how genes and the environment are viewed, and used, to predict the heritability of intelligence has changed over recent years.

Authors such as US psychologists E. E. Maccoby (2000) and Robert Plomin (2004) suggest the additive principle of determining heritability of intelligence (or any phenotype) is not applicable any more. The validity of the additive assumption in computing the relative strength of genetics and environment in determining behaviour has been widely challenged. The first problem is that estimating the environment is usually done without utilising any direct measures of environmental factors. For example, researchers often compute genetic heritability and then subtract that from 100 percent. Obviously, if the estimates of heritability are indeterminate, or prone to error, so are the estimates of E derived by subtracting heritability from 100 percent. A further problem with the additive assumption of computing heritability is that, when genetic heritability is large, it assumes that all environmental factors associated with that behaviour must be small. Therefore, it is better to see human intelligence as a joint result of an interaction between a person's genes and environmental factors. Intelligence should not be seen as the result of 'genetics + environment' but rather of 'genetics × environment'. For example, it is better to view the relative influences of genes and environment on intelligence as the result of a long-term interaction, with environmental factors triggering certain genetic behaviours and the effects of the environment differing between individuals because of their genetic makeup.

What is important for you to note is that these changes and developments in research and thinking have been suggested, encouraged and developed by both theorists and researchers, many of whom we have already mentioned, who support and criticise the idea of genetic heritability in intelligence. So, what has brought about, and resulted from, such a general shift in thinking, from the additive principle of 'genetics + environment' to the later, more integrative, idea of 'genetics × environment'? Well, four considerations surrounding modern-day thinking in behavioural genetics are important when considering any phenotype, particularly intelligence (see Figure 4.12):

- conceptions of heritability and the environment;
- different types of genetic variance;
- the representativeness of twin and adoption studies;
- assortative mating.

Conceptions of genetic heritability and the environment

Gregory Carey (2002) suggests that there are two important contexts within which to consider heritability and environmental influences on intelligence:

- **Abstract concepts** – these are generally theoretical (not applied or practical) concepts. As Carey explains, whatever the numerical estimates of either genetic or environmental influences, they provide us with little information about the specific genes, or specific environmental variables, that influence intelligence.
- **Population concepts** – all of these estimates refer to any group of people considered as a population, but they tell us very little about any single individual. For example, just because intelligence may have a genetic heritability of around 60 percent, it does not mean, for any one individual, that 60 percent of their intelligence is due to genes and 40 percent of their intelligence is due to the environment. Rather, it is estimated across the population that genetic heritability of intelligence is an average of around 40 percent, and individuals will vary around that estimate.

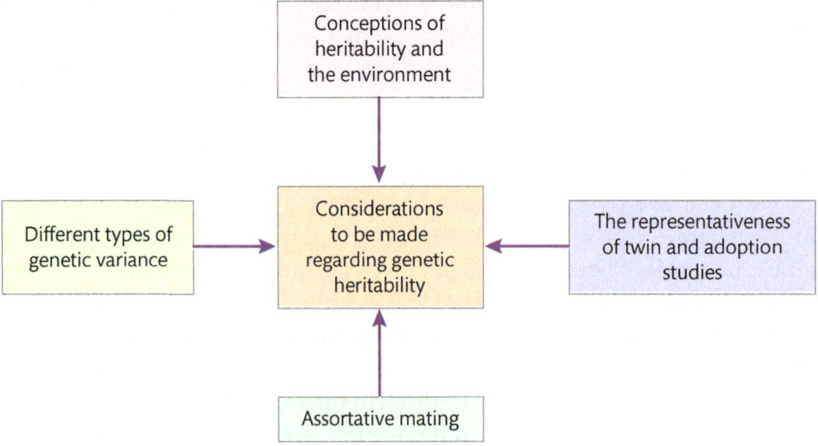

Figure 4.12 Considerations to be made regarding genetic heritability.

Different types of genetic variance

So far in this discussion, we have treated genetic influence on intelligence only as a single entity, namely, the influence of your genes on your intelligence. However, behavioural genetics researchers such as Thomas Bouchard and M. McGue (Bouchard and McGue, 1981) note that genetic influence does not simply comprise one aspect, but in fact three aspects: (1) additive genetic variance; (2) dominant genetic variance; and (3) epistatic genetic variance.

Additive genetic variation is the genetic variance that we have described previously in this discussion; that is, genetic variation in behaviour that is the total of the individual's genes inherited from their parents.

Additive genetic variation
Variation caused by the effects of numerous genes which combine in the defining of phenotypic behaviour.

However, the two other types of genetic variation are known as non-additive genetic variance.

First, **dominant genetic variance** is part of a process by which certain genes are expressed (dominant genes) and other genes are not expressed (recessive genes). Every one of us has two copies of every gene, one inherited from our mother and one from our father. Sometimes the two genes that determine a particular trait (for example, eye colour) will actually code for two types of characteristics (for example, blue eyes and brown eyes). If one of these genes is dominant, then only its character is expressed and not that of the other gene. For example, if blue eyes were a dominant gene, and your mother had brown eyes and your father had blue eyes, you would be likely to inherit blue eyes.

Dominant genetic variance
Part of a process by which certain genes are expressed (dominant) and other genes are not expressed (recessive).

Secondly, **epistatic genetic variance** (known as interactive genetic variance) refers to a process by which genes interact. It is now known that several different genes not only influence physical characteristics and behaviour on their own, but work and interact together. Unlike dominant genetic variance, which just applies to one gene replacing another, epistatic genetic variance is the result of the way certain genes that we inherit determine whether other genes we inherit will be expressed or suppressed (this process is called **epistasis**).

Epistatic genetic variance
Refers to a process by which genes interact. Also known as interactive genetic variance.

Epistatis
The masking or unmasking of the effects of one gene by the action of another.

It is difficult to measure dominant genetic variance and epistatic genetic variance when it comes to intelligence. However, it is now accepted that these three aspects – additive genetic variance, dominant genetic variance and epistatic genetic variance – are thought to make up **total genetic variance** of intelligence.

Total genetic variance
This includes three aspects of genetic variance, additive genetic variance, dominant genetic variance and epistatic genetic variance.

You can see that the genetic side of things is a lot more complicated than just viewing genes as a single entity, as genes interact and suppress other genes. You will see, in the literature, behavioural geneticists referring to terms such as 'narrow heritability' and 'broad heritability'. Narrow heritability is just additive genetic variance. Broad heritability is all three aspects of genetic heritability (additive genetic variance + dominant genetic variance + epistatic genetic variance).

Consequently, authors such as Thomas Bouchard and M. McGue (1981) and US psychologists Heather Chipeur, Michael Rovine and Robert Plomin (1990) have suggested that original estimates of the average percentage of parental genes that children inherit, and siblings share, may have previously been oversimplified. For example, these authors suggest that genetic variations in heritability of any phenotype (including intelligence) should be made in the following terms:

- identical (MZ) twins = additive genetic variance = non-additive genetic variance (where previously it was presumed to be solely additive genetic variance);
- fraternal (DZ) twins = 0.5 of additive genetic variance + 0.25 of non-additive genetic variance (rather than just 0.5 of additive genetic variance).

As you can see, computing the level of genetic variance may be more complicated than previously thought. Today, behavioural geneticists take these factors into account when suggesting the strength of heritability estimates of intelligence.

Problems with the representativeness of twin and adoption studies

One of the considerations put forward by psychologists such as Maccoby and by Leon Kamin and Arthur Goldberger (2002) concerns adoption and twin studies. A significant portion of studies examining heritability effects is devoted to twin and adoption studies. Twin studies are important because they allow the comparison of different types of twins to compare genetic influences; MZ twins who share 100 percent of their genes and DZ twins who share 50 percent of their genes. Adoption studies are important because they include two sets of factors that may account for differences in behaviour: biological parents and environmental parents. Therefore, it is argued that these families aren't necessarily representative of the normal populations. This natural bias in sampling may under- or over-estimate heritability estimates across the general population because genetic influences in these samples may not be representative of the whole population.

This issue is particularly important when considering research that assesses heritability of intelligence using twin and adoption studies. Leon Kamin and Arthur Goldberger (2002) estimate that twin studies might over-estimate the role of genetics, particularly because identical twins have more similar environments than do same-sex fraternal twins. Also, research shows that identical twins are treated more similarly by their parents, spend more time together and more often have the same friends. Their environmental experience comprises a greater proportion of each other's social environment than does that of fraternal siblings. Consequently, if genetic heritability estimates are usually larger in twin studies than in adoption studies, then some of the estimated similarity that is attributed to genetic influence might not be correct. Stoolmiller (1998) has also suggested that adoption studies lead to a similar restriction of the measurement of environmental factors. Stoolmiller argues that the placement strategies of adoption agencies might influence heritability estimates. For example, adoption agencies might always place children in affluent or middle- to high-income families; thus the effects of economic status are never fully explored in these studies, because an adopted child would rarely be placed into a household suffering from poverty.

Assortative mating

Nicholas Mackintosh (Mackintosh, 1998), animal-learning theorist at the University of Cambridge, raises the issue that assortative mating can have an effect on genetic variance and, therefore, on estimates of genetic heritability of intelligence. **Assortative mating** is a complicated name for the simple concept that, when couples mate, they either have several traits in common or contrast wildly in their traits. A lot of the understanding of genetic variation is based on the assumption that two individuals mate quite randomly with random people and, therefore, that any genetic similarity between them is by chance. But we know that this is not true. We know that people mate with people who they perceive to be similar to themselves. For example, we tend to see people mating with people who are of a similar size, or similar in their 'good-lookingness'. This is called positive assortative mating. Equally, we find people mating who are completely the opposite. This is called negative assortative mating. Therefore, in much the same way, the assortative mating principle can be applied to intelligence. That is, individuals may seek to mate with people who are of a similar intelligence. Think about your parents; do they have a similar educational background to each other?

Assortative mating
When individuals mate with individuals that are like themselves (positive assortative mating) or dissimilar (negative assortative mating). These two types of assortative mating are thought to have the effect of reducing and expanding the range of variation of heritable traits.

Modern estimates of the genetic heritability of intelligence

In the light of the considerations just outlined, different researchers have tried to estimate the overall heritability of intelligence across the general population. These estimates tend to be broad estimates of genetic variance (additive and non-additive genetic variance) in intelligence. They break down by what percentage of intelligence is determined by genetics and what percentage can be attributed to the environment. As we have already mentioned, higher estimates of heritability have come from authors like Hans Eysenck (1971; 1991), who once estimated it at 69 percent. There is no evidence to suggest that this is wrong; however, modern-day commentators, given the preceding issues relating to heritability estimates, are more conservative; they suggest that heritability falls into a range. The American Psychological Association Task Force headed by Ulric Neisser, estimates that the heritability of intelligence ranges from 40 to 80 percent (Neisser *et al.*, 1996), while Nicholas Mackintosh (1998) suggests a range of 30 to 75 percent. If you are looking for a more exact figure, Chipeur *et al.* (1990) have suggested the genetic heritability of intelligence at 50 percent which is a commonly – but not always – accepted viewpoint.

All this discussion, and we haven't even considered the extent of environmental effects on intelligence yet!

Environmental influences on intelligence

The list of possible environmental effects on intelligence could be endless. It could range from the effects on intelligence of long-term poverty (for example, never getting the opportunities to develop skills at home, at school and consequently in a career), through to one conversation with one teacher who suggests that the person will never amount to much. Thomas Bouchard and Nancy Segal (1985) list 21 factors that are related to intelligence, including malnutrition, weight at birth, height, years in school, father's economic status, father's and mother's education and influence, average TV viewing, self-confidence, criminality and emotional adaptation. However, the American Psychological Association Task Force (Neisser *et al.*, 1996) identified four main areas of environmental effects on intelligence that can be deemed as the most important. This information allows us to concentrate the debate. Some of these environmental effects you will have come across before (for example, nutrition, schooling and occupation), but we will revisit them so that you can see how they apply directly to the issues of the nature versus nurture debate on intelligence. These four areas are: (1) biological variables; (2) family; (3) school and education; and (4) culture (see Figure 4.13).

Biological variables and maternal effects

It is well acknowledged by the APA Task Force (Neisser *et al.*, 1996) that a number of biological factors influence intelligence. These include nutrition, before- and after-birth factors and substances like alcohol and lead poisoning.

Nutrition

Much of the nutrition hypothesis has already been discussed. Nutrition is the study of food; specifically, the relationship between diet and states of health and disease. You will remember that Lynn (1990) has proposed that nutrition and healthcare improvements are among the

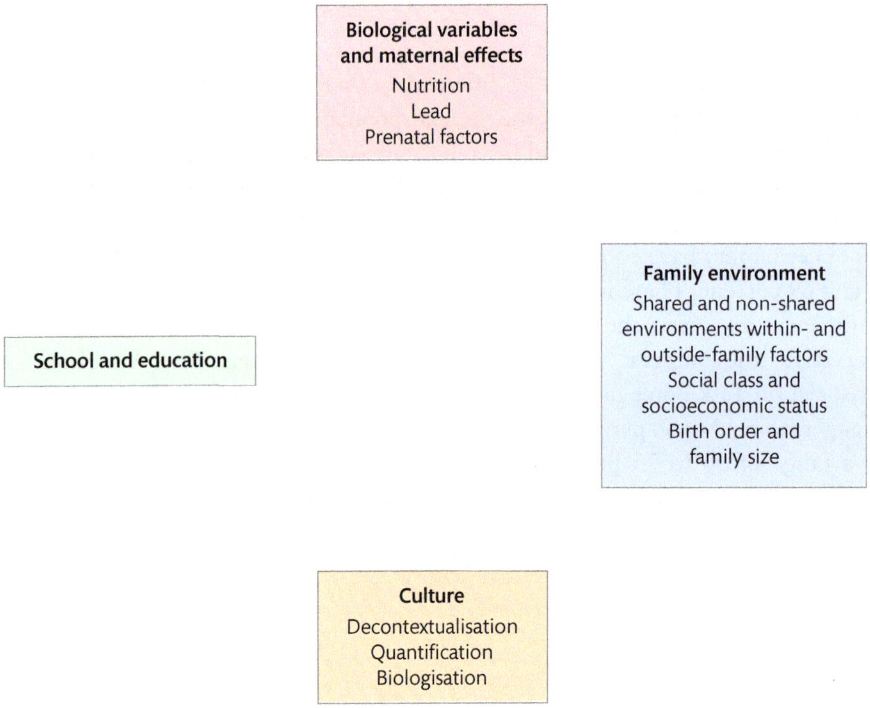

Biological variables and maternal effects
Nutrition
Lead
Prenatal factors

School and education

Family environment
Shared and non-shared environments within- and outside-family factors
Social class and socioeconomic status
Birth order and family size

Culture
Decontextualisation
Quantification
Biologisation

Figure 4.13 Environmental effects on intelligence.

main reasons for the Flynn effect. However, outside Lynn's hypothesis there are findings that nutritional sources can aid aspects of intelligence.

Australian nutritionist Wendy H. Oddy and her colleagues (Oddy *et al.*, 2004) examined over 2,000 Australian children and followed them from birth until the age of 8 years. Oddy and her colleagues found that stopping breast feeding early (at 6 months or less) was associated with reduced verbal intelligence, while children who were fully breast fed for more than 6 months scored between 3 and 6 IQ points higher on a vocabulary intelligence test than did those children who were never breast fed. Similarly, another study conducted by US health psychologist Melanie Smith and her colleagues (Smith *et al.*, 2003) examined 439 school-age, low birthweight children born in the United States. These authors found differences in IQ test scores between breast-fed children and those who did not receive any breast milk. These were 3.6 IQ points for overall intellectual functioning and 2.3 IQ points for verbal ability. You will also remember the debate surrounding the study carried out by two Welsh psychologists, David Benton and Gwilym Roberts (Benton and Roberts, 1988), who found that children given a vitamin–mineral supplement containing several vitamins and minerals were found to show increased IQ scores.

Regardless of the controversy surrounding this work, findings do suggest that nutrition has a positive effect on intelligence. It is important to remember, though, that a number of socioeconomic conditions are often associated with nutrition. You may also remember the words of Lynn (1990): the nutrition hypothesis sees nutrition as a package (or nurturing environment) in which increased intelligence is part of a nurturing environment that includes increased height and lifespan, improved health, decreased rate of infant disease and better vitamin and mineral nutrition. Where those things do not occur – where there is poverty, malnutrition and few economic and social opportunities – there might be lower intelligence scores.

Lead

However, while nutrition is seen as having a positive effect, there are occasions when other biological factors can have a negative effect on IQ. Neisser *et al.* (1996) highlight research concentrating on the effect that exposure to lead can have on intelligence.

The most comprehensive study was carried out in a place called Port Pirie in Australia. In 1986, Australian psychologist Anthony J. McMichael and four colleagues (McMichael *et al.*, 1986) examined the possible relationship between body lead burden and pregnancy outcome among 749 pregnant women in, and around, the largest lead smelting facilities in Australia. Among these women, premature deliveries were statistically significantly associated with higher levels of maternal blood lead concentration at delivery. What followed the initial findings was a series of studies in Port Pirie, which looked at the association between environmental exposure to lead and children's intelligence at 2 years (McMichael *et al.*, 1988), 4 years and 7 years (Baghurst *et al.*, 1992) and 11 and 13 years (Tong *et al.*, 1996). The Port Pirie cohort study started in 1979 and involved 723 children, although only 375 took part in the final study. IQ scores were made on the Bailey IQ scales at 2 years of age, the McCarthy IQ scale at 4 years of age and the Wechsler IQ scale for children at 7 years, 11 years and 13 years of age. At all these ages, IQ scores were significantly associated with lead concentration in people's bodies, even when socioeconomic status, home environment and maternal intelligence were controlled for. This study suggests that there is an association between early exposure to environmental lead and intelligence, and it persists into later childhood.

Prenatal factors

Finally, there are prenatal factors. You are well aware that pregnant women are expected to stop drinking and smo-king. According to many health councils, avoiding smoking and alcohol consumption in pregnancy is crucial. Smoking nearly doubles a woman's risk of having a premature or low birth-weight baby who faces an increased risk of serious health problems. Further, many conditions can arise from the mother's alcohol consumption when she is pregnant; the most common condition is fetal alcohol syndrome (FAS), which is characterised by a pattern of facial abnormalities, growth retardation and brain damage.

Neisser *et al.* (1996) point to these types of consumption by mothers during pregnancy as having an effect on intelligence. Low birth-weight babies, as well as babies suffering from FAS, show reduced intelligence. Danish scientist Erik Lykke Mortensen and colleagues at the University of Copenhagen (Mortensen *et al.*, 2005) examined maternal smoking and subsequent IQ scores among 3,044 males aged between 18 and 19 years. The study found that, regardless of factors such as parental social status and education, single-mother status, mother's height and age, number of pregnancies, the women who smoked 20 or more cigarettes daily late in their pregnancy were likely to have sons who performed less well on standardised IQ tests at age 18 or 19. Evidence also suggests that FAS is related to a number of cognitive functions. US psychologist Sarah Mattson and colleagues at San Diego State University (Mattson and Riley, 1998; Mattson *et al.*, 1996) have found that children prenatally exposed to alcohol exhibit a variety of problems with memory (they found that children with FAS aged 5 years to 16 years had learned fewer words than children of comparable ages) and demonstrate attention problems. Uecker and Nadel (1996) found that children of mothers who drank heavily during pregnancy performed badly in learning spatial relationships among objects. Furthermore, South African psychologist Piyadasa Kodituwakku and her colleagues (Kodituwakku *et al.*, 1995) have shown that children with FAS show deficits in activities that require abstract thinking, such as planning and organising information.

However, research is by no means conclusive. Other research suggests that the links between factors such as smoking, or alcohol consumption, in pregnancy and intelligence might be moderated, disappear or be highlighted by other factors. US psychologists S. W. Jacobson, J. L. Jacobson, R. J. Sokol, L. M. Chiodo and R. Corobana (2004) found, among 337 inner-city African–American children, that prenatal alcohol exposure was not related to IQ scores on the Wechsler Intelligence Test. However, they found that among children who had older mothers, prenatal alcohol was related to IQ scores on the Wechsler Intelligence Test. Bailey *et al.* (2004) examined alcohol use among mothers at a prenatal visit, and then IQ among children at 7 years, among 500 black children. Again, no relationship was found between prenatal alcohol exposure and intelligence, although mothers who binge-drink when pregnant were 1.7 times more likely to have children who had IQ scores in the mentally retarded range.

These findings suggest that age and excess drinking are further factors in the relationship between prenatal drinking and offspring intelligence. But overall, the findings suggest that smoking and alcohol consumption are factors that, to a greater or lesser extent, are connected with IQ.

Maternal effects model

Today, factors such as prenatal nutrition and alcohol consumption are combined into the maternal effects model. US psychiatrist Dr Bernie Devlin and US statistician Michael Daniels (Devlin *et al.*, 1997) showed that prenatal conditions may have substantial effects on the concordance of subsequent scores on IQ for identical twins. Previously, maternal effects had usually been assumed to be small, or non-existent, in terms of affecting genetic variance of intelligence between twins. However, a meta-analysis of 212 studies suggests 20 percent of genetic variance between twins and 5 percent between siblings. These authors suggest that broad heritability estimates when including maternal effect (additive and non-additive genetic variance) might have to be reduced from about 60 to 48 percent. This suggestion indicates that the environmental effects on intelligence may extend to interactions with biological factors.

Family environment

The second environmental factor identified by Neisser *et al.* (1996) is the family environment. There are three sources of related research and evidence that we will concentrate on in this discussion:

- shared and non-shared environments – within- and outside-family factors;
- the social and economic status of the family and the intelligence of the child;
- birth order, family size and child intelligence.

Shared and non-shared environments

Shared environments
Environmental influences that make family members different from each other.

Non-shared environments
Environments that are shared between two individuals.

We saw in the last discussion that the conception of genetics as a single dimension has developed over time. The same could be said of environmental factors. Within behavioural genetics, the conception of how the environment influences intelligence is through two sets of experiences: shared and non-shared. When growing up, siblings (brothers and sisters) are thought to experience both shared and unique environments. **Shared environments** are environments that are shared between two individuals, while **non-shared environments** are environments that are *not* shared between two individuals who share genes. Siblings growing up within the same family will share many environments. These environments may range from minor experiences to more significant ones. Therefore, two siblings having the same parents, living within the same house, going to the same school and experiencing particular times together (e.g. same family relatives, home environment, chaotic mornings before school, dad's awful jokes) have shared environments. A unique environment is an environment that has not been shared by siblings. Again, these environments may range from minor experiences to significant ones. Examples of unique environments might be when two siblings have been raised by different families. However, siblings raised in the same family might also have unique environments from each other. Siblings may have different sets of friends, may go to different schools, may have different types of relationships with their parents and have different interactions with teachers.

What is important in this area is that the theory and research around the differences between environment influences on intelligence has grown in complexity. To begin with, researchers tend to concentrate on comparing how shared and non-shared environmental factors influence intelligence. Early consideration by reviewers such as Bouchard (1994) and Eysenck (1990b) suggested that the environmental influences shared by siblings or twins contribute only marginally to intelligence differences. However, one interesting point to emerge from the literature, carried out by such researchers as US behaviour geneticists Braungart *et al.* (1992a), is that those environmental factors that are unique (non-shared) to family members are influential over *shared* environmental factors. Therefore, non-shared environmental factors, such as different peer friendships, are important mechanisms that explain why members of the same family may differ in their intelligence. This idea is supported by two pieces of research suggesting that the extent of differences in the experiences during childhood among siblings have been found to be related to intelligence differences in adulthood (Baker and Daniels, 1990; Plomin and Daniels, 1987).

Such a finding has led to the development of whole areas of research that have emphasised how important non-shared environmental factors are to intelligence. Most of the research in this area considers how non-shared environmental factors develop: (1) within the family; and (2) outside the family.

Within-family factors

US behavioural geneticist David Reiss (1997) identifies three ways in which inherited genes form phenotypes (behaviours) based on the family environment (see Figure 14.4):

- the passive model
- the child-effects model
- the parent-effects model.

First is the **passive model**. This model suggests that intelligence is generally explained by the 50 percent overlap between a child and their parent. Therefore, intelligence may occur in the child because the child and parent share the same genes that influence a particular type of behaviour. For example, if a child is highly intelligent owing to genetic influences, they are so because one of their biological parents had the genes that cause this high intelligence. The model, very much, just assumes a general genetic overlap and inheritance of behaviour without considering other possible factors and interactions within the family. This is why it is called the passive model. The other two models very much emphasise other dynamic occurrences.

Passive model
Describes genetic transmission of phenotypes, suggesting that the effects of genetics are explained by the 50 percent overlap between a child and their parent.

In the **child-effects model**, the genes cause intelligence in the child, which in turn causes the same or similar behaviour in the parent. Within this model, the parent does not matter in the development of the behaviour, as the child's development of intelligence is the result of genes. An example of this is that the shared genes cause the child to be intelligent (because of their genetic makeup), which in turn causes the parent to act intelligently back to the child (because of their genetic makeup). The parent's own intelligence does not matter in the development of the behaviour, as the child's intelligence is a consequence of the genetic makeup of the child rather than the parent.

Child-effects model
Describes genetic transmission of phenotypes; suggesting that the genes cause the behaviour, which in turn causes the same or similar behaviour in the parent.

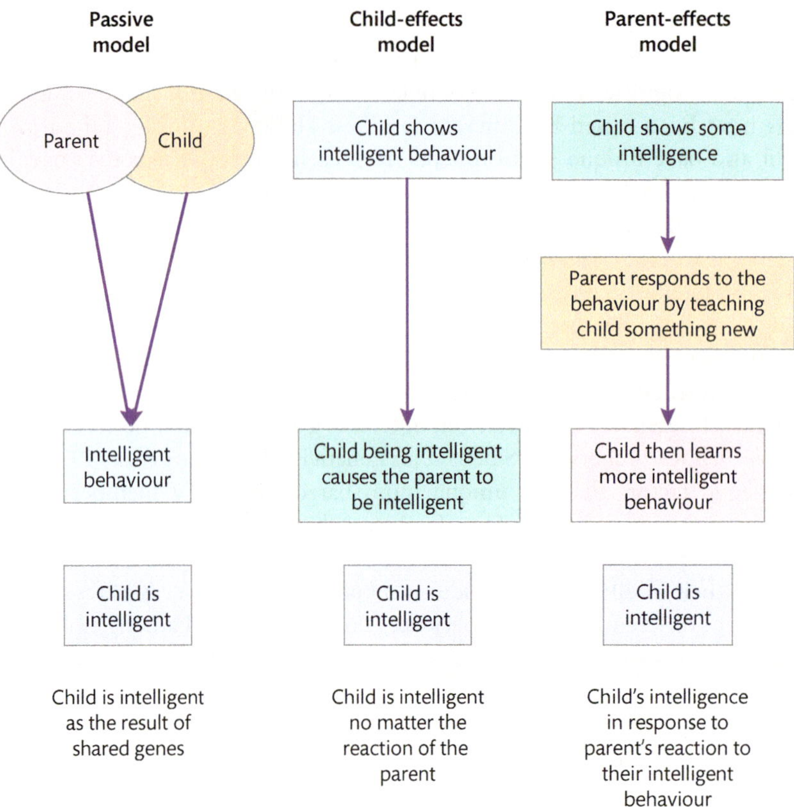

Figure 4.14 Reiss' three models of genetic transmission.

Child-driven effects
How differences between children within the same family will influence different reactions in the parents to how they treat the child.

US psychologist Judith Harris (1995) has expanded this viewpoint to **child-driven effects**, which influence family circumstances that in turn influence the child's intelligence. Harris documents studies showing that adults do not behave in the same way to a child who shows different tendencies. They will treat an attractive child differently to one of their children who is less attractive; they will react differently to the child who shows bad behaviour than to the one who is well behaved. This behaviour will also apply to intelligence. For example, imagine a family with twin children, one of them intelligent and the other not as intelligent. These differences in the children will cause different reactions in the parents. The parents will begin to treat their children differently. The intelligent one may be encouraged to engage in more intelligent activities, while the one perceived to be less intelligent might not be encouraged to do these activities. Harris suggests that these reactions by parents to their children's natural intelligence tendencies can be viewed in two ways: *positive feedback loops* and *negative feedback loops*. Positive feedback loops arise from parents reinforcing children's natural tendencies, as in the example described earlier, where children's natural intelligence abilities are encouraged and any differences between children in their intelligence are developed (the intelligent child is encouraged to be intelligent, while the 'unintelligent' child is encouraged and allowed to engage in other activities). Negative feedback loops occur when children are stopped from behaving in ways consistent with their natural tendencies. Therefore, an intelligent child might be encouraged to stop engaging in merely intelligence-stimulating activities, and an 'unintelligent' child might be encouraged to spend more time engaging in such activities.

In the **parent-effects model**, the behaviour of the child is responded to by the parent, which in turn brings out that behaviour in the child (see Figure 4.14). Within this model, how the parent responds does affect the development of the child's behaviour. For example, a child may begin showing intelligence; this then leads the parent to show intelligence with the child (as it is part of their genetic makeup). This in turn causes the child to become even more intelligent (as it is part of their genetic makeup). Within this model, the parent's behaviour leads to the development of intelligence, which then leads to the development of intelligent behaviour in the child.

Parent-effects model
Describes genetic transmission of phenotypes, suggesting that the behaviour of the child is responded to by the parent, which in turn brings out another behaviour in the child.

Again, Harris extends this idea to within-family situations. In these situations, children might be treated in a particular way by parents, not because of that child's own characteristics, but because of the parents' own beliefs or the characteristics of a child's siblings (brothers or sisters). Let us first look at the example of how the parents' own beliefs shape natural tendencies of children. Again, take our family with the one intelligent twin and the one 'less-intelligent' twin. Our parents of the family may have certain beliefs about behaviour, such as 'children should know the limits of their knowledge and never contradict their parents'. Therefore, the children will be encouraged and directed to behave in such ways. So, in our example of the intelligent and less-intelligent twin, the intelligent child who is likely to contradict their parents will be encouraged not to show their intelligence, and the unintelligent child will be encouraged to gain some knowledge up to their 'limits'. Both children will have had their new behaviour (knowing their limits and not contradicting their parents) driven by their parents' behaviour. Secondly, let us look at how parents might influence children's behaviours in terms of a child's siblings. Harris notes research suggesting that parents who consider their first child to be 'difficult' tend to label their second-born as 'easy'. We can also see how less-intelligent children might be asked, or encouraged, to be more like their intelligent sibling. Equally, the intelligent sibling might be encouraged to spend less time in intelligence-promoting activities and play more like their brother or sister.

What Reiss' and Harris' commentaries do is to suggest that *within-family effects* pose problems when considering genetic heritability. That is, child effects and parent effects can lead to over- and under-estimations of heritability. Remember, behavioural geneticists looking at intelligence are only looking at the concordance between sets of children based on their scores on an intelligence test at some point. However, let us return to our family with one intelligent twin and one less-intelligent twin. Let us imagine that the parents of these twin children have been engaged in a negative feedback loop. They have been trying to encourage both children to be similar; that is, somewhat intelligent. Therefore, the intelligent child has been discouraged from being intelligent all the time, and the less-intelligent child is being discouraged from being too unintelligent. If we then compared these two children, we would find that these twin children have similar intelligence; but this is, in fact, not because of genetic tendencies at all. It is simply because the parents are trying to encourage similar behaviour in both children (i.e. not too active or not too quiet). Therefore, any estimation of similarities in intelligence being caused by genetic heritability of the twins would be an over-estimation. However, if the same pair of twins had been reared differently and both had been in a positive feedback loop – the intelligent child had been encouraged to be more and more intelligent and the less-intelligent child had been encouraged to be more and more unintelligent – then any estimation of the similarities in intelligence being caused by genetic heritability would be an under-estimation because the differences have been exaggerated owing to the parents encouraging the twins to be more and more like themselves. Therefore, as Harris concludes, children's within-family situations not only play an important role in shaping their intelligence but are also an important consideration in estimating the genetic heritability of intelligence.

Outside-family factors

However, Harris (1995) has suggested that non-shared factors outside the family may in fact be more important in developing people's intelligence. Harris presents the group socialisation theory to explain the importance of non-shared environmental factors in determining intelligence.

Group socialisation theory is based largely on the ideas surrounding social identity theory and social categorisation (Tajfel and Turner, 1986). Social psychologists have provided a lot of theoretical and empirical research work that has looked at how individuals perceive their social world as comprising in-groups and out-groups and suggesting that these groups help us form our social identity. Social psychologists argue that one mechanism humans use for understanding the complex social world is social categorisation. In social categorisation, individuals are thought to place other individuals into social groups on the basis of their similarities and differences to the individual. Put simply, individuals who are viewed as similar to the person tend to be placed within their in-group. Individuals who are viewed as different to the person tend to be placed within an out-group. This is a process by which we come to understand our world. As a consequence, the individual's identity (social identity) is based on and derived from the groups they feel they belong to and their understanding of their similarities and differences to different social groups. Social groups can be anything, but common groups could be sex group, ethnic group, your religion, your peers, your interests, your educational status and so on. As such, your identity is based, to a greater or lesser extent, on how much you identify with different social groups. What is also important to our identity is that, when we attach ourselves to certain groups, we also try to fit in with those groups; therefore, our intelligence might begin to reflect the characteristics of a certain group (i.e., you might make friends with people who are highly intelligent; you may then do more intellectual activities than you used to, and you may become more intelligent).

Harris uses this theoretical basis to show how social groups can influence people's intelligence and points out how these non-shared environments that occur in children of the same family can have a huge effect on intelligence. As part of this theory, Harris lists five aspects that are important to consider in how non-shared characteristics might influence our intelligence.

- **Context-specific socialisation** – this aspect refers to the fact that children learn intelligence abilities not only at home but also outside the home. As children get older, they become less influenced by their family life and more influenced by their life outside the family home.
- **Outside-the-home socialisation** – in this aspect Harris makes the point that children may identify with a number of social groups, based on people's age, gender, ethnicity, abilities, interests, personality, intelligence, etc. In other words, we have a range of groups that we identify with and share norms with (attitudes, interests, intelligence), and these groups have different influences on our intelligence.
- **Transmission of culture via group processes** – in this aspect Harris makes two points about the transmission of culture via group processes, which establish norms in our social world that influence our intelligence. First, the shared norms that might influence a child's intelligence aren't necessarily the result of parents sharing them with their children; they are really the result of shared norms among the parents' peers and social groups being passed on to the children. That is, your parents' values, abilities, personality and intelligence are not the result of their parents' norms, but rather of their own social identity, their identification with their own social groups. The second point considers that individual norms, which we have developed from our family, are shared with other people only if they are accepted. For example, an individual might

be intelligent and like reading books. However, unless their friends approve of this behaviour, they may be unlikely to carry on this pastime.

- **Group processes that widen differences between social groups** – it is important to note that with your intelligence, norms are based not just on how you identify with your in-group but also on whether you identify with or reject the out-groups. For example, consider sex roles; your intelligence as a male or female isn't just based on your identification with people of your own sex, but on your rejection of characteristics of the opposite sex. For example, some young women at school believe that subjects such as science and mathematics are men's subjects; consequently, these women become interested in what they perceive to be women's subjects, such as English. This behaviour might have an effect on intelligence.
- **Group processes that widen differences among individuals within the group** – so far, we have assumed that all the groups that we are involved in basically share the same structure. However, we know that within all our social circles we play different roles that might influence, or bring out, different aspects of our intelligence. In our family, as a child, we take a less-senior role; with our friends we might be allowed to be more like ourselves. However, the opposite may be true, and we might not feel we lead a group of friends, but tend to do what others say. It may even be possible that among one group of friends you feel more comfortable than others. Harris' point is that our position in groups changes, and that our intelligence – and influences on our intelligence – change due to the hierarchies within a group. For example, if you are in a group of friends and they all look up to you, your intelligence will be influenced because you might think there is an expectation to come up with ideas for things to do or to solve problems within the group.

What is important to consider in both within-family and outside-family factors is that these aspects can influence intelligence of children to a much greater extent than previously thought. It is not Harris' point that behavioural genetics is wrong and that environmental factors are more important, but rather that behavioural geneticists may sometimes have oversimplified family influences. By ignoring these variables, behavioural geneticists might be under- or over-estimating heritability effects of either genetics or the environment on intelligence.

Socioeconomic status of the family

A family's socioeconomic status is based on its income, parental education level, parental occupation and status in the community. Socioeconomic status is related to various factors, including number of children in the family, opportunities for success in employment, health and area of residence. These factors all might influence intelligence.

Often socioeconomic status is ranked in many countries. For example, in the United Kingdom, one way in which socioeconomic status is measured is by the grading of parents' occupations into five categories:

- Class I: professional occupations;
- Class II: managerial and technical occupations;
- Class III: skilled occupations: manual (M) and unmanual (U);
- Class IV: partly skilled occupations;
- Class V: unskilled occupations.

Socioeconomic status is related to intelligence. Authors such as Linda Gottfredson (Gottfredson, 1986), Arthur Jensen (Jensen, 1993a), Richard Herrnstein and Charles Murray (Herrnstein and Murray, 1994) and J. Phillipe Rushton and C. D. Ankney (Rushton and Ankney, 1996) estimate that in Europe, North America and Japan, socioeconomic status is significantly correlated with scores on standard IQ between $r = 0.3$ and $r = 0.4$, and that there are 45 IQ points between members of the professional occupations (Class I) and those of unskilled occupations (Class V).

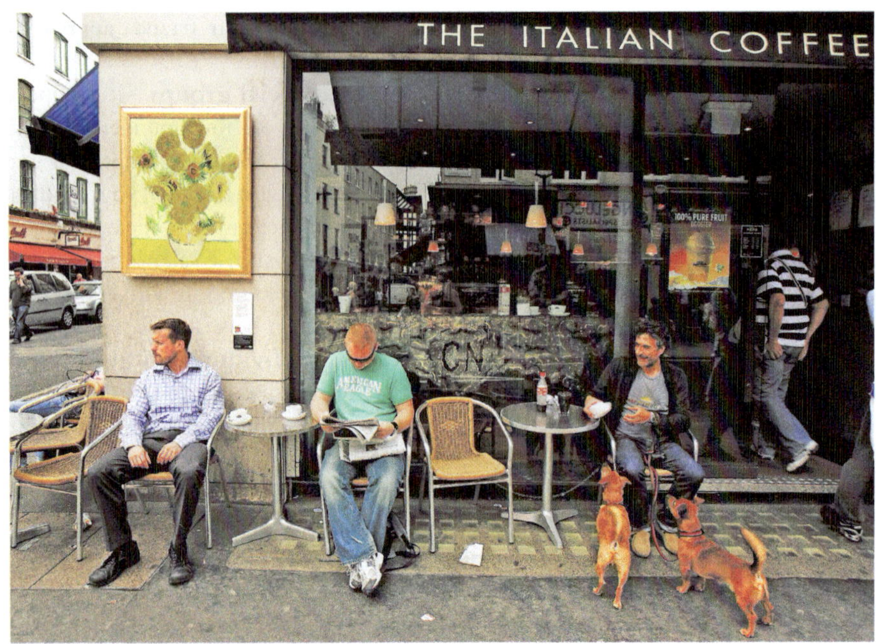

Often evidence of high levels of ability can be found in unexpected places.
Source: Getty Images/Daniel Berehulak

In addition, Nicholas Mackintosh (1998) and Nicholas Mascie-Taylor (1984) presented evidence linking socioeconomic status to intelligence using the British National Child Development Study (NCDS) data. The NCDS examined social and obstetric (care of women during and after pregnancy) factors associated with stillbirth and infant mortality among over 17,000 babies born in Britain in 1958. Surviving members of this birth cohort have been surveyed on five further occasions to monitor their changing health, education, social and economic circumstances, including IQ, in 1965 (age 7), 1969 (age 11), 1974 (age 16), 1981 (age 23) and 1991 (age 33). Mackintosh (1998) and Mascie-Taylor (1984) present evidence that, even when aspects such as financial hardship, birth-weight, size of family, overcrowding, type of accommodation and residence area are taken into account, children who had fathers in Class I (professional occupations) scored 10 IQ points higher than did children who had fathers in Class V (unskilled occupations).

Research also suggests that improved socioeconomic status can improve intelligence. Canadian behavioural geneticist Douglas Wahlsten (Wahlsten, 1997) points to a series of adoption studies in France, in which an infant is moved from a family having low socioeconomic status to a home where parents have high socioeconomic status, and the child's IQ score improves by 12–16 points. Wahlsten also points to studies in the United States that have demonstrated improvements in children's IQ by the same margin, achieved by improving the lives of infants in families with low educational and financial resources and providing them with additional educational day care outside the home, every weekday from the age of 3 months to the start of school.

These types of findings turn our attention to the research that has examined the conditions arising in certain families and how those conditions have influenced intelligence. One interesting and extensive debate has arisen from studies examining the influence on intelligence of birth order and family size.

Birth order, family size and intelligence

In 1973 Dutch psychologists Lillian Belmont and Francis Marolla (Belmont and Marolla, 1973) published a study looking at the birth order of the child, the size of family to which the child belonged and the child's overall IQ score on the Raven Progressive Matrices, among 386 19-year-old Dutch men. What Belmont and Marolla (1973) found was that, even when social class was controlled for, children from larger families had a lower IQ. Furthermore, the authors found that, within each family size, the first-born child always had a better IQ; and to some extent there were declining scores with rising birth order, so that the first-born children scored better than second-born children, second-born children scored better than third-born children and so on. These authors also found that these two factors interacted, and, as family size increased and birth order position increased, IQ scores became lower. So, for example, a second-born child from a family with three children would score higher than would a second-born child from a family containing four children.

Clearly, birth order, family size and intelligence are of interest to parents, politicians and researchers. Furthermore, if such findings are correct, they would have implications for optimum family size and parental choice regarding children's education. Since then, hundreds of research articles have addressed the relationship between family size, birth order and intelligence, and the proposed relationships between family size, birth order and IQ have been found among many cross-section studies. For example, Russian psychologist T. A. Dumitrashku (Dumitrashku, 1996) found that family size and birth order affected intelligence among Russian schoolchildren.

However, this wouldn't be a section about intelligence if debate didn't fiercely surround these findings. The debate, today, on family size, birth order and intelligence centres on the explanation of why, and whether, such effects occur.

FAMILY SIZE AND INTELLIGENCE. In the research area of family size and intelligence, Joseph Lee Rodgers and his colleagues (Rodgers *et al.*, 2000) published a seminal paper that looked at data from the United States. The National Longitudinal Survey of Youth (NLSY) followed 11,406 young people at yearly intervals from ages 14–22 years, and then children born to the original female respondents were surveyed every other year. Rodgers *et al.* found no direct relationship between family size and intelligence. They suggested that previous research has been inaccurate because it combined 'across-family' measures (family size) with 'within-family' (birth order) measures and treated them in the same way. That, is previous authors had treated family size as a within-family effect.

Let us explain what the authors mean. What the authors are highlighting here is a statistical fallacy that occurs when comparing populations of people. Say, for example, that a statistical agency released figures for death rates of the UK Army during the recent Iraq War and for death rates in London (the capital of the United Kingdom). The agency found that, among the army, death rates were 13 per thousand, while deaths in London were 26 per thousand. You perhaps would also not be surprised to find that the announcement of these figures by the statistical agency caught the attention of the media. You might even find a national newspaper running a headline story suggesting that people were safer in the army in Iraq than they were living in London. However, the problem with this sort of statement is that you are comparing two different populations. In the army population you have men and women who are healthy, and most of them are young. In the second population, London, you have a full age range of people – including those people with high mortality rates, such as old people, and people who are terminally ill. The issue is that you are comparing two populations for which a number of different factors determine death rates.

This fallacy applies to the current debate. Rodgers *et al.* illustrate the fallacy with this example. They suggest comparing the intelligence of three children, but these children are:

- a first-born child in a large middle-class white family in Michigan;
- a second-born child in a medium-sized affluent black family in Atlanta;
- a third-born child in a small low-income Hispanic family in California.

If differences are observed in these children's intelligence, Rodgers *et al.* suggest it is impossible to tell whether the differences are down to birth order, family size, socioeconomic status, region of the country or any other variables related to these dimensions.

BIRTH ORDER AND INTELLIGENCE. In the area of birth order and intelligence, research still generally supports Belmont and Marolla's findings. However, other authors have sought to explain that this relationship may be an artefact of another relationship rather than a real relationship. There are three models explaining why birth order may be linked to intelligence: the admixture hypothesis, the confluence model and the resource dilution model.

Admixture hypothesis
A hypothesis used to explain the relationship between birth order and IQ. What this hypothesis suggests is that parental intelligence and socioeconomic status are additional factors to consider in the relationship between birth order and IQ scores, coupled with the fact that parents with lower IQ scores tend to have more children.

The first is the **admixture hypothesis**. E. P. Page and G. Grandon (1979) and, more recently, Joseph Rodgers (2001) suggested an 'admixture hypothesis' that explains the relationship between birth order and IQ. What this hypothesis suggests is that parental intelligence, or socioeconomic status, are additional factors to consider in the relationship between birth order and IQ scores, coupled with the fact that parents with lower IQ scores tend to have more children. This has made findings in previous studies look as if higher birth order causes lower intelligence, when in fact lower intelligence results because parents with lower socioeconomic status and IQ scores tend to have more children. For example, a parent with five children is likely to have a lower IQ score and a lower socioeconomic status. Parents with higher IQ scores and higher socioeconomic status tend to have fewer children. Consequently, any calculation of the relationship between birth order and intelligence is problematic because parents with higher IQ scores and higher socioeconomic status do not tend to have as many children. Thus there cannot be equal measurement of the number of children across the population.

Resource dilution model
A hypothesis used to explain the relationship between birth order and IQ. This model suggests that parental resources (time, energy and financial resources) are finite and that, as the number of children in the family increases, the resources (time, energy and finance) that any one child can gain will decrease.

The second model is the **resource dilution model**. This model was proposed by Judith Blake (Blake, 1981) and elaborated by Douglas Downey (Downey, 2001), but its ideas were first presented by Galton (1874). The resource dilution model of birth order and intelligence test scores suggests that parental resources (time, energy and financial resources) are finite (i.e. *not* endless) and that, as the number of children in the family increases, the resources (time, energy and financial) that can be gained by any single child decreases. Therefore, the first child will get 100 percent of available resources from their parents, the second child will only ever get 50 percent, the third child will only ever get 33 percent and a fourth child will only ever get 25 percent. This model also feeds into the idea that children in larger families have lower intelligence test scores because, as that family grows, the resources that can be accessed also diminish.

Confluence model
A hypothesis used to explain the relationship between birth order and IQ. The model suggests that intellectual development, and thus intelligence, must be understood in the context of the family and an ever-changing intellectual environment within the family.

Third is the **confluence model**, which was originally proposed by US psychologist Robert B. Zajonc (Zajonc, 1976; Zajonc and Markus, 1975) – though, again, Galton (1874) proposed some of these ideas. The confluence model suggests that intellectual development, and therefore intelligence, must be understood within the context of the family, and there is an ever-changing intellectual environment within the family. Zajonc suggests the following factors might influence the relationship between birth order and intelligence:

- First-borns have the advantage of some time in which they do not have to share their parents' attention with any of their siblings.
- Any additional birth automatically limits the amount of attention any of the siblings get, including the first-born.
- First-borns and older siblings have to look after and care for younger siblings to some degree. This means that they undertake some amount of responsibility and may have to explain things to their younger siblings. Zajonc believed that this sort of tutoring helps the older children to develop intelligence abilities, as they have to explain ideas and processes to other people.

- First-born children are exposed to a greater proportion of adult language and ideas from their parents. Those children born later are exposed to less mature speech and ideas because they listen not only to their parents, but to their other siblings. This means they spend a lower proportion of their time listening to adult language and ideas and a greater proportion of time listening to other children's language and ideas.

These last two findings also feed into the idea that children in larger families have lower IQ scores because, as that family grows, the agenda and the context of the family focuses more and more on the children.

Education and intelligence

Education and its relationship to intelligence has already been mentioned. However, we will remind you of some of the findings and extend your view on this area here.

Neisser *et al.* (1996) found that education is both an independent and dependent variable in terms of its relationship to intelligence. Going to school is likely to increase your abilities, particularly those that comprise intelligence (intelligence is a dependent variable), and intelligence is likely to influence your attendance at school and your length of schooling (i.e. whether you end up going to university) and the quality of school you attend (intelligence is an independent variable here). Consequently, intelligence and education are intrinsically linked.

Overall, reviews by US psychologists Alan Kaufman and Elizabeth Lichtenberger (Kaufman, 1990; Kaufman and Lichtenberger, 2005) provide a review of key papers that have looked at the correlation between general intelligence and school attainment and achievement. They conclude that the average correlation between IQ scores and a number of school indicators is around $r = 0.50$, suggesting that intelligence does predict performance at school. Also, two academics of the Hebrew University in Jerusalem, Sorel Cahan and Nora Cohen (1989), compared the effects of a year of school (controlling for age) with those of a year of age on a number of verbal (e.g. verbal and numerical skills) and non-verbal (abstract and reasoning tests, including the Raven's Matrices) intelligence tests. Length of schooling was important in predicting performance, and mattered more than age for all the verbal tests. Length of schooling, however, made a contribution – but a smaller contribution – to performance on some of the non-verbal tests, including the items from the Raven's Matrices.

Other key evidence you need to know when considering education as an environmental factor on intelligence is found in the well-cited papers of US child development psychologist Stephen Ceci (1990; 1991). Ceci did a meta-analysis of studies, and his findings suggest that there are many effects of education on intelligence test scores. The data presented by Ceci includes the overall finding that children who attend school regularly score higher on intelligence tests than do those who attend less regularly, intelligence test scores among pupils decrease over the long summer holidays and there is a rise of 2.7 IQ points for each year of schooling (see also Winship and Korenman, 1997). Douglas Wahlsten (1997) notes that studies have shown that delays in starting school cause intelligence test scores to drop by 5 IQ points a year (i.e. Winship and Korenman, 1997).

Also, it is worth reminding you of Head Start and other similar programmes that have explored the relationship between education and intelligence. You may remember that Head Start, was started in the 1960s by President Lyndon Johnson and was designed to give America's poorest children a head start in preparing them for school and to start to break the cycle of poverty. Evidence was provided to assess the usefulness of such a programme. US individual differences psychologist Charles Locurta (Locurta, 1991) provides a review of this evidence. In 1969, Arthur Jensen suggested that Head Start had failed. The reason for Jensen's pronouncement was that, although children attending the programme showed an initial increase in IQ points – sometimes as much 7–8 points on IQ tests – after 2 or 3 years these higher IQ points were lost (Locurta, 1991). There has been a lot of debate about the effectiveness of Head Start, but in terms of IQ gains, McKey *et al.* (1985) reported that children enrolled in Head Start had significant immediate gains in IQ scores. However, in the longer term (3–4 years), the IQ test scores of Head Start students did not remain higher than those of disadvantaged children who did not attend Head Start.

Finally, there is evidence to suggest that ideas covered in the last discussion regarding socioeconomic status are related to education variables, which, together, are related to intelligence. Socioeconomic status might influence aspects of education, and then intelligence, in a number of ways:

- Families with a high socioeconomic status are often able to prepare their children for school because they have access to resources (e.g. childcare, books and toys) and information (What are the best schools? What aspects are taught to children?) that enhance children's social, emotional and cognitive development and help parents to better prepare their young children for school (Demarest *et al.*, 1993).
- Families of a low economic status face hard challenges when it comes to providing the best care and education for their children. When basic necessities such as money and time are missing, food, housing, clothing and healthcare come first. Educational toys and books, and time searching out the best schools, are luxuries that parents may not have the time or money to pursue (Ramey and Ramey, 1994).
- Parents from poor socioeconomic backgrounds often grew up in poor socioeconomic conditions themselves. Consequently, parents may have inadequate reading skills or may lack knowledge about childhood nutrition (or not be able to afford it), and these benefits aren't passed on to the children before school (Zill *et al.*, 1995).

Culture and intelligence

The final environmental area that Neisser *et al.* (1996) suggest is important to influencing intelligence is the cultural environment in which people live. 'Culture' refers to people's individual values, and the values of their society. Neisser *et al.* suggest culture can have an effect not only on intelligence but also on the type of intelligence that might develop.

Implicit theories of intelligence showed how the definition of what constitutes intelligence shifts across cultures, particularly when you compare western and eastern cultures, and how conceptions of intelligence shift across age and through different disciplines. Well, clearly that discussion of implicit theories of intelligence is relevant here.

However, in addition to implicit theories of intelligence, Serpell (2001) identifies three concepts that explain how intelligence in western societies is set apart from other cultures in the world. These three concepts are decontextualisation, quantification and biologisation.

Decontextualisation

A lot of western thinking is inherited from 3,000 years of classical Greek philosophy. Socrates, Plato and Aristotle were all Greek philosophers who have had a profound impact on the way we think in our culture. In western culture there is a tendency to emphasise mathematics, the scientific method and language. We make clear distinctions between what is right and wrong, what constitutes justice, the need to follow a logical progression and the idea that there are higher and lower planes of ideas and activities – and perhaps a universal truth.

Decontextualisation
The ability to disconnect, or detach oneself, from a particular situation; to think abstractly and then generalise about it.

Decontextualisation is the ability to disconnect, or detach oneself, from a particular situation and think abstractly, and then generalise about it. Serpell (2001) argues that the ability to think abstractly and generalise about things has gained importance in western society because of industrialisation. With the growth of capitalism there is a need for efficiency, some level of bureaucracy and functionality (the ability to come up with abstract principles) to help govern western life, including the markets (financial, housing, consumer), industry and education. These needs become increasingly important. Serpell questions the need to always view decontextualisation as a sign of intelligence, and a failure to decontextualise as a sign of unintelligence.

Quantification

Quantification is the act of discovering, or expressing, the quantity of something. Serpell suggests that the study of intelligence is surrounded by quantification in three ways:

- First is the way that intelligence theory and research is designed to quantify intelligence. That is, when we ask 'what is intelligence?' we are trying to encapsulate a number of meanings and ideas into one word, 'intelligence'.
- Second is a concept called reification (see also Gould, 1981). Reification is the tendency to regard an abstract idea as if it had concrete or material existence. We see intelligence as something that is located in the brain, but we do not know where it is located. Intelligence isn't just about certain processes; but it encapsulates things that are not measurable, such as beauty or sophistication. For many, the invention of the steam engine, or the wheel, are highly intelligent acts; however, they are also acts of beauty to some, and they are certainly of sophistication to many.
- Third is a tendency to quantify intelligence in terms of numbers. We give people intelligence tests, which contain an optimum number of items that should be completed within a certain amount of time. These items have been selected in accordance with studies that have used statistical procedures to determine what aspects of intelligence are out there. The test that is given is determined by the person's age. When participants have finished, they are given scores for their performance, and these scores are then transformed into IQ scores. These IQ scores can then be compared against standardised scores for the tests of people of the same age.

Serpell suggests that consideration of these three points indicates that our understanding of intelligence is surrounded by quantification. All this is not to say that quantification is not a good process to understand intelligence. To produce meaning and conceptual understanding of words; to try to define, measure and locate concepts; and to use numbers as objective criteria are excellent methods by which to ensure the progress and understanding of intelligence. However, Serpell suggests that when we are dealing with something like intelligence, we must be sure that we do not seek to over-quantify this concept.

Biologisation

Serpell (2001) raises our awareness that biological and evolutionary theories have grown in prominence in late twentieth century and early twenty-first century thinking (biologisation). There have been evolutionary psychologists are able to link the evolution of the human species to animals who lived billions of years ago. Many of the arguments put forward by biological and evolutionary psychology are convincing, and inspiring, in the understanding of why we behave the way we do. However, Serpell suggests some caution in over-emphasising these models. It must be remembered that many of these models talk about developments over millions of years, and our advanced study of ourselves is relatively new. Therefore, we must be careful to ensure that our understanding of genetics, evolutions over a long course of history, and genetic variation are not used to explain intelligence within a relatively short period of history.

Final comments on genetic heritability and environmental influences on intelligence

Perhaps the last word in this section goes to Bouchard and Loehlin (2001), who suggest a framework for observing sources of population variance in psychological traits (see Figure 4.15).

To assess population variations in intelligence, Bouchard and Loehlin's framework is not only a good overview of the debate but also sets some prudent criteria in terms of assessing elements such as genetic effects and environmental effects on intelligence. So, in all, we must consider:

- **Genetic influences** – including questions about what gene is involved and what type of genetic variation (for example, additive or non-additive). Is there a sex limitation (e.g. brain size)?
- **Environmental influences** – including to what extent does environment influence the genes, what types of environments are involved (e.g. education, culture) and are there gender effects?
- **Interaction between genetic and environmental influence** – including what type are the interactions between genes and the environment (e.g. nutrition, prenatal causes)?
- **Developmental influences** – including do different genes influence during development, and do different environmental factors influence during development?
- **Assortative mating** – including is assortative mating present in intelligence, and are there sex differences in mating preference for intelligence?
- **Evolution** – including what sort of selective factors were at work during the original evolution of intelligence (e.g. different need for intelligences across different areas of the world)? Are there current selective factors at work?

Genetic

1 To what extent is the trait influenced by genes?
2 What type of gene is involved?
3 How many loci are involved?
4 Is there a sex limitation or sex linkage?
5 Are chromosomal effects involved?

Environmental

1 To what extent is intelligence influenced by the environment?
2 What type of environment is involved?
3 Are there gender effects?
4 Is transmission horizontal, or is it vertical?

Genetic and environmental influence

1 Are there any genetic x environmental interactions on intelligence?
2 What type are the interactions between genes and the environment?

Intelligence

Developmental

1 Do different genes influence during development?
2 Do different environmental factors influence during development?

Assortative mating

1 Is assortative mating present in intelligence?
2 Are there sex differences in mate preference for intelligence?

Evolution

1 What sort of selective factors were at work during the original evolution of intelligence?
2 Are there current selective factors at work?
3 Is intelligence an adaptation?

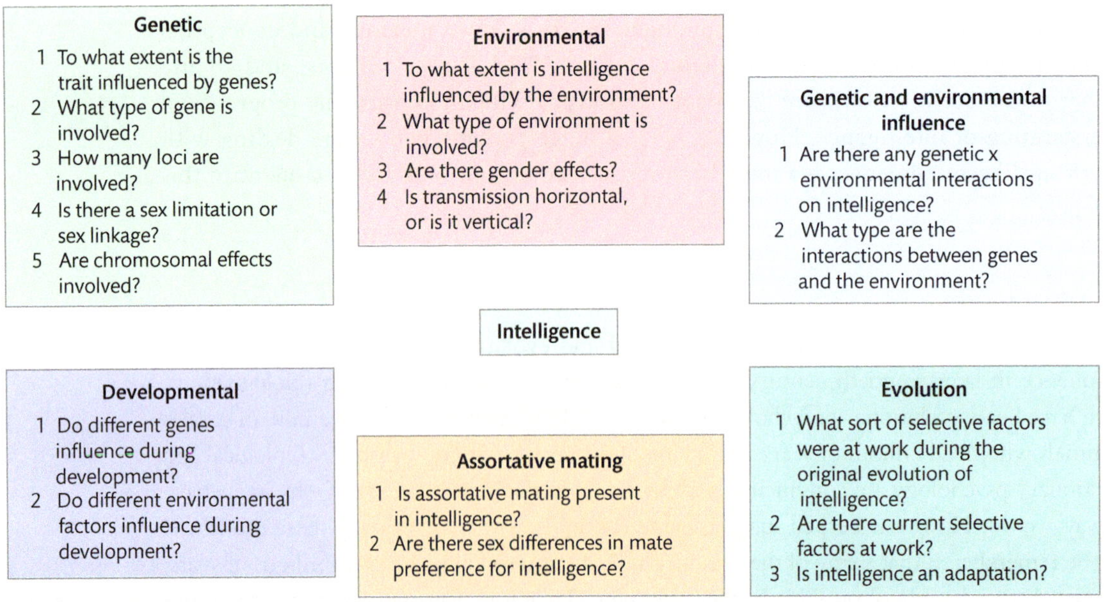

Figure 4.15 Framework and questions regarding sources of population variance in intelligence.
Source: Based on Bouchard and Loehlin (2001).

Clearly, when it comes to intelligence, some of these areas are easier to identify or consider than others. For example, no one has discovered whether there is a gene for intelligence; nor can we be certain about what the different evolutionary demands on intelligence are. However, many of the areas – assessing the level of genetic influence, the types of environmental influence and the possible interactions between genes and the environment – are known, or at least provide sources of evidence that provide evidence for a debate. Applying Bouchard and Loehlin's model to intelligence provides a focus to an area that debates the relative influences of: (1) genes; (2) the environment; and (3) the interactions between genes and the environment on intelligence.[F]

Emotional intelligence

In March 2000 Daniel Goleman published an article, 'Leadership that gets results', in the *Harvard Business Review* (a well-respected business management theory journal). When the chief executive officer (the highest-ranking officer of a company) of the leading worldwide pharmaceutical company read the article, he sent copies of it to the 400 top executives in the company. The article described the theory of emotional intelligence.

Generally, emotional intelligence is the ability to understand your own emotions and those of people around you. In this section we are going to take you through the major theories of emotional intelligence. To some extent the history and the development of theories of emotional intelligence are fragmented; none the less, the literature on emotional intelligence spans a number of perspectives, which certain authors have tried to link together. We will then go on and explore different psychological perspectives on emotional intelligence as well as some of the issues that surround the topic, particularly whether it is a useful concept for psychologists to consider. Finally, we will assess whether women are more 'emotionally intelligent' than men.

Salovey and Mayer's four-branch model of emotional intelligence

In 1990 US psychologists Peter Salovey at Yale University and John D. Mayer at the University of New Hampshire presented the first clear theory of emotional intelligence (Salovey and Mayer, 1990).

In defining emotional intelligence, Salovey and Mayer concentrated on the two words 'emotional' and 'intelligence'. We know it sounds obvious, but it is important that you give equal weight to both words. For these authors emotion is important, as it comprises feelings that encompass physiological responses (for example, sadness, happiness, crying, fear) and cognitions (for example, assessments of the meaning of emotion, learning about ourselves from our emotions). Similarly, intelligence is important because it refers to capacities to think and reason about information. Salovey and Mayer brought these two areas together into one: emotional intelligence.

In their original paper, Salovey and Mayer divided the concept of emotional intelligence into four capacities:

- accurately perceiving emotions;
- using emotions to facilitate thinking;

[F]Maltby, J., Day, L., & Macaskill, A. (2013). The use of intelligence tests: What question emerge from the measurement of intelligence. In *Personality, individual differences and intelligence* (3rd ed., pp. 338–358.). Harlow, Essex: Pearson Education Limited.

- understanding emotional meanings;
- managing emotions.

By 1997 Mayer and Salovey had expanded on their model (Mayer and Salovey, 1997). In this more detailed model, they expanded the four branches as follows:

- **Perceiving branch: perception, appraisal and expression of emotion** – if you were high in this aspect of emotional intelligence, you would be able to recognise emotions in other people, particularly through their use of language (for example, if it is emotionally charged), sound (for example, when the tone of voice changes when they are upset) and behaviour (for example, if they are behaving differently or seem anxious). However, within this branch of emotional intelligence, you would be able to identify accurately your own emotions in relation to your own thoughts and feelings. You would also be able to express emotions properly in accordance with your feelings and thoughts.
- **Facilitating branch: emotional facilitation of thinking** – if you were high in this aspect of emotional intelligence, you would be able to use your emotions as an aid for your memory and to make judgements about certain feelings to prioritise your thinking. You would be able to use emotions to encourage the consideration of multiple viewpoints (for example, not focusing on one emotion, such as being unhappy) and to understand that particular emotions can be used in problem-solving (for example, being happy leads to creativity).
- **Understanding branch: understanding and analysing emotions; employing emotional knowledge** – if you were high in this aspect of emotional intelligence, you would be able to label emotions accurately and recognise the relationships between the emotions (for example, the similarities and differences between dislike and hate). You would also be able to understand the meaning behind emotions and know that some emotions are linked together in a process (for example, to do well in an exam would be accompanied by happiness). You would also understand that there are transitions among emotions (for example, you may have told someone off because you were angry, but later regret it and think you did the wrong thing and feel remorse).
- **Managing branch: reflective regulation of emotion to promote emotional and intellectual growth** – if you were high on this aspect of emotional intelligence, you would have the ability to stay open to feelings that are both pleasant (for example, praise) and unpleasant (for example, criticism). You would have the ability to reflect or detach from a specific emotion to be able to see whether it is informative to you (for example, you may be upset about something, but can you detach yourself from being upset and note that your reaction might have been unreasonable?). You would be able to monitor emotions in yourself and others, and assess whether the emotion expressed is *typical* (for example, asking yourself whether your emotions are a normal reaction to something), is *influencing* you (for example, asking if the emotion is ruling your decision-making) or is *unreasonable* (you might be angry about someone, but realise you are being unfair). Finally, you would show the ability to manage emotion in yourself and others by monitoring emotions and, on some occasions, using them for personal, intellectual or emotional growth (for example, you can do something constructive with your anger).

Furthermore, the authors have further broken these four branches into two main areas:

- **Experiential (relating to, or derived from, experience)** – this area comprises the perceiving branch and the facilitating branch.
- **Strategic (related to intended objective, or plan of action)** – this area comprises the understanding branch and the managing branch.

This model of emotional intelligence is known as an *ability* model because it involves abilities in having and dealing with emotion, using emotion to enhance thought and to reflect and engage with a variety of emotions. Mayer and Salovey arranged the four aspects

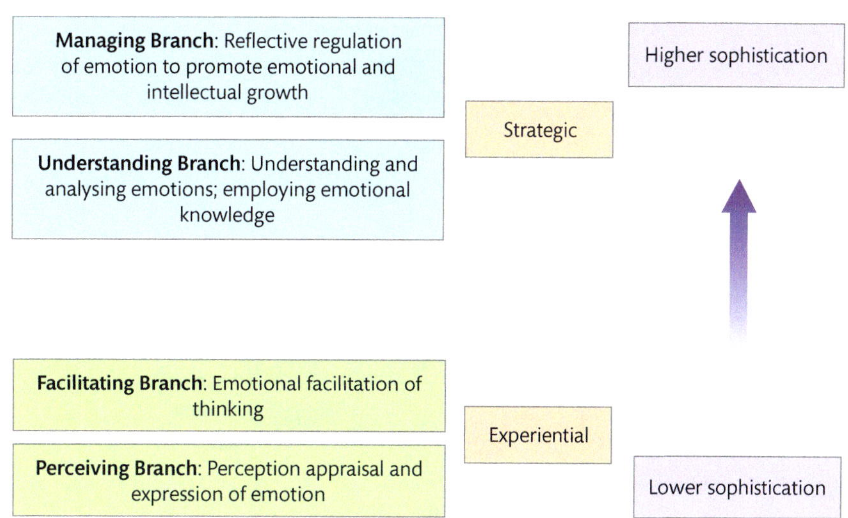

Figure 4.16 Mayer and Salovey's model of emotional intelligence, including the order of sophistication.
Source: From Mayer, J.D., Salovey, P. and Caruso, D.R. (2000). Models of emotional intelligence. In R.J. Sternberg (ed), *The handbook of intelligence* (pp. 398, 404, 415). Cambridge: Cambridge University Press. Reprinted with permission from Cambridge University Press.

of emotional intelligence in an order of sophistication of ability. The order of sophistication, ranging from lowest to highest, is presented in Figure 4.16.

How do Mayer and Salovey measure intelligence? Now in its second edition, The Mayer–Salovey–Caruso Emotional Intelligence Test V2.0 (MSCEIT V2.0; Mayer *et al.*, 2002; 2003) is a 141-item scale used to measure the emotional intelligence abilities described earlier: perception, integration (facilitation), understanding and management.

In this test, the test-taker performs a series of tasks that are designed to assess their ability to perceive, identify, understand and work with emotion. For example, here are some typical items.

- **Ability to identify emotion** – the participant would be shown a picture of a face and asked to assess to what extent different emotions are shown in the face (i.e. happiness, anger, fear, excitement and surprise) (see Figure 4.17a).
- **Ability to use (facilitate) emotion** – the participant would rate on a 5-point scale to what extent a number of moods (i.e. tension, surprise, joy) might be helpful when meeting a partner's family for the very first time (see Figure 4.17b).
- **Ability to understand emotion** – the participant would imagine someone who is stressed about their work and whose boss gave them an additional project. The participant would then be asked to identify which of five emotions (overwhelmed, depressed, ashamed, self-conscious or jittery) they think the person would feel (see Figure 4.17c).
- **Ability to manage emotions** – the participant would be asked to imagine someone coming back from vacation feeling peaceful and content. The test-taker would then be asked to identify the effectiveness of a number of actions for maintaining the feelings of peacefulness and contentment (i.e. making a list of things to do, thinking about where and when to go for the next vacation or deciding whether it is best to ignore the feelings of being peaceful and content as it won't last anyway) (see Figure 4.17d).

Respondents can get overall emotional intelligence scores on the MSCEIT V2.0, as well as subscale scores for the perceiving branch, facilitating branch, understanding branch and managing branch.

(a)
Ability to identify emotion

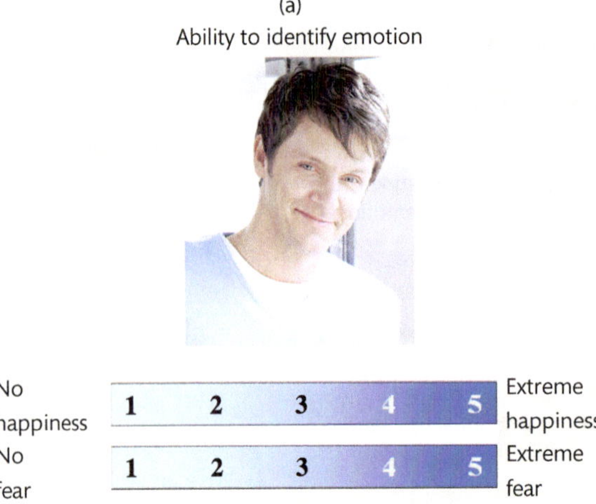

No happiness	1	2	3	4	5	Extreme happiness
No fear	1	2	3	4	5	Extreme fear

(b)
Ability to use (facilitate) emotion

1. What mood(s) might be helpful to feel when meeting in-laws for the very first time?

	Not useful				**Useful**
a. Tension	1	2	3	4	5
b. Surprise	1	2	3	4	5
c. Joy	1	2	3	4	5

(c)
Ability to understand emotion

Tom felt anxious, and became a bit stressed when he thought about all the work he needed to do. When his supervisor brought him an additional project, he felt__________.

a. overwhelmed
b. depressed
c. ashamed
d. self-conscious
e. jittery

(d)

Debbie just came back from vacation. She was feeling peaceful and content.
How well would each action preserve her mood?
Action 1: She started to make a list of things at home that she needed to do.

(a) Very effective (b) Somewhat effective (c) Neutral
(d) Somewhat ineffective (e) Very ineffective

Action 2: She began thinking about where and when she should go on her next vacation.

(a) Very effective (b) Somewhat effective (c) Neutral
(d) Somewhat ineffective (e) Very ineffective

Action 3: She decided it was best ignore the feeling since it wouldn't last anyway.

(a) Very effective (b) Somewhat effective (c) Neutral
(d) Somewhat ineffective (e) Very ineffective

Figure 4.17 Simulated Emotional Intelligence Items from the Mayer–Salovey–Caruso Emotional Intelligence Test 2.0.
(MSCEIT V2.0; Mayer *et al.*, 2002). In the USA: PO Box 950, North Tonawanda, NY 14120-0950, (800) 456-3003. In Canada: 3770 Victoria Park Ave., Toronto, ON M2H 3M6, (800) 268-6011. International Tel: +1-416-492-2627, Fax: 1-800-540-4484 or +1-416-492-3343.

Stop and think

Emotional intelligence qualities

Using Mayer and Salovey's model of emotional intelligence, where do you think your strengths of emotional intelligence lie? Perceiving, facilitating, understanding or managing?

Goleman's model of emotional intelligence

Goleman's development of emotional intelligence (Goleman, 1995), came after Salovey and Mayer's (1990) theory, but is probably the most widely known model of emotional intelligence. Goleman drew on Salovey and Mayer's (1990) work, including an emphasis on physiological and cognitive terms, but he also introduced a number of new ideas.

One of these ideas was that Goleman linked emotional intelligence to a part of the brain called the amygdala. The amygdala is located in the brain's medial temporal lobe and is part of the limbic system of the brain. The limbic system is a group of brain structures that are involved in various emotions, including pleasure, fear and aggression as well as in the formation of memories. The amygdala (the part Goleman was interested in) is involved in aggression and fear, two basic responses that are related to responses to threat. You may recognise this as the 'fight-or-flight' response.

The flight-or-fight response was first described by Walter Cannon, a US physiologist (Cannon, 1929). His theory stated that when animals are faced by threats or danger they have physiological reactions, including the 'firing' of neurons through the sensory cortex of the brain, that are accompanied by increased levels of hormones and neurotransmitters such as epinephrine (adrenaline) and norepinephrine (noradrenaline). These hormones and neurotransmitters are pumped into the body, causing immediate physical reactions such as an increase in heart rate, tensing of muscles and quicker breathing, thereby making the animal alert and attentive to the environment and aware of the danger. This is known as a stress

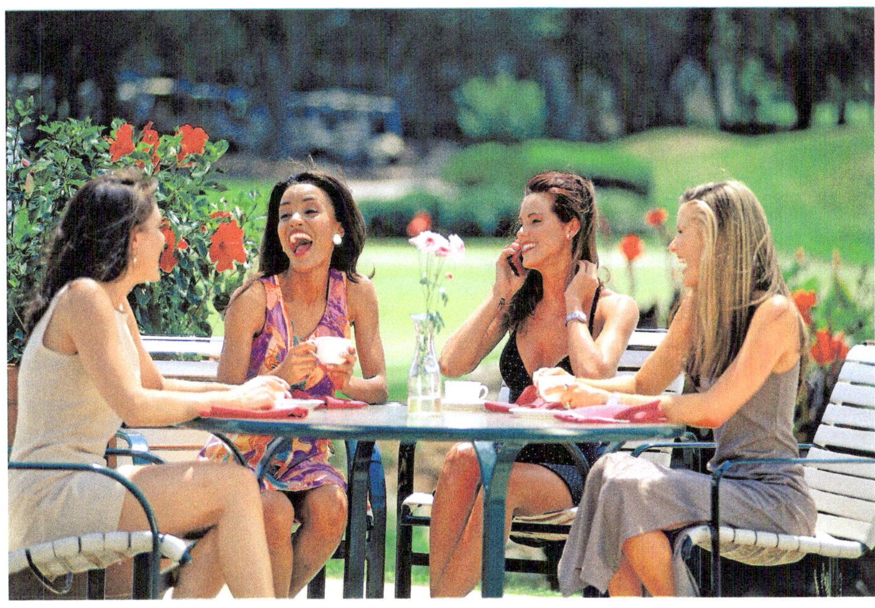

Little do we know it, but this is actually an 'Emotional Intelligence' seminar.
Source: Alamy Images/Ace Stock Ltd.

response. The animal is then faced with two choices. It can either face the threat ('fight') or avoid the threat ('flight').

Goleman uses the processes of the amygdala in his model of emotional intelligence. He argues that the fight-or-flight response is central to emotional intelligence and that, as we develop, we learn to control these two basic emotions. For example, when we were very young and knew we would be told off by our parents, we might have tried to run away to avoid the trouble, or tried to fight (or least have a tantrum) with our parents. As we got older, we would have changed our strategy, and probably have just listened to being told off by our parents and accepted whatever punishment was coming our way. As we got older still, we might have tried to reason with our parents, tried to apologise and reassure our parents that it would never happen again. Goleman suggests that our emotional intelligence reflects a similar process. That is, over time, we learn to control our basic emotional responses (such as fight and flight) to varying degrees. The extent to which we are able to develop, control and use our basic emotional responses is the basis of Goleman's model of emotional intelligence.

Originally in Goleman's (1995) theory, there are five emotional intelligences:

- ability to identify one's emotional states and to understand that there is a connection between emotions, thought and action (for example, you are likely to laugh when you have a happy thought);
- ability to manage and control one's emotions, and to shift undesirable emotions to more adequate ones (for example, to shift the feeling of crying to a feeling of sadness);
- ability to have emotional states that are related with a drive for achievement and be successful (for example, the ability to be happy and for this to drive you on in your work, or in trying to achieve something to make you happy);
- ability to assess, be sensitive and influence other people's emotions (for example, to recognise someone's sadness and cheer them up);
- ability to enter and then sustain good interpersonal relationships (for example, to have good friends and maintain your relationship with them).

Within Goleman's theory, these emotional intelligences form a hierarchy (see Figure 4.18).

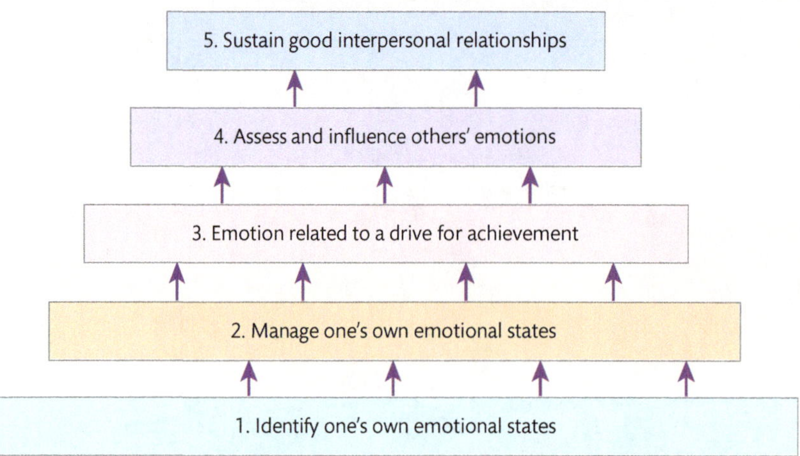

Figure 4.18 Goleman's model of emotional intelligence, arranged in the hierarchy.
Source: From Goleman, D. (2001). An EI-based theory of performance. In C. Cherniss and D. Goleman (eds), *The Emotionally Intelligent Workplace*. New York: Jossey Bass Wiley. Reprinted with permission of John Wiley & Sons Inc.

For example, to be able to manage your emotions (second aspect of emotional intelligence), you must be able to identify them (first aspect of emotional intelligence). To use your emotions in a drive for achievement (third aspect of emotional intelligence), you must be able to identify (first aspect) and manage (second aspect) them. To be able to assess and influence other people's emotions effectively (fourth aspect), you must be able to identify, manage and use them (all the first three aspects). Having all the first four aspects of emotional intelligence leads individuals to enter, and be able to sustain, good interpersonal relationships.

Over the years Goleman refined this model, not only in terms of its theory but also in its application. Goleman's theory and application became popular in the business world, and the development of Goleman's theory centres around the language used in the workplace.

By 2002 (Goleman, 2001; Goleman *et al.*, 2002), Goleman had revised his theory to there being four domains of emotional intelligence. To a great extent he had dropped the third aspect (using your emotions in a drive for achievement) and subsumed it into other aspects. Today, Goleman's theory of emotional intelligence comprises four aspects, which he termed emotional competencies:

- **self-awareness** – which was the old first aspect, the ability to identify one's own emotional states;
- **self-regulation/management** – which was the old second aspect, the ability to manage one's own emotional states;
- **social awareness** – which was the old third aspect, the ability to assess and influence others' emotions;
- **social skills/management** – which was the old fourth aspect, the ability to sustain good interpersonal relationships.

Goleman made two sets of distinctions between these four emotional competencies. The first distinction is between *personal* and *social* competencies. The first two aspects, *self-awareness* and *self-regulation*, are personal competencies, while *social awareness* and *social skills* are social competencies.

The second distinction is between *recognition* and *regulation*. *Self-awareness* and *social awareness* are emotional intelligences that are defined by recognition (identifying one's own emotional state and those of others), and *self-regulation* and *social skills* are emotional intelligences that are defined by regulation (managing one's own emotional states and sustaining good personal relationships).

Additionally, Goleman has identified up to 25 abilities that make up emotional intelligence, though this number changes based on the context of the situation in which emotional intelligence is being applied. For example, some of the abilities are very businesslike because of the model's application to relationships in work. It is difficult to produce a definitive model because Goleman has revised these ideas.

However, Table 4.6 shows how Goleman's emotional intelligence model can be broken down by personal and social competencies and by recognition and regulation competencies, with specific abilities used to illustrate each of the combinations of these competencies.

Goleman's model of emotional intelligence is known as a mixed model of emotional intelligence. The reason for the name 'mixed' is that these models of emotional intelligence combine (mix) central ideas of emotional intelligence with a variety of other personality or behavioural traits. For example, if we look at the abilities listed in Table 4.6, Goleman's model mixes ideas of emotional intelligence (for example, emotional states) with personality and behaviour traits (for example, conscientiousness, adaptability, trustworthiness).

Goleman's model of emotional intelligence is measured by the Emotional Competence Inventory (Goleman and Boyatzis, 2005), which is designed for use in the workplace, and the University Edition, which is designed for use in schools or universities. The Emotional Competence Inventory is a 360-degree instrument. This means that other people evaluate the individuals on their emotional intelligence. The assessor is asked to rate the person in terms

Table 4.6 Goleman's model of emotional intelligence

	Personal competencies	**Social competencies**
Recognition	Self-awareness • Emotional awareness: recognising one's emotions and their possible effects. • Accurate self-assessment: knowing one's strengths and limitations. • Self-confidence: confidence about one's self-worth and capabilities.	Social awareness • Empathy: sensing others' feelings and perspective, and taking an active interest in their feelings and concerns. • Service orientation: anticipating, recognising and meeting people's needs. • Developing others: sensing what others need to develop and improve their abilities. • Leveraging diversity: creating and cultivating opportunities through diverse people. • Political awareness: reading a group's emotional state and understanding power relationships in the group.
Regulation/management	**Self-regulation/management**	**Social skills/management**
	• Self-control: managing disruptive emotions and impulses. • Trustworthiness: maintaining standards of honesty and integrity. • Conscientiousness: taking responsibility for personal performance. • Adaptability: flexibility in handling change. • Achievement drive: self-motivation for achieving excellence. • Innovativeness/initative: being comfortable with and open to novel ideas and new information.	• Developing others: ability to help and improve others. • Influence: having effective tactics for persuasion. • Communication: sending clear and convincing messages. • Leadership: inspiring and guiding people and groups. • Change catalyst: initiating or managing change. • Conflict management: negotiating and resolving disagreements. • Building bonds: nurturing instrumental relationships. • Collaboration and cooperation: working with others towards shared goals. • Teamwork capabilities: creating group energy and synergy in pursuing collective goals.

Sources: Goleman (2001); Goleman *et al.* (2002).

of how characteristic they are of the abilities listed in Goleman's model. Example items in the Emotional Competence Inventory include the assessor determining whether the person:

- presents themselves in an assured, forceful, impressive and unhesitating manner;
- respects, treats with courtesy and relates well to people of diverse backgrounds;
- accurately reads people's moods, feelings or non-verbal cues.

Bar-On's model of emotional intelligence

The third well-recognised model of emotional intelligence was put forward by US psychologist Reuven Bar-On. He names it the emotional–social intelligence model (Bar-On, 1997; 2005).

Like the models of Mayer and Salovey and Goleman, Bar-On's model of emotional intelligence has biological origins. However, rather than emphasising physiological reactions, or part of the brain, Bar-On draws on the evolutionary theory of Darwin. In his book *The Expression of the Emotions in Man and Animals*, Darwin wrote of how animals and humans express and signal to each other with their emotions (Darwin, 1872/1965). Darwin wondered whether human facial expressions are innate, and he set out to show that animals have many of the same ways of physically expressing emotions as humans do. Darwin suggested that the importance of emotional expression was for adaptation and survival. The ability of humans and animals to express emotion (happiness, interest, sadness, fear, anger, surprise) helps animals bond with each other (happiness), is an important process in meeting a mate (interest) and may also act as a protective factor (showing anger to scare people away) or warn others of potential danger (fear). Within this context, Bar-On introduced his model of emotional–social intelligence, which addresses emotionally and socially intelligent behaviour within Darwin's theory of effective adaptation.

Overall, Bar-On saw emotional–social intelligence as a range of interrelated emotional and social competence abilities that allowed individuals to understand and express themselves effectively, understand and relate to others, and cope with environmental demands and pressures. Bar-On based his final model of emotional intelligence on key ideas that had appeared in previous descriptions, definitions and conceptualisations of emotional–social intelligence. In all, he identified five major domains and 15 aspects.

- **Intrapersonal skills** – the ability to recognise, understand and express emotions and feelings. The aspects of intrapersonal skills in this model are emotional self-awareness, assertiveness, self-regard, self-actualisation and independence.
- **Interpersonal skills** – the ability to understand how others feel and relate to them. The aspects of interpersonal skills in this model are interpersonal relationships, social responsibility and empathy.
- **Adaptability scales** – the ability to manage and control emotions. The aspects of adaptability skills in this model are problem-solving, reality testing and flexibility.
- **Stress-management scales** – the ability to manage change, adapt and solve problems of a personal and interpersonal nature. The aspects of stress management skills in this model are stress tolerance and impulse control.
- **General mood** – the ability to generate positive affect and be self-motivated. The aspects of general mood in this model are happiness and optimism.

Bar-On's model of emotional–social intelligence is also known as a mixed model of emotional intelligence. For example, Bar-On mixes ideas of emotional intelligence (i.e. emotional states) and behavioural traits (optimism and flexibility).

Despite developing the theory later, Bar-On was the first of the theorists to develop an emotional intelligence measure, the Emotional Quotient Inventory (EQ-i; Bar-On, 1997). The EQ-i is an estimate of emotional–social intelligence that contains 133 items and employs a five-point response scale format, ranging from 'very seldom or not true of me' (1) to 'very often true of me or true of me' (5). Three things can be computed from the EQ-i: one overall emotional–social intelligence score, five scales representing the main five domains and 15 subscales that make up the five domains.

The five main domains (with the 15 subscales in brackets) are as follows:

- intrapersonal (comprising the self-regard, emotional self-awareness, assertiveness, independence and self-actualisation subscales);
- interpersonal (comprising empathy, social responsibility and interpersonal relationship subscales);
- adaptability (comprising reality-testing, flexibility and problem-solving subscales);
- stress management (comprising stress tolerance and impulse control subscales);
- general mood (comprising optimism and happiness subscales).

However, Bar-On reserves something special for overall scores on the Emotional Quotient Inventory. Those scores can be converted into standard scores based on a mean of 100 and standard deviation of 15, leading to an emotional quotient (EQ) score. This is deliberately meant to resemble IQ (intelligence quotient) scores. High EQ scores suggest that an individual has effective emotional and social functioning in meeting daily demands and challenges. Low EQ scores suggest that an individual has an inability to be effective in meeting daily demands and challenges and suggests the possible existence of emotional and/or social problems.

Providing contexts for understanding the three models of emotional intelligence

So, in considering emotional intelligence, we are presented with three different theories and three different measures of emotional intelligence. One of the major concerns in the emotional intelligence literature is that the theory is not cohesive. However, certain people have set about integrating the theory. This has been done in two ways, by comparing:

- ability and mixed models of emotional intelligence;
- theories of emotional intelligence within a systems of personality approach.

Comparing ability and mixed models of emotional intelligence

The first way in which we can simplify the study of emotional intelligence is to make the distinction between ability models of emotional intelligence and mixed models of emotional intelligence. There is a distinction between psychometric measures of intelligence (based on trying to define intelligence) and cognitive measures of intelligence (which additionally look at some of the cognitive processes that surrounded intelligence; for example, simultaneous and sequential processing). A similar distinction can be made between the models of emotional intelligence.

Authors such as John Mayer, Peter Salovey and David Caruso (Mayer *et al*, 2000) and Robert Emmerling and Daniel Goleman (Emmerling and Goleman, 2003) point out that the model of emotional intelligence that is the most useful depends on what it is trying to achieve. These authors suggest that ability models of emotional intelligence follow the psychometric/measurement tradition by trying to define what the construct is (in this case, what is emotional intelligence). This theory and research are built around trying to identify and define a single theoretical framework that leads to a 'correct' or accurate understanding of what comprises emotional intelligence. Mayer and Salovey's four-branch definition focuses on defining a set of emotional intelligence abilities that are considered unique to emotional intelligence, and it does not include personality or behavioural characteristics that belong to other psychological models (as with the mixed models of emotional intelligence). Mayer *et al.* suggest that following this strategy leads to clear definitions of emotional intelligence. This strategy has a number of advantages:

- Psychologists can clearly identify and communicate what emotional intelligence is.
- Psychologists can understand what emotional intelligence is and how it is related to similar psychological theories by examining the relationship between emotional intelligence and other measures of psychological thinking and feelings (for example, other measures of intelligence and emotion).
- Psychologists can then examine the real applied value of emotional intelligence by looking at its relationship to other variables such as mental health, work and school achievement.

Mayer *et al.* also suggest that, by using such an approach, you can clearly let people know exactly what emotional intelligence is and what it is not, and assure other psychologists that it is not part of some other variable that already exists (for example, personality).

However, Emmerling and Goleman (2003) have made the case for the usefulness of the mixed models of emotional intelligence. It has to be remembered that Goleman's theory and research have been largely developed within the context of applying emotional intelligence to the workplace. Bar-On's model emphasises emotional intelligence as being able to deal best with the demands and stress of the environment. Therefore, with Goleman's and Bar-On's models of emotional intelligence, attention shifts from a focus on defining emotional intelligence to defining the successful 'emotionally intelligent' person. This is done by investigating those abilities that successful emotionally intelligent people have. For example, Goleman's model of emotional intelligence seeks to develop a theory and research around work performance based on social and emotional competencies. He examines how a collection of abilities and behaviour come together in high achievers, or people who do excellently in the workplace (for example, company directors, work leaders), to define emotional intelligence. Emmerling and Goleman argue that this approach is well established in occupational psychology. They suggest that, by following this strategy, mixed ability models of emotional intelligence are able to provide a deeper understanding of people who succeed and of how emotional intelligence, as a sum of a number of new and existing behaviours, is a central part of that success.

Emotional intelligence in the context of a personality system framework

Despite the differences between the various models of emotional intelligence, there has been an attempt to integrate our view of emotional intelligence. John D. Mayer, Peter Salovey and David Caruso (2000) presented the three models of emotional intelligence within a personality systems framework (see Table 4.7).

We will now talk you through Table 4.7. A personality systems framework was introduced by Mayer (1995; 1998; 2005a, b); the framework suggests that there are two dimensions to consider in any set of behaviours:

- **The purpose of a psychological system** – this dimension reflects the contrast between responses to internal needs and experience and responses to the external world.
- **The level of the psychological subsystem** – this dimension reflects the distinction between low, middle and high functions. Mayer defines '**low functions**' as reflecting biological factors (for example, basic biological needs such as eating or physiological factors),

Table 4.7 An overview of personality and its major subsystems with three models of emotional intelligence embedded within it

	Purpose of subsystem			
	Responding to internal needs		**Responding to the external world**	
	High function	**Intrapersonal qualities**	**Interpersonal skills**	
	Learned models culture	*(understanding oneself, having good self-concept and self-esteem)*	*(knowing how to socialise, being comfortable with other people)*	
		(1) Intrapersonal skills	(1) Interpersonal skills	
		(2) Motivating oneself	(2) Handling relationships	
Level of subsystem	**Middle function** Interactive functions	**Motivational and emotional interactions** *(e.g., frustration with something leads to anger)*	**Emotional and cognitive interactions** *(e.g., understanding and perceiving emotions)*	
	Personality, cognitive functions interacting with the environment	(1) Stress management skills	(3) Perception/expression of emotion	(2) Knowing one's emotions
			(3) Facilitating emotion in thought	(2) Recognising emotions in others
			(3) Understanding emotion	(2) Managing emotion
			(3) Regulating emotion	
	Low function	**Motivational directions**	**Emotional qualities**	**Cognitive abilities**
	Biologically related mechanisms	*(satisfying basic needs such as eating)*	*(being emotionally expressive, being happy and calm)*	*(ability to perceive patterns, being analytical)*
	Physiological and neuropsychological functions		(1) General mood	(1) Adaptability skills

Notes:

1 R. Bar-On, *The Emotional Quotient Inventory (EQ-i): A test of emotional intelligence* (Toronto, Canada: Multi-Health Systems, 1997).

2 D. P. Goleman, *Emotional intelligence: Why it can matter more than IQ for character, health and lifelong achievement* (New York: Bantam, 1995).

3 J. D. Mayer and P. Salovey, What is emotional intelligence? In P. Salovey and D. Sluyter (eds), *Emotional development and emotional intelligence: Implications for educators* (New York: Basic Books, 1997), pp. 3–31.

Source: Based on Mayer *et al.* (2000).

'**middle functions**' as reflecting interactive factors (for example, the relationship between personality, cognitive variables and environmental variables) and '**high functions**' as reflecting learned factors (for example, culture).

Mayer drew up a diagram of this system, as outlined in Table 4.7. What Mayer, Salovey and Caruso then did was to divide the different models of emotional intelligence within this framework. As you can see, using this framework emphasises where the different emotional intelligence models are distinct and where they overlap. In terms of each model of emotional intelligence, you can see that:

- Bar-On's model (labelled 1) is divided among the three levels of the personality subsystem: low in terms of adaptability and mood, middle in terms of stress management and high in terms of intrapersonal and interpersonal skills. This reflects Bar-On's intention that emotional intelligence represents successful adaptation to a stressful environment in Darwinian terms, thus involving biological factors combined with learned models of behaviours, involving oneself and others to cope with the stressful environment.

Stop and think

Another emotional intelligence: trait emotional intelligence

Another notable contribution to the emotional intelligence literature is the work of Konstantin Vasily Petrides and colleagues on the concept of trait emotional intelligence. Trait emotional intelligence is different from Salovey and Mayer's ability and Goleman's mixed-models of emotional intelligence and instead conceptualises emotional intelligence as comprising 'emotional self-perceptions' (Petrides and Furnham, 2001). Consequently, trait emotional intelligence centres around one's self-perceived emotional abilities and is sometimes referred to as emotional self-efficacy (belief in our ability to be successful in emotional situations).

- Goleman's model (labelled 2) is split between the middle and high levels, emphasising intrapersonal and interpersonal skills combined with emotional and cognitive interactions, representing his mixed model of abilities in the social world (e.g. the workplace).
- Mayer and Salovey's model (labelled 3) is located entirely within the area of emotional–cognitive interactions, representing the authors' emphasis on emotional intelligence being a set of emotional and cognitive abilities separate from any other aspect of personality.

So, from these two considerations (comparing ability versus mixed models of emotional intelligence, and comparing models of emotional intelligence within a personality subsystems approach), we have a better understanding of how these three different models of emotional intelligence fit together.

The application of emotional intelligence in psychology

So, of what use to psychologists is the concept of emotional intelligence? Well, across a number of psychological domains, emotional intelligence has been found to have mainly positive outcomes, but does it sometimes have a dark side?

One area in which emotional intelligence has been found to be relevant is in health and psychological health. Schutte *et al.* (2007), in a meta-analysis of 44 effect sizes based on the responses of 7,898 participants, found that higher emotional intelligence was associated with better health and psychological health. Emotional intelligence had an average correlation of $r = 0.22$ with physical health, $r = 0.29$ with mental health and $r = 0.31$ with psychosomatic health. In a related area, Mikolajczak and Luminet (2008) examined the relationship between emotional intelligence and self-efficacy and challenge and threat primary appraisals. Self-efficacy is an individual's belief that they can perform some behaviour that will get them a desired positive outcome. Primary appraisals are concerned with how individuals evaluate the nature and meaning of a particular stressful event or situation. A challenge primary appraisal represents the degree to which a stressful event or situation is perceived as allowing for personal growth and development. A threat primary appraisal represents the degree to which a stressful event or situation is perceived as threatening to the person. Mikolajczak and Luminet found that individuals high in emotional intelligence exhibit greater self-efficacy in coping situations (i.e. they can perform some behaviour that will help them cope well with the situation) and appraise a stressful event as a challenge rather than a threat. Also, Externera and Fernandez-Berrocal (2005) found that emotional intelligence was related to life satisfaction and Chamorro-Premuzic *et al.* (2007) found that it was related to higher levels of happiness. Trait emotional intelligence is able to predict a number of successful outcomes, e.g. life satisfaction, lower levels of rumination and better coping, after controlling for personality factors (Petrides *et al.*, 2007).

Emotional intelligence has been found to have a positive benefit in education and the workplace. As we noted above, Goleman's model of emotional intelligence is based around achievement and leadership in the workplace. In terms of other evidence, Downey *et al.* (2008) found that emotional intelligence was significantly associated with higher levels of academic achievement across a range of subjects (mathematics, science, art and geography) among 209 Australian secondary school students, suggesting the usefulness of emotional intelligence in education. Mavroveli *et al.* (2008) found emotional intelligence to correlate positively with teacher-rated positive behaviour and negatively with negative behaviour (e.g. emotional symptoms, conduct problems, peer problems and hyperactivity) among schoolchildren. Rozell *et al.* (2006) examined the relationship between emotional intelligence and individuals working in sales. These authors found that emotional intelligence was positively related to higher levels of performance in a number of sales tasks (e.g. meeting, managing and communicating with customers), which suggests the usefulness of emotional intelligence in the workplace. However, reviews of studies (e.g. Cote and Miners, 2006; Landy, 2005; Zafra *et al.*, 2008) have suggested that there are mixed results, with some studies finding a positive relationship and some studies finding no relationship between emotional intelligence and achievement in education and in the workplace (e.g. Charbonneau and Nicol, 2002; van der Zee *et al.*, 2002). In response to these mixed findings, two studies have suggested that there may be an interesting dynamic between emotional intelligence, general intelligence and academic and workplace achievement. Petrides *et al.* (2004) and, later, Cote and Miners (2006) have presented a 'compensatory' model of emotional intelligence and general intelligence to explain how emotional intelligence may influence achievement. This model suggests that the relationship between emotional intelligence and achievement becomes positive as general intelligence decreases. Together these authors found that, in education (Petrides *et al.*, 2004) and in the workplace (Cote and Miners, 2006), individuals with lower general intelligence demonstrated increased levels of achievement as they demonstrated increased levels of emotional intelligence.

But what about this dark side of emotional intelligence that we mentioned earlier? Well, in 2007, Elizabeth Austin and her colleagues looked at the association between Machiavellianism and emotional intelligence (Austin *et al.*, 2007). Machiavellianism is from the political doctrine of the philosopher Machiavelli, and denies any relevance of morality in political affairs. In psychology, Machiavellianism is generally viewed as a trait which reflects the tendency to be cunning and deceptive in everyday behaviour and interactions with others, particularly in terms of trying to gain advantage for oneself. Austin and her colleagues suggested that, as emotional intelligence comprises traits that enable the individual to manage the emotions of others (such as calming a colleague's angry mood or making someone feel better about oneself), then perhaps the emotional manipulation capability of emotional intelligence might not always be used positively. That is, would someone who was able to manipulate people emotionally, manipulate emotions in other people in a negative way? To examine this idea, Austin *et al.* constructed an emotional manipulation scale and used it to examine the relationship between Machiavellianism and emotional intelligence. Austin *et al.* found that Machiavellianism was found to share a significant negative correlation with emotional intelligence, and emotional manipulation shared a significant positive relationship with Machiavellianism but was unrelated to emotional intelligence. Austin *et al.* concluded that, although people high in Machiavellianism endorse emotionally manipulative behaviour, the evidence did not support the view that such people were successful in emotionally manipulating people owing to the negative relationship between Machiavellianism and emotional intelligence. Furthermore, they found that emotional manipulation was unrelated to emotional intelligence, suggesting that there is no dark side to emotional intelligence.

Sex differences in emotional intelligence

In the light of our discussion earlier regarding sex differences in intelligence, the question arises: 'Do women and men differ in their emotional intelligence?' Well, theoretically, Goleman thinks they do. Goleman (1995) provided separate descriptors of an emotionally intelligent man and woman. Table 4.8 lists these descriptions.

However, the distinctions are not so easy to make when we consider whether women score higher than men do on measures of emotional intelligence. The evidence examining sex differences in emotional intelligence among the samples in the population suggests results are mixed, or that the effect size of any significant difference is small. Remember that we defined an effect size of 0.2 as small, 0.5 as medium and 0.8 as large.

For Mayer and Salovey's ability model of emotional intelligence (and their scores on their Mayer–Salovey–Caruso Emotional Intelligence Test), women are found to score significantly higher than men across the four aspects of emotional intelligence: perception, integration (facilitation), understanding and management. Canadian psychologists Arla L. Day and Sarah A. Carroll found, among 246 undergraduate students (70 men, 176 women), that the effect size for emotional intelligence was higher in women and ranged from 0.18 to 0.30 (Day and Carroll, 2004). Furthermore, US individual difference psychologists Melanie Schulte, Malcolm James Ree and Thomas R. Carretta found an effect size of 0.30 in favour of women scoring higher for overall scores on the MSCEIT than men did (Schulte *et al.*, 2004).

Table 4.8 Goleman's emotional intelligence against IQ and comparing sex differences

	Emotional intelligence
Men	• Outgoing and cheerful • Not prone to fearfulness or worry • Ability to show commitment to people or causes • Takes responsibility • Has an ethical outlook • Sympathetic and caring in relationships • Comfortable with oneself and others
Women	• Assertive and expresses feelings directly • Feels positive about oneself • Life holds meaning • Outgoing • Seeks and enjoys the company of others • Expresses feelings appropriately • Adapts well to stress • Spontaneous • Rarely feels guilty or ruminates

Source: Based on Goleman (1995).

However, findings with Bar-On's Emotional Quotient Inventory (EQ-i) among a US sample of over 3,000 individuals (Bar-On, 1997) suggest a different picture. Bar-On found no significant difference between men and women for overall emotional intelligence scores. However, across the five aspects of emotional intelligence (intrapersonal, interpersonal, adaptability, stress management and general mood) and the 15 subscales that make up the EQ-i, sex differences on emotional intelligence are mixed. Bar-On reports that women score significantly higher on all three aspects of interpersonal skills (empathy, social responsibility and interpersonal relationships) and are more aware of their own emotions than men are. On the other hand, men seem to hold themselves in better self-regard, cope better with stress, are more independent, solve problems better, are more flexible and are more optimistic. These differences are very small, with all but one of the effects being below 0.16; the exception is empathy, where women score higher and the effect size is just under 0.45 (just under medium).

Critical consideration of emotional intelligence theory and research

There are a number of concerns regarding emotional intelligence. One of the first concerns is aimed directly at the mixed models of emotional intelligence. Eysenck (2000) described some of the tendency to mix aspects of intelligence with personality factors as an unscientific approach. Say, for example, that a mixed model of emotional intelligence is found to predict an aspect of work performance. Eysenck suggests that when it comes to understanding this finding, we will be unclear about what is predicting the job performance; that is, is it an aspect of emotional intelligence or is it a personality factor? Eysenck finds it hard to see how this way forward is fruitful for psychology. However, Emmerling and Goleman (2003) argue that such an approach is fruitful. For these authors, mixed models of emotional intelligence allow the researcher to understand how a collection of behaviours come together to define high achievement in people in the workplace. He readily admits that this contrasts with Eysenck's scientific approach, but his method reflects a tradition in occupational psychology of trying to identify competencies that are found in people who achieve highly.

Findings by Melanie Schulte and her colleagues (Schulte *et al.*, 2004) provide evidence that supports Eysenck's view. To define overall ability and competence, the authors looked at the relationships between several measures of intelligence (general intelligence and verbal, quantitative and spatial abilities), the five-factor model of personality (neuroticism, extraversion, openness to experience, agreeableness and conscientiousness), overall scores on the Mayer–Salovey–Caruso Emotional Intelligence Test (a measure of ability-based emotional intelligence) and sex among 102 US university students. In defining human ability, they found that a very large amount of the variance of what can be described as ability was accounted for by general intelligence, personality factors and sex, and that the emotional intelligence measure added very little to our understanding of overall ability and competence. These findings suggest that there is some speculation about the usefulness of emotional intelligence for enhancing the understanding of human ability over and above what is already available, such as general intelligence, the five-factor model of personality and sex.

A second concern voiced by Eysenck is the problem that emotional intelligence has no benchmark by which to assess it. He suggests that, while intelligence has benchmarks of school grades and educational achievement, emotional intelligence has none. However, Goleman would point out that there are several benchmarks by which emotional intelligence could be judged, one of these being success in the world of work.

A third concern arises from the lack of empirical research to confirm some of the biological theories that were proposed alongside the models of emotional intelligence.

Commentators such as individual difference psychologists Gerald Matthews, Moshe Zeidner and Richard Roberts have suggested that, while Goleman and Bar-On link their theories to biological aspects, there is no empirical research to support such assertions (Matthews *et al.*, 2004). Goleman has not sought to link the amygdala and the fight-or-flight response to emotional intelligence. Bar-On proposed that emotional intelligence represents a successful evolutionary adaptation to environmental stress. However, there is no evidence that supports the biological theoretical contexts into which Goleman and Bar-On place their models of emotional intelligence.

Final comments

You should now be able to outline the extent of sex differences between men and women on general intelligence and specific aspects of intelligence, particularly spatial and verbal intelligence. You should be able to describe possible biological and environmental variables that may explain sex differences in intelligence. You should also now be able to outline the major models of emotional intelligence and provide a critical consideration of theory and research in emotional intelligence.[G]

[G]Maltby, J., Day, L., & Macaskill, A. (2013). Further discussions and debates in intelligence: Sex differences in intelligence and emotional intelligence. In *Personality, individual differences and intelligence* (3rd ed., pp. 391–404). Harlow, Essex: Pearson Education Limited.

Summary

- Galton is the forefather of intelligence tests. His central hypothesis was that there are differences in intelligence, and he set out to explore this hypothesis.
- Alfred Binet created the first intelligence test. In 1905, with Theodore Simon, Binet produced the Binet–Simon scale, the first intelligence test, which Simon later described as 'practical, convenient, and rapid'.
- Terman began to recognise the need for 'standardised testing'.
- William Stern developed the idea of the intelligence quotient or, as it is more popularly known today, IQ.
- Yerkes developed a group intelligence test, resulting in the Army Alpha and Army Beta tests.
- Charles Spearman introduced a two-factor theory of intelligence. The first factor of intelligence was specific abilities, 's'. The second factor was what Spearman thought was underlying all the positive correlations between intelligence tests – general ability, 'g'.
- In 1939 Wechsler published the first of the Wechsler tests, the Wechsler–Bellevue Scale. Later he introduced two tests that are still used today: the Wechsler Adult Intelligence Scale (WAIS) and the Wechsler Intelligence Scale for Children (WISC). Alongside these tests, he published a new way of calculating IQ through the use of standard deviations.
- Scottish psychologist John Carlyle Raven first published his Progressive Matrices in 1938. His test was a non-verbal measure of 'g'.
- Thurstone agreed with Spearman's hypothesis of a general factor of intelligence. However, he viewed 'g' differently from Spearman. Thurstone argued that 'g' results from, rather than lies behind, seven primary mental abilities.
- Cattell acknowledged Spearman's work in accepting that there was general intelligence, but he suggested that 'g' comprises two related but distinct components: crystallised intelligence and fluid intelligence.
- Guilford disagreed with the stance of Spearman and, to some extent, with Thurstone and Cattell; he did not acknowledge the existence of 'g'. Instead, Guilford (1977) eventually proposed that intelligence was the result of 150 independent abilities. His theory was named the Structure of Intellect (SI) theory.
- Vernon described intelligence as a hierarchy. Vernon thought that 'g' accounts for the largest amount of variability among humans. The next level in Vernon's hierarchy comprises two major group factors, then minor group factors and then specific factors.
- Carroll (1993) proposed a hierarchical model of intelligence, the Three-Stratum Model of Human Cognitive Abilities. Stratum I comprises specific levels of intelligence, stratum II is made up of eight broad factors arising from these specific abilities and stratum III is the general level of intelligence representing general intellectual ability, similar to 'g'.
- Many intelligence tests in use today reflect theoretical and empirical growth in the understanding of intelligence.
- Sattler (2002) establishes three main aspects in all good intelligence tests: the variety of tasks involved, standardisation of administration and norm referencing. Intelligence tests are used for all sorts of purposes, but mainly for these three: selection, diagnosis and evaluation.
- IQ test scores are important in predicting school and work performance. The average correlation between intelligence and a number of school indicators is around *r* 5 0.50, suggesting that intelligence does predict performance at school. The correlation between intelligence (cognitive ability) and job performance is also around *r* 5 0.50.
- Some psychologists have shown that intelligence in childhood can predict variables across the lifespan; these include death by a certain age and people being diagnosed with certain illnesses, but not all health-related matters.
- At one level the criticisms of and issues with intelligence tests are rather easy to identify. The issues are of reliability, validity and whether the importance of intelligence tests is over-emphasised.

- There is a huge difference between the way that intelligence tests are used and viewed and the modern-day theories and intelligence tests that have been developed in the past 20 years. Naglieri has suggested that, today, intelligence practitioners want not only to test children's intelligence, but to follow it up with interventions that are designed to improve the child's learning in the areas where they have shown weakness.
- Sir Francis Galton suggested that man's natural abilities are inherited under the same conditions as physical features of the animal world that had been described by Darwin. Galton suggested that intelligence is passed down to children through heredity.
- Heritability of intelligence is the estimated assessment of the extent to which intelligence is passed down from parents to children through their genes on average across the population.
- There are largely three types of study that you will regularly see in the heritability of intelligence: family studies, twin studies and adoption studies.
- Heritability estimates of intelligence vary greatly, ranging from an average of 40 percent to an average of 80 percent.
- There are four general issues surrounding genetic heritability estimates: conceptions of heritability and the environment, different types of genetic variance, the representativeness of twin and adoption studies and assortative mating.
- We identify five main areas in which to consider environmental effects on intelligence.
  - The first area is biological variables (nutrition, lead and prenatal factors) and the maternal effects model.
  - The second area is the consideration of family environment and shared and non-shared factors. Non-shared environments consider within-family factors and outside-family factors, including context-specific socialisation, outside-the-home socialisation, transmission of culture via group processes, group processes that widen differences between social groups and group processes that widen differences among individuals within the group.
  - The third area is socioeconomic status variables that also include consideration of birth order, family size and intelligence.
  - The fourth and fifth areas are education and culture, respectively, the latter comprising consideration of factors such as decontextualisation, quantification and biologisation.
- There are three main theories of emotional intelligence: an ability model devised by Mayer and Salovey, called the four-branch model of emotional intelligence; and two mixed ability models, Goleman's model of emotional intelligence and Bar-On's model of emotional–social intelligence.
- Together these three different theories offer two different types of models (ability versus mixed) and three different ways of measuring emotional intelligence. Two contexts can be provided to compare these three models: (1) comparing ability versus mixed models of emotional intelligence; and (2) understanding emotional intelligence in the context of a personality systems approach.
- Research evidence suggests that emotional intelligence is associated with better health, mental health, life satisfaction, happiness and sometimes with achievement in education and in the workplace.
- For sex differences in emotional intelligence based on emotional intelligence ability models, there may be a small effect size in favour of women scoring higher on emotional intelligence. However, findings for mixed models of emotional intelligence suggest no difference between men and women on general emotional intelligence; for specific aspects of emotional intelligence, each sex sometimes scores higher than the other sex – although effect sizes are usually small, except perhaps those for empathy.

Review questions

A. Fill in the missing words to complete the following statements.

1. Galton reasoned that superior intelligence would be a reflection of superior ________________ development of brain and body; thus ______________ measures might provide a reliable index of intelligence.
2. Binet and Simon's test was a measure of ________________ or ________________.
3. The intelligence quotient was a measure of a child's ________________ age to the child's ________________ age.
4. The Wechsler Adult Intelligence Scale contains various measures to assess a full range of abilities. These include ability tests of ________________, ________________, ________________, ________________, ________________, ________________, ________________, ________________, ________________, ________________ and ________________.
5. Intelligence tests are not without their criticisms. Three main considerations of IQ test are based on: ________________________; ________________________; ____.
6. There are numerous environmental influences on intelligence. Thomas Bouchard and Nancy Segal (1985) list 21 factors that are related to intelligence, including: ________________, ________________, ________________, ________________, ________________.
7. Salovey and Mayer's divided the concept of emotional intelligence into four capaci ties: ____________________________; ____________________________; ____________________________; ________________.

B. Read the following statement and answer with the most correct definition.

8. If an individual has an IQ score of 70 – 75 or below, and also demonstrates deficits in areas of adaptive behaviour, e.g., communication, self-care, they can be considered as having an ____________________________.

C. Please select one statement that best answers each of the following questions.

9. Why did Terman adapt the Simon-Binet IQ test in 1916?
   a) because the Simon-Binet test did not work effectively cross-culturally
   b) because the Simon-Binet test did not measure actual intelligence
   c) because the Simon-Binet test was prejudice
   d) because the Simon-Binet test was outdated

10. Which are the main components of Spearman's two factor theory of Intelligence?
   a) visual ability and spatial ability
   b) specific intelligence and general intelligence
   c) emotional abilities and cognitive abilities
   d) primary abilities and secondary abilities

11. What is fluid intelligence?

a) the ability to solve abstract relational problems

b) memories from the past

c) memory of what is happening now

d) both a and c

12. Alzheimer's disease affects what type of intelligence?

a) objective intelligence

b) fluid intelligence

c) systems intelligence

d) crystallised intelligence

13. Raven progressive matrices has several major points. What statement is <u>not</u> correct?

a) can be used with persons ranging from 6 years to adult

b) affects crystallised intelligence

c) measures nonverbal reasoning

d) unlikely to be culturally biased

14. Jayden achieved a score of 100 on the current version of the Wechsler Adult Intelligence Scale. What does his score mean?

a) he completed 100 questions, whether correctly or incorrectly

b) he achieved an average IQ score compared to other people

c) he answered 100 questions correctly

d) he has an above average iq score compared to other people

15. Key factors of emotional intelligence include

a) Self-awareness

b) Self-management

c) Social awareness

d) All of the above

16. Personal competence in emotional intelligence means we must

a) have social awareness and sound social skills

b) have a positive self-concept

c) be aware, regulate our behaviour, and be self-motivated

d) have empathy for others, and be aware of other people

CHAPTER 5

Psychological Disorders

The content in this section has been compiled from:
Lilienfeld, Lynn, Namy, Woolf, Jamieson, Marks & Slaughter, Chapter 16

Lilienfeld, S. O., Lynn, S. J., Namy, L. L., Woolf, N. J., Jamieson, G., Marks, A., & Slaughter, V. (2015). Psychological disorders: When adaptation breaks down. In S. O. Lilienfeld, S. J. Lynn, L. L. Namy, N. J. Woolf, G. Jamieson, A. Marks, & V. Slaughter (Eds.), *Psychology: From inquiry to understanding* (2nd ed., pp. 682–722). Melbourne, VIC: Pearson Australia

CHAPTER 5

Psychological Disorders

Mental health conditions affect a large portion of the population and can affect anyone at any time. People who experience mental health problems experience changes in their thinking, mood, and behaviour. In a hospital or community health setting, you may come across a range of individuals, some of whom may be managing medical comorbidities as well as experiencing a mental health condition. Whether you are working directly or indirectly to treat patient symptomology, it is important to be aware that reduced mental health may affect a number of human functions and interfere with an individual's ability to adapt to change and cope with challenges. This chapter explores the bidirectional connection between mental health and physical health and focuses on some of the most common mental health disorders.

After studying this chapter you should be able to:

- Identify criteria for defining mental health disorders
- Describe historical and cultural concepts of mental illness
- Describe the system for classifying individuals with a mental health disorder: DSM-5
- Identify characteristics of different anxiety disorders
- Identify characteristics of different and mood disorders
- Identify characteristics of borderline and psychopathic personality disorders
- Identify the characteristic symptoms of schizophrenia.

Below are descriptions of five actual patients (with their names changed to safeguard their identity) drawn from real-life clinical experience. Read each description, and ask yourself what these five people have in common.

- Ida, 43 years old, was strolling around a shopping centre by herself. Suddenly, she experienced a burst of incredibly intense anxiety that left her feeling terrified, faint and nauseated. She thought she was having a heart attack and took a taxi to the nearest hospital emergency room. The doctors found nothing wrong with her heart and told her the problem was 'all in her head'. Since then, Ida has refused to leave her house or go anywhere without her husband. Ida's diagnosis: *panic disorder (with agoraphobia).*
- Bill, 45 years old, has not shaved or showered in over 10 years. His beard is more than half a metre long. Bill does not want to shave or shower because he is terrified that tiny 'metal slivers' from the water will find their way into his skin. As much as possible, Bill avoids talking on the telephone or walking through doorways because he is petrified of acquiring germs. Whenever he experiences a thought he feels he should not be having—such as a desire to kiss a married woman—he counts backwards from 100 in sevens. Bill recognises these behaviours as irrational, but has not been able to change them despite about 15 years of treatment. Bill's diagnosis: *obsessive-compulsive disorder.*
- A few days after having a baby at age 30, Ann became incredibly giddy. She felt on top of the world, barely needed any sleep, and soon began sleeping with men she had just met. Ann also became convinced she had turned into a clown—literally. She was even persuaded that she had a bright-red round nose, even though her nose was entirely normal. Looking back on this episode a few weeks later, Ann recognises that her beliefs were out of touch with reality. Ann's diagnosis: *bipolar disorder.*
- Terrell, 28 years old, has just been released from the intensive-care unit of a city hospital. He had shot himself in the stomach after becoming convinced that fish were swimming there. He suspects these fish are part of a government conspiracy to make him physically ill. Terrell's diagnosis: *schizophrenia.*
- Johnny is 18 years old. He is charming, articulate and fun-loving. Yet he is furious that his parents have helped commit him to the inpatient unit of a psychiatric hospital, and he blames his parents, teachers and former friends for his problems. Johnny is well aware that his actions, such as swearing at teachers, holding live cats underwater until they drown, and attempting to blow up his high school with stolen dynamite, are not exactly popular among his peers. But he sees nothing especially wrong with these behaviours and admits that he has never felt guilty about anything. Johnny's diagnosis: *antisocial personality disorder.*

Concepts of mental illness: yesterday and today

These brief sketches do not do justice to the extraordinarily rich and complex lives of these five people, but they give us some sense of the broad scope of *psychopathology*, or mental illness. In almost all mental disorders, we witness a striking failure of adaptation to the environment. In one way or another, people with mental disorders aren't adjusting well to the demands of daily life. Many psychopathology researchers adopt a failure analysis approach to mental disorders (Harkness, 2007). Just as engineers use accidents, such as plane crashes, to help them understand how mechanical systems work properly, psychopathology researchers examine breakdowns in adaptation to help them understand healthy functioning. But what do Ida, Bill, Ann, Terrell and Johnny have in common? Putting it differently, what distinguishes psychological abnormality from normality?

What is mental illness? A deceptively complex question

The answer to this question is not as simple as we might assume, because the concept of mental disorder does not lend itself to a clear-cut dictionary definition (McNally, 2011). Psychologists and psychiatrists have proposed a host of criteria for defining *mental disorder*; we review five of them here. Each criterion captures something important about mental disorder, but each has its shortcomings (Gorenstein, 1984; Wakefield, 1992).

Statistical rarity

Many mental disorders, such as schizophrenia—as in the case of Terrell—are uncommon in the population. Yet we cannot rely on statistical rarity to define mental disorder, because not all rare conditions (such as extraordinary creativity) are pathological, and many mental illnesses (such as mild depression) are quite common (Kendell, 1975).

Subjective distress

Most mental disorders, including mood and anxiety disorders, produce emotional pain for individuals afflicted with them. But not all psychological disorders generate distress. For example, during the manic phases of bipolar disorder, which Ann experienced, people frequently feel better than normal and perceive nothing wrong with their behaviour. Similarly, many adolescents with conduct disorder, like Johnny, experience less distress than the typical adolescent.

Impairment

Most mental disorders interfere with people's ability to function in everyday life. These disorders may destroy marriages, friendships and jobs. Yet the presence of impairment by itself cannot define mental illness, because some conditions, like laziness, can produce impairment but are not mental disorders. Similarly, many medical illnesses that are not mental disorders also cause impairment (for example, traumatic brain injury, diabetes mellitus).

Societal disapproval

Nearly 60 years ago, the psychiatrist Thomas Szasz (1960) argued famously that 'mental illness is a myth' and that 'mental disorders' are nothing more than conditions that society dislikes. He even proposed that psychologists and psychiatrists use diagnoses as weapons of control: by attaching negative labels to people whose behaviours they find objectionable, they are putting these people 'in their place'. Szasz was both right and wrong. He was right that our attitudes towards the seriously mentally ill are often profoundly negative and that deep-seated social prejudices towards them are widespread. He was also right that societal attitudes shape our views of abnormality.

Psychiatric diagnoses are often shaped by the views—and biases—of the historical period. For centuries, some psychiatrists invoked the diagnosis of masturbational insanity to describe individuals whose compulsive masturbation supposedly drove them mad (Hare, 1962). Homosexuality was classified as a mental illness until members of the American Psychiatric Association voted to remove it from their list of disorders in 1973 (Bayer, 1981). As society became more accepting of homosexuality, mental health professionals came to reject the view that such behaviour is indicative of psychological disorder.

But Szasz was wrong that society regards all disapproved conditions as mental disorders (Wakefield, 1992). To take just one example, racism is justifiably deplored by society but is not considered a mental disorder by either laypeople or mental health professionals (Yamey & Shaw, 2002). Neither is messiness or rudeness, even though society considers each of them undesirable. Moral weaknesses and character flaws are not mental disorders.

Biological dysfunction

Many mental disorders probably result from breakdowns or failures of physiological systems. For example, schizophrenia is often marked by an underactivity in the brain's frontal lobes. In contrast, some mental disorders, such as specific *phobias* (intense and irrational fears of objects, places or situations), appear to be acquired largely through learning experiences and may require only a weak genetic predisposition to trigger them.

In fact, it is unlikely that any one criterion distinguishes mental disorders from normality, which explains why mental disorder is difficult or impossible to define (McNally, 2011; Stein et al., 2010). As a consequence, some authors have argued for a *family resemblance view* of mental disorder (Kirmayer & Young, 1999; Lilienfeld & Marino, 1995; Rosenhan & Seligman, 1989). According to this perspective, mental disorders do not all have one thing in common. Just as brothers and sisters within a family look similar but do not all possess exactly the same eyes, ears or noses, mental disorders share a loose set of features. These features include those we have described—statistical rarity, subjective distress, impairment, societal disapproval and biological dysfunction—as well as others, such as a need for treatment, irrationality and loss of control over one's behaviour (Bergner, 1997). So Ida, Bill, Ann, Terrell and Johnny are not alike in precisely the same way. Yet they overlap enough in their features that we recognise each of them as suffering from a mental disorder.

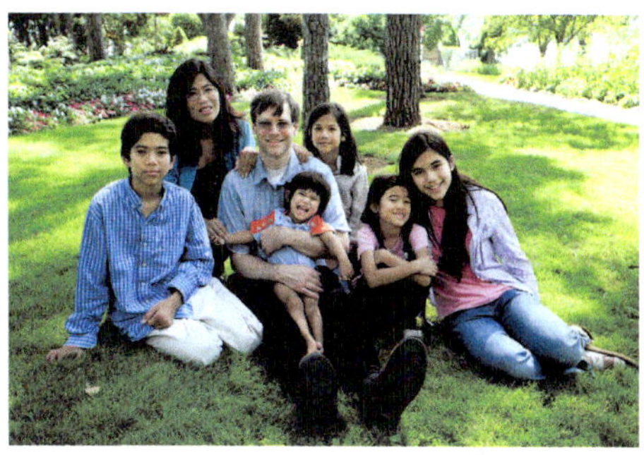

Brothers and sisters share a family resemblance; they look like each other but do not have any one feature in common. The broad category of 'mental disorders' may be similar. Different mental disorders are not alike in the same exact way, but they share a number of features.
(Source: Jarenwicklund/Dreamstime.)

Historical concepts of mental illness: from demons to asylums

Throughout history, people have recognised certain behaviours as abnormal. Yet their explanations and treatments for these behaviours have shifted in tune with prevailing cultural concepts. The history of society's evolving views of mental illness tells the fascinating story of a bumpy road from non-science to science.

The demonic and medical models

During the Middle Ages, many people in Europe viewed mental illnesses through the lens of a **demonic model**. They attributed hearing voices, talking to oneself and other odd behaviours to the actions of evil spirits infesting the body (Hunter & Macalpine, 1963).

Although they rarely refer to demons, many Indigenous peoples around the world explain abnormal behaviour in terms of possession by spirits. Among Australian Aboriginals, spiritual explanations of suffering are often components of holistic explanations that include physical health and community well-being (Parker, 2010; Vicary & Westerman, 2004). These explanations may play a useful role in efforts to treat mental illness in Indigenous communities, rather than being denigrated as wrong or 'primitive'. As the Middle Ages faded and the Renaissance took hold, views of the mentally ill became more enlightened. Over time, more people came to perceive mental illness primarily as a physical disorder requiring medical treatment—a view that some scholars refer to as the **medical model** (Blaney, 1975). Beginning in the fifteenth century,

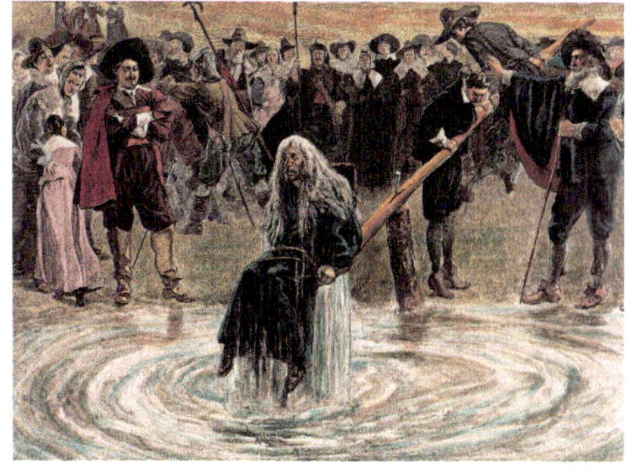

The infamous 'dunking test' for witches, popular during the witch scares of the sixteenth and seventeenth centuries. According to the dunking test, if a woman drowned, it meant she was not a witch. In contrast, if she floated to the top of the water, it meant she was a witch and needed to be executed. Either way, she died.
(Source: Bettman/Corbis.)

Demonic model View of mental illness in which odd behaviour, hearing voices or talking to oneself was attributed to evil spirits infesting the body.

Medical model Perception that regarded mental illness as due to a physical disorder requiring medical treatment.

Asylums Institutions for the mentally ill, first created in the fifteenth century.

Moral treatment Approach to mental illness calling for dignity, kindness and respect for the mentally ill.

Deinstitutionalisation 1960s and 1970s government policy that focused on releasing hospitalised psychiatric patients into the community and closing mental hospitals.

and increasingly in later centuries, European governments began to house psychologically troubled individuals in **asylums**—institutions for the mentally ill (Gottesman, 1991).

Yet the medical treatments of that era were scarcely more scientific than those of the demonic era, and several were equally barbaric. One gruesome treatment was 'bloodletting', which was based on the mistaken notion that excessive blood causes mental illness. In some cases, doctors drained patients of nearly 2 litres of blood, about 40 percent of the body's total. In still other cases, staff tried to frighten patients 'out of their diseases' by tossing them into a pit of snakes, hence the term *snake pit* as a synonym for an insane asylum (Szasz, 2006).

Fortunately, reform was on the way. Thanks to the heroic efforts of Phillippe Pinel (1748–1826) in France, and Dorothea Dix (1802–1887) in America, an approach called **moral treatment** gained a foothold in Europe and America. Advocates of moral treatment insisted that the mentally ill be treated with dignity, kindness and respect. Before moral treatment existed, patients in asylums were often bound in chains; following moral treatment, they were free to roam the halls of hospitals, get fresh air and interact freely with staff and other patients. Still, effective treatments for mental illnesses were virtually non-existent, so many people continued to suffer for years with no hope of relief.

The modern era of psychiatric treatment

It was not until the early 1950s that a dramatic change in society's treatment of the mentally ill arrived on the scene. It was then that psychiatrists introduced a medication imported from France called chlorpromazine (brandname Thorazine) into mental hospitals. Chlorpromazine was not a miracle cure, but it did offer a modestly effective treatment for some symptoms of schizophrenia and other disorders marked by a loss of contact with reality. For the first time, patients with these conditions often became able to function independently, and some returned to their families. Others held jobs for the first time in years, even decades.

By the 1960s and 1970s, the advent of chlorpromazine and similar medications became the primary impetus for a governmental policy known as **deinstitutionalisation**, which

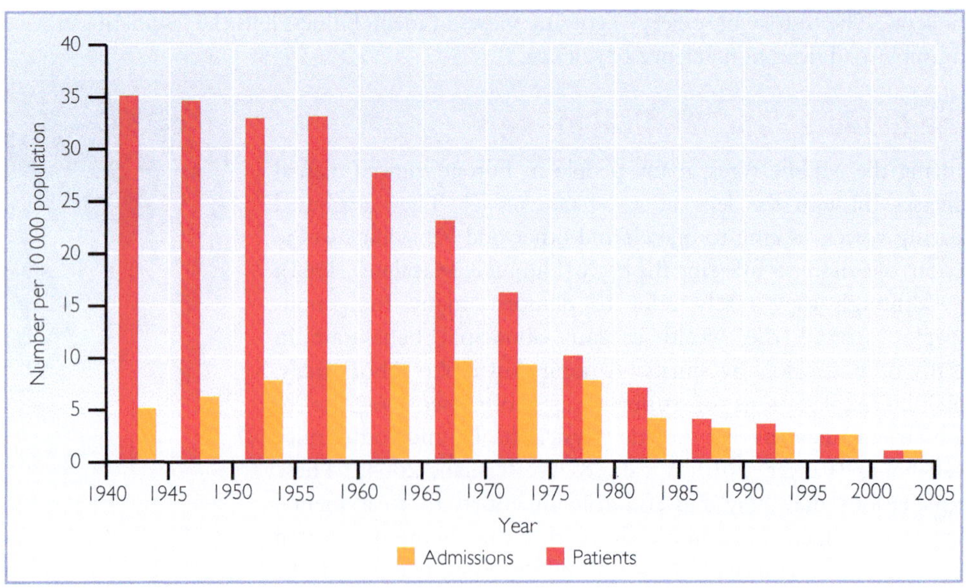

Figure 5.1 Decline in numbers of psychiatric inpatients.

Beginning in the late 1950s, deinstitutionalisation resulted in a massive drop in the number of psychiatric inpatients in Australian hospitals. For example, this graph shows the decline in the number of inpatients in Queensland's public psychiatric institutions. Even while new admissions rose, the number of patients remaining in these institutions dropped. **(Source:** Doessel et al., 2005.)

allowed the release of hospitalised psychiatric patients into the community and contributed to the closure of many mental hospitals (Torrey, 1997). Following deinstitutionalisation, the number of hospitalised psychiatric patients plummeted through the beginning of the twenty-first century (see Figure 5.1). But deinstitutionalisation was a mixed blessing. Some patients returned to a semblance of a regular life, but tens of thousands of others spilled into cities and rural areas without adequate follow-up care. Many went off their medications and wandered the streets aimlessly. Some of the homeless people we can see today on the streets of major cities are a tragic legacy of deinstitutionalisation (Leeper, 1988). Today, psychologists, social workers, and other mental health professionals are working to improve the quality and availability of community care for severely affected psychiatric patients. Among the consequences of these efforts are community mental health centres and halfway houses, free or low-cost care facilities in which people can obtain treatment.

Thankfully, our understanding of mental illness and its treatment today is considerably more sophisticated than it was centuries ago. Still, few of today's treatments are genuine cures.

Psychiatric diagnosis across cultures

Psychiatric diagnoses are shaped not only by history, but by culture (Chentsova-Dutton & Tsai, 2006; Watters, 2010). Psychologists have increasingly recognised that certain conditions are *culture-bound*—that is, specific to one or more societies—although many of these conditions remain poorly researched (see Table 5.1) (Kleinman, 1988; Simons & Hughes, 1986).

Culture-bound syndromes

For example, a disorder specific to Malaysia, the Philippines and some African countries is called 'amok'. This condition is marked by episodes of intense sadness and brooding followed by uncontrolled behaviour and unprovoked attacks on people or animals (American Psychiatric Association, 2000). This condition gave rise to the popular phrase 'running amok', meaning 'going wild'.

Other culture-bound syndromes seem to be variants of conditions in Western culture. Among Aboriginal Australians, for example, a syndrome with many of the same features as depression is understood as 'longing for country' (Westerman, 2003), based on a sense of separation or removal from land or spirit. In Japan, social anxiety is typically expressed as a

Table 5.1 A sampling of common culture-bound syndromes not discussed in the text

Syndrome	Region/population affected	Description
Arctic hysteria	Alaska Natives	Abrupt episode accompanied by extreme excitement and frequently followed by convulsive seizures and coma
Ataque de nervios	Latin America	Symptoms include uncontrollable shouting, attacks of crying, trembling, heat in the chest rising to the head, and verbal or physical aggression
Brain fog	West Africa	Symptoms include difficulties in concentrating, remembering and thinking
Latah	Malaysia and Southeast Asia	Found mostly among women; marked by an extreme startle reaction, followed by a loss of control, cursing and mimicking of others' actions and speech
Mal de ojo (evil eye)	Spain and Latin America	A common term to describe the cause of disease, misfortune and social disruption
Windigo	Native Americans Central and NE Canada	Morbid state of anxiety with fears of becoming a cannibal

(**Source:** Based on Simons, 2001.)

fear of offending others (called *taijin kyofushu),* such as by saying something offensive or giving off a terrible body odour (Kleinknecht et al., 1994; Vriends et al., 2013). In Australia, social anxiety is more commonly generated by fear of public embarrassment, for example when giving a speech. Culture may influence how people express interpersonal anxiety. Because Japanese culture is more collectivistic than Western culture, Japanese people tend to be more concerned about their impact on others than are Westerners. In contrast, Western culture is more individualistic, so people tend to worry more about what may happen to them as individuals.

Cultural universality

Despite the cultural differences we have noted, we should not exaggerate the cultural relativity of mental disorders. Many mental disorders appear to exist in most, perhaps all, cultures. Jane Murphy (1976) conducted a classic study of two isolated societies—a group of Yorubas in Nigeria and a group of Inuit in Alaska—that had experienced essentially no contact with Western culture. These cultures possessed terms for disorders that are strikingly similar to schizophrenia, alcoholism and psychopathic personality, a condition marked by dishonesty, manipulativeness and an absence of guilt and empathy. For example, in Inuit, *kunlangeta* describes a person who lies, cheats, steals, is unfaithful to women and does not listen to elders—a description that fits almost perfectly the Western concept of psychopathic personality. When Murphy asked one of the Inuit how they dealt with such individuals, he replied that 'somebody would have pushed him off the ice when no one was looking'. Apparently, Inuit are not much fonder of psychopaths than we are.

Special considerations in psychiatric classification and diagnosis

There are so many ways in which psychological adaptation can go awry. Thus, we would be hopelessly lost without some system of diagnostic classification. Psychiatric diagnoses serve at least two crucial functions. First, they help us to pinpoint the psychological problem a person is experiencing. Once we have identified this problem, it is often easier to select a treatment. Second, psychiatric diagnoses make it easier for mental health professionals to communicate with each other. When a psychologist diagnoses a patient with schizophrenia, she can be reasonably certain that other psychologists know the patient's principal symptoms. Diagnoses operate as forms of mental shorthand, simplifying complex descriptions of problematic behaviours into convenient summary phrases.

Still, there are a host of misconceptions regarding psychiatric diagnosis. Before turning to our present system of psychiatric classification, we examine the four most prevalent misconceptions.

Misconception 1: *Psychiatric diagnosis is nothing more than pigeonholing; that is, sorting people into different 'boxes'.* According to this criticism, when we diagnose people with a mental disorder, we deprive them of their uniqueness: we imply that all people within the same diagnostic category are alike in all important respects.

Reality. To the contrary, a diagnosis implies only that all people with that diagnosis are alike in at least *one* important respect (Lilienfeld & Landfield, 2008). Psychologists recognise that even within a diagnostic category such as schizophrenia, people differ dramatically in their race and cultural backgrounds, personality traits, interests, cognitive skills and other psychological difficulties. People are far more than their disorders.

Misconception 2: *Psychiatric diagnoses are unreliable.* Reliability refers to consistency of measurement. In the case of psychiatric diagnoses, the form of reliability that matters most is inter-rater reliability: the extent to which different raters (such as different psychologists) agree on patients' diagnoses.

Reality. In fact, for major mental disorders, like schizophrenia, mood disorders, anxiety disorders and alcoholism, inter-rater reliabilities are typically about as high as that for most medical disorders (Matarazzo, 1983)—correlations between raters of .8 or above out of a maximum of 1.0. Still, the picture is not entirely rosy. For many personality disorders (a class of disorders we discuss later), inter-rater reliabilities tend to be considerably lower (Freedman et al., 2013; Zimmerman, 1994).

Misconception 3: *Psychiatric diagnoses are invalid.* From the standpoint of Thomas Szasz (1960) and other critics, psychiatric diagnoses are largely useless because they do not provide us with much, if any, new information. They are merely descriptive labels for behaviours we do not like.

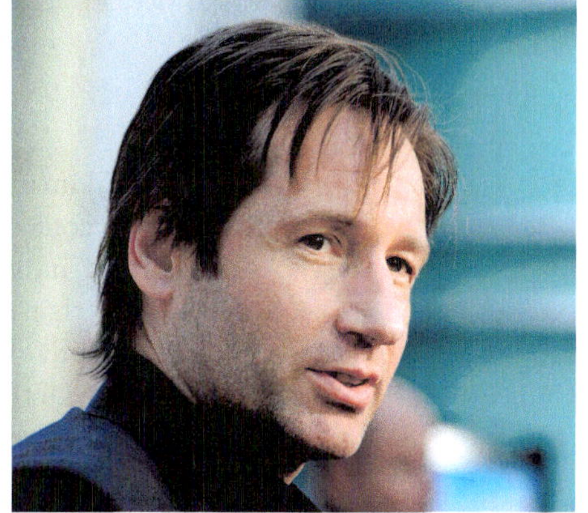

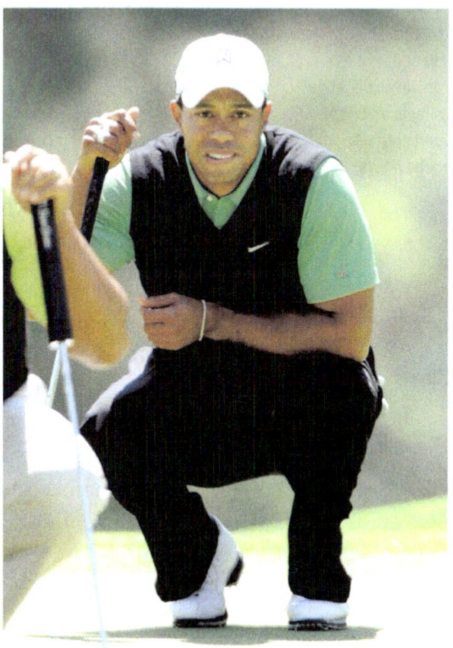

Actor David Duchovny and golfer Tiger Woods are among the many celebrities who have reportedly sought treatment for 'sexual addiction', which is not an official psychiatric diagnosis. Is sexual addiction a genuine condition, or is it merely a descriptive label for problematic behaviour? Many psychologists argue the latter.
(Sources: Jim Ruymen/UPI/Newscom; Kyodo/Newscom.)

Reality. When it comes to some pop psychology labels, Szasz probably has a point. Consider the explosion of diagnostic labels that are devoid of scientific support, such as co-dependency, sexual addiction, internet addiction, road rage disorder, and compulsive shopping disorder (Granello & Beamish, 1998; Kessler et al., 2006; Koran et al., 2006; McCann, Shindler & Hammond, 2003). Although frequently used in talk shows, television programmes, movies and self-help books, these labels are not recognised as formal psychiatric diagnoses.

Yet there is now considerable evidence that many psychiatric diagnoses do tell us something new about the person. In a classic paper, psychiatrists Eli Robins and Samuel Guze (1970) outlined several criteria for determining whether a psychiatric diagnosis is valid. According to Robins and Guze, a valid diagnosis

1. distinguishes that diagnosis from other, similar diagnoses
2. predicts diagnosed individuals' performance on laboratory tests, including personality measures, neurotransmitter levels and brain-imaging findings (Andreasen et al., 1995)
3. predicts diagnosed individuals' family history of psychiatric disorders
4. predicts diagnosed individuals' *natural history*—that is, what tends to happen to them over time; in addition, some authors have argued that a valid diagnosis ideally:
5. predicts diagnosed individuals' response to treatment (Waldman, Lilienfeld & Lahey, 1995).

There is evidence that many mental disorders fulfil Robins and Guze's criteria for validity. Table 5.2 illustrates these criteria using the example of attention-deficit/hyperactivity disorder (ADHD), a disorder we will encounter late in this chapter, which is characterised by inattention, impulsivity and overactivity. ADHD has reasonably good validity, because it is more than a label for behaviours. It tells us something about the diagnosed person we did not already

Table 5.2 Criteria for validity: the case of ADHD. Although controversial in many respects, the diagnosis of attention-deficit/hyperactivity disorder (ADHD) largely satisfies the Robins and Guze criteria for validity.

Robins and Guze criteria	Findings concerning the ADHD diagnosis
1. Distinguishes a particular diagnosis from other similar diagnoses	The child's symptoms cannot be accounted for by other diagnoses, such as substance abuse and anxiety disorders
2. Predicts performance on laboratory tests (personality measures, neurotransmitter levels, brain imaging findings)	The child is likely to perform poorly on laboratory measures of concentration
3. Predicts family history of psychiatric disorders	The child has a higher probability than the average child of having biological relatives with ADHD
4. Predicts what happens to the individual over time	The child is likely to show continued difficulties with inattention in adulthood, but improvements in impulsivity and overactivity in adulthood
5. Predicts response to treatment	The child has a good chance of responding medications, like Ritalin

know (Waldman, Lilienfeld & Lahey, 1995). Still, like many psychiatric diagnoses, ADHD is controversial. Critics have voiced concerns that ADHD is overdiagnosed and applied indiscriminately to children with mild symptoms of distractibility and restlessness that are normal for their age (LeFever, Arcona & Antonuccio, 2004). Indeed, a study of a representative sample of 2996 Australian children and adolescents found that ADHD symptoms occur on a continuum with normality, so there is no sharp distinction between those who have the disorder and those who do not (Haslam et al., 2006).

Labelling theorists
Scholars who argue that psychiatric diagnoses exert powerful negative effects on people's perceptions and behaviours.

Misconception 4: *Psychiatric diagnoses stigmatise people.* According to a group of scholars called **labelling theorists**, psychiatric diagnoses exert powerful negative effects on people's perceptions and behaviours (Scheff, 1984; Slater, 2004). Labelling theorists argue that once a psychologist or psychiatrist gives someone a diagnosis, others come to perceive that person differently. Suddenly, he or she is 'weird', 'strange', even 'crazy.' This diagnosis leads others to treat the person differently, perhaps leading him or her in turn to behave in weird, strange or even crazy ways. The diagnosis thereby becomes a self-fulfilling prophecy.

Reality. In a sensational study, David Rosenhan (1973) got eight normal individuals (himself included) to pose as fake patients in 12 psychiatric hospitals. These 'pseudopatients', as Rosenhan called them, presented themselves to the admitting psychiatrists with a single complaint: they were hearing a voice saying 'empty, hollow and thud'. In all 12 cases, the psychiatrists admitted these pseudopatients to the hospital, almost always with a diagnosis of schizophrenia (one received a diagnosis of manic depression). Remarkably, they remained there for an average of three weeks, despite displaying no further symptoms of mental illness. The diagnosis of schizophrenia, Rosenhan concluded, became a self-fulfilling prophecy, leading doctors and nursing staff to view these normal individuals as disturbed. For example, the nursing staff interpreted one pseudopatient's note-taking as 'abnormal writing behaviour'.

It is true that there is still stigma attached to some psychiatric diagnoses. If someone tells us that a person has schizophrenia, for instance, we may be wary of the individual at first or misinterpret his or her behaviour as consistent with the diagnosis. Yet the negative effects of labels last only so long. Even in Rosenhan's study, all pseudopatients were released from the hospital with diagnoses of either schizophrenia or manic depression 'in remission' ('in remission' means without any symptoms) (Spitzer, 1975). These discharge diagnoses tell us that psychiatrists eventually recognised that these individuals were behaving normally. Overall, there is little evidence that most psychiatric diagnoses themselves generate long-term negative effects (Ruscio, 2003).

Psychiatric diagnosis today: the DSM-5

The official system for classifying individuals with mental disorders is the ***Diagnostic and Statistical Manual of Mental Disorders (DSM)***, which originated in 1952 and is now in its fifth edition, called DSM-5 (APA, 2013). There are 18 different classes of disorders in the DSM-5, several of which we will be discussing in the pages to come.

Diagnostic and Statistical Manual of Mental Disorders (DSM)
Diagnostic system containing the American Psychiatric Association (APA) criteria for mental disorders.

Prevalence
Percentage of people within a population who have a specific mental disorder.

Diagnostic criteria and decision rules

The DSM-5 provides psychologists and psychiatrists with a list of diagnostic criteria for each condition, and a set of decision rules for deciding how many of these criteria need to be met. For example, to diagnose a person with major depressive disorder, DSM-5 requires the person to exhibit at least five of nine symptoms, including fatigue, insomnia, problems concentrating, and significant weight loss over a two-week period, with the requirement that the person experience either depressed mood, diminished interest or pleasure in everyday activities, or both.

'Thinking organic'

DSM-5 warns diagnosticians about physical—or 'organic' (that is, medically induced)—conditions that can simulate certain psychological disorders (Morrison, 1997). DSM-5 notes that certain substance use or medical disorders can mimic the clinical picture of depression. For example, it informs readers that hypothyroidism, a disorder marked by underactivity of the thyroid gland (in our lower necks), can produce depressive symptoms (Tallis, 2011). If a patient's depression appears due to hypothyroidism, the psychologist should not diagnose major depression. It is essential to 'think organic'—that is, to first rule out medical causes of a disorder—when diagnosing psychological conditions.

The DSM-5: other features

DSM-5 is more than a tool for diagnosing mental disorders; it is a valuable source of information concerning the characteristics, such as the prevalence, of many mental disorders. **Prevalence** refers to the percentage of people in the population with a disorder. In the case of major depression, the lifetime prevalence is at least 10 percent among women and at least 5 percent among men (some estimates are even higher). That means that for a woman, the odds are at least 1 in 10 that she will experience an episode of major depression at some point in her life; for a man, the odds are at least 1 in 20 (APA, 2013).

DSM-5 also recognises that there is more to people than their disorders. The manual adopts a biopsychosocial approach, which acknowledges the interplay of biological (e.g. hormonal abnormalities), psychological (e.g. irrational thoughts), and social (e.g. interpersonal interactions) influences. Specifically, it reminds diagnosticians to attend carefully to patients' ongoing life stressors, past and present medical conditions, and overall level of functioning when evaluating their psychological status.

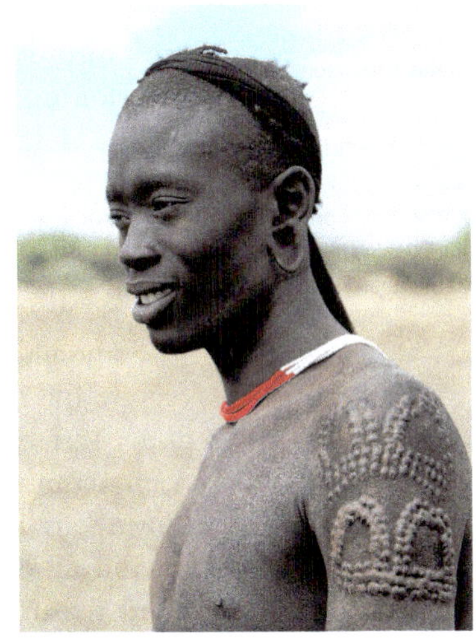
A clinical psychologist would probably perceive cutting oneself as pathological, but DSM-5 reminds clinicians that in some cultures such practices are used to produce tribal scars and should be regarded as normal.
(**Source:** John Warburton Lee/SuperStock.)

Finally, DSM-5 acknowledges that we live in a diverse world filled with people from different ethnic, socioeconomic and cultural backgrounds. Some of them embrace unconventional beliefs, sexual identities, and behaviours that are 'abnormal' from the vantage point of our contemporary Western society. DSM-5 provides information about how differing cultural backgrounds can affect the content and expression of symptoms. This information is vital to

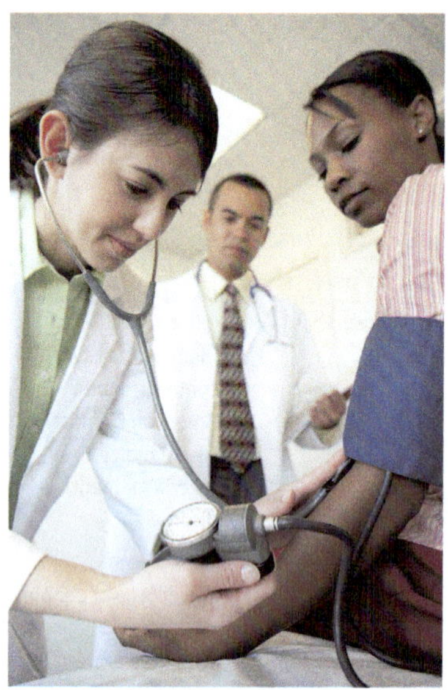

Like some psychological disorders, blood pressure better fits a dimensional than a categorical model, as there is no sharp dividing line between normal and high blood pressure. (**Source:** John Lund/Tiffany Schoepp/Getty Images.)

ensuring that diagnosticians do not incorrectly label someone from a different culture with a mental disorder merely because that person is exhibiting behaviours that those of us in Western culture might find unusual or unfamiliar.

The DSM-5: criticisms

There is little dispute that DSM-5 is a helpful system for slicing up the enormous pie of psychopathology into more meaningful and manageable pieces. Yet DSM-5 and previous versions of the manual have received more than their share of criticism—and sometimes for good reason (Frances & Widiger, 2012; Widiger & Clark, 2000).

There are more than 300 diagnoses in DSM-5, not all of which meet the Robins and Guze criteria for validity. To take only one example, the DSM-5 diagnosis of 'Mathematics Disorder' describes little more than difficulties with performing arithmetic or mathematical reasoning problems. It seems to be more of a label for learning problems than a diagnosis that tells us something new about the person. In addition, although the diagnostic criteria and decision rules for many DSM-5 disorders are based primarily on scientific findings, others are based largely on subjective committee decisions. Another problem with DSM-5 is the high level of **comorbidity** among many of its diagnoses (Angold, 1999; Cramer et al., 2010; Lilienfeld, Waldman & Israel, 1994), meaning that individuals with one diagnosis frequently have one or more additional diagnoses. For example, it is extremely common for people with a major depression diagnosis to meet criteria for one or more anxiety disorders. This extensive comorbidity raises the troubling question of whether DSM-5 is diagnosing genuinely independent conditions as opposed to slightly different variations of one underlying condition (Cramer et al., 2010).

Comorbidity
Co-occurrence of two or more diagnoses within the same person.

Categorical model
Model in which a mental disorder differs from normal functioning in kind rather than degree.

Dimensional model
Model in which a mental disorder differs from normal functioning in degree rather than kind.

Another criticism of DSM-5 is its substantial reliance on a categorical model of psychopathology (Trull & Durett, 2005). In a **categorical model**, a mental disorder—such as major depression—is either present or absent, with no in-between. Categories differ from each other in kind, not degree. Pregnancy fits a categorical model, because a woman is either pregnant or she is not. Yet scientific evidence suggests that many and perhaps most disorders in DSM-5 better fit a **dimensional model**, meaning they differ from normal functioning in degree, not kind (Haslam, Holland & Kuppens, 2012; Krueger & Piasecki, 2002). Height fits a dimensional model because, although people's heights differ, these differences are not all-or-none. The same may be true of many forms of depression and anxiety, which most research suggests lie on a continuum with normality (Kollman et al., 2006; Slade & Andrews, 2005). These findings square with our everyday experience, because we all feel at least a bit depressed and anxious from time to time.

Some authors have proposed that the Big Five, a system of personality dimensions may better capture the true 'state of nature' than many of the categories in DSM-5 (Widiger & Clark, 2000; Wright et al., 2013). For example, depression is typically characterised by high levels of neuroticism and introversion. Indeed, DSM-5 initially planned to include a system of personality dimensions similar to the Big Five in the main text of the manual (Krueger et al., 2007), but this dimensional system was eventually placed in a secondary section of the manual dedicated to future research. Indeed, many psychologists and psychiatrists have resisted a dimensional model, perhaps because they, like the rest of us, are cognitive misers; they strive to simplify the world. Most of us find it easier to think of the world in terms of simple black-or-white categories than complex shades of grey (Lilienfeld & Waldman, 2004; Macrae & Bodenhausen, 2000).

A particular concern voiced regarding DSM-5 is its tendency to 'medicalise normality'—that is, to classify relatively mild psychological disturbances as pathological (Frances & Widiger, 2012). For example, in a sharp break from previous versions of the DSM, DSM-5 now allows individuals to be diagnosed with major depressive disorder following the loss of a loved one (assuming they meet the pertinent DSM-5 criteria), including the death of a spouse. Although research may justify this change (Pies, 2012), critics worry that it will open the floodgates to diagnosing many people with relatively normal grief reactions as disordered (Wakefield & First, 2012).

Like virtually all documents crafted by human beings, DSM-5 is vulnerable to political influences (Kirk & Kutchins, 1992). For example, some researchers have lobbied successfully for the inclusion of their 'favourite' disorder or area of specialty. But like all scientific endeavours, the system of psychiatric classification tends to be self-correcting. Just as homosexuality was struck from the DSM in the 1970s, science will continue to weed out invalid disorders, ensuring that future editions of the DSM will be based on better evidence.

Factoid

People with severe mental illnesses, such as schizophrenia, are much more likely to be victims of violence than perpetrators of it (Teplin et al., 2005), probably because they often experience difficulty defending themselves against attack or avoiding dangerous situations.

Normality and abnormality: a spectrum of severity

As you read case histories or descriptions in this chapter, you may wonder 'Is my behaviour abnormal?' or 'Maybe my problems are more serious than I thought'. At times like this, it is useful to be aware of medical students' syndrome (Howes & Salkovskis, 1998). As medical students first become familiar with the symptoms of specific diseases, they often begin to focus on their bodily processes. Soon, they find it hard to stop wondering whether a slight twinge in their chest might be an early warning of heart trouble or a mild headache the first sign of a brain tumour. Similarly, as we learn about psychological disorders, it is only natural to 'see ourselves' in some patterns of behaviour, largely because in meeting the complex demands of daily life, we all experience disturbing impulses, thoughts and fears from time to time. So do not become alarmed as you learn about these conditions, as many are probably extremes of psychological difficulties we all experience on occasions.

But at some point in your life, you may experience a psychological problem that is so disturbing and persistent that you will want to talk with someone about it. If so, you will probably find it worthwhile to consult with a family member, friend, physician, school counsellor, clergy person, or mental health professional such as a psychologist or psychiatrist.

Mental illness and the law: a controversial interface

Psychological problems not only affect our mental functioning; they can also place us at risk for legal problems. There are few topics about which the general public is certain it knows more, yet actually knows less, than the interface between mental illness and the law. The issues here are as complex as they are controversial.

MENTAL ILLNESS AND VIOLENCE. One of the most pervasive myths in psychology is that mentally ill people are at greatly heightened risk for violence (Martinelli, Binney & Kaye, 2014). In fact, the overwhelming majority of people with schizophrenia and other psychotic disorders are not physically aggressive towards others (Friedman, 2006; Rueve & Welton, 2008). One might have hoped that the seemingly endless parade of 'real crime' shows on television would have helped to combat this misconception, but it has probably done the opposite. Although only a small percentage of mentally ill people commit aggressive acts (Peterson, Skeem, Kennealy, Bray & Zvonkovic, 2014), popular culture often portrays characters with mental illness as violent, perpetuating this idea throughout society.

Still, like many misconceptions, this one contains a kernel of truth. Although most mentally ill people are not at increased risk for violence, some subgroups are. According to Australian forensic psychologist Paul Mullen (2000), these include people who have poor compliance with medication and treatment, who are not engaged with treatment or are resistant to it, and who lack insight into their illness. They also include those who are convinced they are being persecuted (by the government, for example) and those with a substance abuse disorder (Douglas, Guy & Hart, 2009; Monahan, 1992; Steadman et al., 1998).

Stop and think

THE INSANITY DEFENCE: FREE WILL VERSUS DETERMINISM

In courts of law, mental illnesses and the law occasionally collide head-on, often with unpredictable consequences. The best-known example of this clash is the **mental disorder defence** (known in some countries as the **insanity defence**), which is premised on the idea that we should not hold people legally responsible for their crimes if they were not of 'sound mind' when they committed them. This defence comes in many forms in different parts of the world.

Most contemporary forms of this defence are based loosely on the *M'Naghten rule*, formulated during an 1843 British trial. This rule requires that, to be declared insane, persons must have either (1) not known what they were doing at the time of the crime or (2) not known that what they were doing was wrong (Melton et al., 1997). A defendant (accused person) who was so disoriented during an epileptic seizure that he did not even realise he was attacking a police officer might fulfil the first prong of *M'Naghten*; a defendant who believed he was actually murdering Adolf Hitler when he shot his next-door neighbour might fulfil the second. Several other versions of the defence strive to determine whether defendants were incapable of controlling their impulses at the moment of the crime. Because this judgement is exceedingly difficult (how can we know whether a man who murdered his wife in the heat of overwhelming anger *could* have controlled his temper had he really tried?), some courts ignore it.

The mental disorder defence is controversial, to put it mildly. To its proponents, this defence is necessary for defendants whose mental state is so deranged that it impairs their freedom to decide whether to commit a crime (Sadoff, 1992; Stone, 1982). To its critics, this defence is nothing more than a legal cop-out that excuses criminals of responsibility (Lykken, 1982; Szasz, 1991). These divergent perspectives reflect a more deep-seated disagreement about free will versus determinism. The legal system assumes that our actions are freely chosen, whereas scientific psychology assumes that our actions are completely determined by prior variables, including our genetic make-up and learning history. So, lawyers and judges tend to view the defence as a necessary exception for the small minority of defendants who lack free will. In contrast, many psychologists view this defence as illogical, because they see all crimes, including those committed by people with severe mental disorders, as equally 'determined'.

There are numerous misconceptions regarding the mental disorder defence (see Table 5.3). For example, although most people believe that a sizeable proportion, perhaps 15–20 percent, of criminals are acquitted (found innocent) on the basis of the verdict, the actual percentage is less than 1 percent in the United States (Silver, Cirincione & Steadman, 1994). This erroneous belief probably stems from the *availability heuristic*. Because we hear a great deal about a few widely publicised cases of defendants acquitted on the grounds of mental disorder, we overestimate this verdict's prevalence (Butler, 2006). A better appreciation of the facts surrounding the insanity defence may help to dispel unwarranted public views regarding its use.

Table 5.3 Popular misconceptions regarding the mental disorder (or insanity) defence

Myth	Reality
Insanity is a psychological or psychiatric term.	*Insanity* is a purely legal term that refers only to whether the person was responsible for the crime, not to the nature of his or her psychiatric disorder.
The determination of mental disorder rests on a careful evaluation of the person's current mental state.	The determination of mental disorder rests on a determination of the person's mental state at the time of the crime.
A large proportion of criminals escape criminal responsibility by using the mental disorder defence.	The mental disorder defence is raised in only about 1 percent of criminal trials and is successful only about 25% of the time.
Most people acquitted on the basis of a mental disorder defence quickly go free.	The average mental disorder acquittee spends close to three years in a psychiatric hospital, often longer than the length of a criminal sentence for the same crime.
Mental disorder defences are complicated and frequently fool juries as a result.	Most successful mental disorder verdicts are delivered by judges, not juries.
Most people who use the mental disorder defence are faking mental illness.	The rate of faking mental illness among mental disorder defendants appears to be low.

(*Sources:* Butler, 2006; McCutcheon & McCutcheon, 1994; Pasewark & Pantle, 1979; Phillips, Wolf & Coons, 1994; Silver, Cirincione & Steadman, 1994.)

INVOLUNTARY COMMITMENT. We are all familiar with *criminal commitment*, which is just a fancy term for putting someone in jail. Yet society possesses another mechanism for committing individuals against their will. Known as **involuntary commitment**, it is a procedure for protecting society from certain mentally ill people, and certain mentally ill people from themselves. In Australia, mentally ill individuals can be committed against their will only if they are unable to consent to treatment because of their illness, they pose a serious threat to their own or others' health, safety or property, and no less restrictive treatment can be provided. Psychiatrists can recommend involuntary commitment and detain a person in a psychiatric institution temporarily without prior review by a judge.

Involuntary commitment Procedure of placing some mentally ill people in a psychiatric hospital or other facility based on their potential danger to themselves or others, or their inability to care for themselves.

Involuntary commitment raises difficult ethical questions. Advocates of this procedure contend that the government has the right to assume the role of 'parent' over mentally ill individuals who are dangerous and do not possess sufficient insight to appreciate the impact of their actions (Chodoff, 1976; Satel, 1999). In contrast, critics argue that by involuntarily institutionalising people who have not committed any crimes, the government is depriving them of their civil liberties (Schaler, 2004; Szasz, 1978). Critics of involuntary commitment also point out that mental health professionals often do a poor job of forecasting the risk that people will harm themselves or others (Monahan, 1992) and may be biased by the person's race or gender (Garb, 1998). Still, studies show that mental health professionals can predict violence at better-than-chance levels, especially when patients have very recently engaged in, or are immediately threatening, violence (Kramer, Wolbransky & Heilbrun, 2007; Lidz, Mulvey & Gardner, 1993; Monahan et al., 2000).

Assess your knowledge — FACT or FICTION?

1. According to a family resemblance view, no single criterion distinguishes mental disorder from normality. (True/False)
2. Once the medical model began to take hold in the Renaissance, treatments for mental disorders came to be based on strong scientific evidence. (True/False)
3. Almost all deinstitutionalised patients return successfully to their families and communities. (True/False)
4. Some mental disorders appear to be present in most, if not all, cultures. (True/False)
5. Virtually all psychiatric diagnoses are unreliable. (True/False)
6. Most severely mentally ill individuals are not prone to violence. (True/False)

Answers: (1) T; (2) F; (3) F; (4) T; (5) F; (6) T

Anxiety disorders: the many faces of worry and fear

We begin our discussion of psychological disorders with problems stemming from anxiety. Fortunately, most everyday anxieties generally do not last long or feel especially uncomfortable. Anxiety in small doses can even be adaptive. It can permit a lightning-quick response to danger, steer us away from harmful behaviour and inspire us to solve festering problems. Yet sometimes anxiety spirals out of control, and it can become excessive and inappropriate. It may even feel life-threatening (Mendelowicz & Stein, 2000).

Anxiety disorders are among the most prevalent of all mental disorders; a survey of 8841 Australians showed that 14.4 percent had met diagnostic criteria for one or more anxiety disorders within the past year, but only about one-third of these sufferers sought treatment (Slade et al., 2009). The average age of onset for anxiety disorders (11 years) is much earlier

Table 5.4 Lifetime prevalence of mental disorders in Australia (percentage)

Panic disorder	5.2	Dysthymia	1.9
Agoraphobia	6.0	Bipolar I-II disorder	2.9
Social anxiety disorder	10.6	Any mood disorder	15.0
Generalised anxiety disorder	5.9	Alcohol abuse	18.9
Obsessive-compulsive disorder	2.8	Alcohol dependence	3.8
Posttraumatic stress disorder	12.2	Drug use disorders	7.5
Any anxiety disorder	26.3	Any substance use disorder	24.7
Depressive episode	11.6	Any mental disorder	45.5

(**Source:** Australian Bureau of Statistics, 2007.)

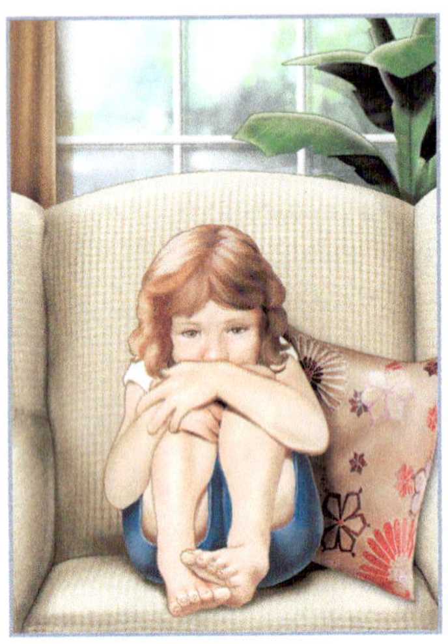

Many anxiety disorders, including phobias, frequently have an initial onset in childhood.

than for most other disorders, including substance use disorders (20 years) and mood disorders (30 years; Kessler et al., 2005). Table 5.4 displays the lifetime prevalence of anxiety disorders, along with many other disorders we consider in this chapter.

Yet anxiety is not limited to anxiety disorders. Anxiety can seep into numerous aspects of our functioning, including concerns regarding our physical health. In a controversial condition called **somatic symptom disorder**, new to DSM-5, anxieties about physical symptoms—that are either medically verified or purely psychological in origin—can become so intense and 'over the top' that they interfere with daily living. In cases of illness anxiety disorder (another new diagnosis that is similar to what was previously called **hypochondriasis**), people become so preoccupied with the idea that they are suffering from a serious undiagnosed illness that no amount of reassurance can relieve their anxiety. Much like radar operators who stay on their toes for signs of incoming planes, people with illness anxiety disorder seem continually on the alert for signs of physical illness, constantly checking the internet, for example, for information about symptoms and signs of diseases. Despite repeated medical reassurance and physical examinations they may insist that their mild aches, pains and twinges are signs of serious diseases such as cancer, AIDS or heart disease.

Somatic symptom disorders
Conditions marked by physical symptoms that suggest an underlying medical illness, but that are actually psychological in origin.

Hypochondriasis
An individual's continual preoccupation with the notion that he or she is suffering from a serious physical disease.

Generalised anxiety disorder (GAD)
Continual feelings of worry, anxiety, physical tension and irritability across many areas of life functioning.

Generalised anxiety disorder: perpetual worry

We all get caught up with worry from time to time. Yet for the 3 percent of us who have **generalised anxiety disorder (GAD)**, worry is a way of life. People with GAD spend an average of 60 percent of each day worrying, compared with 18 percent for the rest of the general population (Craske et al., 1989). Many describe themselves as 'worry warts'. They tend to think anxious thoughts, feel irritable and on edge, have trouble sleeping, and experience considerable bodily tension and fatigue (Andrews et al., 2010; Barlow, Chorpita & Turovsky, 1996). Often they worry too much about the small things in life, like an upcoming meeting at work or a social event. One-third of those with GAD develop it following a major stressful event—such as a wedding, an illness, physical abuse, the death of a relative—or as the result of lifestyle changes, such as completing school and embarking on a career (Mellinger & Lynn, 2003; Hazlett-Stevens, Pruitt & Collins, 2008). People with GAD are more likely to be female than male—as is the case with most anxiety disorders—as well as middle-aged, widowed or divorced, poor, and prone to 'self-medication' with alcohol and drugs to relieve symptoms (Grant et al., 2005; Noyes, 2001).

Asians, Hispanics and African Americans are at relatively low risk for GAD (Grant et al., 2005). GAD may be the core anxiety disorder out of which all others develop (Barlow, 2002). Indeed, people with GAD often experience other anxiety disorders, including phobias and panic disorder, which we consider next.

Panic attacks Brief, intense episodes of extreme fear characterised by sweating, dizziness, light-headedness, racing heartbeat and feelings of impending death or going crazy.

Panic disorder Repeated and unexpected panic attacks, along with either persistent concerns about future attacks or a change in personal behaviour in an attempt to avoid them.

Panic disorder: terror that comes out of the blue

The Greek god Pan was a mischievous spirit who popped out of the bushes to scare the living daylights out of travellers. Pan lent his name to **panic attacks**, which occur when nervous feelings gather momentum and escalate into intense bouts of fear, even terror. Panic attacks can occur only rarely, or they can occur on a daily basis for weeks, months or even years at a time. People are diagnosed with **panic disorder** when they experience panic attacks that are repeated and unexpected, and when they either experience persistent concerns about panicking or change their behaviour to avoid future attacks (for example, change jobs) (APA, 2013). Panic attacks typically peak within 10 minutes and can include sweating, dizziness, light-headedness, a racing or pounding heart, shortness of breath, feelings of unreality, and fears of going crazy or dying (Craske et al., 2010). Because many patients experiencing their initial panic attack believe they are having a heart attack, many first go to the emergency room, only to be sent home and—like Ida, whom we met at the outset of the chapter—told 'it's all in your head'. Some panic attacks are associated with specific situations, such as riding in elevators or shopping in supermarkets, whereas others come entirely out of the blue—that is, without warning—often generating fears of the situations in which they occur.

The term *panic* stems from the name of Pan, the Greek god of shepherds and flocks, who frightened travellers. **(Source:** Danilo Ascione/ Dreamstime.)

First-person account:

PANIC DISORDER

'For me, a panic attack is almost a violent experience. I feel disconnected from reality. I feel like I'm losing control in a very extreme way. My heart pounds really hard, I feel like I can't get my breath, and there's an overwhelming feeling that things are crashing in on me.' *(Dickey, 1994)*

Panic attacks can occur in every anxiety disorder, as well as in mood and eating disorders. Even high-functioning people can experience panic attacks in anticipation of stressful events (Cox & Taylor, 1998): about 20–25 percent of university students report at least one panic attack in a one-year period, with about half that number reporting unexpected attacks (Lilienfeld, 1997). Panic disorder often develops in early adulthood (Kessler et al., 2007) and is associated with a history of fears of separation from a parent during childhood (Lewinsohn et al., 2008). It is unclear, though, whether this correlation means that separation fears predispose to later panic disorder, or whether such fears are merely an early reflection of the same underlying condition that gives rise to panic disorder.

Phobia Intense fear of an object or a situation that is greatly out of proportion to its actual threat..

Phobias: irrational fears

A **phobia** is an intense fear of an object or a situation that is greatly out of proportion to its actual threat. Many of us have mild fears—of things such as spiders and snakes—that are not severe enough to be phobias. For a fear to be diagnosed as a phobia, it must restrict our life, create considerable distress, or do both.

Phobias are the most common of all anxiety disorders. One in nine people has a phobia of an animal, blood or injury, or a situation such as a thunderstorm. Social fears are just as common (Kessler et al., 1994). Agoraphobia, which we examine next, is the most debilitating of the phobias and occurs in about 1 in 20 (Magee et al., 1996) (see Figure 5.2).

Agoraphobia

Agoraphobia
Fear of being in a place or situation from which escape is difficult or embarrassing, or in which help is unavailable in the event of a panic attack

Some 2700 years ago, in the city-states of ancient Greece, agoraphobia acquired its name as a condition in which certain fearful citizens could not pass through the central city's open-air markets (agoras). A common misconception is that agoraphobia is a fear of crowds or public places. But **agoraphobia** actually refers to a fear of being in a place or situation in which escape is difficult or embarrassing, or in which help is unavailable in the event of a panic attack (APA, 2013).

Agoraphobia typically emerges in the mid-teens and is often a direct outgrowth of panic disorder. In fact, most people with panic disorder develop agoraphobia (Cox & Taylor, 1998; Sanderson & Dublin, 2010) and become apprehensive in a host of settings, such as shopping centres, crowded movie theatres, tunnels, bridges or wide-open spaces. The manifestation of agoraphobia seems to differ across cultures. For example, some Inuit in Greenland suffer from a condition called 'kayak angst', marked by a pronounced fear of going out to sea alone in a kayak (Barlow, 2000; Gusow, 1963).

In rare cases, agoraphobia reaches extreme proportions. Two clinicians saw a 62-year-old woman with agoraphobia who had not left her house—even once—for 25 years (Jensvold &

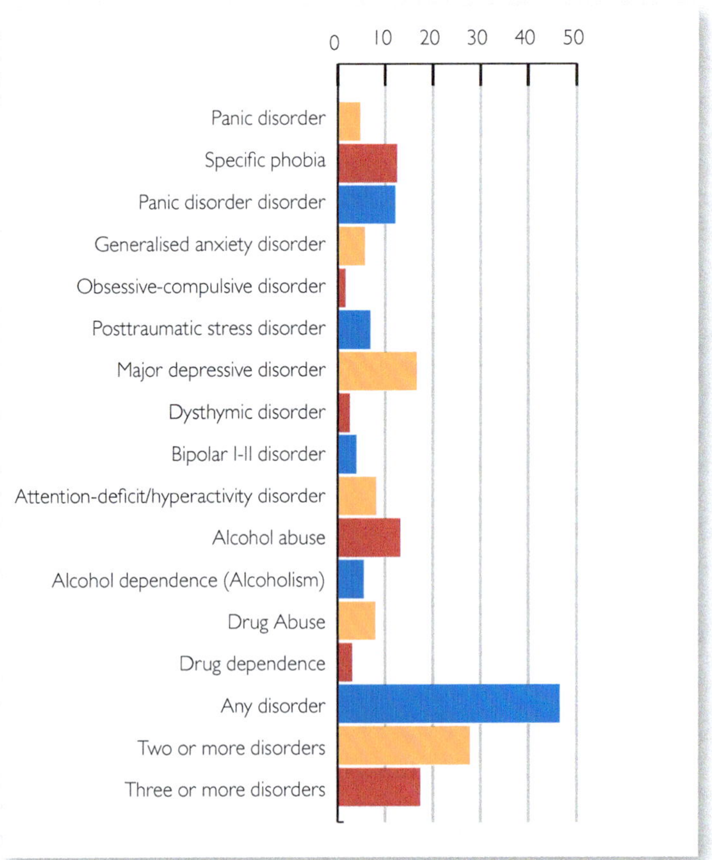

Figure 5.2 Lifetime prevalence estimates of disorders (in percent).
(**Source:** Based on data from Merikangas et al., 2007; Kessler et al., 2005.)

Turner, 1988). Having experienced severe panic attacks and terrified by the prospect of still more, she spent almost all of her waking hours locked away in her bedroom, with curtains drawn. The therapists attempted to treat her agoraphobia by encouraging her to take short trips out of her house, but she repeatedly refused to walk even a few steps past her front door. Nevertheless, cases of agoraphobia and other anxiety disorders are quite treatable.

Specific phobia
Intense fear of objects, places or situations that is greatly out of proportion to their actual threat.

Social anxiety disorder
Intense fear of negative evaluation in social situations.

Posttraumatic stress disorder (PTSD)
Marked emotional disturbance after experiencing or witnessing a severely stressful event.

Specific phobia and social anxiety disorder

Phobias of objects, places or situations—called **specific phobias**—commonly arise in response to animals, insects, thunderstorms, water, elevators and darkness. Many of these fears, especially of animals, are widespread in childhood but disappear with age (APA, 2013). Some of the most common fears involve insects and animals such as spiders and snakes.

SOCIAL ANXIETY DISORDER. Surveys show that most people rank public speaking as a greater fear than dying (Wallechinsky, Wallace & Wallace, 1977). Given that statistic, imagine how people with **social anxiety disorder**—formerly called 'social phobia' in DSM-IV—must feel. They experience an intense fear of negative evaluation in social situations, such as while eating, giving a speech, conversing with others, and performing in public. Their social fears can even extend to swimming, swallowing and signing their checks in the presence of others (Mellinger & Lynn, 2003). Their anxiety goes well beyond the stage fright that most of us feel occasionally (Heimberg & Juster, 1995).

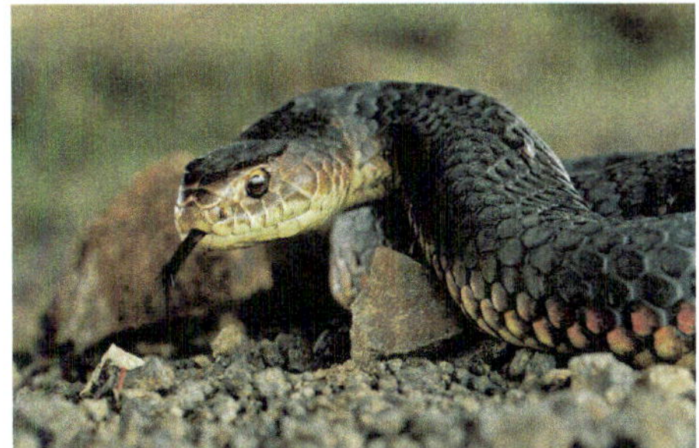

Some of the most common fears involve creatures, such as spiders and snakes.
(**Source:** Robert Gubiani/Dreamstime.)

Posttraumatic stress disorder: the enduring effects of experiencing horror

One of the most significant changes in DSM-5 is that posttraumatic stress disorder and obsessive-compulsive disorders, which were formerly included in the category of anxiety disorders, are now positioned in their own separate diagnostic categories. Yet because both disorders are associated with significant anxiety, we consider them under the heading of anxiety-related disorders.

When people experience or witness a traumatic event, such as front-line combat, an earthquake or sexual assault, they may develop **posttraumatic stress disorder (PTSD)**. In DSM-5, PTSD is in a new class of 'trauma and stressor-related disorders' in which the definition of a traumatic event is broad. It includes direct exposure to a traumatic event, such as a rape, wartime combat, or a natural disaster. Nevertheless, it also includes situations in which people learn about an event from a friend or relative who experienced threatened or actual death or in which people are exposed repeatedly to distressing details of a traumatic event, such as the sexual abuse of an elderly person.

Flashbacks are among the hallmarks of PTSD. The terror of war can return decades after the original trauma and be reactivated by everyday stressful experiences (Foa & Kozak, 1986). In recounting his war experiences, Vietnam veteran Tim O'Brien (1990) commented: 'The hardest part, by far, is to make the bad pictures go away. In war time, the world is

First-person account:

SOCIAL ANXIETY DISORDER

'When I would walk into a room full of people, I'd turn red and it would feel like everybody's eyes were on me. I was embarrassed to stand off in a corner by myself but I couldn't think of anything to say to anybody. It was humiliating. I felt so clumsy, I couldn't wait to get out.' (Dickey, 1994)

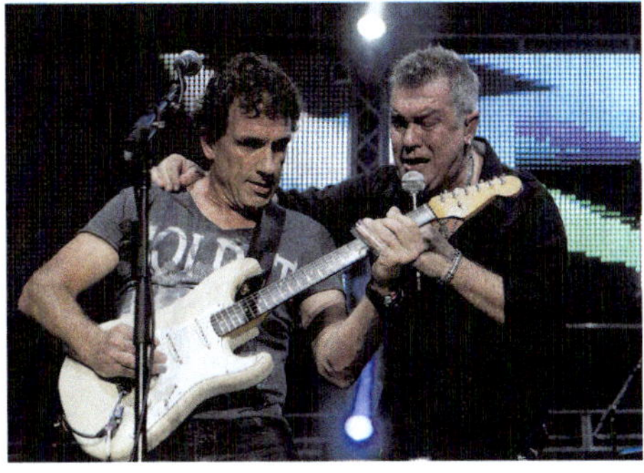

Australian band Cold Chisel's famous song 'Khe Sanh', about a Vietnam veteran, captures some of the symptoms of PTSD beautifully: '... car parks made me jumpy, and I never stopped the dreams, or the growing need for speed and novocaine.'
(**Source:** Robert Cianflone/Getty Images.)

Obsessive-compulsive disorder (OCD) Condition marked by repeated and lengthy (at least one hour per day) immersion in obsessions or compulsions, or both.

Obsessions Persistent ideas, thoughts or impulses that are unwanted and inappropriate, causing marked distress.

one big long horror movie, image after image, and if it's anything like Vietnam, I'm in for a lifetime of wee-hour creeps' (p. 56).

Other symptoms include: efforts to avoid thoughts, feelings, places, objects and conversations that remind the person of the event; recurrent dreams of the trauma; and increased arousal reflected in difficulty sleeping and startling easily (APA, 2013). Reminders of the incident can trigger full-blown panic attacks, as in the case of a Vietnam veteran who hid under his bed whenever he heard a city helicopter in the distance—more than 20 years since the end of the war (Baum, Cohen & Hall, 1993; Foa & Rothbaum, 1998; Jones & Barlow, 1990). PTSD isn't easy to diagnose. Some of its symptoms, such as anxiety and difficulty sleeping, may have been present before the stressful event and commonly occur in other disorders. Moreover, some people malinger (fake) PTSD to obtain government benefits, so diagnosticians must rule out this possibility (Rosen, 2006).

Factoid

Have you ever been unable to get a tune or a snatch of a tune out of your head? Psychologists have a term for this phenomenon: it is called an 'earworm'. A recent study revealed that 98 percent of students have experienced earworms.

First-person account:

OBSESSIVE-COMPULSIVE DISORDER

'I couldn't do anything without rituals. They transcended every aspect of my life. Counting was big for me. When I set my alarm at night, I had to set it to a number that wouldn't add up to a "bad" number. I would wash my hair three times as opposed to once because three was a good luck number and one wasn't. It took me longer to read because I'd count the lines in a paragraph. If I was writing a term paper, I couldn't have a certain number of words on a line if it added up to a bad number. I was always worried that if I didn't do something, my parents were going to die.' (Dickey, 1994)

Obsessive-compulsive and related disorders: trapped in one's thoughts and behaviours

The hallmarks of obsessive-compulsive and related disorders are repetitive and distressing thoughts and behaviours (Hollander et al., 2011). The most common of these disorders are obsessive-compulsive disorder, body dysmorphic disorder, and Tourette's Disorder. Just about all of us have had a thought or even a silly jingle that we just could not get out of our head. Patients with **obsessive-compulsive disorder (OCD)** know all too well what this experience is like, except that their symptoms are more severe. They typically suffer from **obsessions**: persistent ideas, thoughts or urges that are unwanted and inappropriate and cause marked distress. Unlike typical worries, obsessions are not extreme responses to everyday stressors. They usually centre on 'unacceptable' thoughts about such topics as contamination, sex, aggression or religion (Franklin & Foa, 2008). For example, individuals with OCD may be consumed with fears of being dirty or thoughts of killing others. Unlike ordinary worriers, people with OCD typically are disturbed by their thoughts and usually see them as irrational or nonsensical (Fullana et al., 2009). They may even label themselves 'crazy' or dangerous. Despite their best efforts, people with OCD cannot find a way to make these thoughts stop.

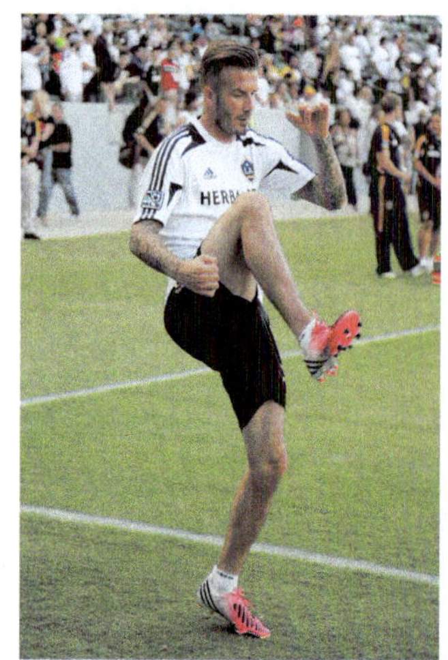

David Beckham, the famous British soccer player, has reported that he feels compelled to count his clothes and cans of cola and to arrange magazines in straight lines (Dolan, 2006).
(**Source:** Allstar Picture Library/Alamy.)

Most OCD patients also experience symptoms linked closely to obsessions, namely **compulsions**: repetitive behaviours or mental acts that they initiate to reduce or prevent distress. In most cases, patients feel driven to perform the action that accompanies an obsession to prevent some dreaded event or 'make things right'. Common OCD-type rituals include:

- repeatedly checking door locks, windows, electronic controls and ovens
- performing tasks in set ways, like putting on shoes in a fixed pattern
- counting the number of dots on a wall or touching or tapping objects
- repeatedly arranging and rearranging objects
- washing and cleaning repeatedly and unnecessarily

- saying a prayer or specific phrase every time an obsession comes to mind
- hoarding newspapers, books, letters, soft-drink cans or other objects.

Individuals with OCD spend an hour or more a day immersed in obsessions, compulsions, or both; one patient spent 15–18 hours per day washing his hands, showering, getting dressed, and cleaning money. Still, many individuals with OCD lead remarkably successful lives. Several celebrities have spoken publicly about their struggles with the disorder. For example, Cameron Diaz avoids touching doorknobs by opening doors with her elbows, Leonardo DiCaprio sidestepped cracks in sidewalks as a child, and Megan Fox is fearful of using restaurant silverware because of concerns about contamination with bacteria (Fisher, Marikar & Shaw, 2013).

Compulsions repetitive behaviours or mental acts performed to reduce or prevent stress.

People with the related condition of body dysmorphic disorder (BDD) become preoccupied with imagined or slight defects in their appearance, such as lips that are perceived to be 'too thin' or ears that are 'too big'. One patient with BDD treated by one of your book's authors was so preoccupied with tiny moles on his forehead that he spent hours every day thinking about them, checking mirrors, and wearing hats in an attempt to cover them up. One-third of patients with BDD also suffer from OCD (Phillips et al., 2005). Some individuals with BDD undergo repeated cosmetic surgeries to correct their perceived body imperfections, yet they receive little comfort from these procedures because their underlying obsession about their appearance remains untreated. Celebrities may be particularly prone to body dysmorphic disorder because our culture places a high premium on physical attractiveness; Michael Jackson and Heidi Montag underwent numerous cosmetic surgeries and may have exhibited features of this condition.

Tourette's Disorder is a condition marked by repeated automatic behaviours—motor tics such as twitching and facial grimacing, and vocal tics such as grunting and throat clearing. A common myth about the disorder is that most individuals with Tourette's Disorder engage in frequent cursing, a symptom known as coprolalia. However, 70 percent or more of patients with Tourette's Disorder do not curse (Goldenberg, Brown & Weiner, 2004).

Factoid

Following birth, perhaps as many as 2–3 percent of new mothers experience a condition called postpartum obsessive-compulsive disorder. In some cases, the infant becomes the focus of the mother's bizarre thoughts and compulsive behaviours. These symptoms can include compulsions: excessively checking the child to ensure his or her safety and hiding knives for fear of stabbing the child, as well as obsessions: picturing the child dying in their sleep (Speisman, Storch & Abramowitz, 2011). Some mothers become so fearful of what they might do to their children that they avoiding taking care of their baby (Durães, Martins, Borralho & Paiva, 2015). Fortunately, such women almost never harm their children, and effective treatments are available.

from inquiry to understanding

MORE THAN A PACK RAT: WHY DO PEOPLE HOARD?

Mark is an art dealer, and he is also a hoarder. Financially well-off, he built an add-on room to his home to store his clutter. From floor to ceiling, the room is filled with books, catalogues, newspapers and comic books, with a tiny footpath (often called a 'goat path') cleared to enter and exit. In the past six months, the clutter has spilled over into his living room, dining room and bedroom. The mere thought of which items to discard paralyses him with indecision and intense anxiety. He dares not invite a woman he recently met on the art circuit to his home for fear she would be turned off by the mess. His bed is so covered with 'stuff' that he has slept in a hotel for the past week. Instead of doing a major clean-up, he approached a realtor about buying a second home so that he could 'store his stuff' in his current home and 'start fresh'.

Mark is a composite of several patients treated by one of your authors. Mark's hoarding behaviour meets all of the DSM-5 criteria for the new disorder of hoarding, which is distinct from its close cousin, OCD. Hoarders often experience a strong urge to acquire possessions, often with little or no actual value, and become convinced that they cannot part with them. Some hoarders harbour large numbers of animals, such as cats and dogs, which they are unable to care for. Compulsive buying or collecting free items can severely limit liveable space and pose a serious fire hazard.

Hoarding disorder and OCD differ in key respects. Only a minority of hoarders— probably less than 20 percent—meet diagnostic criteria for OCD (Frost et al., 2006). Moreover, hoarders do not perform rituals related to their possessions, and typically become anxious only when they encounter a situation in which they feel pressured to discard items they have accumulated. In addition, many hoarders have limited insight and rarely acknowledge that they have a problem unless they are confronted by family members, friends or employers, or, like Mark, become concerned about how others view them (Pertusa et al., 2010).

Hoarding is a curious combination of impulsiveness, reflected in the urge to accumulate, compulsive acquisition of possessions, and anxiety-related avoidance of parting with what is hoarded. Hoarding is associated with indecisiveness, leading hoarders to question whether they might need the item in the future, whether it is valuable, or whether they will regret throwing it away for sentimental reasons (Frost & Gross, 1993).

Researchers are still not sure why people hoard. Brain imaging studies reveal that hoarders show impairments in brain circuits associated with judgement, decision-making and emotional regulation (Pertusa et al., 2010). In addition, research on animal models suggests that some primates, including monkeys and apes, as well some rodents, including rats, engage in hoarding behaviours, and that such behaviours may be associated with similar brain abnormalities as in humans (Andrews-McClymont, Lilienfeld & Duke, 2013). Perhaps hoarding is a case of a basically adaptive behaviour gone terribly awry. In some cases, it makes perfect sense to store up food and possessions, especially when they are important for our survival and we are running short of them. But when this drive becomes rigid and overpowering, pathological hoarding may result.

Nearly 30 percent of individuals with OCD suffer from a tic disorder (Richter et al., 2003). Some researchers suggest that OCD and Tourette's Disorder share biological roots (Mell, Davis & Owens, 2005). A number of children develop OCD or Tourette's Disorder after experiencing strep throat or scarlet fever infections caused by streptococcal (strep) bacteria. Scientists are seeking to determine whether strep triggers an immune system response that affects the brain and brings about OCD symptoms, or whether the relationship between strep and OCD symptoms is coincidental (Gause et al., 2009; Kurlan & Kaplan, 2004; Nicholson et al., 2012). Another possibility is that children with strep feel irritable and uncomfortable, which worsens OCD symptoms.

The roots of pathological anxiety, fear, and repetitive thoughts and behaviours

How do anxiety disorders arise? Different theories propose explanations that focus on the environment, catastrophic thinking and biological influences.

Learning models of anxiety: anxious responses as acquired habits

According to learning theories, fears are—you guessed it—learned. Watson and Rayner's (1920) famous demonstration of classical conditioning of fearing a small furry animal (remember poor Little Albert from Chapter 1?) powerfully conveys how people learn fears.

Operant conditioning, which relies on reinforcements and punishments offers another account of how fears are maintained. If a socially awkward girl repeatedly experiences rejection when she asks boys to go to the movies, she may become shy around them. If this pattern of rejection continues, she could develop full-blown social anxiety disorder. Paradoxically, her avoidance of boys provides negative reinforcement, because it allows her to escape the unpleasant consequences of social interaction. This sense of relief perpetuates her avoidance, and ultimately her anxiety.

Learning theorists (Rachman, 1977) believe that fears can arise in two additional ways. First, we can acquire fears by observing others engaging in fearful behaviours (Mineka &

Cook, 1993). A father's fear of dogs might instil the same fear in his child. Secondly, fears can stem from information or misinformation from others. For example, if a mother tells her children that riding in elevators is dangerous, they may end up taking the stairs. In a study by Australian psychologists Paula Barrett, Ron Rapee, Mark Dadds and Sharon Ryan (1996), anxious children avoided threatening stimuli more after talking about them with a parent.

Table 5.5 Anxiety and interpretation of ambiguity

Selected Homophones	
Threatening meaning/spelling	**Non-threatening meaning/spelling**
Bury	Berry
Die	Dye
Patients	Patience
Bruise	Brews
Flu	Flew
Sword	Soared
Bore	Boar

Anxiety leads us to interpret ambiguous stimuli negatively. Researchers have asked anxious and non-anxious participants to listen to *homophones*—words that sound the same but have two different meanings and spellings—and to write down the word they heard. In these studies, they have used homophone pairs in which one meaning (and spelling) is threatening and the other is non-threatening. Compared with non-anxious subjects, anxious participants are more likely to write down the version of the homophone that is threatening, such as 'bury' as opposed to 'berry' (Blanchette & Richards, 2003; Mathews, Richards & Eysenck, 1989).

Catastrophising and anxiety sensitivity

People with social anxiety disorder predict that many social encounters will be interpersonal disasters, and some people with fears of storms are so fearful that they seek the shelter of a basement when mild thunderstorms are detected on radar 50 kilometres away (Voncken, Bogels & deVries, 2003). As these examples illustrate, catastrophising is a core feature of anxious thinking (Beck, 1976; Ellis, 1962; Ellis & Dryden, 1997). People catastrophise when they predict terrible events—such as contracting a life-threatening illness from touching a doorknob—despite their low probability (A. T. Beck, 1964; Beck, 1995).

As Australian psychologists Colin MacLeod and Ron Rapee have amply demonstrated (for example, Matthews & MacLeod, 2005; Rapee & Heimberg, 1997), anxious people have distinctive ways of processing information. Their attention is biased towards potential threats, and they tend to interpret ambiguous situations in a negative light (see Table 5.5). Many people with anxiety disorders harbour high levels of **anxiety sensitivity**, a fear of anxiety-related sensations (Reiss & McNally, 1985; Stein, Jang & Livesley, 1999). Think of the times your muscles felt tight, you felt a bit dizzy when you stood up quickly or your heart raced after climbing a flight of stairs. You may have dismissed these physical symptoms as harmless. Yet people with high anxiety sensitivity tend to misinterpret them as dangerous—perhaps as early signs of a heart attack or stroke—and react with intense worry (Clark, 1986; Lilienfeld, 1997; McNally & Eke, 1996). As a result, their barely noticeable physical sensations or minor anxiety can spiral into full-blown panic attacks. One patient repeatedly misinterpreted muscular tension in her neck—a normal symptom of anxiety—as evidence that her head would explode, and a panic attack would reliably follow.

Anxiety sensitivity
Fear of anxiety-related sensations.

Anxiety: genetic and biological influences

Numerous twin studies show that many anxiety disorders, including panic disorder, phobias, PTSD and OCD, are genetically influenced (Afifi et al., 2010; Roy et al., 1995; Samuels et al., 2011; Van Grootheest et al., 2007). In particular, genes affect whether we inherit high levels of neuroticism—a tendency to be highly strung and irritable which can set the stage for excessive worry (Anderson, Taylor & McLean, 1996; Zinbarg & Barlow, 1996). On a genetic basis, people who experience GAD are virtually indistinguishable from those who experience major depression, which also is associated with high levels of neuroticism (Kendler & Karkowski-Shuman, 1997). This finding suggests a shared genetic pathway for these disorders.

Studies that have attempted to identify a single gene associated with OCD have provided mixed results at best, although evidence is accumulating that genes that transport serotonin and glutamate probably play some role in the development of OCD (Samuels et al., 2011). Much like a car that is stuck in gear, obsessive people experience problems with shifting thoughts and behaviours (Schwartz & Bayette, 1996). Brain scans also reveal increased activity in portions of the frontal lobes where information is filtered, prioritised and organised. Under these circumstances, people cannot seem to get troubling thoughts out of their minds or inhibit repeated rituals.

Assess your knowledge — FACT or FICTION?

1. Panic attacks typically peak in 10 minutes or less. **(True/False)**
2. According to some theorists, GAD is the core anxiety disorder out of which others develop. **(True/False)**
3. Because PTSD is characterised by dramatic symptoms, it is typically an easy disorder to diagnose. **(True/False)**
4. Catastrophising is a core feature of anxious thinking. **(True/False)**
5. Genes exert little influence on obsessive-compulsive disorder. **(True/False)**

Answers: (1) T; (2) T; (3) F; (4) T; (5) F

Mood disorders and suicide

Imagine you are interviewing someone who has come to you for help. As the client begins to talk about his life, it becomes clear that even the simplest activities, like dressing or driving to work, have become enormous acts of will. He reports difficulty sleeping and unaccountably wakes up before dawn each day. He refuses to answer the telephone, and lies listlessly for hours staring at the television. His mood is downcast, and occasionally tears well up in his eyes. He has recently lost a fair amount of weight. His world is grey, a void. Towards the end of the interview, he tells you he has begun to contemplate suicide.

Major depressive episode
State in which a person experiences a lingering depressed mood or diminished interest in pleasurable activities, along with symptoms that include weight loss and sleep difficulties.

You have just interviewed a person who suffers from a *mood disorder*, so-called because his difficulties centre on his bleak mood, which colours all aspects of his existence. His symptoms meet the criteria for a **major depressive episode**, a key feature of major depressive disorder, which we encountered earlier in our discussion of psychiatric diagnosis. We will soon discuss another mood disorder, *bipolar disorder*, in which people's mood is often the mirror image of depression. We focus on these two disorders because they represent the extremes of a spectrum of mood disorders, ranging from major depressive disorder on one end to bipolar disorder on the other (Angst et al., 2010).

Major depressive disorder: common, but not the common cold

Over the course of their lifetime, about 20 percent of Australians will experience a mood disorder. Due to its frequency, some have called depression the 'common cold' of psychological disorders (Seligman, 1975). Yet this description does not begin to capture the profound depths of suffering that people with this condition experience. Depressive disorders can begin at any age, but are most likely to strike people in their thirties. Contrary to popular misconception, they are less common in elderly adults than in younger people (Klerman, 1986).

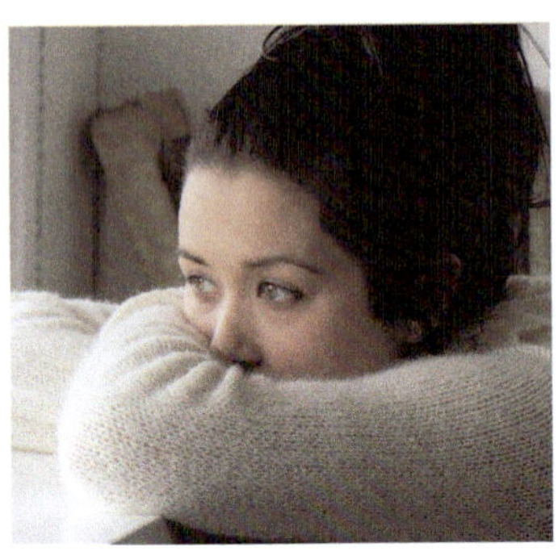

In most cultures, women are generally at greater risk for developing depression than men. The reasons for this difference are not fully understood.
(Source: Rosanne Olson/Digital Vision/Getty Images.)

Women are about twice as likely to be depressed as men. This gender difference may be associated with women's tendency to ruminate more than men (Nolen-Hoeksema, 2002; 2003). Yet it may also be associated with differences between men and women in economic power, sex hormones, social support and history of physical or sexual abuse (Howland & Thase, 1998). The sex difference in depression is widespread but not universal. In some cultures, such as certain Mediterranean populations, Orthodox Jews and the Amish, this sex difference is largely absent (Piccinelli & Wilkinson, 2000), but researchers do not know why. One possibility is that the differences in the rates of depression across genders in Western cultures reflect an under-diagnosis of depression in men. Australian research indicates that women are more willing to seek help for mental health problems and use psychological services than men, who are socialised to be stoical and believe that admitting to psychological problems is shameful (Judd, Komiti & Jackson, 2008).

The symptoms of depression may develop gradually over days or weeks; in other cases, they may surface rather suddenly. Depression, like the common cold, is recurrent. The average person with major depression experiences five or six episodes over the course of their lifetime. Most of these episodes last from six months to a year. However, in as many as a quarter or more of cases, depression is persistent and can be present for as long as decades with no relief (Murphy & Byrne, 2012; Satyanarayana et al., 2009). Generally, the earlier depression strikes the first time, the more likely it will persist or recur (Coryell et al., 2009). In sharp contrast to the common cold, depression can produce severe impairment. In extreme cases, people may fail to feed or clothe themselves or take care of basic health needs like brushing their teeth or showering.

Explanations for major depressive disorder: a tangled web

The multifaceted phenomenon of depression illustrates the biopsychosocial approach, underscoring how different factors can combine to produce psychological symptoms. Let us reconsider the depressed man you imagined interviewing at the beginning of this section. From his severely depressed father and perpetually anxious mother, he may have inherited a tendency to respond to stressful situations with negative emotions (neuroticism). Each day he wasted hours ruminating about losing his job and became convinced that a competitive colleague was trying to undermine his authority. The quality of his work nose-dived. He withdrew socially and began to refuse invitations to go golfing with his buddies. His friends tried to cheer him up, but the black cloud that hung over his head would not budge. Feeling rebuffed, his friends stopped inviting him to do anything. His once-bright social world became a black void, and he moped around doing virtually nothing. He felt helpless. Eventually, his dark thoughts turned to suicide. This example highlights a key point. To fully understand depression, we must appreciate the complex interplay of all of the following: inborn tendencies, stressful events, interpersonal relationships, loss of reinforcers in everyday life, negative thoughts, and feelings of helplessness (Akiskal & McKinney, 1973; Ilardi & Feldman, 2001).

Depression and life events

Sigmund Freud (1917) suggested that early loss can render us vulnerable to depression later in life. He may have been onto something, because the loss of beloved people or even the threat of loss can trigger depression in adulthood. Stressful life events that represent loss or threat of separation are especially tied to depression (Brugha, 1995; Mazure, 1998; Paykel, 2003). The particular relevance of interpersonal stressors to depression may help to account for the sex difference in depression. Research on Australian adolescents found that girls experienced more interpersonal stressors and more problems in their romantic relationships and close friendships than boys, and were more reactive to these stressors (Shih et al., 2006). However, the loss creates a blow to our sense of self-worth and can sting every bit as much as the loss of a relationship (Finlay-Jones & Brown, 1981). A crucial determinant of whether we will become depressed is whether we have lost or are about to lose something we value dearly, like someone we love, financial support or self-esteem (Beck, 1964; Blatt, 1974; Zuroff, Mongrain & Santor, 2004). Recall that in DSM-5, people who become depressed following the loss of a loved one can be formally diagnosed with depression, whereas this was not the case in previous editions of the manual.

Pessimism and other symptoms of depression can set the stage for negative life circumstances, like getting fired from a job or losing a close relationship (Hammen, 1991; Harkness & Luther, 2001). The causal arrow of this association thus points in both directions. Negative life events set us up to bring us down, but depression can create problems in living.

Interpersonal model: depression as a social disorder

James Coyne hypothesised that depression not only reacts to interpersonal problems, but also creates them (Coyne, 1976; Joiner & Coyne, 1999; Rudolph et al., 2000). When people become depressed, he argued, they seek excessive reassurance, which in turn leads others to dislike and reject them. Coyne (1976) asked undergraduates to talk on the telephone for 20 minutes with depressed patients, non-depressed patients or non-patient women drawn from the community. He did not inform students they would be interacting with depressed patients. Yet following the interaction, students who spoke with depressed patients became more depressed, anxious and hostile than those who interacted with non-depressed individuals. Moreover, participants were more rejecting of depressed patients and expressed much less interest in interacting with them in the future. For Coyne, depression is a vicious cycle. Depressed people often elicit hostility and rejection from others, which in turn maintains or worsens their depression.

Many, but not all, studies have replicated Coyne's findings that people with depression seek excessive reassurance and tend to stir up negative feelings in others (Burns et al., 2006; Hames, Hagen & Joiner, 2013; Starr & Davila, 2008). Constant worrying, mistrust, fears of rejection and abandonment, and socially inappropriate behaviours can also be a social turnoff to many people (Wei et al., 2005; Zborowski & Garske, 1993).

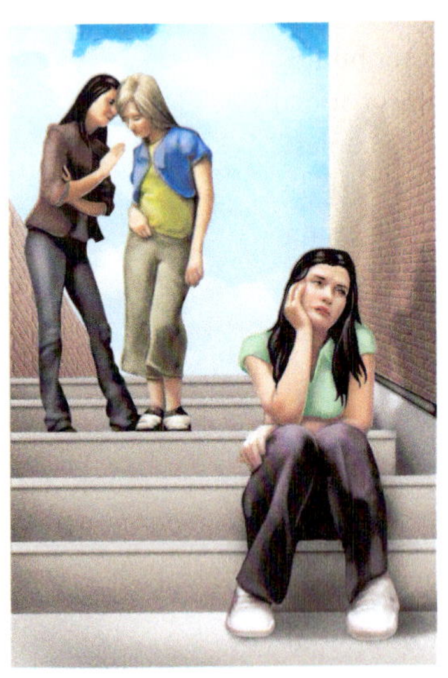

According to James Coyne's interpersonal model of depression, depression can trigger rejection from others, in turn contributing to further depression.

Behavioural model: depression as a loss of reinforcement

Peter Lewinsohn's (1974) behavioural model assumes that depression results from a low rate of response-contingent positive reinforcement. Put in simpler terms, when depressed people try different things and receive no pay-off for them, they eventually give up. They stop participating in many pleasant activities, leaving them little opportunity to obtain reinforcement from others. In time, their personal and social worlds shrink, as depression seeps into virtually every nook and cranny of their lives. Lewinsohn later observed that depressed people sometimes lack social skills (Segrin, 2000; Youngren & Lewinsohn, 1980), making it even harder for them to obtain reinforcement from others. To make matters worse, if people respond to depressed individuals with sympathy and concern, they may reinforce and maintain these individuals' withdrawal. This view implies a straightforward recipe for breaking the grip of depression: pushing ourselves to engage in pleasant activities. Sometimes merely getting out of bed can be the first step towards conquering depression (Dimidjian et al., 2006).

Behavioural model: depression as a disorder of thinking

In contrast, Aaron Beck's influential **cognitive model of depression** holds that depression is caused by negative beliefs and expectations (Beck, 1976; 1987). Beck focused on the cognitive triad, three components of depressed thinking: negative views of oneself, of one's experiences and of the future. These habitual thought patterns, called negative schemas, presumably originate in early experiences of loss, failure and rejection. Activated by stressful events in later life, these schemas reinforce depressed people's negative experiences (Scher, Ingram & Segal, 2005).

Cognitive model of depression
Theory that depression is caused by negative beliefs and expectations.

A depressed person's view of the world is bleak because they put a decidedly negative mental spin on their experiences and they are biased to recall negative, rather than positive, events. They also suffer from *cognitive distortions*, which are skewed ways of thinking. One example is selective abstraction, in which people come to a negative conclusion based on only an isolated aspect of a situation. A man might consistently single out a trivial error he committed in a touch football game and blame himself completely for the loss. It is as though people with depression are wearing glasses that filter out all of life's positive experiences and bring all of life's negative experiences into sharper focus. Moreover, inaccurate perceptions may lead to depression, and depressed feelings may contribute to inaccurate perceptions, bringing about a downward spiral of depression (Kistner et al., 2006).

There is considerable support for Beck's idea that depressed people hold negative views of themselves, the future and the world (Haaga, Dyck & Ernst, 1991; Ingram, 2003). But the evidence for the role of cognitive distortions in non-hospitalised, or not seriously depressed, individuals is not as strong (Disner et al., 2011; Haack et al., 1996). In fact, a review of research suggests that, compared with people without depression, individuals with mild depression actually have a slightly more accurate view of circumstances, a phenomenon called *depressive realism* (Moore & Fresco, 2012). In contrast, people who are not depressed experience *illusory control* over their environments. This surprising conclusion comes from research in which non-depressed people were more likely than depressed people to believe they controlled a light bulb when it came on, even though experimenters rigged when it turned on and off (Alloy & Abramson, 1979; 1988). Thus, depressed people were more realistic in their estimates of personal control, because they had no control over the bulb. Researchers recently replicated this finding, but suggested that depressed individuals experience difficulties attending to and processing information about the light (Msetfi et al., 2005). Rather than being more realistic, depressed people may just be less attentive to 'reality', a finding consistent with cognitive models.

Learned helplessness: depression as a consequence of uncontrollable events

Martin Seligman accidentally stumbled across some unusual findings related to depression in his work with dogs (Seligman, 1975; Seligman & Maier, 1967). He was testing dogs in a shuttle

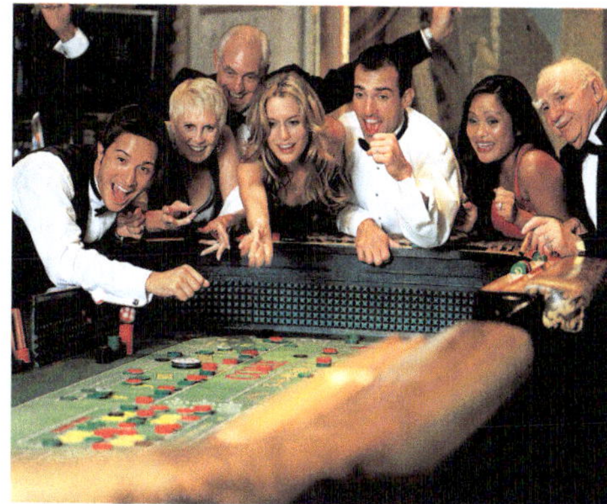

Most people have an illusion of control; for example, they mistakenly believe that they are more likely to win a gamble if they toss the dice than if someone else does. Interestingly, people who are mildly or modestly depressed tend not to fall prey to this thinking error (Golin, Terrell & Johnson, 1977), suggesting they may actually be more realistic than non-depressed people under certain circumstances.
(**Source:** Rob Melnychuk/Digital Vision/Getty Images.)

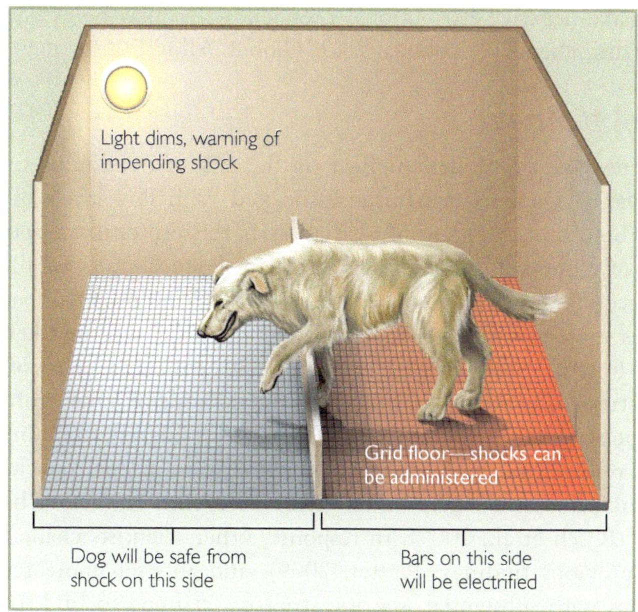

Figure 5.3 The shuttle box. Using an apparatus like this, Martin Seligman found that dogs gave up trying to escape electric shocks. He called this phenomenon 'learned helplessness'.

box, depicted in Figure 5.3; one side of the box was electrified and the other side, separated by a barrier, was not. Ordinarily, dogs avoid painful shocks by jumping over the barrier to the non-electrified side of the box. Yet Seligman found something surprising. Dogs first restrained in a hammock and exposed to shocks they could not escape, later often made no attempt to escape shocks in the shuttle box, even when they could easily get away from them. Some of the dogs just sat there, whimpering and crying, passively accepting the shocks as though they were inescapable. They had learned to become helpless.

Learned helplessness Tendency to feel helpless in the face of events we cannot control.

Bruce Overmier and Martin Seligman (1967) described **learned helplessness** as the tendency to feel helpless in the face of events we cannot control, and argued that it offers an animal model of depression. They noted striking parallels between the effects of learned helplessness and depressive symptoms: passivity, appetite and weight loss, and difficulty learning that one can change circumstances for the better. But we must be cautious in drawing conclusions from animal studies, because many psychological conditions, including depression, may differ in animals and humans (Raulin & Lilienfeld, 1999).

Provocative as it is, Seligman's model cannot account for all aspects of depression. It does not explain why depressed people make internal attributions (explanations) for failure. In fact, the tendency to assume personal responsibility for failure contradicts the notion that depressed people regard negative events as beyond their control.

The original model also doesn't acknowledge that the mere expectation of uncontrollability is not sufficient to induce depression. After all, people do not become sad when they receive large amounts of money in a lottery, even though they have no control over that event (Abramson, Seligman & Teasdale, 1978).

When data do not fit a model, good scientists revise it. Seligman and his colleagues (Abramson et al., 1978) altered the learned helplessness model to account for the attributions people make to explain their worlds. They argued that persons prone to depression attribute failure to internal (as opposed to external) factors, and success to external (as opposed to internal) factors. A person with depression might blame a poor test grade on a lack of ability (an internal factor), and a good score on the ease of the exam (an external factor). The researchers also observed that depression-prone people make attributions that are global and stable: they tend to see their failures as general and fixed aspects of their personalities. Still, internal, global and stable attributions may be more a consequence than a cause of depression (Harvey & Weary, 1984). The depression brought on by undesirable life events may skew our thinking, leading us to make negative attributions, a tendency that may be evident as early as primary school (Fincham, Diener & Hokoda, 2011; Gibb & Alloy, 2006).

Depression: the role of biology

Twin studies indicate that genes exert a moderate effect on the risk of developing major depression (Kendler et al., 1993). Depression is often associated with low levels of the neurotransmitter serotonin (Robinson, 2007). Specific variations in the serotonin transporter gene (which affects the rate of reuptake) seem to play a role in depression, especially in conjunction with life experiences. Research conducted in New Zealand indicates that people who inherit two copies of this stress-sensitive gene are two and a half times more likely to develop depression following four stressful events than people with another version of the gene that is not sensitive to stress (Caspi et al., 2003). The stress-sensitive gene probably affects people's ability to dampen negative emotions in the face of stress (Kendler, Gardner & Prescott, 2003). Nevertheless, researchers who reviewed all the available evidence concluded that there was no basis for a link between the gene and stressful life events, on the one hand, and depression, on the other (Risch et al., 2009). In response, other scientists challenged how these authors analysed previous findings (Rutter, 2009), and an even more recent review, which included studies with substantial, specific stressors, claimed to find strong and consistent evidence for the important part genes play in determining the relationship between negative emotions and stress (Karg et al., 2011).

To resolve questions regarding the role of gene-life events interactions in depression, researchers will need to conduct well-designed studies in which stressful life events are carefully defined to determine whether the positive findings are replicable. The hope is that these studies will clarify whether any genetic irregularities that surface are specific to depression; they may be associated with anxiety, too (Hariri et al., 2002). Depression also appears linked to low levels of the neurotransmitter norepinephrine (Leonard, 1997; Robinson, 2007) and diminished neurogenesis (growth of new neurons), which brings about reduced hippocampal volume (Pittinger & Duman, 2008; Videbech & Ravnkilde, 2004). Many patients with depression have problems in the brain's reward and stress-response systems (Depue & Iacono, 1989; Forbes, Shaw & Dahl, 2007) and decreased levels of dopamine, the neurotransmitter most closely tied to reward (Martinot et al., 2001). This finding may help to explain why depression is often associated with an inability to experience pleasure.

Bipolar disorder: when mood goes to extremes

Ann, the new mother with bipolar disorder we met at the beginning of the chapter, experienced many of the classic symptoms of a **manic episode**. These episodes are typically marked by dramatically elevated mood (feeling 'on top of the world'), decreased need for sleep, greatly heightened energy, inflated self-esteem, increased talkativeness and irresponsible behaviour. People in a manic episode often display 'pressured speech', as though they cannot get their words out quickly enough, and are difficult to interrupt (Goodwin & Jamison, 1990). Their ideas often race through their heads quickly, which may account for the heightened rate of creative accomplishments in some bipolar individuals. Symptoms of a manic episode typically begin with a rapid increase over only a few days.

Bipolar disorder, formerly called 'manic-depressive disorder', is diagnosed when there is a history of at least one manic episode (APA, 2013). In contrast to major depression, bipolar disorder is equally common in men and women. In the great majority of cases—more than 90 percent—people who have had one manic episode experience at least one more (Alda, 1997). Some have episodes separated by many years and then have a series of episodes, one rapidly following the other. More than half the time, a major depressive episode precedes or follows a manic episode (Solomon et al., 2010). Manic episodes often produce serious problems in social and occupational functioning, such as substance abuse and unrestrained sexual behaviour. Because their judgement is so impaired, people in the midst of manic episodes may go on wild spending sprees or drive while intoxicated. One of your book's authors treated a manic patient who passed himself off to a financial company as his own father, gained access to his father's savings for retirement, and gambled away his entire family fortune. Another frittered away most of his life's savings by purchasing more than 100 bowling balls, none of which he needed. The negative effects of a manic episode, including loss of employment, family conflicts and divorce, can persist for many years (Coryell et al., 1993).

Bipolar disorder is among the most genetically influenced of all mental disorders (Miklowitz & Johnson, 2006). Twin studies suggest that its heritability ranges from about 60 percent to as high as 85 percent (Alda, 1997; Lichtenstein et al., 2009; McGuffin et al., 2003). Scientists believe that genes that increase the sensitivity of the dopamine receptors

First-person account:

BIPOLAR DISORDER

'When I start going into a high, I no longer feel like an ordinary [homemaker]. Instead I feel organised and accomplished and I begin to feel I am my most creative self. I can write poetry easily . . . melodies without effort . . . paint . . . I feel a sense of euphoria or elation . . . I don't seem to need much sleep . . . I've just bought six new dresses . . . I feel sexy and men stare at me. Maybe I'll have an affair, or perhaps several . . . However, when I go beyond this state, I become manic . . . I begin to see things in my mind that aren't real . . . One night I created an entire movie . . . I also experienced complete terror . . . when I knew that an assassination scene was about to take place . . . I went into a manic psychosis at that point. My screams awakened my husband . . . I was admitted to the hospital the next day.' *(Fieve, 1976, p. 17)*

Manic episode
Experience marked by dramatically elevated mood, decreased need for sleep, increased energy, inflated self-esteem, increased talkativeness and irresponsible behaviour.

Bipolar disorder
Condition marked by a history of at least one manic episode.

(Willner, 1995) and decrease the sensitivity of serotonin receptors may boost the risk of bipolar disorder (Ogden et al., 2004). Many genes appear to be culprits in increasing the risk of bipolar disorder, and there is at least some genetic overlap between psychotic symptoms in bipolar disorder and schizophrenia (Craddock, O'Donovan & Owen, 2005; Lichtenstein et al., 2009; Purcell et al., 2009).

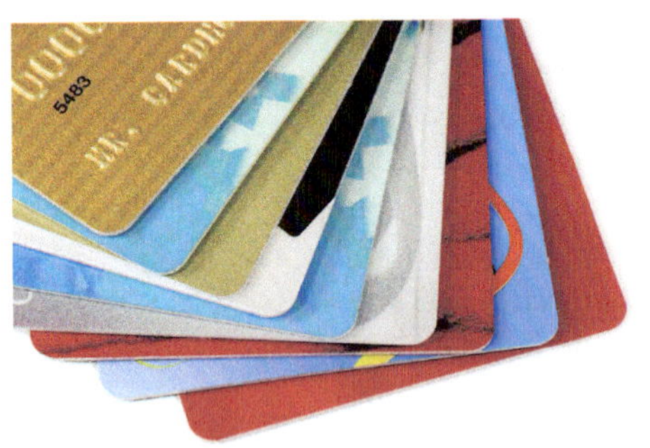

People in the midst of manic episodes frequently go on uncontrolled spending sprees and may 'max out' multiple credit cards in the process.
(Source: Ilya Genkin/Dreamstime.)

Brain-imaging studies suggest that people with bipolar disorder experience increased activity in structures related to emotion, including the amygdala (Chang et al., 2004; Yurgelun-Todd et al., 2000), and decreased activity in structures associated with planning, such as the prefrontal cortex (Kruger et al., 2003). Still, the cause–relationship between physiological findings and mood disorders is not clear. For example, the high levels of norepinephrine and differences in brain activity observed in people with bipolar disorder may be an effect rather than a cause of the disorder (Thase, Jindal & Howland, 2002).

Bipolar disorder is influenced by more than biological factors. Stressful life events are associated with an increased risk of manic episodes, more frequent relapse, and a longer recovery from manic episodes (Johnson & Miller, 1997; Yan-Meier et al., 2011). Interestingly, some manic episodes appear to be triggered by positive life events associated with striving for and achieving goals, such as job promotions or winning poetry contests (Johnson et al., 2000; Johnson et al., 2008). Once again, we can see that psychological disorders arise from the intersection of biological, psychological and sociocultural forces.

Suicide: facts and fiction

Major depression and bipolar disorder are associated with a higher risk of suicide than most other disorders (Miklowitz & Johnson, 2006; Wolfsdorf et al., 2003). Estimates suggest that more than a third of people with bipolar disorder have attempted suicide, and that the suicide rate of people with bipolar disorder is about 15 times higher than that of the general population (Harris & Barraclough, 1997; Novick, Swartz & Frank, 2010). Some anxiety disorders, such as panic disorder, social anxiety disorder, and substance abuse are also associated with heightened suicide risk (Spirito & Esposito-Smythers, 2006). However, suicide itself is not a psychological disorder and its deadly reach extends far beyond any one condition. In 2007, some 1880 suicides were recorded in Australia, a figure that represents 1.4 percent of all deaths and is probably a significant underestimate, because many suicides are reported as accidents (De Leo et al., 2010). This number easily exceeds the national road toll (1616), and dwarfs the number of deaths recorded as due to murder or manslaughter (162) for the same year. In 2007, suicide was the fifteenth-ranked cause of death overall in the country (tenth for men); among Australians in their twenties, approximately one in seven deaths was a suicide. For each completed suicide, there are an estimated 23 suicide attempts. In Table 5.6, we present a number of common myths and misconceptions about suicide.

It is essential to try to predict suicide attempts, because most people are acutely suicidal for only a brief window of time (Schneidman, Farberow & Litman, 1970; Simon, 2006) and intervention during that time can be critical. Unfortunately, the prediction of suicide poses serious practical problems. First, we cannot easily conduct longitudinal studies to determine which people will attempt suicide. It would be unethical to allow people believed to be at high suicide risk to go through with attempts to allow us to pinpoint predictors of suicide. Second, it is difficult to study the psychological states associated with suicide because the period of high risk for a suicide attempt is often very brief. Third, the low prevalence of suicide makes predicting it difficult (Sher, 2011). The rate of completed suicides in Australia is

Table 5.6 Common myths and misconceptions about suicide

Myth	Reality
Talking to depressed people about suicide makes them more likely to commit the act.	Talking to depressed persons about suicide often makes them more likely to obtain help.
Suicide is almost always completed with no warning.	Many or most individuals who commit suicide communicate their intent to others.
As a severe depression lifts, people's suicide risk decreases.	As a severe depression lifts, the risk of suicide may actually increase, in part because individuals possess more energy to attempt the act.
Most people who threaten suicide are seeking attention.	Although attention-seeking motivates some suicidal behaviours, most suicidal acts stem from severe depression and hopelessness.
People who talk a lot about suicide almost never commit it.	Talking about suicide is associated with a considerably greater risk of suicide.

roughly 12.6 per 100 000 people in the general population (Australian Bureau of Statistics, 2016). So if only about one-hundredth of 1 percent of the population completes a suicide, our best guess—with about 99.99 percent accuracy—is that no one will commit suicide. Nevertheless, the social costs of failing to predict a suicide are so great that efforts to accurately predict suicide attempts continue.

The good news is that research has taught us a great deal about risk factors for suicide. The single best predictor of completed suicide is a prior attempt (Hawton, Casanas, Comabella, Haw & Saunders, 2013; Hoyer, Licht & Mortensen, 2009). About three times as many men as women commit suicide, but more women than men attempt suicide (Australian Bureau of Statistics, 2016; McKenna & Harrison, 2012). Interestingly, hopelessness may be an even better predictor of suicide than depression (Klonsky, Kotov, Bakst, Rabinowitz & Bromet, 2012) because people are most likely to try to kill themselves when they see no future escape from their pain. Intense agitation is also a powerful predictor of suicide risk (Fawcett, 1997). People who wished they had died after a suicide attempt are more than twice as likely to later commit suicide as those who are relieved they survived or who were ambivalent about the attempt (Henriques et al., 2005). A list of risk factors for suicide appears in Table 5.7.

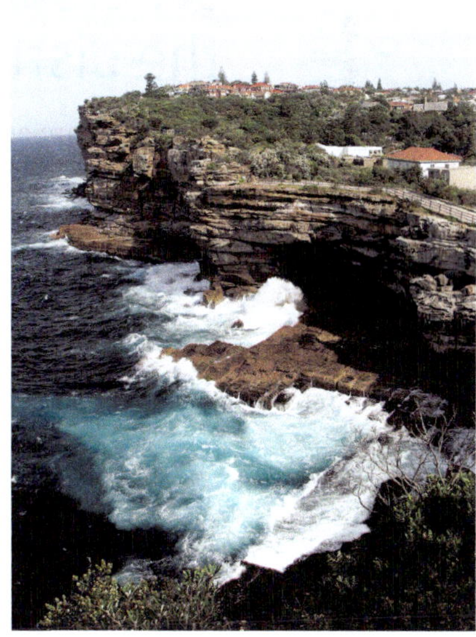

'The Gap' is an ocean cliff in Sydney's east that reportedly witnesses about 50 suicides each year. In an effort to reduce this figure, funding is being sought to install high fences, lights, security cameras and emergency phones with direct connections to the police and counsellors. (**Source:** Tomas Pavelka/Dreamstime.)

Table 5.7 Major suicide risk factors

1. Depression	**8.** Recent loss of a loved one; being divorced, separated or widowed
2. Hopelessness	**9.** Family history of suicide
3. Substance abuse	**10.** Personality disorders, such as borderline personality disorder
4. Schizophrenia	**11.** Anxiety disorders, such as panic disorder and social phobia
5. Homosexuality, probably because of social stigma	**12.** Old age, especially in men
6. Unemployment	**13.** Recent discharge from a hospital
7. Chronic, painful or disfiguring physical illness	

Assess your knowledge — FACT or FICTION?

1. Men and women are equally likely to suffer from major depression. **(True/False)**
2. Depression is associated with stressful life events. **(True/False)**
3. According to Lewinsohn, depression is caused by a low rate of response-contingent positive reinforcement. **(True/False)**
4. According to Seligman, depression-prone people make specific and unstable attributions for negative life events. **(True/False)**
5. Most people who have a manic episode never have another. **(True/False)**
6. Depression is a better predictor of suicide than hopelessness. **(True/False)**

Answers: (1) F; (2) T; (3) T; (4) F; (5) F; (6) F

Personality and dissociative disorders: the disrupted and divided self

Most of us are accustomed to thinking of ourselves as one coherent unified identity. But some individuals—especially those with personality and dissociative disorders—experience a serious disruption in their thoughts or behaviours that prevents them from experiencing a healthy, consistent identity. Identifying personality disorders is not easy, because we all have some variations in personality and sense of self.

Personality disorders

Personality disorder Condition in which personality traits, appearing first in adolescence, are inflexible, stable, expressed in a wide variety of situations, and lead to distress or impairment.

Of all psychological conditions, personality disorders are historically among the least reliably diagnosed (Fowler, O'Donohue & Lilienfeld, 2007; Perry, 1984; Zimmerman, 1994). That is because clinicians sometimes disagree about whether a given patient exhibits certain personality disturbances, such as excessive impulsivity or identity problems. DSM-5 states that we should diagnose a **personality disorder** only when personality traits: first appear by adolescence; are inflexible, stable and expressed in a wide variety of situations; and lead to distress or impairment (APA, 2013). But more than most patterns of behaviour we have described, whether we perceive someone with a personality disorder as abnormal depends on the context in which their behaviour occurs (Price & Bouffard, 1974). The suspiciousness of a person with a paranoid personality disorder may be a liability in a cooperative work group, but an asset in a private investigator.

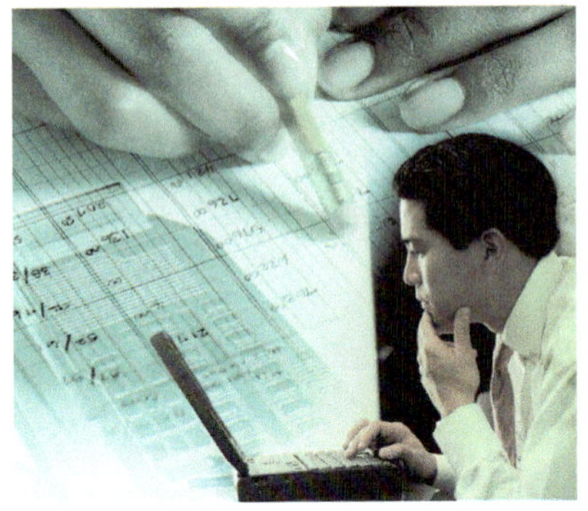

At least in mild doses, features of some personality disorders may be adaptive in certain occupations. For example, the traits of obsessive-compulsive personality disorder, which include attention to detail and perfectionism, may come in handy for accountants. (**Source:** Stockbyte/Getty Images.)

Although the 10 personality disorders in DSM-5 are distinguishable from each other, they often exhibit substantial comorbidity with each other and with other mental disorders, such as major depression and generalised anxiety disorder (Lenzenweger, McLachlan & Rubin, 2007), leading some to question whether they are truly distinct from one another and from other psychological conditions (Harkness & Lilienfeld, 1997). Only a handful of these disorders have been the focus of extensive and systematic research (Blashfield & Intoccia, 2000). As a consequence, in this section we will consider in detail the two most widely investigated personality disorders—borderline personality disorder and psychopathic personality. In many respects, the fascinating issues these extensively studied disorders raise highlight the complexities involved in diagnosing and understanding personality disorders in general.

Borderline personality disorder: stable instability

Estimates suggest that between 2 and 6 percent of adults, most of them women (Swartz et al., 1990; Zanarini et al., 2011), develop **borderline personality disorder**, a condition marked by instability in mood, identity and impulse control. Individuals with borderline personality disorder tend to be extremely impulsive and unpredictable, although many are married and hold down good jobs. They are often unsure of who they are, and their interests and life goals frequently shift dramatically from year to year. Their relationships frequently alternate from extremes of worshipping partners one day to hating them the next. Some scholars have aptly described this disorder as a pattern of 'stable instability' (Grinker & Werble, 1977). The name 'borderline personality' stems from the now outmoded belief that this condition lies on the border between psychotic and 'neurotic'—relatively normal, yet mildly disabled—functioning (Stern, 1938).

Borderline personality disorder
Condition marked by extreme instability in mood, identity and impulse control.

BORDERLINE PERSONALITY: A VOLATILE BLEND OF TRAITS. Persons with borderline personality's impulsivity and rapidly fluctuating emotions often have a self-destructive quality: many engage in drug abuse, sexual promiscuity, overeating and even self-mutilation, like cutting themselves when upset (Salsman & Linehan, 2012). They may threaten suicide to manipulate others, reflecting the chaotic nature of their relationships (Leichsenring et al., 2011). Because many experience intense feelings of abandonment when alone, they may jump frantically from one unhealthy relationship to another.

EXPLANATIONS OF BORDERLINE PERSONALITY DISORDER. Psychoanalyst Otto Kernberg (1967; 1975) traced the roots of borderline personality to childhood problems with developing a sense of self and bonding emotionally to others. According to Kernberg, individuals with borderline personality disorder cannot integrate differing perceptions of people, themselves included. This defect supposedly arises from an inborn tendency to experience intense anger and frustration from living with a cold, unempathetic mother. Kernberg argued that borderline individuals experience the world and themselves as unstable because they tend to 'split' people and experiences into either all good or all bad. Although influential, Kernberg's model of borderline personality remains inadequately researched.

According to Marsha Linehan's (1993) sociobiological model, individuals with borderline personality disorder inherit a tendency to overreact to stress, and experience lifelong difficulties with regulating their emotions (Crowell, Beauchaine & Linehan, 2009). Indeed, twin studies suggest that borderline personality traits are substantially heritable (Carpenter et al., 2013; Torgersen et al., 2000). Difficulties in controlling emotions may be responsible for the rejection many individuals with borderline personality disorder encounter, as well as their excessive concerns about being validated, loved and accepted.

Edward Selby and Thomas Joiner's emotional cascade model holds that intense rumination about negative events or emotional experiences may result in uncontrolled 'emotional cascades', which prompt self-injurious actions like cutting. Although these impulsive and desperate actions succeed in providing brief distraction from rumination, they often fuel further bouts of rumination, creating a vicious cycle of problems with regulating emotions (Selby et al., 2009; Selby & Joiner, 2009).

For many years, psychologists believed that borderline personality was a lifelong condition that was highly resistant to treatment. Yet according to a recent study of treatment-seeking patients with borderline personality disorder, 85 percent improved with treatment over a 10-year period, and only 12 percent relapsed

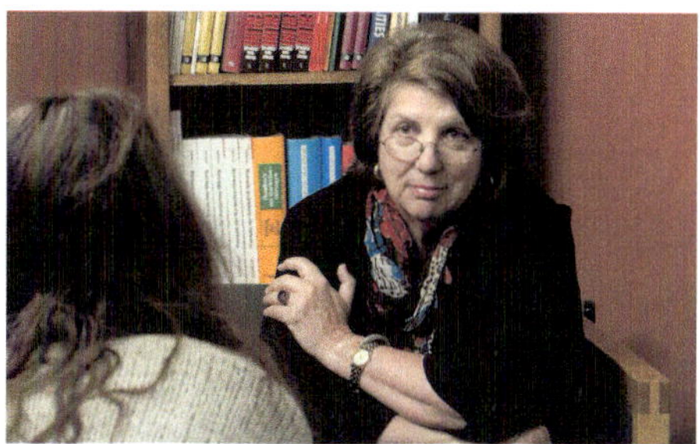

Psychologist Marsha Linehan of the University of Washington is the world's leading expert on the treatment of borderline personality disorder. In 2011, she surprised many people by acknowledging publicly that she had been diagnosed with the condition earlier in life. Linehan's courageous admission may help to dispel some of the unjustified stigma surrounding this personality disorder. **(Source:** Peter Yates/New York Times/Redux.)

(Gunderson et al, 2011). The patients with borderline personality actually showed a lower relapse rate compared with patients with major depression and other personality disorders.

Psychopathic personality: don't judge a book by its cover

We do not intend to alarm you. Yet the odds are high that in your life, you have met—perhaps even dated—at least one person whom psychologists describe as a **psychopathic personality**, which used to be known informally as a 'psychopath' or 'sociopath'.

Psychopathic personality is not formally a psychological disorder and is not listed in DSM-5. Nevertheless, it overlaps moderately to highly with the DSM-5 diagnosis of **antisocial personality disorder (ASPD)**. In contrast to ASPD, which is marked by a lengthy history of illegal and irresponsible actions, psychopathic personality is marked by a distinctive set of personality traits (Lilienfeld, 1994). Because much more psychological research has concentrated on psychopathic personality than on ASPD (Hare, 2003; Patrick, 2006), we focus on psychopathic personality here, as this condition is far better understood.

First-person account:

PSYCHOPATHIC PERSONALITY

'In my lifetime I have murdered 21 human beings. I have committed thousands of burglaries, robberies, larcenies, arsons and last but not least I have committed sodomy on more than 1000 male human beings. For all of these things I am not the least bit sorry. I have no conscience so that does not worry me.'

(Carl Panzram, a serial killer, burglar and arsonist, quoted in King, 1997, p. 169).

PSYCHOPATHIC PERSONALITY: A DANGEROUS MIXTURE OF TRAITS. Those with psychopathic personality—most of them male—are guiltless, dishonest, manipulative, callous and self-centred (Cleckley, 1941/1988; Lykken, 1995). Given these distinctly unpleasant personality traits, one might assume we would all go out of our way to avoid individuals with this disorder—and we would probably be better off if we did. However, many of us seek out people with psychopathic personality as friends and even romantic partners, because they tend to be charming, personable and engaging (Dutton, 2012; Hare, 1993). This was certainly the case with Johnny, whom you will recall from the beginning of the chapter. Like Johnny, many people with this condition have a history of conduct disorder, marked by lying, cheating and stealing in childhood and adolescence.

Psychopathic personality Condition marked by superficial charm, dishonesty, manipulativeness, self-centredness and risk-taking.

Antisocial personality disorder (ASPD) Condition marked by a lengthy history of irresponsible and/or illegal actions.

If the traits we have described fit someone you know to a T, there is no need to panic. Despite popular conception, most people with psychopathic personality are not physically aggressive. Nevertheless, they are at somewhat heightened risk for crime compared with the average person, and a handful—probably a few percent—are habitually violent (Leistico et al., 2008). American mass murderer Ted Bundy, who assaulted and murdered numerous young women and girls during the 1970s, almost certainly met the criteria for psychopathic personality disorder, as do about 25 percent of prison inmates (Hare, 2003). Also, despite scores of movie portrayals of crazed serial killers, people with this disorder typically are not psychotic. To the contrary, most are entirely rational. They know full well that their irresponsible actions are morally wrong; they just do not care (Cima, Tonnaer & Hauser, 2010).

There is reason to suspect that people with this condition populate not only much of the criminal justice system, but also positions of leadership in corporations and politics (Babiak & Hare, 2006). For example, among the US presidents, higher estimated levels of a constellation of traits called fearless dominance, which assess the boldness and adventurousness often found in psychopaths, are linked to superior leadership as rated by expert historians. Indeed, some psychopathic traits, such as interpersonal skills, superficial likability, ruthlessness and risk-taking, may give people with this disorder a leg-up for getting ahead of the rest of the pack. Still, there is surprisingly little research on 'successful psychopaths'—people with high levels of psychopathic traits who function well in society (Hall & Benning, 2006; Widom, 1977).

Factoid

Although the view that individuals with psychopathic personality are 'hopeless cases' who can't be rehabilitated is widely accepted, recent evidence suggests that at least some people with this disorder may improve as a consequence of psychotherapy (Salekin, 2002; Skeem, Monahan & Mulvey, 2002). This may be especially true when treatment is prolonged and intensive (Caldwell, 2011).

CAUSES OF PSYCHOPATHIC PERSONALITY. Despite nearly six decades of research, the causes of psychopathic personality remain largely unknown (Skeem et al., 2011). Classic research shows that individuals with this disorder do not show much classical conditioning to unpleasant unconditioned stimuli such as electric shocks (Lykken, 1957). Similarly, when asked to sit patiently in a chair for an impending electric shock or a loud blast of noise, their levels of skin conductance—an indicator of arousal—increase only about one-fifth as much as those without psychopathic personality (Hare, 1978; Lorber, 2004). These abnormalities probably stem from a deficit in fear, which may give rise to some of the key features of the disorder (Fowles & Dindo, 2009; Lykken, 1995; Patrick, 2006). Perhaps partly as a consequence of this dearth of fear, people with psychopathic personality are not motivated to learn from punishment and so tend to repeat the same mistakes in life (Newman & Kosson, 1986; Zeier et al., 2012).

An alternative explanation is that individuals with this disorder are under-aroused. The Yerkes–Dodson law describes a well-established psychological principle: an inverted U-shaped relationship between arousal, on the one hand, and mood and performance, on the other. As this law reminds us, people who are habitually under-aroused experience stimulus hunger: they are bored and seek out excitement. The under-arousal hypothesis may help to explain why those with psychopathic personality tend to be risk-takers (Zuckerman, 1989), as well as why they frequently get in trouble with the law and abuse all manner of substances (Taylor & Lang, 2006). Nevertheless, the causal arrow between under-arousal and psychopathy may run in the opposite direction: if people with psychopathic traits are fearless, they may experience little arousal in response to stimuli (Lykken, 1995).

Dissociative disorders

When speaking about ourselves, we use the words 'me' and 'I' without giving it a second thought. That is not the case in most **dissociative disorders**, which involve disruptions in consciousness, memory, identity or perception (APA, 2013). The idea that one person can have more than one identity—is an extraordinary claim. So, it is no wonder that dissociative identity disorder (DID) is one of the most controversial of all diagnoses. Before we consider the debate that swirls around this condition, we consider several other dissociative disorders.

Depersonalisation/derealisation disorder

If you have ever felt detached from yourself, as though you are living in a movie or dream or observing your body from the perspective of an outsider, you have experienced depersonalisation. More than half of adults have experienced one brief episode of depersonalisation, and such experiences are especially common among adolescents and university students (APA, 2000; Simeon et al., 1997). Derealisation, the sense that the external world is strange or unreal, often accompanies both depersonalisation and panic attacks. Only if people experience multiple episodes of depersonalisation, derealisation, or both, do they qualify for a diagnosis of **depersonalisation/derealisation disorder**.

Dissociative amnesia

In **dissociative amnesia**, people cannot recall important personal information—most often following a stressful experience—that is not due to ordinary forgetting. Their memory loss is extensive and can include suicide attempts or violent outbursts (Sar et al., 2007). More commonly, psychologists diagnose dissociative amnesia when adults report gaps in their memories for child abuse.

This diagnosis has proven controversial for several reasons. First, memory gaps regarding non-traumatic events are common in healthy individuals and are not necessarily stress-

Dissociative disorder
Condition involving disruptions in consciousness, memory, identity or perception.

Depersonalisation/derealisation disorder
Condition marked by multiple episodes of depersonalisation, derealisation, or both.

Dissociative amnesia
Inability to recall important personal information—most often related to a stressful experience—that can't be explained by ordinary forgetfulness.

Factoid

Sleep disturbances may play a prominent role in symptoms of dissociation such as depersonalisation. When people are deprived of sleep for 24 hours, they report more dissociative-like symptoms, and when they are taught sleep hygiene techniques to improve their sleep, they report fewer dissociative symptoms (van der Kloet et al., 2012). Some researchers propose that a disturbed sleep-wake cycle produces dreamlike thoughts during the daytime that cause or at least fuel dissociative experiences.

related or indicative of dissociation (Belli et al., 1998). Second, most people may not be especially motivated to recall child abuse or other upsetting events. As Richard McNally (2003) pointed out, not thinking about something is not the same as being unable to remember it, which is amnesia. Third, careful studies have turned up no convincing cases of amnesia that cannot be explained by other factors, like disease, brain injury, normal forgetting, or an unwillingness to think about disturbing events (Kihlstrom, 2005; Pope et al., 2007). Fourth, individuals with high levels of dissociation are less likely to forget supposedly threatening (sexual) words, which experimenters direct them to forget (Elzinga, van Dyck & Spinhoven, 2000).

At times, we have all felt like running away from our troubles. In **dissociative fugue**, a type of dissociative amnesia, people not only forget significant events in their lives, but also flee their stressful circumstances ('fugue' is Latin for 'flight'). In some cases, they move to another city or another country, assuming a new identity. Fugues can last for hours or, in unusual cases, years. Dissociative fugue is rare, occurring in about 2 of every 1000 people (APA, 2000), with more prolonged fugue states even rarer (Karlin & Orne, 1996).

Dissociative fugue
Sudden, unexpected travel away from home or the workplace, accompanied by amnesia for significant life events.

In 2006, a 57-year-old husband, father and Boy Scout leader from New York was found living under a new name in a homeless shelter in Chicago after he left his garage near his office and disappeared. When a tip to *America's Most Wanted* uncovered his true identity six months later, his family contacted him, but he claimed to have no memory of who they were (Brody, 2007).

In this and other fugue cases, it is essential to find out whether the fugue resulted from a head injury, a stroke, or another neurological cause. Moreover, some people merely claim amnesia to avoid responsibilities or stressful circumstances, relocate to a different area, and get a fresh start in life. Even when fugues occur shortly after a traumatic event, it is difficult to know whether the trauma caused the amnesia. Scientists don't fully understand the role trauma, psychological factors and neurological conditions play in fugue states (Kihlstrom, 2005).

Dissociative identity disorder (DID)
Condition characterised by the presence of two or more distinct personality states that recurrently take control of the person's behaviour.

Dissociative identity disorder: multiple personalities, multiple controversies

Dissociative identity disorder (DID) is characterised by the presence of two or more distinct personality states (the term 'identities' was deleted in DSM-5) that markedly disrupt the person's usual sense of identity and may be observed by others or reported by the individual. These personality states or 'alters', as they are sometimes called, are often very different from the primary or 'host' personality and may be of different names, ages, genders and even races. In some cases, these features are the opposite of those exhibited by the host personality. For example, if the host personality is shy and retiring, one or more alters may be outgoing or flamboyant. Psychologists have reported the number of alters to range from one (the so-called 'split personality') to hundreds or even thousands, with one reported case of 4500 personalities (Acocella, 1999). In general, women are more likely to receive a DID diagnosis and report more alters than men (APA, 2000).

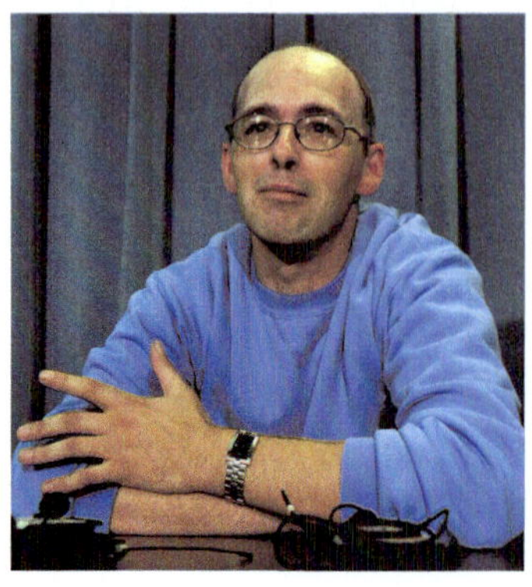

Jeffrey Ingram, age 40, experienced a dissociative fugue in which he claimed for more than a month that he could not remember anything about his life. He was reunited with his fiancée in 2006 only after he appeared on television shows asking the public to identify him. (**Source:** Karl Gehring/The Denver Post/AP Images.)

Researchers have identified intriguing differences among alters in their respiration rates (Bahnson & Smith, 1975), brain wave activity (EEG; Ludwig et al., 1972), eyeglass prescriptions (Miller, 1989), handedness (Savitz et al., 2004), skin conductance responses (Brende, 1984), voice patterns and handwriting (Lilienfeld & Lynn, 2003). Fascinating as these findings are, they do not provide conclusive evidence for the existence of alters. These differences could stem from changes in mood or thoughts over time or to bodily changes, such as muscle tension, that people can produce on a voluntary basis (Allen & Movius, 2000; Merckelbach, Devilly & Rassin, 2002). Moreover, scientists have falsified claims that alters are truly distinct. When psychologists have used objective measures of memory, they have typically found that information presented to one alter is available to the other, providing no evidence for amnesia across alters (Allen & Movius, 2000; Huntjens et al., 2012).

The primary controversy surrounding DID revolves around one question: Is DID a response to early trauma, or is it a consequence of social and cultural factors (Merskey, 1992)? According to the posttraumatic model (Gleaves, May & Cardeña, 2001; Ross, 1997), DID arises from a history of severe abuse—physical, sexual, or both—during childhood. This abuse leads individuals to 'compartmentalise' their identity into distinct alters as a means of coping with intense emotional pain. In this way, the person can feel as though the abuse happened to someone else.

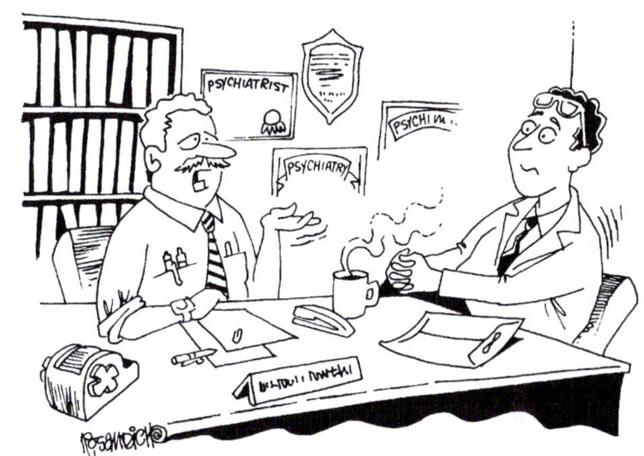

"I HAVE 25 PATIENTS IN MY COUNSELING GROUP--MRS. SHERMAN, MR. MARTIN, AND MR. MARTIN'S 23 OTHER PERSONALITIES."

(Source: Dan Rosandich, www.CartoonStock.com.)

Advocates of the posttraumatic model claim that 90 percent or more of individuals with DID were severely abused in childhood (Gleaves, 1996). Nevertheless, many studies that reported this association did not check the accuracy of abuse claims against objective information such as court records of abuse (Coons, Bowman & Milstein, 1988). Moreover, researchers have not shown that early abuse is specific to DID, as it is present in many other disorders (Pope & Hudson, 1992). These considerations do not exclude a role for early trauma in DID, but they suggest that researchers must conduct further controlled studies before drawing strong conclusions (Gleaves, 1996; Gleaves et al., 2001).

Advocates of the competing sociocognitive model say the claim that some people have hundreds of personalities is extraordinary, but the evidence for it is unconvincing (Giesbrecht et al., 2008; Lilienfeld et al., 1999; McHugh, 1993; Merskey, 1992; Spanos, 1994, 1996). According to this model, people's expectancies and beliefs—shaped by certain psychotherapeutic procedures and cultural influences and a tendency to fantasise and misremember events, rather than early traumas—account for the origin and maintenance of DID. Advocates of this model claim that some therapists use procedures like hypnosis and repeated prompting of alters that suggest to patients that their puzzling symptoms are the products of indwelling identities (Lilienfeld & Lynn, 2003; Lilienfeld et al., 1999). The following observations and findings support this hypothesis:

- Many or most DID patients show few or no clear-cut signs of this condition, such as alters, prior to psychotherapy (Kluft, 1984).

- Mainstream treatment techniques for DID reinforce the idea that the person possesses multiple identities. These techniques include using hypnosis to 'bring forth' hidden alters, communicating with alters and giving them different names, and encouraging patients to recover repressed memories supposedly housed in dissociated selves (Spanos, 1994, 1996).
- The number of alters per DID individual tends to increase substantially when therapists use these techniques (Piper, 1997).
- Researchers have reported a link between dissociation and the tendency to fantasise in everyday life (Giesbrecht et al., 2008), which may be related to the production of false memories, although the interpretation of these findings has proven controversial (Dalenberg et al., 2011).

In 1970, there were 79 documented cases of DID in the world literature. In 1986, the number of DID cases had mushroomed to approximately 6000 (Lilienfeld et al., 1999), and some estimates in the early twenty-first century are in the hundreds of thousands. The sociocognitive model holds that the popular media have played a pivotal role in the DID epidemic (Elzinga, van Dyck & Spinhoven, 1998). Indeed, much of the dramatic increase in DID's prevalence followed closely on the release of the best-selling book *Sybil* (Schreiber, 1973) in the mid-1970s, later made into an Emmy Award–winning television movie starring Sally Field. The book and later film told the heartbreaking story of a young woman with 16 personalities who reported a history of sadistic child abuse. Interestingly, subsequently released audiotapes of Sybil's therapy sessions suggested that she had no alters or memories of child abuse prior to treatment and that her therapist had urged her to behave differently on different occasions (Rieber, 1999).

Over the past two decades, media coverage of DID has skyrocketed (Showalter, 1997; Spanos, 1996; Wilson, 2003), with some celebrities, such as comedian Roseanne Barr and football star Hershel Walker, claiming to suffer from the disorder. Although DID is virtually non-existent in Japan and India, it is now diagnosed with considerable frequency in some countries, such as Holland, in which it has recently received more publicity (Lilienfeld et al., 1999). In summary, there is considerable support for the sociocognitive model and the claim that therapists, along with the media, are creating alters rather than discovering them. The dissociative disorders provide a powerful, although troubling, example of how social and cultural forces can shape psychological disorders.

Assess your knowledge — FACT or FICTION?

1. Personality disorders are almost always reliably diagnosed. **(True/False)**
2. Borderline personality is among the most unstable of the personality disorders. **(True/False)**
3. Most people with psychopathic personality disorder are not habitually violent. **(True/False)**
4. Child abuse clearly causes DID. **(True/False)**
5. The media have played little role in the recent increase in DID diagnoses. **(True/False)**

Answers: (1) F; (2) T; (3) T; (4) F; (5) F

The enigma of schizophrenia

Psychiatrist Daniel Weinberger has called **schizophrenia** the 'cancer' of mental illness: it is perhaps the most severe of all disorders—and the most mysterious (Levy-Reiner, 1996). As we will discover, it is a devastating disorder of thought and emotion associated with a loss of contact with reality.

Schizophrenia
Severe disorder of thought and emotion associated with a loss of contact with reality.

Symptoms of schizophrenia: the shattered mind

Even today, many people confuse schizophrenia with DID (Wahl, 1997). Swiss psychiatrist Eugen Bleuler gave us the modern term 'schizophrenia' in 1911. The term literally means 'split mind', which no doubt contributed to the popular myth that the symptoms of schizophrenia stem from a split personality. You may have even heard people refer to a 'schizophrenic attitude' when explaining that they are 'of two minds' regarding an issue. Don't be misled. As Bleuler recognised, the difficulties of individuals with schizophrenia arise from disturbances in attention, thinking, language, emotion and relationships with others. In contrast to DID, which is supposedly characterised by multiple intact personalities, schizophrenia is characterised by one personality that is shattered.

Schizophrenia causes most of its sufferers' levels of functioning to plunge. More than half suffer from serious disabilities, such as an inability to hold a job and maintain close relationships (Harvey, Reichenberg & Bowie, 2006). Indeed, more than 10 percent of homeless people, with some estimates ranging as high as 45 percent, qualify for a diagnosis of schizophrenia (Folsom & Jeste, 2008). Individuals who experience schizophrenia comprise less than 1 percent of the population, with most estimates ranging from .4–.7 percent (Saha et al., 2005). Yet they make up half of the approximately 100 000 patients in state and county mental institutions in the United States (Grob, 1997). But there is some good news. Today, more than ever, people with schizophrenia can function in society, even though they may need to return periodically to hospitals for treatment (Lamb & Bachrach, 2001; Mueser & McGurk, 2004).

Researchers have struggled with the problem of describing schizophrenia since the eighteenth century, when Emil Kraepelin first outlined the features of patients with dementia praecox, meaning psychological deterioration in youth. But Kraepelin didn't get it quite right. Even though the typical onset of schizophrenia is in the mid-twenties for men and the late twenties for women, schizophrenia can also strike after the age of 45 (APA, 2000).

Delusions: fixed false beliefs

Among the hallmark symptoms of schizophrenia are **delusions**—strongly held fixed beliefs that have no basis in reality. Delusions

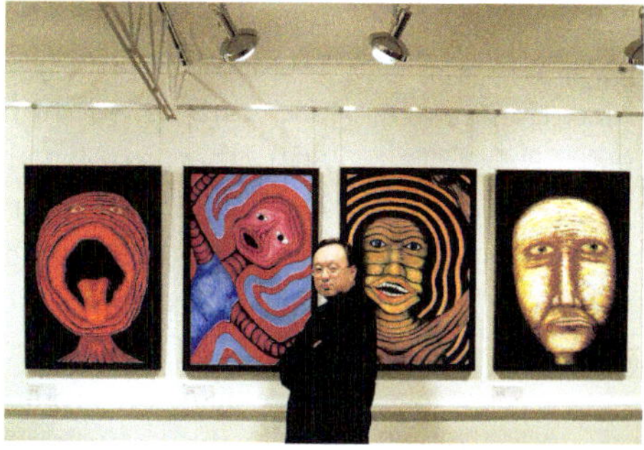

Melbourne's Cunningham Dax Collection contains 12 000 works of art by people who have experienced mental illness, some of whom received a diagnosis of schizophrenia. The collection preserves and exhibits these creative works to promote public understanding of people with mental illness. **(Source:** Michael Potter/Newspix/News Ltd.)

First-person account:

SCHIZOPHRENIA

'The reflection in the store window—it's me, isn't it? I know it is, but it's hard to tell. Glassy shadows, polished pastels, a jigsaw puzzle of my body, face, and clothes, with pieces disappearing whenever I move . . . Schizophrenia is painful, and it is craziness when I hear voices, when I believe people are following me, wanting to snatch my very soul. I am frightened, too, when every whisper, every laugh is about me; when newspapers suddenly contain cures, four-letter words shouting at me; when sparkles of light are demon eyes.' *(McGrath, 1984)*

Factoid

As many as one-half to two-thirds of people with schizophrenia improve significantly, although not completely, and a small percentage recover completely after a single episode (Harrow et al., 2005; Robinson et al., 2004). Researchers found that 20 high-functioning people with schizophrenia—which included doctors, an attorney and a chief executive—used such strategies as taking medication, getting exercise and adequate sleep, avoiding alcohol and crowds, and seeking social support to manage their illness successfully (Marder et al., 2008).

Delusions
Strongly held, fixed beliefs that have no basis in reality.

Psychotic symptoms
Psychological problems reflecting serious distortions in reality.

Hallucinations
Sensory perceptions that occur in the absence of an external stimulus.

are called **psychotic symptoms** because they represent a serious distortion of reality. Terrell, whom you met at the beginning of the chapter, experienced delusions that led to a suicide attempt.

Delusions commonly involve themes of persecution. One man believed that his colleagues had tapped his phone and conspired to get him fired. Another was convinced that a helicopter in the distance beamed the Beatles song 'All You Need Is Love' into his head to make him feel jealous and inadequate. Some patients have reported delusions of grandeur (greatness), including one who believed that she had discovered the cure for cancer, even though she had no medical training. Other delusions centre on the body and may include a firm belief that one is infested with brain parasites or even that one is dead (so-called Cotard's syndrome). Still others involve elaborate themes of sexuality, grandiosity, or guilt for imagined crimes. Australian researchers Langdon, Ward and Coltheart (2010) have proposed that delusions result from reasoning biases to which people with schizophrenia are prone. These include jumping to conclusions from limited information, personalising information (relating it to the self to an excessive degree) and lacking skill at theory of mind tasks. These biases leave delusion-prone people with an impaired capacity to experience a shared social reality with others.

Hallucinations: false perceptions

Among the other serious symptoms of schizophrenia are **hallucinations**: sensory perceptions that occur in the absence of an external stimulus. They can be auditory (involving hearing), olfactory (involving smell), gustatory (involving taste), tactile (involving the sense of touch) or visual. Most hallucinations in schizophrenia are auditory, usually consisting of voices. In some patients, hallucinated voices express disapproval or carry on a running commentary about the person's thoughts or actions. *Command hallucinations*, which tell patients what to do ('Go over to that man and tell him to shut up!') may be associated with a heightened risk of violence towards others (McNiel, Eisner & Binder, 2000). Incidentally, extremely vivid or detailed visual hallucinations—especially in the absence of auditory hallucinations—are usually signs of an organic (medical) disorder or substance abuse rather than schizophrenia (Shea, 1998).

Do your thoughts sound like voices in your head? Many people experience their thoughts as inner speech, which is entirely normal. Some researchers suggest that auditory hallucinations occur when people with schizophrenia believe mistakenly that their inner speech arises from a source outside themselves (Bentall, 2000; Frith, 1992; Thomas, 1997). Brain scans reveal that when people experience auditory hallucinations, brain areas associated with speech perception and production become activated (Jardri et al., 2011; McGuire, Shah & Murray, 1993).

Factoid

One of the more unusual delusion conditions is *folie à deux* (French for the 'folly of two'), known more technically as 'shared psychotic disorder' in DSM-5. In *folie à deux*, one person in a close relationship, often a marriage, induces the same delusion in his or her partner. For example, both partners may end up convinced that the government is poisoning their food (Silveira & Seeman, 1995). Rare cases of *folie à deux* in identical twins, *folie à trois* (involving three people) and *folie à famille* (involving an entire family) have also been reported.

Disorganised speech

Consider this example of the speech of a patient with schizophrenia: 'It was shockingly not of the best quality I have known all such evildoers coming out of doors with the best of intentions' (Grinnell, 2008). We can see that this patient skips from topic to topic in a disjointed way. Most researchers believe that this peculiar language results from thought disorder (Meehl, 1962; Stirk et al., 2008). The usual associations that we forge between two words, such as mother–child, are considerably weakened or highly unusual for individuals with schizophrenia (for example, mother–rug)

(Kuperberg et al., 2006). In severe forms, the resulting speech is so jumbled it is almost impossible to understand, leading psychologists to describe it as 'word salad'. Language problems, like thought disorder, point to fundamental impairments in schizophrenia in the ability to shift and maintain attention, which influence virtually every aspect of affected individuals' daily lives (Cornblatt & Keilp, 1994; Fuller et al., 2006).

Grossly disorganised behaviour or catatonia

When people develop schizophrenia, self-care, personal hygiene and motivation often deteriorate. They may avoid conversation; laugh, cry or swear inappropriately; or wear a warm coat on a sweltering summer day.

Catatonic symptoms involve motor (movement) problems, including holding the body in bizarre or rigid postures, curling up in a foetal position, resisting simple suggestions to move or speak, and pacing aimlessly. Catatonic individuals may also repeat a phrase in conversation in a parrot-like manner, a symptom called *echolalia*. At the opposite extreme, they may occasionally engage in bouts of frenzied, purposeless motor activity.

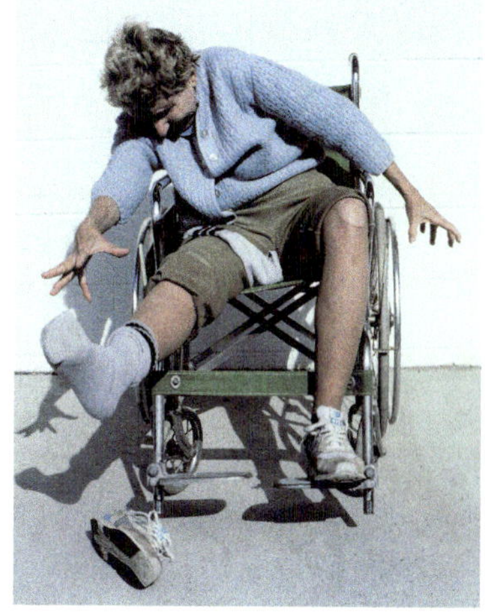

Catatonic individuals, like the person shown here, may permit their limbs to be moved to any position and maintain this posture for lengthy periods of time, a condition called 'waxy flexibility'.
(Source: Grunnitus Studio Photo Researchers.)

Explanations for schizophrenia: the roots of a shattered mind

Today, virtually all scientists believe that psychosocial factors play some role in schizophrenia. For example, there is evidence that immigrants and people living in large cities are at increased risk of developing the disorder (McGrath et al., 2008). Nevertheless, researchers also agree that these factors probably trigger the disorder only in people with a genetic vulnerability.

The family and expressed emotion

Early theories of schizophrenia mistakenly laid the blame for the condition on mothers, with so-called *schizophrenogenic* (schizophrenia-producing) mothers being the prime culprits. Based on informal observations of families of a schizophrenic child, some authors described such mothers as overprotective, smothering, insensitive, rejecting and controlling (Arieti, 1959; Lidz, 1973). Other theorists pointed the finger of blame at the interactions among all family members (Dolnick, 1998).

But as important as clinical experience can be in generating hypotheses, it does not provide an adequate arena for testing them. Indeed, these early studies were severely flawed, largely because they lacked control groups of people without schizophrenia. A now widely accepted rival hypothesis is that family members' responses are not the cause of schizophrenia, but instead are typically a response to the stressful experience of living with a severely disturbed person.

Catatonic symptoms
Motor problems, including extreme resistance to complying with simple suggestions, holding the body in bizarre or rigid postures, or curling up in a foetal position.

It is widely acknowledged that parents and family members do not 'cause' schizophrenia (Gottesman, 1991; Walker et al., 2004). Still, families may play a role in determining whether schizophrenia patients relapse. After leaving hospital, patients experience more than twice the likelihood of relapse (50–60 percent) when their relatives display high *expressed emotion* (EE)—that is, criticism, hostility and over-involvement (Brown et al., 1962; Butzlaff & Hooley, 1998; Kuipers, 2011). Criticism is especially predictive of relapse (Halweg et al., 1989; McCarty et al., 2004) and may result in part from relatives' frustrations in living with a person with schizophrenia who displays disruptive behaviours (Cechnicki et al., 2012). Indeed, EE may reflect family members' reactions to their loved one's schizophrenia as much as contribute to their loved one's relapse (King, 2000).

Schizophrenia: brain, biochemical and genetic findings

Research using a variety of technologies has uncovered intriguing biological clues to the causes of schizophrenia. We focus on three such clues: brain abnormalities, neurotransmitter differences and genetic findings.

BRAIN ABNORMALITIES. Research indicates that one or more of four fluid-filled structures called *ventricles* which cushion and nourish the brain, are typically enlarged in individuals with schizophrenia. This finding is important for two reasons. First, these brain areas frequently expand when others shrink (Barta et al., 1990; Raz & Raz, 1990). Second, deterioration in these areas is associated with thought disorder (Vita et al., 1995).

Other brain abnormalities in schizophrenia include increases in the size of the *sulci*, or spaces between the ridges of the brain (Cannon, Mednick & Parnas, 1989), and decreases in (a) the size of the temporal lobes (Boos et al., 2007; Job et al., 2005), (b) activation of the amygdala and hippocampus (Hempel et al., 2003), and (c) the symmetry of the brain's hemispheres (Luchins, Weinberger & Wyatt, 1982; Zivotofsky et al., 2007). Functional brain-imaging studies show that the frontal lobes of people with schizophrenia are less active than those of non-patients when engaged in demanding mental tasks (Andreasen et al., 1992; Knyazeva et al., 2008), a phenomenon called *hypofrontality*. Still, it is not clear whether these findings are causes or consequences of the disorder. For example, hypofrontality could be due to the tendency of patients with schizophrenia to concentrate less on tasks compared with other individuals. Researchers also need to rule out alternative explanations for brain underactivity that could arise from patients' diet, drinking and smoking habits, and medication use (Hanson & Gottesman, 2005).

Some studies have suggested that marijuana use in adolescence can bring about schizophrenia and other psychotic disorders in genetically vulnerable individuals (Arseneault et al., 2002; Compton et al., 2009; Degenhardt et al., 2009; Degenhardt & Hall, 2006). Nevertheless, it is difficult to pin down a causal relationship between marijuana use and schizophrenia for three reasons: (1) people who use marijuana are likely to use a variety of other drugs, which they may be reluctant to report on surveys; (2) individuals with schizophrenia may be more likely to use marijuana, so the causal arrow may be reversed; and (3) the rates of schizophrenia remained stable between 1970–2005 in the United Kingdom, although marijuana use increased over this period (Frisher et al., 2009). Still, people with a personal or family history of psychotic disorders, including schizophrenia, would be particularly ill advised to use marijuana.

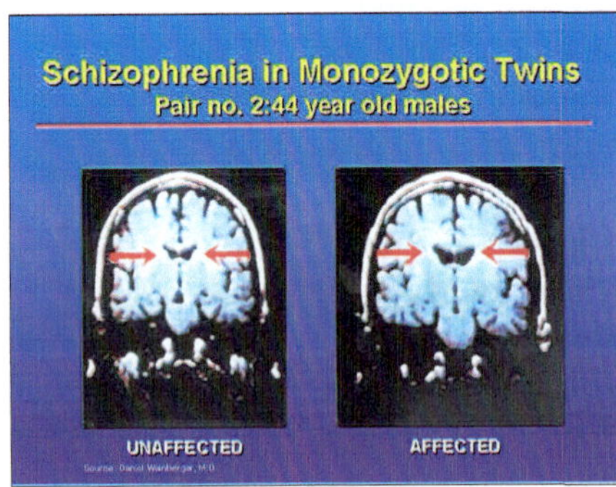

In one monozygotic (identical) twin with schizophrenia, the fluid-filled ventricles of the brain (*see red arrows*) are enlarged relative to his co-twin without schizophrenia. Such enlargement is typical in schizophrenia and probably reflects a deterioration in brain tissue surrounding the ventricles, which expand to fill the missing space.
(Source: Daniel R. Weinberger, MD. Courtesy NIH-Dr Daniel Weinberger, Clinical Brain Disorders Branch.)

NEUROTRANSMITTER DIFFERENCES. The biochemistry of the brain is one of the keys to unlocking the mystery of schizophrenia. One early explanation was the *dopamine hypothesis* (Carlsson, 1995; Keith et al., 1976; Nicol & Gottesman, 1983). The evidence for the role of dopamine in schizophrenia is mostly indirect. First, most anti-schizophrenia drugs block dopamine-receptor sites. To put it crudely, they 'slow down' nerve impulses by partially blocking the action of dopamine. Second, amphetamine, a stimulant drug that blocks the reuptake of dopamine, tends to make the symptoms of schizophrenia worse (Lieberman & Koreen, 1993; Snyder, 1975).

Nevertheless, the hypothesis that a simple excess of dopamine creates the symptoms of schizophrenia does not seem to fit the data. A better-supported rival hypothesis is that abnormalities in dopamine *receptors* produce these symptoms. Receptor sites in the brain appear to be highly specific for dopamine transmission. These sites respond uniquely to drugs designed to reduce psychotic symptoms and are associated with difficulties in attention, memory and motivation (Busatto et al., 1995; Keefe & Henry, 1994; Reis et al., 2004).

These findings provide evidence for a direct tie between dopamine pathways and symptoms of schizophrenia, such as paranoia. As we have seen, some of the symptoms of schizophrenia represent distortions or excesses of normal functions and include hallucinations, delusions and disorganised speech and behaviour. We can contrast these so-called *positive symptoms* with *negative symptoms*, which reflect a decrease in or loss of normal functions. These symptoms include social withdrawal and diminished motivations, decreased expression of emotions, and brief and limited speech (Andreasen et al., 1995). People with schizophrenia are less impaired when their symptoms are predominantly positive rather than negative (Harvey, Reichenberg & Bowie, 2006). There is evidence that positive symptoms result from dopamine excess in some brain regions and negative symptoms from dopamine deficits in other brain regions (Davis et al., 1991). However, the cause of negative symptoms can be difficult to pinpoint, because they may arise from prolonged institutionalisation and medication side-effects. Dopamine is probably only one of several neurotransmitters that play a role in schizophrenia; other likely candidates include noradrenaline, glutamate and serotonin (Cornblatt, Green & Walker, 1999; Grace, 1991).

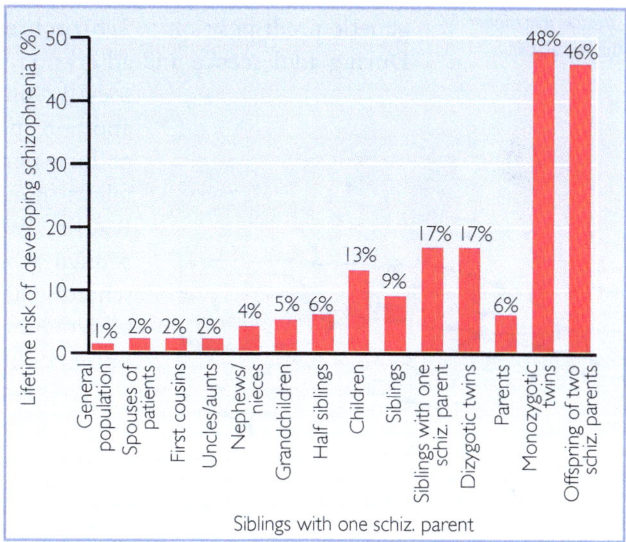

Figure 5.4 Schizophrenia risk and the family. The lifetime risk of developing schizophrenia is largely a function of how closely an individual is genetically related to a person with schizophrenia.
(**Source:** Based on data from Gottesman [1991].)

GENETIC INFLUENCES. Still unresolved is the question of which biological deficits are present prior to schizophrenia and which appear after the disorder begins (Seidman et al., 2003). The seeds of schizophrenia are often sown well before birth and lie partly in individuals' genetic endowment. As can be seen in Figure 5.4, being the offspring of someone diagnosed with schizophrenia greatly increases one's odds of developing the disorder. If we have a sibling with schizophrenia, we have about a 1 in 10 chance of developing the disorder; these odds are about 10 times higher than those of the average person. As genetic similarity increases, so does the risk of schizophrenia

Still, it is possible that the environment accounts for these findings because siblings not only share genes but also grow up in the same family. To eliminate this ambiguity, researchers have conducted twin studies. These studies provide convincing support for a genetic influence on schizophrenia. If we have an identical twin with schizophrenia, our risk rises to about 50 percent. An identical twin of a person with schizophrenia is about three times as likely as a fraternal twin of a person with schizophrenia to develop the disorder, and about 50 times as likely as an average person (Gottesman & Shields, 1972; Kendler & Diehl, 1993; Meehl, 1962). Adoption data also point to a genetic influence. Even when children who have a biological parent with schizophrenia are adopted by parents with no hint of the disorder, their risk of schizophrenia is greater than that of a person with no biological relative with schizophrenia (Gottesman, 1991). Interestingly, scientists have identified structural brain abnormalities, like ventricular enlargement and decreases in brain volume, in the healthy close relatives of patients with schizophrenia, further suggesting that genetic influences produce a vulnerability to schizophrenia (Staal et al., 2000).

Vulnerability to schizophrenia: diathesis-stress models

Diathesis-stress models Perspective proposing that mental disorders are a joint product of a genetic vulnerability, called a diathesis, and stressors that trigger this vulnerability.

Diathesis-stress models incorporate much of what we know about schizophrenia. Such models propose that schizophrenia, along with many other mental disorders, is a joint product of a genetic vulnerability, called a *diathesis*, and stressors that trigger this vulnerability (Meehl, 1962; Walker & DiForio, 1997; Zubin & Spring, 1977).

Paul Meehl (1990) suggested that approximately 10 percent of the population has a genetic predisposition to schizophrenia. What are people with this predisposition like? During adolescence and adulthood, they may strike us as 'odd ducks'. They may seem socially uncomfortable, and their speech, thought processes and perceptions may impress us as unusual. They are likely to endorse items on psychological tests such as 'Occasionally, I have felt as though my body did not exist' (Chapman, Chapman & Raulin, 1978). Such individuals display symptoms of psychosis-proneness or *schizotypal personality disorder*. Most people with schizotypal personality disorder do not develop full-blown schizophrenia, perhaps because they have a weaker genetic vulnerability or because they have experienced fewer stressors.

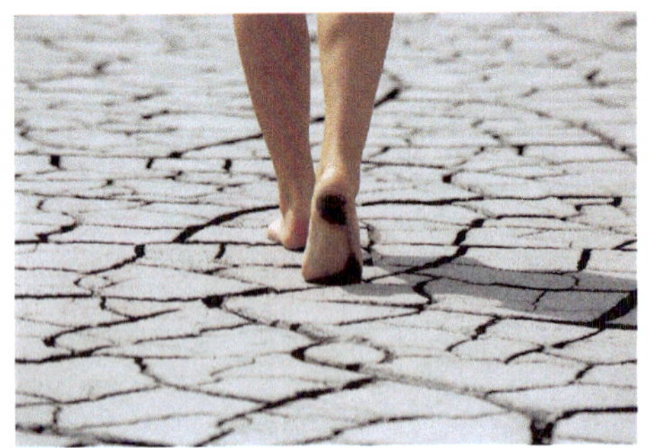

Many people with schizotypal personality disorder are prone to 'magical thinking'—the belief that their thoughts can influence actions through supernatural or otherwise mysterious processes. For example, they may believe that stepping on a crack in the pavement will create misfortune. **(Source:** Monkey Business Images/Dreamstime.)

Factoid

Data show that more people with schizophrenia are born in the winter and spring than at other times of the year (Davies et al., 2003; Torrey et al., 1997). The reason for this strange finding doesn't appear to lie in astrology: certain viral infections that affect pregnant women and that may trigger schizophrenia in vulnerable foetuses are most common in winter months.

Well before people experience symptoms of schizophrenia, we can identify 'early warning signs' or markers of vulnerability to this condition. People with schizotypal personality disorder display some of these markers, which include social withdrawal, thought and movement abnormalities (Mittal et al., 2007; Walker, Baum & DiForio, 1998), learning and memory deficits (Volgmaier et al., 2000), temporal lobe abnormalities (Siever & Davis, 2004), impaired attention (Keefe et al., 1997) and eye-movement disturbances when tracking moving objects (Iacono, 1985; Lenzenweger et al., 2007). Their difficulties extend to the social realm and begin early in life. Elaine Walker and Richard Lewine (1990) found that people who viewed home movies of siblings interacting could identify which children later developed schizophrenia at better-than-chance levels. Even at an early age, vulnerable children's lack of emotions and decreased eye contact and social responsiveness tipped off observers. This design is valuable because it gets around the retrospective bias introduced by asking adults to report on their childhood experiences.

However, most people with a vulnerability to schizophrenia do not develop it. Whether someone ends up with the disorder depends on the impact of events that interfere with normal development. Children of women who had the flu during their second trimester of pregnancy (Brown et al., 2004; Mednick et al., 1988), suffered starvation early in pregnancy (Susser & Lin, 1992) or experienced complications while giving birth (Weinberger, 1987) are at a somewhat heightened risk of schizophrenia. Viral infections in the uterus during pregnancy may also play a key role in triggering certain cases of schizophrenia

(Walker & DiForio, 1997). But the great majority of people exposed to infection or trauma before birth never show signs of schizophrenia. So these events probably create problems only for people who are genetically vulnerable to begin with (Cornblatt, Green & Walker, 1999; Verdoux, 2004).

Assess your knowledge — FACT or FICTION?

1. Delusions are rare in schizophrenia. **(True/False)**
2. Most hallucinations in schizophrenia are visual. **(True/False)**
3. Schizophrenogenic mothers often cause schizophrenia. **(True/False)**
4. The evidence for the dopamine hypothesis is mostly indirect. **(True/False)**
5. There is little support for the genetic transmission of schizophrenia. **(True/False)**

Answers: (1) F; (2) F; (3) F; (4) T; (5) F

Childhood disorders: recent controversies

Although in this chapter we have focused primarily on disorders of adulthood, we now close with a few words about childhood disorders, especially those that have been front and centre in the public eye. Each of the disorders we consider—autism spectrum disorders, attention-deficit/hyperactivity disorder, and early-onset bipolar disorder—have garnered their share of controversy in the popular media and the scientific community.

Autism spectrum disorders

One in 88. According to the Centers for Disease Control (CDC, 2013) that is the proportion of individuals with **autism spectrum disorder (ASD)**, a category in DSM-5 that includes autistic disorder (better known as autism) and Asperger's disorder, a less severe form of autism. DSM-5 contends that the symptoms of autism can best be described as on a continuum of severity, rather than in categorical terms, with many children with Asperger's disorder being able to function effectively in a school or occupational setting.

Autism spectrum disorder (ASD) DSM-5 category that includes autistic disorder and Asperger's disorder.

Although the proportion of people with ASD may not seem all that high, it is remarkably high compared with the figure of 1 in 2000 to 2500, which researchers had until recently accepted for many years (Wing & Potter, 2002). Statistics from the US Department of Education revealed a 657 percent increase in the rates of autism (technically called 'infantile autism') across the country from 1993 to 2003. Figure 5.5 dramatic upsurges in the prevalence of autism have led many researchers and educators, and even some politicians, to speak of an autism 'epidemic' (Kippes & Garrison, 2006). But is the epidemic real?

Individuals with autism are marked by persistent deficits in language, social bonding and imagination, sometimes accompanied by intellectual impairment (APA, 2013). The DSM-5 breaks down the symptoms of autism spectrum disorders into social impairments and repetitive or restrictive behaviours, which can include repetitive speech or movements, resistance to change, and highly specialised and limited interests and preoccupation with certain foods or unusual objects such as light bulbs. The causes of autism remain mysterious, although twin studies suggest that genetic influences play a prominent role (Hallmayer et al., 2011; Rutter, 2000). The children of both the youngest and oldest parents of twins studied in Sweden

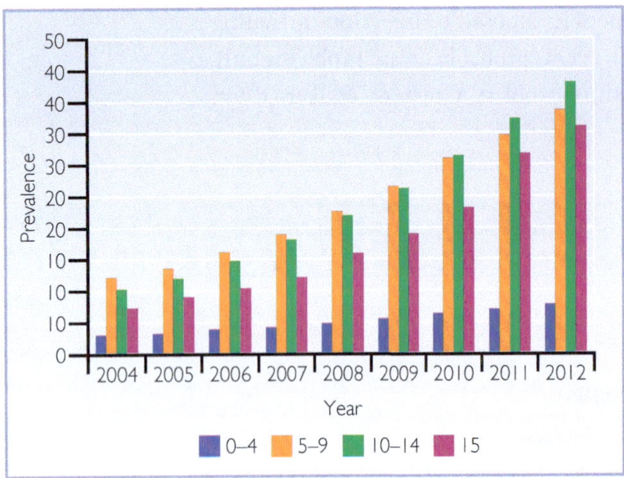

Figure 5.5 The autism epidemic in Australia, 2004–2012, by age group. The fact that autism diagnoses have been skyrocketing is not controversial—but the reasons for the increase are.
(**Source:** Reproduced courtesy of Bob Buckley.)

were at highest risk of developing ASD, but the genetic mechanisms underlying this association between parental age and ASD remain unknown (Lundström et al., 2010). Still, genetic influences alone cannot easily account for an astronomical rise in a disorder's prevalence over the span of a decade. It is therefore not surprising that researchers have looked to environmental variables to explain this bewildering increase. In particular, some investigators have pointed their fingers squarely at one potential culprit: vaccines (Rimland, 2004).

Much of the hype surrounding the vaccine–autism link was fuelled by a study of only 12 children in the late 1990s (Wakefield et al., 1998), demonstrating an apparent linkage between autistic symptoms and the MMR vaccine—the vaccine for mumps, measles, and rubella, also known as German measles. (The journal *Lancet*, which published the study, officially retracted it in 2010, saying that Wakefield never received ethical clearance for the investigation and that the article contained false claims about participant recruitment.) The symptoms of autism usually become most apparent shortly after the age of two, not long after infants have received MMR and other vaccinations for a host of diseases. Indeed, tens of thousands of parents insist that their children developed autism following the MMR vaccine or following vaccines containing a preservative known as *thimerosol*, which is present in many mercury-bearing vaccines.

Nevertheless, studies in the United States, Europe and Japan have failed to replicate the association between the MMR vaccine and autism, strongly suggesting that the seeming correlation between vaccinations and autism was a mirage (Offit, 2008). The results of several large American, European and Japanese studies show that even as the rate of MMR vaccinations remained constant or declined, the rate of autism diagnoses continued to soar (Herbert, Sharp & Gaudiano, 2002; Honda, Shimizu & Rutter, 2005). Moreover, even after the Danish government stopped administering thimerosol-containing vaccines, the prevalence of autism still skyrocketed (Madsen et al., 2002).

Many parents of children with autism probably fell prey to *illusory correlation* they had 'seen' a statistical association that did not exist. Their error was entirely understandable. Given that their children had received vaccines and developed autistic symptoms at around the same time, it was only natural to perceive an association between the two events.

Making matters more complex, recent research calls into question the very existence of the autism epidemic (Grinker, 2007; Wilson, 2005). Most previous investigators had neglected to take into account an alternative explanation—changes in diagnostic practices over time, which have expanded the autism diagnosis to include more mildly affected children, including those with *Asperger's disorder* (which appears to be a mild form of autism). Evidence suggests that more liberal diagnostic criteria rather than vaccines can account for most, if not all, of the reported autism epidemic (Gernsbacher, Dawson & Goldsmith, 2005; Lilienfeld & Arkowitz, 2007).

Of course, at least a small part of the epidemic might be genuine, and some still unidentified environmental cause could account for the increase. But in evaluating the evidence, we should ask ourselves a critical question: which is the more parsimonious explanation of a 657 percent increase within one decade—a vaccine that has yet to be shown to produce any increase in the symptoms of autism, or a simple change in diagnostic practices?

Attention-deficit/hyperactivity disorder and early-onset bipolar disorder

Even the best-adjusted children often appear overactive, energetic and restless. But children with **attention-deficit/hyperactivity disorder (ADHD)** often behave like caricatures of the exuberant child. You probably know or have known someone with ADHD: 7-8 percent of Australian children aged between 4 – 7 years satisfy the diagnostic criteria for the disorder (Lawrence et al., 2015). Males experience a higher prevalence of ADHD (10.4% compared with 4.3% for females) (Lawrence et al., 2015) and approximately sixty percent of children with ADHD continue to display ADHD symptoms into their mid 20's (Sibley et al., 2016). The ADHD diagnosis subsumes two subtypes: (1) with hyperactivity and (2) without hyperactivity, in which inattention is predominant (APA, 2013).

AUTISM
IS JUST
THE TIP OF
THE
ICEBERG
MMR
AND
AUTISM
WHAT IS
WRONG WITH
MY CHILD?

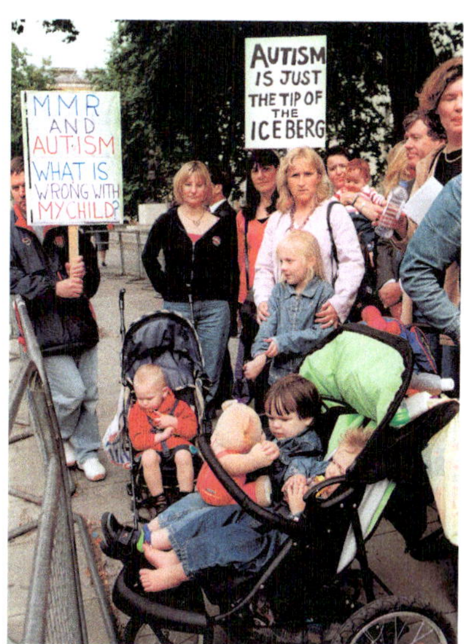

Tens of thousands of parents remain convinced that vaccines trigger autism, despite scientific evidence to the contrary.
(**Source:** Janine Weidel Photolibrary/Alamy.)

Symptoms of ADHD

The first signs of ADHD may be evident as early as infancy. Parents often report that children with ADHD are fussy, cry incessantly, and frequently move and shift their position in the crib (Wolke, Rizzo & Woods, 2002). By three years of age, they are constantly walking or climbing, and are restless and prone to emotional outbursts. But it is not until primary school that their behaviour patterns are likely to be labelled 'hyperactive' and a treatment referral made. Teachers complain that such children will not remain in their seats, follow directions or pay attention, and that they display temper tantrums with little provocation. Such children often struggle with learning disabilities, difficulties with processing verbal information, and poor balance and coordination (Jerome, 2000; Mangeot et al., 2001). By middle childhood, academic problems and disruptive behaviour are frequently evident.

A high level of physical activity often diminishes as children with ADHD mature and approach adolescence. Nevertheless, by adolescence, impulsiveness, restlessness, inattention, problems with peers, delinquency and academic difficulties comprise a patchwork of adjustment problems (Barkley, 2006; Hoza, 2007; Kelly, 2009). Alcohol and substance abuse are frequent (Molina & Pelham, 2003), and many adolescents with ADHD appear in juvenile court as a result of running away from home, skipping school and stealing (Foley, Carlton & Howell, 1996). Adults with ADHD are at increased risk for accidents and injuries (Woodward, Fergusson & Horwood, 2000), divorce (Wymbs et al., 2008), unemployment and contact with the legal system (Hinshaw, 2002).

Factoid

Although attentional problems are a key component of ADHD, many children with the condition can concentrate when sufficiently motivated. Sit with a child with ADHD playing his or her favourite computer game, and you will probably be impressed with the child's intense concentration. This curious phenomenon occurs because children with ADHD can sometimes 'hyperfocus' when something captures their attention; however, they experience difficulty shifting their attention to focus on tasks that are not attention-grabbing, such as homework and chores (Barkley, 1997).

ADHD appears to be genetically influenced in many cases, with estimates of its heritability as high as .80 (Swanson & Castellanos, 2002). What may be inherited are: (a) abnormalities in genes that influence serotonin, dopamine and norepinephrine; (b) a smaller brain volume; and (c) decreased activation in the frontal areas of the brain (Monastra, 2008).

People with ADHD can be treated successfully with stimulant medications. Nevertheless, these medications occasionally have serious side-effects, making accurate diagnosis a serious public health issue. Yet an accurate diagnosis of ADHD can be problematic. A host of conditions that can cause problems in attention and behavioural control, including traumatic brain injuries, diabetes, thyroid problems, vitamin deficiencies, anxiety and depression, must

Attention-deficit/hyperactivity disorder (ADHD)
Childhood condition marked by excessive inattention, impulsivity and activity.

first be ruled out (Monastra, 2008). In addition, there is sometimes a fine line between highly energetic children and children with mild ADHD. As a consequence, some scholars have expressed concerns that ADHD is over-diagnosed in some settings (LeFever, Arcona & Antonuccio, 2003), although others point to evidence that some children with ADHD are actually overlooked by many diagnosticians (Sciutto & Eisenberg, 2007).

Many children have problems concentrating. There can be a fine line between children who have trouble paying attention in class and children who are diagnosed with ADHD.

The controversy over early-onset bipolar disorder

Perhaps the most controversial diagnostic challenge is distinguishing children with ADHD from children with bipolar disorder (Meyer & Carlson, 2008). The diagnosis of early-onset bipolar disorder was once rare, but ballooned from only .42 percent of cases of outpatient mental health visits in the early 1990s to 6.67 percent of such visits in 2003 (Moreno et al., 2007), raising concerns about its over-diagnosis. Children are particularly likely to receive a diagnosis of early-onset bipolar disorder when they show rapid mood changes, reckless behaviour, irritability and aggression (McClellan, Kowatch & Findling, 2007). Popular books like *The Bipolar Child* (Papolos & Papolos, 2007), which list these and other symptoms, catch the eye of many parents with troubled children and raise concerns about bipolar disorder. Yet a moment's reflection suggests that many children fit this description, and surely many children with ADHD can be so characterised. Because 60–90 percent of children with bipolar disorder are also diagnosed with ADHD, a hypothesis to consider is that many children diagnosed with bipolar disorder are merely those with severe symptoms of ADHD, such as extreme temper outbursts and mood swings (Geller et al., 2002; Kim & Miklowitz, 2002). To address concerns about the over-diagnosis of bipolar disorder in children, DSM-5 developed a new category of *disruptive mood dysregulation disorder* to diagnose children with persistent irritability and frequent behaviour outbursts (APA, 2013). Nevertheless, the validity of this condition remains controversial, and some experts have expressed concerns that it may result in labelling children with repeated temper tantrums as pathological (Frances, 2012). A thorough evaluation involving parents, teachers and mental health professionals is essential to an accurate diagnosis of early-onset bipolar disorder, as well as ADHD.[A]

Assess your knowledge — FACT or FICTION?

1. The rates of diagnosed autism have sharply declined in recent years. **(True/False)**
2. Most cases of autism are caused by vaccines. **(True/False)**
3. More boys than girls are diagnosed with ADHD. **(True/False)**
4. Parents first notice their children's attention problems in primary school. **(True/False)**
5. Children with bipolar disorder are likely also to be diagnosed with ADHD. **(True/False)**

Answers: (1) F; (2) F; (3) T; (4) F; (5) T

[A]Lilienfeld, S. O., Lynn, S. J., Namy, L. L., Woolf, N. J., Jamieson, G., Marks, A., & Slaughter, V. (2015). *Psychological disorders: When adaptation breaks down.* In S. O. Lilienfeld, S. J. Lynn, L. L. Namy, N. J. Woolf, G. Jamieson, A. Marks, & V. Slaughter (Eds.), *Psychology: From inquiry to understanding* (2nd ed., pp. 682-722). Melbourne, VIC: Pearson Australia..

Summary

Conceptions of mental illness: yesterday and today

- Psychologists and psychiatrists have proposed many criteria for defining mental disorder, including – statistical rarity, subjective distress, impairment, societal disapproval and biological dysfunction
- Psychiatric diagnoses are shaped not only by history, but by culture
- Psychiatric classification and diagnosis can help to pin point the psychological problem a person is experiencing – enabling treatment.
- The official system for classifying individuals with mental disorders is the *Diagnostic and Statistical Manual of Mental Disorders (DSM)*

Anxiety disorders: the many faces of worry and fear

- Anxiety disorders are among the most prevalent of all mental disorders
- There are different types of anxiety. Some of the most common anxiety disorders include: Generalised anxiety disorder, panic disorder, obsessive compulsive disorder (OCD) and posttraumatic stress disorder (PTSD)

Mood disorders and suicide

- Due to its frequency, depression has been referred to as the 'common cold' of psychological disorders
- There are many explanations for major depressive disorder, including: life events, interpersonal, behavioural and cognitive factors, as well as the role of biology

Personality and dissociative disorders: the disrupted and divided self

- Of all psychological conditions, personality disorders are historically among the least reliably diagnosed
- There are different types of personality disorders, including borderline personality disorder – which can involve an individual being extremely impulsive, taking risks, having an explosive temper and having unstable moods.

The enigma of schizophrenia

- Schizophrenia is thought to be the most severe of all mood disorders - associated with a loss of contact with reality
- When people develop schizophrenia, they can experience grossly disorganised behaviour or catatonia

Childhood disorders: recent controversies

- There are many developmental disorders that present in children, including: autism spectrum disorder, attention-deficit/hyperactivity disorder, and early-onset bipolar disorder
- Individuals with autism are marked by persistent deficits in language, social bonding and imagination, sometimes accompanied by intellectual impairment
- Attention-deficit/hyperactivity disorder (ADHD) is a condition marked by excessive inattention, impulsivity and activity.

Review questions

A. Fill in the missing words to complete the following statements.

1. Psychiatric disorders are not only shaped by history, but also by ____________.
2. The official system for classifying individuals with mental disorders is the ____________.
3. As per the DSM-5, to diagnose a person with major depressive disorder, an individual is required to exhibit at least five of nine symptoms, including fatigue, ____________, problems concentrating, and _______________ over a ____ week period, with the requirement that the individual experience with depressed mood, _____________, or both.

B. Read the following statements and answer with the most correct definition.

4. The co-occurrence of two or more diagnoses within the same person is defined as ________.
5. Marked emotional disturbance after experiencing or witnessing a severely distressing and/or stressful event is known as _______________________.
6. If a child is presents with excessive inattention, impulsivity and activity, they may be diagnosed with ________________________.

C. Please select one statement that best answers each of the following questions.

7. The main distinguishing feature of psychotic disorders is
   a) confusion of fantasy and reality
   b) antisocial conduct
   c) preoccupying anxiety
   d) neurotic behavior
8. An individual who has an extreme lack of self-confidence and who allows others to run his or her life is said to have a(n) ______________ personality.
   a) dependent
   b) narcissistic
   c) unreasonable
   d) disruptive
9. A rare condition in which detached personalities exist in the same individual is called
   a) dissociative identity disorder
   b) split personality
   c) schizophrenia
   d) amnesia
10. Conversion disorder and hypochondriasis are classified as
    a) demonic disorders
    b) somatoform disorders
    c) psychosomatic disorders
    d) somatisation disorders
11. In most anxiety disorders, the person's distress is
    a) focused on a precise situation
    b) related to regular life stresses
    c) greatly out of proportion to the situation
    d) based on a physical cause

12. Simon has been extremely anxious for much of the past year, but can't explain why. There is a good chance that he is experiencing
    a) a generalised anxiety disorder
    b) sociopathy
    c) psychosis
    d) a nervous breakdown

13. Irrational and very specific fears that persist even when there is no real danger to a person are called
    a) anxieties
    b) detachments
    c) phobias
    d) obsessions

14. False beliefs that are held even when the facts contradict them are called
    a) daydreams
    b) hallucinations
    c) illusions
    d) delusions

15. Uneasiness in social situations, fear of judgement, and timidity are characteristic of what personality disorder?
    a) histrionic
    b) obsessive-compulsive
    c) schizoid
    d) avoidant

16. A person who experiences a long series of imagined physical complaints suffers from
    a) a conversion response
    b) somatisation disorder
    c) a traumatic disorder
    d) hysteria

17. Which of the following is characteristic of a dissociative disorder?
    a) phobic disorder
    b) amnesia
    c) paranoia
    d) mood disorder

18. Which of the following is a dissociative disorder?
    a) depression
    b) neurotic disorder
    c) multiple personality
    d) paranoia

19. Sensory experiences that occur in the absence of a stimulus are called
    a.) deceptions.
    b) hallucinations
    c) delusions
    d) substance episodes

20. An individual who is quite concerned with orderliness, perfectionism, and a rigid routine might be classified as a(n) ____________ personality.
    a) moody
    b) obsessive-compulsive
    c) schizoid
    d) avoidant

CHAPTER 6

Health-Risk Behaviours

The content in this section has been compiled from:

Morrison et al., Chapter 3

Morrison, V., Bennet, P., Butow, P., Mullan, B., & White, K. (2015). Health-risk behaviour. In V. Morrison, P. Bennet, P. Butow, B. Mullan, & K. White (Eds.), *Introduction to health psychology in Australia* (2nd ed., p. 63). Melbourne, VIC: Pearson Australia.

Donatelle, Chapter 10

Donatelle, R. J. (2015). Reaching and maintaining a healthy weight. In R. J. Donatelle (Ed.), *Health: The basics* (11th ed., pp. 293–294, 297–298). Upper Saddle River, NJ: Pearson Education.

Donatelle, Chapter 11

Donatelle, R. J. (2015). Improving your personal fitness. In R. J. Donatelle (Ed.), *Health: The basics* (11th ed., pp. 330–332). Upper Saddle River, NJ: Pearson Education.

Donatelle, Chapter 7

Donatelle, R. J. (2015). Recognizing and avoiding addiction and drug abuse. In R. J. Donatelle (Ed.), *Health: The basics* (11th ed., pp. 206–226). Upper Saddle River, NJ: Pearson Education.

Donatelle, Chapter 8

Donatelle, R. J.(2015). Drinking alcohol responsibly and ending tobacco use. In R. J. Donatelle (Ed.), *Health: The basics* (11th ed., pp. 228–258). Upper Saddle River, NJ: Pearson Education.

CHAPTER 6

Health-Risk Behaviours

Health-risk behaviours include behaviours that exert a compelling influence on health. Many health-risk behaviours are established during adolescence, and are often maintained into adulthood, affecting health and wellbeing in later life. Such behaviours that are reviewed in this chapter include tobacco use, alcohol consumption, physical activity and diet.

After studying this chapter, you should be able to:

- Define and describe health behaviour
- Describe what health behaviours are associated with increased health risks
- Describe environmental and psychosocial factors contributing to obesity
- Describe the benefits of regular physical activity in the prevention of chronic health conditions
- Describe drug-related behaviours: misuse and abuse
- Explain the biopsychosocial effects of alcohol and tobacco use on health.

What is health behaviour?

Kasl and Cobb (1966, p. 246) defined health behaviour as 'any activity undertaken by a person believing themselves to be healthy for the purposes of preventing disease or detecting it at an asymptomatic stage'. This definition was influenced by a medical perspective in that it assumes that healthy people engage in particular behaviour, such as exercise or seeking medical attention, purely to prevent their chance of disease onset. However, this very specific definition should be viewed with caution. Many people engage in a variety of apparently health-related behaviour, such as exercise, for reasons other than disease prevention, including weight control, appearance, as a means of gaining social contacts, and pleasure. Nevertheless, whether intentional or not, engaging in health behaviour may prevent disease and may also prevent the progression of disease once it is established. This perspective was acknowledged by Harris and Guten (1979, p. 18), who defined health behaviour as 'behaviour performed by an individual, regardless of his/her perceived health status, with the purpose of protecting, promoting or maintaining his/her health'. According to this definition, health behaviour could include the behaviour of 'unhealthy' people. For example, an individual who has heart disease may change their diet to help to limit its progression, just as a healthy person may change their diet in order to reduce their future risk of heart disease. Further elaboration of definitions of health behaviour was provided by Matarazzo (1984), who distinguished between what he termed **behavioural pathogens** and **behavioural immunogens**. In spite of definitional differences, health behaviour research generally adopts the view that health behaviour is that which is associated with an individual's health status, regardless of current health or motivations.

Behavioural pathogen
A behavioural practice thought to be damaging to health (e.g. smoking).

Behavioural immunogen
A behavioural practice considered to be health-protective (e.g. exercise).

The World Health Organization (2002) defines 'risk' as 'a probability of an adverse outcome, or a factor that raises this probability' (p. 7). Many of these risks are behavioural, although others are environmental, such as pollution or poverty. It is worth remembering that what is considered health-risk behaviour has changed over the past century as medical understanding has developed; for example, we know now that smoking and excessive exposure to the sun carry significant risks for development of some cancers, whereas our ancestors did not. To further muddy the waters, there is also evidence of health benefits of some behaviours considered generally as 'risky'. Perhaps the best example is sun exposure, which is receiving growing attention in relation to skin cancer risk, yet in the early twentieth century sun exposure was considered useful in the treatment of skin tuberculosis and today sunlight therapy may be offered in the treatment of skin disorders. Furthermore, there is some tentative evidence relating vitamin D levels (which are raised with sunlight exposure) to reduced cardiovascular risk (Judd & Tangpricha, 2009; Norman & Powell, 2014). Later in this chapter we also raise the issue of beneficial effects of moderate alcohol consumption.[A]

Factors contributing to overweight and obesity

Although excess calorie intake and too little physical activity are major contributors to excess weight, other factors, including genetics and physiology, also predispose us to excess body fat. Newer thinking about reducing obesity risk involves a more ecological approach that seeks to change obesogenic environmental and contextual factors that contribute to obesity. It isn't just a simple "eat this, not that, and exercise more" mantra for prevention. Learned behaviour in the home, influences at school and in social environments, media influences, and the environments where we live, work, and play are important to our weight profiles

[A]Morrison, V., Bennet, P., Butow, P., Mullan, B., & White, K. (2015). Health-risk behaviour. In *Introduction to health psychology in Australia* (2nd ed., p. 63). Melbourne, VIC: Pearson Australia.

(Spruijt-Metz, 2012; Affenito, Franko, Striegel-Moore & Thompson. 2011). Experts realise that a complex web of interactive factors influences what we eat, how much we eat and when we eat, as well as how we expend energy. Figuring out what these factors are and developing key strategies to reduce risk is key (Spruijt-Metz, 2012; Affenito et al. 2011).[B]

Environmental factors

Environmental factors have come to play a large role in weight maintenance. Automobiles, remote controls, desk jobs, and long sessions on computers and other devices all cause us to sit more and move less, and this lack of physical activity causes a decrease in energy expenditure. Time our grandparents may have spent going for a walk after dinner is now more frequently devoted to watching television, playing video games, texting, or reading online. Coupled with our culture of eating more, it's a recipe for weight gain.

Greater access to high-calorie foods

More foods that are high in calories and low in nutrients exist today compared to the past. There are many environmental factors that can prompt us to consume them:

- Advertising constantly bombards us with messages that promote eating—emphasising good taste over the poor nutritional value of most of what is being sold.
- Super-sized portions are now the norm as larger dishes, cups, and serving utensils mask serving sizes and lead to increased calorie and fat intake.
- Drinks like lattes and extra large sodas add many extra calories.
- Families have increased reliance on restaurant and store-bought convenience foods, which tend to be higher in calories than food made from scratch.
- Bottle-feeding infants may increase energy intake relative to breast-feeding.
- Misleading food labels confuse consumers about serving sizes.
- Fast-food restaurants, cafes, vending machines, and quick-stop markets are everywhere, offering easy access to food at all hours.

The good news is that the consumption of refined and added sugar in Australia has decreased with recent data revealing a 23% reduction in sugar consumption between 1995 and 2011 (Barclay & Brand-Miller, 2011; Ridoutt et al., 2016). Some believe that a greater awareness of the perils of consuming too many high-sugar soft drinks and beverages has caused people to make mindful choices about the foods they are eating. Others worry that we should be seeing weight loss if we are consuming fewer calories. One possibility is that we are exercising less than ever, thereby offsetting any potential weight loss (Dietz et al. 2013).

Early sabotage: a youthful start on obesity

Children have always loved junk food. However, today's youth have easy access to a vast array of high-fat, high-calorie foods, exercise less, have fewer physical education requirements in schools, and are more obese than ever before. Over one in four Australian children and adolescents are now overweight or obese, and rates are two times higher than for their parent's generation (Australian Bureau of Statistics, 2015). Sedentary activities such as social media sites, video games, and television have replaced vigorous physical play for many, and school policies have also been a factor in the growth of childhood obesity. For decades the trend was to eliminate recess and physical education classes while school canteens were much more likely to serve students pizza and fries than healthy food. The classic American suburb, with its high-speed roads and lack of sidewalks, has also impacted childhood obesity.

[B]Donatelle, R. J.(2015). Reaching and maintaining a healthy weight. In *Health: The basics* (11th ed., pp. 293–294). Upper Saddle River, NJ: Pearson Education Inc.

Even when parks or schools are near home, it may be too dangerous for children to walk to them. Similarly, the availability of transport in Australia, has impacted on the increase in childhood obesity, with more children opting to travel by motorised transport to and from school (Gerrard, 2009).

In addition, youth are at risk because of factors that are only beginning to be understood. Several studies have suggested that maternal nutrition, diabetes, and obesity—particularly where there is high fat consumption during pregnancy—may play a role in predisposing the fetus to becoming overweight or obese prior to puberty and early onset puberty (Poston.,Harthoorn & Van Der Beek., 2011; Connor et al., 2012). Research also shows that race and ethnicity seem to be intricately interwoven with environmental factors in increasing risks to young people (Schuster et al., 2012; Odgen et al., 2012).

On top of potential physical problems of obesity, obese kids often face weight-related stigma and vicious comments about their size from their peers. Obesity stigma is a major threat to overweight and obese children's self-esteem; it increases risk of suicidal thoughts, anxiety, and depression, contributes to low grades in school, and decreases likelihood of physical activity. Obese youth may feel a lack of social acceptance, be bullied by classmates, and develop feelings of mistrust and fear of others (Puhl & King, 2013; Schafer & Ferraro, 2011).

Psychosocial and socioeconomic factors

The relationship of weight problems to emotional insecurities, needs, and wants remains difficult to assess. What we do know is that eating tends to be a focal point of people's lives and is in part a social ritual associated with companionship, celebration, and enjoyment. It can also be used to soothe fears, sadness, and worry—hence the term *comfort food*. What's more, your weight can even be linked to your friends and partners. The psychosocial aspect of the eating experience can be a major obstacle to successful weight control.

Socioeconomic status can have a significant effect on risk for obesity. When tough economic times hit, people tend to eat more inexpensive, high-calorie foods. People living in poverty may live in communities with less access to fresh, nutrient-dense foods and have less time to cook nutritious meals owing to shiftwork, longer commutes, or multiple jobs (Gillespie et al., 2012). Additionally, unsafe neighborhoods and poor infrastructure, such as lack of sidewalks or parks, can make it difficult for less-affluent people to exercise (Sallis et al., 2012).[C]

Physical activity for health

Physical activity
Refers to all body movements produced by skeletal muscles resulting in substantial increases in energy expenditure.

Physical activity refers to all body movements produced by skeletal muscles that result in substantial increases in energy expenditure. Walking, swimming, strength training, dancing, and doing yoga are examples of physical activity. Physical activities can vary by light, moderate, or vigorous intensity. For example, walking on a flat surface at a casual pace requires little effort (light), whereas walking uphill is more intense and harder to do (moderate). Jogging and running are examples of vigorous intensity physical activities. There are three general categories of physical activity defined by the purpose for which they are done: leisure-time physical activity, occupational physical activity, and lifestyle physical activity.

[C]Donatelle, R. J.(2015). Reaching and maintaining a healthy weight. In *Health: The basics* (11th ed., pp. 293-294, 297–298). Upper Saddle River, NJ: Pearson Education Inc.

Exercise refers to a particular kind of physical activity that fits into the leisure-time category. Although all exercise is physical activity, not all physical activity would be considered exercise. For example, walking from your car to class is physical activity, whereas going for a brisk 30-minute walk or jog is considered exercise. **Exercise** is defined as planned, structured, and repetitive bodily movements done most often to improve or maintain one or more components of physical fitness, such as cardiorespiratory endurance, muscular strength or endurance, or flexibility.

Exercise
Planned, structured, and repetitive bodily movement done to improve or maintain one or more components of physical fitness.

From a major review of research on physical activity and health, researchers concluded that "there is irrefutable evidence of the effectiveness of regular physical activity in the primary and secondary prevention of several chronic diseases (e.g., cardiovascular disease, diabetes, cancer, hypertension, obesity, depression, and osteoporosis) (Kokkinos, Sheriff & Kheirbek, 2011)." Adding more physical activity to your day, like walking or cycling to school, can benefit your health. In fact, if all Americans followed the 2008 Physical Activity Guidelines (see Table 6.1), it is estimated that about one third of deaths related to coronary heart disease; one quarter of deaths related to stroke and osteoporosis; one fifth of deaths related to colon cancer, high blood pressure, and type 2 diabetes; and one seventh of deaths related to breast cancer could be prevented (Warburton et al., 2007).

Regular participation in physical activity improves more than 50 different physiological, metabolic, and psychological aspects of human life. Figure 6.1 in two pages summarises some of these major health-related benefits.

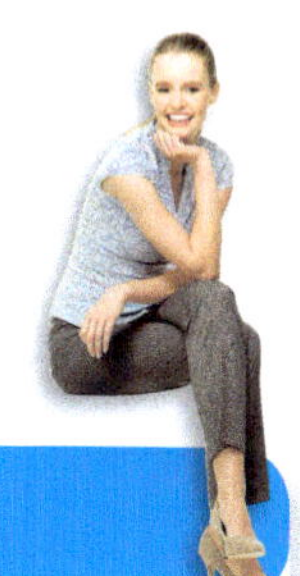

"Why Should I Care?"

Being physically active reduces your risk for many chronic diseases. That may not seem like an immediate concern, but there are a lot more immediate benefits: Becoming physically fit can help improve your physical appearance and sense of self-esteem, boost your resistance to diseases like colds and flus, reduce your stress level, improve your sleep, and help you concentrate. All that, and it's fun, too!

Table 6.1 2008 Physical Activity Guidelines for Americans

	Key Guidelines for Health*	For Additional Fitness or Weight Loss Benefits*	Additional Exercises
Adults	150 min/week moderate-intensity physical activity **OR** 75 min/week of vigorous-intensity physical activity **OR** Equivalent combination of moderate- and vigorous-intensity physical activity (i.e., 100 min moderate intensity + 25 min vigorous intensity)	300 min/week moderate-intensity physical activity **OR** 150 min/week of vigorous-intensity physical activity **OR** Equivalent combination of moderate- and vigorous-intensity physical activity (i.e., 200 min moderate intensity + 50 min vigorous intensity) **OR** More than the previously described amounts	Muscle strengthening activities for **all** the major muscle groups at least 2 days/week
Older Adults	If unable to follow above guidelines, then as much physical activity as their condition allows	If unable to follow above guidelines, then as much physical activity as their condition allows	In addition to muscle strengthening activities, exercise to improve balance
Children and Youth	60 min or more of moderate- or vigorous-intensity physical activity at least 3 days/week	At least 60 min of moderate- or vigorous-intensity physical activity on every day of the week	Include muscle strengthening activities at least 3 days/week Include bone-strengthening activities at least 3 days/week

*Accumulate this physical activity in sessions of 10 minutes or more at one time.

Source: Office of Disease Prevention and Health Promotion, U.S. Department of Health and Human Services, *2008 Physical Activity Guidelines for Americans: Be Active, Healthy, and Happy!*, ODPHP Publication no. U0036 (Washington, DC: U.S. Department of Health and Human Services, 2008), www.health.gov

Reduced risk of cardiovascular diseases

Aerobic exercise is good for the heart and lungs and reduces the risk for heart-related diseases. It improves blood flow and eases the performance of everyday tasks. Regular exercise makes the cardiovascular and respiratory systems more efficient by strengthening the heart muscle, enabling more blood to be pumped with each stroke, and increasing the number of *capillaries* (small blood vessels that allow gas exchange between blood and surrounding tissues) in trained skeletal muscles, which supply more blood to working muscles. Exercise also improves the respiratory system by increasing the amount of oxygen that is inhaled with each breath and distributed to body tissues (Plowman & Smith. 2011).

Regular physical activity can reduce hypertension, or chronic high blood pressure, a cardiovascular disease itself and a significant risk factor for other coronary heart diseases and stroke (Grover et al., 2011). Regular aerobic exercise also improves the blood lipid profile. It typically increases high-density lipoproteins (HDLs, or "good" cholesterol), which are associated with lower risk for coronary artery disease because of their role in removing plaque built up in the arteries (American Heart Association, 2013). Triglycerides (a blood fat) typically decrease with aerobic exercise. Low-density lipoproteins (LDLs, or "bad" cholesterol) and total cholesterol are often improved with exercise due to weight loss and the improvements in HDL and triglycerides.

Reduced risk of metabolic syndrome and type 2 diabetes

Being regularly physically active reduces the risk of metabolic syndrome, a combination of risk factors that produces a synergistic increase in risk for heart disease and diabetes (Mehta, 2010). Metabolic syndrome includes high blood pressure, abdominal obesity, low levels of HDLs, high levels of triglycerides, and impaired glucose tolerance (Mehta 2010). Regular participation in moderate-intensity physical activities reduces risk for each factor individually and collectively (Lee, 2012).

Research indicates that a healthy dietary intake combined with sufficient physical activity could prevent many of the current cases of type 2 diabetes (Uusitupa,Tuomilehto, & Puska, 2011). In a major national clinical trial, researchers found that exercising 150 minutes per week and eating fewer calories and less fat could prevent or delay the onset of type 2 diabetes (National Diabetes Information Clearinghouse, 2008).

Reduced cancer risk

After decades of research, most cancer epidemiologists believe that the majority of cancers are preventable and can be avoided by healthier lifestyle and environmental choices (Kendall et al., 2015; Nagle et al., 2015; Olsen et al., 2015). In fact, a report released by the World Cancer Research Fund in conjunction with the American Institute for Cancer Research stated that two thirds of all cancers could be prevented based on lifestyle changes (World Cancer Research Fund/American Institute for Cancer Research, 2009). A recent Australia study established that 32% of all cancer diagnoses in 2010 were attributed to 13 different modifiable lifestyle factors (Whiteman et al., 2015). The three leading factors contributing to cancer diagnoses were tobacco smoke (13.4%), exposure to solar radiation (6.2%) and an inadequate diet (6.1%). More specifically, one third of cancers could be prevented by being physically active and eating well. Regular physical activity appears to lower the risk for some specific cancers, particularly colon and rectal cancer (Clarke & Lockett, 2014). Regular exercise is also associated with lower risk for breast cancer. Research on exercise and breast cancer risk has found that the earlier in life a woman starts to exercise, the lower her breast cancer risk (Colditz & Bohlke, 2015).[D]

[D]Donatelle, R. J.(2015). Improving your personal fitness. In *Health: The basics* (11th ed., pp. 330–332). Upper Saddle River, NJ: Pearson Education Inc.

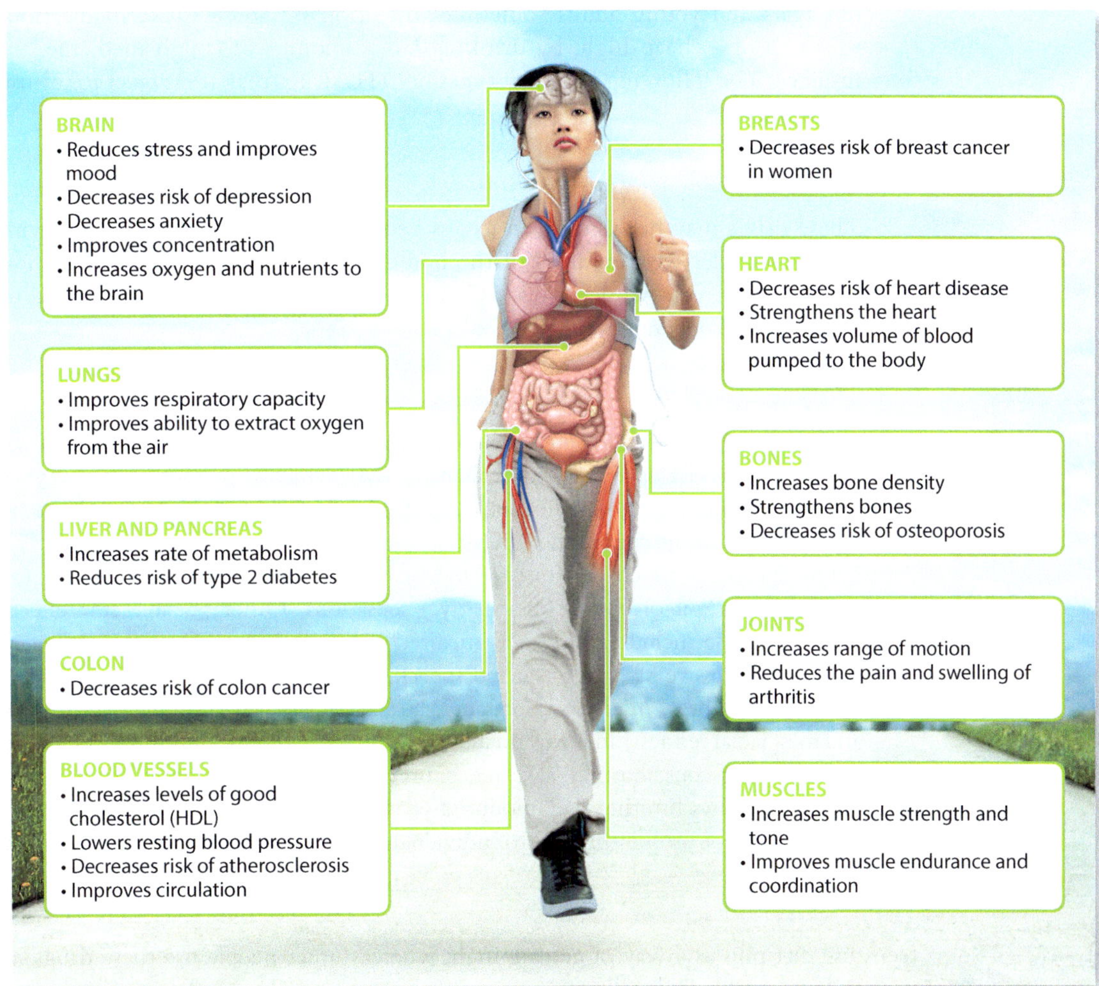

Figure 6.1 Some Health Benefits of Regular Exercise

Drug misuse and abuse

Although drug abuse is usually referred to in connection with illicit psychoactive drugs, many people also abuse and misuse prescription, over-the-counter (OTC), and recreational drugs. We now discuss these drug-related behaviours and focus on university students' drug use.

Abuse of over-the-counter drugs

Over-the-counter medications come in many different forms, including pills, liquids, nasal sprays, and topical creams. Although many people assume that no harm can come from drugs that are not illegal or regulated, OTC medications can be abused, with resultant health complications and potential addiction. High doses of certain OTC drugs may cause hallucinations, bizarre sleep patterns, mood changes, and in extreme cases, can lead to death. People who appear to be most vulnerable to abusing OTC drugs are teenagers, young adults, and people over the age of 65.

OTC drugs are abused when taken in more than the recommended dosage or for longer than is recommended. Abuse of and addiction to OTC drugs can be accidental. A person may develop tolerance from continued use, creating an unintended dependence. However,

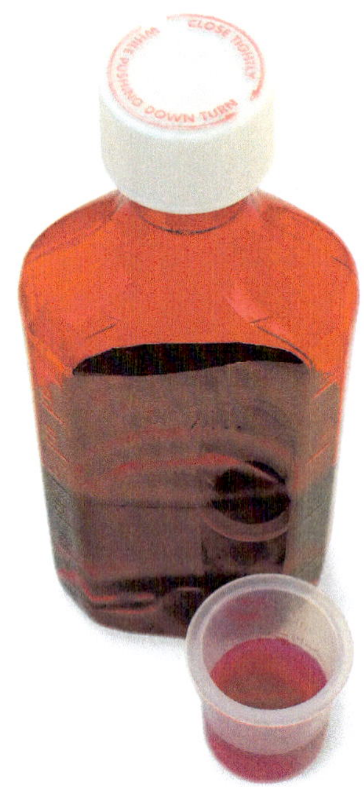

Over-the-counter cough syrup is frequently abused by young people seeking a high from the ingredient DXM.
(**Source:** Lori Sparkia/Shutterstock)

teenagers and young adults sometimes intentionally abuse OTC medications in search of a cheap high, by drinking large amounts of cough medicine, for instance. The following are a few types of OTC drugs that are subject to misuse and abuse:

Sleep aids

These drugs may be harmful in excess because they can cause problems with the sleep cycle, weaken areas of the body, or induce narcolepsy (a condition of excessive, intrusive sleepiness). Continued use of these products can lead to tolerance and dependence.

Cold medicines (cough syrups and tablets)

There are many different ingredients in cough and cold medicines, but one of particular concern is dextromethorphan (DXM), which is present in many types of OTC cold and cough medications. As many as 5 percent of high school seniors report taking drugs containing DXM in order to get high (Johnston et al., 2011). Large doses of products containing DXM can cause hallucinations, loss of motor control, and "out-of-body" (dissociative) sensations. Other possible side effects of DXM abuse include confusion, impaired judgement blurred vision, dizziness, paranoia, excessive sweating, slurred speech, nausea, vomiting, abdominal pain, irregular heartbeat, high blood pressure, headache, lethargy, numbness of fingers and toes, facial redness, and dry and itchy skin. In extreme cases, abuse of DXM can lead to loss of consciousness, seizures, brain damage, and even death. Some states have passed laws limiting the amount of products containing DXM that a person can purchase or prohibiting sale to individuals under age 18 (EROWID, 2011).

Diet pills

Some teens use diet pills as a way of getting high, whereas other people use these drugs in an attempt to lose weight. Diet pills often contain a stimulant such as caffeine or an herbal ingredient claimed to promote weight loss, such as *Hoodia gordonii*. Although they can sometimes cause serious side effects, many diet pills are marketed as dietary supplements and so are regulated by the Food and Drug Administration (FDA) as food, not as drugs. This means their manufacturers may make unsubstantiated claims of effectiveness or use untested and unsafe ingredients.

Prescription drug abuse

In Australia at present, the abuse of prescription medications is at an all-time high (Dobbin, 2014). Individuals abuse prescription medications because they are an easily accessible and inexpensive means of altering a user's mental and physical state. Some people also have the mistaken idea that prescription drugs are a "safer high." The latest data available from the 2010 National Drug Strategy Household Survey (Australian Institute of Health and Welfare, 2011) found that 7.4% of Australians aged 14 years and over had used prescription medications for nonmedical reasons at least once in their lifetime. The mortality and morbidity rates associated with prescription pharmaceuticals in Australia is also increasing steadily (AIHW, 2014).

Prescription drug abuse is particularly common among teenagers and young adults. In the United States in 2011, 3 percent of teenagers (aged 12 to 17) and 5 percent of 18- to 25-year-olds reported abusing prescription drugs in the past month. Comparatively, in Australia in 2010, 10.3% percent of 20- to 29-year-old reported abusing prescription pharmaceuticals at least once in their lifetime (AIHW, 2011). Recent research indicates that the problem may be getting worse, particularly among the youngest segments of society (AIHW, 2014).

The risks associated with prescription drug abuse vary. They can be as mild as decreased or irregular heart rate or as severe as death. Individuals who inject prescription drugs expose themselves to additional risks, including contracting HIV, hepatitis B and C, and other bloodborne viruses.

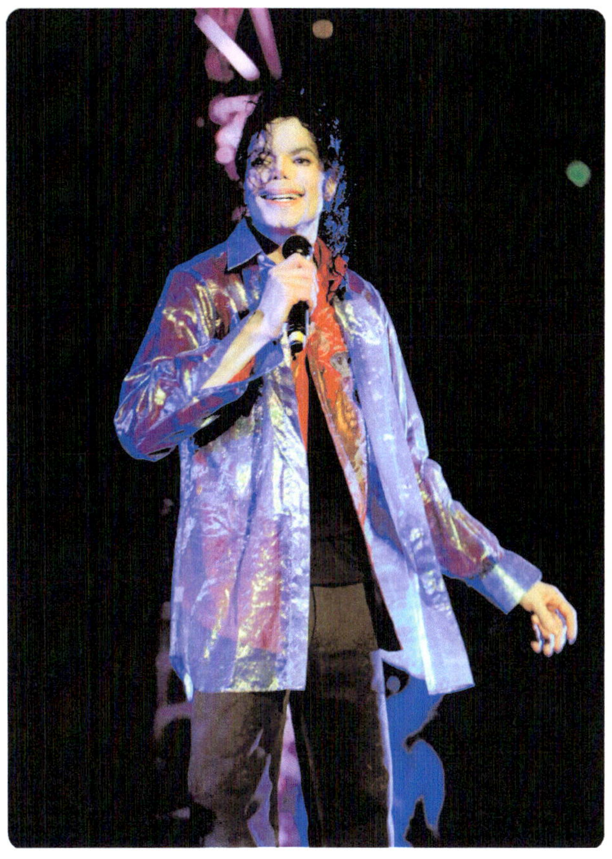

Why is prescription drug abuse on the rise?

Prescription drugs have legitimate and legal uses, which makes them more readily available than illicit drugs. The fact that prescription drugs are regulated and approved by the FDA leads to the impression that they are safer than illicit drugs. This is a fallacy, as was tragically demonstrated by the 2010 death of pop star Michael Jackson. Although his death was ruled a homicide, it ultimately stemmed from his abuse of numerous prescription medications.
(Source: AF Archive/Alamy)

University students and prescription drug abuse

Prescription drug abuse among students has increased dramatically over the past decade. Because they are prescribed by doctors and approved by the Therapeutic Goods Administration, many university students seem to perceive prescription drugs as safer and more socially acceptable than illicit drugs. Nothing could be further from the truth when these drugs are misused. Some students who abuse prescription drugs believe that such use will enhance their well-being or performance (Housden, Morein-Zamir & Sahakian, 2011; Partridge, Bell, Lucke & Hall, 2013). Painkillers are among the most popular prescription drugs used on campus. Students who abuse prescription painkillers such as Vicodin, OxyContin, or Percocet say they do so to relax or get high.

A concern on college campuses in the United States is the increased abuse of stimulant drugs such as Adderall and Ritalin, which are intended to treat attention-deficit/hyperactivity disorder (ADHD). Students primarily report using ADHD drugs for academic gain. Studies in the United States reveal that between 3% and 6% of college students had used stimulants at some point during their academic studies (Bogle & Smith, 2009; McCabe, 2008). Another American study found that friends with prescriptions were the most commonly reported source of prescription stimulants and that most students obtained their drugs for free or at a cost of $1 to $5 (Garnier-Dykstra et al., 2012). Users generally believed that the drugs were beneficial, despite frequent reports of adverse reactions. The most commonly reported adverse effects were sleeping difficulties, irritability, and reduced appetite. On the other hand, a recent study of Australian university students revealed that the use of prescription stimulant drugs was uncommon, with participants reporting that they were hesitant to use prescription stimulants to boost in their alertness due to potential side effects (Partridge et al., 2013).

Illicit drugs

The problem of illicit (illegal) drug use touches us all. We may use illicit substances ourselves, watch someone we love struggle with drug abuse, or become the victim of a drug-related

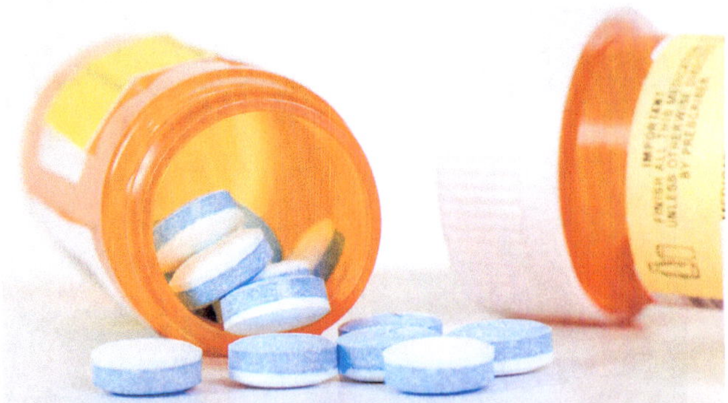

Painkillers such as OxyContin, Percocet, Percodan, Vicodin, and others are highly addictive; if they are taken daily for several weeks, that is enough time for addiction to develop. OxyContin, in particular, can be a highly addictive and dangerous narcotic when abused.
(Source: Thomas M Perkins/Shutterstock.)

crime. At the very least, we are forced to pay increasing taxes for law enforcement and drug rehabilitation. When our coworkers use drugs, the effectiveness of our own work is diminished. If the car we drive was assembled by drug-using workers at the plant, we are in danger. A drug-using bus driver, surgeon, or pilot jeopardise our safety, too.

Illicit drug users span all age groups, genders, ethnicities, occupations, and socioeconomic groups. Illicit drug use in the United States peaked at around 25 million users between 1979 and 1986, then declined until 1992, and has since remained stable at somewhere between 22 and 23 million users per year in the United States. Among youth, however, illicit drug use, notably use of marijuana, has been rising in recent years. In comparison, data from the National Drug and Alcohol Research Centre established that illicit drug use in Australia declined between the years of 1998 and 2007, but significantly increased in 2010 (Roxburgh, Ritter, Slade & Burns, 2013). While marijuana use is popular among youth, data reveals that significantly less secondary school students in Australia were using cannabis in 2011 (12.7%) as compared to 1996 (32.4%) (Roxburgh et al., 2013).

Illicit drug use on campus

Illicit drug use has seen a resurgence on university campuses in recent years. Even so, it is not the norm. Close to 50 percent of university-aged students nationwide have tried an illicit drug at some point in their lives. The vast majority of those people reported using marijuana. The increase over the past decade in the percentage of university students using illicit drugs is due to an increase in marijuana use (see Table 6.2) (Johnston et al., 2011).

University administrators, staff, and faculty are concerned about the link between substance abuse and poor academic performance, depression, anxiety, suicide, property damage, vandalism, fights, serious medical problems, and death. Students who use marijuana and/or other illicit drugs are at increased risk for disruptions in university attendance (Arria et al., 2013). A longer-term consequence of illicit drug use among university students is a significantly increased chance of unemployment after university. The most recent research shows that 10 percent of people who were persistent drug users during university experienced unemployment after university compared with 1.7 percent of students who did not use drugs and 4.8 percent of those who used drugs sporadically (Arria et al., 2013).

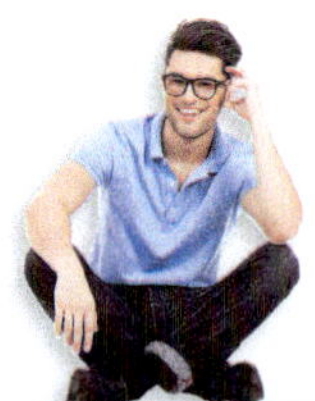

"Why Should I Care?"

Addictions of any kind limit your ability to make good decisions and maintain your focus, making it hard for you to meet your full potential as a student and as a member of the community. A seemingly harmless habit may actually be progressing into an addiction that prevents you from attending classes, meeting new people, or participating in other activities that you might find enjoyable.

Table 6.2 30-Day Drug Use Prevalence, Full-Time University Students vs. Respondents 1–4 Years beyond High School

	Full-Time University (%)	Others (%)
Any illicit drug	21.4	25.8
Any illicit drug other than marijuana	8.2	8.7
Marijuana	19.4	24.0
Inhalants	0.3	0.2
Hallucinogens	1.2	1.5
LSD	0.5	1.0
Hallucinogens other than LSD	0.8	0.8
Ecstasy (methylene-dioxymethamphetamine, MDMA)	0.7	1.0
Cocaine	1.2	1.6
Crack	0.1	0.3
Other cocaine	1.2	1.5
Heroin	less than 0.05 %	0.3
Narcotics other than heroin	2.1	3.9
Amphetamines, adjusted	4.5	2.4
Crystal methamphetamine	less than 0.05%	0.5
Sedatives (barbiturates)	0.8	1.2
Tranquillisers	1.6	2.3

Source: L. D. Johnston et al., *Monitoring the Future National Survey Results on Drug Use, 1975–2011*, Volume 2, *College Students and Adults Ages 19–50* (Ann Arbor: Institute for Social Research, The University of Michigan, 2012), Available at http://monitoringthefuture.org

Factors that can increase the risk of substance use

Research has identified the following factors in a student's life that increase the risk of substance abuse; the more factors, the greater the risk.

POSITIVE EXPECTATIONS. As mentioned previously, some students take drugs such as Adderall and Ritalin believing that the drugs will help their ability to study. But the vast majority of students say they take drugs in order to relax, reduce stress, and forget problems.

GENETICS AND FAMILY HISTORY. Genetics and family history play a significant role in the risk for developing an addiction.

SUBSTANCE USE IN HIGH SCHOOL. Two-thirds of university students who use illicit drugs began doing so in high school.

MENTAL HEALTH PROBLEMS. Students who report being diagnosed with depression are more likely to have abused prescription drugs, to have used marijuana or other illicit drugs, and to be current or frequent smokers.

SORORITY AND FRATERNITY MEMBERSHIP. Being a member of a sorority or fraternity increases the likelihood of using alcohol, marijuana, or cocaine and makes one twice as likely to abuse prescription drugs.

Protective factors that can reduce the risk of substance use

Many protective factors can influence a student to avoid drugs. Some of the most commonly reported include the following (National Center on Addiction and Substance Abuse at Columbia University, 2007):

PARENTAL ATTITUDES AND BEHAVIOUR. Students who say they are more influenced by their parents' concerns or expectations drink less, use marijuana less, and smoke significantly less than do students who are less influenced by parents.

RELIGION AND SPIRITUALITY. The greater the student's level of religiosity (hours in prayer, attendance at services), the less likely he or she is to drink, smoke, or use other drugs.

STUDENT ENGAGEMENT. The more a student is involved in the learning process and extracurricular activities, the less likely he or she is to binge drink, use marijuana, or abuse prescription drugs.

UNIVERSITY ATHLETICS. University athletes drink at higher rates than do nonathletes, but are less likely to use illicit drugs.

HEALTHY SOCIAL NETWORK. Having a wide range of friends and supports to help cope with the challenges of life is a well-known protective factor against many negative behaviours, including drug use.

Common drugs of abuse

Hundreds of drugs are subject to abuse—some are legal, such as recreational drugs and prescription medications, whereas many others are illegal and classified as "controlled substances." For general purposes, drugs can be divided into the following categories: stimulants, marijuana and other cannabis products, opioids, depressants, hallucinogens, inhalants, and steroids. These categories are discussed in subsequent sections; Table 6.3 summarises the categorisation, uses, and effects of various drugs of abuse, both licit (prescription) and illicit.

Stimulants

Stimulants
Drugs that increase activity of the central nervous system.

A **stimulant** is a drug that increases activity of the central nervous system. Its effects, therefore, usually involve increased activity, anxiety, and agitation; users often seem jittery or nervous while high. Commonly used stimulants include cocaine, amphetamines, methamphetamine, and caffeine. (Nicotine, the addictive substance in tobacco products is another common stimulant.)

Cocaine

A white crystalline powder derived from the leaves of the South American coca shrub (not related to cocoa plants), *cocaine* ("coke") has been described as one of the most powerful naturally occurring stimulants.

METHODS OF USE AND PHYSICAL EFFECTS. Cocaine can be taken in several ways, including snorting, smoking, and injecting. The powdered form is snorted through the nose, which can damage mucous membranes and cause sinusitis. It can destroy the user's sense of smell, and occasionally it even eats a hole through the septum. The effects of cocaine are felt rapidly. When snorted, the drug enters the bloodstream through the lungs in less than 1 minute and reaches the brain in less than 3 minutes. Cocaine binds at receptor sites in the central nervous system, producing intense pleasure. The euphoria quickly abates, however, and the desire to regain the pleasurable feelings makes the user want more cocaine.

Table 6.3 Drugs of Abuse: Uses and Effects (continues)

Category	Drugs	Trade or Street Names	Dependence	Usual Method	Possible Effects	Overdose Effects	Withdrawal Syndrome
Stimulants	Cocaine	Coke, Flake, Snow, Crack, *Coca, Blanca, Perico*	*Physical:* Possible *Psychological:* High *Tolerance:* Yes	Snorted, smoked, injected	Increased alertness, excitation, euphoria, increased pulse rate and blood pressure, insomnia, loss of appetite	Agitation, increased body temperature, hallucinations, convulsions, possible death	Apathy, long periods of sleep, irritability, depression, disorientation
	Amphetamine, methamphetamine	Crank, Ice, Cristal, Crystal Meth, Speed, Adderall, Dexedrine	*Physical:* Possible *Psychological:* High *Tolerance:* Yes	Oral, injected, smoked			
	Methylphenidate	Ritalin (Illys), Concerta, Focalin, Metadate	*Physical:* Possible *Psychological:* High *Tolerance:* Yes	Oral, injected, snorted, smoked			
Cannabis	Marijuana	Pot, Grass, Sinsemilla, Blunts, *Mota, Yerba, Grifa*	*Physical:* Possible *Psychological:* High *Tolerance:* Yes	Oral, smoked	Euphoria, relaxed inhibitions, increased appetite, disorientation	Fatigue, paranoia, possible psychosis	Hyperactivity, decreased appetite, insomnia
	Hashish, hashish oil	Hash, Hash oil	*Physical:* Unknown *Psychological:* Moderate *Tolerance:* Yes	Smoked, oral			
Narcotics	Heroin	Diamorphine, Horse, Smack, Black tar, *Chiva*	*Physical:* High *Psychological:* High *Tolerance:* Yes	Injected, snorted, smoked	Euphoria, drowsiness, respiratory depression, constricted pupils, nausea	Slow and shallow breathing, clammy skin, convulsions, coma, possible death	Watery eyes, runny nose, yawning, loss of appetite, irritability, tremors, panic, cramps, nausea, chills and sweating
	Morphine	MS-Contin, Roxanol	*Physical:* High *Psychological:* High *Tolerance:* Yes	Oral, injected			
	Hydrocodone, oxycodone	Vicodin, OxyContin, Percocet, Percodan	*Physical:* High *Psychological:* High *Tolerance:* Yes	Oral			
	Codeine	Acetaminophen w/ Codeine, Tylenol w/ Codeine	*Physical:* Moderate *Psychological:* Moderate *Tolerance:* Yes	Oral, injected			
Depressants	Gamma-hydroxybutyrate	GHB, Liquid Ecstasy, Liquid X	*Physical:* Moderate *Psychological:* Moderate *Tolerance:* Yes	Oral	Slurred speech, disorientation, drunken behaviours without odor of alcohol, impaired memory of events, interacts with alcohol	Shallow respiration, clammy skin, dilated pupils, weak and rapid pulse, coma, possible death	Anxiety, insomnia, tremors, delirium, convulsions, possible death
	Benzodiazepines	Valium, Xanax, Halcion, Ativan, Rohypnol (Roofies, R-2), Klonopin	*Physical:* Moderate *Psychological:* Moderate *Tolerance:* Yes	Oral, injected			
	Other depressants	Ambien, Sonata, Barbiturates, Methaqualone (Quaalude)	*Physical:* Moderate *Psychological:* Moderate *Tolerance:* Yes	Oral			

Table 6.3 Drugs of Abuse: Uses and Effects (continued)

Category	Drugs	Trade or Street Names	Dependence	Usual Method	Possible Effects	Overdose Effects	Withdrawal Syndrome
Hallucinogens	Methylene-dioxymethamphetamine (MDMA), analogs	Ecstasy, XTC, Adam, MDA (Love Drug), MDEA (Eve)	*Physical:* None *Psychological:* Moderate *Tolerance:* Yes	Oral, snorted, smoked	Heightened senses, teeth grinding, dehydration	Increased body temperature, electrolyte imbalance, cardiac arrest	Muscle aches, drowsiness, depression, acne
	LSD	Acid, Microdot, Sunshine, Boomers	*Physical:* None *Psychological:* Unknown *Tolerance:* Yes	Oral		Longer, more intense "trips"	None
	Phencyclidine, analogs	PCP, Angel Dust, Hog, Ketamine (Special K)	*Physical:* Possible *Psychological:* High *Tolerance:* Yes	Smoked, oral, injected, snorted	Hallucinations, altered perception of time and distance	Unable to direct movement, feel pain, or remember	Drug-seeking behaviour
	Other hallucinogens	Psilocybe mushrooms, Mescaline, Peyote, Dextromethorphan	*Physical:* None *Psychological:* None *Tolerance:* Possible	Oral			
Inhalants	Amyl and butyl nitrite	Pearls, Poppers, Rush, Locker Room	*Physical:* Unknown *Psychological:* Unknown *Tolerance:* No	Inhaled	Flushing, hypotension, headache	Methemo-globinemia	Agitation
	Nitrous oxide	Laughing gas, Balloons, Whippets	*Physical:* Unknown *Psychological:* Low *Tolerance:* No	Inhaled	Impaired memory, slurred speech, drunken behaviour, slow-onset vitamin deficiency, organ damage	Vomiting, respiratory depression, loss of consciousness, possible death	Trembling, anxiety, insomnia, vitamin deficiency, confusion, hallucinations, convulsions
	Other inhalants	Adhesives, spray paint, hairspray, lighter fluid	*Physical:* Unknown *Psychological:* High *Tolerance:* No	Inhaled			
Anabolic Steroids	Testosterone	Depo Testosterone, Sustanon, Sten, Cypt	*Physical:* Unknown *Psychological:* Unknown *Tolerance:* Unknown	Injected	virilisation, edema, testicular atrophy, gynecomastia, acne, aggressive behaviour	Unknown	Possible depression
	Other anabolic steroids	Parabolan, Winstrol, Equipose, Anadrol, Dianabol	*Physical:* Unknown *Psychological:* Yes *Tolerance:* Unknown	Oral, injected			

Source: Adapted from U.S. Department of Justice Drug Enforcement Administration, "DEA Drug Fact Sheets," 2011, www.justice.gov

Cocaine alkaloid, or *freebase*, is obtained from removing the hydrochloride salt from cocaine powder. In this base form, the cocaine is much more suitable for smoking. Smoked freebase cocaine reaches the brain within seconds and produces an intense high that disappears quickly, leaving a powerful craving for more. *Crack* is identical pharmacologically to freebase, but the hydrochloride salt is still present and is processed with baking soda and water. It is a cheap, widely available drug that is smokable and very potent. Because crack is such a pure drug, it takes little time to achieve the desired high, and a crack user can become addicted quickly.

Some cocaine users occasionally inject the drug intravenously, which introduces large amounts into the body rapidly, creating a brief, intense high, and a subsequent crash. Injecting users place themselves at risk not only for contracting HIV and hepatitis (a severe liver disease) through shared needles, but also for skin infections, vein damage, inflamed arteries, and infection of the heart lining.

Cocaine is both an anesthetic and a central nervous system stimulant. In tiny doses, it can slow the heart rate. In larger doses, the physical effects are dramatic: increased heart rate and blood pressure, loss of appetite that can lead to dramatic weight loss, convulsions, muscle twitching, irregular heartbeat, and even death resulting from an overdose. Other effects of cocaine include temporary relief of depression, decreased fatigue, talkativeness, increased alertness, and heightened self-confidence. However, as the dose increases, users become irritable and apprehensive, and their behaviour may turn paranoid or violent.

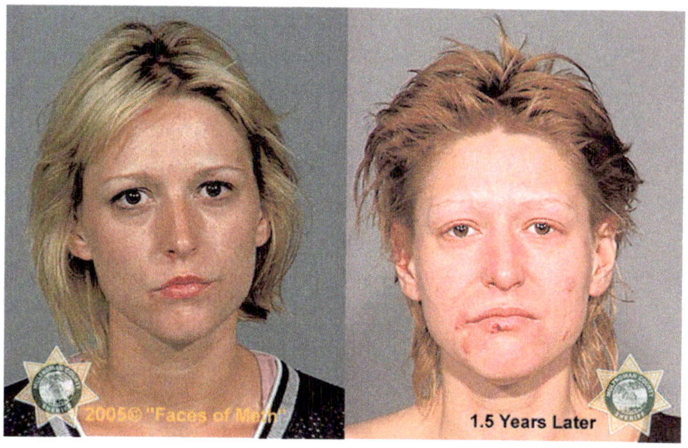

The physical consequences of methamphetamine use are often dramatic. The photo at left shows a person before she began using methamphetamine. The photo at right shows the same person just 1.5 years after methamphetamine use.
(Source: Faces of Meth; p. 214 Karen Mower/E+/Getty Images.)

Amphetamines

The **amphetamines** include a large and varied group of synthetic agents that stimulate the central nervous system. Small doses of amphetamines improve alertness, lessen fatigue, and generally elevate mood. With repeated use, however, physical and psychological dependence develops. Sleep patterns are affected (insomnia); heart rate, breathing rate, and blood pressure increase; and restlessness, anxiety, appetite suppression, and vision problems are common. High doses over long time periods can produce hallucinations, delusions, and disorganised behaviour.

Amphetamines
A large and varied group of synthetic agents that stimulate the central nervous system.

Certain types of amphetamines or amphetamine-like drugs are used for medicinal purposes. As discussed earlier, drugs prescribed to treat ADHD are stimulants and are increasingly abused on campus.

METHAMPHETAMINE. An increasingly common form of amphetamine, *methamphetamine* (commonly called "meth") is a potent, long-acting, inexpensive drug that is highly addictive. In 2011, about 2 percent of high school seniors reported using methamphetamine in their lifetime (Johnston et al., 2011).

Australian researchers estimate that during 2013–14 there were 268,000 regular methamphetamine users (Degenhardt et al., 2016). In the short term, methamphetamine produces increased physical activity, alertness, euphoria, rapid breathing, increased body temperature, insomnia, tremors, anxiety, confusion, and decreased appetite.

Methamphetamine can be snorted, smoked, injected, or orally ingested. When snorted, the effects can be felt in 3 to 5 minutes; if orally ingested, effects occur within 15 to 20 minutes. The pleasurable effects of methamphetamine are typically an intense rush lasting only a few minutes when snorted; in contrast, smoking the drug can produce a high lasting more than 8 hours. Users often experience tolerance after the first use, making methamphetamine a highly addictive drug. Methamphetamine increases the release of and blocks the reuptake of the brain chemical (or neurotransmitter) dopamine, leading to high levels of the chemical in the brain. This action occurs rapidly and produces the intense euphoria, or "rush," that many users feel after snorting, smoking, or injecting the drug. But over time, meth destroys dopamine receptors, making it impossible to feel pleasure. Researchers have now established that due to destructive action on nerves, people who abuse methamphetamine (or cocaine) are at increased risk for developing Parkinson's disease later in life (CPDD Community Website, 2011).

Other problems resulting from long-term use include reduced motor skills and impaired verbal learning, severe weight loss, cardiovascular damage, anxiety, confusion, and insomnia. Methamphetamine abuse causes destruction of tissues and blood vessels, inhibiting the body's ability to repair itself. Acne appears, sores take longer to heal, and the skin loses its luster and elasticity, making users appear years or even decades older. Increased risk of heart attack and stroke, liver damage, hallucinations, violence, paranoia, psychotic behaviour, and even death are also associated with long-term methamphetamine use. Recent studies of chronic methamphetamine abusers have revealed severe structural and functional changes in areas of the brain associated with emotion and memory, which may account for many of the emotional and cognitive problems observed in chronic methamphetamine abusers. Some of these changes persist after the methamphetamine abuse has stopped. Other changes reverse after sustained periods of abstinence from methamphetamine, lasting typically longer than a year, but problems can remain.

Abusers of methamphetamine can also develop a side effect called "meth mouth." Within a short period of time, teeth can turn greyish brown. Further damage occurs when users obsessively grind their teeth, binge on sugary food and drinks, and neglect to brush or floss for long periods of time. In addition, meth causes the salivary glands to dry out, which allows the mouth's acids to eat away at tooth enamel, causing cavities.

Meth users are at increased risk for transmission of HIV, hepatitis B and C, and other sexually transmitted diseases. Meth can alter judgement increase libido, and lessen inhibitions, leading users to engage in unsafe behaviours, including risky sexual behaviour. Among meth users who inject the drug, HIV and other infectious diseases can be spread through sharing of contaminated needles, syringes, and other injection equipment that is used by more than one person.

Caffeine

Caffeine
A stimulant drug that is legal in the United States and found in many coffees, teas, chocolates, energy drinks, and certain medications.

Almost half of all Australians (46%) drink coffee every day, and many others consume caffeine in some other form, making it the most widely consumed drug in Australia (Australian Bureau of Statistics, 2014). Coffee, tea, soft drinks, chocolate, and other caffeine-containing products are legal, popular, and loved for their wake-up effects. Caffeine may be commonplace, but excessive consumption is associated with addiction and certain health problems.

Caffeine is derived from the chemical family called *xanthines,* which are found in plant products such as coffee, tea, and chocolate. The xanthines are mild central nervous system stimulants that enhance mental alertness and reduce feelings of fatigue. Other stimulant effects include increased heart muscle contractions, oxygen consumption, metabolism, and urinary output. A person feels these effects within 15 to 45 minutes of ingesting a caffeinated product. It takes 4 to 6 hours for the body to metabolise half of the caffeine ingested, so, depending on the amount of caffeine taken in, it may continue to exert effects for a day or longer. Figure 6.2 compares the caffeine content of various products.

As the effects of caffeine wear off, frequent users may feel let down—mentally or physically depressed, exhausted, and weak. To counteract this, they commonly choose to drink another cup of coffee or tea, or another soda. Habitually engaging in this practice leads to tolerance and psychological dependence. Symptoms of excessive caffeine consumption include chronic insomnia, jitters, irritability, nervousness, anxiety, and involuntary muscle twitches. Withdrawing from caffeine may compound the effects and produce severe headaches, fatigue, and nausea. Because caffeine meets the requirements for addiction—tolerance, psychological dependence, and withdrawal symptoms—it can be classified as addictive.

No strong evidence exists to suggest that moderate caffeine use (less than 300 mg daily, or approximately three cups of regular coffee) produces harmful effects in healthy, nonpregnant people. For most people, caffeine poses few health risks and may actually have some benefits, such as lower risk of depression among women, a lower risk of prostate cancer among men, and lower risk of stroke among both men and women (Havard Health Letter, 2012).

Marijuana and other cannabinoids

Although archaeological evidence documents the use of *marijuana* ("grass," "weed," or "pot") as far back as 6,000 years, the drug did not become popular in the United States until the 1960s. Today marijuana is the most commonly used illicit drug in both Australia and the United States. The 2013 National Drug Strategy Household Survey found that approximately 35% of Australians over the age of 14 had tried marijuana at least once in their lifetime, while 10.2% reported using marijuana in the previous 12 months (AIHW, 2014). In comparison, approximately 41 percent of Americans over the age of 12 have tried marijuana at least once (Substance Abuse and Mental Health Services Administration, 2012). Some 29 million people have reported using marijuana in the past year, and more than 18.1 million have reported using marijuana within the past month. Marijuana use is also on the rise on university campuses, following the trend of increased use in the general population (Substance Abuse and Mental Health Services Administration, 2012).

Methods of use and physical effects

Marijuana is derived from either the *Cannabis sativa* or *Cannabis indica* (hemp) plant. Most of the time, marijuana is smoked, although it can also be ingested, as in brownies baked with marijuana in them. When marijuana is smoked, it is usually rolled into cigarettes (joints) or placed in a pipe or water pipe (bong). Current American-grown marijuana is a turbocharged version of that grown in the late 1960s. **Tetrahydrocannabinol (THC)** is the psychoactive substance in marijuana and the key to determining how powerful a high it will produce. More potent forms of the drug can contain up to 27 percent THC, but most average 10 percent (Substance Abuse and Mental Health Services Administration, 2012). *Hashish,* a potent cannabis preparation derived mainly from the plant's thick, sticky resin, contains high THC concentrations. Hash oil, a substance produced by percolating a solvent such as ether through dried marijuana to extract the THC, is a tar-like liquid that may contain up to 300 mg of THC in a dose.

Tetrahydrocannabinol (THC) The chemical name for the active ingredient in marijuana.

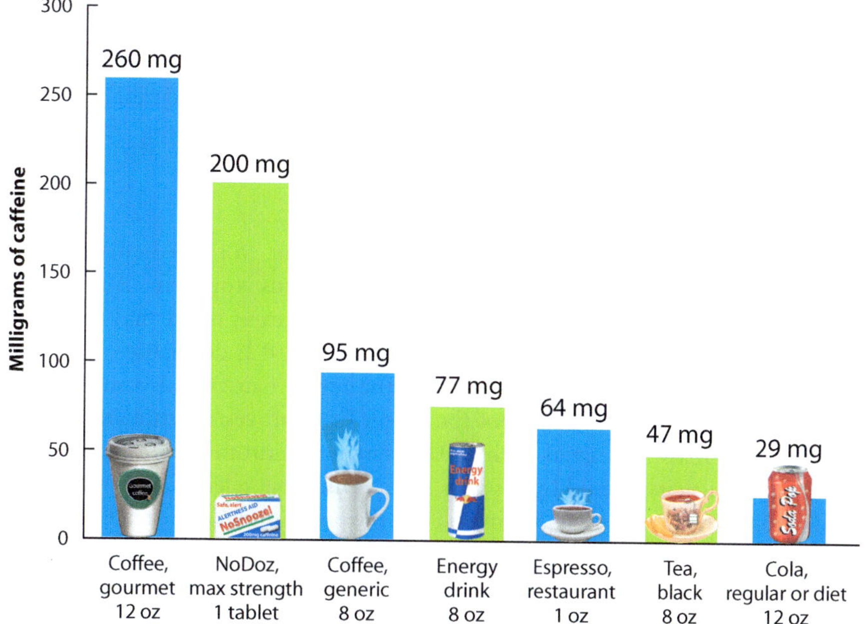

Figure 6.2 Caffeine Content Comparison

Source: Data from USDA National Nutrient Database for Standard Reference, Release 25 (2012), www.ars.usda.gov

Skills for Behaviour Change

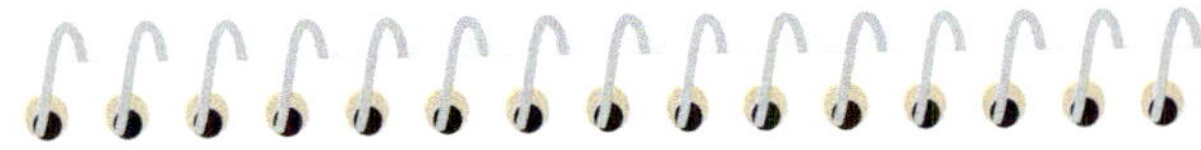

Responding to Offer of Drugs

No matter what your experience has been up until now, it is likely that you will be invited to use drugs at some point in your life. Here are some questions to consider *before* you find yourself in a situation in which you have the opportunity or feel pressure to use illicit drugs:

- Why am I considering trying drugs? Am I trying to fit in or impress my friends? What does this say about my friends if I need to take drugs to impress them? Are my friends really looking out for what is best for me?
- Am I using this drug to cope or feel different? Am I depressed?
- What could taking drugs cost me? Will this cost me my career if I am caught using? Could using drugs prevent me from getting a job?
- What are the long-term consequences of using this drug?
- What will this cost me in terms of my friendships and family? How would my close family and friends respond if they knew I was using drugs?

Even when you make the decision not to use drugs, it can be difficult to say no gracefully. Some good ways to turn down an offer:

- "Thanks, but I've got a big test (game, meeting) tomorrow morning."
- "I've already got a great buzz right now. I really don't need anything more."
- "I don't like how (insert drug name here) makes me feel."
- "I'm driving tonight. So I'm not using."
- "I want to go for a run in the morning."
- "No."

The effects of smoking marijuana are generally felt within 10 to 30 minutes and usually wear off within 3 hours. The most noticeable effect of THC is the dilation of the eyes' blood vessels, which produces the smoker's characteristic bloodshot eyes. Marijuana smokers also exhibit coughing; dry mouth and throat ("cotton mouth"); increased thirst and appetite; lowered blood pressure; and mild muscular weakness, primarily exhibited in drooping eyelids. Users can also experience severe anxiety, panic, paranoia, and psychosis, and may have intensified reactions to various stimuli; colour, sounds, and the speed at which things move may seem altered. High doses of hashish may produce vivid visual hallucinations.

Marijuana and Driving. Marijuana use presents clear hazards for drivers of motor vehicles and others on the road with them. The drug substantially reduces a driver's ability to react and make quick decisions. Perceptual and other performance deficits resulting from marijuana use may persist for some time after the high subsides. Users who attempt to drive, fly, or operate heavy machinery often fail to recognise their impairment. Recent research indicates you are two and a half times more likely to be involved in a motor vehicle accident if you drive under the influence of marijuana (Asbridge et al., 2012). Combining even a small amount of marijuana and alcohol enhances the impairing effects of both drugs even more.

Marijuana as Medicine. The use of marijuana for medicinal purposes is a contentious topic in Australia despite some evidence suggesting that marijuana, when used with care, is safe and has therapeutic benefits (Barbosa, Mizumoto, Bogenschutz & Strassman, 2012; dos Santos et al., 2012). It has been shown to help control side effects such the severe nausea and vomiting produced by chemotherapy, the chemical treatment for cancer. It improves appetite and forestalls the loss of lean muscle mass associated with AIDS-wasting syndrome. Marijuana reduces the muscle pain and spasticity caused by diseases such as multiple sclerosis. At present, patients in Australia can access marijuana for medicinal purposes under the strict supervision of their general practitioner, nevertheless, patients often have difficulty sourcing safe and suitable products (Parliament of Australia, 2016). The Australian Federal Parliament, in 2016, introduced the Narcotic Drugs Amendment Act 2016 which included amendments to the Narcotic Drugs Act 1967 to allow for the cultivation of safe and legal marijuana for medicinal and scientific purposes. Marijuana's legal status for medicinal purposes continues to be hotly debated.

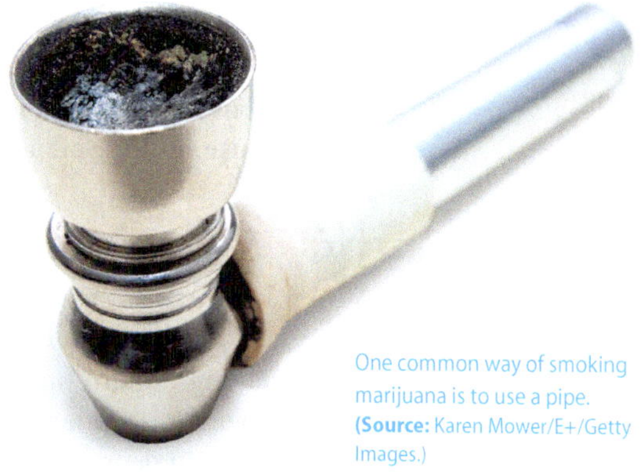

One common way of smoking marijuana is to use a pipe. **(Source:** Karen Mower/E+/Getty Images.)

EFFECTS OF CHRONIC MARIJUANA USE. Because marijuana has typically been illegal in Australia and most parts of the United States and has been widely used only since the 1960s, the long-term studies of its effects have been difficult to conduct. Studies conducted in the 1960s involved marijuana with THC levels that were only a fraction of those of today, so their results may not apply to the stronger forms now available.

Numerous studies have shown that marijuana smoke contains 50 to 70 percent more carcinogenic hydrocarbons than does tobacco smoke. Because marijuana smokers typically inhale more deeply and hold their breath longer than do tobacco smokers, the lungs are exposed to more carcinogens. As well, effects from irritation (e.g., cough, excessive phlegm, and increased lung infections) similar to those experienced by tobacco smokers can occur (National Institute on Drug Abuse, 2012). Lung conditions such as chronic bronchitis, emphysema, and other lung disorders are also associated with smoking marijuana.

Inhaling marijuana smoke introduces carbon monoxide into the bloodstream. Because the blood has a greater affinity for carbon monoxide than it does for oxygen, its oxygen-carrying capacity is diminished, and the heart must work harder to pump oxygen to oxygen-starved tissues. Smoking marijuana also results in three times more tar inhalation and retention in the respiratory tract than does smoking tobacco.

Recent research has found that frequent and/or long-term marijuana use may significantly increase a man's risk of developing testicular cancer. The risk was particularly elevated (about twice that of those who never smoked marijuana) for those who used marijuana at least weekly or who had long-term exposure to the substance beginning in adolescence. The results also suggested that the association with marijuana use might be limited to *nonseminoma*, an aggressive, fast-growing testicular malignancy that tends to strike early, between ages 20 and 35, and accounts for about 40 percent of all testicular cancer cases (National Institute on Drug Abuse, 2012).

According to the National Survey on Drug Use and Health, teens and young adults who use marijuana are more likely to develop serious mental health problems. A number of studies have shown an association between marijuana use and increased rates of anxiety, depression, suicidal ideation, and schizophrenia Alcohol and Drug Abuse Institute, 2012). Some of these studies have shown age at first use as an indicator of vulnerability to later problems.

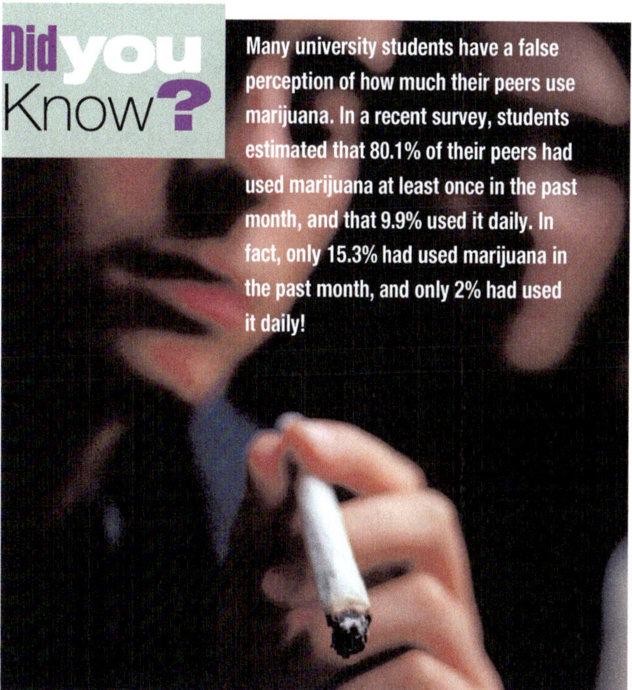

Many university students have a false perception of how much their peers use marijuana. In a recent survey, students estimated that 80.1% of their peers had used marijuana at least once in the past month, and that 9.9% used it daily. In fact, only 15.3% had used marijuana in the past month, and only 2% had used it daily!

Source: Data from American College Health Association, *American College Health Association-National College Health Assessment (ACHA-NCHA): Reference Group Data Report, Fall 2012* (Hanover, MD: American College Health Association, 2013).
(Source: Bubbles Photolibrary/Alamy)

Other risks associated with marijuana use include suppression of the immune system, blood pressure changes, and impaired memory function. Recent studies suggest that pregnant women who smoke marijuana may have children who have subtle brain changes that can cause difficulties with problem-solving skills, memory, and attention, and can more than double the risk of giving birth prematurely (National Institute on Drug Abuse, 2011; Science Daily, (2012).

Narcotics and depressants

Whereas central nervous system stimulants increase muscular and nervous system activity, **depressants** slow down neuromuscular activity and cause sleepiness or calmness. If the dose is high enough, brain function can be slowed to the point of causing death. Forms include opioids, benzodiazepines, and barbiturates, although alcohol is the most widely used central nervous system depressant.

Opioids cause drowsiness, relieve pain, and produce euphoria. Also called *narcotics,* opioids are derived from the parent drug *opium*, a dark, resinous substance made from the milky juice of the opium poppy seedpod, and they are all highly addictive. Opium and heroin are both illegal in Australia and the United States, but some opioids are available by prescription for medical purposes: Morphine is sometimes prescribed for severe pain, and codeine is found in prescription cough syrups and other painkillers. Several prescription drugs, including Vicodin, Percodan, OxyContin, Demerol, and Dilaudid, contain synthetic opioids.

Depressants
Drugs that slow down the activity of the central nervous and muscular systems and cause sleepiness or calmness.

Opioids
Drugs that induce sleep, relieve pain, and produce euphoria; includes derivatives of opium and synthetics with similar chemical properties; also called *narcotics.*

Endorphins
Opioid-like hormones that are manufactured in the human body and contribute to natural feelings of well-being.

Physical effects of opioids

Opioids are powerful depressants of the central nervous system. In addition to relieving pain, these drugs lower heart rate, respiration, and blood pressure. Side effects include weakness, dizziness, nausea, vomiting, euphoria, decreased sex drive, visual disturbances, and lack of coordination.

The human body's physiology could be said to encourage opioid addiction. Opioid-like hormones called **endorphins** are manufactured in the body and have multiple receptor sites, particularly in the central nervous system. When endorphins attach themselves at these points, they create feelings of painless well-being; medical researchers refer to them as "the body's own opioids." When endorphin levels are high, people feel euphoric. The same euphoria occurs when opioids or related chemicals are active at the endorphin receptor sites. Of all the opioids, heroin has the greatest notoriety as an addictive drug. The following section discusses the progression of heroin addiction; addiction to any opioid follows a similar path.

HEROIN ADDICTION. *Heroin* is a white powder derived from morphine. *Black tar heroin* is a sticky, dark brown, foul-smelling form of heroin that is relatively pure and inexpensive. Once considered a cure for morphine dependence, heroin was later discovered to be even more addictive and potent than morphine. Today heroin has no medical use.

Heroin is a depressant that produces drowsiness and a dreamy, mentally slow feeling. It can cause drastic mood swings, with euphoric highs followed by depressive lows. Heroin slows respiration and urinary output and constricts the pupils of the eyes. Symptoms of tolerance and withdrawal can appear within 3 weeks of first use.

In 2011, 620,000 Americans reported using heroin in the past year, a considerable increase since 2002 (Substance Abuse and Mental Health Services Administration, 2010). Comparatively, Australia reports similar statistics with over 40,000 Australians, or 0.2% of the population in 2010 reporting using heroin in the past year, somewhat higher than 2001 (AIHW, 2014). Positive results from more recent statistics reveal that in 2013, heroin use was almost half that of 2010 with approximately 20,000 Australians, or 0.1% of the population reporting using heroin (AIHW, 2014) Although heroin is usually injected, the contemporary version of heroin is so potent that users can get high by snorting or smoking the drug. This has attracted a more affluent group of users who may not want to inject, for reasons such as the increased risk of contracting diseases, for example, HIV.

The most common route of administration for heroin addicts is "mainlining"—intravenous injection of powdered heroin mixed in a solution. Many users describe the "rush" they feel when injecting themselves as intensely pleasurable, whereas others report unpredictable and unpleasant side effects. The temporary nature of the rush contributes to the drug's high potential for addiction—many addicts shoot up four or five times a day. Mainlining can cause veins to scar and eventually collapse. Once a vein has collapsed, it can no longer be used to introduce heroin into the bloodstream. Addicts become expert at locating new veins to use: in the feet, the legs, the temples, under the tongue, or in the groin.

Treatment for Heroin Addiction. Programs to help people addicted to heroin and other opioids have not been very successful. Some addicts resume drug use even after years of drug-free living because the craving for the injection rush is very strong. It takes a great deal of discipline to seek alternative, nondrug highs.

Heroin addicts experience a distinct pattern of withdrawal. Symptoms of withdrawal include intense desire for the drug, sleep disturbance, dilated pupils, loss of appetite, irritability, goose bumps, and muscle tremors. The most difficult time in the withdrawal process occurs 24 to 72 hours following last use. All of the preceding symptoms continue, along with nausea, abdominal cramps, restlessness, insomnia, vomiting, diarrhea, extreme anxiety, hot and cold flashes, elevated blood pressure, and rapid heartbeat and respiration. Once the peak of withdrawal has passed, all these symptoms begin to subside. Still, the recovering addict has many hurdles to jump.

Methadone maintenance is one treatment available for people addicted to heroin or other opioids. This synthetic narcotic blocks the effects of opioid withdrawal. It is chemically similar enough to opioids to control the tremors, chills, vomiting, diarrhea, and severe abdominal pains of withdrawal. Methadone dosage is decreased over a period of time until the addict is weaned off it.

Methadone maintenance is controversial because of the drug's own potential for addiction. Critics contend that the program merely substitutes one addiction for another. Proponents argue that people on methadone maintenance are less likely to engage in criminal activities to support their habits than heroin addicts are. For this reason, many methadone maintenance programs are financed by state or federal government and are available free of charge or at reduced cost.

A number of new drug therapies for opioid dependence are emerging. Naltrexone (Trexan), an opioid antagonist, has been approved as a treatment. While on naltrexone, recovering addicts do not have the compulsion to use heroin, and if they do use it, they don't get high, so there is no point in using the drug. More recently, researchers have reported promising results with Temgesic (buprenorphine), a mild, nonaddicting synthetic opioid that, like heroin and methadone, bonds to certain receptors in the brain, blocks pain messages, and persuades the brain that its cravings for heroin have been satisfied.

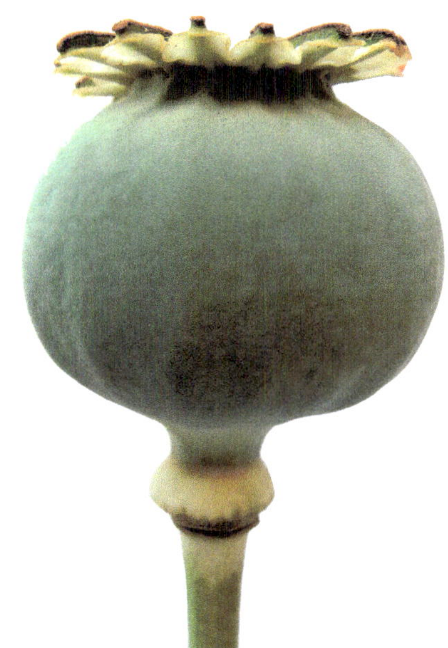

Opium is extracted from opium poppy seed pods like this one.
(Source: Gregor/Shutterstock)

Benzodiazepines and barbiturates

Benzodiazepines A class of central nervous system depressant drugs with sedative, hypnotic, and muscle relaxant effects; also called *tranquillisers*.

Barbiturates Drugs that depress the central nervous system, have sedative and hypnotic effects, and are less safe than benzodiazepines.

A *sedative* drug promotes mental calmness and reduces anxiety, whereas a *hypnotic* drug promotes sleep or drowsiness. The most common sedative-hypnotic drugs are **benzodiazepines**, more commonly known as *tranquillisers*. These include prescription drugs such as Valium, Ativan, and Xanax. Benzodiazepines are most commonly prescribed for tension, muscular strain, sleep problems, anxiety, panic attacks, and alcohol withdrawal. **Barbiturates** are sedative-hypnotic drugs that include Amytal and Seconal. Because they are less safe than benzodiazepines, barbiturates are not typically prescribed for medical conditions that call for sedative-hypnotic drug therapy. Today, benzodiazepines have largely replaced barbiturates, which were used medically in the past for relieving tension and inducing relaxation and sleep.

Sedative-hypnotics have a synergistic effect when combined with alcohol, another central nervous system depressant. Taken together, these drugs can lead to respiratory failure and death.

All sedative or hypnotic drugs can produce physical and psychological dependence in several weeks. A complication specific to sedatives is cross-tolerance, which occurs when users develop tolerance for one sedative or become dependent on it and develop tolerance for others as well. Withdrawal from sedative or hypnotic drugs may range from mild discomfort to severe symptoms, depending on the degree of dependence.

ROHYPNOL. One benzodiazepine of concern is Rohypnol, a potent *tranquillisers* similar in nature to Valium but many times stronger. The drug produces a sedative effect, amnesia, muscle relaxation, and slowed psychomotor responses. The most publicise "date rape" drug, Rohypnol has gained notoriety as a growing problem on university campuses. The drug has been added to punch and other drinks at parties, where it is reportedly given to women in hopes of lowering their inhibitions and facilitating potential sexual conquests.

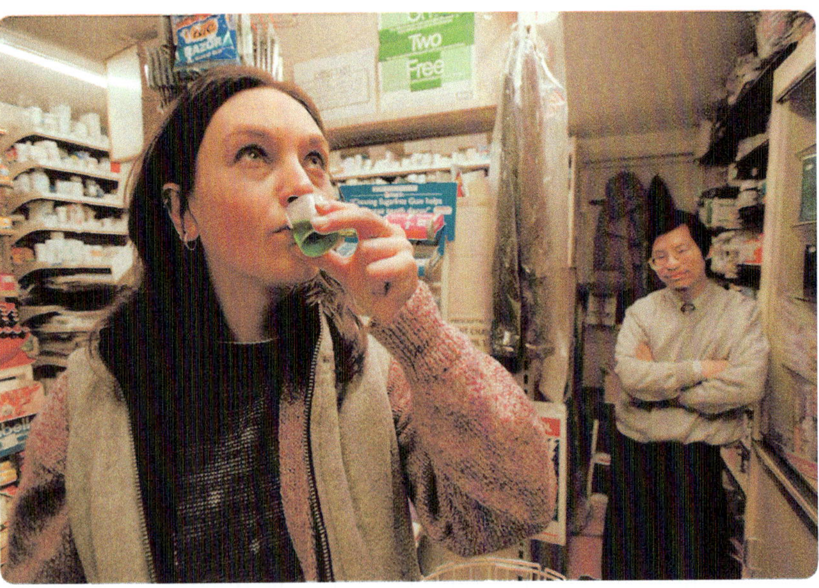

Why is it so hard to quit using heroin?

Heroin's effect on the body is similar to the well-being created by endorphins. Stopping heroin use causes withdrawal symptoms that can be very difficult to manage, which keeps many addicts from attempting to quit. Methadone is a synthetic narcotic that blocks the effects of withdrawal. Although it is still a narcotic and must be administered under the supervision of clinic or pharmacy staff, methadone allows many heroin addicts to lead somewhat normal lives.
(Source: David Hoffman Photolibrary/Alamy)

GHB

Gamma-hydroxybutyrate (GHB) is a central nervous system depressant known to have euphoric, sedative, and anabolic (bodybuilding) effects. It was originally sold over the counter to bodybuilders to help reduce body fat and build muscle. Concerns about GHB led the FDA in the United Stated to ban OTC sales in 1992, and GHB is now a Schedule I drug (Schedule I drugs are classified as having a high potential for abuse, with no currently accepted medical use in the United States) (The Partnership at Drugfree.org, 2012). Similarly, GHB is considered an illegal drug in Australia with penalties for using, making, selling, possessing or driving under the influence (The Australian Drug Foundation, 2016). GHB is an odorless, tasteless fluid. Like Rohypnol, GHB has been slipped into drinks without being detected, resulting in loss of memory, unconsciousness, amnesia, and even death. Other dangerous side effects include nausea, vomiting, seizures, hallucinations, coma, and respiratory distress.

Hallucinogens

Hallucinogens, or *psychedelics,* are substances that are capable of creating auditory or visual hallucinations and unusual changes in mood, thoughts, and feelings. The major receptor sites for most of these drugs are in the reticular formation (located in the brain stem at the upper end of the spinal cord), which is responsible for interpreting outside stimuli before allowing these signals to travel to other parts of the brain. When a hallucinogen is present at a reticular formation site, messages become scrambled, and the user may see wavy walls instead of straight ones or may "smell" colours and "hear" tastes. This mixing of sensory messages is known as **synesthesia**. Users may also become less inhibited or recall events long buried in the subconscious mind. The most widely recognised hallucinogens are LSD, Ecstasy, PCP, mescaline, psilocybin, and ketamine. All are illegal and carry severe penalties for manufacture, possession, transportation, or sale.

Hallucinogens
Substances capable of creating auditory or visual distortions and unusual changes in mood, thoughts, and feelings.

Synesthesia
An effect, which can be created by a drug, in which sensory messages are incorrectly assigned—for example, the user "hears" a taste or "smells" a sound.

LSD

Of all the psychedelics, *lysergic acid diethylamide* (*LSD*) is the most notorious. First synthesised in the late 1930s by Swiss chemist Albert Hoffman, LSD received media attention in the 1960s when young people used the drug to "turn on, tune in, drop out." Use was banned in the 1970s and had tapered off until recently, when it made a comeback.

Most commonly known as "acid," LSD especially attracts younger users. It's estimated that about 6 percent of Americans between ages 18 and 25 have used LSD at least once in their lifetime (Substance Abuse and Mental Health Services Administration, 2012). As a comparison, a national survey of university students showed that 5 percent had used the drug at some point in their lives (Johnston et al;, 2012).

The most common and most popular form of LSD is blotter acid—small squares of blotter-like paper that have been impregnated with a liquid LSD mixture. The blotter is swallowed or chewed briefly. LSD also comes in tiny thin squares of gelatin called *windowpane* and in tablets called *microdots,* which are less than an eighth of an inch across (it would take 10 or more to add up to the size of an aspirin tablet). One of the most powerful drugs known to science, LSD can produce strong effects in doses as low as 20 micrograms. (To give you an idea of how small a dose this is, the average postage stamp weighs approximately 60,000 micrograms.) As with any illegal drug, purchasers run the risk of buying an impure product.

In addition to its psychedelic effects, LSD produces several physical effects, including increased heart rate, elevated blood pressure and temperature, goose bumps (roughened skin), increased reflex speeds, muscle tremors and twitches, perspiration, increased salivation, chills, headaches, and mild nausea. The drug also stimulates uterine muscle contractions, so it can lead to premature labor and miscarriage in pregnant women. Research into long-term effects has been inconclusive.

The psychological effects of LSD vary. Euphoria is the common psychological state produced by the drug, but *dysphoria* (a sense of evil and foreboding) may also be experienced. The drug also shortens attention span, causing the mind to wander. Thoughts may be interposed and juxtaposed, so the user experiences several different thoughts simultaneously. Users become introspective, and suppressed memories may surface, often taking on bizarre symbolism. Many more effects are possible, including decreased aggressiveness and enhanced sensory experiences.

LSD causes distortions of ordinary perceptions, such as the movement of stationary objects. "Bad trips," the most publicise risk of LSD, are commonly related to the user's mood. The person, for example, may interpret increased heart rate as a heart attack.

Although there is no evidence that LSD creates physical dependence, it may create psychological dependence. Many LSD users become depressed for 1 or 2 days following a trip and turn to the drug to relieve this depression. The result is a cycle of LSD use to relieve post-LSD depression, which often leads to psychological addiction.

Ecstasy

Ecstasy is the most common street name for the drug *methylene-dioxymethamphetamine (MDMA),* a synthetic compound with both stimulant and mildly hallucinogenic effects. It is one of the most well-known **club drugs** or "designer drugs," a term applied to synthetic analogs of existing illicit drugs that tend to be popular among teens and young adults at nightclubs, bars, raves, and other all-night parties. Ecstasy creates feelings of extreme

Club drugs
Synthetic analogs that produce similar effects of existing drugs.

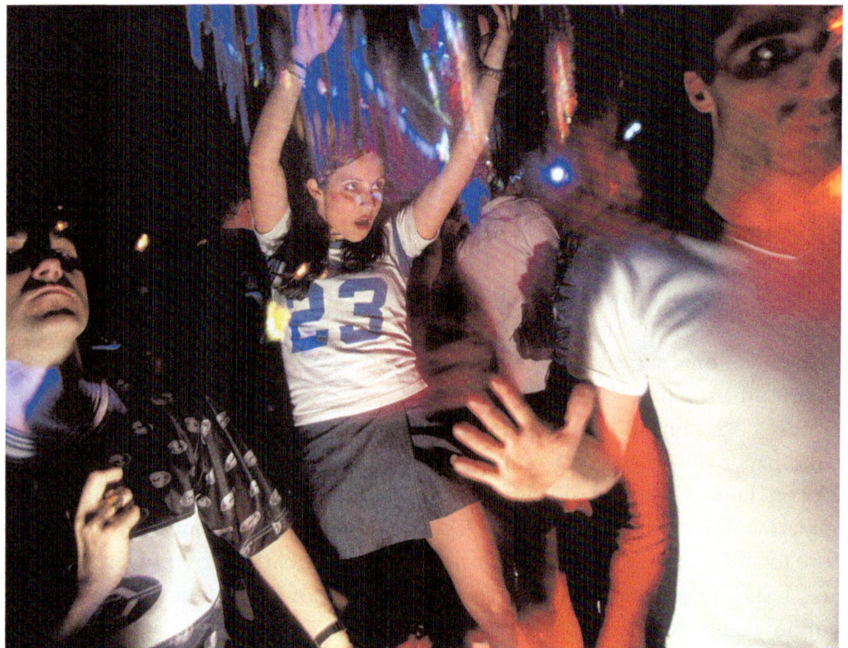

So-called club drugs are often abused by teens and young adults at nightclubs, bars, or all-night dances. Although users may think them relatively harmless, they can produce hallucinations, paranoia, amnesia, dangerous increases in heart rate and blood pressure, coma, and, in some cases, death.
(Source: PeerPoint/Alamy.)

euphoria, openness and warmth, an increased willingness to communicate, feelings of love and empathy, increased awareness, and heightened appreciation for music. Young people may use Ecstasy initially to improve their mood or get energised. Like other hallucinogenic drugs, Ecstasy can enhance the sensory experience and distort perceptions, but it does not create visual hallucinations. Effects begin within 20 to 90 minutes and can last for 3 to 5 hours.

Some of the risks associated with Ecstasy use are similar to those of other stimulants. Because of the nature of the drug, Ecstasy users are at greater risk of inappropriate and/or unintended emotional bonding and have a tendency to say things they might feel uncomfortable about later. Physical consequences of Ecstasy use may include mild to extreme jaw clenching, tongue and cheek chewing; short-term memory loss or confusion; increased body temperature as a result of dehydration and heat stroke; and increased heart rate and blood pressure. Individuals with high blood pressure, heart disease, or liver trouble are at greatest danger when using this drug. As the effects of Ecstasy begin to wear off, the user can experience mild depression, fatigue, and a hangover that can last from days to weeks. Chronic use appears to damage the brain's ability to think and to regulate emotion, memory, sleep, and pain. Combined with alcohol, Ecstasy can be extremely dangerous and sometimes fatal. Some studies indicate that the drug may cause long-lasting neurotoxic effects by damaging brain cells that produce serotonin (National Institute on Drug Abuse, 2010; American College Health Association, 2013).

PCP

Phencyclidine, or *PCP,* is a synthetic substance that became a black-market drug in the early 1970s. PCP was originally developed as a dissociative anesthetic, which means that patients receiving this drug could keep their eyes open and apparently remain conscious but feel no pain during a medical procedure. Afterward, patients would experience amnesia for the time the drug was in their system. Such a drug had obvious advantages as an anesthetic, but its unpredictability and drastic effects (postoperative delirium, confusion, and agitation) made doctors abandon it, and it was withdrawn from the legal market.

On the illegal market, PCP is a white, crystalline powder that users often sprinkle onto marijuana cigarettes. It is dangerous and unpredictable regardless of the method of administration. Common street names for PCP are "angel dust" for the crystalline powdered form and "peace pill" and "horse tranquillisers" for the tablet form. The effects of PCP depend on the dose. A dose as small as 5 mg will produce effects similar to those of strong central nervous system depressants—slurred speech, impaired coordination, reduced sensitivity to pain, and reduced heart and respiratory rate. Doses between 5 and 10 mg cause fever, salivation, nausea, vomiting, and total loss of sensitivity to pain. Doses greater than 10 mg result in a drastic drop in blood pressure, coma, muscular rigidity, violent outbursts, and possible convulsions and death.

Psychologically, PCP may produce either euphoria or dysphoria. It also is known to produce hallucinations as well as delusions and overall delirium. Some users experience a prolonged state of "nothingness." The long-term effects of PCP use are unknown.

Mescaline

Mescaline is one of hundreds of chemicals derived from the peyote cactus, a small, button-like plant that grows in the southwestern United States and in Latin America. Natives of these regions have long used the dried peyote "buttons" for religious purposes.

Users typically swallow 10 to 12 buttons. They taste bitter and generally induce immediate nausea or vomiting. Long-time users claim that the nausea becomes less noticeable with frequent use. Those who are able to keep the drug down begin to feel the effects within 30

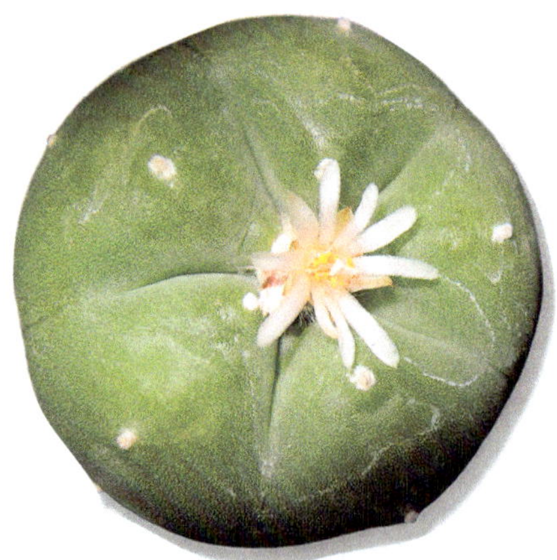

Mescaline comes from "buttons" of the peyote cactus, like this one.
(**Source:** ©Bob Cheung/Shutterstock.)

to 90 minutes, when mescaline reaches maximum concentration in the brain. (It may persist for up to 9 or 10 hours.) Mescaline is both a powerful hallucinogen and a central nervous system stimulant.

Products sold on the street as mescaline are likely to be synthetic chemical relatives of the true drug. Street names of these products include DOM, STP, TMA, and MMDA. Any of these can be toxic in small quantities.

Psilocybin

Psilocybin and *psilocin* are the active chemicals in a group of mushrooms sometimes called "magic mushrooms." *Psilocybe* mushrooms, which grow throughout the world, can be cultivated from spores or harvested wild. When consumed, these mushrooms can cause hallucinations. Because many mushrooms resemble the *Psilocybe* variety, people who harvest wild mushrooms for any purpose should be certain of what they are doing. Mushroom varieties can be easily misidentified, and mistakes can be fatal. Psilocybin is similar to LSD in its physical effects, which generally wear off in 4 to 6 hours.

Ketamine

The liquid form of *ketamine,* or Special K, as it is commonly called, is used as an anesthetic in some hospitals and veterinary clinics. After stealing it from hospitals or medical suppliers, dealers typically dry the liquid (usually by cooking it) and grind the residue into powder. Special K causes hallucinations, because it inhibits the relay of sensory input; the brain fills the resulting void with visions, dreams, memories, and sensory distortions. The effects of ketamine are similar to those of PCP—confusion, agitation, aggression, and lack of coordination—and less predictable. Aftereffects of ketamine are less severe than those of ecstasy, so it has grown in popularity as a club drug.

Inhalants
Chemical vapors that are sniffed or inhaled to produce highs.

Inhalants

Inhalants are chemicals that produce vapors that, when inhaled, can cause hallucinations and create intoxicating and euphoric effects. Not commonly recognise as drugs, inhalants are legal to purchase and universally available, but dangerous when used incorrectly. They generally appeal to young people who can't afford or obtain illicit substances. Some products often misused as inhalants include rubber cement, model glue, paint thinner, lighter fluid, varnish, wax, spot removers, and gasoline. Most of these substances are sniffed or "huffed" by users in search of a quick, cheap high. Amyl nitrite and nitrous oxide ("laughing gas") are also sometimes abused.

Because they are inhaled, the volatile chemicals in these products reach the bloodstream within seconds. An inhaled substance is not diluted or buffered by stomach acids or other body fluids and thus is more potent than it would be if swallowed. This characteristic, along with the fact that dosages are extremely difficult to control because everyone has unique lung and breathing capacities, makes inhalants particularly dangerous.

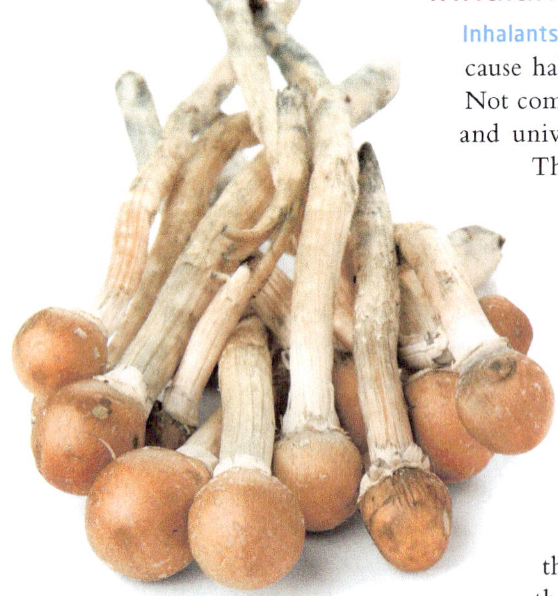

Psilocybe mushrooms produce hallucinogenic effects when ingested.
(**Source:** Martyn Vickery/Alamy.)

The effects of inhalants usually last fewer than 15 minutes and resemble those of central nervous system depressants. Users may experience dizziness, disorientation, impaired coordination, reduced judgement, and slowed reaction times. Combining inhalants with alcohol produces a synergistic effect and can cause severe liver damage that can be fatal.

An overdose of fumes from inhalants can cause unconsciousness. If the user's oxygen intake is reduced during the inhaling process, death can result within 5 minutes. Whether a user is a first-time or chronic user, *sudden sniffing death* syndrome can be a consequence. This syndrome can occur if a user inhales deeply and then participates in physical activity or is startled.

Anabolic steroids

Anabolic steroids are artificial forms of the male hormone testosterone that promote muscle growth and strength. Steroids are available in two forms: injectable solutions and pills. These **ergogenic drugs** are used primarily by people who believe the drugs will increase their strength, power, bulk (weight), speed, and athletic performance.

Anabolic steroids Artificial forms of the hormone testosterone that promote muscle growth and strength.

Ergogenic drugs Substances believed to enhance athletic performance.

It was once estimated that up to 20 percent of university athletes used steroids. Now that stricter drug-testing policies have been instituted by the National Collegiate Athletic Association (NCAA), reported use of anabolic steroids among intercollegiate athletes has decreased; only about .2 percent of university students report taking them in the past 30 days (The National Collegiate Athletic Association, 2012). Comparatively, a 2011 study of over 22,000 Australian high school students revealed that 2.4% of 12-17-year-old students had used anabolic steroids in their lifetime and 1.8% in the past year (Dunn & White, 2011). Interestingly, anabolic steroid use was more common among 12-15-year-olds than 16-17-year-olds. Among both adolescents and adults, steroid abuse is higher among men than it is among women. However, steroid abuse is growing most rapidly among young women (National Institute on Drug Abuse, 2010). The use of steroids among athletes periodically makes the news. Recently, much focus has been placed on Major League Baseball, Australia Football League, cycling, and the 2016 Rio Summer Olympic Games where 100 Russian athletes were barred for illegal drug use (Oksman, 2016).

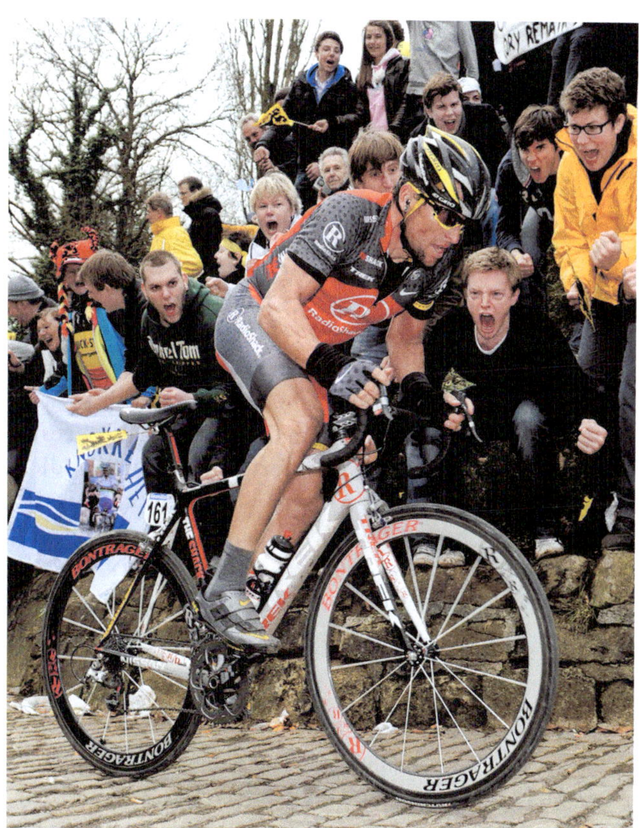

After being stripped of seven Tour de France titles in 2012 and an Olympic medal in 2013, cyclist Lance Armstrong publicly ended his years of denial and admitted to doping. He was banned from cycling for life and has been sued by the U.S. federal government and others for fraud.
(**Source:** PCN/Corbis.)

Physical effects of steroids

Although their primary effects are not psychotropic, anabolic steroids can produce a state of euphoria and diminished fatigue in addition to increased bulk and power in both sexes. These qualities give steroids an addictive quality. When users stop, they can experience psychological withdrawal and sometimes severe depression, in some cases leading to suicide attempts. If untreated, depression associated with steroid withdrawal has been known to last for a year or more after steroid use stops.

Men and women who use steroids experience a variety of adverse effects. These drugs cause mood swings (aggression and violence), sometimes known as "roid rage"; acne; liver tumors; elevated cholesterol levels; hypertension; kidney disease; and immune system disturbances. There is also a danger of transmitting AIDS and hepatitis (a serious liver disease) through shared needles. In women, large doses of anabolic steroids may trigger the development of masculine attributes such as lowered voice, increased facial and body hair, and male-pattern baldness; they may also result in an enlarged clitoris, smaller breasts, and changes in or absence of menstruation. When taken by healthy men, anabolic steroids shut down the body's production of testosterone, causing men's breasts to grow and testicles to atrophy.

Treatment and recovery

An estimated 21.6 million Americans aged 12 or older needed treatment for an illicit drug or alcohol use problem in 2011. Of these, only 2.3 million—approximately 11 percent—received treatment (Substance Abuse and Mental Health Services Administration, 2012).This gap between needing and receiving treatment occurs because the most difficult step in the treatment and recovery process is for the substance abuser to admit that he or she is an addict. Admitting to addiction is difficult because of the power of *denial*—the inability to see the truth. Denial is the hallmark of addiction. It can be so powerful that a planned intervention is sometimes necessary to break down the addict's defenses against recognising the problem. In Australia, the extent to which a substance abuser accesses treatment depends on a multitude of individual and social determinants such as preferred drug of choice, geographical location and availability of treatment and maintenance programs. Statistics suggest that heroin users are more likely to be in treatment, with approximately 50% of heroin users engaged in treatment, when compared to methamphetamine and marijuana users, with approximately 20% and 5% in treatment respectively (Ritter, Lancaster, Grech & Reuter, 2011). This difference can be attributed to the widespread availability of pharmacological maintenance programs (e.g., methadone and buprenorphine) in Australia.

Recovery from drug addiction or addiction to a behaviour is a long-term process and frequently requires multiple episodes of treatment. The first step generally begins with abstinence—refraining from the behaviour. **Detoxification** refers to an early abstinence period during which an addict adjusts physically and cognitively to being free from the addiction's influence. It occurs in virtually every recovering addict, and although it is uncomfortable for most addicts, it can be dangerous for some. This is primarily true for those addictedto chemicals, especially alcohol and heroin, and painkillers such as OxyContin. For these people, early abstinence may involve profound withdrawals that require medical supervision. Because of this, most inpatient treatment programs provide a pretreatment component of supervised detoxification to achieve abstinence safely before treatment begins.

Detoxification The process, which involves abstinence, of freeing a drug user from an intoxicating or addictive substance in the body or from dependence on such a substance.

Treatment approaches

Outpatient behavioural treatment encompasses a wide variety of programs for addicts who visit a clinic at regular intervals. Most of the programs involve individual or group drug counselling. Some programs also offer other forms of behavioural treatment, such as the following:

- Cognitive behavioural therapy, which seeks to help patients recognise, avoid, and cope with the situations in which they are most likely to abuse drugs
- Multidimensional family therapy, which addresses a range of influences on the drug abuse patterns of adolescents and is designed for them and their families

- Motivational interviewing, which is a client-centred, direct method for enhancing intrinsic motivation to change by exploring and resolving ambivalence
- Motivational incentives (contingency management), which uses positive reinforcement to encourage abstinence from drugs

Residential treatment programs can also be very effective, especially for those with more severe problems. For example, therapeutic communities (TCs) are highly structured programs in which addicts remain at a residence, typically for 6 to 12 months. The focus of the TC is on the resocialisation of the addict to a drug-free lifestyle.

12-Step programs

The first 12-step program, Alcoholics Anonymous (AA), began in 1935 in Akron, Ohio. Since its inception, the 12-step program has become the most widely used approach around the world, including Australia. The 12-step program deals not only with alcoholism, but also drug abuse and various other addictive or dysfunctional behaviours. There are more than 200 different recovery programs based on the program, including Narcotics Anonymous, Cocaine Anonymous, Crystal Meth Anonymous, Gamblers Anonymous, and Pills Anonymous.

The 12-step program is nonjudgemental and based on the idea that a program's only purpose is to work on personal recovery. Working the 12 steps includes admitting to having a serious problem, recognising there is an outside power that could help, consciously relying on that power, admitting and listing character defects, seeking deliverance from defects, apologising to those individuals one has harmed in the past, and helping others with the same problem. The 12-step meetings are held at a variety of times and locations in almost every city. There is no membership cost, and the meetings are open to anyone who wishes to attend.

Addressing drug misuse and abuse

Around the globe, the public is alarmed by the persistent problem of illegal drug use. Respondents in public opinion polls feel that the most important strategy for fighting drug abuse is educating young people. They also endorse strategies such as stricter border surveillance to reduce drug trafficking; longer prison sentences for drug dealers; increased government spending on prevention; antidrug law enforcement; and greater cooperation among government agencies, private groups, and individuals providing treatment assistance.

To address safety concerns, many employers have instituted mandatory drug testing. Despite controversies over accuracy of urinalysis tests, this practice is becoming more common.

All of these approaches will probably help up to a point, but they do not offer a total solution to the problem. Drug abuse has been a part of human behaviour for thousands of years, and it is not likely to disappear in the near future. For this reason, it is necessary to educate ourselves and to develop the self-discipline necessary to avoid dangerous drug dependence.

In general, researchers in the field of drug education agree that a multimodal approach is best. Young people should be taught the difference between drug use, misuse, and abuse. Factual information that is free of scare tactics must be presented; lecturing and moralising have proven not to work.

Harm reduction strategies

Harm reduction is a set of practical approaches to reducing negative consequences of drug use, incorporating a spectrum of strategies from safer use to managed use to abstinence. Harm reduction approaches have been widely used in needle exchange programs, where injection drug users receive clean needles and syringes and bleach for cleaning needles; these efforts help reduce the number of HIV and hepatitis B cases. Harm reduction may also involve changing the legal sanctions associated with drug use, increasing the availability of treatment services to drug abusers, and/or attempting to change drug users' behaviour through education. Harm reduction strategies meet drug users "where they're at," addressing conditions of use along with the use itself. This strategy recognises that people always have and always will use drugs and, therefore, attempts to minimise the potential hazards associated with drug use rather than the use itself. [E]

Alcohol: an overview

When many of us think of dangerous drugs, illegal substances such as heroin or cocaine often come to mind. But in reality, two socially accepted drugs—alcohol and tobacco—kill far more people. In Australia, tobacco is the single most preventable cause of death with more drug-related deaths and hospitalisations attributable to tobacco than illicit drugs and alcohol combined (AIWF, 2010). Alcohol is also a major cause of morbidity and mortality in Australia through road accidents, violence and crime (Ministerial Council on Drug Strategy, 2011). In the United States, excessive use of alcohol is responsible for about 80,000 deaths annually—twice as many as illicit drugs (Centers for Disease Control and Prevention, 2008)—and tobacco is the single largest preventable cause of death in the United States, claiming a whopping 443,000 lives a year (CDCP, 2008).

Throughout history, humans have used alcohol during social gatherings, religious ceremonies, and everyday life. The consumption of alcoholic beverages is interwoven with many traditions, and moderate use of alcohol can enhance celebrations or special times. Research shows that very low levels of alcohol consumption, particularly red wine, may actually lower some health risks in older adults (Marrone et al., 2012; Stockley, 2012; Klatsky, 2009). Even though alcohol can play a positive role in some people's lives, it is first and foremost a chemical substance that affects physical and mental behaviour. The fact is, alcohol is a drug, and if it is not used responsibly, it can be dangerous.

It is estimated that half of Americans consume alcoholic beverages regularly, and about 21 percent abstain from drinking alcohol altogether (National Center for Health Statistics, 2010).Among those who drink, consumption patterns vary. More men are regular drinkers, and men typically drink more than do women. White drinkers are more likely to drink daily or nearly daily than are nonwhites. As age increases, the number of people who consume alcohol regularly decreases (NCHS, 2010).

Alcohol and students

Binge drinking
A binge is a pattern of drinking alcohol that brings blood alcohol concentration (BAC) to 0.08 gram-percent or above; for a typical adult, this pattern corresponds to consuming five or more drinks (male) or four or more drinks (female) in about 2 hours.

The heavy consumption of alcohol among students has been documented globally (Karam, Kypri & Salamoun, 2007; Wechsler & Nelson, 2008; Wicki, Kuntsche & Gmel, 2010; Hallett et al., 2012). In the United States, Alcohol is the most popular drug on university campuses: 62 percent of students report having consumed alcoholic beverages in the past 30 days (Figure 6.3) (American College Health Association, 2013). Approximately 39 percent of all university students engage in binge drinking (Substance Abuse and Mental Health Services Administration, 2012)—a pattern of drinking that brings blood alcohol concentration (BAC) to 0.08 gram-percent or above. Students who might go out and drink only once a week are considered binge drinkers if they consume five or more drinks (for men) or four or more drinks (for women) within 2 hours (National Institute on Alcohol Abuse and Alcoholism, 2012). Comparatively, in Australia, a large scale study of undergraduate university students aged 17 to 25 years found that 94% of participants had consumed alcohol in the

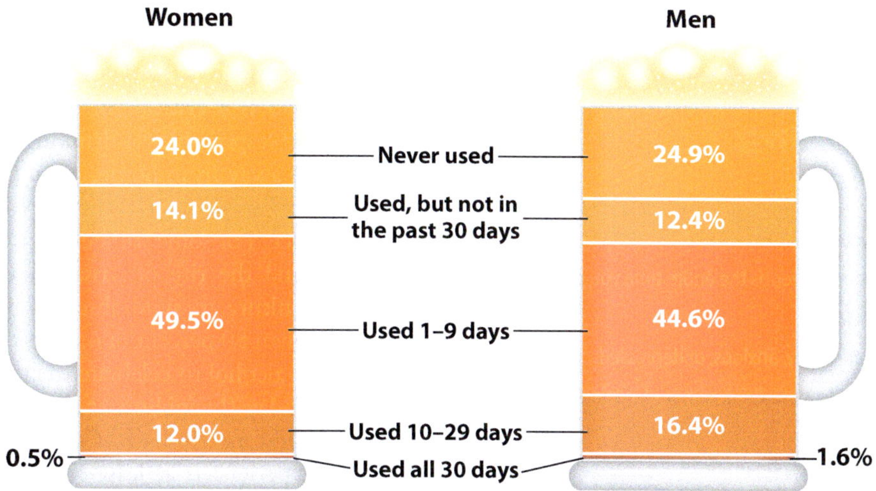

Figure 6.3 University Students' Patterns of Alcohol Use in the Past 30 Days
Source: Data from American College Health Association, *American College Health Association—National College Health Assessment II: Reference Group Executive Summary, Fall 2012* (Hanover, MD: American College Health Association, 2013).

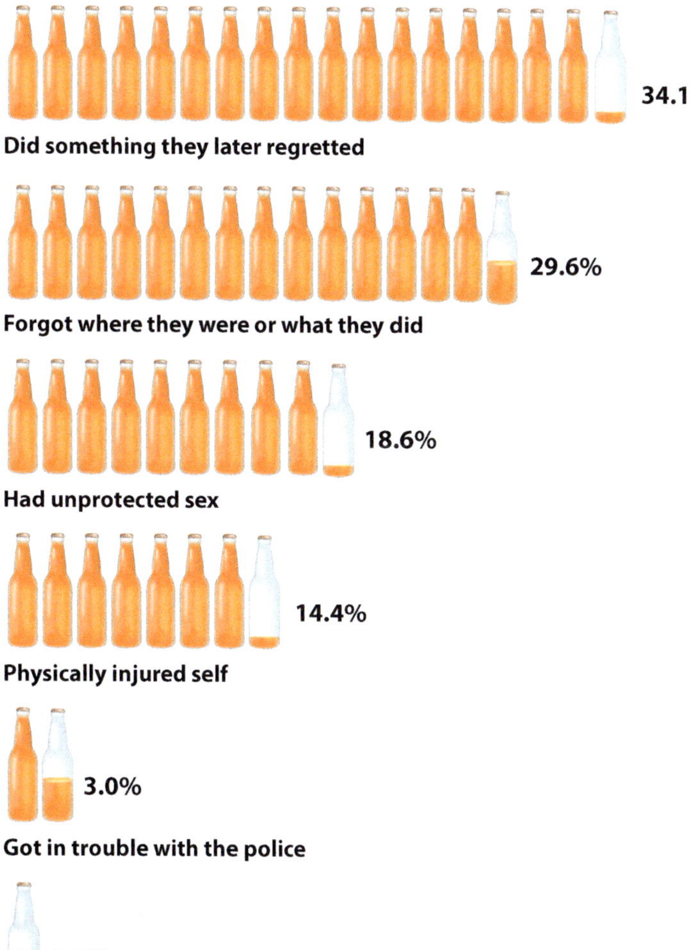

Figure 6.4 Prevalence of Negative Consequences of Drinking among College Students, Past Year
Source: Data from American University Health Association, *American College Health Association—National College Health Assessment II: Reference Group Executive Summary, Fall 2012* (Hanover, MD: American College Health Association, 2013).

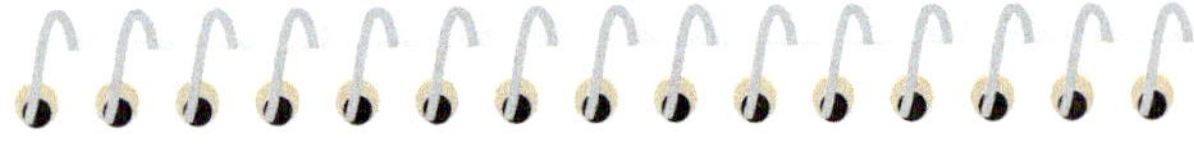

Skills for Behaviour Change

Tips for Drinking Responsibly

- Eat before and while you drink.
- Stay with the same group of friends the entire time you drink.
- Don't drink before the party.
- Avoid drinking if you are angry, anxious, or depressed.
- Pace yourself. Drink one alcoholic drink an hour (or add even more time between drinks).
- Alternate alcoholic and nonalcoholic drinks.
- Determine ahead of time the number of drinks you will have for the evening.
- Avoid drinking games.
- Keep track of the number of drinks you drink.
- Don't drink and drive. Volunteer to be the sober driver.

last 12 months, while 34% drank alcohol at hazardous levels (greater than 6 standard drinks in one sitting) (Hallett et al., 2012).

University is a critical time to become aware of and responsible for drinking. Many students are away from home, often for the first time, and are excited by their newfound independence. For some students, this independence and the rite of passage into the university culture are symbolised by alcohol use. More than 80 percent of university students drink alcohol to celebrate their twenty-first birthday (Neighbors et al., 2011). In a recent study, nearly half of students celebrating experienced at least one negative consequence of drinking alcohol (e.g., headache, feeling very sick to their stomach, etc.) (Lewis et al., 2012).

The transition into university itself may put first-year students at risk for alcohol misuse. During high school, students who are university bound drink less than their classmates who aren't headed to university, and those students who report a difficult transition to university are more likely to engage in high-risk drinking (NIAAA, 2012). Many students say they drink to have fun, but may really be coping with stress, boredom, anxiety, or pressures created by academic and social demands. For other students alcohol lowers inhibitions and is a way to manage social anxiety and shyness.

A significant number of students experience negative consequences as a result of their alcohol consumption (Figure 6.4). Nearly 2 percent reported having sex with someone without giving consent, and 0.6 percent reported having sex with someone without getting consent. Women are more likely to have someone use force or the threat of force to have sex with them when alcohol is involved.

Alcohol use among university students also has consequences related to academic performance.[E] Alcohol consumption tends to disrupt sleep, particularly the second half of the night's sleep, and these disruptive effects increase daytime sleepiness and decrease alertness. Research shows that daytime sleepiness as a result of alcohol use and disruptive sleep negatively impacts students' academic performance and puts them at risk for greater alcohol-related consequences (Ompyer, 2012;Kenney et al., 2012).

Fortunately, many university students report practicing protective behaviours when consuming alcohol to reduce the risk of negative consequences as a result of their alcohol use. The Skills for Behaviour Change box provides some of these strategies for drinking responsibly.

High-risk drinking and university students

According to a recent study, 1,825 university students die each year because of alcohol-related unintentional injuries, including car accidents in the United States (Hingson et al., 2009). Consumption of alcohol is the number one cause of preventable death among undergraduate

---

[E]Donatelle, R. J.(2015). Recognizing and avoiding addiction and drug abuse. In *Health: The basics* (11th ed., pp. 206-223). Upper Saddle River, NJ: Pearson Education Inc.

university students in the United States today (Hingson et al., 2009). Similarly, excessive alcohol consumption and alcohol related harm is a concern for Australian university students. Hughes (2012) reported that university students living at on campus consume hazardous amounts of alcohol and normalise their heavy consumption despite knowing the consequences of alcohol misuse.

Although everyone who drinks is at some risk for alcohol-related problems, university students seem to be particularly vulnerable for the following reasons:

- Alcohol exacerbates their already high risk for suicide, automobile crashes, and falls.
- Many university students' customs and celebrations encourage certain dangerous practices and patterns of alcohol use.
- Advertising and promotions from the alcoholic beverage industry heavily target university campuses.
- Beer and other drink specials enable students to consume large amounts of alcohol cheaply.
- University students are particularly vulnerable to peer influence.
- University administrators often deny that alcohol problems exist on their campuses.

University students are also more likely than their noncollegiate peers to drink recklessly, play drinking games, and engage in other dangerous practices. One such practice is **pre-gaming** (also called pre-loading or front-loading), which involves planned heavy drinking with friends over brief periods of time prior to going out to a bar, party, or sporting event. It is estimated that about 55 percent of both university men and women pre-game before going to a bar or nightclub (Wells, Graham & Purcell, 2008; Johnston et al., 2012). Pre-gamers also have higher alcohol consumption during the evening and suffer more negative consequences.

Pre-gaming
A strategy of drinking heavily, usually with friends, before going out to parties or bars.

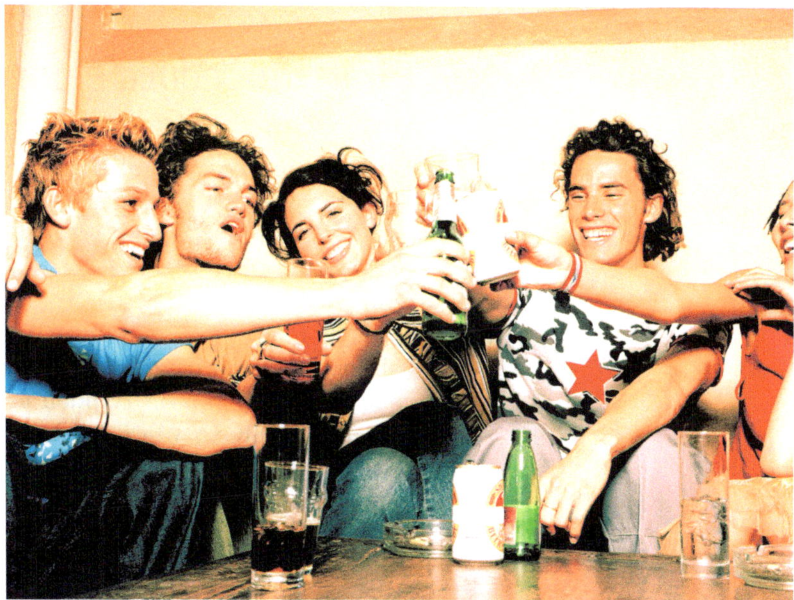

How much do university students really drink?

It may sometimes seem like your campus is crowded with heavy drinkers, but, in fact, most university students—about 60%—drink only occasionally, and 24% don't drink at all. However, university students have high rates of binge drinking; when they do drink, they tend to drink a lot. Irresponsible consumption of alcohol can easily result in disaster, so it is important for you to take control of when you drink, and how much.

Source: American College Health Association, *American College Health Association—National College Health Assessment II (ACHA-NCHA II) Reference Group Data Report, Fall 2012* (Hanover, MD: American College Health Association, 2013).

(**Source:** Stockbyte/ Getty Images.)

Two-thirds of university students engage in drinking games that involve binge drinking (Ahern et al., 2010). Those who participate in drinking games are much less likely to monitor or regulate how much they are drinking and are at risk for extreme intoxication. Men more often than women participate in drinking games to consume larger amounts of alcohol (Cameron et al., 2010), and drinking games have been associated with alcohol-related injuries and deaths from alcohol poisoning. You may want to ask yourself whether your own alcohol consumption or your own drinking patterns might be a problem.

Unfortunately, recent studies confirm what students have been experiencing for a long time—binge drinkers cause problems not only for themselves, but also for those around them. One study indicated that more than 696,000 students between the ages of 18 and 24 were assaulted by another student who had been drinking. Other students report sleep and study disruptions, vandalism of personal property, sexual abuse, and other unwanted sexual advances. Women from colleges with medium to high binge-drinking rates are 1.5 times more at risk of being raped than those from schools with low binge-drinking rates.

Some people use extreme measures to control their eating and/or exercise excessively so that they can save calories, consume more alcohol, and become intoxicated faster (Hingson et al., 2009). "**Drunkorexia**" is a colloquialism currently being use to describe the combination of two dangerous behaviours: disordered eating and heavy drinking. Early studies have found that university students who restrict the number of calories they consume prior to drinking are more likely to binge drink (Burke at al., 2010). One study found that 16 percent of women surveyed "saved" calories for drinking by restricting normal caloric intake (Giles et al., 2009). Motivations for drunkorexia include preventing weight gain, getting drunk faster, and saving money that would be spent on food to buy alcohol. Potential risks of drunkorexia include risk of black outs, forced sexual activity, unintended sexual activity, and alcohol poisoning.

Drunkorexia A colloquial term to describe the combination of disordered eating, excessive physical activity and heavy alcohol consumption.

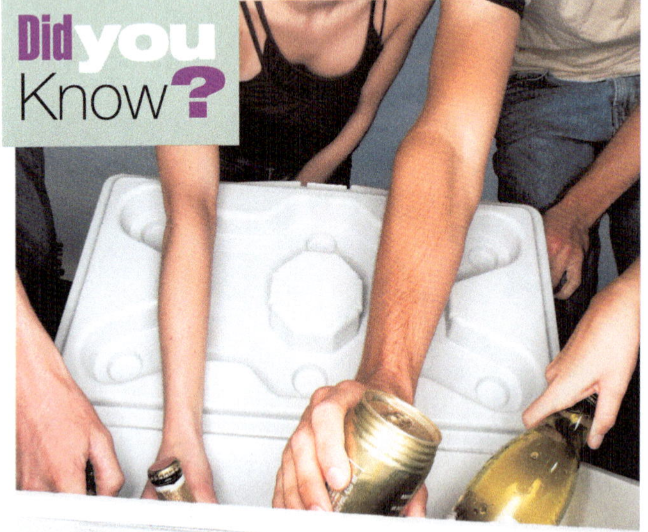

The average college student spends about $900 per year on alcohol—compared to spending an average of about $450 a year on books.

Source: Data from Phoenix House's Facts on Tap, "School Daze?" Accessed 2011, www.factsontap.org
(**Source:** Corbis/Photolibrary, Inc.)

Efforts to reduce student drinking

What are universities currently doing to address the problem of drinking on campus? Programs that have proven particularly effective use cognitive-behavioural skills training with *motivational interviewing*, a nonjudgemental approach to working with students to change behaviour. One of these programs is Brief Alcohol Screening and Intervention for College Students (BASICS), which has been effective for heavy-drinking students with already existing or risk for problems related to alcohol. A recent study found that both male and female students significantly changed their behaviour with regards to drinking after participating in the program (DiFulvio et al., 2012). E-interventions—electronically based alcohol education interventions using text messages, e-mails, and podcasts—and Web interventions such as the Alcohol e-Check Up to Go (e-Chug) have shown promise in reducing alcohol-related problems among first-year students.

Web-based education for first-year students, particularly those who are incoming, has become an increasingly important intervention used by universities to reduce both hazardous drinking and alcohol-related problems. Because first-year students are at increased risk for alcohol-related problems, schools ensure that students are made aware of risks and effects of alcohol. Universities have been using a *social norms* approach to reducing alcohol consumption, sending a consistent message to students about actual drinking behaviour on campus. Many students perceive that their peers drink more than they actually do, which may cause them to feel pressured to drink more themselves.

Ethyl alcohol (ethanol) An addictive, intoxicating drug produced by fermentation and the main ingredient in alcoholic beverages.

Fermentation The process whereby yeast organisms break down plant sugars to yield ethanol.

Distillation The process whereby alcohol vapors are condensed and mixed with water to make hard alcohol.

Alcohol in the body

Learning about the metabolism and absorption of alcohol can help you understand how it affects each person differently and how it is possible to drink safely. It is also key in understanding how to avoid life-threatening circumstances such as alcohol poisoning.

The chemistry and potency of alcohol

The intoxicating substance found in beer, wine, liquor, and liqueurs is **ethyl alcohol**, or **ethanol**. It is produced during a process called **fermentation**, in which yeast organisms break down plant sugars, yielding ethanol and carbon dioxide. Hard liquor is produced through further processing called **distillation**, during which alcohol vapors are condensed and mixed with water to make the final product.

The **proof** of an alcoholic drink is a measure of the percentage of alcohol in the beverage and therefore the strength of the drink. Alcohol percentage is half of the given proof. For example, 80 proof whiskey or scotch is 40 percent alcohol by volume, and 100 proof vodka is 50 percent alcohol by volume. Lower-proof drinks will produce fewer alcohol effects than the same amount of higher-proof drinks. Most wines are between 12 and 15 percent alcohol, and most beers are between 2 and 8 percent, depending on state laws and type of beer.

When discussing alcohol consumption, researchers usually talk in terms of "standard drinks." As defined by the National Institute on Alcohol Abuse and Alcoholism, a **standard drink** is any drink that contains about 14 grams of pure alcohol (about 0.6 fluid ounce or 1.2 tablespoons; see Figure 6.5). The actual size of a standard drink depends on the proof: A 12-oz can of beer and a 1.5-oz shot of vodka are both considered one standard drink because they contain the same amount of alcohol—about 0.6

Standard drink equivalent (and % alcohol)	Approximate number of standard drinks in:
Beer = 12 oz (~5% alcohol)	12 oz = 1 16 oz = 1.3 22 oz = 2 40 oz = 3.3
Malt liquor = 8.5 oz (~7% alcohol)	12 oz = 1.5 16 oz = 2 22 oz = 2.5 40 oz = 4.5
Table wine = 5 oz (~12% alcohol)	750-mL (25-oz) bottle = 5
80 proof spirits (gin, vodka, etc.) = 1.5 oz (~40% alcohol)	mixed drink = 1 or more* pint (16 oz) = 11 fifth (25 oz) = 17 1.75 L (59 oz) = 39

Figure 6.5 What Is a Standard Drink?

*Note: It can be difficult to estimate the number of standard drinks in a single mixed drink made with hard liquor. Depending on factors such as the type of spirits and the recipe, a mixed drink can contain from one to three or more standard drinks.

Source: Adapted from National Institute on Alcohol Abuse and Alcoholism, *Rethinking Drinking: Alcohol and Your Health*, NIH Publication no. 10-3770 (Bethesda, MD: National Institutes of Health, Revised 2010).

fluid ounce. If you are estimating your blood alcohol concentration using standard drinks as a measure (see the following sections), you need to keep in mind the size of your drinks as well as their proof. For example, you may have bought only one beer while you were at the ballpark last weekend, but if that beer came in a 22-oz cup, then you actually consumed two standard drinks.

Proof
A measure of the percentage of alcohol in a beverage. Proof is double the percentage of alcohol in the drink.

Standard drink
The amount of any beverage that contains about 14 grams of pure alcohol.

Absorption and metabolism

Unlike the molecules found in most foods and drugs, alcohol molecules are sufficiently small and fat soluble to be absorbed throughout the entire gastrointestinal system. Approximately 20 percent of ingested alcohol diffuses through the stomach lining into the bloodstream, and nearly 80 percent passes through the lining of the upper third of the small intestine. A negligible amount of alcohol is absorbed through the lining of the mouth.

Several factors influence how quickly your body will absorb alcohol: the alcohol concentration in your drink, the amount of alcohol you consume, the amount of food in your stomach, pylorospasm (spasm of the pyloric valve in the digestive system), your metabolism, weight and body mass index, and your mood.

The higher the concentration of alcohol in your drink, the more rapidly it will be absorbed. As a rule, wine and beer are absorbed more slowly than distilled beverages. "Fizzy" alcoholic beverages—such as champagne and carbonated wines—are absorbed more rapidly than those containing no sparkling additives. Carbonated beverages and drinks served with mixers cause the pyloric valve—the opening from the stomach into the small intestine—to relax, thereby emptying the contents of the stomach more rapidly into the small intestine. Because the small intestine is the site of the greatest absorption of alcohol, carbonated beverages increase the rate of absorption.

The more alcohol you consume, the longer absorption takes. Alcohol can irritate the digestive system, which causes pylorospasm. When the pyloric valve is closed, nothing can move from the stomach to the upper third of the small intestine, which slows absorption. If the irritation continues, it can cause vomiting. Alcohol also takes longer to absorb if there is food in your stomach, because the surface area exposed to alcohol is smaller, and because a full stomach retards the emptying of alcoholic beverages into the small intestine. The **Student Health Today** box on the following page discusses the effects of mixing energy drinks with alcohol.

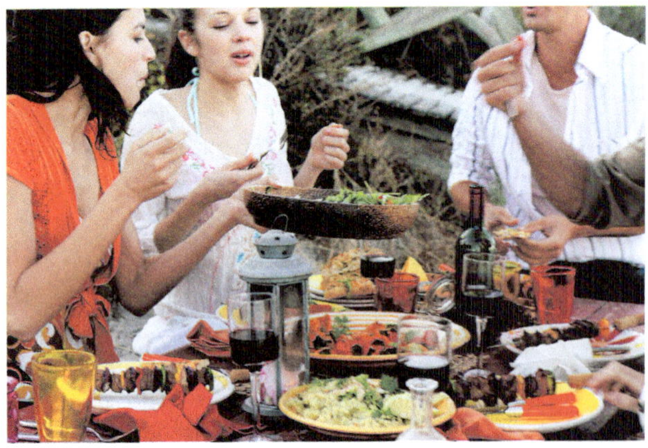

Why do people feel the effects of alcohol differently?

Many factors influence how rapidly a person's body absorbs alcohol, and thus how quickly that person feels the effects of the alcohol. For example, eating while drinking slows down the absorption of alcohol into your bloodstream. Other relevant factors include gender, body weight, body composition, and mood.
(Source: Goodshoot/Jupiter Images.)

Mood is another factor in absorption, because emotions affect how long it takes for the contents of the stomach to empty into the intestine. Powerful moods like stress and tension are likely to cause the stomach to dump its contents into the small intestine, meaning alcohol is absorbed much more rapidly when people are tense than when they are relaxed.

Once it has been absorbed into the bloodstream, alcohol circulates throughout the body and is metabolised in the liver, where it is converted to *acetaldehyde*—a toxic chemical that can cause nausea and vomiting as well as long-term effects such as liver damage—by the enzyme *alcohol dehydrogenase.* It is then rapidly oxidised to *acetate,* converted to carbon dioxide and water, and eventually excreted from the body. A very small portion of alcohol is excreted unchanged by the kidneys, lungs, and skin.

Student Health Today

Alcohol and Energy Drinks: A Dangerous Mix

Thirty-four percent of 18- to 24-year-olds are regular energy drink consumers, and the alcohol industry has used the popularity of energy drinks to promote its own caffeinated alcoholic beverages (CABs)—premixed alcohol and energy drink products like Sparks, Rockstar 21, and Tilt. In addition, energy drink companies promote mixing energy drinks with alcohol products. Red Bull, for example, promotes a top drinks list suggesting "Jaegerbombs" and "Tucker Death mix."

Because students often mix energy drinks with alcohol for the sake of masking the taste or effects, these drinks can be particularly dangerous. One study found that students drinking alcohol with energy drinks consumed more than those who drank other types of alcoholic beverages (8.3 drinks vs. 6.1 drinks, respectively).

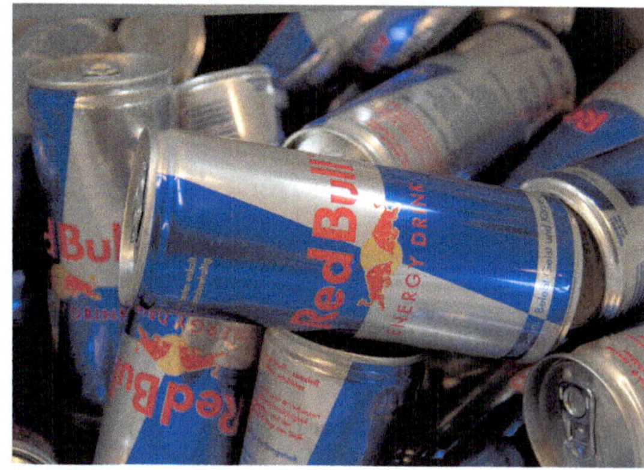

Mixing alcohol with energy drinks, such as Red Bull, can have serious consequences.

Students also report not noticing the signs of intoxication (dizziness, fatigue, headache, or lack of coordination) when they had consumed alcohol-mixed energy drinks. Caffeine may delay the onset of normal sleepiness, increasing the amount of time a person would normally stay awake and drink. The caffeine in energy drinks also reduces the subjective feeling of drunkenness without actually reducing alcohol-related impairment. Students who reported drinking alcohol-mixed energy drinks were more likely to be taken advantage of sexually; they were also twice as likely to take advantage of someone sexually, ride with a drunk driver, be hurt or injured, or require medical treatment. They were more than twice as likely than non–energy drink drinkers to meet the criteria for alcohol dependency. Weekly or daily energy drink consumption is also strongly associated with alcohol dependency.

More than 20,000 emergency room visits related to highly caffeinated beverages were reported in the past year, according to researchers from the U.S. Substance Abuse and Mental Health Services Administration (SAMHSA). Approximately 42 percent of the cases involving energy drinks were in combination with alcohol or drugs, such as Ritalin or Adderall, and 18- to 25-year-olds were the most common age group seeking emergency treatment for energy drink emergencies.

Sources: D. L. Thombs et al., "Event-level Analyses of Energy Drink Consumption and Alcohol Intoxication in Bar Patrons," *Addictive Behaviors* 35, no. 4 (2010): 325–330; S. Snipes et al., "High-Risk Cocktails and High Risk Sex: Examining the Relation between Alcohol Mixed with Energy Drink Consumption, Sexual Behavior, and Drug Use in College Students," *Addictive Behaviors* 38 (2013): 1418–1423 (in press); Join Together, "Combining Energy Drinks with Alcohol More Dangerous Than Drinking Alcohol Alone," The Partnership at Drug Free.org, www.drugfree.org; A.M. Arria et al., "Energy Drink Consumption and Increased Risk for Alcohol Dependence," *Alcoholism: Clinical and Experimental Research* 35, no. 2 (2011): 365–375; W. I. William et al., "Energy Drinks: Psychological Effects and Impact on Well-Being and Quality of Life: A Literature Review," *Innovations in Clinical Neuroscience* 9, no. 1 (2012): 25–34; Substance Abuse and Mental Health Services Administration, Center for Behavioral Health Statistics and Quality, *The DAWN Report: Update on Emergency Department Visits Involving Energy Drinks: A Continuing Public Health Concern.* (Rockville, MD: Substance Abuse and Mental Health Services Administration, January 10, 2013).
(Source: INSADCO Photography/Alamy.)

Alcohol contains 7 calories (kcal) per gram. This means that the average regular beer contains about 150 calories. Mixed drinks may contain more if they are combined with sugary soda or fruit juice. The body uses the calories in alcohol in the same manner it uses those found in carbohydrates: for immediate energy or for storage as fat if not immediately needed.

The breakdown of alcohol occurs at a fairly constant rate of 0.5 ounce per hour (approximately equivalent to one standard drink). This amount of alcohol is equivalent to 12 ounces of 5 percent beer, 5 ounces of 12 percent wine, or 1.5 ounces of 40 percent (80 proof) liquor. Unmetabolised alcohol circulates in the bloodstream until enough time passes for the body to break it down.

Blood alcohol concentration (BAC) The ratio of alcohol to total blood volume; the factor used to measure the physiological and behavioural effects of alcohol.

Blood alcohol concentration

Blood alcohol concentration (BAC) is the ratio of alcohol to total blood volume. It is the factor used to measure the physiological and behavioural effects of alcohol. Despite individual differences, alcohol produces some general behavioural effects, depending on BAC (see Figure 6.6). At a BAC of 0.02 percent, a person feels slightly relaxed and in a good mood. At 0.05, relaxation increases, there is some motor impairment, and a willingness to talk becomes apparent. At 0.08, the person feels euphoric, and there is further motor impairment. The legal limit for BAC is 0.08 percent in all states and the District of Columbia. At 0.10, the depressant effects of alcohol become apparent, drowsiness sets in, and motor skills are further impaired, followed by a loss of judgement. Thus, a driver may not be able to estimate distance or speed, and some drinkers may do things they would not do when sober. As BAC increases, the drinker suffers increasingly negative physiological and psychological effects.

A drinker's BAC depends on weight and body fat, the water content in body tissues, the concentration of alcohol in the beverage consumed, the rate of consumption, and the volume of alcohol consumed. Heavier people have larger body surfaces through which to diffuse alcohol; therefore, they have lower concentrations of alcohol in their blood than do thin people after drinking the same amount. Because alcohol does not diffuse as rapidly into body fat as into water, alcohol concentration is higher in a person with more body fat. Because a woman is likely to have proportionately more body fat and less water in her body tissues than does a man of the same weight, she will be more intoxicated than a man after drinking the same amount of alcohol.

Body fat is not the only contributor to the differences in alcohol's effects on men and women. Compared with men, women have half as much *alcohol dehydrogenase,* the enzyme that breaks down alcohol in the stomach before it reaches the bloodstream and the brain. Therefore, if a man and a woman drink the same amount of alcohol, the woman's BAC will be approximately 30 percent higher than the man's, leaving her more vulnerable to slurred speech, careless driving, and other drinking-related impairments. Hormonal differences can also play a role: Certain points in the menstrual cycle and the use of oral contraceptives are likely to contribute to longer periods of intoxication. Figure 6.7 compares blood alcohol levels in men and women by weight and consumption.

Blood Alcohol Concentration (BAC)	Psychological and Physical Effects
Not Impaired	
<0.01%	Negligible
Sometimes Impaired	
0.01–0.04%	Slight muscle relaxation, mild euphoria, slight body warmth, increased sociability and talkativeness
Usually Impaired	
0.05–0.07%	Lowered alertness, impaired judgment, lowered inhibitions, exaggerated behaviour, loss of small muscle control
Always Impaired	
0.08–0.14%	Slowed reaction time, poor muscle coordination, short-term memory loss, judgment impaired, inability to focus
0.15–0.24%	Blurred vision, lack of motor skills, sedation, slowed reactions, difficulty standing and walking, passing out
0.25–0.34%	Impaired consciousness, disorientation, loss of motor function, severely impaired or no reflexes, impaired circulation and respiration, uncontrolled urination, slurred speech, possible death
0.35% and up	Unconsciousness, coma, extremely slow heartbeat and respiration, unresponsiveness, probable death

Figure 6.6 The Psychological and Physical Effects of Alcohol

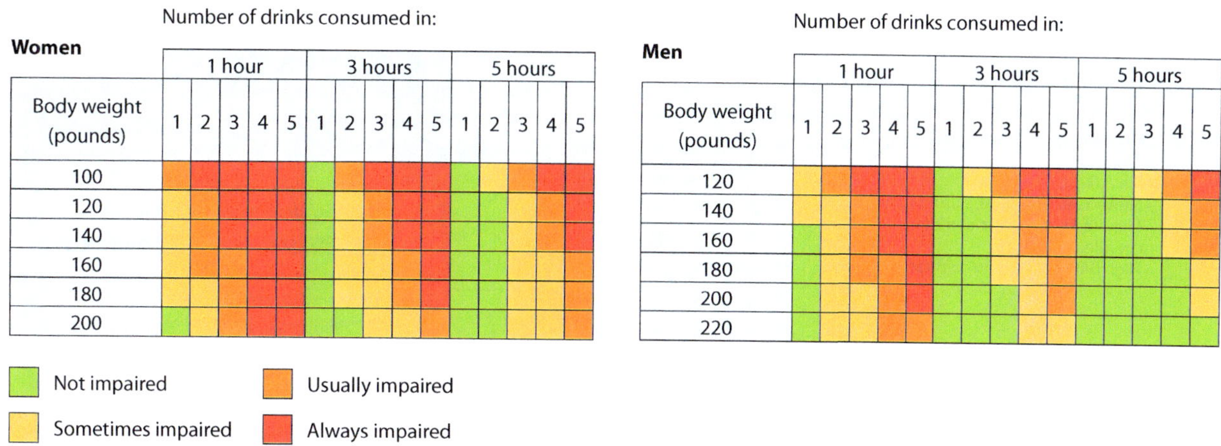

Figure 6.7 Approximate Blood Alcohol Concentration (BAC) and the Physiological and Behavioural Effects

Remember that there are many variables that can affect BAC, so this is only an estimate of what your BAC would be.

Both breath analysis (breathalyser tests) and urinalysis are used to determine whether an individual is legally intoxicated, but blood tests are more accurate measures of BAC. An increasing number of states are requiring blood tests for people suspected of driving under the influence of alcohol. In some states, refusal to take the breath or urine test results in immediate revocation of a person's driver's license.

People can develop physical and psychological tolerance to the effects of alcohol through regular use. The nervous system adapts over time, so greater amounts of alcohol are required to produce the same physiological and psychological effects. Though BAC may be quite high, the individual has learned to modify his or her behaviour to appear sober. This ability is called **learned behavioural tolerance**.

Learned behavioural tolerance The ability of heavy drinkers to modify behaviour so that they appear to be sober even when they have high BAC levels.

Alcohol and your health

The immediate and long-term effects of alcohol consumption can vary greatly (Figure 6.8). Whether or not you experience any immediate or long-term consequences as a result of your alcohol use depends on you as an individual, the amount of alcohol you consume, and your circumstances.

Immediate and short-term effects of alcohol

The most dramatic effects produced by ethanol occur within the central nervous system (CNS). Alcohol depresses CNS functions, which decreases respiratory rate, pulse rate, and blood pressure. As CNS depression deepens, vital functions become noticeably affected. In extreme cases, coma and death can result.

Alcohol is a diuretic that causes increased urinary output. Although this effect might be expected to lead to automatic **dehydration**, the body actually retains water, most of it in the muscles or in the cerebral tissues. Because water is usually pulled out of the *cerebrospinal fluid* (fluid within the brain and spinal cord), drinkers may suffer symptoms that include "morning-after" headaches.

Dehydration Loss of water from body tissues.

Alcohol irritates the gastrointestinal system and may cause indigestion and heartburn if consumed on an empty stomach. In addition, people who engage in brief drinking sprees during which they consume unusually high amounts of alcohol put themselves at risk for irregular heartbeat or even total loss of heart rhythm, which can disrupt blood flow and damage the heart muscle.

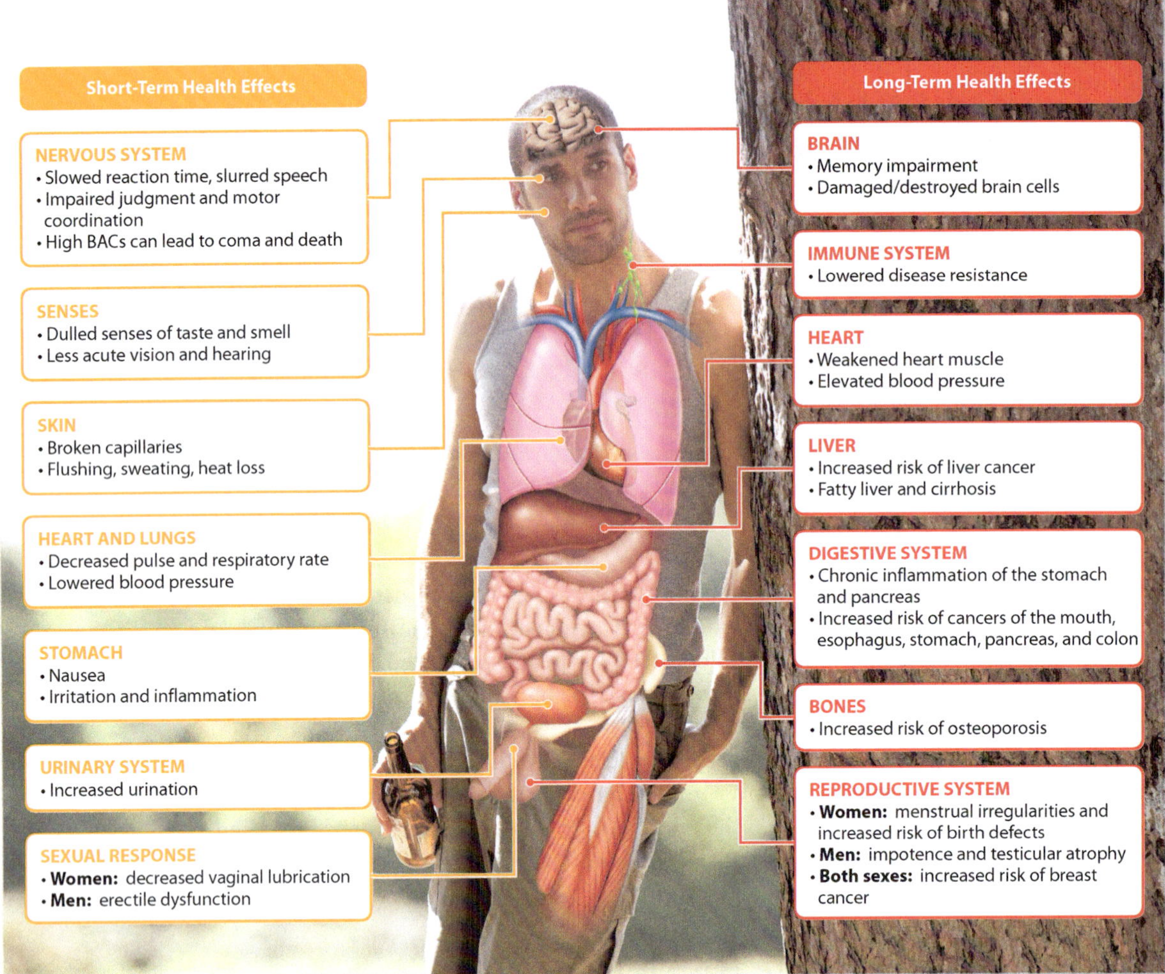

Figure 6.8 Effects of Alcohol on the Body and Health
(**Source:** I Love Images/Getty Images.)

Hangover

Hangover
The physiological reaction to excessive drinking, including headache, upset stomach, anxiety, depression, diarrhea, and thirst.

Congeners
Forms of alcohol that are metabolised more slowly than ethanol and produce toxic by-products.

A **hangover** is often experienced the morning after a drinking spree. Its symptoms are familiar to most people who drink: headache, muscle aches, upset stomach, anxiety, depression, diarrhea, and thirst. Hangovers kick in for more than half of people after their blood alcohol content reaches 0.11. Approximately 20 to 25 percent of those who drink enough to get a hangover do not experience them (Rohsenow et al., 2012). Smoking while drinking may also worsen hangovers. The more people smoke on the day they drink alcohol heavily, the more likely they are to have a hangover, and heavy drinking paired with heavy smoking leads to more intense hangovers (Jackson et al., 2013). **Congeners**, forms of alcohol that are metabolised more slowly than ethanol and are more toxic, are thought to play a role in the development of a hangover. The body metabolises the congeners after the ethanol is gone from the system, and their toxic by-products may contribute to the hangover. Alcohol also upsets the water balance in the body, which results in excess urination, dehydration, and thirst the next day. Increased production of hydrochloric acid can irritate the stomach lining and cause nausea. Recovery from a hangover usually takes 12 hours. Bed rest, solid food, and aspirin or ibuprofen may help relieve a hangover's discomforts, but the only sure way to avoid one is to abstain from excessive alcohol use in the first place.

Alcohol and injuries

Alcohol use plays a significant role in the types of injuries people experience. Hospitalisations for alcohol overdoses among 18- to 24-year-olds rose by 25 percent over the last 10 years, and about 30 percent of young adults hospitalised for overdoses involve excessive alcohol consumption (White et al., 2001). Alcohol use is involved in approximately 70 percent of fatal injuries during activities such as swimming and boating. A person with a BAC over 0.1 who operates a boat is 16 times more likely to be killed in an accident than a person who had not been drinking (NIAAA, 2012; CDCP, 2012). Alcohol is involved in 40 percent of fatal injuries due to house fires (CDCP, 2011).

Alcohol use is also a key risk factor for suicide—playing a role in approximately one third of suicides in the United States. Alcohol may increase suicide risk by increasing the intensity of depressive thoughts, lowering inhibitions to harm oneself, and interfering with the ability to assess future consequences of one's actions (U.S. Department of Health and Human Services (HHS) Office of the Surgeon General and National Action Alliance for Suicide Prevention, 2012).

Alcohol and sexual decision making

Alcohol has a clear influence on one's ability to make good decisions about sex because it lowers inhibitions, and you may do things you might not do when sober. Students who are intoxicated are less likely to use safer sex practices and are more likely to engage in high-risk sexual activity. About 1 in 5 university students reports engaging in sexual activity, including having sex with someone they just met and having unprotected sex, after drinking (Davis, 2010). The chance of acquiring a sexually transmitted infection or experiencing an unplanned pregnancy also increases as students drink more heavily.

Alcohol and sexual assault and violence

In a recent survey, almost 20 percent of undergraduate women reported experiencing some type of sexual assault since entering university—with most incidents involving alcohol or unknowingly consuming a drug placed in their drinks (Lawyer et al., 2010). Another study of university students showed heavy drinking to be associated with dating violence by men in their first year of university. Among women, heavy drinking in their sophomore year predicted dating violence in their junior year (Stappenbeck, 2010; Nielsen et al., 2012).

Alcohol and weight gain

The "freshman 15" and other university-year weight gain may have more to do with alcohol consumption than the food served in the dining halls. Alcohol has 7 calories per gram—nearly as much as fat (9 calories per gram) and more than carbohydrates or protein (4 calories per gram)—and the calories from alcohol provide few nutrients. A standard drink contains 12 to 15 grams of alcohol, meaning a single drink can add about 100 calories to your daily intake. By drinking an extra 150 calories a day more than you need, you can gain 1 pound a month and up to 12 pounds a year (Nielsen et al., 2012).

Alcohol poisoning

Alcohol poisoning (also known as **acute alcohol intoxication**) occurs much more frequently than people realise and can all too often be fatal. Alcohol, used either alone or in combination with other drugs, is responsible for more toxic overdose deaths than any other substance.

The amount of alcohol that causes a person to lose consciousness is dangerously close to the lethal dose. Death from alcohol poisoning can be caused by either central nervous system and respiratory depression or by the inhalation of vomit or fluid into the lungs. Al-

Alcohol poisoning (acute alcohol intoxication)
A potentially lethal blood alcohol concentration that inhibits the brain's ability to control consciousness, respiration, and heart rate; usually occurs as a result of drinking a large amount of alcohol in a short period of time.

cohol depresses the nerves that control involuntary actions such as breathing and the gag reflex (which prevents choking). As BAC levels reach higher concentrations, eventually these functions can be completely suppressed. If a drinker becomes unconscious and vomits, there is a danger of asphyxiation through choking to death on one's own vomit.

Blood alcohol concentration can continue rising even after a drinker becomes unconscious, because alcohol in the stomach and intestine continues to empty into the bloodstream. Signs of alcohol poisoning include inability to be roused; a weak, rapid pulse; an unusual or irregular breathing pattern; and cool (possibly damp), pale, or bluish skin. If you are with someone who has been drinking heavily and who exhibits these symptoms, or if you are unsure about the person's condition, call your local emergency number (9-1-1 in most areas) for immediate assistance.

Long-term effects of alcohol

Alcohol is distributed throughout most of the body and may affect many organs and tissues. Problems associated with long-term, habitual use of alcohol include diseases of the nervous system, cardiovascular system, and liver, as well as some cancers.

Effects on the nervous system

The nervous system is especially sensitive to alcohol. Even people who drink moderately experience shrinkage in brain size and weight and a loss of some degree of intellectual ability.

Research suggests that developing brains in adolescents are much more prone to brain damage than was previously thought. Alcohol appears to damage the frontal areas of the adolescent brain, which are crucial for controlling impulses and thinking through consequences of intended actions (Silveri, 2012). In addition, researchers suggest that people who begin drinking at an early age are at much higher risk of experiencing alcohol abuse or dependence, drinking five or more drinks per drinking occasion, and at least weekly driving under the influence of alcohol (Silveri, 2012).

Cardiovascular effects

Alcohol affects the cardiovascular system in a number of ways. Numerous studies have associated light to moderate alcohol consumption (no more than two drinks a day) with a reduced risk of coronary artery disease (Arriola et al., 2010; Wilson et al., 2010; The American Heart Association, 2011). Several mechanisms have been proposed to explain how this might happen. The strongest evidence points to an increase in high-density lipoprotein (HDL) cholesterol, which is known as "good" cholesterol. Studies have shown that moderate drinkers have higher levels of HDL (Arriola et al., 2010; Wilson et al., 2010; The AHA, 2011). Alcohol's effects on blood clotting, insulin sensitivity, and inflammation are also thought to play a role in protecting against heart disease.

However, alcohol consumption is not a preventive measure against heart disease—it causes many more cardiovascular health hazards than benefits. Drinking too much alcohol contributes to high blood pressure and higher calorie intake, both of which are risk factors for cardiovascular disease (AHA, 2011).

Liver disease

One result of heavy drinking is that the liver begins to store fat—a condition known as *fatty liver.* If there is insufficient time between drinking episodes, this fat cannot be transported to storage sites, and the fat-filled liver cells stop functioning. Continued drinking can cause a further stage of liver deterioration called *fibrosis,* in which the damaged area of the liver develops fibrous scar tissue. Cell function can be partially restored at this stage with proper nutrition and abstinence from alcohol. If the person continues to drink, however,

Cirrhosis
The last stage of liver disease associated with chronic heavy use of alcohol, during which liver cells die and damage becomes permanent.

Alcoholic hepatitis
Condition resulting from prolonged use of alcohol, in which the liver is inflamed; can be fatal.

cirrhosis results (Figure 6.9). Among the top 10 causes of death in the United States, cirrhosis occurs as liver cells die and damage becomes permanent. **Alcoholic hepatitis** is another serious condition resulting from prolonged use of alcohol. A chronic inflammation of the liver develops, which may be fatal in itself or progress to cirrhosis

Cancer

Alcohol is considered a carcinogen. The repeated irritation caused by long-term use of alcohol has been linked to cancers of the esophagus, stomach, mouth, tongue, and liver. In one study, National Institute on Alcohol Abuse and Alcoholism scientists discovered a possible link between acetaldehyde and DNA damage that could help explain the connection between drinking and certain types of cancer (Seitz & Becker, 2007).

There is substantial evidence that women who consume even low levels of alcohol (three to six drinks per week) have a higher risk of breast cancer compared with those who abstain, and the risk is even higher for women who consume more than 2 drinks per day (Chen et al;, 2011). Girls and young women who drink alcohol also increase their risk of benign (noncancerous) breast disease, which in turn increases the risk for developing breast cancer. In a recent study, girls and young women who drank 6 or 7 days a week were 5.5 times more likely to have benign breast disease than those who didn't drink or who had less than one drink per week (Berkey et al., 2010).

Other effects

Alcohol abuse is a major cause of chronic inflammation of the pancreas, the organ that produces digestive enzymes and insulin. Chronic abuse of alcohol inhibits enzyme production, which further inhibits the absorption of nutrients. Drinking alcohol can block the absorption of calcium, a nutrient that strengthens bones. This should be of particular concern to women because of their risk for osteoporosis, as heavy consumption of alcohol worsens this condition. Evidence also suggests that alcohol impairs the body's ability to recognise and fight foreign bodies, such as bacteria and viruses.

Alcohol and pregnancy

Teratogenic substances cause birth defects. Of the 30 known teratogens in the environment, alcohol is one of the most dangerous and common. If a woman ingests alcohol while

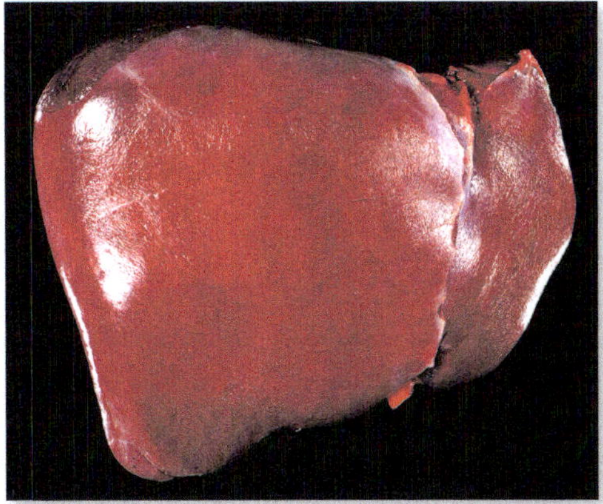

(a) A normal liver

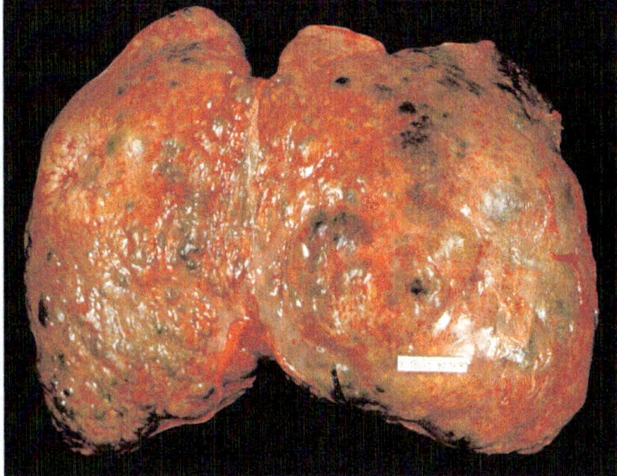

(b) A liver with cirrhosis

Figure 6.9 Comparison of a Healthy Liver with a Cirrhotic Liver

In cirrhosis, healthy liver cells are replaced with scar tissue that interferes with the liver's ability to perform its many vital functions. **(Source:** left: CNRI/SPL/Science Source; right: Martin M. Rotker/Science Source.)

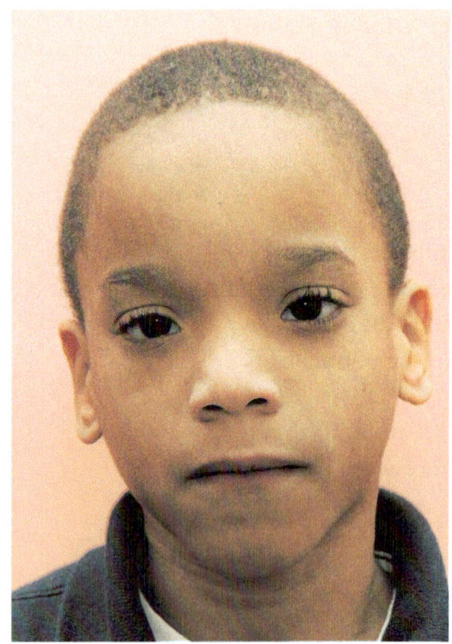

Characteristic facial features of FAS include a small, upturned nose with a low bridge and a thin upper lip. **(Source:** Centers for Disease Control and Prevention.)

pregnant, it will pass through the placenta and enter the growing fetus's bloodstream. A global study of alcohol consumption in pregnant mothers in Australia, New Zealand, Ireland and the United Kingdom revealed alarming results. Forty percent of Australian women, 56% of New Zealand women, 75% of women in the UK and 82% of Irish women reported consuming alcohol while pregnant (O'Keeffe et al., 2015). These percentages significantly dropped in the second and third trimesters indicating that the vast majority of most women consumed alcohol during the period in when they were not yet aware of their pregnancy. Nevertheless, there was a small minority of women who reported drinking four or more alcoholic beverages in one sitting, during their second trimester: 1% of Australian women, 0.1% of New Zealand women, 1% of women in the UK and 0.4% of Irish women. It is well-known that consuming four or more drinks a day during pregnancy may significantly increase the risk of childhood mental health and learning problems. There is more research now that points to even moderate use (small glass of wine, half a pint of beer or shot of liquor) of alcohol once or twice a week during pregnancy can cut a baby's intelligence by several points (Lewis et al, 2012). The best advice to women who are pregnant is that any use may result in varying degrees of effects, ranging from mild learning disabilities to major physical, mental, and intellectual impairment. Alcohol consumed during the first trimester poses the greatest threat to organ development; exposure during the last trimester, when the brain is developing rapidly, is most likely to affect CNS development.

Fetal alcohol syndrome (FAS) A disorder involving physical and mental impairment that may affect the fetus when the mother consumes alcohol during pregnancy.

A disorder called **fetal alcohol syndrome (FAS)** is associated with alcohol consumption during pregnancy and is the most common, preventable cause of mental impairment in the Western world. FAS is the third most common birth defect and the second leading cause of mental retardation in the United States, with an estimated incidence of 1 to 2 in every 1,000 live births (CDCP, 2010). At present, there are no reliable Australian estimates of FAS due to data being sourced from multiple, unreliable sources such as case notes, clinical records and the birth defects register. However, the pattern of analyses on FAS reveals that more indigenous children are diagnosed with FAS than non-indigenous children (Elliott, Payne, Morris, Haan & Bower, 2008; Rothstein, Heazlewood & Fraser, 2007).

Among the symptoms of FAS are mental retardation, small head, tremors, and abnormalities of the face, limbs, heart, and brain. Children with FAS may experience problems such as poor memory and impaired learning, reduced attention span, impulsive behaviour, and poor problem-solving abilities, among others.

Children who do not have all of the physical or behavioural symptoms of FAS may be diagnosed with disorders such as partial fetal alcohol syndrome or alcohol-related neurodevelopmental disorder; all of these disorders (including FAS) fall under the umbrella term *fetal alcohol spectrum disorders* (FASD). An estimated 40,000 infants in the United States are affected by FASD each year—more than those affected by spina bifida, Down syndrome, and muscular dystrophy combined (Fetal Alcohol Spectrum Disorders (FASD) Center for Excellence, 2013). Infants whose mothers habitually consumed more than 3 oz of alcohol (approximately six drinks) in a short time period when pregnant are at high risk for FASD. Risk levels for babies whose mothers consume smaller amounts are uncertain. To avoid any chance of harming her fetus, any woman of childbearing age who is or may become pregnant is advised to refrain from consuming any amount of alcohol.

Drinking and driving

Traffic accidents are the leading cause of accidental death for all age groups from 1 to 44 years old (CDCP, 2010). Approximately 31 percent of all traffic fatalities in 2010 involved at least one alcohol-impaired driver (having a BAC of 0.08 percent or higher) (National Highway Traffic Safety Administration, 2010). These statistics are not surprising given that Australian research has found that 52% of drivers reported drinking driving at least once in their life, with 72% of individuals reporting driving after consuming at least two alcoholic beverages in the previous year (Owens & Boorman, 2011). Males are overrepresented in alcohol-attributable motor vehicle accidents with 103 males losing their lives in alcohol-attributable motor vehicle accidents, as compared to 17 females (Gao, Ogeil & Lloyd, 2014).

In 2010, there were 10,228 alcohol-impaired driving fatalities in the United States in Australia, land transport accidents were the leading cause of premature death for individuals aged 1-14 years (AIHW, 2016; National Highway Traffic Safety Administration, 2012), and in the same year, there were 1,495 alcohol-impaired driving fatalities in Australia (Gao et al., 2014). Over the past 20 years, the percentage of intoxicated drivers involved in fatal crashes decreased for all age groups (Figure 6.10). Laws that raised the drinking age to 21, stricter law enforcement, laws prohibiting anyone under 21 from driving with any detectable BAC, increased automobile safety, and educational programs designed to discourage drinking and driving all likely contributed to the reduction in fatalities. Furthermore, all states have zero-tolerance laws for driving while intoxicated, and the penalty is usually suspension of the driver's license (National Highway Traffic Safety Administration, 2012). Similarly, in order to combat drink driving and reduce alcohol-attributable motor vehicle accidents in Australia, random breath testing (RBT), media campaigns, rehabilitation programs, ignition interlocks and drink driving penalties are employed as countermeasures (Terer & Brown, 2014).

Despite all these measures, the risk of being involved in an alcohol-related automobile crash remains substantial. Laboratory and test track research shows that the vast majority of drivers are impaired even at 0.08 BAC with regard to critical driving tasks. The likelihood of a driver being involved in a fatal crash rises significantly with a BAC of 0.05 percent and even more rapidly after 0.08 percent (Insurance Institute for Highway Safety, 2010).

Alcohol-related fatal crashes occur more often at night than during the day, and the hours between 9:00 P.M. and 6:00 A.M. are the most dangerous. Seventy-five percent of fatally injured drivers involved in nighttime single-vehicle crashes had detectable levels of alcohol in their blood (Insurance Institute for Highway Safety, 2010). The risk of being involved in an alcohol-related crash also varies with the day of the week. In 2010, 26 percent of all fatal crashes during the week were alcohol related, compared with 45 percent on weekends (IIHS, 2010).

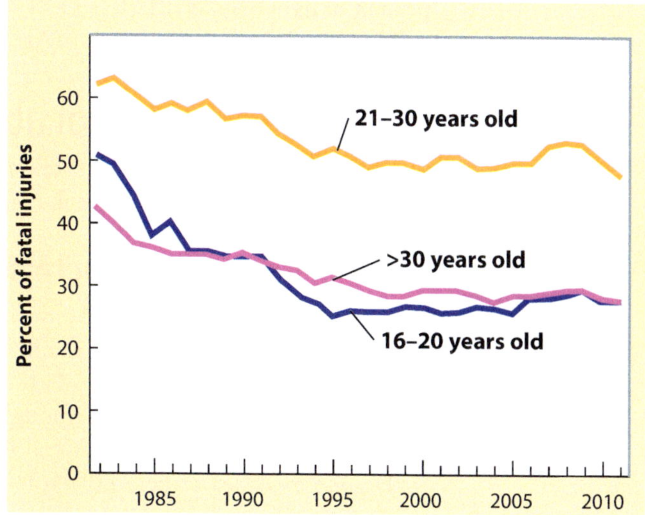

Figure 6.10 Percentage of Fatally Injured Drivers with BACs Greater Than 0.08%, by Driver Age, 1982–2011

Source: Insurance Institute for Highway Safety, "Fatality Facts 2011: Alcohol," Copyright © 2013. Reprinted by permission of Insurance Institute of Highway Safety.

Abuse and dependence

Alcohol use becomes **alcohol abuse** when it interferes with work, school, or social and family relationships, or when it entails any violation of the law, including driving under the influence (DUI). **Alcoholism**, or **alcohol dependence**, results when personal and health problems related to alcohol use are severe, and stopping alcohol use results in withdrawal symptoms.

Identifying an alcoholic

As with other drug addictions, craving, loss of control, tolerance, psychological dependence, and withdrawal symptoms must be present to qualify a drinker as an addict. Irresponsible and problem drinkers, such as people who get into fights or embarrass themselves or others when they drink, are not necessarily alcoholics. Alcoholics can be found at all socioeconomic levels and in all professions, ethnic groups, geographical locations, religions, and races. Data indicate that about 15 percent of people in the United States are problem drinkers, and about 5 to 10 percent of male drinkers and 3 to 5 percent of females would be diagnosed as alcohol dependent (Medline Plus, 2011). In Australia, 18.2% of people surveyed in 2010 over the age of 14 years were identified as risky drinkers (consuming on average more than two standard drinks per day) (AIHW, 2014). Thirty-eight percent of people aged 14 years or old reported that they had consumed alcohol at a level placing them at high risk of injury (consuming on average more than four standard drinks on a single occasion), with 26% of these individuals reporting high risk drinking monthly (AIHW, 2014).

Alcohol abuse Use of alcohol that interferes with work, school, or personal relationships or that entails violations of the law.

Alcoholism (alcohol dependence) Condition in which personal and health problems related to alcohol use are severe and stopping alcohol use results in withdrawal symptoms.

Recognising and admitting the existence of an alcohol problem is often extremely difficult. Alcoholics deny their problem, often making statements such as, "I can stop any time I want to. I just don't want to right now." The fear of being labeled a "problem drinker" often prevents people from seeking help. People who recognise alcoholic behaviours in themselves may wish to seek professional help to determine whether alcohol has become a controlling factor in their lives. (The **Skills for Behaviour Change** box on the following page gives tips for cutting down on drinking.)

Among full-time American college students, 1 in 4 experienced alcohol abuse or dependence in the past year (Center of Behavioral Health Statistics and Quality, 2012). In a recent study in the United States, the progression to alcohol dependency based on university students' drinking patterns when they entered showed that 1.9 percent of nondrinkers, 4.3 percent of light drinkers, 12.8 percent of moderate drinkers, and 19 percent of heavy drinkers developed alcohol dependency (Arria, 2013).

The causes of alcohol abuse and alcoholism

We know that alcoholism is a disease with biological and social/environmental components, but we do not know what role each component plays in the disease.

Biological and family factors

Research into the hereditary and environmental causes of alcoholism has found higher rates of alcoholism among children of alcoholics than in the general population. The development of alcoholism among individuals with a family history of alcoholism is about four to eight times more common than it is among individuals with no such family history (National Institute on Alcohol Abuse and Alcoholism, 2007).

Despite evidence of heredity's role in alcoholism, scientists do not yet understand the precise role of genes in increased risk for alcoholism, nor have they identified a specific "alcoholism" gene. Alcohol use disorders are between 50 percent and 60 percent heritable. Anxiety and depression, by comparison, are around 20 to 40 percent heritable, respectively (Levin, 2012).Adoption studies have helped demonstrate a strong link between biological parents' substance use and their children's risk for addiction. Recently, scientists have found a gene that, by controlling the way that alcohol stimulates the brain to release dopamine, can trigger feelings of reward. Alcohol gives individuals with the gene a stronger sense of reward from alcohol, making it more likely for them to be heavy drinkers (Stacey, 2012). However, there is nothing deterministic about the genetic basis for addiction. Although no single gene causes addiction, multiple genes can affect the ability to develop addiction.

Social and cultural factors

Some people begin drinking as a way to dull the pain of an acute loss or an emotional or social problem even if they are not genetically predisposed to alcoholism. Unfortunately, they become even sadder as the depressant effect of the drug begins to take its toll, sometimes causing them to antagonise friends and other social supports. Eventually, the drinker becomes physically dependent on the drug.

Family attitudes toward alcohol also seem to influence whether a person will develop a drinking problem. It has been clearly demonstrated that people who are raised in cultures where drinking is a part of religious or ceremonial activities or part of the family meal are less prone to alcohol dependence. In contrast, societies where alcohol purchase is carefully controlled and drinking is regarded as a rite of passage to adulthood appear to have greater tendency for abuse. The Health in a Diverse World box on the following page discusses some of the patterns of alcohol use and abuse around the world.

The amount of alcohol a person consumes seems to be directly related to the drinking habits of that individual's social group. A recent study found that those whose friends and relatives drank heavily were 50 percent more likely to drink heavily themselves (Niels Rosenquist et al., 2010). Moreover, even having friends of friends who drank heavily appeared to influence individual alcohol consumption. The opposite

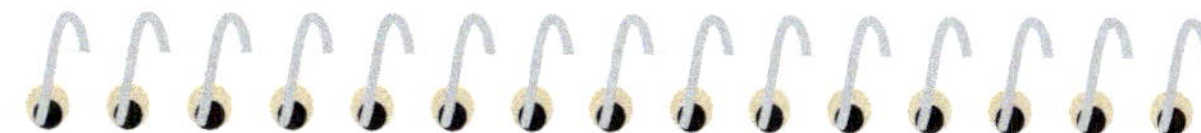

Skills for Behavioural Change

Cut Down on Your Drinking

If you have a severe drinking problem, alcoholism in your family, or other medical problems, you should stop drinking completely. If you need to cut down on your drinking, these steps can help you:

- **If you suspect that you drink too much, talk with a counsellor or a clinician at your student health centre.** That person can advise you about what is right for you.
- **Write your reasons for cutting down or stopping.** You may want to improve your health, sleep better, or get along better with your family or friends.
- **Set a drinking limit.** Determine a limit for how much you will drink. If you aren't sure what goal is right for you, talk with your counsellor. Once you determine your goal, write it down and put it where you can see it, such as on your refrigerator or bathroom mirror.
- **Keep a diary of your drinking.** Write down every time you have a drink. Try to keep your diary for 3 or 4 weeks. This will show you how much you drink and when.
- **Keep little or no alcohol at home.** You don't need the temptation.
- **Drink slowly.** When you drink, sip slowly. Take a break of 1 hour between drinks. Drink a nonalcoholic beverage after every alcoholic drink you consume.
- **Learn how to say no.** You do not have to drink when other people are or take a drink when offered one. Practice ways to say no politely. Stay away from people who give you a hard time about not drinking.
- **Stay active.** Use the time and money once spent on drinking to do something fun with your family or friends.
- **Get support.** Ask your family and friends for support to help you reach your goal. Talk to your counsellor if you are having trouble cutting down.
- **Avoid temptations.** Watch out for people, places, or times that make you drink, even if you do not want to. Plan ahead of time what you will do to avoid drinking when you are tempted.
- **Remember, don't give up!** Most people don't give up drinking all at once. If you don't reach your goal the first time, try again. Get support from people who care about you and want to help.

Source: National Institutes of Health from National Institute on Alcohol Abuse and Alcoholism, "How to Cut Down on Your Drinking," NIH Pub no. 96-3770, 1996, www.niaaa.nih.gov

is also true, that people who were friends with abstinent individuals or had family members who were abstinent were less likely to drink themselves. This finding has increased importance for individuals who are in treatment or have been in treatment and their need to sever ties with heavy drinkers to successfully maintain their abstinence.

Women and alcoholism

Women tend to become alcoholics at later ages and after fewer years of heavy drinking than do men. With greater risks for cirrhosis, excessive memory loss and shrinkage of the brain, heart disease, and cancers of the mouth, throat, esophagus, liver, and colon than male alcoholics, women suffer the consequences of alcoholism more profoundly and become addicted faster with less alcohol use (CDCP, 2012).

Highest risks for alcoholism occur among women who are unmarried but living with a partner, are in their twenties or early thirties, or have a husband or partner who drinks heavily. Other risk factors for women include a family history of drinking problems, pressure to drink from a peer or spouse, depression, and stress.

Alcohol and prescription drug abuse

When alcohol and prescription drugs are taken together, severe medical problems can result, including alcohol poisoning, unconsciousness, respiratory depression, and death. The greatest risks from drug mixing occur when alcohol is mixed with prescription painkillers. Both drugs slow breathing rates in unique ways and inhibit the coughing reflex; when combined, they can stop breathing altogether. Alcohol also interacts with antianxiety medications (e.g., Xanax), antipsychotics, antidepressants, sleep medications, and muscle relaxants, causing dizziness and drowsiness and making falls and unintentional injuries more likely. The prescription drugs that are most commonly combined with alcohol include opioids (e.g., Vicodin, OxyContin, Percocet), stimulants (e.g., Ritalin, Adderall, Concerta), sedative/anxiety medications (e.g., Ativan, Xanax), and sleeping medications (e.g., Ambien, Halcion).

Costs to society

Alcohol-related costs to American society are estimated to be well over $223.5 billion when health insurance, criminal justice costs, treatment costs, and lost productivity are considered (CDCP, 2011). Reportedly, alcoholism is directly or indirectly responsible for over 25 percent of the nation's medical expenses and lost earnings (CDCP, 2011). One recent study estimated that underage drinking alone costs society $61.9 billion annually (Miller et al., 2006). The largest costs were related to violence ($35 billion) and drunken driving accidents ($9.5 billion), followed by high-risk sex (nearly $5 billion), property crime ($3 billion), and addiction treatment programs (nearly $2.5 billion). By dividing the cost of underage drinking by the estimated number of underage drinkers, the study estimated that every underage

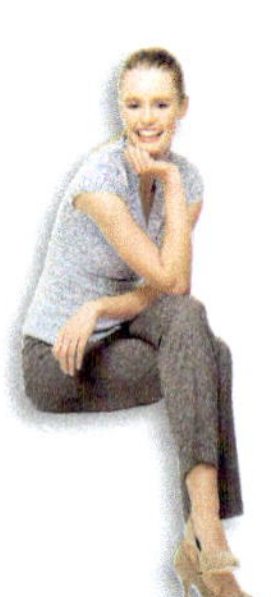

"Why Should I Care?"

Being physically active reduces your risk for many chronic diseases. That may not seem like an immediate concern, but there are a lot more immediate benefits: Becoming physically fit can help improve your physical appearance and sense of self-esteem, boost your resistance to diseases like colds and flus, reduce your stress level, improve your sleep, and help you concentrate. All that, and it's fun, too!

(**Source:** Edyta Pawlowska/Shutterstock.)

Health in a Diverse World

Global Health and Alcohol Use

Alcohol consumption comes with many serious social and developmental issues, including violence, child neglect and abuse, and absenteeism in the workplace. Throughout the world, alcohol is a factor in 60 types of diseases and injuries and a component cause in 200 others. Almost 4 percent of all deaths worldwide are attributed to alcohol, greater than deaths caused by HIV/AIDS, violence, or tuberculosis. Worldwide, the impact of alcohol use is as follows:

* The use of alcohol results in 2.5 million deaths each year.
* 320,000 people ages 15 to 29 die from alcohol-related causes annually—9 percent of all deaths for that age group.
* Alcohol is the world's third largest risk factor for disease burden.
* It is the leading risk factor for disease burden in the Western Pacific and the Americas and the second leading risk factor in Europe.

A large variation exists in adult per capita consumption. The highest consumption levels can be found in the developed world, mostly the Northern Hemisphere, but also in Argentina, Australia, and New Zealand. Medium consumption levels can be found in southern Africa, with Namibia and South Africa having the highest levels, and in North and South America. Low consumption levels can be found in the countries of North Africa and sub-Saharan Africa, the Eastern Mediterranean region, and southern Asia and the Indian Ocean. These regions represent large populations of Muslims, who have high rates of abstention.

Source: World Health Organization, *Global Status Report on Alcohol and Health*, (Geneva: WHO Press, 2011) Available at www.who.int

drinker costs society an average of over $2,000 a year (Underage Drinking Enforcement Training Center, 2011).

In Australia in 2010, the direct cost of alcohol related problems was estimated at $14.33 billon (Manning, Smith & Mazerolle, 2013). Of this $14.33 billion, $6.05 billion represents costs to Australian productivity, $3.66 billion represents costs associated with traffic accidents and $1.69 billion represents costs to the health care system. (Manning et al., 2013). The remaining $2.96 billion represents costs to the criminal justice system which includes costs to police, courts, prisons, insurances administrations, violence, loss of life, child protection and support services, out of home expenses and intense family support. When taking into consideration the harm caused by others' drinking (e.g., street noise, petty costs from damaged property or more seriously, costs such as child abuse or physical violence), this number dramatically increases to an estimated $36 billion (Laslett et al., 2010).

Treating alcoholism

Despite growing recognition of our national alcohol problem, only a very small percentage of alcoholics ever receive care in special treatment facilities. Numerous factors contribute to this low treatment utilisation, including high costs or inability to pay for treatment, lack of insurance, inability or unwillingness to admit to an alcohol problem, the social stigma attached to alcoholism, potential loss of income, breakdowns in referral and delivery systems, and failure of the professional medical establishment to recognise and diagnose alcoholic symptoms among patients (Substance Abuse and Mental Health Services Administration). Student efforts to fit in by drinking can escalate into alcohol abuse behaviour and put their health, well-being, and chances of academic success at risk. Of the nearly 12,000 university students admitted into treatment for substance abuse, approximately 47 percent report alcohol as their primary substance of abuse (Center of Behavioral Health Statistics and Quality, 2012).

Alcoholics who decide to quit drinking will experience *detoxification,* the process by which addicts end their dependence on a drug. Withdrawal symptoms include hyperexcitability, confusion and agitation, sleep disorders, convulsions and tremors of the hands, depression, headache, and seizures. For a small percentage of people, alcohol withdrawal results in a severe syndrome known as **delirium tremens (DTs)**, characterised by confusion, delusions, agitated behaviour, and hallucinations.

Delirium tremens (DTs) A state of confusion, delusions, and agitation brought on by withdrawal from alcohol.

Alcoholics Anonymous (AA) An organisation whose goal is to help alcoholics stop drinking; includes auxiliary branches such as Al-Anon and Alateen.

Treatment programs

The alcoholic who is ready for help has several avenues of treatment: psychologists and psychiatrists specialising in the treatment of alcoholism, private treatment centres, hospitals specifically designed to treat alcoholics, community mental health facilities, and support groups such as **Alcoholics Anonymous (AA)**.

Private treatment facilities

Upon admission to a private treatment facility, the patient receives a complete physical exam to determine whether underlying medical problems will interfere with treatment. Shortly after detoxification, alcoholics begin their treatment for psychological addiction. Most treatment facilities keep their patients from 3 to 6 weeks. Treatment at private centres can cost several thousand dollars, but some insurance programs or employers will assume most of this expense.

Therapy

Several types of therapy, including family therapy, individual therapy, and group therapy, are commonly used in alcoholism recovery programs. In family therapy, the person and family members examine the psychological reasons underlying the addiction and environmental factors enabling it. In individual and group therapy with fellow addicts, alcoholics learn positive coping skills for situations that have regularly caused them to turn to alcohol.

On some university campuses, the problems associated with alcohol abuse are so great that student health centres are opening their own treatment programs. For example, the University of Texas offers a support service called Complete Recovery 101, and at other schools students in recovery live together in special housing. Because it can be difficult to recover from an alcohol abuse problem in university, support programs such as these hope to offer the support and comfortable environment recovering students need.

Relapse

Success in recovery varies with the individual. Over half of all alcoholics relapse (resume drinking) within the first 3 months of treatment. Why is the relapse rate so high? Treating an addiction requires more than getting the addict to stop using a substance; it also requires getting the person to break a pattern of behaviour that has dominated his or her life. Many alcoholics refer to themselves as "recovering" throughout their lifetime; they never use the word *cured*.

People who are seeking to regain a healthy lifestyle must not only confront their addiction, but must also guard against the tendency to relapse. Identifying situations in their lives that could trigger relapse—such as becoming angry or frustrated, or being around others drinking—are important for alcoholics. It can help to join a support group; maintain stability (resisting the urge to move, travel, assume a new job, or make other drastic life changes); set aside time each day for reflection; and assume responsibility for their own actions. To be effective, recovery programs must offer alcoholics ways to increase self-esteem and resume personal growth.

Tobacco use

Tobacco use is the single most preventable cause of death in Australia and the United States (AIHW, 2010; CDCP, 2012). Nearly 443,000 American and 15,000 Australians die each year of tobacco-related diseases (Begg, Vos, Barker, Stevenson, Stanley & Lopez, 2007). Moreover, another 10 million people will suffer from health disorders caused by tobacco. To date, tobacco is known to cause about 20 diseases, and about half of all regular smokers die of smoking-related diseases.

While tobacco usage has steadily declined in the past decades, millions of people continue to light up. In 2011, approximately 43 million or 13.9% of U.S. adults smoked cigarettes (CDCP, 2012). In Australia in 2013, just under 3 million people, or approximately 12.8% of the population, aged 14 years over, smoked cigarettes daily (AIHW, 2014). A particular bright spot in the fight against smoking is the declining prevalence of the habit among 18- to 24-year-olds. In 2001, almost 25% of 18- to 24-year-olds were smoking daily, while in 2013, this number reduced to 13% (AIHW, 2014). Moreover, it is also positive to note that less young people are taking up smoking. In 2013, 95% of 12- to 17 year olds reported having never smoked (AIHW, 2014). Nonetheless, tobacco is a stubborn problem throughout the world due to its highly addictive nature and the environmental and social factors that make quitting difficult.

Tobacco and social issues

U.S. and state governments have waged a long war on tobacco. But production and distribution of tobacco products involve many political and economic issues. Tobacco-growing states derive substantial income from tobacco production, and federal, state, and local governments benefit enormously from cigarette taxes.

Advertising

The tobacco industry spends an estimated $36 million per day on advertising and promotional material (Campaign for Tobacco-Free Kids, 2012). With the number of smokers declining by about 1 million each year, the industry must actively recruit new smokers. Tobacco advertising also plays an important role in encouraging young people to begin a lifelong addiction to smoking before they are old enough to fully understand its long-term health risk (American Lung Association, 2013). Ninety percent of adults who smoke started by the age of 21, and half of them became regular smokers by their eighteenth birthday. Tobacco companies also target children and teens with tobacco products that are candy, fruit, or alcohol flavored, thus making them more palatable to young people (Tobacco Free Providence, 2012).

Advertisements in women's magazines imply that smoking is the key to financial success, thinness, independence, and social acceptance—and they have apparently been working. From the mid-1970s through the early 2000s, cigarette sales to women increased dramatically. Not coincidentally, by 1987 cigarette-induced lung cancer had surpassed breast cancer as the leading cancer killer among women and has remained the leading cancer killer in every year since (American Cancer Society, 2013).

Women are not the only targets of gender-based cigarette advertisements. Men are depicted in locker rooms, charging over rugged terrain in off-road vehicles, or riding stallions into the sunset in blatant appeals to a need to feel and appear masculine. Minorities are also often targeted. Recent studies have shown a higher concentration of tobacco advertising in magazines aimed at African Americans, such as *Jet* and *Ebony*, than in similar magazines aimed at broader audiences, such as *Time* and *People*. Billboards and posters aiming the cigarette message at Latinos have dotted the landscape and store windows in

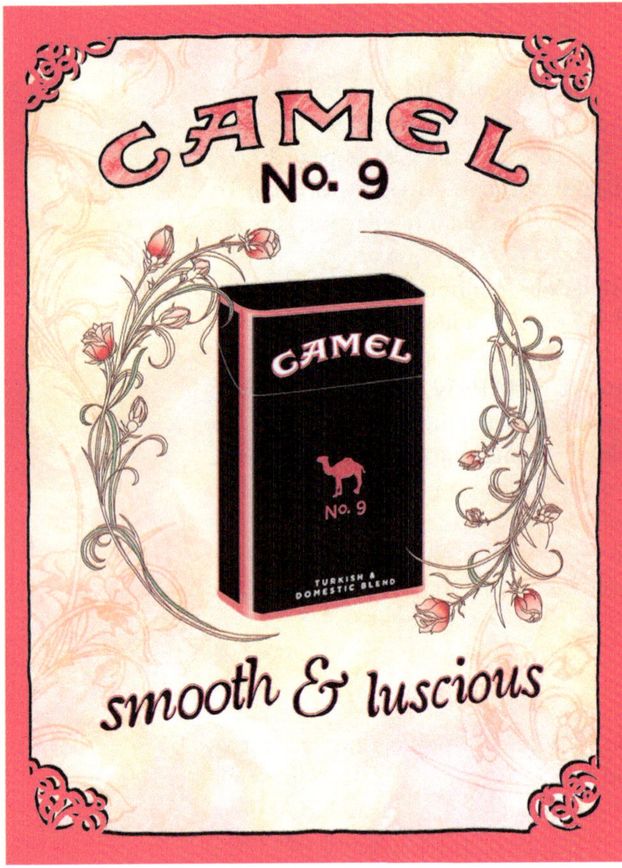

Cigarette companies market to women with glamorous packaging and ad campaigns borrowed from cosmetics, perfume (such as the famous Chanel scents evoked by this Camel No. 9 brand), and the fashion industry.
(Source: Handout/MCT/Newscom.)

Latino communities for many years, especially in low-income areas. Recent innovations by tobacco companies have included sponsorship of community-based events such as festivals and annual fairs.

Financial costs to society

Estimates show that tobacco use causes more than $193 billion in annual health-related economic losses. The economic burden of tobacco use totals more than $96 billion in medical expenditures and $97 billion in indirect costs (absenteeism, added cost of fire insurance, training costs to replace employees who die prematurely, disability payments, etc.) (American Lung Association, 2011). The economic costs of smoking are estimated to be about $3,100 per smoker per year (CDCP, 2008; CDCP, 2010). These costs far exceed the tax revenues on the sale of tobacco products, even though the average cigarette tax in 2012 was $1.48 per pack and is rising in some states (Campaign for Tobacco-Free Kids, 2012).

University students and tobacco use

Being placed in a new and often stressful social and academic environment makes university students especially vulnerable to outside influences. On top of targeted advertising, peer influence can prompt students to start smoking, and many universities still sell tobacco products in campus stores. University men and women have nearly identical rates of cigarette smoking, but men use more cigars and smokeless tobacco (Johnston et al., 2012). On the plus side, cigarette smoking among U.S. university students has decreased in recent years (see Figure 6.11) (Johnston et al., 2012).

See the Points of View box on the following page for a discussion of banning smoking on campuses.

Why do university students smoke?

Some of the reasons students smoke are to relax or to reduce stress. Smokers are more likely to have higher levels of perceived stress than nonsmokers. Other key reasons students smoke are to fit in or because they are addicted.

For some students weight control is an important motivator, and fear of weight gain is a common reason for smoking relapse among those who quit. Students diagnosed or treated for depression are much more likely to use tobacco compared to students who are not.

Social smoking

Many university smokers identify themselves as "social smokers"—those who smoke only when they are with people, rather than alone. Half of university smokers deny being smokers, even though they reported smoking in the past 30 days. Many of these students smoke in social situations where they also drink alcohol. Like regular smokers, social smokers engage in more alcohol use, illicit drug use, and higher sexual risk-taking behaviours than do nonsmokers (Sutfin, et al., 2012). Even occasional smoking is not without risks of damaging health effects. Social smoking in university can lead to a complete dependence on nicotine and all the associated health risks.

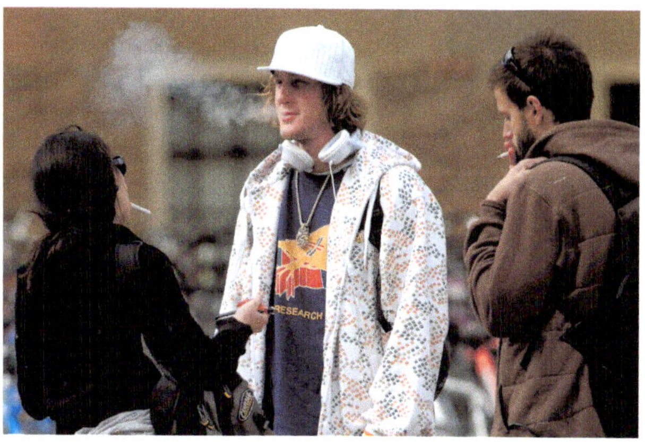

Is social smoking really that bad for me?

An occasional puff once in a while when you are out with friends can't hurt, right? Wrong! There is no "safe" amount of tobacco use—any smoking or exposure to smoke increases your risks for negative health effects such as heart disease and lung cancer. And even if you only smoke once or twice a week and consider yourself a social smoker, chances are you're on the road to dependence and a more frequent smoking habit.
(Source: Helen H. Richardson/Denver Post/Getty Images.)

Tobacco and its effects

Smoking, the most common form of tobacco use, delivers a strong dose of nicotine, as well as 7,000 other chemical substances, including arsenic, formaldehyde, and ammonia, directly to the lungs. Among these chemicals are more than 69 known or suspected carcinogens (U.S. Department of Health and Human Services, 2010). The heat from tobacco smoke is also harmful. Inhaling hot toxic gases exposes sensitive mucous membranes to irritating chemicals that weaken the tissues and contribute to cancers of the mouth, larynx, and throat.

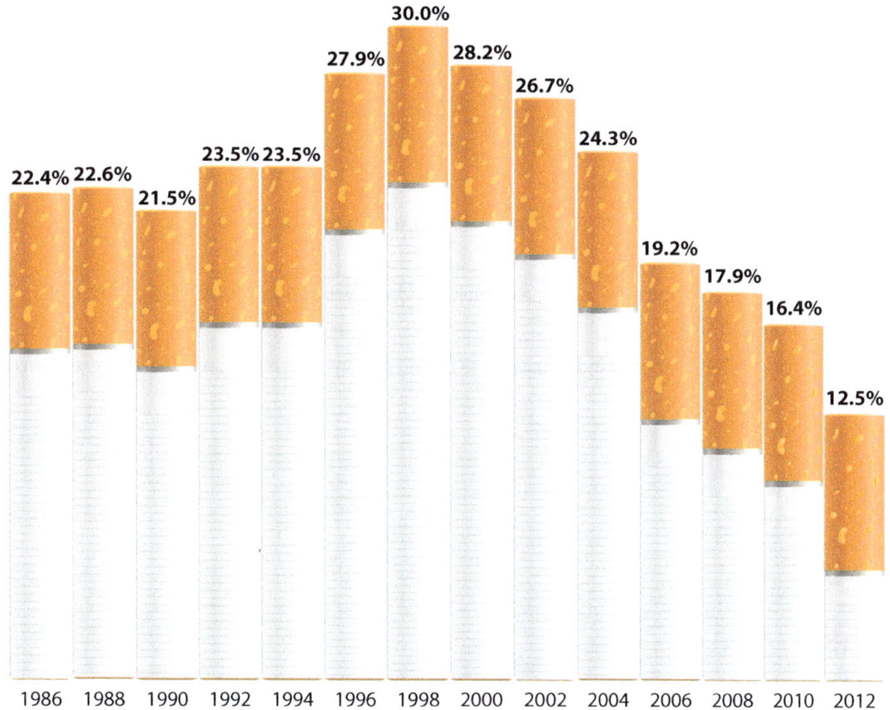

Figure 6.11 Trends in Prevalence of Cigarette Smoking in the Past Month among College Students
Source: Data from L. D. Johnston et al., "Monitoring the Future National Survey Results on Drug Use, 1975–2011, Volume II: College Students and Adults Ages 19–50" (Ann Arbor: Institute for Social Research, The University of Michigan, 2013).

Points of View

Smoking on University & University Campuses:

Should it be Banned?

City Campus
This is a smoke free area.
Smoking is prohibited
on University land.
Thank you for not smoking
on the University Campus.

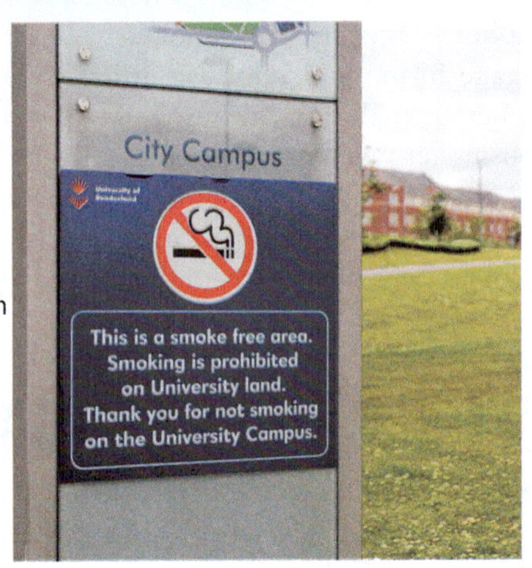

In recent years hundreds of campuses implemented all-out prohibitions or significant restrictions on tobacco use, with many more campuses pursuing becoming smoke-free. It is estimated that currently 17 percent of all U.S. campuses are tobacco or smoke-free, and the number is rapidly growing. The debate regarding tobacco-free campuses is contentious at many schools. Below are some of the major points for both sides of the question.

Arguments for Banning Tobacco on Campuses

- The majority of university students—4 out of 5—do not smoke.
- Two thirds of students and most employees prefer to attend classes held on a smoke-free campus.
- One in five students say they have experienced some immediate health impact from exposure to environmental tobacco smoke.
- Nonsmokers are 40 percent less likely to become smokers if they live in smoke-free dorms.

Arguments against Banning Tobacco on Campuses

- There are so many other causes of potentially harmful fumes on campus—from diesel trucks, for example—that banning smoking wouldn't really affect the overall health and air quality on campus.
- The policy would be difficult if not impossible to enforce.
- Smokers forced outside to light up are possibly being put in danger at night or in other situations when they would have to leave residence halls.
- Smoking bans in public and private places violate the rights of smokers and encourage discriminatory treatment of people addicted to nicotine.

Where Do You Stand?

- Is smoking on a university campus a threat to public health?
- Do you think that smokers have the right to smoke in dorms, in campus buildings, in adjacent parks, or in other public places on campus? Why or why not?
- How do you feel when you are walking across campus and someone is smoking close to you? Do you feel as though you could or should ask smokers to put out their cigarettes?
- Would banning smoking be discriminatory? A violation of individual rights? Should student smokers be singled out for exclusion on university campuses?

Sources: University of Michigan, National Tobacco Free Campus Initiative, http://sph.umich.edu; American Smokers' Rights Foundation, U.S. Colleges and Universities with Smoke-free and Tobacco-Free Policies, January 2, 2013, U.S. Surgeon General's June 2012 webinar on tobacco-free college campuses.
(Source: Elvele Images Ltd/Alamy.)

Nicotine

Nicotine
The primary stimulant chemical in tobacco products; nicotine is highly addictive.

The highly addictive chemical stimulant **nicotine** is the major psychoactive substance in all tobacco products. In its natural form, nicotine is a colourless liquid that turns brown upon exposure to air. When tobacco leaves are burned in a cigarette, pipe, or cigar, nicotine is released and inhaled into the lungs. Sucking or chewing tobacco releases nicotine into the saliva, and the nicotine is then absorbed through the mucous membranes in the mouth.

Nicotine is a powerful central nervous system stimulant that produces a variety of physiological effects. In the cerebral cortex, it produces an aroused, alert mental state. Nicotine stimulates the adrenal glands, which increases the production of adrenaline. It also increases heart and respiratory rates, constricts blood vessels, and, in turn, increases blood pressure because the heart must work harder to pump blood through the narrowed vessels.

Tar and carbon monoxide

Cigarette smoke is a complex mixture of chemicals and gases produced by the burning of tobacco and its additives. Particulate matter condenses in the lungs to form a thick, brownish sludge called **tar**, which contains various carcinogenic agents, such as benzopyrene, and chemical irritants, such as phenol. Phenol has the potential to combine with other chemicals that contribute to developing lung cancer.

In healthy lungs, millions of tiny hairlike projections (*cilia*) on the surfaces lining the upper respiratory passages sweep away foreign matter, which is expelled from the lungs by coughing. However, the cilia's cleansing function is impaired in smokers' lungs by nicotine, which paralyses the cilia for up to 1 hour following a single cigarette. This allows tars and other solids in tobacco smoke to accumulate and irritate sensitive lung tissue.

Cigarette smoke also contains poisonous gases, the most dangerous of which is **carbon monoxide**, the deadly gas that comes out of exhaust pipes in cars. In the human body, carbon monoxide reduces the oxygen-carrying capacity of the red blood cells by binding with the receptor sites for oxygen; this causes oxygen deprivation in many body tissues. It is at least partly responsible for increased risk of heart attacks and strokes in smokers.

Tar
A thick, brownish sludge condensed from particulate matter in smoked tobacco.

Carbon monoxide
A gas found in tobacco smoke that reduces the ability of blood to carry oxygen.

Tobacco addiction

Smoking is a complicated behaviour. Somewhere between 60 and 80 percent of people have tried a cigarette. Of those who try smoking, there is a 68 percent chance that sooner or later they will become nicotine dependent (C. Quintero-Lopez et al., 2011). Why do some walk away from cigarettes while others get hooked?

Beginning smokers usually feel the effects of nicotine with their first puff. Smoking is a very efficient drug-delivery system, getting the drug to the brain in just a few seconds. These symptoms, called **nicotine poisoning**, include dizziness, light-headedness, rapid and erratic pulse, clammy skin, nausea, vomiting, and diarrhea. These unpleasant effects cease as tolerance to the chemical develops, which happens almost immediately in new users, perhaps after the second or third cigarette. In contrast, tolerance to most other drugs, such as alcohol, develops over a period of months or years. Regular smokers often no longer experience the "buzz" of smoking, but continue to smoke simply because stopping is too difficult

A pack-a-day smoker experiences 300 "hits," or **pairings**, a day. In pairing, an environmental cue triggers a craving for nicotine (National Institute on Drug Abuse Research Report Series, 2012). Simple pairings, such as drinking a cup of coffee, sitting in a car, finishing a meal, or sipping a beer, induce nicotine craving. The brain gets used to these pairings and cries out in displeasure when the association is missing.

Nicotine poisoning
Symptoms often experienced by beginning smokers, including dizziness, diarrhea, light-headedness, rapid and erratic pulse, clammy skin, nausea, and vomiting.

Pairing
An environmental cue that triggers nicotine cravings.

Tobacco products

Tobacco comes in several forms.

Cigarettes

Filtered cigarettes, which are designed to reduce levels of gases such as hydrogen cyanide and carbon monoxide, may actually deliver more hazardous gases to the user than do nonfiltered brands. Some smokers use low-tar and low-nicotine products as an excuse to smoke more cigarettes. This practice is self-defeating because they wind up exposing themselves to more harmful substances than they would with regular-strength cigarettes.

Clove cigarettes contain about 40 percent ground cloves (a spice) and about 60 percent tobacco. Many users mistakenly believe that these products are made entirely of ground cloves and that smoking them eliminates the risks associated with tobacco. In fact, clove cigarettes contain higher levels of tar, nicotine, and carbon monoxide than do regular cigarettes—and the numbing effect of eugenol, the active ingredient in cloves, allows smokers to inhale the smoke more deeply. The same effect is true of *menthol cigarettes:* The throat-numbing effect of the menthol allows for deeper inhalation.

Cigars

Many people believe that cigars are safer than cigarettes, when in fact nothing could be further from the truth. Cigar smoke contains 23 poisons and 43 carcinogens. Most cigars contain as much nicotine as several cigarettes, and when cigar smokers inhale, nicotine is absorbed as rapidly as it is with cigarettes. For those who don't inhale, nicotine is still absorbed through the mucous membranes in the mouth.

While cigar use has declined in recent years, the sale of little cigars has increased approximately 240 percent (ACS, 2013). About the same size and shape as cigarettes, little cigars come in packs of 20, can be candy or fruit flavored, and cost much less than cigarettes. In a recent study, users of little cigars were more likely to be younger, male, black, and current cigarette, cigar, hookah, or marijuana smokers. Users also tended to have a lower perception of harm, greater sensation-seeking behaviours, and higher perceived levels of stress (Sterling et al., 2013).

Bidis

Bidis
Hand-rolled flavored cigarettes.

Generally made in India or Southeast Asia, **bidis** are small, hand-rolled cigarettes that come in a variety of flavors, such as vanilla, chocolate, and cherry. They have become increasingly popular with university students, because they are viewed to be safer and cheaper than cigarettes. However, they are far more toxic than cigarettes. A study found that bidis produced three times more carbon monoxide and nicotine and five times more tar than cigarettes (CDCP, 2011). The leaf wrappers are nonporous, which means that smokers have to pull harder to inhale and inhale more to keep the bidi lit. During testing, it took an average of 28 puffs to smoke a bidi, compared to only 9 puffs for a regular cigarette. This results in much more exposure to higher amounts of tar, nicotine, and carbon monoxide (CDCP, 2011).

Pipes and Hookahs

Pipes have had a long history of use throughout the world, including ritualistic and ceremonial use in many cultures. Hookahs—a type of water pipe with a long hose for inhaling—originated in the Middle East, but has become particularly popular among university-aged adults in the United States recently. While water pipes may cut down on the throat irritation users feel by cooling smoke before it is inhaled, it's important to realise two things: first, the main ingredient in hookahs remains tobacco; and second, a hookah does not filter out any harmful chemicals found in tobacco smoke. According to the National Cancer Institute and the American Cancer Society, pipe smoking carries risks similar to cigar smoking (ACS, 2013).

Smokeless Tobacco

There are two types of smokeless tobacco: chewing tobacco and snuff.

Chewing tobacco comes in three forms—loose leaf, plug, or in a pouch—and contains tobacco leaves treated with molasses and other flavorings. The user dips the tobacco by placing a small amount between the lower lip and teeth to stimulate the flow of saliva and release the nicotine. Dipping rapidly releases nicotine into the bloodstream. Use of chewing tobacco by teenagers, especially white males, has increased in recent years (CDCP, 2012).

Snuff is a finely ground form of tobacco that can be inhaled, chewed, or placed against the gums. It comes in dry or moist powdered form or sachets (tea bag–like pouches). In 2009, "snus" became the latest form of smokeless tobacco to hit the market in the United States. Popular for more than 100 years in Sweden, these small sachets of tobacco are placed inside the cheek and sucked. Some people prefer snus to chewing tobacco because it doesn't require the user to spit frequently.

Smokeless tobacco is just as addictive as cigarettes and actually contains more nicotine—holding an average-sized dip or chew in the mouth for 30 minutes delivers as much nicotine as smoking four cigarettes. A two-can-a-week snuff user gets as much nicotine as a ten-pack-a-week smoker.

Dental problems are common among users of smokeless tobacco. Contact with tobacco juice causes receding gums, tooth decay, bad breath, and discoloured teeth. Damage to both the teeth and jawbone can contribute to early loss of teeth.

Chewing tobacco
A stringy type of tobacco that is placed in the mouth and then sucked or chewed.

Dipping
Placing a small amount of chewing tobacco between the lower lip and teeth for rapid nicotine absorption.

Snuff
A powdered form of tobacco that is sniffed and absorbed through the mucous membranes in the nose or placed inside the cheek and sucked.

Health hazards of tobacco products

Each day, cigarettes contribute to approximately 1,170 deaths from cancer, cardiovascular disease, and respiratory disorders (Campaign for Tobacco Free Kids, 2013). In addition, tobacco use can negatively impact the health of almost every system in your body. Figure 6.12 summarise some of the physiological and health effects of smoking.

Cancer

Lung cancer is the leading cause of cancer deaths in Australia and the United States. The American Cancer Society estimates that tobacco smoking causes 85 to 90 percent of all cases of lung cancer; fewer than 10 percent of cases occur among nonsmokers. There were an estimated 228,190 *new* cases of lung cancer in the United States in 2013 alone, and an estimated 159,480 Americans died from the disease in 2013 (AMC, 2013). The most recent Australian statistics reveal that there were estimated 10,926 new lung cancer diagnoses in 2012 and an estimated 8,256 deaths from lung cancer in the same year (AIHW, 2016). The AIHW, 2016 estimate that an Australian's risk of being diagnosed with lung cancer before their 85th birthday will be 1 in 17 (1 in 22 females and 1 in 13 males). Figure 6.13 illustrates how tobacco smoke damages the lungs.

Lung cancer can take 10 to 30 years to develop, and the outlook for its victims is poor. Most lung cancer is not diagnosed until it is fairly widespread in the body; at that point, the 5-year survival rate is only 16 percent. When a malignancy is diagnosed and recognise while still localised, the 5-year survival rate rises to 52 percent (AMC, 2013).

If you are a smoker, your risk of developing lung cancer depends on several factors. First, the amount you smoke per day is important. Someone who smokes two packs a day is 15 to 25 times more likely to develop lung cancer than a nonsmoker. Also, smoking as little as one cigar per day can double the risk of several cancers, including that of the oral cavity (lip, tongue, mouth, and throat), esophagus, larynx, and lungs. A second factor is when you started smoking; if you started in your teens, you have a greater chance of

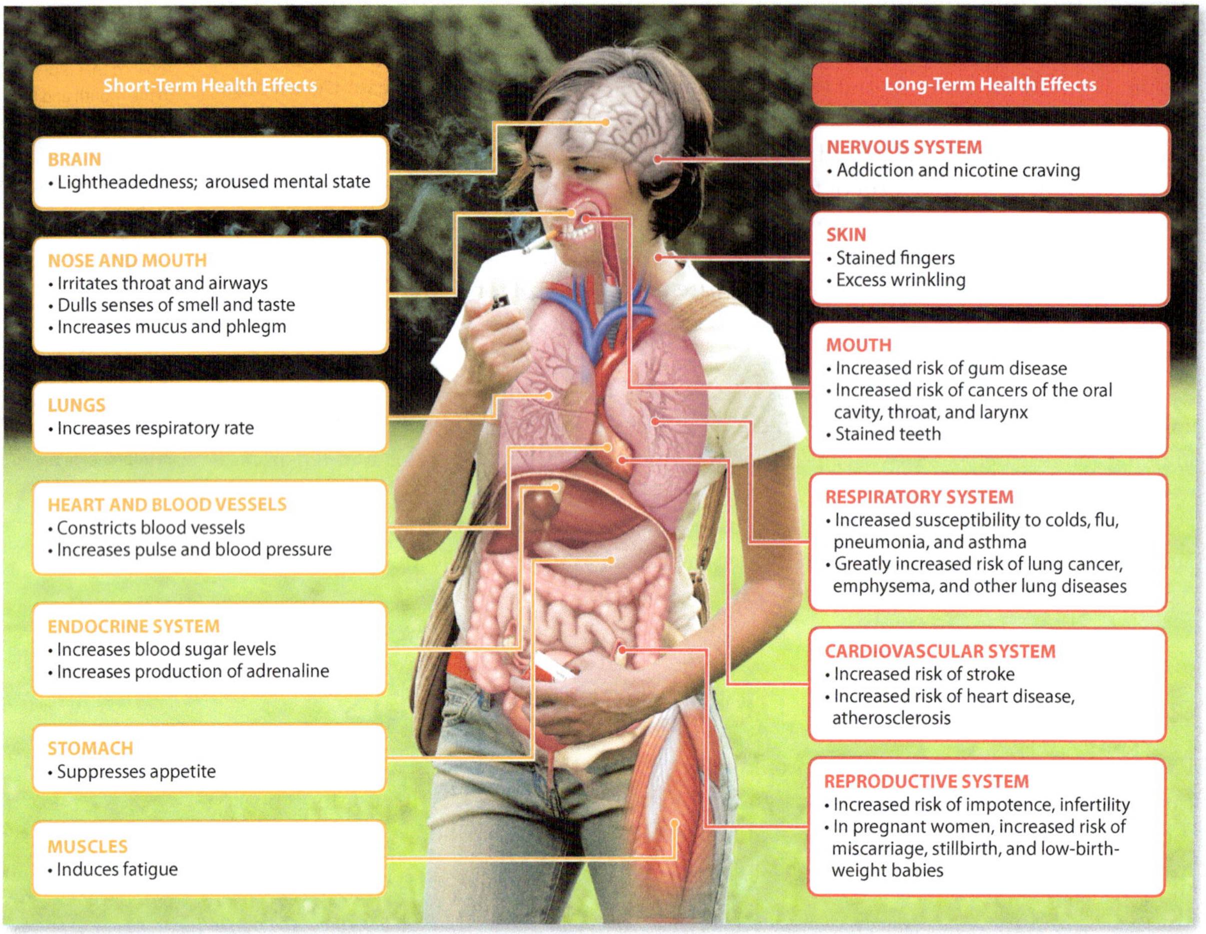

Short-Term Health Effects

BRAIN
- Lightheadedness; aroused mental state

NOSE AND MOUTH
- Irritates throat and airways
- Dulls senses of smell and taste
- Increases mucus and phlegm

LUNGS
- Increases respiratory rate

HEART AND BLOOD VESSELS
- Constricts blood vessels
- Increases pulse and blood pressure

ENDOCRINE SYSTEM
- Increases blood sugar levels
- Increases production of adrenaline

STOMACH
- Suppresses appetite

MUSCLES
- Induces fatigue

Long-Term Health Effects

NERVOUS SYSTEM
- Addiction and nicotine craving

SKIN
- Stained fingers
- Excess wrinkling

MOUTH
- Increased risk of gum disease
- Increased risk of cancers of the oral cavity, throat, and larynx
- Stained teeth

RESPIRATORY SYSTEM
- Increased susceptibility to colds, flu, pneumonia, and asthma
- Greatly increased risk of lung cancer, emphysema, and other lung diseases

CARDIOVASCULAR SYSTEM
- Increased risk of stroke
- Increased risk of heart disease, atherosclerosis

REPRODUCTIVE SYSTEM
- Increased risk of impotence, infertility
- In pregnant women, increased risk of miscarriage, stillbirth, and low-birth-weight babies

Figure 6.12 Effects of Smoking on the Body and Health
(**Source:** TPH/allOver photography/Alamy.)

Figure 6.13 Lung Damage from Chemical in Tobacco Smoke

Smoke particles irritate lung pathways, causing extra mucus production, and nicotine paralyses the cilia that normally function to keep the lungs clear of excess mucus. The result is difficulty breathing, "smoker's cough," and chronic bronchitis. At the same time, tar collects within the alveoli (air sacs), ultimately causing their walls to break, leading to emphysema. Tar and other carcinogens in tobacco smoke also cause cellular mutations that lead to cancer.
(**Source:** James Stevenson/Science Source.)

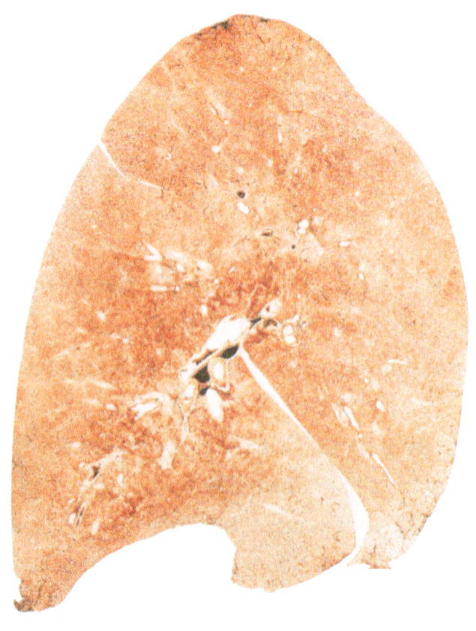

(a) A healthy lung

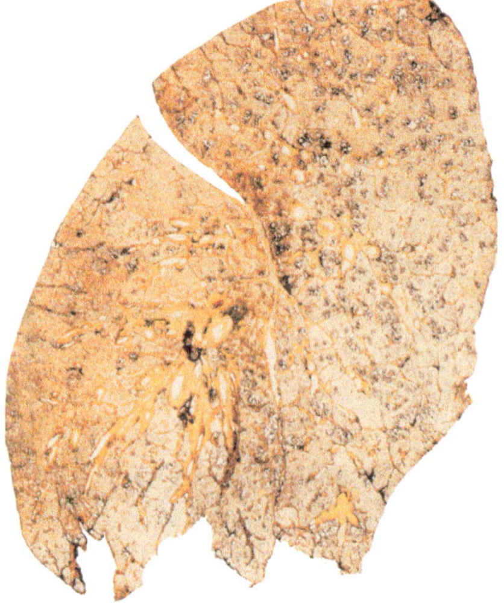

(b) A smoker's lung permeated with deposits of tar

developing lung cancer than do people who start later. And a third risk factor is if you inhale deeply when you smoke. Smokers are also more susceptible to the cancer-causing effects of exposure to other irritants, such as asbestos and radon, than are nonsmokers.

A major health risk of chewing tobacco is **leukoplakia**, a condition characterised by leathery white patches inside the mouth that are produced by contact with irritants in tobacco juice. Three to 17 percent of diagnosed leukoplakia cases develop into oral cancer. There were over 41,000 cases of oral cancer diagnosed in 2013—the vast majority of which were caused by smokeless tobacco or cigarettes (ACS, 2013). Users of smokeless tobacco are 50 times more likely to develop oral cancers than are nonusers (International Agency for Research on Cancer, 2007). Warning signs include lumps in the jaw or neck; colour changes or lumps inside the lips; white, smooth, or scaly patches in the mouth or on the neck, lips, or tongue; a red spot or sore on the lips or gums or inside the mouth that does not heal in 2 weeks; repeated bleeding in the mouth; and difficulty or abnormality in speaking or swallowing.

Leukoplakia
A condition characterised by leathery white patches inside the mouth; produced by contact with irritants in tobacco juice.

The lag time between first use and contracting cancer is shorter for smokeless tobacco users than for smokers, because absorption through the gums is the most efficient route of nicotine administration. Many smokeless tobacco users eventually "graduate" to cigarettes and further increase their risk for developing additional problems.

Tobacco is linked to other cancers as well. The rate of pancreatic cancer is more than twice as high for smokers as nonsmokers. Typically, people diagnosed with pancreatic cancer live only about 3 months after their diagnosis. Cancers of the lip, tongue, salivary glands, and esophagus are five times more likely to occur among smokers than among nonsmokers. Smokers are also more likely to develop kidney, bladder, and larynx cancers. A growing body of evidence suggests that long-term use of smokeless tobacco also increases the risk of cancer of the larynx, esophagus, nasal cavity, pancreas, colon, kidney, and bladder (Zhao et al., 2010).

Cardiovascular disease

Over a third of all tobacco-related deaths occur from heart disease (American Heart Association, 2013). Smokers have a 70 percent higher death rate from heart disease than nonsmokers do, and heavy smokers have a 200 percent higher death rate than moderate smokers do. In fact, smoking cigarettes poses as great a risk for developing heart disease as high blood pressure and high cholesterol levels do. Daily cigar smoking, especially for people who inhale, also increases the risk of heart disease (cigar smokers double their risk of heart attack and stroke) (American Heart Association, 2013).

Smoking contributes to heart disease by adding the equivalent of 10 years of ageing to the arteries (American Heart Association, 2013). One explanation for the mechanism behind this is that smoking and exposure to environmental tobacco smoke (ETS) encourage and accelerate the buildup of fatty deposits (plaque) in the heart and major blood vessels (*atherosclerosis*). Smokers can experience a 50 percent increase in plaque accumulation in the arteries, compared with ex-smokers, and a 20 percent increase in plaque buildup for nonsmokers regularly exposed to ETS. For unknown reasons, smoking decreases blood levels of HDLs, the "good cholesterol" that helps protect against heart attacks.

Smoking also contributes to **platelet adhesiveness**, the sticking together of red blood cells that is associated with blood clots. The oxygen deprivation associated with smoking decreases the oxygen supplied to the heart and can weaken tissues. Smoking also contributes to irregular heart rhythms, which can trigger a heart attack. Both carbon monoxide and nicotine in cigarette smoke can precipitate angina attacks (pain spasms in the chest when the heart muscle does not get the blood supply it needs).

Platelet adhesiveness
Stickiness of red blood cells associated with blood clots.

A stroke occurs when a small blood vessel in the brain bursts or is blocked by a blood clot, denying oxygen and nourishment to vital portions of the brain, and smokers are twice as likely to suffer strokes as nonsmokers (American Heart Association, 2012). Depending on the area of the brain affected, stroke can result in paralysis, loss of mental functioning, or death. Smoking contributes to strokes by raising blood pressure, which increases the stress on vessel walls, and platelet adhesiveness contributes to blood clot formation.

Respiratory disorders

Smoking quickly impairs the respiratory system. Smokers can feel its impact in a relatively short period of time—they are more prone to breathlessness, chronic cough, and excess phlegm production than are nonsmokers their age. Over time, cumulative lung damage can lead to chronic obstructive pulmonary disease (COPD), including chronic bronchitis and emphysema. Ultimately, smokers are up to 18 times more likely to die of lung disease than are nonsmokers (ACS, 2013).

Chronic bronchitis may develop in smokers because their inflamed lungs produce more mucus, which they constantly try to expel along with foreign particles. This results in the persistent cough known as "smoker's hack." Smokers are also more prone than nonsmokers to respiratory ailments such as influenza, pneumonia, and colds.

Emphysema
A chronic lung disease in which the tiny air sacs in the lungs are destroyed, making breathing difficult.

Emphysema is a chronic disease in which the alveoli (the tiny air sacs in the lungs) are destroyed, impairing the lungs' ability to obtain oxygen and remove carbon dioxide. Where healthy people expend only about 5 percent of their energy in breathing, people with advanced emphysema expend nearly 80 percent. Because the heart has to work harder to do even the simplest tasks, it may become enlarged, and death from heart damage may result. There is no known cure for emphysema, and the damage is irreversible. Approximately 80 percent of all cases are related to cigarette smoking (Johns Hopkins Health Alerts, 2012).

Sexual dysfunction and fertility problems

Despite attempts by tobacco advertisers to make smoking appear sexy, research shows it can actually cause impotence in men. Studies have found that male smokers are much more likely to experience erectile dysfunction than are nonsmokers (Haarte et al., 2013). Toxins in cigarette smoke damage blood vessels, reducing blood flow to the penis and leading to an inadequate erection. It is thought that impotence may indicate oncoming cardiovascular disease.

In women, smoking can lead to infertility and problems with pregnancy. Women who smoke increase their risk for infertility, ectopic pregnancy, miscarriage, and stillbirth. Smoking during pregnancy also increases risk of sudden infant death syndrome and the chances of the baby being born with a cleft lip or cleft palate (CDCP, 2012). Smoking while pregnant accounts for approximately 30 percent of premature births and increases the risk of low birth weight (less than 5.5 pounds), which in turn increases babies' likelihood of illness or death (CDCP, 2013).

Unique risks for women

Today, 16.5 percent of women—slightly more than 1 in 6—smoke, compared with 21.6 percent of men. Women who smoke now are just as likely to die of cancer and other smoking related diseases as men, and both active and passive smoking increase chances of breast cancer (Thun et al., 2013). Accordingly, women have assumed a much larger burden of smoking-related diseases than they did in the past. Women are 26 times more likely to die from lung cancer than non-smoking women compared to 30 years ago (Thun et al., 2013).

Higher rates of osteoporosis, depression, and thyroid-related diseases are just some of the risks that women who smoke take. Women who smoke (particularly those who also use oral contraceptives) are also at increased risk for blood clots, on top of heavier menstrual bleeding, longer duration of cramps, and less predictable length of menstrual cycle.

Other health effects

Studies have shown tobacco use to be a serious risk factor in the development of gum disease (American Academy of Periodontology, 2013). In addition, smoking increases risk of macular degeneration, one of the most common causes of blindness in older adults. It also causes premature skin wrinkling, staining of the teeth, yellowing of the fingernails, and bad breath. Nicotine speeds up the process by which the body uses and eliminates drugs, making medications less effective. In addition, recent research suggests that smoking significantly increases the risk for Alzheimer's disease (Cataldo et al., 2013).

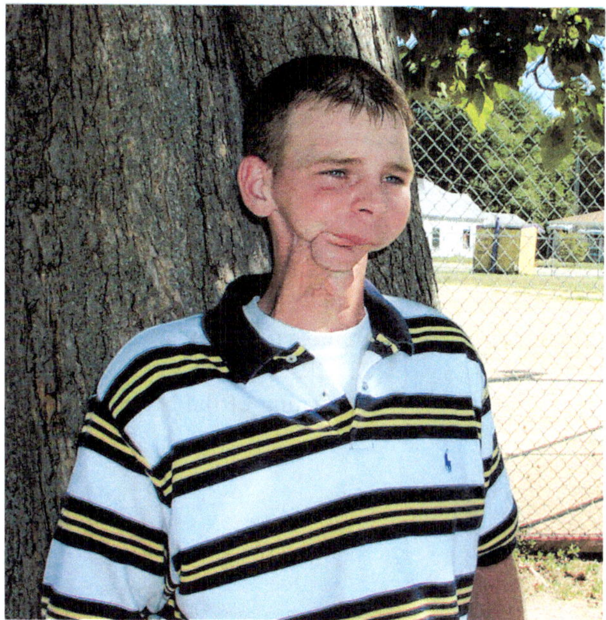

Is chewing tobacco as harmful as smoking?

No matter in what form you use it—cigar, pipe, bidi, dip, snuff, or cigarette—tobacco is hazardous to your health. Chewing tobacco and snuff actually contain more nicotine than cigarettes and just as many toxic and carcinogenic chemicals. This young cancer survivor began using smokeless tobacco at age 13; by age 17, he was diagnosed with squamous cell carcinoma. He has undergone surgery to remove neck muscles, lymph nodes, and his tongue, and he now educates others about the dangers of chewing tobacco.

(Source: James Stevenson/Science Source; p. 250 NSTEP® (National SpitTobacco Education Program), an Oral Health of America program.)

Environmental tobacco smoke

Even though fewer than 14 percent of Australians smoke, air pollution from smoking in public places continues to be a problem. **Environmental tobacco smoke (ETS)** is divided into two categories: mainstream and sidestream smoke. **Mainstream smoke** refers to smoke drawn through tobacco while inhaling; **sidestream smoke** (commonly called *secondhand smoke*) refers to smoke from the burning end of a cigarette or smoke exhaled by a smoker. People who breathe smoke from someone else's smoking product are said to be *involuntary* or *passive* smokers. Over the past 20 years, nicotine exposure in nonsmoking Australians has declined significantly due to to increased public awareness of health dangers associated with secondhand smoke and the multitude of legislative changes that ban smoking in certain public places (such as beaches, railway platforms, skate parks, play grounds) and the workplace (AIHW, 2010).

Environmental tobacco smoke (ETS) Smoke from tobacco products, including secondhand and mainstream smoke.

Mainstream smoke Smoke that is drawn through tobacco while inhaling.

Sidestream smoke The cigarette, pipe, or cigar smoke breathed by nonsmokers; commonly called *secondhand smoke*.

Children are more heavily exposed to ETS than adults. Over 53 percent of U.S. children aged 3 to 11 years—or 22 million children—are exposed (CDCP, 2012). Disparities in ETS also occur among ethnic and racial lines and among income levels. African Americans have been found to have higher levels of exposure to ETS than whites and Latinos. ETS exposure is also higher among low-income persons (CDCP, 2012). In Australia from 1995 and 2007, childhood exposure to secondhand smoke in the home decreased significantly. In 1995, 31% of households with dependent children were smoking in the home, whereas in 2007, only 8% of households with dependent children reported smoking in the home (AIHW, 2010).

Risks from environmental tobacco smoke

Although involuntary smokers breathe less tobacco than active smokers do, they still face risks from exposure. According to the American Lung Association, secondhand smoke has about 2 times more tar and nicotine, 5 times more carbon monoxide, and 50 times more ammonia than mainstream smoke. Every year, ETS is estimated to be responsible for approximately 3,400 lung cancer deaths in nonsmoking adults, 46,000 coronary and heart disease deaths in nonsmoking adults who live with smokers, and higher risk of death in newborns from sudden infant death syndrome (CDCP, 2012).

The Environmental Protection Agency has designated secondhand smoke as a known carcinogen. There are more than 50 cancer-causing agents found in secondhand smoke (CDCP, 2012). There is also strong evidence that secondhand smoke interferes with normal functioning of the heart, blood, and vascular systems, significantly increasing the risk for heart disease and having immediate effects on the cardiovascular system. Studies indicate that nonsmokers exposed to secondhand smoke were 20 to 30 percent more likely to have coronary heart disease than those who were not (CDCP, 2012).

WARNING:
Cigarettes are addictive.
© U.S. HHS
1-800-QUIT-NOW
BRAND
20 Class A Cigarettes

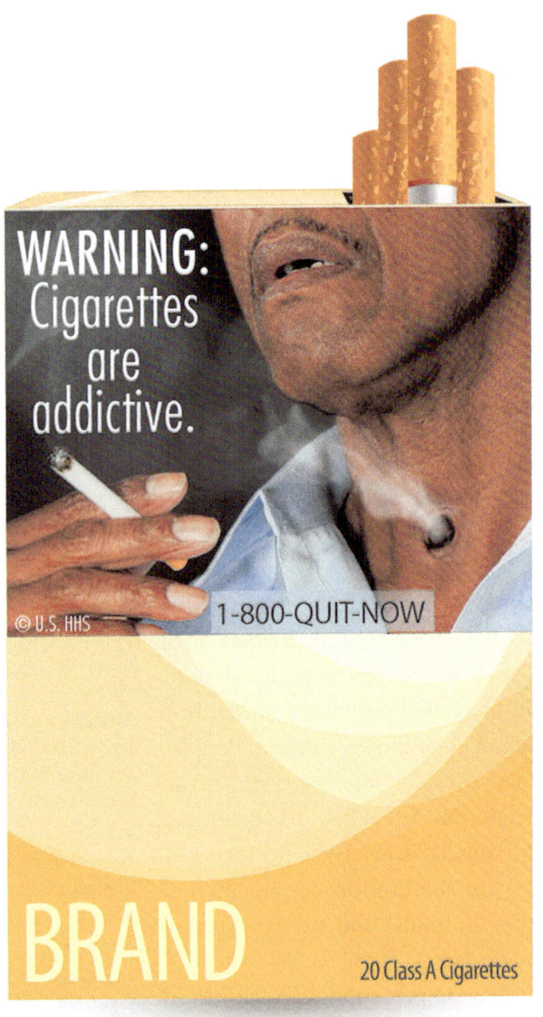

Figure 6.14 Proposed New Cigarette Product Warning Labels

The U.S. Food and Drug Administration proposed that graphic warning images, such as this one, be placed on all cigarette packages and advertisements. However, lawsuits prevented their implementation, and the FDA is now in the process of creating new warning labels.

Source: U.S. Food and Drug Administration, "Proposed Cigarette Product Warning Labels," Accessed May 23, 2011, www.fda.gov

(**Source:** imago stock&people/Newscom.)

Tobacco use and prevention policies

It has been more than 40 years since the government began warning that tobacco use is hazardous to the health of the nation. Despite all the education on the health hazards of tobacco use, health care spending and lost productivity associated with smoking still exceeds $193 billion each year (CDCP, 2011).

In the late 1990s, the tobacco industry reached a Master's Settlement Agreement with 40 states: This legal agreement requires tobacco companies to pay out approximately $206 billion over 25 years. The agreement also included a variety of measures to support antismoking education and advertising and to fund research to determine effective smoking cessation strategies.

Unfortunately, most of the money designated for tobacco control and prevention at the state level has not been used for this purpose. Facing budget woes, many states have drastically cut spending on antismoking programs. In the few states that have spent the settlement money on smoking cessation programs, there has been some reported success in decreasing cigarette use (Tobacco-Free Kids, 2011). The Family Smoking Prevention and Tobacco Control Act signed into law in 2009 allows the U.S. Food and Drug Administration (FDA) to forbid advertising geared

Table 6.5 Coping Strategies for Common Smoking Withdrawal Problems

Withdrawal Challenge	Estimated Length of Symptoms	Coping Strategies*
Anger, frustration, and irritability	Peaks in first week after quitting, but can last 2–4 weeks.	Avoid caffeine, which can amp up an already agitated mood. Get a massage; try deep breathing or exercise.
Anxiety	Builds over the first 3 days and may last up to 2 weeks.	Same strategies as above. Also remind yourself that the symptoms usually pass by themselves over time.
Mild depression	One month or less.	Be with supportive friends, increase physical activity, make a list of things that are upsetting you and write down possible solutions. If depression lasts longer than a month, seek medical advice.
Weight gain	Usually begins in the early weeks and continues through the first year after quitting.	Studies show nicotine replacement products such as gum and lozenges can help counter weight gain. You may also ask your doctor about the drug bupropion (brand names Wellbutrin or Zyban), which has also been shown to counter weight gain.

*Asking your doctor for nicotine replacement products or other medications is a valid coping strategy for any of the withdrawal challenges listed here.

Source: Adapted from National Cancer Institute, "Handling Withdrawal Symptoms When You Decide to Quit," National Cancer Institute Fact Sheet, 2010, www.cancer.gov

toward children, to lower the amount of nicotine in tobacco products, to ban sweetened cigarettes that appeal to young people, and to prohibit labels such as "light" and "low tar." (111th Congress of the United States of America, 2009) One of the most significant impacts of the law is that it requires more prominent health warnings on advertising of tobacco products. Smokeless tobacco ads now must contain a warning that fills 20 percent of the advertising space. Cigarette packages and advertising were required to have bigger, stronger warnings that must cover the top half of the front and back of each package and include "colour graphics depicting the negative health consequences of smoking" (Figure 6.14). The FDA created graphics modeled after ads already used in Canada, Australia, and New Zealand, but lawsuits brought on by tobacco companies prevented their implementation in 2012.

Quitting

Smokers must break both the physical addiction to nicotine and the habit of lighting up at certain times of day. Approximately 70 percent of adult smokers in the United States want to quit smoking, and up to 44 percent make a serious attempt to quit each year. However, only somewhere between 4 and 7 percent succeed (CDCP, 2011). The most recent data available in Australia reveals that 86% of the smoking population aged 14 years or older reported actively attempting to change their smoking behaviour in the past 12 months (AIHW, 2014). Thirty percent reported

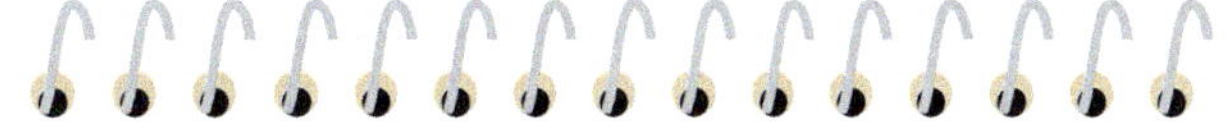

Tips for Quitting Smoking

Skills for Behaviour Change

If you're a smoker and you're ready to quit, try these tips to help kick the habit:

- Use the four Ds to fight the urge to smoke:
- Delay—put off smoking for 10 minutes; when the 10 minutes are up, put it off for another 10 minutes.
- Deep breathing.
- Drink water.
- Do something else.
- Keep "mouth toys" handy: hard candy, gum, toothpicks, and carrot sticks can help.
- If you've had trouble stopping before, ask your doctor about nicotine chewing gum, patches, nasal sprays, inhalers, or lozenges.
- Make an appointment with your dental hygienist to have your teeth cleaned.
- Examine those associations that trigger your urge to smoke.
- Tell your family and friends that you've stopped smoking so they won't offer you a cigarette.
- Aim to spend your time in places that don't allow smoking.
- Take up a new sport, exercise program, hobby, or organisational commitment. This will help shake up your routine and distract you from smoking.

Tech & Health

E-Cigarettes: Health Risks and Concerns

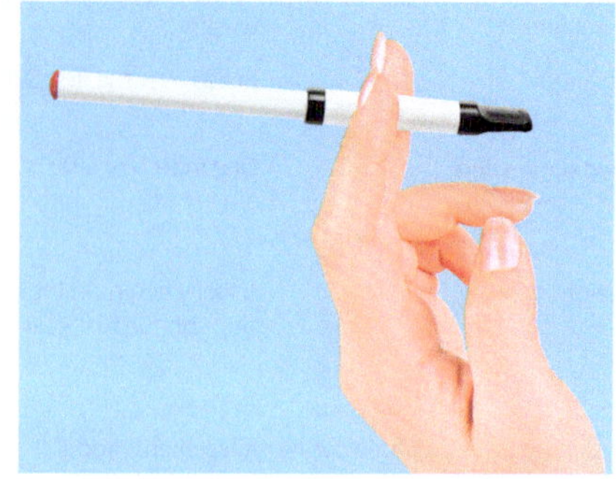
Electronic cigarette, or e-cigarette.

Electronic cigarettes, also called e-cigarettes, are increasingly popular worldwide. They consist of a battery, atomiser, and a cartridge containing nicotine and other chemicals. The cartridge vaporises the nicotine and allows users to inhale it. Because there is no smoke, some feel e-cigarettes must be safe compared to regular cigarettes. They are often marketed as antismoking devices. Unfortunately, e-cigarettes still have a host of worries associated with them.

While the lack of smoke may reduce some risks, nicotine—the main component of cigarettes that causes cardiovascular damage—makes e-cigarettes far from healthy. The U.S. Food and Drug Administration (FDA) analysed samples of two popular brands and found variable amounts of nicotine and traces of known carcinogens. Almost always manufactured in China, the devices are built without real safety or quality controls. Defective parts and leaky cartridges are par for the course. There is also no safe way to dispose of e-cigarette products and accessories, potentially resulting in nicotine exposure to children, other adults, or pets, as well as contamination of water or soil. Currently, e-cigarettes do not contain any health warnings, and health professionals continue to urge for more action to regulate these products.

Sources: University of California, Riverside, "Electronic Cigarettes Are Unsafe and Pose Health Risks, UC Riverside Study Finds," 2010, http://newsroom.ucr.edu; U.S. Food and Drug Administration, "FDA and Public Health Experts Warn about Electronic Cigarettes," 2010, www.fda.gov; L. Dale, Mayo Clinic, "Electronic Cigarettes: A Safe Way to Light Up?" 2011, www.mayoclinic.com; E. Sohn, Discovery News, "How Safe Are E-Cigarettes?" 2011, http://news.discovery.com; A. Norton, "Are E-Cigarettes Bad for Health?" 2012, www.huffingtonpost.com

trying to quit with no success, 36% reported reducing the amount smoked per day and 20% gave up smoking for at least one month (AIHW, 2014). Quitting is often a lengthy process involving several unsuccessful attempts before success is finally achieved; even successful quitters suffer occasional slips. For those smokers unable to quit, they can expect to lose at least one decade of life compared to those who do not smoke. Cessation before the age of 40 years reduces the risk of death associated with continued smoking by about 90 percent (Jha et al., 2013).

The person who wishes to quit smoking has several options. Most people who are successful quit "cold turkey"—that is, they decide simply not to smoke again. Others focus on gradual reduction in smoking levels, which can reduce risks over time. Still others resort to short-term programs, such as those offered by the American Cancer Society, which are based on behaviour modification and a system of self-rewards. Treatment centres community outreach plans sponsored by a local medical clinic, and telephone quit lines are helpful for some, whereas some people work privately with their physicians to reach their goal. Programs that combine several approaches have shown the most promise.

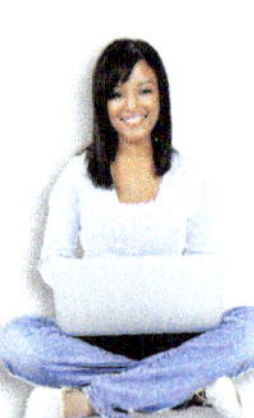

"Why Should I Care?"

If the life-threatening health consequences aren't enough to make you give up smoking, consider the negative impact smoking can have on your social (and romantic!) life. Popular media may make smoking seem glamorous and sexy, but in reality, smoking makes your breath, hair, and clothing smell bad; it causes your skin to age prematurely; it yellows your teeth; and it can interfere with a man's ability to achieve and maintain an erection.

(**Source:** Elena Elisseeva/Shutterstock.)

Breaking the nicotine addiction

Nicotine addiction may be one of the toughest addictions to overcome. Symptoms of nicotine withdrawal include irritability, restlessness, nausea, vomiting, and intense cravings for tobacco (see Table 6.5). The evidence is strong that consistent pharmacological treatments can help a smoker quit: An estimated 25 to 33 percent of people who have used nicotine replacement therapy or smoking-cessation medications continue to abstain from cigarettes for over 6 months (American Cancer Society, 2010). The Skills for Behaviour Change box presents one of the American Cancer Society's approaches for quitting smoking.

Nicotine withdrawal Symptoms, including nausea, headaches, irritability, and intense tobacco cravings, suffered by nicotine-addicted individuals who cease using tobacco.

Nicotine replacement products

Nontobacco products that replace depleted levels of nicotine in the bloodstream have helped some people stop using tobacco. The two most common are nicotine chewing gum and the nicotine patch, both of which are available over the counter. The FDA has also approved a nicotine nasal spray, a nicotine inhaler, and nicotine lozenges. Another product called an e-cigarette is also available, although it comes with its own health concerns.

Nicotine gum delivers about as much nicotine as a cigarette does, but because it is absorbed through the mucous membrane of the mouth, it doesn't produce the same rush. Users experience no withdrawal symptoms and fewer cravings for nicotine as the dosage is reduced until they are completely weaned—users chew up to 20 pieces of gum a day for 1 to 3 months. Nicotine-containing lozenges are available in two strengths, and a 12-week program of use is recommended to allow users to taper off the drug.

The nicotine patch is generally used in conjunction with a comprehensive smoking-behaviour cessation program. A small, thin patch placed on the smoker's upper body delivers a continuous flow of nicotine through the skin, helping to relieve cravings. Patches can be bought with or without a prescription and are available in different dosages. The FDA recommends using the patch for a total of 3 to 5 months. During this time, the dose of nicotine is gradually reduced until the smoker is fully weaned from the drug. The patch costs less than a pack of cigarettes—about $4—and some insurance plans will pay for it (Everyday Health, 2011).

The nasal spray, which requires a prescription, is much more powerful and delivers nicotine to the bloodstream faster than gum or the patch. Patients are warned to be careful not to overdose; as little as 40 mg nicotine taken at once could be lethal. The FDA has advised that it should be used for no more than 3 months and never for more than 6 months, so that smokers don't find themselves as dependent on nicotine in spray form as they were on cigarettes. The FDA also advises that no one who experiences nasal or sinus problems, allergies, or asthma should use it.

The nicotine inhaler, which also requires a prescription, consists of a mouthpiece and cartridge. By puffing on the mouthpiece, the smoker inhales air saturated with nicotine, which is absorbed through the lining of the mouth, not the lungs. This nicotine enters the body much more slowly than the nicotine in cigarettes does. Using the inhaler mimics the hand-to-mouth actions used in smoking and causes the back of the throat to feel as it would when inhaling tobacco smoke.

Smoking cessation medications

Bupropion (brand names Zyban and Wellbutrin), an antidepressant, is FDA approved as a smoking-cessation aid. Varinicline (brand name Chantix) reduces nicotine cravings and the urge to smoke, and blocks the effects of nicotine at nicotine receptor sites in the brain. Both these drugs may sometimes cause changes in behaviour such as agitation, depression, hostility, and suicidal thoughts. If someone experiences these things while on a smoking cessation drug, they should stop taking it and contact their health care professional (U.S. Food and Drug Administration, 2009).

Benefits of quitting

Many tissues damaged by smoking can repair themselves. As soon as a smoker stops, the body begins the repair process (Figure 6.15). Within 8 hours, carbon monoxide and oxygen levels return to normal, and "smoker's breath" disappears. Circulation and the senses of taste and smell improve within weeks. Often, within a month of quitting, the mucus that clogs airways is broken up and eliminated. The risk of dying from a heart attack falls by half after only 1 year without smoking and declines steadily thereafter. At the end of 10 smoke-free years, the ex-smoker can expect to live out his or her normal life span, and after about 15 years without smoking, the ex-smoker's risk of coronary heart disease is similar to that of people who have never smoked (American Lung Association, 2012).

A recent study suggested women who quit smoking before age 40 may avoid more than 90 percent of the added risk of dying early. Women who quit before 30 could avoid 97 percent of that risk (Pirie et al., 2013). Women who quit are also less likely to bear babies with low birth weight.

Another significant benefit of quitting smoking is the money saved. A pack of cigarettes averages $6.00, including taxes (Campaign for Tobacco-Free Kids, 2012). Using this number, a pack-a-day smoker burns through about $42.00 per week, or $2,184.00 per year. That is money that could otherwise have gone toward a car payment or a much-earned vacation over spring break.[F]

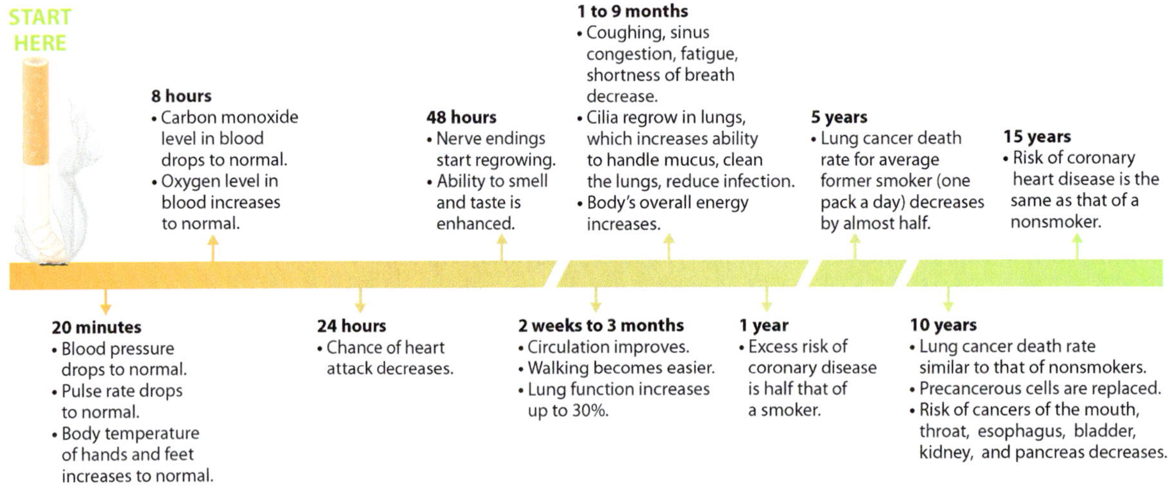

Figure 6.15 When Smokers Quit

Within 20 minutes of smoking that last cigarette, the body begins a series of changes that continues for years. However, by smoking just one cigarette a day, the smoker loses all these benefits, according to the American Cancer Society.

[F] Donatelle, R. J.(2015). Drinking alcohol responsibly and ending tobacco use. In *Health: The basics* (11th ed., pp. 228-254). Upper Saddle River, NJ: Pearson Education Inc.

Summary

What is health behaviour?

- Harris and Guten (1979, p. 18), define health behaviour as 'behaviour performed by an individual, regardless of his/her perceived health status, with the purpose of protecting, promoting or maintaining his/her health'
- A person's health can be influenced by a number of factors related to biological, lifestyle, societal and environmental factors – many of which can be modified to some extent
- Common behavioural risk factors include tobacco, alcohol and illicit drug use, and excess body weight (an outcome of dietary and exercise behaviours)

Factors contributing to overweight and obesity

- Although excess calorie intake and too little physical activity are major contributors to excess weight, there are other complex factors that can contribute such as learned behaviours in the home, influences at school and in social environments, and media influences

Physical activity for health

- There is overwhelming evidence of the effectiveness of regular physical activity in the primary and secondary prevention of several chronic diseases (e.g., cardiovascular disease, diabetes, cancer, hypertension, obesity, depression, and osteoporosis)

Drug misuse and abuse

- Over-the-counter drugs are abused when taken in more than the recommended dosage or for longer than is recommended
- There are varying types of over-the-counter drugs that are subject to misuse and abuse, e.g., sleep aids, cold medications and diet pills
- The risks associated with prescription drug abuse can vary from being as mild as decreased or irregular heart rate or as severe as death
- Illicit drug users span all age groups, genders, ethnicities, occupations, and socioeconomic groups

Alcohol: an overview

- Alcohol is responsible for a considerable burden of death, disease and injury
- Any level of drinking increases the risk of ill-health and injury
- Problems associated with long-term, habitual use of alcohol include diseases of the nervous system, cardiovascular system, and liver, as well as some cancers

Tobacco and its effects

- Smoking, the most common form of tobacco use, delivers a strong dose of nicotine, as well as 7,000 other chemical substances
- There is no "safe" amount of tobacco use—any smoking or exposure to smoke increases your risks for negative health effects such as heart disease and lung cancer
- Despite all the education on the health hazards of tobacco use, health care spending and lost productivity associated with smoking remains high

Review questions

A. Fill in the missing words to complete the following statements.

1. The ________________ is associated with health and longevity in terms of behaviour.
2. The psychological and physical effects of blood alcohol concentration reading of ______________ may include: lowered alertness, impaired judgement, lowered inhibitions, exaggerated behaviour, loss of muscle control. While, the psychological and physical effects of blood alcohol reading of ______________ may include: impaired consciousness, loss of motor function, slurred speech, uncontrolled urination, impaired circulation and respiration and possible death.
3. Some of the biological factors related to alcohol abuse include a ____________________ ____________________________. Whereas, some of the social and cultural factors related to alcohol abuse include one's ______________ and ______________________________.
4. Drinking ______________________ a day during pregnancy may significantly increase the risk of childhood mental health and learning problems. The condition associated with alcohol consumption during pregnancy is called ____________________________.

B. Fill in the missing words and/or key concepts to complete the following table.

5. There are various types of drugs and they have varying impacts on the body. Fill in the missing words to complete the following table.

Class of drug	Effect on body	Example
Stimulants		Nicotine, caffeine, cocaine, ecstasy, ritalin
Depressants	Slows down brain and nerve activity OR (Central nervous system depressants)	
Hallucinogens		LSD, Ketamine, mushrooms
Narcotics	Blocks nerve impulses	

6. The five main treatment approaches for drug and alcohol users that involve both individual and group counselling. Fill in the missing treatment modalities and aims of each therapy.

Treatment modality	Aim of therapy
Cognitive behavioural therapy	
	Includes the client and their family in addressing the patterns and influences of drug and alcohol abuse
Motivational interviewing	
Motivational incentives (contingency management)	
	Meetings are open to anyone at no membership cost. Work is focused on personal recovering using the 12-step approach.

C. Please select one statement that best answers each of the following questions.

7. The national physical activity recommendations for a healthy adult is
   a) 60 mins/week vigorous-intensity physical activity
   b) 150 mins/week moderate intensity physical activity
   c) 75 min/week of vigorous-intensity physical activity
   d) both b) and c)

8. Which of the following statements is correct?
   a) 1 in 2 Australian children and adolescents are now overweight or obese, and rates are 2 times higher than for their parent's generation.
   b) 1 in 2 Australian children and adolescents are now overweight or obese, and rates are 3 times higher than for their parent's generation.
   c) over 1 in 4 Australian children and adolescents are now overweight or obese, and rates are 2 times higher than for their parent's generation.
   d) over 1 in 4 Australian children and adolescents are now overweight or obese, and rates are 3 times higher than for their parent's generation.

9. Harm reduction for drug users includes which of the following strategies?
   a) explore "where they're at" in terms of their drug addition, explore the conditions of use along with the frequency and intensity of use.
   b) needle exchange program where injecting drug users receive clean needles/syringes and bleach for cleaning needles in an attempt to help reduce HIV and hepatitis B cases.
   c) include the modification of relevant legal sanctions associated with drug use and increasing the availability of treatment services.
   d) all the above

10. Alcohol abuse is defined as
   a) interfering with social, occupational and educational functioning
   b) any violation of the law, including driving under the influence
   c) when ceasing alcohol consumption results in alcohol withdrawal symptoms
   d) all the above

CHAPTER 7

Motivation

The content in this section has been compiled from:
Zimbardo, Chapter 9

Zimbardo, P. G., Johnson, R. L., & McCann, V. (2014). Motivation and emotion. In P. G. Zimbardo, R. L. Johnson, & V. McCann (Eds.), *Psychology: Core concepts* (7th ed., pp. 363–387, 407-408). Upper Saddle River, NJ: Pearson Education.

CHAPTER 7

Motivation

Motivation refers to the drives – particularly wants and needs – that propel us in specific directions. Many health conditions are associated with modifiable lifestyle behaviours, such as a poor diet and physical inactivity. However, existing behaviour patterns are especially difficult to change, even when the individual recognises that their health is at risk. Health care professionals have a vital role in motivating their clients and/or patients to adopt healthier lifestyles. For example, compliance with a task may be required to help clients and/or patients achieve optimal and systemic health. To obtain compliance, existing unhelpful behaviours must be altered. To modify behaviour, it is vital to understand the basic concepts of human motivation before you are able to help patients achieve their goals. This chapter examines types of motivation, theories and components of motivation, all of which can be applied in practice to gain increased levels of patient motivation and compliance.

After studying this chapter you should be able to:

- Describe internal and external factors that motivate individuals
- Identify and describe theories of motivation:
  - Instinct theory
  - Drive theory
  - Freud's psychodynamic theory
  - Maslow's hierarchy of needs
- Describe influences that can change motivational priorities.

What motivates Cathy Freeman? Ever since she was little, Cathy had one dream – to win a gold medal at the Olympics. And win a gold medal she did! Under the watchful eye of over 9 million fellow Australians who tuned in on the TV, Cathy Freeman, Australia's best-known female sprinter, won gold in the 400m final at the 2000 Summer Olympic games in Sydney. But this was certainly not the first time Cathy came first in a race. When she was only eight years old, Cathy won her first race in the 80m sprint at her school athletics carnival. Nonetheless, disappointingly, Cathy never received a trophy. Instead, she watched on in sorrow as her non-indigenous peers, who she had beaten, received trophies.

Did her competitive spirit originate from her experiences of racial discrimination, or perhaps from her tumultuous childhood? Cathy was born in Mackay Far North Queensland on the 16th of February 1973 to indigenous parents, Cecelia and Norman Freeman. Cathy and her family of three brothers (Gavin, Garth and Norman) and younger sister (Anne-Marie) grew up in commission housing. While Cathy was close to her sister, Anne-Marie spent most of her life in disability housing as she needed ongoing care for cerebral palsy. Norman, an ex-Rugby League player, was a heavy drinker and often engaged in violent outbursts so severe that Cathy's mother would have to take her children out of the family home to ensure their safety. When she was 5 years old, Cathy's parents divorced and her father moved out of the family home and at the age of 10, Cathy experienced an assault.

Despite showing athletic talent from an early age, winning most state and national titles, Cathy was significantly disadvantaged. Financial hardship made it difficult for her to access the resources required to pursue her dreams. Moreover, as member of a minority group that historically was not afforded the same opportunities as non-indigenous individuals, Cathy experienced many roadblocks. These roadblocks however played an integral role in Cathy's success, only stimulating her desire to reach for the stars.

With the little money they had, Cathy's mother Cecilia and her stepfather Bruce Barber, did what they could to support Cathy's athletic talent. Bruce saw talent in young Cathy early on, commenting that she had the movement and symmetry in her body of a champion racehorse. When she was 10 years old, Cathy began training with Bruce and despite having little money or the experience necessary to coach her, Bruce worked tirelessly to support and encourage his step-daughter in her athletic pursuit. He requested assistance from state school sporting officials in order to set up a training programme for Cathy to further develop her awe-inspiring talent.

When she was in her early teens, Cathy was awarded a scholarship to Fairholme College in Toowoomba. During her time at the prestigious and impressive boarding school, Cathy felt extremely out of place being only one of three indigenous children in a population of over 600 students. Following her time at Fairholme, Cathy received another scholarship, but this time to Kooralbyn International School, renowned for generating successful athletes. It was here that Cathy's strength and stamina in running was developed through her first professional training experience with Mike Danila.

In 1990, Cathy was afforded the opportunity to participate in the 4 x 100m relay at the Commonwealth Games in Auckland. Her team came first! Nonetheless, upon returning home, Cathy was confronted with the devastating news that her beloved sister, Anne-Marie, had passed away. While Cathy was shattered by the news, she decided to rise above and dedicate her future victories to her sister.

Against all the odds, in 1992, Cathy was the first indigenous woman to represent Australia, at the Barcelona Olympics. Although her results were disappointing, she learned a lot from her experience. Post-Barcelona, tragically Cathy was faced with more terrible news. Her father had passed away of a stroke and she was unable to fly home to attend his funeral.

Despite her adversities, in the subsequent years, Cathy won numerous international championships with her athletic success exploding her into the limelight. Cathy's childhood dreams finally came true when she won gold at the 2000 Sydney Olympics. But what role did her adversities play in her motivation to excel? Freeman is quoted as saying, "You got to try and reach for the stars or try and achieve the unreachable." (Freeman, 2007; Freeman & Scott, 2004).

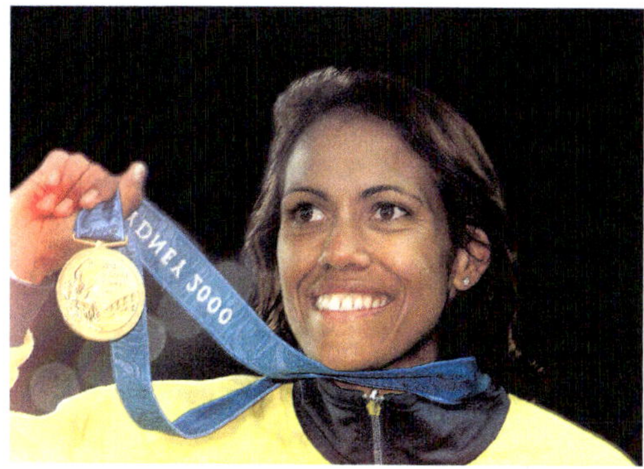

(**Source:** Olivier Labalette/DPPI/Icon SMI/Newscom.)

PROBLEM. Motivation is largely an internal and subjective process: How can we determine what motivates people like Cathy Freeman to work so hard at becoming the best in the world at what they do?

Throughout this chapter, we will use Cathy Freeman's case to illustrate the basic concepts involved in motivation and emotion. We begin by defining what we mean by motivation, followed by consideration of what motivates people to work—or, like Cathy Freeman, to push herself physically and mentally in order to pursue her dreams of winning gold at the Olympic games. Is it for some external (*extrinsic*) reward, or is it done for personal (*intrinsic*) satisfaction?

What motivates us?

In everyday conversation, we use many terms that refer to motivation: *drive, instinct, energy, purpose, goal, intensity, perseverance, desire, want,* and *need.* You will note that all these terms refer to internal psychological "forces" that presumably make us do what we do. But the fact that we cannot observe these internal forces is what makes the psychology of motivation so challenging.

Questions about motivation seldom arise when people behave predictably: getting up in the morning, answering the phone, stopping for red lights, or greeting their friends. On the other hand, we *do* wonder what motivates people whose behaviour falls outside the bounds of the ordinary, such as those who seem obsessed with food or sex, those who gamble away their life savings, those who rob banks—and those celebrities who behave indiscreetly.

Core Concept
Motives are internal dispositions to act in certain ways, although they can be influenced by multiple factors, both internal and external.

Yet another part of the problem of motivation involves motivating people. If you are also an employer, you probably want to motivate your employees to work hard. If you are a coach, you want to motivate your players to train hard so the team can win. But let's bring it closer to home: As a student, you probably also want to learn how to motivate yourself to study a bit more.

So, how do we go about understanding and controlling motivation? Let's begin with the basics, by defining what we mean by *motivation.*

More broadly, the concept of **motivation** refers to all the processes involved in (a) *sensing a need or desire,* and then (b) *activating and guiding the organism* by selecting, directing, and sustaining the mental and physical activity aimed at meeting the need or desire; and finally, when the need is met, (c) *reducing the sensation of need.* Take thirst, for example: On a warm day, you may sense a biological need for fluids that causes you to feel thirsty. That feeling of thirst then focuses your behaviour on getting something to drink. When you have drunk your fill, the uncomfortable sensation of thirst diminishes, and the motive fades into the background.

Motivation
Refers to all the processes involved in initiating, directing, and maintaining physical and psychological activities.

Sometimes, of course, students drink beer not to quench their thirst, but because their friends are drinking or because TV ads have primed them to associate beer drinking with fun. In this case, the need is said to be purely *psychological,* not a *biological* need. In fact, many of our motives involve a complex combination of biological and psychological needs, especially those involving our social interactions, emotions, and goals. Take, for example, the complex processes that underlie our motivation for work.

Extrinsic motivation

The desire to engage in an activity to achieve an external consequence, such as a reward.

Intrinsic motivation

The desire to engage in an activity for its own sake rather than for some external consequence, such as a reward.

Why people work: McClelland's theory

Most people work to make money, of course. Psychologists refer to money and other incentives as *extrinsic motivators,* because they come from outside the person. In general, **extrinsic motivation** involves external stimuli that goad an organism to action. For students, grades are one of the most powerful extrinsic motivators. Other examples of extrinsic motivators include food, drink, praise, awards, and sex.

People can also have *intrinsic motives* for working—motives that arise from within the person. You are intrinsically motivated when you enjoy meeting a new challenge on the job. More generally, **intrinsic motivation** involves engaging in an activity—work or play—for its own sake, regardless of an external reward or threat. You just do it because it meets a psychological need. In short, an intrinsically motivated activity is its own reward.

So, how could we assess a person's motivation for work? Psychologist David McClelland (1958) suspected that the stories people would tell to describe a series of ambiguous pictures could reveal their motives—using the *Thematic Apperception Test (TAT),* developed by Henry Murray (1938). You can see one such picture in Figure 7.1, but before you read the caption, imagine what might be happening with the boy and the violin. Initially, McClelland rated the stories for what they described as the **need for achievement (n Ach)**, defined as the desire to attain a difficult, but desired goal.

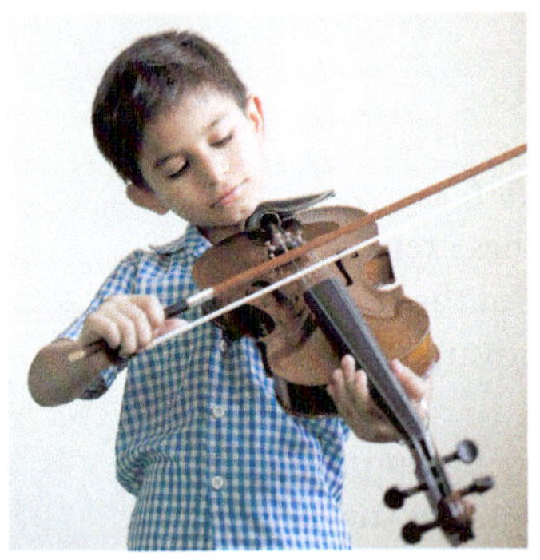

Figure 7.1 Alternative Interpretations of an ambiguous picture
(Source: PhotosIndia.com LLC/Alamy.)

Story Showing High *n Ach:* The boy has just finished his violin lesson. He's happy at his progress and is beginning to believe that all his sacrifices have been worthwhile. To become a concert violinist, he will have to give up much of his social life and practice for many hours each day. Although he knows he could make more money by going into his father's business, he is more interested in being a great violinist and giving people joy with his music. He renews his personal commitment to do all it takes to make it.

Story Showing Low *n Ach:* The boy is holding his brother's violin and wishing he could play it. But he knows it isn't worth the time, energy, and money for lessons. He feels sorry for his brother, who has given up all the fun things in life to practice, practice, practice. It would be great to wake up one day and be a top-notch musician, but it doesn't happen that way. The reality is boring practice, no fun, and the likelihood that he'll become just another guy playing a musical instrument in a small-town band.

Now read the caption for Figure 7.1 if you haven't already done so: It gives examples of how a high–*n Ach* individual and a low–*n Ach* individual might interpret the same picture. With these examples in mind, you can judge whether your own story is low or high in *n Ach.*

Indeed, McClelland found that certain characteristics distinguish people with a high need for achievement, as measured by the stories they told about ambiguous pictures. They not only work harder and become more successful at their work than those lower in achievement motivation, but they also show more persistence on difficult tasks (McClelland, 1987b; Schultz & Schultz, 2006). In school, those with high *n Ach* tend to get better grades (Raynor, 1970), perhaps because they also tend to have higher IQ scores (Harris, 2004). In their career paths, they take more competitive jobs (McClelland, 1965), assume more leadership roles, and earn more rapid promotions (Andrews, 1967). If they go into business, they are more successful than those with low *n Ach* (McClelland, 1987a, 1993).

I/O psychology: putting achievement motivation in perspective

Worker motivation is the domain of industrial/organisational (I/O) psychologists, who know that not everyone has a high need for achievement, nor does every job offer intrinsic challenges. At least two other motives propel us to work (McClelland, 1985). For some of us, work meets a *need for affiliation,* while for others work satisfies a *need for power.* (The need for power should not necessarily be construed as negative but rather in the more positive sense of wanting to plan projects and manage people to get a job done.) Given these three needs for work—achievement, affiliation, and power—it becomes the manager's task to structure jobs so that workers simultaneously meet their own needs as well as the manager's goal for productivity. (Managers, themselves, are usually motivated both by the needs for achievement and power.)

There are, of course, other reasons why we work beyond achievement, affiliation, and power needs. As we have said, work is a way to make a living. It is also a means to a desired lifestyle. But most of all, work is wrapped up in a person's identity: I am a teacher, a surgeon, a farmer, a park ranger, and so on. We focus on achievement, affiliation, and power here because those are the motives that have received the most attention so far by psychologists.

Need for achievement (n Ach) In McClelland's theory, a mental state that produces a psychological motive to excel or to reach some goal.

Should you find yourself in a management position, here are some need-specific pointers that come out of the research on motivating employees:

- Give those high in *n Ach* tasks that challenge them, but with achievable goals. Even though high–*n Ach* employees are not primarily motivated by extrinsic rewards, you can use bonuses, praise, and recognition effectively with them as feedback for good performance.
- A cooperative, rather than competitive, environment is best for those high in the need for *affiliation*. Find opportunities for such employees to work with others in teams rather than at socially isolated workstations.
- For those high in *power*, give them the opportunity to manage projects or work teams. You can encourage power-oriented workers to become leaders who help their subordinates satisfy their own needs. Again—although power motivation can be purely self-serving—don't fall into the trap of thinking that the need for power is necessarily bad.

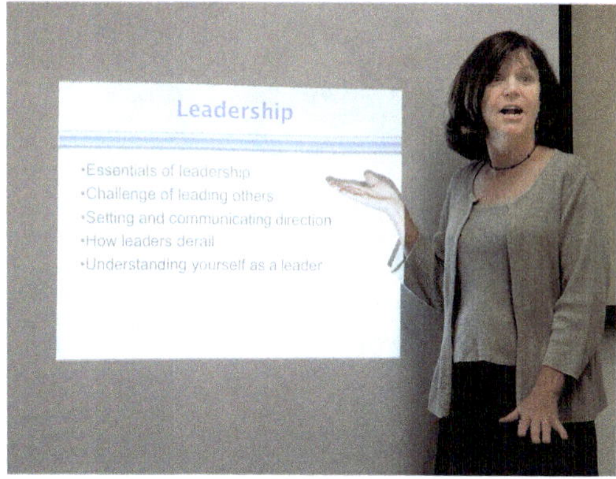

According to McClelland, people have different patterns of motivation for work. Some are motivated by affiliation, some by power, and some by the need for achievement (*n Ach*). A good leader knows how to capitalise on each of these.
(Source: David Young-Wolff/PhotoEdit, Inc.)

Satisfying people's needs should make them happier with their jobs and more motivated to work. I/O psychologists call this *job satisfaction*. But does job satisfaction actually lead to better employee performance? Studies show that higher job satisfaction indeed correlates with lower absenteeism, lower employee turnover, and increased productivity—all of which are reflected in increased profits for any business (Schultz & Schultz, 2006).

It is also worth noting that the need for achievement is not limited to work. It can also boost performance in art, science, literature—and in athletics. Let's explore two instructive cases in point.

A cross-cultural view of achievement

When she won the Olympic gold medal in the women's 200-meter butterfly, American swimmer Misty Hyman said:

> I think I just stayed focused. It was time to show the world what I could do. I am just glad I was able to do it. I knew I could beat Susie O'Neil, deep down in my heart I believed it, and I know this whole week the doubts kept creeping in, they were with me on the blocks, but I just said, "No, this is my night" (Neal, 2000).

Contrast that with Naoko Takahashi's explanation of why she won the women's marathon:

> Here is the best coach in the world, the best manager in the world, and all of the people who support me—all of these things were getting together and became a gold medal. So I think I didn't get it alone, not only by myself (Yamamoto, 2000).

Individualism The view, common in the Euro-American world, that places a high value on individual achievement and distinction.

As you can see from these distinctively different quotes, the American's perspective on achievement motivation reflects a distinctively Western bias. Americans tend to see achievement as the result of individual talent, determination, intelligence, or attitude. Much of the world, however, sees achievement differently—in a broader context, as a combination of personal, social, and emotional factors (Markus et al., 2006).

Collectivism The view, common in Asia, Africa, Latin America, and the Middle East, that values group loyalty and pride over individual distinction.

This observation fits with Harry Triandis's (1990) distinction between cultures that emphasise *individualism* or *collectivism*. Western cultures, including the United States, Canada, Britain, and Western Europe, emphasise **individualism**. People growing up in these cultures learn to place a premium on individual performance. By contrast, says Triandis, the cultures

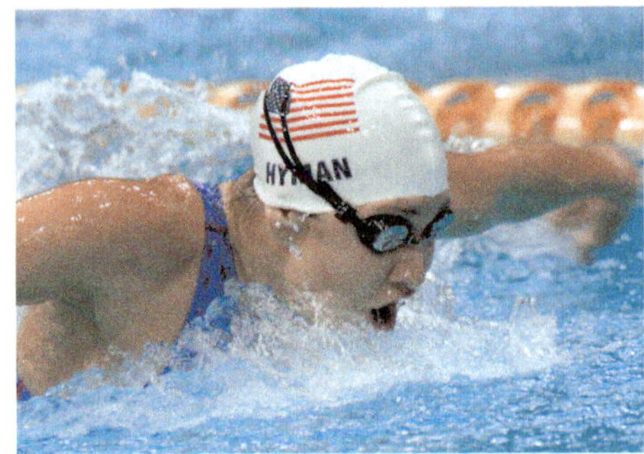

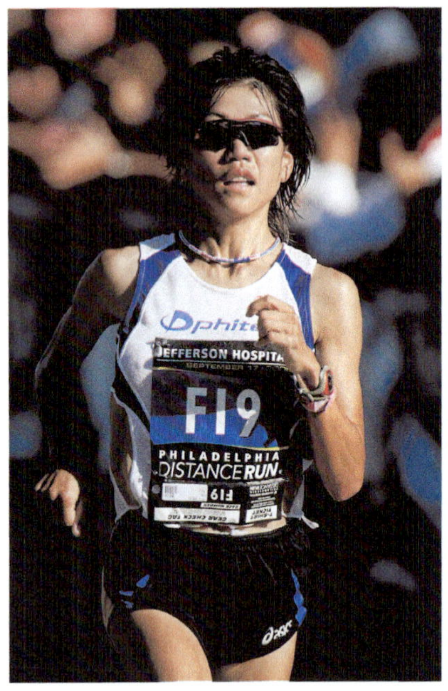

Misty Hyman (top) and Naoko Takahashi (bottom) have very different perspectives on their athletic achievements—perspectives that reflect their cultural differences. **(Source:** Top: Antonio Scorza/AFP/Newscom; bottom: Matt Rourke/AP Images.)

of Latin America, Asia, Africa, and the Middle East often emphasise **collectivism**, which values group loyalty and subordination of self to the group. Even in the collectivist cultures of Japan, Hong Kong, and South Korea, where high values are placed on doing well in school and business, the overarching goal is not achieving individual honors but bringing honor to the family, team, or other group.

Without a cross-cultural perspective, it would be easy for Americans to jump to the erroneous conclusion that motivation for individual achievement is a "natural" part of the human makeup. But Triandis's insight suggests that *n Ach* has a strong cultural component. In collectivist cultures, the social context is considered just as important for achievement as are talent, intelligence, or other personal characteristics in individualistic cultures.

The unexpected effects of rewards on motivation

We have suggested that extrinsic rewards are among the many reasons people work. But what do you suppose would happen if people were given extrinsic rewards (praise, money, or other incentives) for leisure activities—rewards for doing things that they find *intrinsically* enjoyable? Would the reward make the activity more—or less—enjoyable? Would a reward affect motivation?

Overjustification

To find out, Mark Lepper and his colleagues (1973) performed a classic experiment using two groups of schoolchildren who enjoyed drawing pictures. One group agreed to draw pictures for a reward certificate, while a control group made drawings without any expectation of reward. Both groups made their drawings enthusiastically. Some days later, however, when given the opportunity to draw pictures again, without a reward, the previously rewarded children were much less enthusiastic about drawing than those who had not been rewarded. In fact, the group that had received no rewards were actually *more* interested in drawing than they had been the first time!

Lepper's group concluded that external reinforcement had squelched the internal motivation in the reward group, an effect they called **overjustification**. As a result of overjustification, they reasoned, the children's motivation had changed from intrinsic to extrinsic. Consequently, the children were less interested in making pictures in the absence of reward. It appears that a reward can sometimes take the fun out of doing something for the sheer pleasure of it.

Overjustification The process by which extrinsic (external) rewards can sometimes displace internal motivation, as when a child receives money for playing video games.

When do rewards work?

But do rewards *always* have this overjustification effect? If they did, how could we explain the fact that many professionals both love their work and get paid for it? Subsequent experiments have made it clear that rewards can interfere with intrinsic motivation, but only under certain conditions (Covington, 2000; Eisenberger & Cameron, 1996).

Specifically, the overjustification effect occurs when a reward is given *without regard for quality of performance*. This explains what happened to the children who were given certificates for their drawings. The same thing can happen in the business world, when employees are given year-end bonuses regardless of the quality of their work or in the classroom when all students get As.

The lesson is this: Rewards can be used effectively to motivate people—but only if the rewards are given for a job well done, contingent on quality of performance, not as a bribe. In general, rewards can have three major effects on motivation, depending on the conditions:

- Rewards can be an effective way of motivating people *to do things they would not otherwise want to do*—such as mowing the lawn or taking out the garbage.
- Rewards can actually add to intrinsic motivation, *if given for good performance:* We saw this clearly in the case of Cathy Freeman.
- And, as we have also seen, rewards can *interfere* with intrinsic motivation, *if given without regard for the quality of the work*—as Lepper's study showed.

So, if a child doesn't like to practice the piano, wash the dishes, or do homework, no amount of reward is going to change her attitude. On the other hand, if she enjoys piano practice, you can feel free to give praise or a special treat for a job well done. Such rewards can make a motivated person even more motivated. Similarly, if you have disinterested employees, don't bother trying to motivate them with pay raises (unless, of course, the reason they're unmotivated is that you are paying them poorly). But when it is deserved, impromptu praise, an unexpected award, or some other small recognition may make good employees perform even better. The danger of rewards seems to occur only when the rewards are extrinsic and are given without regard to the level of performance.

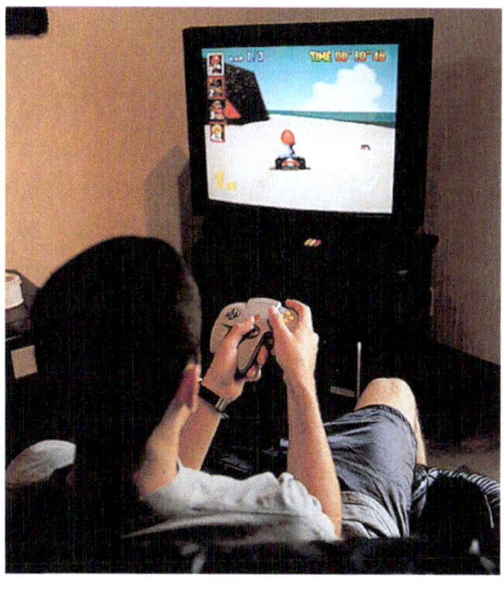

Overjustification occurs when extrinsic rewards for doing something enjoyable take the intrinsic fun out of the activity. It is likely that this person would not enjoy video games as much if he were paid for playing. (**Source:** David Young-Wolff/PhotoEdit, Inc.)

So, how do you think professors should reward students in order to encourage their best work?

Flow
In Csikszentmihalyi's theory, an intense focus on an activity accompanied by increased creativity and near-ecstatic feelings. Flow involves intrinsic motivation.

Using psychology to learn psychology

The world's greatest achievements in music, art, science, business, and countless other pursuits usually arise from intrinsically motivated people pursuing ideas or goals in which they are deeply interested. People achieve this state of mind when absorbed by some problem or activity that makes them lose track of time and become oblivious to events around them. Psychologist Mihaly Csikszentmihalyi (1990, 1998) calls this special state of mind **flow**. And although some people turn to drugs or alcohol to experience an artificial flow feeling, meaningful work produces far more satisfying and sustained flow experiences. Athletes, such as Cathy Freeman, could probably not endure their intense daily training regimens without entering the flow state.

What is the link with studying and learning? If you find yourself lacking in motivation to learn the material for a particular class, the extrinsic promise of eventual good grades may not be enough to prod you to study effectively tonight. You may, however, be able to trick yourself into developing intrinsic motivation and flow by posing this question: What do people who are specialists in this field find interesting? Among other things, the experts are fascinated by an unsolved mystery, a theoretical dispute, or the possibility of an exciting practical application. A psychologist, for example, might wonder: What motivates violent behaviour? Or, how can we increase people's motivation to achieve? Once you find such an issue, try to discover what solutions have been proposed. In this way, you will share the mindset of those who are leaders in the field. And—who knows?—perhaps you will become fascinated too.

How are our motivational priorities determined?

Until recently, psychology had no comprehensive explanation or theory that successfully accounted for the whole range of motivation. Hunger seemed so different from the need for achievement. Fears often have roots hidden from consciousness. Most biological drives feel unpleasant, but sexual arousal is pleasurable. The result was that some psychologists concentrated on the most basic survival motives, such as hunger and thirst, while other psychologists tried to explain sex, affiliation, creativity, and a variety of other motives. No one, however, managed to put together a motivational "theory of everything" that could encompass all our motives and, at the same time, be consistent with real-world observations.

But now, a new contender has emerged that, many psychologists say, may be able to do it all.

Core Concept

A new theory combining Maslow's hierarchy with evolutionary psychology solves some long-standing problems by suggesting that functional, proximal, and developmental factors set our motivational priorities.

About a half-century ago, Abraham Maslow proposed one of the most influential ideas ever to come out of psychology: that different motives have different priorities, based on a *hierarchy of needs*. For example, a threat to one's life usually trumps thirst. But thirst takes priority over the needs for affiliation or respect. But what about the artist who, in the *flow* state, disregards the need for food or warmth, sometimes for days at a time? And what about those "instincts" that drive animal migrations and, perhaps, some human behaviours, such as nursing in newborn infants? Let's see how a new hierarchy of needs incorporates these concepts.

Instinct theory

Instinct theory The now-outmoded view that certain behaviours are completely determined by innate factors. The instinct theory was flawed because it overlooked the effects of learning and because it employed instincts merely as labels rather than as explanations for behaviour.

Since the early days of William James, psychologists have realise that all creatures, humans included, possess an inborn set of behaviours that promotes survival. According to **instinct theory**, these built-in behaviours account reasonably well for the regular cycles of animal activity, found in essentially the same form across a species. We see these cycles in bird migrations, in the mating rituals of antelope, and in the return of salmon to the streams in which they were hatched only to spawn and die after a journey of more than 1,000 miles.

Although such so-called "instinctive" behaviour patterns do not depend heavily on learning, experience can modify them. Thus, we see a combination of instinctive behaviour and learning when bees communicate the location of food to each other or a mother cat helps her kittens hone their hunting skills. Such examples show that "instincts" involve both a lot of nature (genetically determined) and a little nurture (learning).

Because the term *instinct* seemed to explain so much, it migrated quickly from the scientific vocabulary to the speech of everyday life. Unfortunately, it lost precision in the process. So we now speak casually of "maternal instincts" or of an athlete who "instinctively catches the ball" or of an agent who has an "instinct" for picking new talent. In fact, we use the term in so many ways that its meaning has become almost meaningless—a mere label rather than an explanation for behaviour.

Fixed-action patterns Genetically based behaviours, seen across a species, that can be set off by a specific stimulus. The concept of *fixed-action patterns* has replaced the older notion of instinct.

As a result, the term *instinct* has long since dropped out of favor among scientists (Deckers, 2001). Ethologists, who study animal behaviour in natural habitats, now prefer the term **fixed-action patterns**, more narrowly defined as unlearned behaviour patterns that are triggered by identifiable stimuli and that occur throughout a species. Examples of fixed-action patterns include not only the "instinctive" behaviours described earlier but also such diverse behaviours as nest building in birds, suckling responses in newborn mammals, and dominance displays in baboons.

Do instincts—perhaps in their new guise as fixed-action patterns—explain any part of human behaviour? The question raises the nature–nurture controversy under a new name. Biology *does* seem to account for some human behaviours, such as nursing, that we see in newborns. But instincts or fixed-action patterns are not very useful in explaining the array of more complex behaviours found in people at work and play. For example, while we might speculate that the motivation of a hard-driving executive could involve some basic "killer" instinct, such an explanation is no better than attributing Cathy Freeman's success to a running instinct.

Drive theory

The concept of *drive* originated as an alternative to instinct for explaining behaviour with a strong biological basis, as in eating, drinking, and mating. Psychologists defined a **biological drive** as the state of energy or tension that moves an organism to meet a biological need (Woodworth, 1918). Thus, thirst drives an animal in need of water to drink. Likewise, a need for food arouses a hunger that drives organisms to eat. So, in **drive theory**, a biological **need** produces a drive state that, in turn, channels behaviour toward meeting the need. When the need is satisfied, drive level subsides—a process called *drive reduction*. You have experienced drive reduction when you feel satisfied after a big meal or when you get in a warm bath after being chilled.

Biological drive A motive, such as thirst, that is based primarily in biology. A *drive* is a state of tension that motivates an organism to satisfy a biological *need*.

Drive theory Developed as an alternative to instinct theory, drive theory explains motivation as a process in which a biological *need* produces a *drive* that moves an organism to meet the need. For most drives this process returns the organism to a balanced condition, known as *homeostasis*.

Need In drive theory, a need is a biological imbalance (such as dehydration) that threatens survival if the need is left unmet. Biological needs are believed to produce drives.

Homeostasis The body's tendency to maintain a biologically balanced condition, especially with regard to nutrients, water, and temperature.

According to drive theory, what organisms seek is a balanced condition in the body, known as **homeostasis** (Hull, 1943, 1952). So, creatures that have an *un*balanced condition (caused, say, by lack of fluids) are driven to seek a homeostatic balance (by drinking). Similarly, we can understand hunger as an imbalance in the body's energy supply. It is this imbalance that drives, or motivates, a food-deprived animal to eat in order to restore a condition of equilibrium.

Unfortunately for drive theory, the story of motivation has proved not to be that simple. In particular, drive theory faltered when cognitive, social, and cultural forces were at work, as we will see later in our discussion of hunger. Moreover, drive theory cannot explain why, in the absence of any apparent deprivation or obvious needs, organisms sometimes act merely to *increase* stimulation. It is hard to imagine, for example, a basic need or a biological drive that could prompt people to go skiing or jump out of airplanes. Even at an animal level, laboratory rats that are hungry or thirsty and given opportunity to eat or drink in a new maze environment do not initially eat or drink. Rather, they explore the novel setting first: Curiosity trumps hunger and thirst (Zimbardo & Montgomery, 1957).

Cognitive psychologists also pointed out that biological drives could not explain behaviour motivated by goals, such as getting a promotion at work or an A in psychology. Nor will drives explain why laboratory rats will cross an electrified grid merely to reach a novel environment to explore or why Cathy Freeman endured thousands of hours of grueling training to win glory. Psychologists call these *psychological motives.* In contrast to *biological drives,* psychological motives serve no immediate biological need but, rather, are strongly rooted in learning, incentives, threats, or social and cultural pressures. The human need for achievement is another good example of a psychological motive. Obviously, many motivated behaviours, especially in humans, can stem from a combination of biological and cognitive or environmental factors. We will see the practical side of the biological versus psychological distinction later when we dissect hunger, the quintessential example of a combined biological drive and psychological motive.

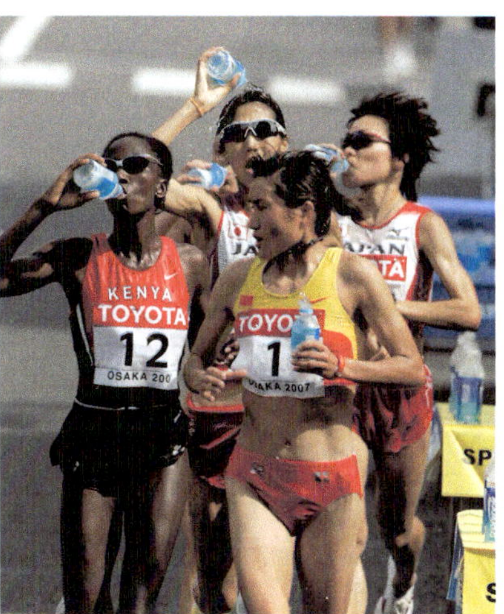

According to drive theory, a need for fluids motivates (drives) us to drink. A homeostatic balance is reached when the need is satisfied. **(Source:** Bobby Yip/Reuters/Landov.)

For these reasons, psychologists have concluded that drive theory holds some—but not all—answers to the riddle of motivation. Still, they have been reluctant to abandon the concept of *drive*, which has come to mean a biologically based motive that plays an important role in survival or reproduction. We now look on drive theory as a useful but incomplete theory of motivation.

Freud's psychodynamic theory

Sigmund Freud challenged the view that we know what motivates our own behaviour. Instead, Freud proposed, most human motivation stems from the murky depths of the unconscious mind, which he called the *id*. There, he said, lurked two basic desires: *eros,* the erotic desire; and *thanatos,* the aggressive or destructive impulse. Virtually everything we do, said Freud, is based on one of these urges or on the maneuvers that the mind uses to keep these desires in check. To avoid mental problems, we must continually seek acceptable outlets for our sexual and aggressive needs. Freud believed that work, especially creative work, indirectly satisfied the sex drive, while aggressive acts like swearing and shouting or playing aggressive games serve as a psychologically safe outlet for our deeper destructive tendencies.

It is important to realise that Freud developed his ideas in the heyday of instinct theory, so eros and thanatos are often thought of as instincts. But it would oversimplify Freud's theory to think of it as just another instinct theory. He wasn't trying to explain the everyday, biologically based behaviours that we find in eating, drinking, mating, nursing, and sleeping. Rather, he was trying to explain the symptoms we find in mental disorders such as phobias or depression.

The new evolutionary theory of motivation borrows Freud's notion that two main motives underlie all we do. Evolutionary psychologists agree that just two fundamental motives underlie everything we do. But in place of sex and aggression, the new theory posits the Darwinian needs for survival and reproduction.

Modern-day psychologists also agree that Freud had put his finger on another important idea: Much mental activity, including motivation, *does* occur outside of consciousness. However, contemporary psychologists stand divided on the details of the Freudian unconscious, (Bornstein, 2001; Westen, 1998).

One more of Freud's ideas was also on target, according to the evolutionary theorists. Among the principal theories of motivation discussed in this chapter, Freud's is the only one that takes a *developmental* approach to motivation. That is, Freud taught that our motives undergo change as we move from childhood to adulthood. With maturity, he said, our sexual and aggressive desires become less conscious. We also develop more and more subtle and sophisticated ways of meeting our needs—particularly desires for sex and aggression—without getting into trouble (see Table 7.1).

Table 7.1 Theories of motivation compared

Theories	Emphasis	Examples
Instinct Theory	Biological processes that motivate behaviour patterns specific to a species	bird migration, fish schooling
Drive Theory	Needs produce drives that motivate behaviour until drives are reduced	hunger, thirst
Freud's Theory	Motivation arises from unconscious desires; developmental changes in these urges appear as we mature	sex, aggression
Maslow's Theory	Motives result from needs, which occur in a priority order (a needs hierarchy)	esteem needs, self-actualisation
Evolutionary Theory	Priority of motives determined by functional, proximal, and developmental factors	Food odor (proximal stimulus) may raise the priority of hunger drive

Maslow's hierarchy of needs

What happens when you must choose between meeting a biological need and fulfilling a desire based on learning—as when you choose between sleeping and staying up all night to study for an exam? Abraham Maslow (1970) said that you usually act on your most pressing needs, which occur in a natural *hierarchy* or priority order, with biological needs taking precedence. Unlike the other theories of motivation we have considered, Maslow's perspective attempts to span the whole gamut of human motivation from biological drives to social motives to creativity (Nicholson, 2007).

Maslow's most memorable innovation, then, was his **hierarchy of needs**, which posited six classes of needs listed in priority order (see Figure 7.2). The "higher" needs exert their influence on behaviour only when the more basic needs are satisfied:

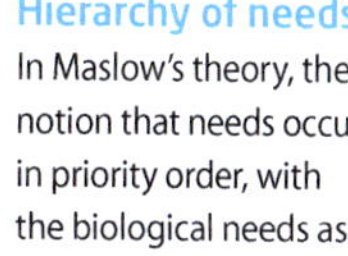

Hierarchy of needs In Maslow's theory, the notion that needs occur in priority order, with the biological needs as the most basic.

- *Biological needs,* such as hunger and thirst, lie at the base of the hierarchy and must be satisfied before higher needs take over.
- *Safety needs* motivate us to avoid danger, but only when biological needs are reasonably well satisfied. Thus, a hungry animal may risk its physical safety for food until it gets its belly full, at which point the safety needs take over.
- *Love, attachment, and affiliation needs* energise us when we are no longer concerned about the more basic drives such as hunger, thirst, and safety. These "higher" needs make us want to affiliate with others, to love, and to be loved.
- *Esteem needs,* following next in the hierarchy, include the needs to like oneself, to see oneself as competent and effective, and to do what is necessary to earn the respect of oneself and others.
- *Self-actualisation,* the "highest" need, but with the lowest priority, motivates us to seek the fullest development of our creative human potential. Self-actualising persons are self-aware, self-accepting, socially responsive, spontaneous, and open to novelty and challenge.

In his original formulation, Maslow put self-actualisation at the peak of the needs hierarchy. But late in his life, Maslow suggested yet another highest order need, which he called *self-transcendence.* This he conceptualised as going beyond self-actualisation, seeking to further some cause beyond the self (Koltko-Rivera, 2006). Satisfying this need could involve anything from volunteer work to absorption in religion, politics, music, or an intellectual pursuit. What distinguishes self-transcendence from self-actualisation is its shift beyond personal pleasure or other egocentric benefits.

But how does Maslow's theory square with observation? It explains why we may neglect our friends or our career goals in favor of meeting pressing biological needs signaled by pain, thirst, sleepiness, or sexual desire. Yet—in contradiction to Maslow's theory—people may sometimes neglect their basic biological needs in favor of higher ones, as we might see in a father risking his life to rescue his child from a burning building. To Maslow's credit, he recognised these problems. Just as important, he called attention to the role of social motivation in our lives at a time when these motives were being neglected by psychology (Nicholson, 2007). As a result, a great body of work now demonstrates this need we have for relationships with others.

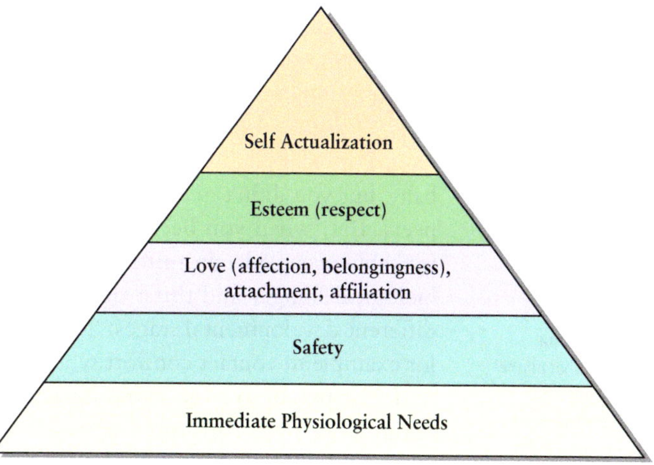

Figure 7.2 Maslow's Hierarchy of Needs

Critics point out that Maslow's theory also fails to explain other important human behaviours: why you might miss a meal when you are absorbed in an interesting book or why sensation seekers would pursue risky interests (such as rock climbing or auto racing) that override their safety needs. The theory also fails to explain the behaviour of people who deliberately take their own lives. And it ignores the powerful sex drive.

Cross-cultural psychologists have also criticised Maslow's theory and other "self theories," noting that an emphasis on self-actualisation applies primarily to individualistic cultures, which emphasise individual achievement (Gambrel & Cianci, 2003). In contrast, group-oriented (collectivistic) cultures emphasise success of the group rather than *self*-actualisation (Shiraev & Levy, 2006). In fairness to Maslow, however, we should note that he recognised that there could be cultural differences in motivation (1943). And even the severest critics will acknowledge that, with all its flaws, Maslow's theory was an important step toward a comprehensive theory of motivation.

Putting it all together: a new hierarchy of needs

In the face of such criticism, can we find something in Maslow's theory worth saving? Douglas Kenrick and his colleagues (2010) point to the idea of a *motivational hierarchy* as Maslow's singular great insight. But, they note, its major difficulty is that our motivational priorities are not rigidly fixed—as Maslow himself realised. Indeed, an individual may change motivational priorities from time to time. Nor do different people necessarily have the same motivational priorities. The solution, said Kenrick's group, is to understand that we must view the needs hierarchy as fluid—subject to change by three sorts of influences, seen as what they call the *functional, proximal,* and *developmental levels of analysis.*

The **functional level of analysis** looks at the *function* of a motive, which (from an evolutionary perspective) relates to survival and reproductive success. Functional influences arrange our motives in a kind of "default" hierarchy, grounded in the basic needs, such as hunger and thirst. These needs motivate us to seek such things as food drink, warmth, and shelter, without which we could not live. Similarly, sexual motivation arises from the evolutionary mandate to propel one's genes into future generations. This need for sexual gratification and reproduction, then, gives rise to a whole range of social needs, including not only the physical urge for sex but also needs for affiliation, esteem, and parenting. These "higher" reproductive needs, however, generally have lower priority than the survival needs.

Functional level of analysis Concerns the adaptive function of a motive in terms of the organism's survival and reproduction.

Proximal level of analysis Concerns stimuli in the organism's immediate environment, which can change motivational priorities. (In humans, *proximal* could also refer to things that the individual is thinking about.)

Developmental level of analysis Concerns changes in the organism's developmental progress that might change motivational priorities, as when hormones heighten sexual interest in adolescence.

Proximal means "nearby"—so the **proximal level of analysis** focuses on immediate events, objects, incentives, and threats that influence motivation. For example, the aroma of freshly baked bread is a proximal stimulus that can suddenly arouse the hunger motive. Or imagine that you are at a theater enjoying a movie when someone yells, "Fire!" Your motivation suddenly shifts from relaxation and enjoyment of the movie to fear and self-preservation. In more formal terms, an important *proximal* stimulus can trigger a temporary modification in your usual motivational hierarchy.

Your stage of life can also affect your motivational profile. Thus, the **developmental level of analysis** shows how the order in which motives appear changes throughout your life span. For example, hunger, thirst, and contact comfort held centre stage when you were a baby, but you didn't give a whit about reproduction or about garnering the esteem of your peers. But, when you became a teenager, sexual motives and the need for social approval probably occupied a prominent place in your needs hierarchy, sometimes trumping even the biological hunger and thirst drives. Likewise, proximal cues may affect you differently at different developmental stages. So, you may be most sensitive to different proximal cues—for example to contact comfort when you are young or to a comely peer in your teens.

Less obvious are the evolutionary foundations for artistic creativity, athletic pursuits, stamp collecting, or any of a thousand other human pursuits. And this is where the new theory proposed by Kenrick and his group becomes controversial: They push self-actualisation off the pinnacle of Maslow's hierarchy and replace it with needs for mating and parenting (which

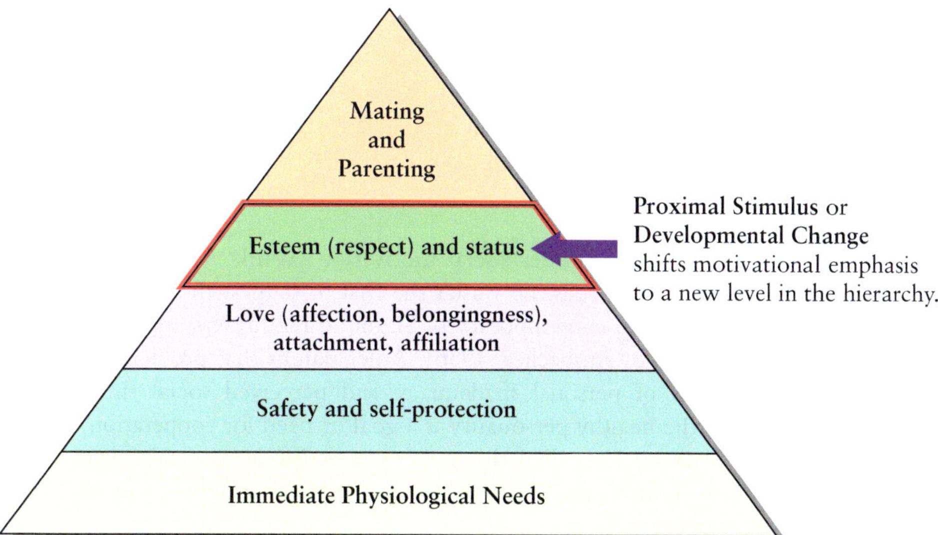

Figure 7.3 Evolutionary Psychology's Revision of Maslow's Hierarchy

Maslow had neglected). All the productivity and creativity that Maslow thought of as self-actualisation is really just a means to the real ends of reproduction and assuring the survival of one's genetic offspring. As you might expect, critics have raised objections (Ackerman & Bargh, 2010; Kesebir et al., 2010; Lyubomirsky & Boehm, 2010; Peterson & Park, 2010).

What Kenrick's group may have overlooked is the possibility that "higher" motives—including a need to be creative or to satisfy one's curiosity—may have become functionally independent of their evolutionary roots. Certainly, creative persons—famous entertainers, for example—have an advantage in the mating game. Nevertheless, evolution may also have taken a shortcut by wiring our creative urges directly to our pleasure centres. If that is true—and it remains to be explored by researchers—people may pursue their interests just for the pure joy of doing so (Peterson & Park, 2010). This *intrinsic motivation* may have become functionally independent of its original biological aims.

Where does all this leave us? A consensus seems to be emerging on a few ideas that may bring some unity to the field of motivation at long last (Schaller et al., 2010). Most psychologists would likely agree that:

- Our motives have a "default" hierarchy or priority order that is essentially the same from person to person—much as Maslow described.
- This default hierarchy of motives must be understood in a functional or evolutionary context, with the most basic motives being related to survival, followed by motives related to reproduction and to survival of offspring.
- An individual's motivational hierarchy is not rigid but can be influenced by proximal stimuli and by the person's developmental level.

As we have noted, there remains some disagreement as to whether the "higher" motives (such as creativity) are always based on the reproductive urge or can instead become independent *intrinsic* motives.

What this new hybrid approach to motivation does for us, then, is to bring together Maslow's hierarchy and evolutionary psychology to make a big tent that can encompass motivation of all sorts—from hunger and thirst to affiliation, status, and creativity. All must be ultimately understood in terms of a hierarchy and in terms of their evolutionary roots. We still don't know precisely how the brain manages to arrange and rearrange the motivational hierarchy, but at last we may have a framework within which the theoretical details can be worked out.

Determining what motivates others

Where do you start when you want to know what motivates a person's behaviour—perhaps someone who has been self-destructive or hurtful to you? We suggest caution before deciding that the source is some immutable personality trait. Instead, we recommend first looking for any external incentives or threats—extrinsic motivators—that might be at work. Many times, these will tell the whole story.

Beyond that, we suggest you consider social motivation. While Maslow emphasised social motives in his hierarchy of needs, he wasn't the first to suggest their importance in human behaviour. Alfred Adler, a contemporary of Sigmund Freud, was arguably the first social psychologist (Ansbacher & Ansbacher, 1956). Adler taught that problem behaviour often grows out of feelings of personal inadequacy and perceived social threats. The counterbalancing trend in the healthy personality is a goal or need for cooperation and the desire for acceptance by others. He called this *social interest*. Modern social psychologists combine the notions of social motivation with extrinsic incentives and threats in what they call the "power of the situation."

Applying these notions to Cathy Freeman, it is not a stretch to suspect that her motivation involves a highly competitive desire to win. But whether that is a "neurotic" goal growing out of deep feelings of inferiority, we do not have enough information to know. Should she ever seek psychological help, the therapist would certainly raise that question—to which Cathy Freeman may or may not know the answer.

Adler's ideas are much more complex than we can detail here. Suffice it to say that a person who feels threatened may respond defensively, with annoying behaviour or aggression. If you are that person's parent, teacher, employer, or friend, the trick is not to respond in kind. Don't give attention to an attention getter. Don't respond aggressively to an aggressor. Don't try to "get even" with a vengeful person. And don't smother a withdrawn individual with pity. Instead, treat the person with respect—and an understanding of the social motives behind the unwanted behaviour.

Where do hunger and sex fit into the motivational hierarchy?

Core Concept

Although dissimilar in many respects, hunger and sex both have evolutionary origins, and each has an essential place in the motivational hierarchy.

In this section of the chapter, we focus on hunger and sex, two quite different motives that represent the twin forces that evolution has used to shape the human species: the drives to *survive* and *reproduce*. Everyone reading this book inherited the genes of ancestors who managed to do both. Here's the big idea around which this section is organised.

Ultimately, our task is to show how an evolutionary new perspective on motivation manages to bring both of these motives together under one theoretical umbrella.

Hunger: a homeostatic drive and a psychological motive

You will probably survive if you don't have sex, but you will die if you don't eat. Unlike sex, hunger is one of our personal biological survival mechanisms (Rozin, 1996). When food is available, the hunger drive leads quite naturally to eating. Yet there is more to hunger than biology: It has social and cognitive foundations, too, as we will see in the *multiple-systems approach* to hunger and weight control (see Figure 7.4).

The multiple-systems approach to hunger

Your brain generates hunger by combining biological and psychological information of many kinds, including your body's energy requirements and nutritional state, your food

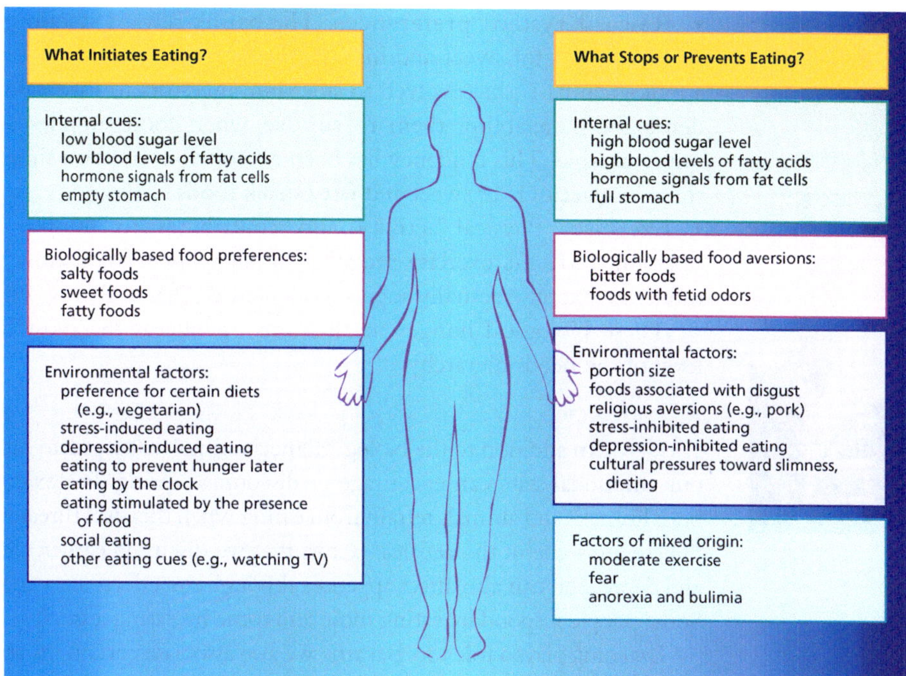

Figure 7.4 Multiple-Systems Model of Hunger and Eating

Hunger isn't just a matter of an empty stomach. The multiple-systems model combines all the known influences on hunger and eating.

preferences, food cues in your environment, and cultural demands. For example, your readiness to eat a slice of bacon depends on factors such as your blood sugar level, how long it has been since you last ate, whether you like bacon, what time of day it is (breakfast?), whether a friend might be offering you a slice, and whether bacon is an acceptable food in your culture. Assembling all this data, the brain sends signals to neural, hormonal, organ, and muscle systems to start or stop bacon seeking and eating (DeAngelis, 2004b; Flier & Maratos-Flier, 2007). As you may have surmised, the multiple-systems approach is another way of saying that hunger operates at many levels of the motivational hierarchy, meeting many needs that do not necessarily stem from the biological hunger drive.

BIOLOGICAL FACTORS AFFECTING HUNGER AND EATING. In the brain, the stomach, the blood, and fat cells stored all over the body, a host of biological factors work to regulate hunger and eating behaviour. Among the most important are these:

- **Brain mechanisms controlling hunger.** The hypothalamus is literally a "nerve centre" for hunger, with one region activating feelings of hunger and another dampening hunger. But the hypothalamus does not operate alone. Other regions, particularly in the brain stem, work with the hypothalamus to monitor the status of blood sugar, nutrients in the gut, and fat stores, using a suite of receptors and chemical messengers (Flier, 2006).
- **Set point (homeostatic) mechanisms.** An internal biological "scale" continually assesses the body's fat stores and informs the central nervous system of the result. Whenever deposits stored in specialised fat cells fall below a certain level, or **set point**, signals trigger eating behaviour—a homeostatic process. Research suggests that obesity may result when this homeostatic balance gets off kilter. Studies implicate certain chemicals (such as the hormone *ghrelin*) that signal hunger, along with others (such as *leptin*) that signal when the set point has been reached. Animals lacking leptin, for example, continue to eat even when not hungry (Grimm, 2007).

Set point Refers to the tendency of the body to maintain a certain level of body fat and body weight.

- **Sensors in the stomach.** Pressure detectors in the stomach signal fullness or a feeling of emptiness. These messages are sent to the brain, where they combine with information about blood nutrients and the status of the body's fat cells.

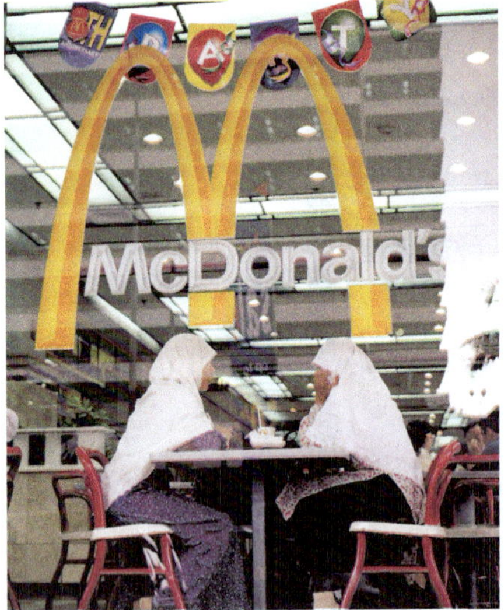

In the global economy, calorie-dense fast foods have become readily available, changing dietary habits and contributing to a worldwide epidemic of obesity. (**Source:** Eightfish/Getty Images.)

- **Reward system preferences.** The brain's reward system gives us preferences for sweet and high-fat foods. These preferences have a biological basis that evolved to steer our ancestors toward calorie-dense foods, enabling them to survive when food supplies were unpredictable. This tendency has been exploited in modern times by the manufacturers of sweet and fatty snack foods.
- **Exercise.** Physical activity also contributes to hunger and satiation. Extreme exercise provokes hunger, but studies show that moderate exercise actually suppresses appetite (Hill & Peters, 1998).

These biological hunger mechanisms operate at the most basic level of the needs hierarchy.

PSYCHOLOGICAL FACTORS AFFECTING HUNGER AND EATING. In addition to the biological mechanisms that regulate eating, our emotional state can encourage or discourage eating. For example, both humans and animals refrain from eating when they feel threatened. (These are some of the *proximal* factors that we discussed earlier.) Stress and depression can also affect appetite, although the effects are variable: Some people respond by eating more and some by eating less.

Learning plays a role too. Because we also associate certain situations with food, we may feel hungry regardless of our biological needs. This explains why you suddenly want to eat when you notice that the clock says lunchtime. It also explains why you snack while watching TV or dish up a second helping at Thanksgiving dinner.

Culture can have a huge effect too. This can be seen in societies, such as the United States, where media influences and social norms promote a thin body type. On the other hand, in Oceania, where larger figures are often considered more attractive, social norms promote heftier bodies (Newman, 2004).

While the ideal promoted in movies, magazines, and on TV is one of thinness, Americans receive a different message from commercials that encourage eating. That message, combined with an abundance of cheap, tasty junk food results in a growing obesity problem in a population obsessed with weight. Moreover, as the influence of U.S. culture becomes more global, American eating habits have become more universal, with the result that calorie-dense snacks and fast foods are making people fatter all over the world (Hébert, 2005; Popkin, 2007).

Eating disorders

Anorexia nervosa
An eating disorder involving persistent loss of appetite that endangers an individual's health and stemming from emotional or psychological reasons rather than from organic causes.

Bulimia nervosa
An eating disorder characterised by eating binges followed by "purges," induced by vomiting or laxatives; typically initiated as a weight-control measure.

Only rarely does the condition called *anorexia* (persistent lack of appetite) result from a physical disorder, such as shock, nausea, or an allergic reaction. More commonly, the cause has psychological roots—in which case the syndrome is called **anorexia nervosa**. "Nervous anorexia" typically manifests itself in extreme dieting. It can be so extreme, in fact, that the disorder posts the highest mortality rate of any recognised psychological condition (Agras et al., 2004; Park, 2007). In the following discussion, we will revert to common usage by calling the disorder simply *anorexia*.

What qualifies as anorexia? When a person weighs less than 85 percent of her desirable weight and still worries about being fat, anorexia is the likely diagnosis. People with anorexia may also face a problem called *bulimia* or **bulimia nervosa**, characterise by periods of binge eating followed by drastic purging measures, which may include vomiting, fasting, or using laxatives. In many cases, depression and obsessive-compulsive disorder further complicate the clinical picture.

Commonly, a person with anorexia acts as though she is unaware of her condition and continues dieting, ignoring other danger signs that may include cessation of menstruation, osteoporosis, bone fractures, and shrinkage of brain tissue. Over time, bulimic vomiting, done to purge the food she has eaten, results in damage to her esophagus, throat, and teeth caused by stomach acid.

What causes anorexia? A strong hint comes from the finding that most persons with the disorder are young females. Significantly, such eating disorders are most prevalent in Western cultures, particularly among middle- and upper-middle-class young women (Striegel-Moore & Bulik, 2007). Clearly, it is not a hunger disorder caused by lack of resources.

Those with anorexia commonly have histories of good behaviour, as well as academic and social success, but they nevertheless starve themselves, hoping to become more acceptably thin and attractive (Keel & Klump, 2003). In an effort to lose imagined "excess" weight, the person with anorexia rigidly suppresses her appetite, feeling rewarded for such self-control when she does lose pounds and inches—but never feeling quite thin enough (see Figure 7.5).

Work focusing on genetic factors has complicated the assumption that social pressures cause anorexia and bulimia (Novotney, 2009; Striegel-Moore & Bulik, 2007). This makes sense from an evolutionary standpoint, says clinical psychologist Shan Guisinger (2003). She points out the hyperactivity often seen in individuals with anorexia—as opposed to the lethargy common in most starving persons—suggesting that hyperactivity under conditions of starvation may have been an advantage that motivated the ancestors of modern-day individuals with anorexia to leave famine-impoverished environments.

All in all, it is beginning to appear that anorexia—like hunger itself—is a condition caused by multiple factors that stem from biology, cognition, and social pressures.

Obesity and weight control

At the other extreme of weight control, the problem of obesity has grown at an alarming rate since the early 1980s, with the result that 65 percent of Americans are overweight and 30 percent are now classified as obese (DeAngelis, 2004b; Mann et al., 2007). Comparatively, the most recent Australian data indicates that in 2014–15, 35.5% of adults were considered

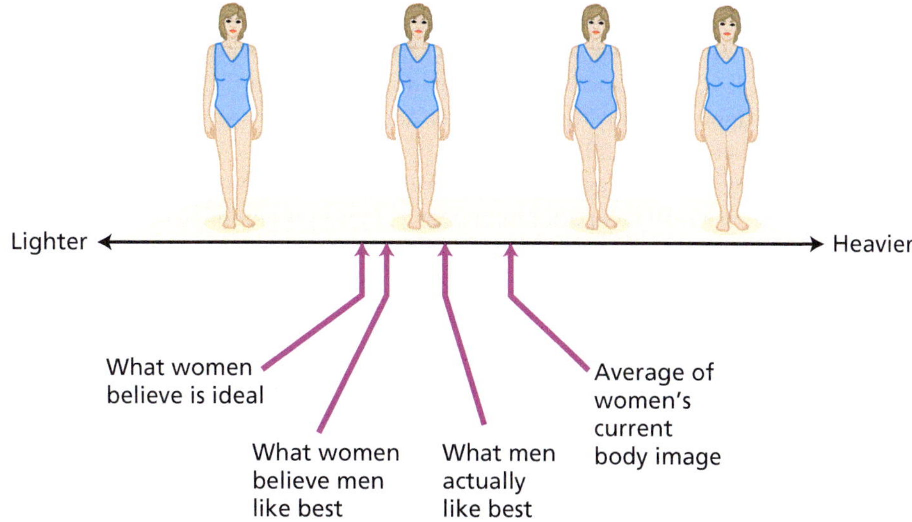

Figure 7.5 Women's Body Images

April Fallon and Paul Rozin (1985) asked female university students to give their current weight, their ideal weight, and the weight they believed men would consider ideal. The results show that the average woman felt that her current weight was significantly higher than her ideal weight—and higher than the weight she thought men would like. To make matters worse, women also see their bodies as looking larger than they actually are (Thompson, 1986). When men were asked to rate themselves on a similar questionnaire, Fallon and Rozin found no such discrepancies between ideal and actual weights. But, when asked what they saw as the ideal weight for women, they chose a higher weight than women did. No wonder women go on diets more often than men and are more likely to have a major eating disorder (Mintz & Betz, 1986; Striegel-Moore et al., 1993).

overweight while 27.9% of adults were considered obese (Australian Bureau of Statistics, 2015). This equates to over 11.2 million Australians falling within the overweight or obese category, with more men (70.8%), considered overweight or obese, than women (56.3%) (Australian Bureau of Statistics, 2015). The real problem, of course, is not obesity but the associated health risks for such problems as heart disease, stroke, and diabetes—although experts disagree on just how much of a problem this is among those who are only slightly overweight (Couzin, 2005; Gibbs, 2005). Unfortunately, the fundamental causes of this obesity epidemic are not well understood (Doyle, 2006).

No one in the field of obesity research believes that the condition results from the lack of "will power"—a simplistic and scientifically useless concept, as we will see in the next section (Friedman, 2003). Rather, most experts believe that obesity results from multiple factors. Prominent among them are poor diet, including super-size portions and an increasing prevalence of food high in fat and sugar. In one laboratory experiment, rats given a diet of sausage, Ho Hos, pound cake, bacon, and cheesecake lost the ability to control their eating and quickly became obese (Johnson & Kenny, 2010).

Genetics also have a role (Bell, 2010; DeAngelis, 2004a; Flier & Maratos-Flier, 2007), but so does activity level. For example, the long-term Nurses' Health Study showed that every two-hour increase in daily TV watching translated into a 23-percent increase in obesity among the nurses in the sample (Hu et al., 2003). Finally, one study suggests not getting enough sleep may trigger eating and a resulting weight gain, perhaps because the body mistakes sleepiness for hunger (Hasler et al., 2004).

From an evolutionary viewpoint, humans are still Stone Age creatures biologically adapted to deal with periods of feast and famine. So we tend to eat more than we need when food is abundant as a hedge against future periods of starvation. Unfortunately, this Stone-Age strategy is not well suited to life in a modern world—where most people in developed countries also have no need to expend energy running down game or digging roots. Nor are we well suited for a world of French fries, deep-dish pizzas, donuts, Snickers, and nachos, which appeal to our deeply ingrained tastes for salty, fatty, and sweet foods—which just happen to be rich in calories (Parker-Pope, 2009; Pinel et al., 2000).

The problem is also not lack of awareness. Americans, especially, seem obsessed by weight and weight loss, as a glance at the magazine headlines on the newsstand will show. At any given time, approximately three out of ten adult Americans say they are on some sort of weight-control diet (Gallup, 2010).

Yet, despite all we know about hunger and weight control, no one has yet discovered a weight-loss scheme that really works for most people. Notwithstanding nationally advertised claims, no diet, surgical procedure, drug, or other weight-loss gimmick has ever produced long-term weight loss for a majority of the people who have tried it. At this point, the best odds for most people lie in cognitive-behavioural therapies (Institute of Medicine, 2002; Rich, 2004). And for those struggling with weight, it is encouraging to know that some potentially effective weight-control chemicals are being tested as you read this, although it may be several years before anything both safe and effective comes to market (Flier & Maratos-Flier, 2007). In the meantime, experts suggest that the best pathway to long-term weight control involves maintaining a well-balanced diet, a program of moderate exercise and, if you want some extra help, cognitive-behavioural therapy.

The problem of will power and chocolate cookies

Psychologists don't talk much about "will power," although the term can be heard in everyday conversation, where it usually refers to resisting food, drink, or some other temptation. In particular, psychologists don't like the archaic assumption of the "will" as a special faculty of the mind—a throwback to 19th-century phrenology. Thus, "will power" is like the term "instinct"—merely a label rather than an explanation. Psychologists also object to the term "will power" because it is often used as a moral judgement, suggesting that a person has a deficiency in character—a "weak will."

Alternatives to will power

Modern psychologists usually prefer terms such as *self-control* or *impulse control*—terms that carry less baggage and can be related to environmental influences and to known brain mechanisms. For example, we know that controlling one's eating is more difficult during the holiday season, with its abundance of food. Similarly, damage to parts of the limbic system is known to make control of eating more difficult.

Psychologists have also contrived devilish tests to measure impulse control. What have they found? To nobody's surprise, the ability to control one's impulses correlates with all sorts of positive outcomes, including better mental health, more effective coping skills, better relationships, and higher academic achievement. But such findings still leave the big question unanswered: What *is* self-control—or "will power"?

The biology of self-control

A team of researchers at Florida State University seems to have placed the ability to resist temptation on a solid scientific footing (Gailliot et al., 2007). What they found is that self-control has a biological basis. And it also has a price.

The Florida group first placed undergraduate psychology students in one of several onerous situations in which they were asked to exercise self-control—such as resisting a tempting plate of warm, freshly baked chocolate cookies or watching a funny video clip without laughing. Then the researchers gave the students a second task, such as a scrambled-word problem or a hand–eye coordination test. A control group also performed the second task, but they were not first asked to stifle their laughter, nor were they exposed to plates of tempting cookies.

Before we go any further, see if you can predict who did better on the second task. Was it those in the experimental group, who had to resist their impulses? Or was it the control group, who had been allowed to indulge themselves?

You were right if you guessed that those who had to face down temptation (resisting the cookies or soberly watching the funny video) were *less* successful on the second task. Apparently self-control is a cognitive resource that, like physical stamina, can become temporarily depleted. And, surprisingly, self-control seems to have a physical presence in the blood, as well as in behaviour. The study found that those who had been asked to control their urges had lower blood-sugar levels than those who had not restrained themselves. Because sugar (glucose) is an energy source for the body, the researchers speculate that exerting will power used up some of that energy, making people less efficient on the second task (Baumeister et al., 1998, 2007; Wargo, 2009).

But there is hope for those weak of will! A sugared drink not only brought blood glucose back up to its original level, but it brought the performance of the self-controllers back to the level of the indulgers. Apparently, what we call "will power" is based, at least in part, on the body's ready energy reserves.

So, should you have a cola and a candy bar to boost your "will" before the next psychology test? Probably not such a good idea, says Matthew Gaillot, leader of the Florida study—especially if you are trying to control your weight. Better, he says, to keep your energy level up with a diet that includes longer-lasting proteins or complex carbohydrates (Cynkar, 2007).

And some additional advice from a cognitive perspective: If you want to insure that you are mentally sharp, moderation is a better strategy than denial.

Sexual motivation: an urge you can live without

No one enjoys being hungry or thirsty. But we can't say the same for sex: Unlike hunger or thirst, *arousal* of the sex drive can be pleasurable. And even though sexually aroused individuals may seek to reduce the tension by mating or other sexual activity, the sex drive is not homeostatic—again unlike hunger and thirst. That is, having sex does not return the body to an equilibrium condition. Moreover, sexual motivation can serve diverse goals, including pleasure, reproduction, and social bonding. In other words, sex—like hunger—is linked with diverse motives in the hierarchy.

In one other respect, sexual motivation has a kinship with hunger and thirst: It has its roots in survival. But even in this respect, sex is unique among biological drives because lack of sex poses no threat to the *individual's* survival. We can't live for long without food or water, but some people live their lives without sexual activity (although some would say that that's not really living!). Rather, sexual motivation involves the survival of the species, not the individual.

All the biological drives—sex included—exert such powerful influences on behaviour that they have led to numerous social constraints and taboos, such as prohibitions on eating certain meats or drinking alcohol. In the realm of sexuality, we find extensive culture-specific rules and sanctions involving a wide variety of sexual practices. In fact, all societies regulate sexual activity, but the restrictions vary widely. For example, homosexuality has been historically suppressed in the United States and in Arab cultures, but it is widely accepted in many Asian and Pacific Island nations. Rules about marriage among relatives and exposure of genitals and breasts also vary from culture to culture.

Even the discussion of sex can become mired in taboo, misinformation, and embarrassment. Scientists who study human sexuality have felt intense social and political pressures, which show no signs of abating in the present. The result is that the scientific understanding of sexuality, which we will survey below, has been hard won.

Sex, hunger, and the hierarchy of needs

Maslow said almost nothing about sex. The new evolution-based needs hierarchy, however, corrects this omission. Kenrick's group still gives priority to hunger, thirst, and other survival needs at the base of the hierarchy. Sex and related motives follow at the "higher" levels: attachment, affiliation, belongingness, and parenting. But this doesn't mean that a pizza always wins over the opportunity for sex. As we have seen, the hierarchy is fluid, not rigid. In addition, hunger and sex are both biological drives *and* psychological motives. Because biological drives generally have priority over psychological motives, the attraction of sex can sometimes take precedence over eating—in which case proximal sex overpowers proximal pizza.

The what and why of sexual orientation

Sexual orientation One's erotic attraction toward members of the same sex (a homosexual orientation), the opposite sex (heterosexual orientation), or both sexes (a bisexual orientation).

Ever since Kinsey's first reports were published, we have known that human **sexual orientation** is a complex issue relating to sexual attraction, along with several other aspects of human relating, including our sexual behaviour, desired intimate relationships, affiliation with gay or straight (or other) communities, and how we personally identify our sexual orientation (Herek et al., 2010).

Heterosexuality and homosexuality represent the two major forms of sexual orientation: A *heterosexual orientation* is to the opposite sex; a *homosexual orientation* is to the same sex. Another common variation is *bisexuality*, which refers to sexual interest in both males and females

(Diamond, 2008). But to complicate matters, cross-cultural studies reveal considerable variability in sexual orientation. In parts of New Guinea, for example, the culture dictates that homosexual behaviour is universal among young males, who then switch to a heterosexual orientation when they marry (Money, 1987). Among American adults, various estimates put the percentage of homosexuality at 1 to 9 percent, more or less, depending on whether homosexuality is defined as (a) feelings of attraction to persons of the same sex, (b) one's primary orientation or, (c) having *ever* engaged in same-sex erotic behaviour (Diamond, 2007; Savin-Williams, 2006). As Table 7.2 indicates, the incidence of homosexuality among females is about half that of males. Incidentally, homosexual behaviour is quite common among animals—particularly bonobos (pigmy chimpanzees), who are genetically close relatives to humans (Driscoll, 2008).

Transsexualism refers to people who view themselves as persons of the sex opposite to their biological sex. Thus, a transsexual person with the phenotype of a male thinks of him/herself as a female. Such persons should not be confused with cross-dressers, who indulge in a sexual fetish known as *transvestism*. (Those who cross-dress for nonsexual reasons are not classified under transvestism.) It is also important to realise that none of these variations predicts sexual orientation. That is, knowing that a person is transsexual or a cross-dresser does not tell us whether he or she is gay, lesbian, bisexual, or straight (Devor, 1993).

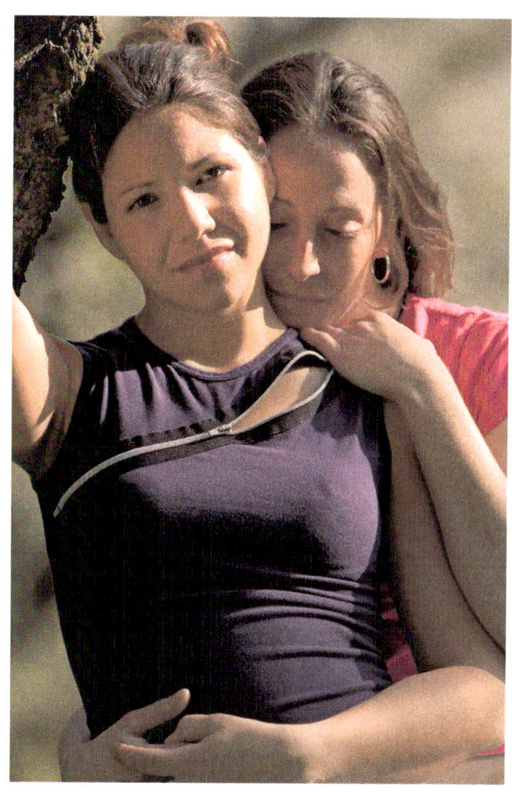

The origins of sexual orientation are unclear, although some evidence points to biological factors. What is clear is that research on sexual orientation often generates controversy.
(Source: First Light/Alamy.)

Origins of sexual orientation

So, what does the available evidence tell us about the factors that determine sexual orientation? We know several things that are *not* involved. Speaking biologically, we know that sexual orientation in adults is *not* related to testosterone levels—although the issue of testosterone or estrogen influences on the fetus is still an open question (McAnulty & Burnette, 2004). From a social perspective, we also know that parenting styles or family configurations do *not* cause children to identify as straight or gay (Golombok & Tasker, 1996). Similarly, researchers have come up empty handed in their attempts to link human sexual orientation to early sexual experiences, such as molestation or other abuse.

Although much of the work has focused on biology, most experts have concluded that a combination of biological, environmental, and social factors are at play. To illustrate this research, let's look at a famous study of male identical twins. Richard Pillard and Michael Bailey (1991) discovered that when one twin is homosexual, the chance of the other being homosexual is about 50 percent. This compares with an incidence of roughly 5 or 6 percent in the general population. The same study also found that the rate drops to 22 percent for fraternal twins and 11 percent for adoptive brothers of homosexuals. A later study of female twin pairs produced essentially the same results (Bower, 1992).

One of the more puzzling findings links sexual orientation in males (but not females) to birth order, specifically how many older brothers one has (Abrams, 2007; Blanchard, 2008; Bogaert, 2005). The more older brothers a boy has, the more likely he is to have a same-sex orientation. This effect occurs whether or not boys are raised with their biological brothers, according to a study of adopted versus biological brothers—a finding that apparently rules out environmental influences after birth (Bogaert, 2006). While no one knows what the causative factor is, some scientists believe that some aspect of the prenatal environment tips the balance one way or the other. (Bower, 2006a).

Again, research shows that social and environmental factors must also be taken into account. While few studies examine how adolescents develop a sexual orientation, some scholars theorise that social influences such as peers, the media, schools, and parenting can affect the direction of sexual development. Hyde and Jaffee (2000) reviewed numerous large studies that suggest adolescent girls who become heterosexual often develop their identities and social roles amidst messages that disparage homosexuality and promote heterosexuality.

Turning to the earlier preadolescent period, a longitudinal study of 182 children in fourth to eighth grade looked at the ways some children enter into a period of sexual questioning (Carver et al., 2004). Specifically, the researchers found that girls and boys who, for various reasons, question whether they will marry someone of the other sex and whether they will fulfill typical gender roles come to feel distressed about their competence in peer relationships (although this turmoil seems not to affect how much they are liked and accepted by their peers).

Research in this area remains controversial because of the strong feelings, political issues, and prejudices involved (Herek, 2000). Further, it has attracted scientific criticism because much of it is correlational—rather than experimental—so the data cannot establish cause and effect with certainty. Moreover, some observers object to this whole line of research, saying that gay men and lesbians should not feel pressured to justify their behaviour by seeking a "cause" for it (Byne, 1995).

Not a disorder

We should also note that, until the 1970s, the diagnostic manual of the American Psychiatric Association listed homosexuality as a mental disorder—a classification that has since been removed and repudiated by both psychologists and psychiatrists (Greenberg, 1997). Then, more recently, the American Psychological Association passed a resolution advising against therapies aimed at changing sexual orientation, on the grounds that they are ineffective, unnecessary, and potentially harmful (Munsey, 2009).

And what does the evidence say about sexual orientation and mental health? The message coming through numerous studies says that mental disorders and relationship problems occur in about the same proportion in heterosexuals and homosexuals (DeAngelis, 2002c; Kurdek, 2005). As we might expect, the only exception involves stress-related problems—e.g., anxiety and depression—associated with discrimination against homosexuals. The research also shows no differences in adjustment or development of children raised by heterosexual or homosexual parents (APA, 2010; Patterson, 2006).

So, where does this leave us in our understanding of sexual orientation? Attitudes toward minority forms of sexual orientation, such as homosexuality, differ sharply among cultures around the world, with Americans among the most divided on issues such as gay marriage. Most experts—but not all—would say that the research strongly supports some biological influence on sexual orientation. Just how biology might influence our behaviour in the bedroom, however, remains a major puzzle and a topic for continuing research.[A]

[A]Zimbardo, P. G., Johnson, R. L., & McCann, V. (2014). Motivation and emotion. In P. G. Zimbardo, R. L. Johnson, & V. McCann (Eds.), *Psychology: Core concepts* (7th ed., pp. 363–387). Upper Saddle River, NJ: Pearson Education.

[B]Zimbardo, P. G., Johnson, R. L., & McCann, V. (2014). Motivation and emotion. In P. G. Zimbardo, R. L. Johnson, & V. McCann (Eds.), *Psychology: Core concepts* (7th ed., pp. 407–408). Upper Saddle River, NJ: Pearson Education.

Summary

Motivation is largely an internal and subjective process: How can we determine what motivates people like Cathy Freeman to work so hard at becoming the best in the world at what they do?

- The subjective nature of motivation has forced psychologists to study the underlying processes indirectly, using a variety of methods, including animal studies, the *TAT*, and brain scans.
- Psychologists have identified many important influences on motivation, including culture, goals, unconscious processes, various biological factors, and social pressures. Rewards, both *intrinsic* and *extrinsic* are also important for world-class athletes like Cathy Freeman.
- One of the biggest questions involves the priorities we give to our motives—an issue that Maslow addressed in his famous *hierarchy of needs*. Recently, evolutionary psychologists have proposed an updated needs hierarchy. Many athletes, performers and artists apparently do much of their work in a state of *flow*—a mental state in which the person focuses on an intrinsically rewarding task to the exclusion of all other needs.
- Understanding motivation also requires understanding a person's emotions—because emotions are a class of motives aroused by persons, objects, and situations in the individual's external world. Emotions serve as the "values" we place on alternatives when we make choices and decisions.

What motivates us?

Core concept

Motives are internal dispositions to act in certain ways, although they can be influenced by multiple factors, both internal and external.

The concept of motivation refers to inferred internal processes that select and direct behaviour toward a goal. Motivation also helps explain behaviour that cannot be explained by the circumstances alone. Psychologists find it useful to distinguish intrinsic motivation from extrinsic motivation.

David McClelland pioneered the study of the need for achievement (n Ach), a motive important for I/O psychologists concerned about worker motivation and job satisfaction. The need for achievement also correlates with academic success and other accomplishments in life. But just as important as n Ach are the needs for power and affiliation, according to McClelland. Cross-cultural research also shows that societies vary in the intensity of their need for achievement, depending on their tendencies toward individualism or collectivism.

Psychologists have found that extrinsic rewards can destroy motivation for intrinsically rewarding tasks through overjustification. This is not always the case, however, but rather when rewards are given without regard for the quality of performance.

Great achievements usually come from people in a state of flow. Those in a flow state are intrinsically motivated by some problem or activity. The use of drugs or alcohol to achieve an artificial flow feeling is not usually effective.

How are our motivational priorities determined?

Core concept

A new theory combining Maslow's hierarchy with evolutionary psychology solves some long-standing problems by suggesting that functional, proximal, and developmental factors set our motivational priorities.

Psychology has no successful theory that accounts for all of human motivation. Psychologists have explained biologically based motivation in terms of instinct theory, fixed-action patterns, and drive theory, and homeostasis. Cognitive psychologists have emphasised biological motives. Freud called attention to unconscious motivation and thought that all our motives derive from unconscious sexual and aggressive desires. None of these approaches successfully explains the full range of human motivation however.

With his influential hierarchy of needs, Maslow attempted to explain the priorities in which human motives appear. Critics have, however, pointed out many exceptions to his hierarchy. Recently, evolutionary psychologists have proposed a revision of Maslow's theory suggesting that our "default" motivational priorities can change, depending on developmental factors and on important (proximal) stimuli.

In trying to understand another person's motivation, a good place to start is with extrinsic incentives and threats. In addition, Alfred Adler taught that social motives explain many problem behaviours. Social psychologists combine these notions under the heading of the *power of the situation*.

Where do hunger and sex fit into the motivational hierarchy?

Core concept

Although dissimilar in many respects, hunger and sex both have evolutionary origins, and each has an essential place in the motivational hierarchy.

Hunger is both a biological drive and a psychological motive, best understood by a multiple-systems approach. Americans receive mixed messages from the media, promoting both thinness and calorie-dense foods, which may play a role in disorders such as obesity, anorexia nervosa, and bulimia nervosa. None of these problems is completely understood, although both social and biological factors are thought to be involved. The problem of obesity has become an epidemic in America and is rapidly being exported throughout the world. Many people seek to control their appetite and body weight, although no weight-loss scheme is effective for most people over the long run.

Will power is a common term in everyday language, although psychologists avoid it because it suggests a separate faculty of the mind. They prefer *impulse control* or *self-control,* terms that can be explained in terms of brain mechanisms and environmental influences. Recently, researchers have found that impulse control takes a cognitive toll and is reflected in blood sugar levels.

Unlike hunger and weight control, the sex drive is not homeostatic, even though sexual motivation is heavily influenced by biology, but learning also plays a role, especially in humans. As Maslow's hierarchy did, the new evolution-based hierarchy generally gives hunger priority over sex, although the hierarchy is fluid.[B]

Review questions

A. Fill in the missing words to complete the following statements.

1. The concept of motivation refers to all the processes involved in ____________________, and then ____________________ by selecting, directing, and sustaining the mental and physical activity aimed at meeting the need or desire; and finally, when the need is met, ____________________ .
2. David McClelland proposed that an individual's specific needs are acquired over time and are shaped by one's life experiences. Most of these needs can be classed as either ________________, ________________, or ________________.
3. In McClelland's theory, people with a high need for achievement (n Ach) seek to excel and thus tend to avoid both ______________ and high-risk situations. Achievers avoid low-risk situations because the ____________________ success is not a genuine achievement. In high-risk projects, achievers see the outcome as one of chance rather than one's own effort. High n Ach individuals prefer work that has a moderate probability of success, ideally a 50% chance.
4. In Maslow's, 'hierarchy of needs', there are classes of needs listed in order. They include: ________________; ________________; ________________________________; ________________; ________________.
5. Most organisms seem to try and maintain ________________ - a state of physiological equilibrium.

B. Read the following sentences and answer with the most correct definition.

6. The desire to engage in an activity to achieve an external consequence, such as a reward is defined as ____________________.
7. The desire to engage in an activity for its own sake rather than for some external consequence, such as a reward is defined as ________________________.

C. Fill in the missing words and/or key concepts to complete the following table.

8.

Theories	Emphasis	Examples
______________	Biological processes that motivate behaviour patterns specific to a species	Bird migration, fish schooling
______________	Needs produce drives that motivate behaviour until drives are reduced	Hunger, thirst
______________	Motivation arises from unconscious desires; developmental changes in these urges appear as we mature	Sex, aggression
______________	Motives result from needs, which occur in a priority order (a need hierarchy)	Esteem needs, self-actualisation
______________	Priority of motives determined by functional, proximal, and developmental factors	Food odor (proximal stimulus) may raise the priority of hunger drive

D. Please select one statement that best answers each of the following questions.

9. Needs and expectations at work are sometimes dived into two types
   a) external/internal
   b) social/spiritual
   c) effort/reward
   d) extrinsic/intrinsic

10. Maslow suggests that human needs are arranged in a series of levels, a hierarchy of importance. Which of the following statements are relevant to Maslow's hierarchy of needs theory?
    a) a need is not necessarily fully satisfied before a subsequent need arises
    b) the hierarchy is not necessarily in a fixed order
    c) a satisfied need is no longer a motivator
    d) all of the above

11. McClelland's achievement motivation theory states that people with a high achievement need have a preference for:
    a) clear and unambiguous feedback
    b) non-competitive situations
    c) attaining success through their own efforts rather than through teamwork
    d) both (a) and (c)

12. Motivation that is due to factors within students or inherit to the task is called:
    a) intrinsic motivation
    b) extrinsic motivation
    c) behavioural motivation
    d) intent motivation

13. The term used to describe humans' desire for life-sustaining supports such as food and water is:
    a) motivation
    b) self-esteem
    c) primary need
    d) secondary need

14. According to Maslow's hierarchy of needs, if a person's esteem needs have been satisfied, then it is safe to assume that all of the following needs have also been satisfied EXCEPT:
    a) knowing
    b) belonging
    c) safety
    d) psychological

15. According to Hull, what is reinforcing?
    a) drive reduction
    b) drive induction
    c) incentive reduction
    d) incentive deduction

CHAPTER 8

Behaviour Change: Motivation, Adherence and Collaborative Treatment Planning

The content in this section has been compiled from:
Drench Chapter 6

Drench, M. E., Noonan, A. C., Sharby, N., & Ventura, S. H. (2012). Motivation, adherence and collaborative treatment planning. In M. E. Drench, A. C. Noonan, N. Sharby, & S. H. Ventura (Eds.), *Pyschosocial aspects of health care* (3rd ed., pp. 114–141). Upper Saddle River, NJ: Pearson Education.

CHAPTER 8

Behaviour Change: Motivation, Adherence and Collaborative Treatment Planning

Behaviour, the result of individual or collective action, is a key determinant of an individuals' health. As outlined in Chapter six, behaviour plays an important role in people's wellbeing (for example, smoking, poor diet, lack of exercise and sexual risk-taking can cause a large number of diseases). As health professionals, you may be expected to support a client and/or patient to change a behaviour, which may mean changing long standing habits. Whether you are working towards implementing health promotion programmes, or with individual clients and/or patients there is substantial evidence that the use of theory in designing and implementing behaviour change strategies improves the effectiveness of interventions and therapeutic outcomes. In this chapter we build on concepts of motivation (chapter seven) and examine theories of behaviour change of which can be applied in treatment planning.

After studying this chapter you should be able to:

- Describe factors that can affect motivation and adherence
- Describe models to enhance motivation and adherence:
- Health belief model
- Transtheoretical model
- Five A's behavioural intervention protocol
- Motivational interviewing
- Identify techniques to promote effective interpersonal communication in facilitating behaviour change.

As clinicians, we ask clients to adhere to many things, such as monitoring blood glucose levels, taking prescribed medications, using orthoses, and doing exercises. The more motivated and willing clients are to be actively involved in their therapeutic intervention, the more adherent they will be and the better their outcomes. Most clients are highly motivated to get well. However, many of us have had the experience of working with clients who feel sorry for themselves, feel the world is against them, and want to spend the rest of their lives moping around or staying in bed. In addition, some clients are unwilling to make changes. Why do clients with the same diagnosis, age, gender, and socioeconomic status act so differently?

Motivation is a two-part multifactorial phenomenon. The client first has to possess a desire to achieve a goal and then commit to an action to accomplish it. If the clinicians singularly set the goals, the clients may not be adherent because the goals are not their own, a considerable barrier to motivation. In addition, clients may feel they face too many barriers to be adherent, such as lack of transportation, time, finances, pain, fatigue, family conflicts, and differences in health beliefs and culture.

The phenomenon presented here as adherence is known in some fields as compliance. Studies generally define adherence as the degree to which clients follow a treatment regimen (Rand, 1993; World Health Organization [WHO], 2003). The treatment program could be in a clinic or at home and might include activities such as a diet, exercise plan, or other lifestyle changes.

Many factors affect therapeutic adherence. Some are motivators that enhance it; others are barriers that thwart adherence (King et al., 2002; Resnick & Spellbring, 2000). Examples of factors that impact therapeutic adherence include the characteristics of a disease or condition, the financial cost of treatment, the nature and duration of treatment, availability of the health care services where treatment takes place, patient perception of the condition and treatment and patient characteristics such as age, socioeconomic status and living arrangements (Banerjee & Varma, 2013). In fact, the WHO (2003) uses a model of five dimensions of adherence: patient-related factors, social/economic factors, therapy-related factors, condition-related factors, and health system-related factors. This chapter discusses theoretical concepts that influence motivation and adherence, describes collaborative relationships, identifies common barriers to collaborative treatment planning, and explores strategies that health care practitioners can use to enhance client motivation and adherence.

The phenomenon presented here as adherence is known in some fields as compliance. Studies generally define adherence as the degree to which clients follow a treatment regimen (Rand, 1993; World Health Organization [WHO], 2003). The treatment program could be in a clinic or at home and might include activities such as a diet, exercise plan, or other lifestyle changes. In fact, the WHO (2003) uses a model of five dimensions of adherence: patient-related factors, social/economic factors, therapy-related factors, condition-related factors, and health system-related factors.

Some studies use clinic attendance or self-reports to assess adherence. In others, the clinician evaluates the degree to which clients adhere with specific programs. The Sport Injury Rehabilitation Adherence Scale (SIRAS) (Bassett & Prapavessis, 2007) is an example. This 5-point scale measures three items: intensity of exercises, extent that recommendations and directions are followed, and receptiveness to changes in the program. Another example uses a multivariate approach, integrating several kinds of measurements. The 4-item subscale from the Situation Motivational Scale (Guay, Vallerand, & Blanchard, 2000) was used to examine clients' beliefs about the intrinsic and extrinsic benefits of a physical therapy program by asking them "Why are you starting physical therapy?"

The importance of motivation and adherence in improving outcomes has been well documented in the literature. For example, adults with osteoarthritis who adhered to a community-based aquatic exercise program showed improvements in physical function and quality of life and well-being (Belza, Topolski, Kinne, Patrick, & Ramsey, 2002). Long-term independent adherence by clients with chronic low back pain, after supervised rehabilitation ended, resulted in significant improvements in many parameters, including scales of perception of disability and pain (Hartigan, Rainville, Sobel, & Hipona, 2000).

Now that you've read about how motivation and adherence benefit the client, consider how nonadherence might influence you as a practitioner. Think about how you might feel or react when a client does not adhere to your therapeutic regimen. Think about how frequent nonadherence, over time, could influence what you prescribe for future clients. Could you see yourself ever "giving up" on some clients or prescribing a different program based on how you "read" them?

Physical therapists during their first year of clinical practice defined the "difficult patient" as one who is not open to therapy, is opposed to therapy, or lacking in motivation (Greenfield, Anderson, Cox, & Tanner, 2008). Sometimes, therapists blame their clients, which affects both parties. As one novice therapist said, "I shut off a little bit . . . if you don't care about yourself, then why should I care about you" (Greenfield et al., 2008, p. 1159)? This inexperienced therapist's attitude was judgemental and unethical, failing to respect the dignity and autonomy of the client to make his or her own choices. If we listen to clients, we can better assess how ready, willing, and able they are to make changes, to understand actual or perceived obstacles, and to help them become successful.

von Korff and coworkers (1997) identified important principles regarding increasing motivation and adherence for us to consider when working with clients. First, *illness management skills are learned, and behaviour is self-directed.* Most clients grow and develop without concerns related to illness or disability. Until a need arises, these illness management skills cannot be practiced. Clients who have survived previous hardships will adapt to illness or disability more readily. Those who have not will benefit from additional counselling and education. However, until clients value the information as necessary for their own health, independent management is not likely to occur. Patience and individualised education are needed with those learning these skills for the first time.

Second, *motivation and self-confidence are important determinants of behaviour.* As we will discuss, clients must be motivated to make changes in their health behaviour. They also must believe that they are capable of achieving success. It is critical to identify what is most important in their lives, what they enjoy doing, and what they find easy to do. Goals established with these elements in mind are more likely to be motivating and achievable. For example, if the goal is to quit smoking, it might be motivating to focus the client's attention on a child or spouse who would be left alone should he or she die from lung disease.

Finally, *the process of monitoring and responding to changes, symptoms, emotions, and functions improves adaptation to illness.* Learning to adapt to an illness or disability requires the acquisition of many new skills. The process of monitoring and responding to changes related to the illness or disability provides a natural and incremental method for learning to deal with all that is entailed. Consider the life of Sebastian, a 22-year-old man who sustained a cervical 7 spinal cord injury approximately 14 months ago. His initial recovery was hampered by the involvement of his well-meaning, but overprotective, mother. Over time, family counselling has helped both Sebastian and his mother understand the importance of separation. Recently, he has assumed full responsibility for managing his new life.

Education and persuasion can be used to help motivate clients, but strategies to overcome barriers toward progress must be continually refined. Rewards, such as recognition and praise, may be helpful in encouraging the maintenance of positive changes, but the recognition and praise have to be authentic. Health care professionals need to be more than "cheerleaders" who praise clients for the slightest changes. The client must feel praiseworthy for this to be effective.

Factors affecting motivation and adherence

Locus of control

Psychologists and other health care providers have long been interested in determining why individuals behave the way they do. Why do some people practice "wellness" behaviours, eating a balanced diet and exercising regularly, while others smoke and overindulge in food and alcohol, even though they know it is detrimental to their health? Why do some clients with chronic pain manage well, while others develop maladaptive behaviours?

One of the early researchers to study behaviour was Julian Rotter. He described a theory that he called "locus of control," which is based on life experiences and influenced by one's culture and family. According to Rotter's seminal 1966 work, people develop preconceived expectations about what will happen to them in the future. Those who believe they can influence what will happen to them are described as having an internal locus of control. They tend to be self-motivated and follow suggested treatment protocols because they believe they can make a difference in their lives. Other individuals have an external locus of control, believing that what happens to them is a result of outside influences or events. They may be less adherent to treatment protocols because they believe that their efforts will not make a difference.

Many studies have examined the relationship between locus of control and health-related behaviours. Hussey and Gilliland (1989) report that individuals with an internal locus of control are more health oriented and more likely to follow suggested health care plans than those whose locus of control is external. In reviewing the nursing literature, Oberle (1991) found that some studies support the Hussey-Gilliland findings, whereas others contradict them. This may be due to the fact that locus of control is a dynamic concept with many points on its continuum. It can range from strongly internal to strongly external. In addition, the measures of locus of control assess tendencies that can vary and even change (Wallston, 1992).

Clients with chronic pain who have a strong internal locus of control are better able to deal with their pain than those with a strong external locus of control (Toomey, Mann, Abashian, & Thompson-Pope, 1991). However, because of its dynamic nature, locus of control can shift. Evidence of this was generated when clients with chronic pain were treated in multidisciplinary pain management clinics and were able to increase their internal locus of control and, as a result, better manage their pain (Coughlin, Bandura, Fleischer, & Guck, 2000).

Clients' beliefs in the benefits and effects of treatment strongly affect adherence. Engstrom and Oberg (2005) found that clients with chronic pain who had lower expectations of therapy did not fully adhere to treatment recommendations and, as a result, experienced more pain, more disability, and deficient overall health. To facilitate treatment adherence habits, clinicians need to explore the client's beliefs about the benefits of the proposed therapy. The good news for clients and health care providers is that locus of control is a fluid concept. Even clients with a strong external locus of control can learn to take control of their situations. Note, however, that although health care providers need to understand the importance of locus of control, we must recognise that other factors also influence motivation and adherence.

Self-efficacy

Why do some clients improve, while others, with similar problems, do not? This happens for many reasons, and one of them is the client's own perception of his or her reality. Sometimes, there is a gap between what clients can actually do and what they think they can do. This can be particularly true if clients have not been able to do for a long duration what they had previously been able to do. This becomes their new reality and can hamper improvements. As clinicians, you can help change perceptions and emphasise clients' assets to facilitate a more realistic self-perception of what they should be able to achieve.

This phenomenon of a client's perception of reality is known as self-efficacy (Burton, Shapiro, & German, 1999; Conn, 1998), which was first introduced by Bandura (1977). It is a sense of competence and ability that is related to how successful people believe they can be in accomplishing a task. The idea that people believe that they are able to control their actions and behaviour can affect their rehabilitation (Jensen & Lorish, 2005; Schenkman, Hall, Kumar, & Kohrt, 2008; Woodard & Berry, 2001).

Some people avoid a task if they do not believe they can adequately participate or complete it. In contrast, those who believe they will ultimately succeed continue their efforts, even if they are having difficulty. People judge their own abilities, which, in turn, affects their behaviour, level of motivation, and adherence to health care regimens. This self-judgement can also determine how long someone persists with a difficult task. It is important to note that these personal judgements are not always accurate.

When people misjudge their abilities, they may become angry and frustrated and lose their focus on the task. They believe things are more difficult than they really are. However, people with a strong sense of self-efficacy may see a difficult situation as more of a challenge, causing them to try even harder (Bandura, 1997). This may partly explain why clients may react differently to the same circumstances.

Individuals with a strong sense of self-efficacy are better able to cope following a disability or illness (Maciejewski, Prigerson, & Mazure, 2000; Robinson-Smith, Johnston, & Allen, 2000). For instance, women who survived breast cancer and participated in a strength/weight training program for 6 months demonstrated a high degree of self-efficacy and adhered to their exercise programs (Ott et al., 2004). In a study of people with chronic low back pain before and 2 years following treatment, 80 percent exercised regularly because they believed that their actions could be successful. In fact, they did show improvements in flexibility, strength, pain levels, and disability scores (Mailloux, Finno, & Rainville, 2006).

A corollary of self-efficacy and a key motivator for adherence is outcome expectation. Adults in a retirement community who adhered to a walking program reported that they did so because they believed they were able to participate (self-efficacy) and that their actions would result in specific health benefits (outcome expectation) (Resnick & Spellbring, 2000). Fortunately, like locus of control, self-efficacy is a dynamic concept. People can improve their sense of efficacy by observing others accomplishing tasks and by learning to successfully complete tasks themselves (Bandura, 1997; Resnick, Palmer, Jenkins, & Spellbring, 2000). This is important information for health care professionals. We can assist our clients by introducing them to clients with similar diagnoses who have functionally integrated their illness or disability into their lives. Experienced survivors can serve as role models for those who have recently been diagnosed or injured. In addition, we can assist our clients by establishing reasonable short-term goals. Clients develop a sense of accomplishment, improve their sense of self-efficacy, and become motivated to comply with future treatments as they successfully achieve goals.

Self-esteem

Like locus of control and self-efficacy, self-esteem affects motivation. Self-esteem describes how individuals feel about themselves. Do they accurately assess their self-worth in comparison to others? Do they have pride in their abilities? A person with strong self-esteem is more likely to feel in control of his or her life and be more motivated to be an active participant in health care than a person with low self-esteem (Turner, 1999).

Many factors affect self-esteem. What may appear to be insignificant to us might be extremely important to a client. People in a rehabilitation setting or skilled nursing facility may feel better if they are able to wear their own clothing rather than hospital attire. A woman who uses a wheelchair may feel better about herself if a hairdresser is available to cut, colour, and style her hair. Someone with burns might improve his self-esteem if he learns to apply cosmetics to mask his injuries. It may also help to have personal items nearby to remind clients of their homes and families. A simple compliment from a health care provider can also help boost a client's self-esteem.

Self-esteem is often negatively impacted by alterations in body image. For example, children who had amputations of limbs to treat primary malignant bone tumors reported significantly lower levels of self-esteem than their counterparts who could be treated with surgical limb-sparing procedures (Marchese et al., 2007). Similarly, low self-esteem, anxiety, difficulty with social relationships, changes in body image, and depression are seen in clients with craniofacial conditions, facial injuries, facial cancer, and conditions to surgically correct face and jaw problems (DeSousa, 2008). One symptom of depression is low self-esteem. The lowered self-esteem can affect a client's motivation to participate in treatment.

Social determinants of health

In addition to locus of control, self-efficacy, and self-esteem, a number of social determinants play a significant role in determining a client's motivation and treatment adherence. Factors such as race/ethnicity, literacy, education, income, and place of residence can influence lifestyle decisions about whether clients do things like exercise, take their medications, and eat healthy diets. Behaviour change occurs where our clients live—at home, work, and school—but some communities fail to offer the infrastructure needed to modify lifestyle (Woolf, 2008). For instance, if a plan entails healthier nutrition, is there a store with fresh fruit nearby? Can clients or members of their support system get there? Is the food affordable (Woolf, 2008, 2009)?

Adherence to medical regimens, whether they involve medication, diets, exercise programs, or stress management, requires that clients be both willing and able to make the desired changes. Often a client faces barriers to change that are difficult for health care providers to detect. Some cultural issues may affect health care. However, it is important to mention here that a culturally sensitive and knowledgeable provider will communicate with clients in ways that respect their beliefs and values when making recommendations. For example, it is important to consider the role of the family and community in decision making and support, the desire to use alternative medicine, and the amount of trust the client places in the providers' advice (White et al., 2007). When clients are comfortable with medical recommendations, they are more likely to be adherent. The information needed is most likely to be elicited and negotiated in a skillful client interview.

Community resources

Intensive counselling is often required to change poor habits, for example, addictions to substances such as alcohol or cigarettes. This takes a considerable amount of time and usually occurs outside of medical encounters in programs available at community locations, such as the YMCA or Weight Watchers®. Unfortunately, clinicians generally lack adequate knowledge of existing programs outside of formal medical environments to make referrals. When such information is available, however, lack of ability to pay for nonmedical programs and lack of transportation can be deterrents. It is crucial for health providers to avoid underestimating the difficulty of changing behaviour and adhering to treatment programs. We must not assume that providing information and support will always be sufficient (Woolf, 2008).

Social support

The presence of social support, which shows people that they are loved, cared about, and valued, can enhance well-being. Clients who are supported are more optimistic, experience less depression and anxiety, have higher self-esteem and a better quality of life, and adhere more to treatment interventions (Platt et al., 2001; Symister & Friend, 2003). Social support leads to a winning combination: The more supported people feel, the more satisfied they are with their care, resulting in greater adherence (Bylund & Makoul, 2002). Lack of social support has been associated with low levels of motivation and may lead to nonadherence; therefore, it is beneficial to consider social support mechanisms when developing plans of care.

Another principle of von Korff and coworkers (1997) regarding motivation and adherence is that *social factors influence health behaviours*. The social environments at home, work, and in the health care system can support or impede health behaviours. Changes in these environments may be necessary to promote optimal health. Consider Jon, a university sophomore who has been diagnosed with hepatitis C. His liver biopsy shows early signs of cirrhosis. He lives near campus with a group of friends who host "keg" parties nearly every weekend night. Because he finds it impossible to avoid drinking in this environment, his health care provider might help him to see that moving into a new setting would be a healthy choice, though it would come at the expense of cutting ties with close friends.

It is important for health providers to determine clients' histories and what they bring to their current circumstances. People with illness or injury may find that they are unable to perform many of their activities of daily living. Frustration, anger, and lack of motivation may follow. A social support system can make it easier for clients to function. For example, people may be able to keep medical appointments if they have transportation. Members of a social support system may encourage a client to adhere to treatment plans, such as reminding a client to take medication, eat healthy meals, and exercise. This support can motivate a client to remain hopeful and adherent, even in difficult times.

Clients who live with a spouse or another adult have somewhat greater adherence to medical treatment than adults who live alone (DiMatteo, 2004a). A study of caregivers for clients discharged from an outpatient geriatric assessment centre found that those caregivers who agreed with health provider recommendations had greater adherence to treatment protocols and were more likely to help clients reach the goals (Bogardus et al., 2004). In a broader sense, when caregivers and health providers work together and caregivers believe in the efficacy of recommendations, clients are the winners.

The stress that caregivers experience can significantly impact adherence. One study involving children with disabilities showed that as family stress increased, children's adherence to home exercises decreased, resulting in a loss of functional skills (Rone-Adams, Stern, & Walker, 2004). Health care professionals can help reduce family stress by recommending appropriate resources for assistance, such as stress management programs, caregiver support groups, and respite care.

If clients do not have support systems in place, they can be referred to appropriate community resources. For example, Meals-on-Wheels can provide nourishment. Transportation may be provided by local councils. A home health aide might assist with activities of daily living. Health care providers are responsible for knowing about the programs and resources that are available in their clients' community, so they can inform them about these services.

Information can empower clients, providing they have the resources needed to act on the information learned. With the information and resources required to make health behaviour changes, clients are able to gain control over what they are experiencing and, therefore, may be in a better position to adhere to a recommended therapeutic regimen. Empowerment is a strong motivator. It helps to strengthen relationships between clients and health care professionals, building trust and reducing anxiety so that goals can be achieved. A sense of empowerment strengthens confidence and self-efficacy, which may also result in participatory decision making and self-management (Heisler, Bouknight, Hayward, Smith, & Kerr, 2002).

In addition to locus of control, self-efficacy, self-esteem, and social determinants, other factors that affect a client's motivation and ability to participate with health care include coping styles. In one study of people with cystic fibrosis, their coping style influenced how adherent they were to treatments, such as physical therapy, enzymes, and vitamins (Abbott, Dodd, Gee, & Webb, 2001).

Motivation and adherence go hand in hand. In a study investigating why children do not take their asthma medication (that is to say, lack of adherence to the treatment regimen), the children gave reasons of lack of motivation, difficulty remembering to do so, and social barriers. This occurs even in the face of the perceived consequences of nonadherence, such as feeling sick and not being able to participate in peer activities (Penza-Clyve, Mansell, & McQuaid, 2004).

Barriers to adherence

Just as there are motivators that increase therapeutic adherence, there are also barriers that decrease it. These barriers may predict inadequate adherence with a therapeutic regimen and, as a result, negatively impact achievement of goals. Health professionals need to address barriers before expecting people to change their behaviour. We have already discussed many barriers, such as lack of finances, transportation, interest, and social support. In addition, the impact of an illness can affect one's ability to adhere to treatment regimens. This lack of ability is manifested as pain, fatigue, and feeling overwhelmed. There are also psychosocial barriers that can influence self-assessment of function, such as secondary gain; secondary loss; emotional distress (i.e., anger, anxiety, depression); psychopathology; somatisation, symptom magnification, and malingering; and comprehension and mental status (Gatchel, 2004).

Traditionally, health care practitioners believed that education about the value and importance of exercise and other healthy behaviours, in and of itself, would be ample motivation for clients to alter their actions. We now understand, however, that changing human behaviour is a far more complicated process. Identifying barriers is a by-product of good communication. Once you identify barriers, you can work to mitigate them.

Role of health care providers in promoting motivation and adherence

Mrs. Menendez is at home recuperating from total hip replacement surgery. She fractured her hip when she fell on the ice in front of her home. Recently discharged from the hospital, she will receive services from the Visiting Nurses Association.

My supervisor and I visited Mrs. Menendez to evaluate her home to eliminate falling hazards. I was appalled! She had numerous scatter rugs throughout her home. I suggested she remove them immediately so that she wouldn't trip on them. She refused. The rugs had belonged to her mother, and she enjoys having them in her home; they make her feel comfortable and connected to her family. In addition, she has a 20-pound Boston Terrier, who has a habit of jumping on people. I was concerned that he would knock her over. I really thought she should put him in a kennel while she recuperated. She said, "No way! I love my dog and missed him when I was in the hospital." She likes to have him sit on her lap in the evening because he helps her "relax and calm down."

Her husband is another problem. While I was trying to encourage Mrs. Menendez to do things for herself, he wanted to wait on her "hand and foot." He didn't want her to move from her comfortable chair in the living room. I tried to explain that she needed to walk to become stronger, to improve her balance, and increase her endurance. He didn't want to listen to me. He was afraid that she might fall again, and he didn't want to "lose her." They've been married for over 50 years. What was I to do?

—*From the journal of Samantha Marino, physical therapist student*

The interaction between Samantha and the Menendez family illustrates the importance of the health provider in motivating clients to comply with care. Health providers need to recognise clients' values and priorities and incorporate them into a care plan to establish reasonable and effective outcomes. Flexibility is also an important component of the interaction. For example, Mrs. Menendez might have considered removing the scatter rugs, if she knew she could replace them once she was more stable on her feet. Samantha could suggest that the dog be put into a closed room while Mrs. Menendez is walking and be present when she is seated. In addition, Samantha could also work with Mr. Menendez to establish goals to increase his wife's strength and endurance. With these strategies, she would include him as a valued team member. Perhaps he could record his wife's daily progress. Samantha needs to understand and respect that Mr. Menendez, the dog, and the scatter rugs are all part of Mrs. Menendez's frame of reference. Samantha could utilise these resources to motivate her client to comply with treatments.

Strategies to enhance motivation and adherence

Modifying health behaviours

Various approaches to changing or modifying health behaviours are documented in the medical literature. Treatment interventions based on behaviour theory seem most likely to have positive outcomes, particularly when clients and providers work together toward shared goals (Hirano, Laurent, & Lorig, 1994; Lorish & Gale, 1999, 2002; Meyer & Mark, 1995; von Korff et al., 1997). Multiple factors need to be addressed to improve adherence, such as those associated with the individualised behavioural, cognitive, emotional, and technical needs of the client (DiMatteo, 2004b; Haynes, McKibbon, & Kanani, 1996; Herborg, Haugbolle, Sorensen, Rossing, & Dam, 2008; McDonald, Garg, & Haynes, 2002; Pampallona, Bollini, Tibaldi, Kupelnick, & Munizza, 2002; Schroeder, Fahey, & Ebrahim, 2004; Weingarten et al., 2002).

Therapeutic interventions can be developed that foster motivation and adherence by modifying health behaviours. To effectively promote motivation and adherence, health care professionals need to understand basic theories of behaviour and change. Several models have been designed to change health behaviours, and there are too many to include in this chapter. We will provide information here about four models that are frequently utilised and illustrate how they can be applied: the health belief model, the transtheoretical model for health behaviour change, the five A's behavioural intervention protocol, and motivational interviewing.

Health belief model

The *health belief model*, developed by Hochbaum, Leventhal, Kegeles, and Rosenstock, utilises psychological theories of decision making to determine what actions individuals might choose when presented with various health care choices (Rosenstock, 1966).

This model is based on the earlier seminal work of Lewin and colleagues (1944), who believed that health behaviours and choices are influenced by the value people place on a potential outcome and their belief that a certain course of action would result in that desired outcome.

Wallston (1992) suggests that health-related behaviour also depends on the value that people place on their health. People who perceive that they can control their illness may place a higher value on health and comply with treatments in order to improve. In contrast, those who believe they have no control over their illness may place less emphasis on their health. They may be nonadherent with treatment, believing that their actions will not positively influence their health. These perceptions and beliefs, either positive or negative or accurate or not, can influence therapeutic outcomes. In fact, a comprehensive meta-analysis of 18 studies investigating the health belief model's effectiveness in predicting and explaining behaviour ascertained that perceived benefits and perceived barriers were the strongest predictors of health outcomes (Carpenter, 2010). Expectations and apprehensions of being able to participate and reap benefits from treatment also play an integral role (Bouglanger, Campo, Glanville, Lowe & Yang, 2012; Constantino, Arnkoff, Glass, Amertrano & Smith, 2011; Schenkman et al., 2008). Clients tend to adhere to treatment interventions and have higher attendance levels if they perceive that their clinician is accurately justifies treatment and listens carefully to their opinions and experiences regarding treatment (Escolar-Reina et al., 2010; Kauppi, Hatonen, Adams & Valimaki, 2015).

The health belief model is intricately entwined with people's perceptions of their health status. As such, it is based on subjective beliefs, as opposed to objective measurements. According to the health belief model, in order for people to change behaviour, they must be ready to make a change. This readiness is based on their health beliefs and includes an understanding of what causes the problem. If clients believe that health is given by a higher power, then they will also believe that they have no ability to make a change in their status. Some clients believe that they are capable of making the change but also believe that the barriers that have to be overcome are not worth it. For instance, if we ask the "cook in the family" to change his or her diet, this can affect the way he or she cooks for the whole family. If that client believes the family will be highly resistant to this change, he or she may be reluctant to make the change because of the conflict it is likely to create.

Clients must also believe that the value of making the change is stronger than the consequences of not making the change. Hypertension typically has no noticeable symptoms and is rarely detected by the client. Therefore, asking a client to take a medication that causes side effects will not be valuable if the client sees no benefit in controlling blood pressure. Health beliefs can also affect clients' sense of self-efficacy and whether or not they believe that they have the ability to be successful in achieving their goal.

To help motivate clients to make the changes we suggest, clients' beliefs must align with our view that Western medicine provides appropriate solutions. Different cultures have different common health beliefs. It is important to elicit these beliefs so that they can be discussed and form the basis for a truly collaborative plan of care to which the client is willing to adhere.

Transtheoretical model for health behaviour change

The *transtheoretical model for health behaviour change* focuses on motivation. Although this is a heavily utilised and often discussed model, few guidelines are available for applying it. In addition, evidence of efficacy in the short term is greater than that which exists for long-term behavioural change (Adams & White, 2005). "There is abundant evidence that other external and social factors, such as age, gender, and socioeconomic position, influence exercise behaviour, motivation to participate in physical activity, and stage of activity" (Adams & White, 2005, p. 239).

Change in health behaviour is a process that takes time. The transtheoretical model for health behaviour change, also called the stages of change model (Prochaska, DiClimente, & Norcross, 1992; Prochaska, Redding, & Evers, 2002; Prochaska & Velicer 1997), recognises that change does not happen easily and that people move through various stages of readiness to change. Identifying the signs of these stages will help us tailor our interventions to current needs. Further, even when progress toward change occurs, clients are likely to relapse into earlier stages. In fact, relapse appears to be a necessary element in the process and must be addressed so clients can begin anew. As described in Table 8.1, clients are likely to pass through six nonlinear stages on their way to change, including the following:

- **Pre-contemplation** An abundance of clients are in this stage when we first encounter them and have no plans to begin to make a change. During pre-contemplation, clients are not expecting to make any changes within the next 6 months. At this stage, people may be uninformed as to the consequences of their behaviours or may have given up, having been unsuccessful at earlier attempts to change. These clients tend to refuse to discuss or consider consequences of their actions. Although they may be perceived and labeled as unmotivated, they may just not be *ready* to change. Providing them with additional information regarding the positive aspects of change can help them progress to the next stage, known as contemplation.
- **Contemplation** In the contemplation stage, clients are aware of the need to change and are considering doing so within the next 6 months. They have "done their homework" and have learned the pros and cons of their situation. However, these clients can sometimes feel overwhelmed with information and become stuck in this stage for months. They are not ready for action, but encouraging them, providing additional resources, and reducing their barriers to change may help them move to the next stage, known as preparation.
- **Preparation** During the preparation stage, people plan to take action in the near future. They know what they need to do and have a plan as to how they will achieve their goals. In addition, they recognise that the positive aspects of change outweigh the negative elements. They are prepared and tend to quickly move to the action stage where observable changes can be measured.
- **Action** Health professionals perceive clients in the action stage as highly motivated. When clients adhere to home programs, lose weight, and join gyms or health clubs, the health providers feel a sense of satisfaction for having helped them achieve their goals.
- **Maintenance** Once people achieve their goals, they progress to the maintenance stage and can remain there for 6 months to 5 years. During this period, they continue to develop self-confidence and are less tempted to relapse to their former behaviour. However, clients often do relapse and may return to any of the earlier stages.
- **Termination** The final stage, termination, occurs when clients have reached their goals, incorporated positive lifestyle changes, and are confident that they will not return to their "old ways."

Table 8.1 Transtheoretical model for health behaviour change/stages of change model

Pre-contemplation	No thought of change	"I'm not changing my diet; why should I?"
Contemplation	Considering change	"I'm not changing my diet now but may begin at some point."
Preparation	Preparing to change	"I will make changes in the next year."
Action	Implementing change	"I've been exercising for 30 minutes, three times a week, for the past few months."
Maintenance	Maintaining change	"I've been exercising for 30 minutes, three times a week, for over 6 months now."
Termination	Change is integrated	"I test my blood sugar four times a day, like clockwork."

Health care professionals who understand where clients are in the process of change can better provide appropriate support and help them move forward. Attempting to force a person who is in the pre-contemplation stage to the action phase can be frustrating for both the client and the health provider and will usually result in only short-term success and a high dropout or relapse rate.

Five A's behavioural intervention protocol

Lorish and Gale (2002) built on the theoretical components of the models discussed above and developed the *five A's behavioural intervention protocol*. The five steps are easy to follow, take little time to complete, and have been shown to be more successful in promoting client motivation and adherence than information and advice alone. This model is also closely aligned with the transtheoretical model and motivational interviewing.

The five A's model provides a structure and format for interacting with clients capable of developing a collaboration that will support them to make behavioural changes to improve health. The first A is to *address the issue*. We need to make sure that we have the clients' attention and that we are also fully attentive. We name the problem and present the need for intervention. Second, we *assess the clients*. In this step, we determine where they are in the stages of change, as well as identifying any barriers preventing them from engaging in more healthful behaviours. We can ask the clients what they would like to change and how prepared they are to implement changes. It will be helpful to determine any previous attempts to change behaviour. Third, we *advise the clients*. This is where we include the traditional medical role of providing information and educating the clients about their illness and the reasons why changes are needed. We can help the clients understand the benefits of change and the consequences of not changing. Fourth, we *assist the clients* to make change. This is where we negotiate an agreeable plan of care. Finally, we *arrange for follow-up*. Behaviour change is a long and difficult journey, and one appointment will typically not result in change. Schedule another appointment to review progress, address barriers, and renegotiate the protocol.

In order for clients to change, they must be knowledgeable about their situation, motivated to change, and have the resources to make it happen. The five A's address all of these issues and involve a dialogue between the health care provider and the clients to reduce barriers and negotiate positive behavioural changes.

Numerous other behavioural techniques have been found to improve health management among clients who have chronic illnesses (Beresford et al., 1992; Ignacio-Garcia & Gonzalez-Santos, 1995; Woodard & Berry, 2001). These include the following: collaborative goal setting; assessing readiness for new behaviours in small, manageable steps; providing personalised education, observation, and feedback; self-monitoring of changes and symptoms; and counselling in techniques to obtain appropriate social support. Health care providers must design structured behavioural interventions that incorporate these behaviour techniques to facilitate clients' independence in using important health management skills.

Motivational interviewing

Motivational interviewing is predicated on the belief that clients are responsible for their own actions and health and, consequently, for changing their health behaviours. It epitomise client autonomy and self-determination. Because self-efficacy and outcome expectations shape actions, motivational interviewing can be a valuable strategy to enhance motivation and adherence. Initially used with the treatment of addictions and alcohol use, it is a client-centred, directive counselling approach first developed by Miller (1983) and later expanded by Miller and Rollnick (1995). It is now used in medical, public health, and other health promotion arenas (Britt, Hudson, & Blampied, 2004; Resnicow et al., 2002) for promoting physical activity in clients with chronic heart failure (Brodie & Inoue, 2005), promoting public health (Shinitzky & Kub, 2001), changing behaviour in clients with chronic obstructive pulmonary disease (Rollnick, Miller, Butler, & Aloia, 2008), and weight reduction in women with type 2 diabetes (West, DiLillo, Bursac, Gore, & Greene, 2007).

An evidence-based, directive, client-centred counselling approach, motivational interviewing helps a client's intrinsic motivation to change by delving into ambivalence and working to end it (Levensky, Forcehimes, O'Donohue, & Beitz, 2007); that is to say, it help clients adhere to treatment recommendations. Building on the transtheoretical model for health behaviour change (Prochaska et al., 1992, 2002; Prochaska & Velicer 1997), motivational interviewing follows four key counselling principles (Levensky et al., 2007; Miller & Rollnick, 2002):

- **Express empathy** The health care provider communicates an understanding of what clients are experiencing and accepts their ambivalence. "Readiness to change" comes from within the client and can ebb and flow. Clients are helped to overcome their "ambivalence or lack of resolve" to change.
- **Develop a discrepancy** The provider helps clients become aware of the discrepancies between their present unhealthy behaviours and the goals and values that they would be striving to achieve. The responsibility to self-determine and reach a commitment to change rests with the client.
- **Roll with resistance** Because motivation to change ultimately comes from the client rather than the provider, the health provider does not directly interfere with any client resistance. Coercion, persuasion, and confrontation are counterproductive and contradictory to the core concepts of motivational interviewing.
- **Support self-efficacy** The health provider supports and communicates the belief that clients are able to effect change. A partnership exists between the client and clinician rather than a paternalistic relationship (Miller & Rollnick, 1995).

Important skills for motivational interviewing include reflective listening, asking open-ended questions, affirming, and summarising. Because the premise is to help clients become aware of their problems, for example, nonadherence, and what consequences can ensue from lack of following the recommended course of behaviour, we ask key questions to elicit inherent motivation rather than provide the information. Four important questions to ask are listed in Box 8.1.

Patient education looks different with motivational interviewing because it uses an ask–tell–ask approach. For example, "Tell me what you already know about diabetes and how it is treated" (*ask* the question). Ask for permission to provide more information as needed (*tell* the information). For instance, "It sounds like you know that drinking is not good for your liver. I have some specific information that I would like to share with you. Is that all right?" *Ask* what the client thinks about the new information you provided.

As an "interpersonal style," clinicians facilitate alternate thinking, a new picture with better results, which can help motivate the client to change behaviour and instill commitment to that change. To do that, they work with clients to negotiate a plan of action. With information

Box 8.1 Key questions to elicit motivation

- What is the best thing that can happen to you if you do not change?
- What is the worst thing that can happen to you if you do not change?
- What is the best thing that can happen to you if you do change?
- What is the worst thing that can happen to you if you do change?

you have already elicited from the clients, you can then ask questions, such as "Are there things that you think you could change, even if they are small things?" "Can you think of one thing that you are able to change?" "What else would you be willing to change?" "What might you be willing to change later if this change is successful?" "What do you need to help you change?" Health professionals affirm and support all facets of the conversation to change.

Goal setting

"Goal-setting has long been regarded as a cornerstone of effective rehabilitation" (Lawler, Dowswell, Hearn, Forster, & Young, 1999, p. 402) and is important in treatment success. Goals need to be negotiated between clients and providers, participating as equals, and clients' needs, not those of health providers, should be the focus. Goals that are important in clients' lives tend to be functional, meaningful, and motivating (Randall & McEwen, 2000; von Korff et al., 1997). Because the goals have relevancy in their lives, clients tend to be more committed to them. When clients are involved in establishing goals, they become partners in their care (Playford et al., 2000; Skinner, 2004).

Ideally, the client not only sets short-term and long-term goals but also enters into a contract to reach these goals by adhering to healthy behaviours (Bodenheimer, Lorig, Homan, & Grumbach, 2002). Clients are most successful in achieving treatment outcomes when their goals are specific, challenging, and achievable, and they have the opportunity to successfully practice the skills (Bandura, 1977, 1997; Locke, Shaw, Saari, & Latham, 1981). Therefore, we must be careful to agree on goals that are neither too high nor too low. If a goal is set too high, clients will be unable to achieve success. If a goal is too low, clients may achieve success but will lack a sense of accomplishment. In either case, this may lead to frustration and nonadherence.

Clinicians should review the goals with the client and mutually revise them as needed. This is also a good opportunity to discuss concerns and barriers and explore strategies to mitigate them (Schenkman et al., 2008). Clients' involvement should be active enough that they realise their collaborative role. This means that if clients are asked to identify their goals for treatment, responses should mirror the goals recorded in their health care records. Incorporating clients' goals into the plan of care requires active listening to ensure that we fully understand what clients are conveying. Their ideas then need to be developed into attainable and measurable goals that not only meet the criteria for standards of professional documentation but also maximise the chance of health insurance reimbursement (Chinman et al., 1999).

Once goals have been established, it can be helpful for clients to write out their goals in their own words. They may record them in a journal or calendar so that they can regularly review them. You can help clients establish realistic time frames for completing these goals. It is important to note, though, that goals do not always indicate forward progress. Some goals may be to maintain function or to slow the rate of decline that occurs with some long-term illnesses (Cott & Finch, 1991). In addition, having clients sign personal contracts stating they will adhere to treatment plans has been shown to improve motivation and adherence (Jones & Kovalcik, 1988).

Health care professionals and clients need to recognise that most people will not adhere to treatment programs 100 percent of the time. For example, clients occasionally forget to take medications or follow dietary recommendations. These minor lapses are considered normal. According to Barsa del Alcazar (1998), clients who are "moderately adherent" are demonstrating adaptive behaviour. This is especially true of clients who are undergoing long-term treatments, such as dialysis. Health care professionals need to recognise and accept this adaptive behaviour because it allows clients to continue to have control of their own lives. They can also help clients' family members understand this behaviour so they will continue to be supportive, rather than critical, of the behaviour of their loved ones.

Following illness or injury, clients' goals frequently include returning immediately to their previous state of health. Health care professionals need to discuss prognosis and anticipated time frames for recovery. Educating clients about the importance of short-term goals and their relationship to long-term goals is critical (Adams & White, 2005; Bradley, Bogardus, Tinetti, & Inouye, 1999). Health practitioners need to provide sufficient education so that clients can make constructive, informed decisions (Daily Mock, 2001). They also need to integrate the clients' viewpoints and work from a perspective that realistically conforms to the clients' perspective (Herborg et al., 2008).

Long-term goals are sometimes more important to patients than short-term goals. In a study of patients with osteoarthritis, long-term instead of short-term goals, as well as being actively involved in the process, were strongly associated with long-term adherence to the therapeutic intervention (Veenhof et al., 2006). When clients understand and appreciate the link between short- and long-term goals, they may be more motivated to adhere to programs. In addition, early and continued involvement in goal setting promotes active participation, and clients take responsibility for their own care.

Clients expect clinicians to know what questions to ask to retrieve important information regarding concerns, goals, resources, treatment ideas, and outcomes. Although this may occur in long-term care, professionals working in fast-paced environments may have only one opportunity to ask clients to identify their goals. Asking one question about goals during the initial examination, however, is not enough. In addition, clients may rely on health care professionals to share established goals with other members of the team. This may not happen. Even clients who are ill enough to require care in an intensive care unit may move from that setting to transitional care and, finally, to outpatient or home care, sometimes after only a few days in each setting. Transfers of service are likely to be accompanied by a complete change in the members of the health care team, with little or no continuity other than what is provided by written reports. Ideally, these reports should relay all details that are important to consider.

Education and empowerment

Client education is an important component of health care (Jensen, Gwyer, Shepard, & Hack, 2000; Mostrom & Shepard, 1999; Vanderhoff, 2005). Studies have shown that educated clients practice wellness behaviours and, if ill or injured, remain motivated and adhere to treatment programs (Sluijs, 1991). Client education needs to be culturally sensitive and utilise the components of effective communication. Ask clients if they will be able to adhere to the program that you have both agreed on. If not, ask why and make appropriate modifications. Attempt to eliminate any barriers that might interfere with adherence.

According to an early study by Treichler (1967), classroom students remember only 10 percent of what they read, but the retention increases as they are more engaged in this experience, climbing to 80 percent of what they personally experience and 90 percent of what they teach to others. In the clinical setting, clients and families are also learners. Providing clients with written directions, pictures, and time to discuss instructions and ask questions will help them remember prescribed treatment programs. All treatment adjuncts need to be clear and easy to understand, customised to meet the needs of the clients, and relevant to them. To be beneficial, clinicians need to review any form of documentation and share feedback.

Various educational approaches have been found useful, including treatment booklets with clear graphics; videotapes, DVDs, iPods®, iPhones®, and YouTube; informational conversations with clinicians, and equipment (i.e., for exercise) and adjunct equipment (i.e., inhalers or oxygen) (Bassett & Prapavessis, 2007; Moore, von Korff, Cherkin, Saunders, & Lorig, 2000; Stelzner, Rodriguez, Krapfl, Jordan, &Schenkman, 2003; Sweeney, Taylor, & Calin, 2002).

Have clients repeat directions or demonstrate tasks to ensure they understand. In addition, according to Treichler's model, giving clients the opportunity to teach their program to significant others, under your guidance, may aid in their retention.

Sluijs (1991) noted that the more information clients are given at one time, the more likely they are to forget. They will forget even more if they are worried, concerned, or in pain when they receive information. When possible, try to mitigate anxiety and discomfort at the outset. Yet, how often do we overload clients with information during our first encounter? Ideally, provide clients with basic information during the initial meeting, emphasising the most important components of the instruction. More complex information can be given at a later time. During subsequent sessions, determine whether clients correctly remember instructions. If a client has only one treatment session, however, you should communicate only the most essential information. Encourage clients to contact you with questions or concerns and provide your telephone number and e-mail address.

People have different teaching and learning styles. Most people tend to teach the way they prefer to learn (Brock & Allen, 2000; Mostrom & Shepard, 1999). However, this may not always be effective. Our teaching approach may not match the client's learning style. Some individuals prefer to hear only the facts, whereas others prefer a more personable approach. Allow time for clients to tell you how they feel and to ask questions. This strategy may instill comfort and prepare clients to absorb the information you are prepared to communicate. Whereas some people learn best by watching a demonstration and listening to instructions, others prefer trying things immediately. Recognising and making adjustments for individual learning styles can make health care professionals more effective teachers and clinicians (Lawrence, 1997; Vanderhoff, 2005).

Today, a great deal of information on health care is available. Clients can open a newspaper, watch television, or listen to the radio to hear about the latest medical research. In addition, more people have access to the Internet, at home or through local libraries and schools. Clients need to be educated on how to evaluate all sources of information because some are unreliable (Vanderhoff, 2005). As health care professionals, we need to be well informed so that we can answer questions appropriately and ensure that clients receive accurate information. Motivation and adherence can be enhanced if clients are well educated regarding their diagnosis and prognosis.

Feedback and follow-up

Positive feedback has been shown to improve self-esteem, enhance individuals' perceptions of their own competency, and improve motivation and adherence (Goudas, Minardou, & Kotis, 2000; Mulvaney, 2009). Health care professionals track clients' progress in medical records, but do we adequately share this information with clients? Understanding the progress they have made can give clients a sense of control and motivate them to continue (Lawler et al., 1999). It is important to give feedback in a timely manner. Positive feedback may be provided whenever clients follow through with program guidelines or make progress toward their goals. For example, clients with multiple myeloma and bone lesions who received encouragement and support were able to adhere to an aerobic and strengthening exercise program, in spite of the discomfort they experienced while they were receiving high-dose chemotherapy and stem cell transplantation (Coleman, Hall-Barrow, Coon, & Stewart, 2003). Other forms of feedback are also useful. Clients with heart failure who had already completed a supervised exercise program had greater adherence to exercise when they received graphic feedback and used goal setting and guidance (Duncan & Pozehl, 2002).

Clients can give themselves positive self-feedback. For example, they may track their own progress in journals or calendars. Reviewing this information can be a motivator. Consider Mrs. Thompson, who was trying to lose weight and increase her endurance following cardiac surgery. She had been in a cardiac rehabilitation program for several months and had become discouraged. As a result, she started "forgetting" about her exercise and walking program and no longer made time to adhere to other aspects of her treatment plan. Her exercise physiologist suggested she review the progress she had recorded in her journal. Reading the entries, Mrs. Thompson was surprised at how far she had come. Identifying her accomplishments enhanced her self-esteem and motivated her to return to her program with renewed energy.

Feedback to clients depends on consistent follow-up, can enhance adherence (Hall, 1999), and can take many forms, such as telephone calls, e-mails, group attendance, and personal counselling. In addition, scheduled assessment visits with clinicians may be helpful to review information, discuss how the client is progressing, and identify any barriers that have arisen. Follow-up contact is an opportunity to bolster sagging adherence, identify challenges early, and modify programs as necessary. Just as introducing the concept of adherence and setting mutual goals at the outset of a therapeutic program are key elements, supervised training with follow-up checks and feedback are continuing critical ingredients.

Health care practitioners need to encourage, support, educate, communicate, and build sustaining therapeutic alliances with clients. Having information, and being able to use it, and being involved in partnerships increases the clients' self-efficacy, which, in turn, may result in greater adherence to their therapeutic intervention. This is why the last of the five A's behavioural intervention protocol is to *arrange for follow-up*.

Peer support groups

Peer group participation has been shown to help people clarify values, improve self-esteem, increase knowledge, develop coping strategies, maintain healthy lifestyle habits, and reduce or eliminate addictions (Bernard, 1991). In fact, groups are so beneficial and popular, it seems as though they exist for almost any problem, condition, or diagnosis. Interacting with others who have gone through or are going through similar experiences may assist clients in understanding their own limitations or impairments and give them greater confidence in their ability to succeed (Resnick et al., 2000; Turner, 1999). Support groups also benefit family members who are learning to live with an individual who has been diagnosed with an illness or who has sustained an injury. Groups offer social support and provide a forum for sharing stories and strategies for success. Clients with ankylosing spondylitis who were in a self-help group exercised more frequently, strengthened their own locus of control, utilised external support more freely, and continued to improve outcome measurements over time (Barlow, Macey, & Struthers, 1993).

Peer support groups can be especially effective in promoting positive health and wellness behaviours. For example, Turner (1999) described peer-led initiatives as a social support system for adolescents. Teens often feel more comfortable talking to one another rather than discussing their concerns with adults. Turner cautions, however, that when teen peer groups are developed, peer leaders need extensive training in listening and basic counselling skills in order to be effective. He emphasises the need for adequate training, adult support, and the availability of appropriate referral resources. There must also be a trained adult available whom they can contact immediately if the need arises. Developing effective peer support programs can be quite time consuming, but the results are worth the effort.

Health care professionals direct some peer support groups, but group members direct others, as in the teen group noted above. Such programs can be a positive adjunct to professional health care services. However, when developing these programs, health care providers must remember that peer leaders have the same concerns and problems as group members. Therefore, it is important to provide professional social support mechanisms for all peer leaders if their problems begin to overwhelm them (Sherman, Sanders, & Yearde, 1998).

Information regarding peer group meetings is often available from local newspapers, hospitals, libraries, or churches. National resources, such as the Muscular Dystrophy Association and the United Cerebral Palsy Association, can be found on the Internet. Practitioners may consider developing peer support groups at their own facilities if none are available in the community.

Functional programs

Following illness or injury, many clients are concerned with their ability to be independent. Studies have shown that clients are more motivated to adhere to treatment programs that are related to functionality (Brody, 2005). In addition, clients are more likely to comply with programs that cause the least disruption in their lifestyles. Finding ways to fit treatment plans into a client's normal routine helps ensure long-term adherence (Brody, 2005).

Keep programs realistic and avoid complex instructions. Provide variety and choice when possible to prevent clients from becoming disinterested. Develop functional programs based on daily routines. For example, if a client needs to follow a complicated medication schedule, suggest the client purchase a weekly medication dispenser. Guide the client to identify the best time each week to fill the dispenser and establish a realistic strategy for remembering to take the medication on time. If the medication needs to be taken with food, he or she may want to leave the dispenser on the table where meals are eaten.

Be sure that home programs are functional in nature. Consider Mrs. Farrari, who slipped in the supermarket and fractured her shoulder. The therapist first suggested a nonfunctional exercise program. Mrs. Farrari stated the exercises were "boring" and did not interest her. After careful questioning about her home environment, where she lived alone, the therapist suggested that Mrs. Farrari move frequently used items to higher shelves. The client relocated teacups and glasses in the kitchen cabinets and towels and facecloths in the bathroom closet. As a result, as her day progressed, so did her accomplishments of her treatment goals. While a more structured exercise program might have accelerated her progress, she would not have made any progress if she did not adhere to the therapeutic program.

It is especially beneficial for families with children who have disabilities to integrate home exercise programs with a functional routine, such as bathing, dressing, and playing. It is incumbent upon the health provider to collaborate with caregivers to simplify activities so that stress is minimised, and limited time and energy are used most effectively (Rone-Adams et al., 2004).

Primary and secondary control-enhancing strategies

Some clients start out motivated but lose their impetus over time. This is especially true for clients dealing with a chronic impairment or terminal illness. No matter how hard they work, their condition is not likely to significantly change or improve. Maintaining motivation can also be difficult for elderly people. Even healthy people experience decreased hearing acuity and loss of muscle tone, strength, flexibility, and memory as they age. They cannot participate in activities the way they could when they were younger.

How can we help these clients sustain their motivation to adhere to programs and achieve therapeutic outcomes? Studies have shown that a two-step approach, involving primary and secondary control-enhancing strategies, can be very effective (Chipperfield & Perry, 2006; Wrosch, Heckhausen, & Lachman, 2000). These strategies allow clients to feel in control of their lives, maintain their self-esteem, and remain motivated.

Primary control-enhancing strategies allow people to accomplish desired goals in new ways by modifying the environment. Consider Mrs. McKenzie, who loved to walk to the corner store to get her daily newspaper. As her rheumatoid arthritis progressed, she purchased a motorise scooter that allowed her to continue her routine. When primary control-enhancing strategies no longer achieve the goals, secondary strategies can be utilised to retain a form of personal control. Clients who use secondary control-enhancing strategies modify their internal environment by altering their expectations and reframing what is important. As her condition worsened, Mrs. McKenzie found that she could not control the scooter and began to have her newspaper delivered to her home. Both types of strategies require the client to be cognitively flexible and to be able to adjust to changing circumstances. This can be difficult and require the support of both health care professionals and the social network.

Creative strategies to support motivation and adherence

In addition to goal setting, other techniques that promote adherence and healthy behaviours include individualised action plans (Moore et al., 2000) and contracts with built-in incentives for goal achievement. Peer support with spouses and exercise partners has helped with smoking cessation, improving eating habits, and exercise/walking (Prochaska & Velicer, 1997). Reminders, such as laminated cue cards and exercise clothes, if applicable, can be placed in strategic locations in the client's environment (Bassett & Prapavessis, 2007; Sweeney et al., 2002).

The use of technology also fosters motivation and adherence. Clients with chronic stroke who participated in a program of physical therapy plus robotic devices showed high scores on the Intrinsic Motivation Inventory, sustained their interest, and received specific feedback (Colombo et al., 2007). Virtual reality systems, such as the Nintendo Wii™ system, are being used in many health care settings, including private practices, extended care facilities, and hospital-based rehabilitation units (Coyne, 2008). In addition, Dance Dance Revolution® is being used for aerobic conditioning and airway clearance for patients with cystic fibrosis (Coyne, 2008).

Collaboration

I had a terrible experience in the clinic today. I was working in the gym with Mrs. Swanson, a woman who had her left leg amputated above the knee because of complications related to her diabetes. Just as she was finishing her exercises, one of the medical residents came by. Apparently, Mrs. Swanson agreed to participate in a study that was designed to examine how well clinicians at our hospital collaborate with patients on establishing goals and treatment plans. I asked for permission to sit in on the interview. What a mistake! This is how the interview went:

Interviewer: Who decides what you are going to do in physical therapy?

Mrs. Swanson: Well, Suzy does, of course! She's so smart. I don't know how I would have gotten this far without everything she has taught me.

Interviewer: Do you ever suggest to Suzy that you would like to try a different exercise or work on something specific that you need to be able to do at home?

Mrs. Swanson: Oh, no. She really knows just what I need to learn. After all the schooling she's had, how would I know anything more?

At first, I felt touched and kind of proud, but as the interview continued, I became embarrassed. The questioning continued about Mrs. Swanson's home situation. She mentioned how sad she was that she probably wouldn't be able to participate in her weekly line dancing class now that she was missing a leg. She started sobbing and talking about how she would be no good to anyone any more. I really thought that I had done a good job of incorporating her goals into my treatment plan. Today, I realised I had not.

—*From the journal of Suzanne Ballis, physical therapist student*

We have discussed the importance of establishing therapeutic partnerships with our clients that are based on genuine concern and mutual respect and trust. A healthy client–provider relationship involves understanding clients' perspectives and leads to explicitly shared expectations for outcomes. Collaborative goal setting is an important step toward empowering clients to take responsibility for their own recovery. Providing opportunities to make real choices in treatment goals and planning stimulates clients to utilise their own skills and resources to achieve positive outcomes. In addition, client satisfaction is positively associated with the degree of client involvement in the collaborative design and implementation of health care plans (Daily Mock, 2001; Green et al., 2008).

This is true even when the collaboration involves end-of-life care. A hematologist-oncologist said: "A patient may relapse and die of his disease. But, in the effort that he and I both put into this as partners in fighting his disease, there's a great solace. . . . I hope to do my very best in helping him die with ease" (Kearney, Weininger, Vachon, Harrison, & Mount, 2009, p. 1158).

Health practitioners agree that care plans should be client centred and established and managed in collaboration with clients and all of their care providers (Baker, Marshak, Rice, & Zimmerman, 2001; Randall & McEwen, 2000). In early intervention, for instance, transdisciplinary teams consist of the child's parents, along with professionals from a variety of disciplines (King et al., 2009; Rapport, McWilliams, & Smith, 2004). Ideas and expertise are shared among team members to evaluate and meet the needs of the child. Once the collaborative plan has been established, team members train each other to provide hands-on interventions. For example, a special education teacher may train the child's parents in behavioural techniques to obtain their child's attention and cooperation. An occupational therapist may instruct a special educator in the principles of positioning to facilitate the child's involvement in classroom activities that require upright sitting. Professional members of the team assume a consultative role, providing assistance to bring about changes in the care plan as needed. Active family involvement is central to the process, and this helps to ensure that a holistic approach is maintained.

Consider the case of Lisa Marie, a 2-year-old girl with a diagnosis of cerebral palsy. She has been treated by the same physical therapist (PT), occupational therapist (OT), and speech/language pathologist (SLP) since she came home from the neonatal intensive care unit. The individualised family service plan (IFSP) was coordinated by a case manager and involved Lisa Marie's parents and all health care professionals who would be involved in her care. Although only one member of the health care team can visit each month, collaborative planning occurs, involving all team members, especially the family. Occasional tension does exist between the practitioners and Lisa Marie's parents regarding what is "right" for her care, but this tension forces periodic reexamination of the goals and the progress being made.

Because family involvement is essential, team members have established bonds with Lisa Marie, her parents, and two older siblings. All family members have learned how they can help facilitate Lisa Marie's development. Her parents use effective handling skills, which were taught by the PT and OT. Her brother, Eric, helps position her in the seating system she uses for eating meals and participating in family activities. The SLP taught Eric to position Lisa Marie in a way that minimises the risk of aspiration when she is eating. Lindsay, Lisa Marie's sister, plays videogames with her, prerequisites for power-mobility training, which Lisa will begin once she makes the transition to her new school-based program next year.

Lisa Marie will soon be 3 years old, and the therapists have been helping prepare everyone for the transition to a public preschool program in the fall. She will be entering an innovative program, in which children with special needs are integrated with neighborhood children who have no identified special needs. Each of Lisa Marie's therapists has participated in the development of her individualised education plan (IEP). In addition to submitting written reports of all aspects of Lisa Marie's life, they also participated in a team meeting with the family and school-based personnel. Her services must be linked to educational goals, so part of the work of both teams of professionals has been to help the family understand which services would be "appropriate."

Barriers to collaboration

Chinman and colleagues (1999) conducted a needs assessment in a large mental health clinic to determine the levels of interest and willingness of both clients and providers to participate in collaborative treatment planning. They identified the most significant barriers to collaboration as clients' disabilities, nonadherence, and clients' lack of interest in collaboration. Conversely, clients perceived the main barriers as providers' lack of time, uncertainty that treatment goals would be helpful, and inadequate knowledge about how to collaborate in treatment planning. The researchers suggested two additional reasons why some practitioners fail to provide this opportunity. First, they must relinquish some power in the relationship if they are going to empower clients. Second, they feel that *they* know what is best for their clients. For collaborative treatment planning to be successful, practitioners need to provide clients with opportunities for participation and may need to educate them in the actual techniques of collaborative planning.

Another potential barrier to collaboration is failure to take clients' premorbid lifestyle and history into account, except in a very superficial way. Clients may feel "stripped" of their previous identity. Their former lifestyle may seem somewhat irrelevant in light of significantly altered physical or cognitive function. On the other hand, when important aspects of the premorbid lifestyle are considered, motivating factors can be identified and used to develop an effective treatment plan.

Consider the case of Jenny, whose story of successful recovery from traumatic brain injury was summarised by Price-Lackey and Cashman (1996). Hers was actually a story of self-recovery. When the therapists involved in her rehabilitation failed to capture and incorporate Jenny's life history, she became frustrated, discharged herself from her residential treatment program, and struggled to develop her own, eventually successful program. Had the therapists fully examined Jenny's history, they would have discovered that she had always been remarkably independent and self-disciplined. She sought out progressively greater challenges and worked diligently until she mastered them. Throughout her life, Jenny reframed adverse situations, enabling her to view potentially negative experiences as opportunities for change and growth and strive for completion in the face of adversity. She eventually incorporated these skills into her self-directed therapy, which she described as a long and lonely process. Counselling that emphasised cognitive restructuring would have been extremely helpful to Jenny in the early stages of recovery, but failure to identify this important aspect of her history prevented this from happening.

Clients conceptualise their needs in terms of the functional abilities and resources needed to help them return to their premorbid lifestyles. Therefore, providers need to conceptualise clients in terms of more than diagnoses and symptoms that must be matched with appropriate treatment options. Coordination and integration of both perspectives through effective collaboration are beneficial.

Strategies for improving collaboration

Asking clients to identify the biggest problems they are facing in managing their illness may provide the basis for improved collaboration. Consider the following example:

> I tried something new with my patients this month. About one week prior to each client's appointment, I sent out a brief questionnaire. Clients were asked to answer a few basic, open-ended questions before coming in for their visits. The questions addressed concerns or problems they might be experiencing with their health or lifestyle. I was amazed at the results. I had expected the majority would respond, but every one of my clients did! The other expectation I had was that this simple reflection would help focus our sessions. It did, but other benefits occurred, too. Patients reported feeling more relaxed during the visit because they knew all their concerns would be addressed. One of my clients suggested that I add a section to record my answers to concerns discussed during the visit. They'll be given a copy of this to take home.
>
> —*From the journal of Cathy Smith-Peterson, nurse practitioner student*

In addition to asking clients to identify questions or problems, it may be helpful to ask them other pointed questions at various intervals in the treatment process. For example, they could be asked to define their own role in maintaining and improving their health, how they perceive the role of the health care professional, and how they define concepts, such as help, therapy, rehabilitation, goals, and outcomes. This type of discussion not only provides baseline information about client beliefs, it can also provide an opportunity to clarify any confusion the client may be experiencing (von Korff et al., 1997).

As discussed earlier, client education is an essential element of health care. In addition to information about a specific illness or disability, some clients may have to learn how to be more active participants in goal setting and taking charge of their health. This might require instruction in helpful concepts and terminology (Daily Mock, 2001). By modeling the process of evaluation and task analysis and communicating in terms that clients can easily understand, health providers can help their clients learn how to independently solve functional problems. For example, if a client tends to identify problems in broad-based terms such as "I want to be able to provide for my family," you may need to help him or her reframe the problem in terms of specific functions. This will facilitate achievement of the ultimate goal of every health plan—independent health care management.

It is important for providers to identify clients' health beliefs, values, and practices because these can be key determinants of motivation and behaviour. For example, if a client believes that herbal supplements offer more benefit than the insulin that has been prescribed as a treatment for diabetes, a change in this belief must be encouraged before a successful outcome can be achieved.

Forms designed to guide treatment planning tend to include information required by payers but may be relatively void of prompts to record client beliefs, strengths, resources, hopes, dreams, and practical needs. Including this information on these forms can enhance collaborative care by providing data of value to the entire health care team.

[A]Drench, M. E., Noonan, A. C., Sharby, N., & Ventura, S. H. (2012). Motivation, adherence and collaborative treatment planning. In M. E. Drench, A. C. Noonan, N. Sharby, & S. H. Ventura (Eds.), *Pyschosocial aspects of health care* (3rd ed., pp. 114–141). Upper Saddle River, NJ: Pearson Education.

Summary

This chapter discussed the theoretical concepts related to motivation and adherence, including locus of control, self-efficacy, self-esteem, and the role of important social determinants of health. Strategies to enhance motivation and adherence involved understanding the importance of shared goal setting; developing realistic and functional goals and treatment plans that are relevant, meaningful, and mutually valued by both the clients and the health provider; ensuring that clients understand instructions; developing and adjusting educational programs to meet clients' learning styles; and providing clients with positive feedback. In addition, methods to help clients adjust goals to effectively deal with chronic illness and impairments were presented. Barriers to motivation were discussed, and principles of behaviour theory, which may be helpful in modifying health behaviours, were reviewed.

The concept of collaboration was discussed from both client and provider perspectives, and common barriers to collaborative planning were identified. When working with clients, we need to remember that many feel a loss of control as a result of illness or injury. We can empower them by facilitating a move toward independent management of their care. Even if complete independence of a task is not possible, many people are able to direct aides, nurses, therapists, and others to assist in a way that is comfortable for the clients. Regaining control of even small tasks can provide motivation to adhere to established programs so that long-range goals can be realised.[A]

Review questions

A. Fill in the missing words to complete the following statements.

1. Non-adherence to medication, lack of trust in the working relationships with medical practitioners, financial issues, limited interest and emotional distress are all examples of ____________________________.
2. In the _________________________ stage of change, an individual has no desire to change and does not see their issue as problematic. Whereas, clients are generally considering change and weighing up of the con's and pro's of changing in the ________________ stage of change.
3. In the _________________________ stage of change, clients typically begin to see the 'cons' of changing as outweighing the 'pros'. Clients might be taking some small steps towards changing behaviour. While others decide to not yet do anything about their behaviour.
4. In the __________________ stage of change, clients are actively taking steps to change their behaviour and making great steps towards significant change. They may try several different techniques to assist in their change process. Additionally, individuals are at the greatest risk of relapse in this stage.
5. Clients are able to successfully manage any temptations and are able to employ new ways of coping. They may have a temporary slip (or lapse), but don't tend to see this as failure. This is known as being in the _______________________ stage of change.

B. Please select one statement that best answers each of the following questions.

6. Identify the stage of change for the following case scenario. Nadia is a 24-year-old female who is engaging in a drug and alcohol program. She has a lengthy history of poly-drug use. Nadia has been trying to stay off cocaine and speed while in rehab. She continues to drink heavily a couple of times a week and also takes benzos as she says this helps her to sleep. Nadia's latest urinalysis reveals cannabis and benzodiazepines. She is concerned that she will be exited from the Drug Program and she states she really wants to stay out of trouble.
   a) pre-contemplation
   b) contemplation
   c) preparation
   d) action
7. Which of the following statements is FALSE?
   a) locus of control is dynamic
   b) locus of control can shift
   c) individuals with internal locus of control are typically more successful than those with an external locus of control
   d) none of the above
8. Which of the following statements defines self-efficacy?
   a) describes how a personal feels about themselves
   b) describes an individual's belief related to their ability to successfully cope with a particular task or situation.
   c) describes an individual's motivation to participate in treatment
   d) all of the above

9. There are many behaviour change models used to increase client motivation and adherence to various treatments in order to facilitate change. According to the Health Belief Model, which statement/s are representative of the model when trying to change health-related behaviours?
   a) focuses on the individual's motivation and ambivalence
   b) is based on the individual's subjective personal beliefs
   c) in order for people to change behaviour, they must be ready to make a change
   d) both b and c

10. The transtheoretical model or the stages of change model consists of six stages. These stages include:
   a) preparation, pre-contemplation, contemplation, action, maintenance and termination
   b) preparation, contemplation, pre-contemplation, maintenance , action and termination
   c) pre-contemplation, contemplation preparation, action, maintenance and termination
   d) action, pre-contemplation, preparation, contemplation, maintenance and termination

11. The five A's behavioural intervention protocol involves which of the following processes?
   a) address the issue, assess the client, advise the client and arrange for a follow-up
   b) assess the client, address the issue, advise the client and arrange for a follow-up
   c) meet the client, assess the client, address the issue, advise the client and arrange for a follow-up
   d) none of the above

12. Motivational interviewing was developed by Miller and Rollnick (1995) and is a widely used approach in public health, psychology and medicine in terms of behaviour change. Which of the following is correct in regards to motivational interviewing?
   a) it was initially used as a treatment for drug and alcohol clients
   b) it is a client-centered approach
   c) the main goal is to facilitate client empowerment by collaborating with the client to develop a sense of autonomy
   d) all of the above

13. In motivational interviewing, helping a client develop awareness of the inconsistencies between their present self, goals and values is called:
   a) expressing empathy
   b) developing discrepancy
   c) rolling with resistance
   d) supporting self efficacy

14. In motivational interviewing, rather than arguing, coercing and persuading your client, the aim is to empower the client and elicit their own motivation to change. This is called:
   a) expressing empathy
   b) developing discrepancy
   c) rolling with resistance
   d) supporting self efficacy

CHAPTER 9

Social Psychology

The content in this section has been compiled from:

Vaughan & Hogg, Chapter 2

Vaughan, M. G., & Hogg, M. A. (2014). Social cognition and social thinking. In Social psychology (7th ed., pp. 38–43, 45–46, 56–69). Frenchs Forest, NSW: Pearson Australia.

Vaughan & Hogg, Chapter 3

Vaughan, M. G., & Hogg, M. A. (2014). Attribution and social explanation. In Social psychology (7th ed., pp. 74–78, 80–99). Frenchs Forest, NSW: Pearson Australia.

Vaughan & Hogg, Chapter 5

Vaughan, M. G., & Hogg, M. A. (2014). Attitudes. In Social psychology (7th ed., pp. 136–155, 159–163). Frenchs Forest, NSW: Pearson Australia.

Vaughan & Hogg, Chapter 6

Vaughan, M. G., & Hogg, M. A. (2014). Persuasion and attitude change. In Social psychology (7th ed., pp. 174–209). Frenchs Forest, NSW: Pearson Australia.

Vaughan & Hogg, Chapter 7

Vaughan, M. G., & Hogg, M. A. (2014). Social Influence. In Social psychology (7th ed., pp. 214–233). Frenchs Forest, NSW: Pearson Australia.

Vaughan & Hogg, Chapter 9

Vaughan, M. G., & Hogg, M. A. (2014). Leadership and decision making. In Social psychology (7th ed., pp. 312–313). Frenchs Forest, NSW: Pearson Australia.

CHAPTER 9

Social Psychology

Social psychology is the study of how people influence others' behaviour, beliefs and attitudes. As we have seen in earlier chapters, knowledge of psychological concepts can be relevant to the maintenance of health, the prevention of illness, and/or the adjustment to illness. Social psychology makes an important contribution to individual determinants of health, because lifestyles are likely to be determined by health attitudes and health beliefs. Clearly clients' and patients' health related attitudes and beliefs contribute to individual differences in their responses to health maintenance behaviours. This chapter discusses the integral tenets of social psychology (e.g. attributions, attitudes and compliance) and examines the role such concepts play in not only health care settings (e.g., compliance with medical procedures), but also our everyday lives. We explore the interaction between our view of self and others, types of social influence (e.g. obedience), and how groups, or the people with whom we interact, affect our decision making processes.

After studying this chapter you should be able to:

- Define social psychology
- Identify and describe social schemas and categories
- Describe social encoding
- Describe social inference
- Describe how people seek the causes of behaviour (attribution)
- Describe attribution theory and the process of attributing behaviour
- Identify and describe biases in attribution
- Identify and describe the function of attitudes and how they predict behaviour
- Describe persuasive communication
- Describe compliance and conformity
- Describe cognitive dissonance and attitude change
- Describe types of social influence.

Cognitive development

Social psychology studies 'how human thought, feeling and behaviour is influenced by and has influence on other people'. Within this broad definition, thought has occupied a pivotal role: people think about their social world, and on the basis of thought they act in certain ways. Psychologists use another term in their treatment of our thinking processes. While thought and cognition are often used interchangeably in popular language, there are some differences in emphasis made within psychology. *Thought* is very much the internal language and symbols we use. It is often conscious, or at least something we are or could be aware of. The term *cognition* has another connotation since it also refers to mental processing that can be largely automatic. We are unaware of it and only with some effort notice it, let alone characterise it in language or shared symbols. In this sense, cognition acts like a computer program: it operates in the background, running all the functions of the computer that we are aware of.

Cognition and thought occur within the human mind. They are the mental activities that mediate between the world out there and what people subsequently do. Their operation can be inferred from what people do and say—from people's actions, expressions, sayings and writings. If we can understand cognition, we may gain some understanding of how and why people behave the way they do. **Social cognition** is an approach in social psychology that focuses on how cognition is affected by wider and more immediate social contexts and on how cognition affects our social behaviour.

Social cognition
Cognitive processes and structures that influence and are influenced by social behaviour.

During the 1980s there was an explosion in social cognition research. According to Taylor (1998), during social cognition's heyday 85 percent of submissions to the *Journal of Personality and Social Psychology,* social psychology's flagship journal, were social cognition articles. Social cognition remains healthy and vibrant as the dominant perspective on the explanation of social behaviour (e.g. Dijksterhuis, 2010; Fiske & Taylor, 2008; Macrae & Quadflieg, 2010; Moskowitz, 2005). It has taught us much about how we process and store information about people, and how this information affects the way we perceive and interact with others. It has also taught us new methods and techniques for conducting social psychological research—methods and techniques borrowed from cognitive psychology, and more recently neuroscience, and then refined for social psychology. Social cognition has had, and continues to have, an enormous impact on social psychology (Devine, Hamilton & Ostrom, 1994).

A short history of cognition in social psychology

Wilhelm Wundt (1897) was one of the founders of modern empirical psychology. He used self-observation and introspection to gain an understanding of cognition (people's subjective experience), which he believed to be the main purpose of psychology. This methodology became unpopular because it was not scientific. Data and theories were idiosyncratic, and because they were effectively autobiographical they were almost impossible to refute or generalise.

Because psychologists felt that theories should be based on publicly observable and replicable data, there was a shift away from studying internal (cognitive) events towards external, publicly observable events. The ultimate expression of this change in emphasis was American **behaviourism** of the early 20th century (e.g. Skinner, 1963; Thorndike, 1940; Watson, 1930)—cognition became a dirty word in psychology for almost half a century. Behaviourists focused on overt behaviour (e.g. a hand wave) as a response to observable stimuli in the environment (e.g. an approaching bus), based on past punishments and rewards for the behaviour (e.g. being picked up by the bus).

Behaviourism
An emphasis on explaining observable behaviour in terms of reinforcement schedules.

By the 1960s, psychologists had begun to take a fresh interest in cognition. This was partly because behaviourism seemed terribly cumbersome and inadequate as an explanation of human language and communication (see Chomsky, 1959); some consideration of how people represent the world symbolically and how they manipulate such symbols was needed. Moreover, the manipulation and transfer of information was beginning to dominate the world: information processing became an increasingly important focus for psychology (Broadbent, 1985; Wyer & Gruenfeld, 1995). This development continued with the computer revolution, which has encouraged and enabled psychologists to model or simulate highly complex human cognitive processes. The computer has also become a metaphor for the human mind, with computer software/programs standing in for cognition. Cognitive psychology, sometimes called cognitive science, re-emerged as a legitimate scientific pursuit (e.g. Anderson, 1990; Neisser, 1967).

In contrast to general psychology, social psychology has almost always been strongly cognitive (Manis, 1977; Zajonc, 1980). This emphasis can be traced at least as far back as Lewin, who is often referred to as the father of experimental social psychology. Drawing on **Gestalt psychology**, Kurt Lewin (1951) believed that social behaviour is most usefully understood as a function of people's perceptions of their world and of their manipulation of such perceptions. As such, cognition and thought are placed centre stage in social psychology. The cognitive emphasis in social psychology has had at least four guises (Jones, 1998; Taylor, 1998): cognitive consistency, naive scientist, cognitive miser and motivated tactician.

After the Second World War, in the 1940s and 1950s there was an enormous amount of research on attitude change. This produced a number of theories sharing an assumption that people strive for **cognitive consistency**: that is, people are motivated to reduce perceived discrepancies between their various cognitions because such discrepancies are aversive (e.g. Abelson et al., 1968; Festinger, 1957; Heider, 1958). Consistency theories gradually lost popularity in the 1960s as evidence accumulated that people are in fact remarkably tolerant of cognitive inconsistency.

In its place there arose in the early 1970s a **naive scientist** model, which characterised people as needing to attribute causes to behaviour and events in order to render the world a meaningful place in which to act. This model underpins the **attribution** theories of behaviour that dominated social psychology in the 1970s. The naive scientist model assumes that people are basically rational in making scientific-like cause–effect analyses. Any errors or biases that creep in are departures from normality that can be traced to limited or inaccurate information and to motivational considerations such as self-interest.

In the late 1970s, however, it became clear that even in ideal circumstances people are not very careful scientists at all. The 'normal' state of affairs is that people are limited in their capacity to process information, and take numerous cognitive shortcuts: they are **cognitive misers** (Nisbett & Ross, 1980; Taylor, 1981). The various errors and biases associated with social thinking are not motivated departures from some ideal form of information processing but are intrinsic to social thinking. Motivation is almost completely absent from the cognitive miser perspective. However, as this perspective has matured, the importance of motivation has again become evident (Gollwitzer & Bargh, 1996; Showers & Cantor, 1985)—the social thinker has become characterised as a **motivated tactician**:

> *a fully engaged thinker who has multiple cognitive strategies available and chooses among them based on goals, motives, and needs. Sometimes the motivated tactician chooses wisely, in the interests of adaptability and accuracy, and sometimes … defensively, in the interests of speed or self-esteem. (Fiske & Taylor, 1991, p. 13)*

The most recent development in social cognition is **social neuroscience**, sometimes called cognitive neuroscience or social cognitive neuroscience (Harmon-Jones & Winkielman, 2007; Lieberman, 2010). Social neuroscience is largely a methodology in which cognitive activity can be monitored by the use of functional magnetic resonance imaging (fMRI), which detects and localises electrical activity in the brain associated with cognitive activities

Gestalt psychology
Perspective in which the whole influences constituent parts rather than vice versa.

Cognitive consistency
A model of social cognition in which people try to reduce inconsistency among their cognitions, because they find inconsistency unpleasant.

Naive psychologist (or scientist)
Model of social cognition that characterises people as using rational, scientific-like, cause–effect analyses to understand their world.

Attribution
The process of assigning a cause to our own behaviour, and that of others.

Cognitive miser
A model of social cognition that characterises people as using the least complex and demanding cognitions that are able to produce generally adaptive behaviours.

Motivated tactician
A model of social cognition that characterises people as having multiple cognitive strategies available, from which they choose on the basis of personal goals, motives and needs.

Social neuroscience
Exploration of brain activity associated with social cognition and social psychological processes and phenomena.

or functions. In this way, different parts of the brain 'light up' when people are, for example, thinking positively or negatively about friends or strangers or social categories, or when they are attributing causality to different behaviours. Social neuroscience is now widely applied to social psychological phenomena—for example, interpersonal processes (Gardner, Gabriel & Diekman, 2000), attributional inference (Lieberman, Gaunt, Gilbert & Trope, 2002), prejudice and dehumanisation (Harris & Fiske, 2006), the experience of being socially excluded (Eisenberger, Lieberman & Williams, 2003) and even religious conviction (Inzlicht, McGregor, Hirsh & Nash, 2009).

Forming impressions of other people

We are very quick to use personality traits when we describe other people, even those we have just met (Gawronski, 2003). People spend an enormous amount of time thinking about other people. We form impressions of the people we meet, have described to us or encounter in the media. We communicate these impressions to others, and we use them as bases for deciding how we will feel and act. Impression formation and person perception are important aspects of social cognition (Schneider, Hastorf & Ellsworth, 1979). However, the impressions we form are influenced by some bits of information more than others.

Which impressions are important?

Configural model
Asch's Gestalt-based model of impression formation, in which central traits play a disproportionate role in configuring the final impression.

Central traits
Traits that have a disproportionate influence on the configuration of final impressions, in Asch's configural model of impression formation.

Peripheral traits
Traits that have an insignificant influence on the configuration of final impressions, in Asch's configural model of impression formation.

According to Solomon Asch's (1946) **configural model**, in forming first impressions we latch on to certain pieces of information, called **central traits**, which have a disproportionate influence over the final impression. Other pieces of information, called **peripheral traits**, have much less influence. Central and peripheral traits are ones that are more or less intrinsically correlated with other traits, and therefore more or less useful in constructing an integrated impression of a person. Central traits influence the meanings of other traits and the perceived relationship among traits: that is, they are responsible for the integrated configuration of the impression.

To investigate this idea, Asch had students read one of two lists of seven adjectives describing a hypothetical person (see Figure 9.1). The lists differed only slightly—one contained the word *warm* and the other the word *cold*. Participants then evaluated the target person on a number of other bipolar evaluative dimensions, such as generous/ungenerous, happy/unhappy, reliable/unreliable. Asch found that participants exposed to the list containing *warm* generated a much more favourable impression of the target than did those exposed to the list containing the trait *cold*. When the words *warm* and *cold* were replaced by *polite* and *blunt*, the difference in impression was far less marked. Asch argued that warm/cold is a central trait dimension that has more influence on impression formation than polite/blunt, which is a peripheral trait dimension. Subsequent research has confirmed that warmth is indeed a fundamental dimension of social perception and impression formation (Fiske, Cuddy & Glick, 2007; Kervyn, Yzerbyt & Judd, 2010). Warmth is also closely connected to how a person can become attached to another (Williams & Bargh, 2008).

Asch's experiment was replicated in a naturalistic setting by Kelley (1950), who ended his introduction of a guest lecturer to students with: 'People who know him consider him to be a rather *cold* [or very *warm*] person, *industrious*, *critical*, *practical* and *determined*.' The lecturer gave identical lectures to a number of classes, half of which received the *cold* and half the *warm* description. After the lecture, the students rated the lecturer on a number of dimensions. Those who received the *cold* trait rated the lecturer as more *unsociable*, *self-centred*, *unpopular*, *formal*, *irritable*, *humourless* and *ruthless*. They were also less likely to ask questions and to interact with the lecturer. This seems to support the Gestalt view that impressions are formed as integrated wholes based on central cues.

However, critics have wondered how people decide that a trait is central. Gestalt theorists believe that the centrality of a trait rests on its intrinsic degree of correlation with other traits. Others have argued that centrality is a function of context (e.g. Wishner, 1960; Zanna & Hamilton, 1972). In Asch's experiment, warm/cold was central because it was distinct from the other trait dimensions and was semantically linked to the response dimensions. People tend to employ two main and distinct dimensions for evaluating other people: good/bad social, and good/bad intellectual (Rosenberg, Nelson & Vivekanathan, 1968), or what Fiske and colleagues call warmth and competence (Fiske, Cuddy & Glick, 2007). Warm/cold is clearly good/bad social, and so are the traits that were used to evaluate the impression (*generous, wise, happy, good-natured, reliable*). However, the other cue traits (*intelligent, skilful, industrious, determined, practical, cautious*) are clearly good/bad intellectual.

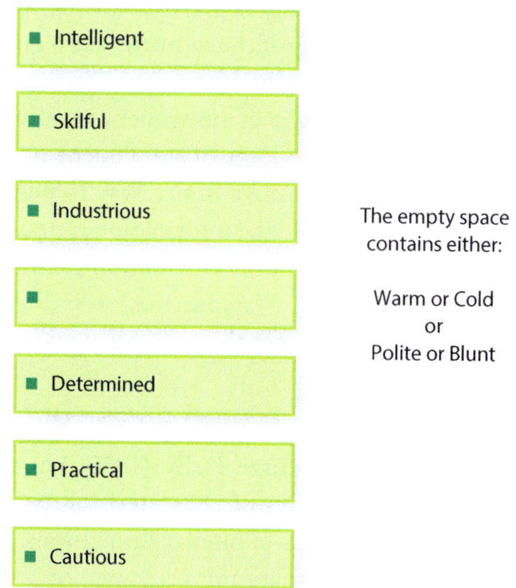

% assigning additional traits as function of focal trait inserted:

Additional traits	Focal traits inserted in the list			
	Warm	Cold	Polite	Blunt
Generous	91	8	56	58
Wise	65	25	30	50
Happy	90	34	75	65
Good-natured	94	17	87	56
Reliable	94	99	95	100

Figure 9.1 Impressions of a hypothetical person, based on central and peripheral traits

Asch (1946) presented participants with a seven-trait description of a hypothetical person in which either the word *warm* or *cold*, or *polite* or *blunt* appeared. The percentage of participants assigning other traits to the target was markedly affected when *warm* was replaced by *cold*, but not when *polite* was replaced by *blunt*

(**Source:** based on Asch (1946))

Biases in forming impressions

Primacy and recency

The order in which information about a person is presented can have profound effects on the subsequent impression. Asch (1946), in another experiment, used six traits to describe a hypothetical person. For half the participants, the person was described as *intelligent, industrious, impulsive, critical, stubborn, envious* (i.e. positive traits first, negative traits last). The order of presentation was reversed for the other group of participants. Asch found a **primacy** effect: the traits presented first disproportionately influenced the final impression, so that the person was evaluated more favourably when positive information was presented first than when negative information was presented first. Perhaps early information acts much like central cues, or perhaps people simply pay more attention to earlier information.

A **recency** effect can emerge where later information has more impact than earlier information. This might happen when you are distracted (e.g. overworked, bombarded with stimuli, tired) or when you have little motivation to attend to someone. Later, when you learn, for example, that you may have to work with this person, you may attend more carefully to cues. All other things being equal, however, primacy effects are more common (Jones & Goethals, 1972), with the clear implication that first impressions do indeed matter.

Primacy
An order of presentation effect in which earlier presented information has a disproportionate influence on social cognition.

Recency
An order of presentation effect in which later presented information has a disproportionate influence on social cognition.

Positivity and negativity

Research indicates that, in the absence of information to the contrary, people tend to assume the best of others and form a positive impression (Sears, 1983). However, if there is any negative information, this tends to attract our attention and assume disproportionate significance in the subsequent impression—we are biased towards negativity (Fiske, 1980). Furthermore, once formed, a negative impression is much more difficult to change in the light of subsequent positive information than is a positive impression likely to change in the light of subsequent negative information (e.g. Hamilton & Zanna, 1974). We may be sensitive in this way to negative information for two reasons:

1 The information is unusual and distinctive—unusual, distinctive or extreme information attracts attention (Skowronski & Carlston, 1989).
2 The information indirectly signifies potential danger, so its detection has survival value for the individual and ultimately the species.

Personal constructs and implicit personality theories

Personal constructs Idiosyncratic and personal ways of characterising other people.

Implicit personality theories Idiosyncratic and personal ways of characterising other people and explaining their behaviour.

George Kelly (1955) has suggested that individuals can develop their own idiosyncratic ways of characterising people. These **personal constructs** can, for simplicity, be treated as sets of bipolar dimensions. For example, I might consider *humour* the single most important organising principle for forming impressions of people, while you might prefer *intelligence*. We have different personal construct systems and would be likely to form different impressions of the same person. Personal constructs develop over time as adaptive forms of person perception and so are resistant to change.

We also tend to develop our own **implicit personality theories** (Bruner & Tagiuri, 1954; Schneider, 1973; Sedikides & Anderson, 1994), *lay theories of personality* (Plaks, Levy & Dweck, 2009), or *philosophies of human nature* (Wrightsman, 1964). These are general principles concerning what sorts of characteristics go together to form certain types of personality. For instance, Rosenberg and Sedlak (1972) found that people assumed that intelligent people are also friendly but not self-centred. Implicit personality theories are widely shared within cultures but differ between cultures (Markus, Kitayama & Heiman, 1996). Like personal constructs, they are resistant to change, and can be idiosyncratically based on personal experiences (Smith & Zárate, 1992).

Physical appearance counts

Although we would probably like to believe that we are way too sophisticated to be swayed in our impressions by mere physical appearance, research suggests this is not so. Because appearance is often the first information we have about people, it is very influential in first impressions; and, as we have seen above, primacy effects are influential in enduring impressions (Park, 1986). This is not necessarily always a bad thing—according to Zebrowitz and Collins (1997), appearance-based impressions can be surprisingly accurate. One of the most immediate appearance-based judgements we make is whether we find someone physically attractive or not. Research confirms that we tend to assume that physically attractive people are 'good' (Dion, Berscheid & Walster, 1972)—they are interesting, warm, outgoing, socially skilled and have what the German poet Friedrich Schiller (1882) called an 'interior beauty, a spiritual and moral beauty'.

Physical attractiveness has a marked impact on affiliation, attraction and love, but can also affect people's careers. For example, in the United States where being taller, for men, is generally considered attractive, Knapp (1978) also found that professional men taller than 1.88 m received 10 percent higher starting salaries than men under 1.83 m. In another study, Heilman and Stopeck (1985) found that attractive male executives were considered more able than less attractive male executives. Interestingly, attractive female executives were considered less able than less attractive female executives; participants suspected that attractive females had been promoted because of their appearance, not their ability.

Stereotypes

Impressions of people are also strongly influenced by widely shared assumptions about the personalities, attitudes and behaviours of people based on group membership: for example, ethnicity, nationality, gender, race and class. These are **stereotypes**. One of the salient characteristics of people we first meet is their category membership (e.g. ethnicity), and this tends to engage a stereotype-consistent impression. Haire and Grune (1950) found that people had little difficulty composing a paragraph describing a 'working man' from stereotype-consistent information, but enormous difficulty incorporating one piece of stereotype-inconsistent information—that the man was *intelligent*. Participants ignored the information, distorted it, took a very long time and even promoted the man from worker to supervisor.

Stereotype
Widely shared and simplified evaluative image of a social group and its members.

Social judgeability

People form impressions to make judgements about other people: whether they are mean, friendly, intelligent or helpful. Research by Leyens and Yzerbyt and their colleagues suggests that people are unlikely to form impressions and make judgements if the target is deemed not to be **socially judgeable** in the specific context: that is, if there are social rules (norms, conventions, laws) that proscribe making judgements (Leyens, Yzerbyt & Schadron, 1992; Yzerbyt, Leyens & Schadron, 1997; Yzerbyt, Schadron, Leyens & Rocher, 1994). However, if the target is deemed to be socially judgeable, then judgements are more polarised and are made with greater confidence the more socially judgeable the target is considered to be. One implication is that people will not make stereotype-based judgements if conventions or legislation proscribe such behaviour as 'politically incorrect', but will readily do so if conventions encourage and legitimise such behaviour.[A]

Social judgeability
Perception of whether it is socially acceptable to judge a specific target.

Social schemas and categories

A **schema** is a 'cognitive structure that represents knowledge about a concept or type of stimulus, including its attributes and the relations among those attributes' (Fiske & Taylor, 1991, p. 98). It is a set of interrelated cognitions (e.g. thoughts, beliefs, attitudes) that allows us quickly to make sense of a person, situation, event or place on the basis of limited information. Certain cues activate a schema. The schema then 'fills in' missing details.

Schema
Cognitive structure that represents knowledge about a concept or type of stimulus, including its attributes and the relations among those attributes.

For example, imagine you are visiting Paris. Most of us have a place schema about Paris, a rich repertoire of prior knowledge about what one does when in Paris—sauntering along boulevards, sitting in parks, sipping coffee at pavement cafés, browsing through bookshops, or eating at restaurants. The reality of life in Paris is more diverse, yet this schema helps to interpret events and guide choices about how to behave. While in Paris you might visit a restaurant. Arrival at a restaurant might invoke a 'restaurant schema', which is a set of assumptions about what ought to take place (e.g. someone ushers you to a table, you study the menu, someone takes your order, you eat, talk and drink, you pay the bill, you leave). An event schema such as this is called a **script** (see below). While at the restaurant, your waiter may have a rather unusual accent that identifies him as English—this would engage a whole set of assumptions about his attitudes and behaviour. A schema about a social group, particularly if it is widely shared, is a stereotype.

Script
A schema about an event.

[A]Vaughan, M. G., & Hogg, M. A. (2014). Social cognition and social thinking. In *Social psychology* (7th ed., pp. 38–43). Frenchs Forest, NSW: Pearson Australia.

Once invoked, schemas facilitate top–down, concept-driven or theory-driven processing, as opposed to bottom–up or data-driven processing (Rumelhart & Ortony, 1977). We tend to fill in gaps with prior knowledge and preconceptions, rather than seek information gleaned directly from the immediate context. The concept of cognitive schema first emerged in research by Bartlett (1932) on non-social memory, which focused on how memories are actively constructed and organised to facilitate understanding and behaviour. It also has a precedent in Asch's (1946) *configural model* of impression formation (discussed above), Heider's (1958) *balance theory* of person perception and, more generally, in Gestalt psychology (Brunswik, 1956; Koffka, 1935). These are all approaches in which simplified and holistic cognitive representations of the social world act as relatively enduring templates for the interpretation of stimuli and the planning of action.

The alternative to a schema approach is one in which perception is treated as an unfiltered, veridical representation of reality (e.g. Mill, 1869); impression formation is, as discussed above, the cognitive algebra of trait combination (e.g. Anderson, 1981); and memory is laid down passively through the repetitive association of stimuli (e.g. Ebbinghaus, 1885).

Types of schema

There are many types of schema; however, they all influence the encoding (internalisation and interpretation) of new information, memory of old information and inferences about missing information. The most common schemas, some of which have been used as examples above, are person schemas, role schemas, event schemas or scripts, content-free schemas and self-schemas.

Person schemas

Person schemas are individualised knowledge structures about specific people. For example, you may have a person schema about your best friend (e.g. that she is kind and intelligent but is silent in company and would rather frequent cafés than go mountain climbing), or about a specific politician, a well-known author or a next-door neighbour.

Role schemas

Role schemas are knowledge structures about role occupants: for example, airline pilots (they fly the plane and should not be seen swigging whisky in the cabin) and doctors (although often complete strangers, they are allowed to ask personal questions and get you to undress). Although role schemas can quite properly apply to **roles** (i.e. types of function or behaviour in a group), they can sometimes be better understood as schemas about social groups, in which case if such schemas are shared, they are, in effect, social stereotypes.

Roles
Patterns of behaviour that distinguish between different activities within the group, and that interrelate to one another for the greater good of the group.

Scripts

Schemas about events are generally called scripts (Abelson, 1981; Schank & Abelson, 1977). We have scripts for attending a lecture, going to the cinema, having a party, giving a presentation or eating out in a restaurant. For example, people who often go to football matches might have a very clear script for what happens both on and off the pitch. This makes the entire event meaningful. Imagine how you would fare if you had never been to a football match and had never heard of football. The lack of relevant scripts can often be a significant contributor to feelings of disorientation, frustration and lack of efficacy encountered by sojourners in foreign cultures.

Content-free schemas

Content-free schemas do not contain rich information about a specific category but rather a limited number of rules for processing information. Content-free schemas might specify that if you like John and John likes Tom, then in order to maintain balance you should also like Tom (see balance theory, Heider, 1958), or they might specify how to attribute a cause to someone's behaviour (e.g. Kelley's 1972a idea of causal schemata).

Self-schemas

Finally, people have schemas about themselves. They represent and store information about themselves in a similar but more complex and varied way than information about others. Self-schemas form part of people's concept of who they are, the self-concept.[B]

Social encoding

Social encoding refers to the process whereby external social stimuli are represented in the mind of the individual. There are at least four key stages (Bargh, 1984):

1 *Pre-attentive analysis*—an automatic and non-conscious scanning of the environment.
2 *Focal attention*—once noticed, stimuli are consciously identified and categorised.
3 *Comprehension*—stimuli are given meaning.
4 *Elaborative reasoning*—the stimulus is linked to other knowledge to allow for complex inferences.

Social encoding depends heavily on what captures our attention. In turn, attention is influenced by salience, vividness and accessibility.

Salience

Attention-capturing stimuli are salient stimuli. In social cognition, **salience** refers to the property of a stimulus that makes it stand out relative to other stimuli. Consider the second focus question. For example, a single male is salient in an all-female group but not salient in a gender-balanced group; a woman in the late stages of pregnancy is salient in most contexts except at the obstetrician's clinic; and someone wearing a bright T-shirt is salient at a funeral but not on the beach. Salience is 'out there'—a property of the stimulus domain. People can be salient because:

Salience
Property of a stimulus that makes it stand out in relation to other stimuli and attract attention.

- they are novel (single man, pregnant woman) or figural (bright T-shirt) in the immediate context (McArthur & Post, 1977)
- they are behaving in ways that do not fit prior expectations of them as individuals, as members of a particular social category or as people in general (Jones & McGillis, 1976), or
- they are important to your specific or more general goals, they dominate your visual field, or you have been told to pay attention to them (Erber & Fiske, 1984; Taylor & Fiske, 1975; see Figure 9.2).

Salient people attract attention and, relative to non-salient people, tend to be considered more influential in a group. They are also more personally responsible for their behaviour and less influenced by the situation, and they are generally evaluated more extremely (McArthur, 1981; Taylor & Fiske, 1978; see Figure 9.2). Because we attend more to salient people, they dominate our thoughts and, consequently, increase the coherence (i.e. organisation and consistency) of our impressions. People do not necessarily recall more about salient people;

[B]Vaughan, M. G., & Hogg, M. A. (2014). Social cognition and social thinking. In *Social psychology* (7th ed., pp. 45-46). Frenchs Forest, NSW: Pearson Australia.

Figure 9.2 Some antecedents and consequences of social salience

For social cognition, salience is mainly a property of the stimulus in relation to other stimuli in the social context. It has predictable consequences for perception, thought and behaviour

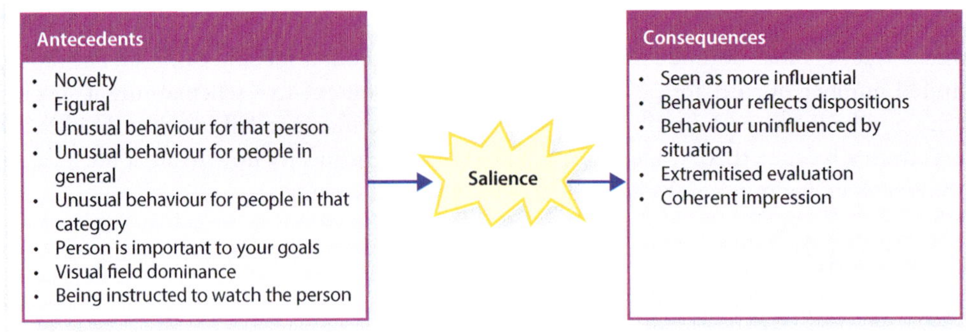

rather, they find it easier to access a coherent impression of the person. For example, imagine you generally do not like very tall men. If you now go to a party where one particularly tall man stands out, you may feel very negative about him and feel that he dominated conversation and was relatively uninfluenced by others. Although you will not necessarily recall much accurate information about his behaviour, you will have formed a fairly coherent impression of him as a person.

Vividness

Vividness An intrinsic property of a stimulus on its own that makes it stand out and attract attention.

Priming Activation of accessible categories or schemas in memory that influence how we process new information.

While salience is a property of the stimulus in relation to other stimuli in a particular context, **vividness** is an intrinsic property of the stimulus itself. Vivid stimuli are those that are:

- emotionally interesting (e.g. a violent crime)
- concrete and image-provoking (e.g. a gory and detailed description of a violent crime), or
- close to you in time and place (e.g. a violent crime committed yesterday in your street) (Nisbett & Ross, 1980).

Vivid stimuli ought to attract attention, just like salient stimuli, and ought therefore to have similar social cognitive effects. However, research has not confirmed this (Taylor & Thompson, 1982). Vividly presented information (e.g. through direct experience or colourful language accompanied by pictures or videos) may be more entertaining, though not more persuasive, than pallidly presented information. Apparent effects of vividness can often be attributed to other factors that co-occur with vividness. For example, vivid stimuli may convey more information, and thus it may be the information and not the vividness that influences social cognition.

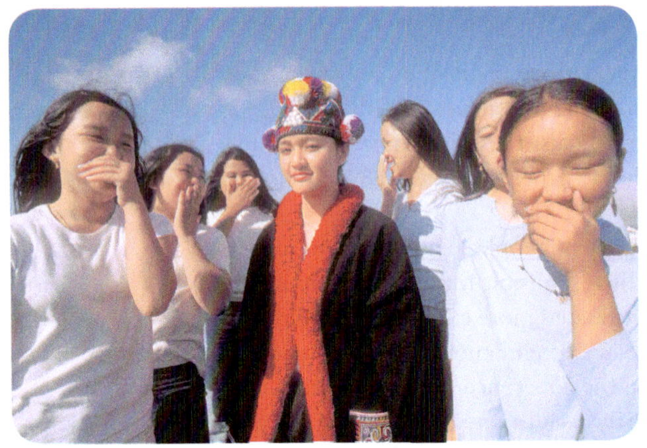

Standing out Salient stimuli capture our attention. This teenager is salient because she is, for a short time at least, in the minority (**Source:** © Francisco Villaflor/Alamy/Photolibrary.)

Accessibility

Attention is often directed not so much by stimulus properties 'out there' but by the accessibility, or ease of recall, of categories or schemas that we already have in our heads (Higgins, 1996). Accessible categories are readily and automatically **primed** by features of the stimulus domain to make sense of the intrinsically ambiguous nature of social information. They are categories that we often use, have recently used, and are consistent with current goals, needs and expectations (Bruner, 1957, 1958). For example, people who are very concerned about sex discrimination (i.e. it is an accessible category) may find that they see sexism almost everywhere: it is readily primed and used to interpret the social world. Some categories are chronically accessible; they are habitually primed in many contexts (Bargh, Lombardi & Higgins, 1988), and this can have pervasive effects. Bargh and Tota (1988) suggest that depression may be attributed in part to chronic accessibility of negative self-schemas.

Research on accessibility exposes people to cues that prime particular categories. This is done in such a way that people do not consciously detect the cue/category link. Participants then interpret ambiguous behaviour (Higgins, Bargh & Lombardi, 1985). Participants could be exposed to words such as *adventurous* or *reckless* and then be asked to interpret behaviour such as 'shooting rapids in a canoe'. The interpretation of the behaviour would be different depending on the category primed by the cue word. For example, studies in the United States have shown that racial categories can be primed by words relating to African Americans. Caucasian participants so primed interpreted ambiguous behaviour as being more hostile and aggressive, which is consistent with racial stereotypes (Devine, 1989).

Once primed, a category tends to encode stimuli by assimilating them into the primed category: that is, interpreting them in a *category-consistent* manner. This is particularly true of ambiguous stimuli. However, when people become aware that a category has been primed, they often contrast stimuli with the category: that is, they interpret them in a *category-incongruent* manner (Herr, Sherman & Fazio, 1983; Martin, 1986). For example, gender is often an accessible category that is readily primed and used to interpret behaviour (Stangor, 1988); but if you knew that gender had been primed, you might make a special effort to interpret behaviour in a non-sexist way.

Memory for people

Social behaviour depends very much on how we store information about other people: that is, on what we remember about other people (Fiske & Taylor, 2008; Martin & Clark, 1990; Ostrom, 1989). Social psychological approaches to person memory draw on cognitive psychological theories of memory and mainly adopt what is called an associative network or *propositional* model of memory (e.g. Anderson, 1990). The general idea is that we store *propositions* (e.g. 'The student reads the book', 'The book is a social psychology text', 'The student has a ponytail') that consist of nodes or ideas (e.g. book, ponytail, student, reads) that are linked by relationships between ideas. The links are *associative* in so far as nodes are associated with other nodes (e.g. *student* and *ponytail*), but some associative links are stronger than others. Links become strengthened the more they are activated by cognitive rehearsal (e.g. recalling or thinking about the propositions), and the more different links there are to a specific idea (i.e. alternative retrieval routes) the more likely it is to be recalled.

Recall is a process in which nodes become activated and the activation spreads to other nodes along established associative links: for example, the node *student* activates the node *ponytail* because there is a strong associative link. Finally, a distinction is made between *long-term memory*, which is the vast store of information that can potentially be brought to mind, and *short-term memory* (or working memory), which is the much smaller amount of information that you actually have in consciousness, and is the focus of your attention, at a specific time.

This sort of memory model has been applied to person memory. In terms of our general impression of someone, we are more likely to recall information that is inconsistent, rather than consistent, with our impression (Hastie, 1988; Srull & Wyer, 1989; Wyer & Carlston,

1994). This is because inconsistent information attracts attention and generates more cognition and thought, and this strengthens linkages and retrieval routes. However, better recall of inconsistent information does not occur when:

- we already have a well-established impression (Fiske & Neuberg, 1990)
- the inconsistency is purely descriptive and not evaluative (Wyer & Gordon, 1982)
- we are making a complex judgement (Bodenhausen & Lichtenstein, 1987)
- we have time afterwards to think about our impression (Wyer & Martin, 1986).

Contents of person memory

Consider your best friend for a moment. No doubt, an enormous amount of detail comes to mind—her likes and dislikes, her attitudes, beliefs and values, her personality traits, the things she does, what she looks like, what she wears, or where she usually goes. This array of information varies in terms of how concrete and directly observable it is: it ranges from appearance, which is concrete and directly observable, through behaviour, to traits that are not directly observable but are based on inference (Park, 1986). Cutting across this continuum is a general tendency for people to cluster together features that are positive and desirable and, separately, those that are negative and undesirable.

Most person-memory research concerns *traits*. Traits are stored in the usual propositional form ('Mary is mean and nasty') but are based on elaborate inferences from behaviour and situations. The inference process rests heavily on making causal attributions for people's behaviour. The storage of trait information appears to be organised with respect to two continua: social desirability (e.g. *warm*, *pleasant*, *friendly*) and competence (e.g. *intelligent*, *industrious*, *efficient*); see Fiske, Cuddy & Glick, 2007). Trait memories can be quite abstract and can colour more concrete memories of behaviour and appearance.

Behaviour is usually perceived as purposeful action, so memory for behaviour may be organised with respect to people's goals: the behaviour 'Michael runs to catch the bus' is stored in terms of Michael's goal to catch the bus. In this respect, behaviour, although more concrete and observable than traits, also involves some inference—inference of purpose (Hoffman, Mischel & Mazze, 1981).

Memory for *appearance* is usually based on directly observable concrete information ('Winston has long blond hair and an aquiline nose') and is stored as an analogue rather than a proposition. In other words, appearance is stored directly, like a picture in the mind, which retains all the original spatial information, rather than as a deconstructed set of propositions that have symbolic meaning. Laboratory studies reveal that we are phenomenally accurate at remembering faces: we can often recall faces with 100 percent accuracy over very long periods of time (Freides, 1974). However, we tend to be less accurate at recognising the faces of people who are of a different race from our own (Malpass & Kravitz, 1969). One explanation of this effect is that we simply pay less attention to, or process more superficially, outgroup faces (Devine & Malpass, 1985). Indeed, superficial encoding undermines memory for faces in general, and one remedy for poor memory for faces is simply to pay more attention (Wells & Turtle, 1988).

Different people witnessing the same event can see very different things, especially when the situation is fast-moving, confusing and frightening. Eyewitness testimony can be highly unreliable.

We are also remarkably inaccurate at remembering appearances in natural contexts where eyewitness testimony is required: for example, identifying or describing a stranger we saw commit a crime (Kassin, Ellsworth & Smith, 1989; Loftus, 1979). This is probably because witnesses or victims often do not get a good, clear look at the offender: the offence may be frightening, unexpected, confusing and over quickly, and the offender may only be glimpsed through a dirty car window or may wear a mask or some other disguise. More broadly, eyewitness testimony, even if confidently given, should be treated with caution (see Box 9.1). However, eyewitness testimony is more accurate if certain conditions are met (Shapiro & Penrod, 1986; see Box 9.2).

Organising person memory

In general, we remember people as a cluster of information about their traits, behaviour and appearance. However, we can also store information about people in a very different way. We can cluster people under attributes or groups. Social memory, therefore, can be organised by *person* or by *group* (Pryor & Ostrom, 1981; see Figure 9.3 on p. 408). In most settings, the preferred mode of organisation is by person, probably because it produces richer and more accurate person memories that are more easily recalled (Sedikides & Ostrom, 1988). (Recall that Julie and Rosa have different memories of Aaron in the third focus question.) Organisation by person is particularly likely when people are significant to us because they are familiar, real people with whom we expect to interact across many specific situations (Srull, 1983).

Research and applications 9.1

Eyewitness testimony is often highly unreliable

On 22 July 2005, two weeks after the 7 July London bombings and the day after the 21 July failed bombing, a Brazilian electrician who had been under surveillance by the police entered Stockwell tube station in London dressed in a bulky winter coat. It was a hot midsummer's day. Plain-clothes police followed him into the station and ordered him to stop. Instead, he ran—vaulting barriers and jumping on to a tube. The police brought him to the ground and shot him five times in the head. There were many witnesses—they gave very different accounts of what had happened. According to the *Guardian* (23 July 2005, p. 3) one eyewitness reported that the man had been pursued by three plain-clothes police, and that there were five shots; another reported 10 policemen armed with machine-guns and that there were six to eight shots; another reported shots from a 'silencer gun'; another reported 20 cops carrying big black guns; another reported that the man had a bomb belt with wires, and that there were two shots.

Research and applications 9.2

Factors that makes eyewitness testimony more accurate

Although eyewitness testimony is often unreliable, there are various ways to improve its accuracy.

The witness:

- mentally goes back over the scene of the crime to reinstate additional cues
- has already associated the person's face with other symbolic information
- was exposed to the person's face for a long time
- gave testimony a very short time after the crime
- is habitually attentive to the external environment
- generally forms vivid mental images.

The person:

- had a face that was not altered by disguise
- was younger that 30 years old
- looked dishonest.

Source: based on Shapiro & Penrod, 1986; Valentine, Pickering & Darling, 2003; Wells, Memon & Penrod, 2006

Figure 9.3 Person memory organised by person or by group

We can organise information about people in two quite different ways. We can cluster attributes under individual people, or we can cluster people under attributes or groups

(**Source:** based on Fiske & Taylor (1991))

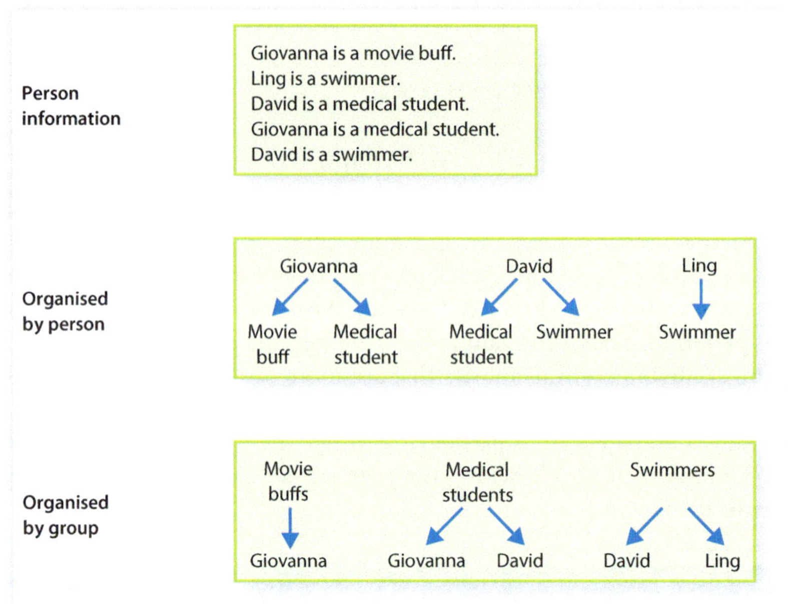

Organisation by group membership is likely in first encounters with strangers: the person is pigeonholed, described and stored in terms of stereotypical attributes of a salient social category (e.g. age, ethnicity, gender). Over time, the organisation may change to one based on the person. For example, your memory of a lecturer you have encountered only a few times lecturing on a topic you are not very interested in will most likely be organised in terms of the stereotypical properties of the group 'lecturers'. If you should get to know this person a little better, you might find that your memory gradually or suddenly becomes reorganised in terms of the lecturer as a distinct individual person.

There is an alternative perspective on the relationship between person-based and group-based person memory, and that is that they can coexist as essentially distinct forms of representation (Srull & Wyer, 1989; Wyer & Martin, 1986). These distinct forms of representation may be associated with different sorts of identity that people may have, based on either interpersonal relationships or group memberships. This idea is consistent with *social identity theory*, which is a theory of group behaviour as something quite distinct from interpersonal behaviour (e.g. Hogg & Abrams, 1988; Tajfel & Turner, 1979).

Person memory
How accurate might you be as a court witness giving detailed evidence about this crime scene?
(**Source:** © Ocean/ Corbis.)

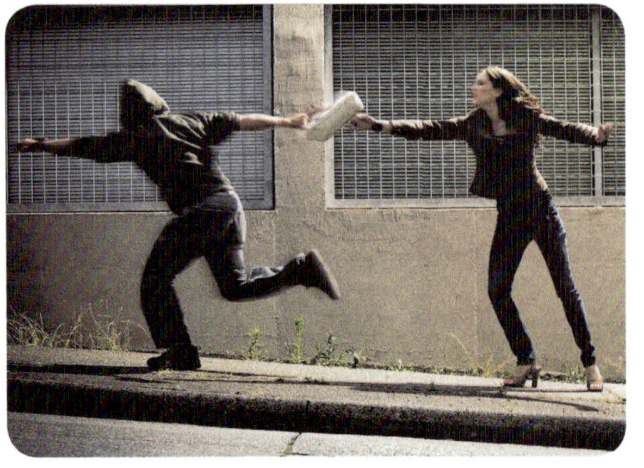

Using person memory

Presumably, in making social judgements we draw upon person memory. In fact, it appears that sometimes we do, but sometimes we do not. Hastie and Park (1986) integrated the findings from a large number of studies to conclude that, by default, people tend to form impressions of people *on-line*: that is, they rely disproportionately on incoming data, which are assimilated by schemas to produce an impression. There is little correlation between memory and judgement. It is more unusual for people to draw on memory and make *memory-based* judgements, but when they do there is a stronger correlation between memory and judgement. Whether people make on-

Research and applications 9.3

Goals and their effects on person memory

People's information processing and social interactive goals affect their memory for other people.

Goal	Effect
Comprehension	Limited memory
Memorising	Variable memory, organised in an *ad hoc* manner, often by psychologically irrelevant categories
Forming impressions	Good memory, organised by traits
Empathising	Good memory, organised by goals
Comparing with oneself	Excellent memory, organised by psychological categories (traits or goals)
Anticipated interaction	Excellent, well-organised memory, type of organisation not yet clear
Actual interaction	Variable memory, depending on concurrent goal

Source: based on Fiske & Taylor (1991)

line or memory-based judgements or impressions is influenced by people's goals and purposes in the interaction or judgement task.

The general principle is that recall of information about other people improves as the purpose of the interaction becomes more psychologically engaging and less superficial (Srull & Wyer, 1986, 1989; Wyer & Srull, 1986). Psychologically engaging interactions entail information processing at a deeper level that involves the elaboration of more complex and more varied links between elements and, consequently, a more integrated memory (Greenwald & Pratkanis, 1984). Paradoxically, then, instructing someone to memorise another person (psychologically not very engaging) will be less effective than asking someone to form an impression, which in turn will be less effective than asking someone to empathise. Box 9.3 shows a number of goals and how they affect person memory.

Social inference

Social inference is, in many respects, the core of social cognition. It addresses the inferential processes (which can be quite formal and abstract, or intuitive and concrete) that we use to identify, sample and combine information to form impressions and make judgements. There are two distinct ways in which we process social information: (a) we can rely automatically on general schemas or stereotypes in a top–down deductive fashion; or (b) we can deliberatively rely on specific instances in a bottom–up inductive fashion. This distinction is a theme that runs through social cognition, and it surfaces in different guises.

We have already discussed the distinction between Asch's configural model (impressions are based on holistic images) and Anderson's cognitive algebra model (impressions are based on integration of pieces of information) earlier. More recently, Brewer (1988, 1994) has proposed a dual-process model that contrasts relatively automatic category-based processing of social information with more deliberate and personalised attribute-based processing. Closely related is Fiske and Neuberg's (1990; Fiske & Dépret, 1996) continuum model, which makes a similar distinction between schema-based and data-based inferences. From research into attitudes come two other related distinctions (Eagly & Chaiken, 1993). Petty and Cacioppo's (1986b) elaboration–likelihood model distinguishes between *central route processing*, where people carefully and deliberately consider information, and *peripheral route processing*, where people make rapid top-of-the-head decisions based on stereotypes, schemas and other cognitive shortcuts. Almost identical is Chaiken's (Bohner, Moskowitz & Chaiken, 1995; Chaiken, Liberman & Eagly, 1989) heuristic–systematic model: people process information carefully and systematically, or they rather automatically rely on cognitive heuristics.

Normative models Ideal processes for making accurate social inferences.

Behavioural decision theory Set of normative models (ideal processes) for making accurate social inferences.

Generally, social cognition researchers have studied inferential processes in comparison with ideal processes, called **normative models**, which produce the best possible inferences. Collectively, these normative models are known as **behavioural decision theory** (Einhorn & Hogarth, 1981). The intuitive strategies of social inference involve a range of biases and errors, which produce suboptimal inferences—inferences that fall short of those dictated by the principles of behavioural decision theory (e.g. Fiske & Taylor, 2008; Nisbett & Ross, 1980).

Departures from normality

Gathering and sampling social information

The first stage in making an inference involves the gathering of data and the sampling of information from those data. In doing this, people tend to rely too heavily on schemas. This can cause them to overlook information that is potentially useful, or to exaggerate the importance of information that is misleading. For example, members of selection committees believe they are assessing candidates objectively on the basis of information provided by the candidate. However, what often happens is that person schemas are quickly, and often unconsciously, activated and used as the basis for candidate assessment. This reliance on person schemas is referred to as 'clinical judgement' and, although by no means all bad, it can produce suboptimal inferences and judgements (Dawes, Faust & Meehl, 1989).

People can also be unduly influenced by extreme examples and small samples (small samples are rarely representative of larger populations: this is called the *law of large numbers*); and they can be inattentive to biases in samples and to how typical a sample is of its population. For example, in Australia and New Zealand there is substantial media coverage of hate-speech by radical 'Islamists' who promote anti-Western violence and terrorism. From this, people may infer that Muslims in general behave like this. However, this inference is based on unrepresentative information (most mass media present extreme, not ordinary, cases) that portrays a small sample of atypical Muslims behaving in an extreme manner.

Regression

Regression Tendency for initial observations of instances from a category to be more extreme than subsequent observations.

Individual cases or instances are often more extreme than the average of the population from which they are drawn: over a number of cases or instances, there is a **regression** to the population mean. For example, a restaurant you have just visited for the first time may have been truly excellent, causing you to extol its virtues to all your friends. However, the next time you go it turns out to be mediocre. On the next visit, it is moderately good, and on the next fairly average. This is an example of regression. The restaurant is probably actually moderately good, but this would not become apparent from one visit: a number of visits would have to be made. The way to control for regression effects in forming impressions is to be conservative and cautious in making inferences from limited information (one or a few cases or instances). However, people tend not to do this: they are generally ignorant of regression, and do not control for it in forming impressions and making judgements (Kahneman & Tversky, 1973).

People can, however, be induced to make more conservative inferences if the initial information is made to seem less diagnostic by the presence of other information. For example, knowing that Hans shoots cats may generate an extreme and negative impression of him: shooting cats is relatively diagnostic of being a nasty person. However, if this piece of information is *diluted* (Nisbett, Zukier & Lemley, 1981) by other information that he is a committed conservationist who writes poetry, collects antiques, drives a hybrid and cares for his infirm mother, the impression is likely to become less extreme, because the tendency to use the diagnosis 'he shoots cats' is weakened.

Base-rate information

Base-rate information is general information, usually factual and statistical, about an entire class of events. For instance, if we knew that only 5 percent of university lecturers gave truly awful lectures, or that only 7 percent of social security recipients preferred being on the dole to working, this would be base-rate information. Research shows that people chronically under-use this information in making inferences, particularly when more concrete anecdotal case studies exist (Bar-Hillel, 1980; Taylor & Thompson, 1982). So, on the basis of vivid and colourful media exposés of dull lecturers or social security cheats, people would tend to infer that these are stereotypical properties of the parent categories, even if they have the relevant base-rate information to hand.

Base-rate information
General, factual, statistical information about an entire class of events.

The main reason that base-rate information is ignored is not so much that it is pallid and uninteresting in comparison with vivid individual instances, but rather that people often fail to see the relevance of base-rate information, relative to other information, to the inference task (Bar-Hillel, 1980). People increase their use of base-rate information when it is made clear that it is more relevant than other information (e.g. case studies) to the inferential task.

Covariation and illusory correlation

Judgements of covariation are judgements of how strongly two things are related. They are essential to social inference and form the very basis of schemas (schemas, as we saw above, are beliefs about the covariation of behaviour, attitudes or traits). To judge covariation accurately—for example, the relationship between hair colour and how much fun one has—we should consider the number of blondes having fun and not having fun, and the number of brunettes having fun and not having fun. The scientific method provides formal statistical procedures that we could use to assess covariation.

However, in making covariation judgements, people fall far short of normative prescriptions (Alloy & Tabachnik, 1984; Crocker, 1981). In general, this is because they are influenced by prior assumptions (i.e. schemas) and tend to search for or recognise only schema-consistent information: people are generally not interested in disconfirming their cherished schemas. So, in assessing the relationship between hair colour and fun, people may have available the social schema that 'blondes have more fun', and instances of blondes who have fun will come to mind much more readily than blondes who are having a miserable time or brunettes who are having a ball.

When people assume that a relationship exists between two variables, they tend to overestimate the degree of correlation or see a correlation where none actually exists. This phenomenon, called **illusory correlation**, was demonstrated by Chapman (1967), who presented students with lists of paired words such as *lion/tiger*, *lion/eggs*, *bacon/eggs*, *blossoms/notebook* and *notebook/tiger*. The students then had to recall how often each word was paired with each other word. Although every word was paired an equal number of times with every other word, participants overestimated meaningful pairings (e.g. *bacon/eggs*) and distinctive pairings (e.g. *blossoms/notebook*—words that were much longer than all the other words in the list).

Chapman reasoned that there are two bases for illusory correlation: **associative meaning** (items are seen as belonging together because they 'ought' to, on the basis of prior expectations) and **paired distinctiveness** (items are thought to go together because they share some unusual feature).

Illusory correlation
Cognitive exaggeration of the degree of co-occurrence of two stimuli or events, or the perception of a co-occurrence where none exists.

Associative meaning
Illusory correlation in which items are seen as belonging together because they 'ought' to, on the basis of prior expectations.

Paired distinctiveness
Illusory correlation in which items are seen as belonging together because they share some unusual feature.

Distinctiveness-based illusory correlation may help to explain stereotyping, particularly negative stereotypes of minority groups (Hamilton, 1979; Hamilton & Sherman, 1989; Mullen & Johnson, 1990). Hamilton and Gifford (1976) had participants recall statements describing two groups, A and B. There were twice as many statements about group A as there were about group B, and there were twice as many positive as negative statements about each group. Participants erroneously recalled that more negative statements (the less common statements) were paired with group B (the less common group). When the experiment was replicated but with more negative than positive statements, participants now overestimated the number of positive statements paired with group B.

In real life, negative events are distinctive, as they are perceived to be more rare than positive events (Parducci, 1968), and minority groups are distinctive, as people often have relatively few contacts with them. Thus, the conditions for distinctiveness-based illusory correlation are met. There is also evidence for an associative-meaning basis to negative stereotyping of minority groups: people have preconceptions that negative attributes go with minority groups (McArthur & Friedman, 1980).

Although illusory correlation may be involved in the formation and use of stereotypes, its role may be limited to conditions where people make memory-based rather than on-line judgements (McConnell, Sherman & Hamilton, 1994)—after all, they have to remember distinctiveness or associative information in order to make illusory correlations.

More radically, it can be argued that stereotypes are not 'illusory' at all. Rather, they are rational, even deliberate, constructs that differentiate ingroups from outgroups in ways that evaluatively favour the ingroup (Leyens, Yzerbyt & Schadron, 1994; McGarty, Haslam, Turner & Oakes, 1993; Oakes, Haslam & Turner, 1994). In this sense, stereotypical differences are functionally adaptive to the stereotyper—they are 'real'—and the process of stereotyping is one in which these differences are automatically (and strategically; for example, through rhetoric) accentuated as a consequence of categorising oneself as a member of one of the groups.

Heuristics

We have now seen how bad we are, in comparison with standards from behavioural decision theory, at making inferences. Perhaps the reason for this is that we have limited short-term memory available for on-line processing but enormous capacity for long-term memory—using the analogy of a computer, the former is RAM, random access memory, and the latter hard-drive capacity. It pays, then, to store information schematically in long-term memory and call up schemas to aid inference. Social inference is thus likely to be heavily theory/schema driven, with the consequence that it is biased towards conservative, schema-supportive inferential practices. Despite doing this, and being so poor at social inference, human beings seem to muddle through. Perhaps the process is adequate for most of our inferential needs most of the time, and we should study these 'adequate' rather than optimal processes in their own right.

Heuristics
Cognitive shortcuts that provide adequately accurate inferences for most of us most of the time.

With just this idea in mind, Tversky and Kahneman (1974; Kahneman & Tversky, 1973) detail the sorts of cognitive shortcut, called **heuristics**, that people use to reduce complex problem solving to simpler judgemental operations. Three principal heuristics have been researched: (1) representativeness, (2) availability and (3) anchoring and adjustment.

Representativeness heuristic
A cognitive shortcut in which instances are assigned to categories or types on the basis of overall similarity or resemblance to the category.

Representativeness heuristic

In deciding how likely it is that a person or an event is an instance of one category or another, people often simply estimate the extent to which the instance superficially represents or is similar to a typical or average member of the category. The **representativeness heuristic** is basically a relevance judgement that disregards base-rate information, sample size, quality of information and other normative principles. Nevertheless, it is fast and efficient and produces inferences that are accurate enough for our purposes most of the time. For example, consider the following information: 'Steve is very shy and withdrawn, invariably helpful, but with little interest in people, or in the world of reality. A meek and tidy soul, he has a need for order and structure, and a passion for detail' (Tversky & Kahneman, 1974). The representativeness heuristic would very quickly lead to the inference that Steve is a librarian rather than, say, a farmer, surgeon or trapeze artist, and in general that would probably be correct.

Availability heuristic

The **availability heuristic** is used to infer the frequency or likelihood of an event on the basis of how quickly instances or associations come to mind. Where instances are readily available, we tend to inflate frequencies. For example, exposure to many media reports of violent Muslim extremists will make that information available and will tend to inflate our estimate of the overall frequency of violent Muslims. Similarly, in forming an impression of a stranger, who has short hair, wears big boots and carries a cane, you might overestimate the likelihood that he will be violent because you have just seen the film *A Clockwork Orange*.

Availability heuristic
A cognitive shortcut in which the frequency or likelihood of an event is based on how quickly instances or associations come to mind.

Under many circumstances, availability is adequate as a basis for making inferences—after all, things that come to mind easily are probably fairly plentiful. However, availability is subject to bias, as it does not control for such factors as idiosyncratic exposure to unusual samples.

Anchoring and adjustment

In making inferences we often need a starting point—an anchor—from which, and with which, we can adjust subsequent inferences (e.g. Wyer, 1976). **Anchoring and adjustment** is a heuristic that ties inferences to initial standards. So, for example, inferences about other people are often anchored in beliefs about ourselves: we decide how intelligent, artistic or kind someone else is with reference to our own self-schema. Anchors can also come from the immediate context. For example, Greenberg, Williams and O'Brien (1986) found that participants in a mock jury study who were instructed to contemplate the harshest verdict first used this as an anchor from which only small adjustments were made. A relatively harsh verdict was rendered. Participants instructed to consider the most lenient verdict first likewise used this as an anchor, subsequently rendering a relatively lenient verdict.

Anchoring and adjustment
A cognitive shortcut in which inferences are tied to initial standards or schemas.

Improving social inference

Social inference is not optimal. We are biased, we misrepresent people and events, and we make mistakes. However, many of these shortcomings may be more apparent than real (Funder, 1987). Social cognition and social neuroscience experiments may provide unnatural contexts, for which our inference processes are not well suited. Intuitive inference processes may actually be well suited to everyday life. For example, on encountering a pit bull terrier in the street, it might be very adaptive to rely on availability (media coverage of attacks by pit bull terriers) and to flee automatically rather than adopt more time-consuming normative procedures: what is an error in the laboratory may not be so in the field.

Nevertheless, inferential errors can sometimes have serious consequences. For example, negative stereotyping of minority groups and suboptimal group decisions may be partly caused by inferential errors. In this case, there may be something to be gained by considering ways in which we can improve social inference. The basic principle is that social inference will improve to the extent that we become less reliant on intuitive inferential strategies. This may be achieved through formal education in scientific and rational thinking as well as in statistical techniques (Fong, Krantz & Nisbett, 1986; Nisbett, Krantz, Jepson & Fong, 1982).

Affect and emotion

Traditionally, social cognition has focused on thinking rather than feeling, but in recent years there has been an 'affective revolution' (e.g. Forgas, 2006; Forgas & Smith, 2007; Haddock & Zanna, 1999; Keltner & Lerner, 2010; Wetherell, 2012). Research has focused on how feelings (affect, emotion, mood) influence and are influenced by social cognition. Different situations (funeral, party) evoke different emotions (sad, happy), but also the same situation (examination) can evoke different emotions (threat, challenge) in different people (weak student, competent student).

Antecedents of affect

Research suggests that people process information about the situation and their hopes, desires and abilities, and on the basis of these cognitive *appraisals* different affective reactions and physiological responses follow. Because affective response (emotion) is, fundamentally, a mode of action readiness tied to appraisals of harm and benefit, the appraisal process is continuous and largely automatic (see Box 9.4).

Based on a distinction between simple primary and more complex secondary appraisals, research has shown that primary appraisals related to whether something is good/bad, or perhaps harmless/dangerous, occur in the amygdala. This is the part of the 'old brain' linked

Research highlight 9.4

How we decide when to respond affectively

According to Richard Lazarus and Craig Smith, affective response rests on seven appraisals, which can be framed as questions that people ask themselves in particular situations. There are two sets of appraisal dimensions, primary and secondary, that are relevant to all emotions.

Primary appraisals

1. How relevant (important) is what is happening in this situation to my needs and goals?
2. Is this congruent (good) or incongruent (bad) with my needs or goals?

Secondary appraisals

These appraisals relate to accountability and coping.

1. How responsible am I for what is happening in this situation?
2. How responsible is someone or something else?
3. Can I act on this situation to make or keep it more like what I want?
4. Can I handle and adjust to this situation however it might turn out?
5. Do I expect this situation to improve or to get worse?

Together, these seven appraisal dimensions produce a wide array of affective responses and emotions. For example, if something were important and bad and caused by someone else, we would feel anger and be motivated to act towards the other person in a way that would fix the situation. If something were important and bad, but caused by ourselves, then we would feel shame or guilt and be motivated to make amends for the situation.

Source: Lazarus, 1991; Smith & Lazarus, 1990

to fast, autonomic system-related emotional reactions. These have survival value (Baxter & Murray, 2002; Russell, 2003).

Hence, primary appraisals generate emotions blindingly quickly, well before conscious recognition of the target of the appraisal (Barrett, 2006). For example, people with a snake phobia showed physiological signs of terror even when they saw photos of snakes so quickly that the images could not even be recognised (Öhman & Soares, 1994). Further, when a person is focused on negative stimulus rather than a positive one, brain activity may even be greater (Ito, Larsen, Smith & Cacioppo, 1998).

Jim Blascovich and his colleagues have studied how challenge and threat act to motivate performance, noting that appraisals which generate emotion are linked approach versus avoidance actions. These in turn have survival value, according to their *biopsychosocial model of arousal regulation* (Blascovich, 2008; Blascovich & Tomaka, 1996). When people feel there is a demand on them, they appraise their resources for dealing with the demand—if perceived resources equal or exceed the demand, people experience a feeling of challenge that motivates approach behaviours (fight); if perceived resources are inadequate to meet the demand, people experience a feeling of threat that motivates avoidance behaviours (flight).

Consequences of affect

Emotion and mood influence thought and action. Affect infuses and therefore affects thinking, judgement and behaviour. In his **Affect Infusion model**, Joe Forgas describes the effects of mood on social cognition (Forgas, 1994, 1995, 2002). The core prediction is that affect infusion occurs only where people process information in an open and constructive manner that involves active elaboration of stimulus details and information from memory.

Affect infusion model
Cognition is infused with affect such that social judgements reflect current mood.

According to Forgas, there are four distinct ways in which people can process information about one another:

- Direct access—they can directly access schemas or judgements stored in memory.
- Motivated processing—they can form a judgement on the basis of specific motivations to achieve a goal or to 'repair' an existing mood.
- Heuristic processing—they can rely on various cognitive shortcuts or heuristics.
- Substantive processing—they can deliberately and carefully construct a judgement from a variety of informational sources.

Current mood states do not influence judgements involving direct access or motivated processing, but they do affect judgements involving heuristic processing or substantive processing. In the latter cases, cognition is infused with affect such that social judgements reflect current mood, either indirectly (affect primes target judgement) or directly (affect acts as information about the target). For example, under heuristic processing mood may itself be a heuristic that determines response—being in a bad mood would produce a negative reaction to another person (i.e. mood-congruence). Under substantive processing, the more we deliberate, the greater the mood-congruence effect. This model fares well in predicting the effects of affect on social cognition.

Affect influences social memory and social judgement—for example, people tend to recall current mood-congruent information more readily than current mood-incongruent information, and judge others and themselves more positively when they themselves are in a positive mood. In line with the affect infusion model, the effect of mood on self-perception is greater for peripheral than central aspects of self—peripheral aspects are less firmly ensconced and therefore require more elaboration and construction than central aspects (e.g. Sedikides, 1995). Stereotyping is also affected by mood. Being in a good mood can increase reliance on stereotypes when group membership is not very relevant (Forgas & Fiedler, 1996), but negative affect can encourage people to correct hastily made negative evaluations of outgroups (Monteith, 1993).

Beyond cognition and neuroscience

Although research on affect and emotion has come a long way in recent years, a number of questions remain and some critical issues have been raised. For example, self-report measures of people's appraisals of a stimulus may be unreliable (Parkinson & Manstead, 1992) as they are based on semantics and influenced by an array of communicative motivations and goals. As a result, we need to know more about how primary appraisals are tied to the valence, novelty, salience or intensity of a stimulus. We also need to understand how primary appraisals give rise to conscious experiences (Keltner & Lerner, 2010).

Social cognition research on affect and emotion, which is what we have discussed in this section, tends to focus on cognitive processes, and increasingly on the underlying neuroscience of basic primary emotions. However, affect and emotion are critical aspects of intergroup relations, and there is now a growing literature on collective and intergroup emotions, (e.g. Branscombe & Doosje, 2004; Brown, Gonzalez, Zagefka, Manzi & Cehajic, 2008; Doosje, Branscombe, Spears & Manstead, 1998, 2006; Mackie, Maitner & Smith, 2009).

Margaret Wetherell (2012) has similarly worried that the contemporary social psychology of affect and emotion is too tied to exploration of cognitive and neurological processes associated with simple or basic emotions. She reminds us that our emotional life is significantly impacted by a vast range of complex and nuanced emotions that may be much more closely tied to language and semantics embedded in everyday discourse. Emotions, both felt and expressed, serve to communicate with others and to 'get things done'.

Where is the 'social' in social cognition?

Social psychology has always described the cognitive processes and structures that influence and are influenced by social behaviour, and there is no doubt that modern social cognition, which really only emerged in the late 1970s, has made enormous advances in this direction. However, some critics have wondered if social cognition has been *too* successful. It may have taken social psychology too far in the direction of cognitive psychology, and more recently neuroscience, while it has diverted attention from many of social psychology's traditional topics. There has been a worry that there may not be any 'social' in social cognition (Kraut & Higgins, 1984; Markus & Zajonc, 1985; Moscovici, 1982; Zajonc, 1989).

Many of the social cognitive processes and structures that are described seem to be little affected by social context and seem more accurately to represent *asocial* cognition operating on social stimuli (i.e. people). In this respect, critics have characterised social cognition as **reductionist** and have focused on three main areas of concern—a failure to deal properly with language and communication—which are two fundamentally social variables, a failure to deal with processes of human interaction, and a failure to articulate properly cognitive processes with wider interpersonal, group and societal processes. However, there are exceptions; for example, Maass and Arcuri's (1996) research on language and stereotyping, and self-categorisation research on collective self and group behaviour (Turner, Hogg, Oakes, Reicher & Wetherell, 1987). It is also the case that more recently there has been a more systematic attempt to (re)-socialise social cognition (e.g. Abrams & Hogg, 1999; Levine, Resnick & Higgins, 1993; Moskowitz, 2005; Nye & Bower, 1996; Wyer & Gruenfeld, 1995).

Reductionism
A phenomenon in terms of the language and concepts of a lower level of analysis, usually with a loss of explanatory power.

One strand of social cognition has, however, moved in the opposite direction towards greater reductionism—in the guise of social neuroscience (e.g. Harmon-Jones & Winkielman, 2007; Lieberman, 2010; Ochsner, 2007; Ochsner & Lieberman, 2001). Social neuroscience, which focuses on brain correlates of behaviour, would seem to suffer all the problems of traditional social cognition, but even more so—mapping complex social behaviour onto localised electrical activity in the brain. Although advocates for social neuroscience see much of value and a central contribution to social psychology in this particular form of reductionism, many other social psychologists are wary, wondering how knowledge of what part of the brain 'lights up' can help us understand complex social behaviours such as negotiation, social dilemmas and conformity—for a discussion of pros and cons of social neuroscience in explaining group processes and intergroup relations, see Prentice and Eberhardt (2008).[C]

Seeking the causes of behaviour

People are preoccupied with seeking, constructing and testing explanations of their experiences. We try to understand our world to make it orderly and meaningful enough for adaptive action, and we tend to feel uncomfortable if we do not have such an understanding. In particular, we need to understand people. Through life most of us gradually construct adequate explanations (i.e. theories) of why people behave in certain ways; in this respect, we are all 'naive' or lay psychologists. This is extraordinarily useful, because it allows us (with varying accuracy) to predict how someone will behave, and possibly to influence whether someone will behave in that way or not. Thus, we gain some control over our destiny.

People construct explanations for both physical phenomena (e.g. earthquakes, the seasons) and human behaviour (e.g. anger, a particular attitude), and in general such explanations are *causal* explanations, in which specific conditions are attributed a causal role. Causal explanations are particularly powerful bases for prediction and control (Forsterling & Rudolph, 1988).

In this section, we discuss how people make inferences about the causes of their own and other people's behaviour, and the antecedents and consequences of such inferences. Social psychological theories of causal inference are called *attribution theories* (Harvey & Weary, 1981; Hewstone, 1989; Kelley & Michela, 1980; Ross & Fletcher, 1985). There are seven main theoretical emphases that make up the general body of **attribution** theory:

1 Heider's (1958) theory of naive psychology
2 Jones and Davis' (1965) theory of correspondent inference
3 Kelley's (1967) covariation model
4 Schachter's (1964) theory of emotional lability
5 Bem's (1967, 1972) theory of self-perception
6 Weiner's (1979, 1985) attributional theory
7 Deschamps' (1983), Hewstone and Jaspars' (1982, 1984) and Hewstone's (1989) intergroup perspective.

We discuss some of these in this section.

Attribution
The process of assigning a cause to our own behaviour and that of others.

How do we attribute causality, and why is it important?

People as naive psychologists

Fritz Heider (1958) believed it was crucially important for social psychologists to study people's naive, or commonsense, psychological theories, because such theories influenced ordinary people's everyday perceptions and behaviour. For example, people who believe in

[C]Vaughan, M. G., & Hogg, M. A. (2014). Social cognition and social thinking. In *Social psychology* (7th ed., pp. 56–69). Frenchs Forest, NSW: Pearson Australia.

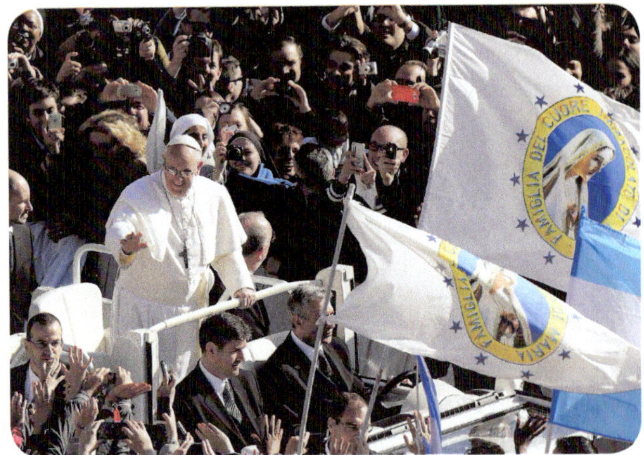

In search of the meaning of life Religions are one expression of our most basic need to understand the world we live in. Millions of Catholics hope that their new Pope will satisfy this need
(**Source:** © Dan Kitwood/Getty Images)

astrology are likely to have different expectations and are likely to act in different ways from those who do not. Heider believed that people are intuitive psychologists who construct causal theories of human behaviour, and because such theories have the same form as systematic scientific social psychological theories, people are actually intuitive or **naive psychologists**.

Heider based his ideas on three principles:

1 Because we feel that our own behaviour is motivated rather than random, we tend to look for the causes and reasons for other people's behaviour in order to discover their motives. The search for causes does seem to pervade human thought, and indeed it can be difficult to explain or comment on something without using causal language. Heider and Simmel (1944) demonstrated this in an ingenious experiment in which people who were asked to describe the movement of abstract geometric figures described them as if they were humans with intentions to act in certain ways. Nowadays, we can witness the same phenomenon in people's often highly emotional ascription of human motives to inanimate figures in video and computer games. The pervasive need that people have for causal explanation reveals itself most powerfully in the way that almost all societies construct an origin myth, an elaborate causal explanation for the origin and meaning of life that is often a centrepiece of a religion.

Naive psychologist (or scientist)
Model of social cognition that characterises people as using rational, scientific-like, cause–effect analyses to understand their world.

2 Because we construct causal theories in order to be able to predict and control the environment, we tend to look for stable and enduring properties of the world around us. We try to discover personality traits and enduring abilities in people, or stable properties of situations, that cause behaviour.

3 In attributing causality for behaviour, we distinguish between personal factors (e.g. personality, ability) and environmental factors (e.g. situations, social pressure). The former are examples of an **internal (or dispositional) attribution** and the latter of an **external (or situational) attribution**. So, for example, it might be useful to know whether someone you meet at a party who seems aloof and distant is an aloof and distant person or is acting in that way because she is not enjoying that particular party. Heider believed that, because internal causes, or intentions, are hidden from us, we can only infer their presence if there are no clear external causes. However, as we see below, people tend to be biased in preferring internal to external attributions even in the face of evidence for external causality. It seems that we readily attribute behaviour to stable properties of people. Klaus Scherer (1978), for example, found that people made assumptions about the stable personality traits of complete strangers simply on the basis of hearing their voices on the telephone.

Internal (or dispositional) attribution
Process of assigning the cause of our own or others' behaviour to internal or dispositional factors.

External (or situational) attribution
Assigning the cause of our own or others' behaviour to external or environmental factors.

Heider identified the major themes and provided the insight that forms the blueprint for all subsequent, more formalised, theories of attribution.

From acts to dispositions

Ned Jones and Keith Davis' (1965; Jones & McGillis, 1976) theory of **correspondent inference** explains how people infer that a person's behaviour corresponds to an underlying disposition or personality trait—how we infer, for example, that a friendly action is due to an underlying disposition to be friendly. People like to make correspondent inferences (attribute behaviour to underlying disposition) because a dispositional cause is a stable cause that renders people's behaviour predictable and thus increases our own sense of control over our world.

Correspondent inference
Causal attribution of behaviour to underlying dispositions.

To make a correspondent inference, we draw on five sources of information, or cues (see Figure 9.4):

1 *Freely chosen* behaviour is more indicative of a disposition than is behaviour that is clearly under the control of external threats, inducements or constraints.
2 Behaviour with effects that are relatively exclusive to that behaviour rather than common to a range of other behaviours (i.e. behaviour with **non-common effects**) tells us more about dispositions. People assume that others are aware of non-common effects and that the specific behaviour was performed intentionally to produce the non-common effect—this tendency has been called **outcome bias** (Allison, Mackie & Messick, 1996). So, for example, if a person has to choose between behaviour A and behaviour B, and both produce roughly the same effects (i.e. no non-common effects) or a very large number of different effects (i.e. many non-common effects), the choice tells us little about the person's disposition. However, if the behaviours produce a small number of different effects (i.e. few non-common effects—e.g. behaviour A produces only terror and behaviour B produces only joy), then the choice does tell us something about that person's disposition.
3 *Socially desirable* behaviour tells us little about a person's disposition, because it is likely to be controlled by societal norms. However, socially undesirable behaviour is generally counter-normative and is thus a better basis for making a correspondent inference.
4 We make more confident correspondent inferences about others' behaviour that has important consequences for ourselves: that is, behaviour that has **hedonic relevance**.
5 We make more confident correspondent inferences about others' behaviour that seems to be directly intended to benefit or harm us: that is, behaviour that is high in **personalism**.

Experiments testing correspondent inference theory provide some support. Jones and Harris (1967) found that American students making attributions for speeches made by other students tended to make more correspondent inferences for freely chosen socially unpopular positions, such as freely choosing to make a speech in support of Cuba's president at the time, Fidel Castro.

In another experiment, Jones, Davis and Gergen (1961) found that participants made more correspondent inferences for out-of-role behaviour, such as friendly, outer-directed

Non-common effects
Effects of behaviour that are relatively exclusive to that behaviour rather than other behaviours.

Outcome bias
Belief that the outcomes of a behaviour were intended by the person who chose the behaviour.

Hedonic relevance
Refers to behaviour that has important direct consequences for self.

Personalism
Behaviour that appears to be directly intended to benefit or harm oneself rather than others.

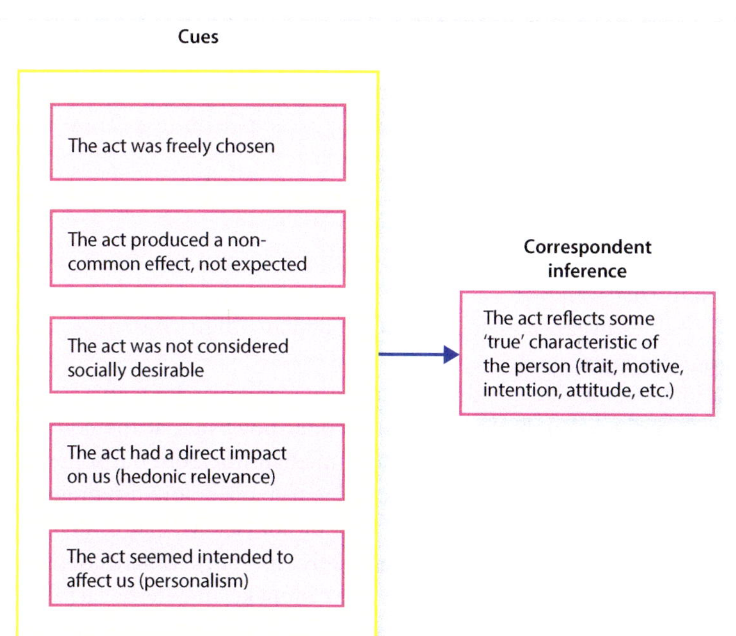

Figure 9.4 How we make a correspondent inference

To make an inference that a person's behaviour corresponds to an underlying disposition, we draw on five sources of information

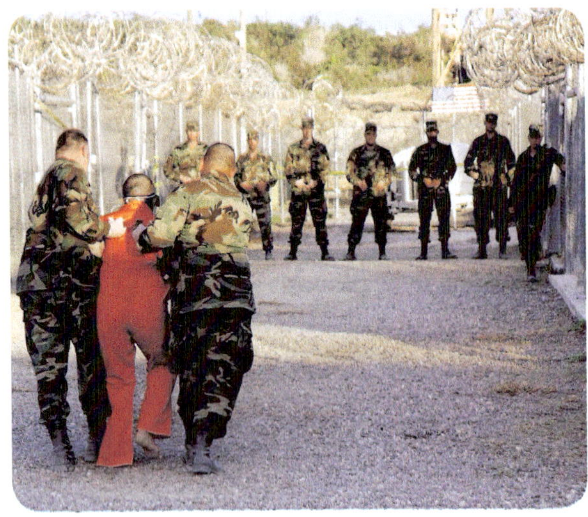

Freely chosen behaviour? Information based on a confession under duress contravenes the Third Geneva Convention of 1949 for the treatment of prisoners. It is also unreliable
(**Source:** Petty Officer 1st class Shane T. McCoy/Corbis Australia Pty Ltd.)

behaviour by someone who was applying for an astronaut job, in which the required attributes favour a quiet, reserved, inner-directed person.

Correspondent inference theory has some limitations and has declined in importance as an attribution theory (Hewstone, 1989; Howard, 1985). For instance, the theory holds that correspondent inferences depend to a great extent on the attribution of intentionality, yet unintentional behaviour (e.g. careless behaviour) can be a strong basis for a correspondent inference (e.g. that the person is a careless person).

There is also a problem with the notion of non-common effects. While correspondent inference theory maintains that people assess the commonality of effects by comparing chosen and non-chosen actions, other research indicates that people simply do not attend to non-occurring behaviours and so would not be able to compute the commonality of effects accurately (Nisbett & Ross, 1980; Ross, 1977). More generally, although we may correct dispositional attributions in the light of situational factors, this is a rather deliberate process, whereas correspondent inferences themselves are relatively automatic (Gilbert, 1995).

Covariation model Kelley's theory of causal attribution—people assign the cause of behaviour to the factor that covaries most closely with the behaviour.

Consistency information Information about the extent to which a behaviour Y always co-occurs with a stimulus X.

Distinctiveness information Information about whether a person's reaction occurs only with one stimulus, or is a common reaction to many stimuli.

Consensus information Information about the extent to which other people react in the same way to a stimulus X.

Discount If there is no consistent relationship between a specific cause and a specific behaviour, that cause is discounted in favour of some other cause.

People as everyday scientists

The best known attribution theory is Harold Kelley's (1967, 1973) covariation model. Kelley believed that in trying to discover the causes of behaviour people act much like scientists. They identify what factor covaries most closely with the behaviour and then assign that factor a causal role. The procedure is similar to that embodied by the statistical technique of analysis of variance (ANOVA), and for this reason Kelley's model is often referred to as an ANOVA model. People use this covariation principle to decide whether to attribute a behaviour to internal dispositions (e.g. personality) or external environmental factors (e.g. social pressure).

In order to make this decision, people assess three classes of information associated with the co-occurrence of a certain action (e.g. laughter) by a specific person (e.g. Tom) with a potential cause (e.g. a comedian):

1 Consistency information—does Tom always laugh at this comedian (high consistency) or only sometimes laughs at this comedian (low consistency)?
2 Distinctiveness information—does Tom laugh at everything (low distinctiveness) or only at the comedian (high distinctiveness)?
3 Consensus information—does everyone laugh at the comedian (high consensus) or is it only Tom who laughs (low consensus)?

Where consistency is low, people discount the potential cause and search for an alternative (see Figure 9.5). If Tom sometimes laughs and sometimes does not laugh at the comedian, then presumably the cause of the laughter is neither the comedian nor Tom but some other covarying factor: for example, whether or not Tom smoked marijuana before listening to the comedian or whether or not the comedian told a funny joke or not (see McClure, 1998, for a review of the conditions under which discounting is most likely to occur). Where consistency is high, and distinctiveness and consensus are also high, one can make an external attribution to the comedian (the cause of Tom's laughter was the comedian), but where distinctiveness

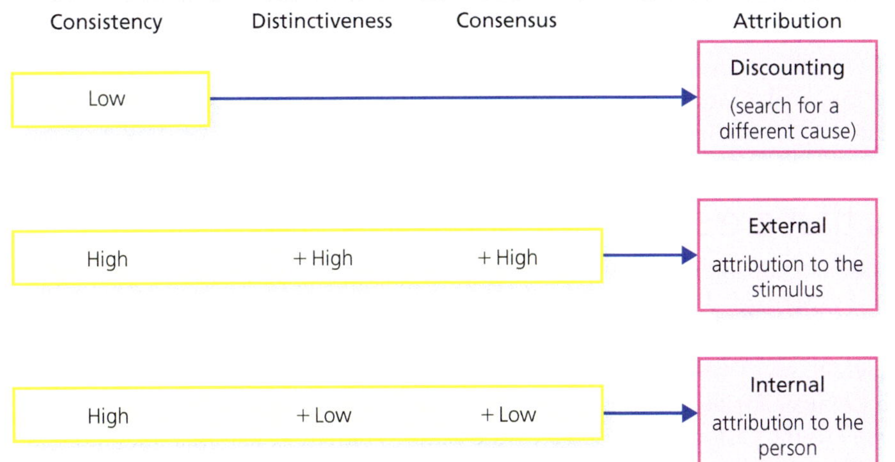

Figure 9.5 Kelley's attribution theory

Kelley's covariation model states that people decide what attributions to make after considering the consistency, distinctiveness and consensus of a person's behaviour

and consensus are low, one can make an internal attribution to Tom's personality (Tom laughed at the comedian because Tom is simply the sort of person who tends to laugh a lot).

McArthur (1972) tested Kelley's theory by having participants make internal or external attributions for a range of behaviours, each accompanied by one of the eight possible configurations of high or low consistency, distinctiveness and consensus information. Although the theory was generally supported (see review by Kassin, 1979), there was a tendency for people to under-use consensus information. There are also some general issues worth considering:

- Just because people can use pre-packaged consistency, distinctiveness and consensus information to attribute causality (the case in experimental tests of Kelley's model), this does not mean that in the normal course of events they do.
- There is evidence that people are actually poor at assessing the covariation of different events—they are poor statisticians (Alloy & Tabachnik, 1984).
- There is no guarantee that people are using the covariation principle—they may attribute causality to the most salient feature or to whatever causal agent appears to be similar to the effect (Nisbett & Ross, 1980).
- If people do attribute causality on the basis of covariance or correlation, then they certainly are *naive* scientists (Hilton, 1988)—covariation is not causation.

Another drawback of the covariation model is that consistency, distinctiveness and consensus information require multiple observations. Sometimes we have this information: we may know that Tom does indeed laugh often at almost anything (low distinctiveness), and that others do not find the comedian particularly amusing (low consensus). At other times, we may have, at best, incomplete information or even no information from multiple observations. How do we attribute causality under these circumstances? To deal with this, Kelley (1972a) introduced the notion of **causal schemata**—beliefs or preconceptions, built up from experience, about how certain kinds of cause interact to produce a specific effect. One such schema is that a particular effect requires at least two causes (called the 'multiple necessary cause' schema): for example, someone with a drink-driving record must have consumed a certain amount of alcohol and have been in control of a vehicle. Although the notion of causal schemata does have some empirical support (Kun & Weiner, 1973) and does help to resolve attributional problems raised by the case of a single observation, it is by no means uncritically accepted (Fiedler, 1982).[D]

Causal schemata
Experience-based beliefs about how certain types of cause interact to produce an effect.

[D]Vaughan, M. G., & Hogg, M. A. (2014). Social cognition and social thinking. In *Social psychology* (7th ed., pp. 74–78). Frenchs Forest, NSW: Pearson Australia.

Attributions for our own behaviour

One far-reaching implication of treating emotion as cognitively labelled arousal is that people may make more general attributions for their *own* behaviour. This idea has been elaborated by Daryl Bem (1967, 1972) in his **self-perception theory**

Self-perception theory Bem's idea that we gain knowledge of ourselves only by making self-attributions: for example, we infer our own attitudes from our own behaviour.

Acts that are stable and controlled

Attributional dimensions of task achievement are the focus of another extension of attribution theory, by Bernard Weiner (1979, 1985, 1986). Weiner was interested in the causes and consequences of the sorts of attribution made for people's success or failure on a task—for example, success or failure in a social psychology examination. He believed that, in making an achievement attribution, we consider three performance dimensions:

1 *Locus*—is the performance caused by the actor (internal) or the situation (external)?
2 *Stability*—is the internal or external cause a stable or an unstable one?
3 *Controllability*—to what extent is future task performance under the actor's control?

These produce eight different types of explanation for task performance (see Figure 9.6). For example, failure in a social psychology examination might be attributed to 'unusual hindrance from others' (the top right-hand box in Figure 9.6) if the student was intelligent (therefore, failure is external) and was disturbed by a nearby student sneezing from hay fever (unstable and controllable, because in future examinations the sneezing student might not be present or have taken an antihistamine, and/or one could choose to sit in a place away from the sneezing student).

Weiner's model is a dynamic one, in that people first assess whether someone has succeeded or failed and accordingly experience positive or negative emotion. They then make a causal attribution for the performance, which produces more specific emotions (e.g. pride for doing well due to ability) and expectations that influence future performance.

The model is relatively well supported by experiments that provide participants with performance outcomes and locus, stability and controllability information, often under role-playing conditions (e.g. de Jong, Koomen & Mellenbergh, 1988; Frieze & Weiner, 1971). However, critics have suggested that the controllability dimension may be less important than was first thought. They have also wondered to what extent people outside constrained laboratory conditions really analyse achievement in this way. Subsequently, Weiner (1995) extended his model to place an emphasis on judgements of responsibility. On the basis of causal attributions people make judgements of responsibility, and it is these latter judgements, not the causal attributions themselves, that influence affective experience and behavioural reactions.

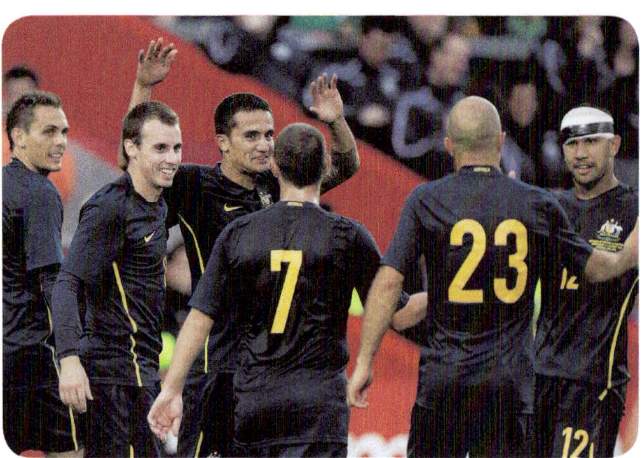

Controllability According to Weiner's attribution model, these Socceroos may attribute their success to unusually hard training—an internal but unstable attribution
(**Source:** AAP Image/Tim Clayton.)

Applying attribution theory

Application of the idea that people need to discover the cause of their own and others' behaviour in order to plan their own actions has had a significant impact on social psychology. We have already seen two examples—achievement

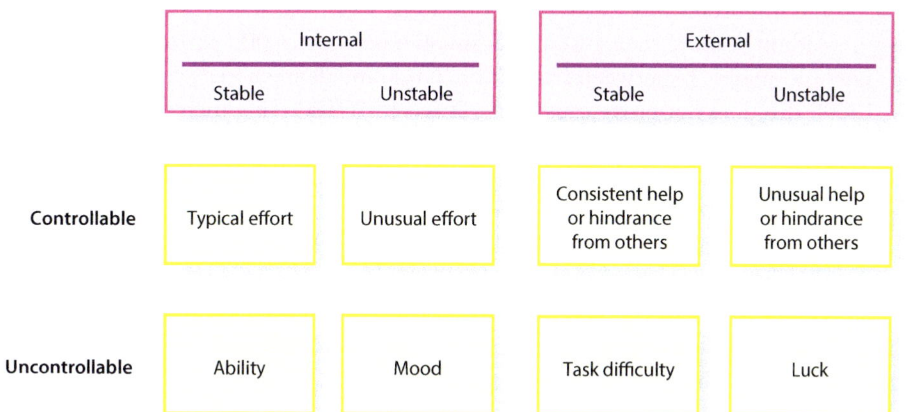

Figure 9.6 Achievement attributions as a function of locus, stability and controllability

How we attribute someone's task achievement depends on:

- *Locus*—is the performance caused by the actor (internal) or the situation (external)?
- *Stability*—is the internal or external cause a stable or an unstable one?
- *Controllability*—to what extent is future task performance under the actor's control?

attributions and the reattribution of arousal as a therapeutic technique. In this section, we explore two further applications: attributional styles, and interpersonal relationships.

Individual differences and attributional styles

Research suggests there are enduring individual differences in the sorts of attributions that people make: their **attributional style**. According to the clinical psychologist Julian Rotter (1966), those of us who are *internals* believe we have some control over the reinforcements and punishments we receive, and therefore over our destiny—things happen because we make them happen. However, those of us who are *externals* are more fatalistic: we believe we have little control over what happens to us—things simply occur by chance, luck or the actions of powerful external agents. To measure people's locus of control Rotter devised a 29-item scale. This scale has been used to relate locus of control to a range of behaviours, including political beliefs, achievement behaviour and reactions to illness. One problem with the scale is that it may not measure a unitary construct (i.e. a single personality dimension) but, rather, a number of relatively independent beliefs to do with control (Collins, 1974).

Attributional style An individual (personality) predisposition to make a certain type of causal attribution for behaviour.

A number of other questionnaires have been devised to measure attributional styles—a tendency for individuals to make particular kinds of causal inference, rather than others, over time and across different situations (Metalsky & Abramson, 1981). Of these, the attributional style questionnaire or ASQ (Peterson et al., 1982; Seligman, Abramson, Semmel & von Baeyer, 1979) is perhaps the most widely known. It measures the sorts of explanation that people give for aversive (i.e. unpleasant) events on three dimensions: internal/external, stable/unstable, global/specific. The global/specific dimension refers to how wide or narrow a range of effects a cause has—'the economy' is a global explanation for someone being made redundant, whereas the closing of a specific company is a specific explanation. People who view aversive events as being caused by internal, stable, global factors have a 'depressive attributional style' (i.e. the glass is half empty), which may promote helplessness and depression and may have adverse health consequences (Abramson, Seligman & Teasdale, 1978; Crocker, Alloy & Kayne, 1988).

Another slightly different scale, called the attributional complexity scale (ACS), has been devised by Fletcher, Danilovics, Fernandez, Peterson and Reeder (1986) to measure individual differences in the complexity of attributions that people make for events.

The notion of attributional style as a personality trait is not without problems: for instance, the ASQ and the ACS provide only limited evidence of cross-situational individual consistency in causal attribution (e.g. Cutrona, Russell & Jones, 1985). Also not without problems is the important link between attributional style, learned helplessness and clinical depression. Although more than 100 studies involving about 15 000 participants confirm an average correlation of 0.30 between attributional style and depression (Sweeney, Anderson & Bailey, 1986), this does not prove causation—it is a correlation in which one factor explains 9 percent of variance in the other.

More useful are diachronic studies, which show that attributional style measured at one time predicts depressive symptoms at a later date (Nolen-Hoeksma, Girgus & Seligman, 1992), but again causality is not established. Causality is difficult to establish because it is, of course, unethical to induce clinical depression in experimental settings. We are largely left with experimental evidence from studies of transitory mood, which is a rather pale analogue of depression. Is it justified to generalise from feelings about doing well or poorly on a trivial laboratory task to full-blown clinical depression?

Interpersonal relationships

Attributions play an important role in interpersonal relationships, particularly close interpersonal relationships (e.g. friendship and marriage) where attributions are *communicated* to fulfil a variety of functions: for instance, to explain, justify or excuse behaviour, as well as to attribute blame and instil guilt (Hilton, 1990).

John Harvey (1987) suggests that interpersonal relationships go through three basic phases: formation, maintenance and dissolution (see also Moreland & Levine's (1982, 1984) model of group socialisation). Fincham (1985) explains that during the formation stage, attributions reduce ambiguity and facilitate communication and an understanding of the relationship. In the maintenance phase, the need to make attributions wanes because stable personalities and relationships have been established. The dissolution phase is characterised by an increase in attributions in order to regain an understanding of the relationship.

A notable feature of many interpersonal relationships is attributional conflict (Horai, 1977), in which partners proffer divergent causal interpretations of behaviour and disagree over what attributions to adopt. Often partners cannot even agree on a cause–effect sequence, one exclaiming, 'I withdraw because you nag', the other, 'I nag because you withdraw'. From research mainly on heterosexual couples, attributional conflict has been shown to be correlated strongly with relationship dissatisfaction (Kelley, 1979; Orvis, Kelley & Butler, 1976; Sillars, 1981).

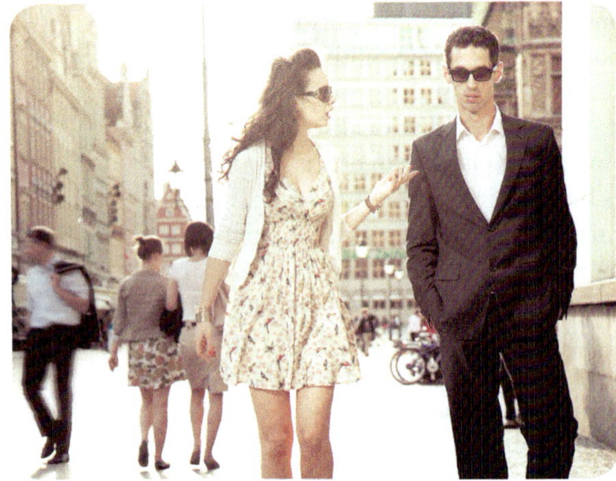

Attributing blame
Couples sometimes cannot agree on what is cause and what is effect. For example, does nagging cause withdrawal or vice versa?
(**Source:** © Konradbak | Dreamstime.com.)

However, the main thrust of research has focused on the role of attributions in heterosexual marital satisfaction (e.g. Fincham & Bradbury, 1993; Fletcher & Thomas, 2000; Noller & Ruzzene, 1991). An important aim has been to distinguish between distressed and non-distressed spouses in order to provide therapy for dysfunctional marital relationships. Correlational studies (e.g. Fincham & O'Leary, 1983; Holtzworth-Munroe & Jacobson, 1985) reveal that happily married (or non-distressed) spouses tend to credit their partners for positive behaviour by citing internal, stable, global and controllable factors to explain them. Negative behaviour is explained away by ascribing it to causes viewed as external, unstable, specific and uncontrollable. Distressed couples behave in exactly the opposite way.

While women tend fairly regularly to think in causal terms about the relationship, men do so only when the relationship becomes dysfunctional. In this respect, and contrary to popular opinion, men may be the more diagnostic barometers of marital dysfunction—when men start analysing the relationship alarm bells should ring!

Do attributional dynamics produce dysfunctional marital relationships, or do dysfunctional relationships distort the attributional dynamic? This important causal question has been addressed by Frank Fincham and Thomas Bradbury (1987; see overview by Hewstone, 1989), who obtained responsibility attributions, causal attributions and marital satisfaction measures from 39 married couples on two occasions 10–12 months apart. Attributions made on the first occasion were found reliably to predict marital satisfaction 10–12 months later, but only for wives.

Another longitudinal study (although over only a two-month period) confirmed that attributions do have a causal impact on subsequent relationship satisfaction (Fletcher, Fincham, Cramer & Heron, 1987). Subsequent, more extensive and better controlled longitudinal studies have replicated these findings for both husbands and wives (Fincham & Bradbury, 1993; Senchak & Leonard, 1993).

Biases in attribution

The attribution process, then, is clearly subject to bias: for example, it can be biased by personality, biased by interpersonal dynamics or biased to meet communication needs. We do not approach the task of attributing causes for behaviour in an entirely dispassionate, disinterested and objective manner, and the cognitive mechanisms that are responsible for attribution may themselves be subject to imperfections that render them suboptimal.

Accumulating evidence for attributional biases and 'errors' occasioned a shift of perspective. Instead of viewing people as naive scientists or even statisticians (in which case biases were largely considered a theoretical nuisance), we now think of people as **cognitive misers** or **motivated tacticians** (Moskowitz, 2005; Fiske & Taylor, 2008). People use cognitive shortcuts (called heuristics) to make attributions that, although not objectively correct all the time, are quite satisfactory and adaptive. Sometimes the choice of shortcut and choice of attribution can also be influenced by personal motives.

Biases are entirely adaptive characteristics of ordinary, everyday social perception (Fiske & Taylor, 2008; Nisbett & Ross, 1980; Ross, 1977). In this section, we discuss some of the most important attributional biases.

Cognitive miser
A model of social cognition that characterises people as using the least complex and demanding cognitions that are able to produce generally adaptive behaviours.

Motivated tactician
A model of social cognition that characterises people as having multiple cognitive strategies available, from which they choose on the basis of personal goals, motives and needs.

Correspondence bias and the fundamental attribution error

One of the best known attribution biases is **correspondence bias**—a general tendency for people to overly attribute behaviour to stable underlying personality dispositions (Gilbert & Malone, 1995). This bias was originally called the **fundamental attribution error**, and although the correspondence bias and fundamental attribution errors are not identical (Gawronski, 2004), the terms are often used interchangeably—the change in the preferred label mainly reflects accumulating evidence that this bias or error may not be quite as 'fundamental' as originally thought (see below).

The fundamental attribution error, originally identified by Lee Ross (1977), refers to a tendency for people to make dispositional attributions for others' behaviour, even when there are clear external/environmental causes. For example, in the Jones and Harris (1967) study mentioned earlier, American participants read speeches about Cuba's President Fidel Castro ostensibly written by fellow students. The speeches were either pro-Castro or anti-Castro, and the writers had ostensibly either freely chosen to write the speech or been instructed to do so. Where there was a choice, participants not surprisingly reasoned that those who

Correspondence bias
A general attribution bias in which people have an inflated tendency to see behaviour as reflecting (corresponding to) stable underlying personality attributes.

Fundamental attribution error
Bias in attributing another's behaviour more to internal than to situational causes.

had written a pro-Castro speech were in favour of Castro, and those who had written an anti-Castro speech were against Castro—an internal, dispositional attribution was made (see Figure 9.7).

However, a dispositional attribution was also made even when the speech writers had been *instructed* to write the speech. Although there was overwhelming evidence for an exclusively external cause, participants seemed largely to overlook this and to still prefer a dispositional explanation—the fundamental attribution error. (Bearing these points in mind, how would you account for the different views held by Helen and Lewis? See the first focus question.)

Other studies furnish additional empirical evidence for the fundamental attribution error (Jones, 1979; Nisbett & Ross, 1980). Indeed, the fundamental attribution error, or correspondence bias, has been demonstrated repeatedly both inside and outside the social psychology laboratory (Gawronski, 2004; Gilbert, 1998; Jones, 1990). Correspondence bias may also be responsible for a number of more general explanatory tendencies: for example, the tendency to attribute road accidents unduly to the driver rather than to the vehicle or the road conditions (Barjonet, 1980); and the tendency among some people to attribute poverty and unemployment to the person rather than to social conditions.

Tom Pettigrew (1979) has suggested that the fundamental attribution error may emerge in a slightly different form in intergroup contexts where groups are making attributions about ingroup and outgroup behaviour—he calls this the *ultimate attribution error* (see below). Correspondence bias and the fundamental attribution error are closely related to two other biases: the *outcome bias* (e.g. Allison, Mackie & Messick, 1996), in which people assume that a person behaving in some particular way intended all the outcomes of that behaviour; and **essentialism** (Haslam, Rothschild & Ernst, 1998; Medin & Ortony, 1989), in which behaviour is considered to reflect underlying and immutable, often innate, properties of people or the groups they belong to.

Essentialism
Pervasive tendency to consider behaviour to reflect underlying and immutable, often innate, properties of people or the groups they belong to.

Nick Haslam and his colleagues have noted that essentialism can be troublesome, particularly when it causes people to attribute stereotypically negative attributes of outgroups to essential and immutable personality attributes of members of that group (e.g. Bain, Kashima & Haslam, 2006; Haslam, Bastian, Bain & Kashima, 2006; Haslam, Bastian & Bissett, 2004). For example, the stereotype of an outgroup as being laid-back, liberal and poorly educated becomes more pernicious if these attributes are considered immutable,

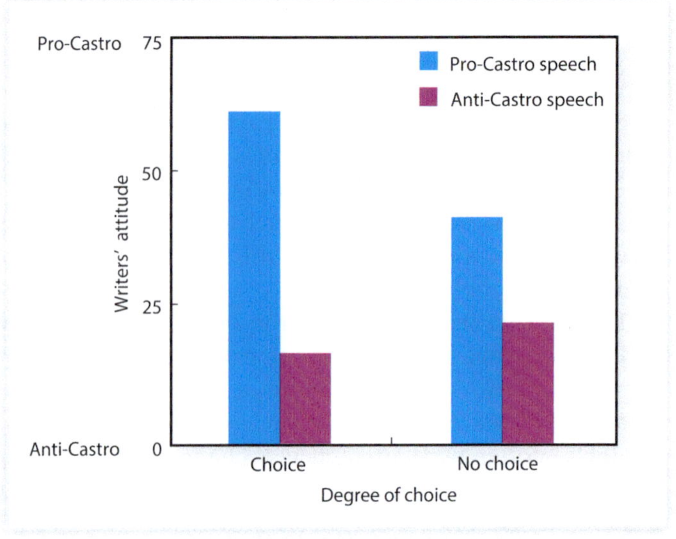

Figure 9.7 The fundamental attribution error: attributing speech writers' attitudes on the basis of their freedom of choice in writing the speech

- Students who freely chose to write a pro- or an anti-Castro speech were attributed with a pro- or anti-Castro attitude respectively
- Although less strong, this same tendency to attribute the speech to an underlying disposition (the fundamental attribution error) prevailed when the writers had no choice and were simply instructed to write the speech

(**Source:** based on data from Jones and Harris (1967))

perhaps genetically induced, properties of the group's members—the people themselves are considered to have personalities that are immutably lazy, immoral and stupid.

Different explanations of the fundamental attribution error have been proposed (as follow).

Focus of attention

The actor's behaviour attracts more attention than the background: it is disproportionately salient in cognition, stands out as the figure against the situational background, and is therefore overrepresented causally (Taylor & Fiske, 1978). Thus the actor and the actor's behaviour form what Heider (1958) called a 'causal unit'. This explanation makes quite a lot of sense. Procedures designed to focus attention away from the actor and on to the situation have been shown to increase the tendency to make a situational rather than dispositional attribution (e.g. Rholes & Pryor, 1982). When people really want to find out about a situation from a person's behaviour, they focus on the situation and are less likely to leap to a dispositional attribution—the fundamental attribution error is muted or reversed (e.g. Krull, 1993).

Differential forgetting

Attribution requires the representation of causal information in memory. There is some evidence that people tend to forget situational causes more readily than dispositional causes, thus producing a dispositional shift over time (e.g. Moore, Sherrod, Liu & Underwood, 1979; Peterson, 1980). Other studies show the opposite effect (e.g. Miller & Porter, 1980), and Funder (1982) has argued that the direction of shift depends on the focus of information processing and occurs immediately after the behaviour being attributed.

Cultural and developmental factors

The correspondence bias was originally called the fundamental attribution error because it was considered to be an automatic and universal outcome of perceptual experience and cognitive activity (e.g. McArthur & Baron, 1983). However, there is evidence that both developmental factors and culture may affect the correspondence bias. For example, in Western cultures, young children explain action in concrete situational terms and learn to make dispositional attributions only in late childhood (Kassin & Pryor, 1985; White, 1988). Furthermore, this developmental sequence itself may not be universal. Norman Miller (1984; see Figure 3.8) reports data showing that Hindu Indian children do not drift towards dispositional explanations at all, but rather towards increasingly situational explanations.

These differences quite probably reflect different cultural norms for social explanation, or more basic differences between Western and non-Western conceptions of self—the autonomous and independent Western self and the interdependent non-Western self (Chiu & Hong, 2007). The fundamental attribution error is a relatively ubiquitous and socially valued feature of Western cultures (Beauvois & Dubois, 1988; Jellison & Green, 1981), but, although present, it is less dominant in non-Western cultures (Fletcher & Ward, 1988; Morris & Peng, 1994).

The fundamental attribution error may not be as fundamental as was first thought. It may, to some extent, be a normative way of thinking. This is one reason why Daniel Gilbert and his colleagues (e.g. Gilbert & Malone, 1995) recommend that the term 'correspondence bias' be used in preference to the term 'fundamental attribution error'. Indeed, according to Bertram Gawronski (2004), the two constructs are subtly different: technically, he argues, the fundamental attribution error is the tendency to underestimate the impact of situational factors; and the correspondence bias is the tendency to draw correspondent dispositional inferences from behaviour that is constrained by the situation.

Linguistic factors

One final, rather interesting, observation by Nisbett and Ross (1980) is that the English language is so constructed that it is usually relatively easy to describe an action and the actor in the same terms, and much more difficult to describe the situation in the same way. For example, we can talk about a kind or honest person, and a kind or honest action, but not a kind or honest situation. The English language may facilitate dispositional explanations (Brown & Fish, 1983; Semin & Fiedler, 1991).

The actor-observer effect

Actor-observer effect Tendency to attribute our own behaviours externally and others' behaviours internally.

Imagine the last time a shop assistant was rude to you. You probably thought, 'What a rude person!' though perhaps put less politely—in other words, you made an internal attribution to the shop assistant's enduring personality. In contrast, how did you explain the last time *you* snapped at someone? Probably not in terms of your personality, more likely in terms of external factors such as time pressure or stress. The **actor-observer effect** (or the self–other effect) is really an extension of the correspondence bias. It refers to the tendency for people to attribute others' behaviour internally to dispositional factors and their own behaviour externally to environmental factors (Jones & Nisbett, 1972). Twenty years of research has provided substantial evidence for this effect (Watson, 1982), and some extensions and qualifications. For example, not only do we tend to attribute others' behaviour more dispositionally than our own, but we also tend to consider their behaviour to be more stable and predictable than our own (Baxter & Goldberg, 1988).

A number of factors can influence the actor–observer effect. People tend to make more dispositional attributions for socially desirable than socially undesirable behaviour, irrespective of who the actor is (e.g. Taylor & Koivumaki, 1976), and there is a tendency for actors to be more dispositional in attributing positive behaviour and more situational in attributing negative behaviour than are observers (e.g. Chen, Yates & McGinnies, 1988).

The actor–observer effect can be inverted if the actor knows that his or her behaviour is dispositionally caused. For example, you may 'adopt' an injured hedgehog in the full knowledge that you are a sucker for injured animals and you have often done this sort of thing in the past (Monson & Hesley, 1982). Finally, the actor–observer effect can be abolished or reversed if the actor is encouraged to take the role of the observer regarding the behaviour to be attributed, and the observer the role of the actor. Under these circumstances, the actor becomes more dispositional and the observer more situational (e.g. Frank & Gilovich, 1989).

There are two main explanations for the actor–observer effect:

1 *Perceptual focus*. This explanation is almost identical to the 'focus of attention' explanation for the correspondence bias (see above). For the observer, the actor and the actor's behaviour are figural against the background of the situation. However, an actor cannot 'see' him/herself behaving, so the background situation assumes the role of figure against the background of self. The actor and the observer quite literally have different perspectives on the behaviour and thus explain it in different ways (Storms, 1973). Perceptual salience does indeed seem to have an important role in causal explanation. For example, McArthur and Post (1977) found that observers tended to make more dispositional attributions for an actor's behaviour when the actor was strongly illuminated than when dimly illuminated.

2 *Informational differences*. Another reason that actors tend to make external attributions and observers internal ones is that actors have a wealth of information to draw on about how they have behaved in other circumstances. They may actually know that they behave differently in different contexts and thus quite accurately consider their behaviour to be under situational control. Observers are not privy to this autobiographical information. They tend simply to see the actor behaving in a certain way in one context, or a limited

range of contexts, and have no information about how the actor behaves in other contexts. It is therefore not an unreasonable assumption to make a dispositional attribution. This explanation, first suggested by Jones and Nisbett (1972), does have some empirical support (Eisen, 1979; White & Younger, 1988).

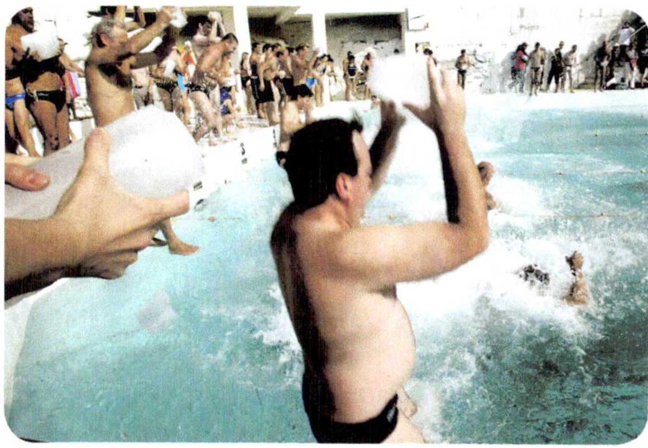

The false consensus effect These mid-winter dippers discover a major attributional bias. Who else would join the 'Icebergs' before breakfast? (**Source:** Brianne Makin/Newspix.)

The false consensus effect

Kelley (1972b) identified consensus information as being one of the three types of information that people used to make attributions about others' behaviour. One of the first cracks in the naive scientist model of attribution was McArthur's (1972) discovery that attributors in fact under-used or even ignored consensus information (Kassin, 1979).

Subsequently, it became apparent that people do not ignore consensus information—they provide their own. People see their own behaviour as typical and assume that under similar circumstances others would behave in the same way. Ross, Greene and House (1977) first demonstrated this **false consensus effect**. They asked students if they would agree to walk around campus for 30 minutes wearing a sandwich board carrying the slogan 'Eat at Joe's'. Those who agreed estimated that 62 percent of their peers would also have agreed, while those who refused estimated that 67 percent of their peers would also have refused.

False consensus effect
Seeing our own behaviour as being more typical than it really is.

There are well over 100 studies that bear testimony to the robust nature of the false consensus effect (see Marks & Miller, 1987; Mullen et al., 1985; Wetzel & Walton, 1985). The effect can arise in several ways:

- We usually seek out similar others and so should not be surprised to find that other people are similar to us.
- Our own opinions are so salient to us, at the forefront of our consciousness, that they eclipse the possibility of alternative opinions.
- We are motivated to ground our opinions and actions in perceived consensus in order to validate them and build a stable world for ourselves.

Other research indicates that the false consensus effect is stronger for important beliefs, ones that that we care a great deal about (e.g. Granberg, 1987), and for beliefs about which we are very certain (e.g. Marks & Miller, 1985). External threat, positive qualities, the perceived similarity of others and minority group status all also inflate perceptions of consensus (e.g. Sanders & Mullen, 1983; Sherman, Presson & Chassin, 1984; van der Pligt, 1984).

Self-serving biases

In keeping with the motivated tactician model of social cognition (Fiske & Taylor, 1991) discussed earlier, attribution is influenced by our desire for a favourable image of ourselves. We are very good at producing **self-serving biases**. Overall, we take credit for our positive behaviours and successes as reflecting who we are and our intention and effort to do positive things (the *self-enhancing bias*). At the same time, we explain away our negative behaviours and failures as being due to coercion, normative constraints and other external situational factors that do not reflect who we 'really' are (the *self-protecting bias*). This is a robust effect that holds across many cultures (Fletcher & Ward, 1988).

Self-serving biases
Attributional distortions that protect or enhance self-esteem or the self-concept.

Self-serving biases are clearly ego-serving (Snyder, Stephan & Rosenfield, 1978). However, Miller and Ross (1975) suggest that there may also be a cognitive component, particularly for the self-enhancing aspect. People generally expect to succeed and therefore accept responsibility for success. If they try hard to succeed, they associate success with their own effort, and they generally exaggerate the amount of control they have over successful performances. Together, these cognitive factors might encourage internal attribution of success. In general, however, it seems likely that both cognitive and motivational factors have a role (Anderson & Slusher, 1986; Tetlock & Levi, 1982) and that they are difficult to disentangle from one another (Tetlock & Manstead, 1985; Zuckerman, 1979).

Self-enhancing biases are more common than self-protecting biases (Miller & Ross, 1975)—partly because people with low self-esteem tend not to protect themselves by attributing their failures externally; rather, they attribute them internally (Campbell & Fairey, 1985). However, self-enhancement and self-protection can sometimes be muted by a desire not to be seen to be boasting over our successes and lying about our failures (e.g. Schlenker, Weingold & Hallam, 1990)—but not totally extinguished (Riess, Rosenfield, Melburg & Tedeschi, 1981). A fascinating self-serving bias, which most of us have used from time to time, acts in anticipation—**self-handicapping**, a term described by Jones and Berglas:

Self-handicapping
Publicly making advance external attributions for our anticipated failure or poor performance in a forthcoming event.

> *The self-handicapper, we are suggesting, reaches out for impediments, exaggerates handicaps, embraces any factor reducing personal responsibility for mediocrity and enhancing personal responsibility for success. (Jones & Berglas, 1978, p. 202)*

People use this bias when they anticipate failure, whether in their job performance, in sport, or even in therapeutic settings when being 'sick' allows one to drop out of life. What a person often will do is to intentionally and publicly make external attributions for a poor showing even before it happens.

Another self-serving instance is the attribution of responsibility (Weiner, 1995), which is influenced by an outcome bias (Allison, Mackie & Messick, 1996). People tend to attribute greater responsibility to someone who is involved in an accident with large rather than small consequences (Burger, 1981; Walster, 1966). For example, we would attribute greater responsibility to the captain of a tanker that spills millions of litres of oil than to the captain of a small fishing boat that spills only a few litres, although the degree of responsibility may actually be the same.

Illusion of control
Belief that we have more control over our world than we really do.

We can link this effect to the tendency for people to cling to an **illusion of control** (Langer, 1975) by believing in a *just world* (Furnham, 2003; Lerner, 1977). People like to believe that bad things happen to 'bad people' and good things to 'good people' (i.e. people get what they deserve), and that people have control over their outcomes. This pattern of attributions makes the world seem a controllable and secure place in which we can determine our own destiny.

Belief in a just world
Belief that the world is a just and predictable place where good things happen to 'good people' and bad things to 'bad people'.

The **belief in a just world** can result in a general pattern of attribution in which victims are deemed responsible for their misfortune—poverty, oppression, tragedy and injustice all happen because victims deserve it. Examples of the just world hypothesis in action are such views as the unemployed are responsible for being out of work, and rape victims are responsible for the violence against them. Another example is the belief, still held by some people, that the six million Jewish victims of the Holocaust were responsible for their own fate—that they deserved it (Davidowicz, 1975). Refer back to the second focus question. Just world beliefs are also an important component of many religious ideologies (Hogg, Adelman & Blagg, 2010).

The belief in a just world may also be responsible for self-blame. Victims of traumatic events such as incest, debilitating illness, rape and other forms of violence can experience a strong sense that the world is no longer stable, meaningful, controllable and just. One way to reinstate an illusion of control is, ironically, to take some responsibility for the event (Miller & Porter, 1983).

Intergroup attribution

Attribution theories are concerned mainly with how people make dispositional or situational attributions for their own and others' behaviour, and the sorts of bias that distort this process. The perspective is very much tied to interpersonal relations: people as unique individuals make attributions for their own behaviour or the behaviour of other unique individuals. However, there is another attributional context—intergroup relations—where individuals as group members make attributions for the behaviour of themselves as group members and others as either ingroup or outgroup members (Deschamps, 1983; Hewstone, 1989; Hewstone & Jaspars, 1982, 1984).

Examples of **intergroup attributions** abound. One example is the attribution of economic ills to minority outgroups (e.g. North African immigrants and refugees in Italy, Romani immigrants in France). Another is the explanation of behaviour in terms of stereotypical properties of group membership—for example, attributions for performance that are consistent with gender stereotypes (Deaux, 1984) or racial stereotypes (Steele, Spencer & Aronson, 2002).

Intergroup attributions
Process of assigning the cause of one's own or others' behaviour to group membership.

Ethnocentrism
Evaluative preference for all aspects of our own group relative to other groups.

Ultimate attribution error
Tendency to attribute bad outgroup and good ingroup behaviour internally, and to attribute good outgroup and bad ingroup behaviour externally.

Intergroup attributions serve two functions, the first relating to ingroup bias and the second to self-esteem.

We have noted in the preceding section several attributional biases that are self-serving. By extension and by taking an intergroup perspective, we can now view **ethnocentrism** as an ingroup-serving bias. Socially desirable (positive) behaviour by ingroup members and socially undesirable (negative) behaviour by outgroup members are internally attributed to dispositions, and negative ingroup and positive outgroup behaviour are externally attributed to situational factors (Hewstone & Jaspars, 1982; Hewstone, 1989, 1990). This effect is more prevalent in Western than in non-Western cultures (Fletcher & Ward, 1988). It is common in team sports contexts, where the success of one's own team is attributed to internal stable abilities rather than effort, luck or task difficulty—we are skilful, they were lucky. This *group-enhancing* bias is stronger and more consistent than the corresponding *group-protective* bias (Mullen & Riordan, 1988; Miller & Ross, 1975).

Pettigrew (1979) has described a related bias, called the **ultimate attribution error**. This is an extension of Ross' (1977) fundamental attribution error, and takes us into the domain of attributions for outgroup behaviour. Pettigrew argued that negative outgroup behaviour is dispositionally attributed, whereas positive outgroup behaviour is externally attributed or explained away so that we preserve our unfavourable outgroup image. The ultimate attribution error refers to attributions made for outgroup behaviour only, whereas broader intergroup perspectives focus on ingroup attributions as well.

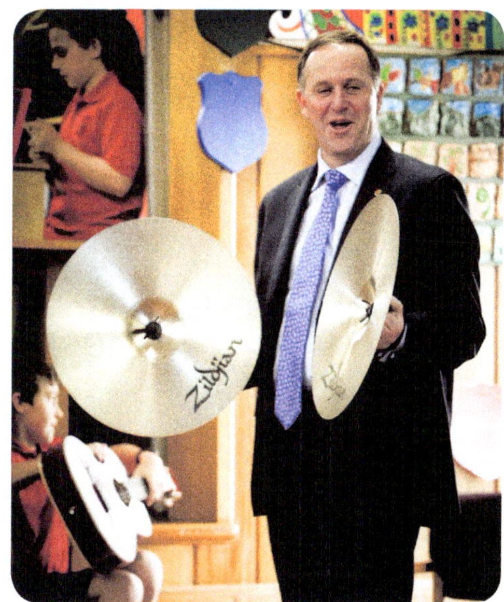

Stereotypical behaviour New Zealand's Prime Minister tries hard to be a regular bloke
(**Source:** NPA/Bethelle McFedries.)

Taylor and Jaggi (1974) conducted an early study of intergroup attributions in southern India against a background of intergroup conflict between Hindus and Muslims. Hindu participants read vignettes describing Hindus or Muslims acting in a socially desirable way (e.g. offering shelter from the rain) or socially undesirable way (e.g. refusing shelter) towards them, and then chose one of a number of explanations for the behaviour. The results were as predicted. Hindu participants made more internal attributions for socially desirable than socially undesirable acts by Hindus (ingroup). This difference disappeared when Hindus made attributions for Muslims (outgroup).

Miles Hewstone and Colleen Ward (1985) conducted a more complete and systematic follow-up, with Malays and Chinese in Malaysia and Singapore. Participants made internal or external attributions for desirable or undesirable behaviour described in vignettes as being performed by Malays or by Chinese. In Malaysia, Malays showed a clear ethnocentric attribution bias—they attributed a positive act by a Malay more to internal factors than a similar act by a Chinese, and a negative act by a Malay less to internal factors than a similar act by a Chinese (see Figure 9.8). The ingroup enhancement effect was much stronger than the outgroup derogation effect. The Chinese participants showed no ethnocentric bias—instead, they showed a tendency to make similar attributions to those made by Malays. In Singapore, the only significant effect was that Malays made internal attributions for positive acts by Malays.

Hewstone and Ward explain these findings in terms of the nature of intergroup relations in Malaysia and Singapore. In Malaysia, Malays are the clear majority group and Chinese an ethnic minority. Furthermore, relations between the two groups were tense and relatively conflictual at the time, with Malaysia pursuing a policy of ethnic assimilation. Both Malays and Chinese generally shared an unfavourable **stereotype** of Chinese and a favourable stereotype of Malays. In contrast, Singapore has been ethnically more tolerant. The Chinese are in the majority, and ethnic stereotypes are markedly less pronounced.

Stereotype
Widely shared and simplified evaluative image of a social group and its members.

The important implication of this analysis is that ethnocentric attribution is not a universal tendency that reflects asocial cognition; rather, it depends on intergroup dynamics in a sociohistorical context. The sorts of attribution that group members make about ingroup and outgroup behaviour are influenced by the nature of the relations between the groups.

This is consistent with Hewstone's (1989) argument that a proper analysis of attribution, more accurately described as social explanation, requires careful articulation (i.e. theoretical integration or connection) of different **levels of analysis (or explanation)** (see Doise, 1986). In other words, we need to know how individual cognitive processes, interpersonal interactions, group membership dynamics and intergroup relations all affect, are affected by and are interrelated with one another.

Level of analysis (or explanation)
The types of concepts, mechanisms and language used to explain a phenomenon.

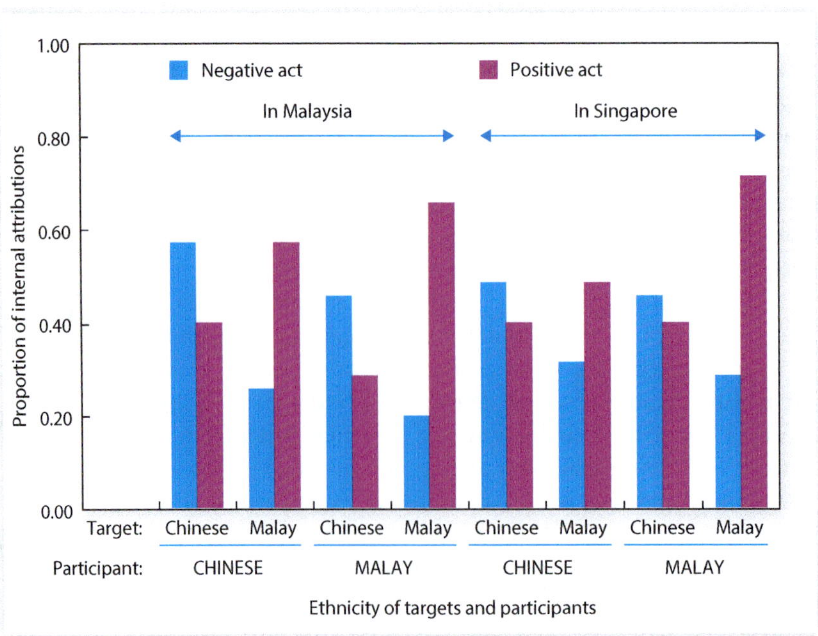

Figure 9.8 Internal attribution of positive and negative acts by Malays or Chinese as a function of attributor ethnicity

Malays showed an ethnocentric attributional bias in which a positive act was more internally attributed to a Malay than a Chinese, and a negative act less internally attributed to a Malay than a Chinese: the effect was more pronounced in Malaysia, where Malays are the dominant group and Chinese the ethnic minority, than in Singapore. Chinese did not show an ethnocentric attribution bias
(**Source:** based on data from Hewstone & Ward (1985))

Further evidence for ethnocentric intergroup attributions comes from studies of interracial attitudes in educational settings in the United States (Duncan, 1976; Stephan, 1977); from studies of inter-ethnic relations between Israelis and Arabs (Rosenberg & Wolfsfeld, 1977) and between Hindus and Muslims in Bangladesh (Islam & Hewstone, 1993); and from studies of race, gender and social class-based attributions for success and failure (Deaux & Emswiller, 1974; Feather & Simon, 1975; Greenberg & Rosenfield, 1979; Hewstone, Jaspars & Lalljee, 1982).

More recently, Diane Mackie and Mi Na Ahn (1998) found that the *outcome bias,* the assumption that the outcomes of behaviour were intended by the person who chose the behaviour, is affected by whether the actor is a member of your group or not, and whether the outcome was desirable or not. Mackie and Ahn found that there was an outcome bias in the case of an ingroup member and a desirable outcome but not when the outcome was undesirable.

There are at least two processes that may be responsible for ethnocentric intergroup attributions:

1 *A cognitive process.* Social categorisation generates category-congruent expectations in the form of expectancies (Deaux, 1976), schemas (e.g. Fiske & Taylor, 1991), or group prototypes or stereotypes (e.g. Hogg & Abrams, 1988; Turner, Hogg, Oakes, Reicher & Wetherell, 1987). Behaviour that is consistent with our stereotypes or expectancies is attributed to stable internal factors, whereas expectancy-inconsistent behaviour is attributed to unstable or situational factors (e.g. Bell, Wicklund, Manko & Larkin, 1976; Rosenfield & Stephan, 1977). When people explain behaviour that confirms their expectancy, they may simply rely on dispositions implied by a stereotype, with little or no effort to consider additional factors (Kulik, 1983; Pyszczynski & Greenberg, 1981).
2 *A self-esteem process.* People's need for secure self-esteem can be nurtured by making comparisons between their ingroup and relevant outgroups. This process is a fundamental aspect of **social identity theory** (e.g. Tajfel & Turner, 1979; also Hogg & Abrams, 1988). Because people derive their social identity from the groups to which they belong (a description and evaluation of themselves in terms of the defining features of the group), they have a vested interest in maintaining or obtaining an ingroup profile that is more positive than that of relevant outgroups. The ethnocentric attributional bias quite clearly satisfies this aim: it internally attributes good things about the ingroup and bad things about the outgroup, and it externally attributes bad things about the ingroup and good things about the outgroup.

Social identity theory
Theory of group membership and intergroup relations based on self-categorisation, social comparison and the construction of a shared self-definition in terms of ingroup-defining properties.

Attribution and stereotyping

Attribution processes operating at the societal level in an intergroup context may play an important role in shaping the profile and dominance of the stereotypes we have of specific groups. Stereotyping is not only an individual cognitive activity; it can also serve ego-defensive functions (making one feel good in contrast to others) and social functions (allowing one to fit in with other people's world views) (Snyder & Miene, 1994).

According to Henri Tajfel (1981a), social groups may activate or accentuate existing stereotypes in order to attribute large-scale distressing events to the actions of specific outgroups—that is, scapegoats. For instance, during the 1930s in Germany the Jews were blamed for the economic crisis of the time. It was convenient to activate the 'miserly Jew' stereotype to explain in simplistic terms the lack of money: there is no money because the Jews are hoarding it. Stereotypes may also be elaborated to justify actions committed or planned against an outgroup (e.g. Crandall, Bahns, Warner & Schaller, 2011). For instance, a group might develop a stereotype of an outgroup as dull-witted, simple, lazy and incompetent in order to explain or justify the economic and social exploitation of that group.

Social representations

Social representations
Collectively elaborated explanations of unfamiliar and complex phenomena that transform them into a familiar and simple form.

One way in which cultural knowledge about the causes of things may be constructed and transmitted is described by Serge Moscovici's theory of **social representations** (e.g. Farr & Moscovici, 1984; Lorenzi-Cioldi & Clémence, 2001; Moscovici, 1961, 1981, 1988; Purkhardt, 1995). Social representations are consensual understandings shared among group members. They emerge through informal everyday communication. They transform the unfamiliar and complex into the familiar and straightforward, and thus provide a commonsense framework for interpreting our experiences.

An individual or a specialist interest group develops a sophisticated, non-obvious, technical explanation of a commonplace phenomenon (e.g. explaining mental illness in terms of biological or social factors rather than spiritual forces). This attracts public attention and becomes widely shared and popularised (i.e. simplified, distorted and ritualised) through informal discussion among non-specialists. It is now a social representation—an accepted, unquestioned commonsense explanation that ousts alternatives to become the orthodox explanation.

Moscovici's original formulation focused on the development of the theory of psychoanalysis, but it is just as applicable to other formal theories and complex phenomena that have been transformed and simplified to become part of popular consciousness: for example, evolutionary theory, relativity theory, dietary and health theories, Marxist economics and AIDS. The theory of social representations has come under some criticism, often for the rather imprecise way in which it is formulated (e.g. Augoustinos & Innes, 1990). Nonetheless, it does suggest a way in which ordinary social interaction in society constructs commonsense or 'naive' causal theories that are widely used to explain events (Heider, 1958).

One source of criticism is that it has been difficult to know how to analyse social representations quantitatively. However, steps have been taken towards the development of appropriate quantitative techniques (Doise, Clémence & Lorenzi-Cioldi, 1993), and Breakwell and Canter (1993) have assembled a collection of chapters describing in practical terms the variety of ways that different researchers have approached the measurement of social representations. These methods include qualitative and quantitative analyses of interviews, questionnaires, observational data and archival material. A good example of this methodological pluralism is Jodelet's (1991) classic description of social representations of mental illness in the small French community of Ainay-le-Chateau, in which questionnaires, interviews and ethnographic observation were all used.

Social representations, like norms tend to be grounded in groups and differ from group to group, such that intergroup behaviour can often revolve around a clash of social representations (Lorenzi-Cioldi & Clémence, 2001). For example, in Western countries attitudes and behaviour that promote healthy lifestyles are associated with higher social status, and health promotion messages tend to emanate from middle-class professional groups (Salovey, Rothman & Rodin, 1998). A social representations analysis suggests that these messages are relatively ineffective in promoting healthy lifestyles for non-middle-class people because they are inconsistent with the wider representational framework of a good life for such people.

The development of the European Union (EU) has provided fertile ground for social representation research (e.g. Chryssochoou, 2000) that connects with the study of European identity dynamics (e.g. Cinnirella, 1997; Huici et al., 1997). The EU is, in many respects, a prototypical social representation—a relatively new and quite technical idea that has its roots in complex economic matters such as free trade and subsidies. But the EU is now an accepted and commonplace part of European discourse which often emphasises more emotive issues of national and European identity—although the recent global and European economic crisis has refocused attention on economic and trade issues associated with the single currency and the concept of a European Central Bank.

Rumour

The process through which social representations are constructed has more than a passing resemblance to the way in which rumours develop and are communicated (Allport & Postman, 1947; DiFonzo & Bordia, 2007). One of the earliest studies of rumour was conducted by Gordon Allport and Leo Postman (1945), who found that if experimental participants described a photograph to someone who had not seen the photo, and then this person described it to another person, and so on, only 30 percent of the original detail remained after five retellings. Allport and Postman identified three processes associated with rumour transmission:

1 *Levelling*—the rumour quickly becomes shorter, less detailed and less complex.
2 *Sharpening*—certain features of the rumour are selectively emphasised and exaggerated.
3 *Assimilation*—the rumour is distorted in line with people's pre-existing prejudices, partialities, interests and agendas.

More naturalistic studies have found rather less distortion as a consequence of rumour transmission (e.g. Caplow, 1947; Schachter & Burdeck, 1955).

Whether or not rumours are distorted, and even whether rumours are transmitted at all, seems to depend on the anxiety level of those who hear the rumour (Buckner, 1965; Rosnow, 1980). Uncertainty and ambiguity increase anxiety and stress, which leads people to seek out information with which to rationalise anxiety, which in turn enhances rumour transmission. (Check the third focus question. Here is one reason why Rajna wanted to pass a rumour on.) Whether the ensuing rumour is distorted or becomes more precise depends on whether people approach the rumour with a critical or uncritical orientation. In the former case the rumour becomes refined, while in the latter (which often accompanies a crisis) the rumour becomes distorted.

Rumours always have a source, and often this source purposely elaborates the rumour for a specific reason. The stock market is a perfect context for rumour elaboration—and, of course, the consequences for ordinary people's everyday lives can be enormous. At the end of the 1990s, rumour played a clear role in inflating the value of 'dot-com' start-up companies, which then crashed in the NASDAQ meltdown early in 2000. More recently, there was enormous build-up and hype surrounding the launching of Facebook as a public company on the stock market in May 2012—Facebook shares lost 25% of their value in the two weeks following the launch. Rumour also played a significant role in the global stock-market crash at the end of 2008 and beginning of 2009 (the market lost more than half its value), and in reports about Greece's economic collapse that depressed the stock market in August 2011 and May 2012.

Another reason that rumours are purposely elaborated is to discredit individuals or groups. An organisation can spread a rumour about a competitor in order to undermine the competitor's market share (Shibutani, 1966), or a group can spread a rumour to blame another group for a widespread crisis. A good example of this is the fabrication and promulgation of conspiracy theories (Graumann & Moscovici, 1987).

Conspiracy theory
Explanation of widespread, complex and worrying events in terms of the premeditated actions of small groups of highly organised conspirators.

Conspiracy theories

Conspiracy theories are simplistic and exhaustive causal theories that attribute widespread natural and social calamities to the intentional and organised activities of certain social groups that are seen to form conspiratorial bodies set on ruining and then dominating the rest of humanity. One of the best documented conspiracy theories is the myth, dating from the

Middle Ages, of the Jewish world conspiracy (Cohn, 1966), which surfaces periodically and often results in massive systematic persecution. Other conspiracy theories include the belief that immigrants are intentionally plotting to undermine the economy, that homosexuals are intentionally spreading HIV, and that witches (in the Middle Ages) and Al-Qaeda (most recently) are behind virtually every world disaster you care to mention (e.g. Cohn, 1975).

Conspiracy theories wax and wane in popularity. They were particularly popular from the mid-17th to the mid-18th century:

> *Everywhere people sensed designs within designs, cabals within cabals; there were court conspiracies, backstairs conspiracies, ministerial conspiracies, factional conspiracies, aristocratic conspiracies, and by the last half of the eighteenth century even conspiracies of gigantic secret societies that cut across national boundaries and spanned the Atlantic. (Wood, 1982, p. 407)*

The accomplished conspiracy theorist can, with consummate skill and breathtaking versatility, explain even the most arcane and puzzling events in terms of the devious schemes and inscrutable machinations of hidden conspirators. Mick Billig (1978) believes it is precisely this that can make conspiracy theories so attractive—they are incredibly effective at reducing uncertainty (Hogg, 2007b, 2012). They provide a causal explanation in terms of enduring dispositions that can explain a wide range of events, rather than complex situational factors that are less widely applicable. Furthermore, worrying events become controllable and easily remedied because they are caused by small groups of highly visible people rather than being due to complex sociohistorical circumstances (Bains, 1983).

Not surprisingly, conspiracy theories are almost immune to disconfirming evidence. For example, in December 2006 the outcome of a three-year, £3.5 million enquiry into the death in 1997 of Princess Diana was reported—although there was absolutely no evidence that the British Royal family had conspired with the British Government to have her killed to prevent her marrying an Egyptian Muslim, this conspiracy theory still persists. There are also conspiracy theories about the 9/11 terrorist attacks in the United States in 2001—some Americans are absolutely convinced it was the doing of the US government, while historian Bernard Lewis (2004) reported that many Muslims believe that the same attacks were perpetrated by Israel (Lewis, 2004).

Societal attributions

The emphasis on attributions as social knowledge finds expression in research into the explanations that people give for large-scale social phenomena. In general, this research supports the view that causal attributions for specific phenomena are located within and shaped by wider, socially constructed belief systems.

For example, research into explanations for poverty reveals that both the rich and the poor tend to explain poverty in terms of poor people's behaviour rather than the situation that those people find themselves in (e.g. Feagin, 1972; Feather, 1974). This individualistic tendency is not so strong for people with a more left-wing or socialist ideology, or for people living in developing countries, where poverty is widespread (Pandey, Sinha, Prakash & Tripathi, 1982).

Explanations for wealth tend to depend on political affiliation. In Britain, Conservatives often ascribe it to positive individual qualities of thrift and hard work, while Labour supporters attribute it to the unsavoury individual quality of ruthless determination (Furnham, 1983). Not surprisingly, there are also cross-cultural differences: for example, individualistic explanations are very common in Hong Kong (Forgas, Morris & Furnham, 1982; Furnham & Bond, 1986).

Similarly, the sorts of explanation given for unemployment are influenced by people's wider belief and value systems. Norm Feather (1985) had Australian students give their explanations of unemployment on a number of dimensions. They preferred societal over individualistic explanations: for example, defective government, social change and economic recession were seen as more valid causes of unemployment than lack of motivation and personal handicap (see also Feather & Barber, 1983; Feather & Davenport, 1981). However, students who were politically more conservative tended to place less emphasis on societal explanations. Studies conducted in Britain also reveal that societal explanations are more prominent than individualistic explanations, and that there is a fair amount of agreement between employed and unemployed respondents (Furnham, 1982; Gaskell & Smith, 1985; Lewis, Snell & Furnham, 1987).

Other research has focused on the sorts of explanation that people give for riots. Riots are enormously complicated social phenomena in that there are both proximal and distal causes—a specific event or action might trigger the riot, but only because of the complex conjunction of wider conditions. For instance, the proximal cause of the 1992 Los Angeles riots may have been the acquittal of Caucasian police officers charged with the beating of an African American motorist, Rodney King; however, this alone would have been unlikely to promote a riot without the background of racial unrest and socioeconomic distress in the United States at the time.

As with explanations of poverty, wealth and unemployment, the sorts of explanation that people give for a specific riot seem to be influenced by the person's sociopolitical perspective (e.g. Litton & Potter, 1985; Reicher, 1984, 2001; Reicher & Potter, 1985; Schmidt, 1972). More conservative members of the establishment tend to identify deviance, or personal or social pathology, while people with more liberal social attitudes tend to identify social circumstances.

For example, Charles Schmidt (1972) analysed print media explanations of the spate of riots that occurred in American cities during 1967. The explanations could be classified on three dimensions:

1 legitimate–illegitimate
2 internal–external cause
3 institutional–environmental cause.

The first two dimensions were strongly correlated, with legitimate external causes (e.g. urban renewal mistakes, slum conditions) going together and illegitimate internal causes (e.g. criminal intent, belief that violence works) going together. Media sources on the political right tended to identify illegitimate internal causes, whereas those classified as 'left–centre' (i.e. liberal) emphasised legitimate external causes.

Finally, Paul Sniderman and his colleagues investigated the way in which people give explanations for racial inequality and have preferences for different government policies (Sniderman, Hagen, Tetlock & Brady, 1986). They used a national sample of Caucasians in the United States (in 1972) and were interested in investigating the influence of level of education. They found that less educated Caucasians employed an 'affect-driven' reasoning process. They started with their (mainly negative) feelings about African Americans, then proceeded directly to advocate minimal government assistance. Having done this, they 'doubled back' to fill in the intervening link to justify their advocacy—namely that African Americans were personally responsible for their own disadvantage. In contrast, better educated Caucasians adopted a 'cognition-driven' reasoning process, in which they reasoned both forwards and backwards. Their policy recommendations were based on causal attributions for inequality, and in turn their causal attributions were influenced by their policy preference.

Culture's contribution

The causal attributions and explanations that people proffer for events and behaviours are influenced not only by the nature of the information available, but also by people's wider belief and value systems. We have already seen, for example, the influence of sociopolitical

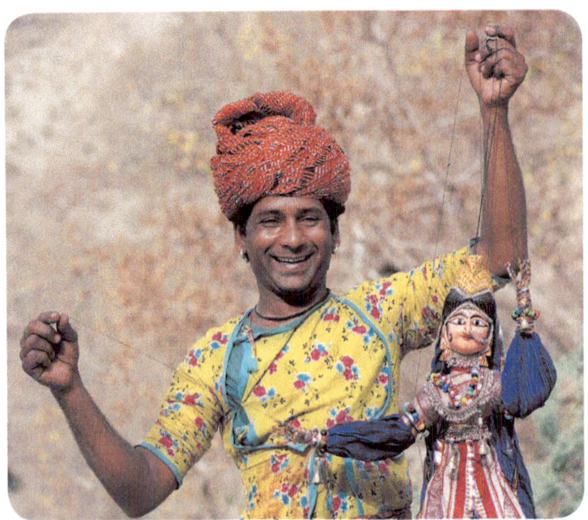

Culture and attribution Is the puppet responsible for its own actions? Easterners are less likely than Westerners to make dispositional attributions about people — let alone about puppets! (**Source:** © Free Agents Limited/CORBIS.)

values, educational status, group membership and ethnicity; and some evidence for the impact of culture.

People from different cultures often make very different attributions, make attributions in different ways or approach the entire task of social explanation in different ways (Chiu & Hong, 2007; Heine, 2012; Smith, Bond & Kağitçibaşi, 2006). Consequently, the potential for cross-cultural interpersonal misunderstanding is enormous. For example, the Zande people of West Africa have a dual theory of causality, where commonsense proximal causes operate within the context of witchcraft as the distal cause (Evans-Pritchard, 1937; see also Jahoda, 1979)—which is, ironically, not really that different from moderate Christians' belief in the proximal operation of scientific principles within the context of God as the distal cause. For the Zande, an internal–external distinction would make little sense.

Another example: the anthropologist Lucien Lévy-Bruhl (1925) reported that the natives of Motumotu in New Guinea attributed a pleurisy epidemic to the presence of a specific missionary, his sheep, two goats and, finally, a portrait of Queen Victoria. Although initially quite bizarre, these sorts of attribution are easily explained as social representations. How much more bizarre are they than, for example, the postulation in physics of other universes and hypothetical particles shaped like strings or membranes as part of a unified theory to explain the origin and structure of the cosmos (Hawking, 1988; Hawking & Mlodinow, 2010)—the science journalist John Horgan exclaimed that 'This isn't physics any more. It's science fiction with mathematics' (Horgan, 2011, p. B7).

One area of cross-cultural attribution research is the correspondence bias, as explained earlier. We have seen that in Western cultures people tend to make dispositional attributions for others' behaviour (Gilbert & Malone, 1995; Ross, 1977). There is also evidence that such dispositional attributions become more evident over ontogeny (e.g. Pevers & Secord, 1973). In non-Western cultures, however, people are less inclined to make dispositional attributions (Carrithers, Collins & Lukes, 1986; Morris & Peng, 1994). This is probably partly a reflection of the more pervasive and all-enveloping influence of social roles in more collectivist non-Western cultures (Fletcher & Ward, 1988; Jahoda, 1982) and partly a reflection of a more holistic world view that promotes context-dependent, occasion-bound thinking (Shweder & Bourne, 1982).

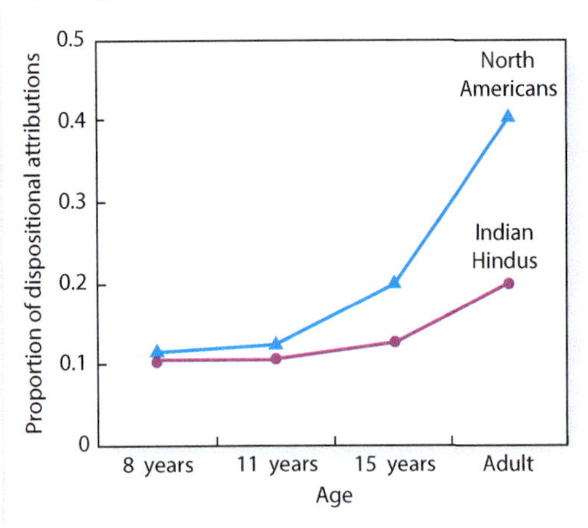

Figure 9.9 Dispositional attributions as a function of age and cultural background

North Americans and Indian Hindus initially do not differ in the proportion of dispositional attributions made for behaviour. However, by the age of 15 there is a clear difference that strengthens in adulthood, with Americans being significantly more dispositional than Indians in their attributions
(**Source:** based on data from Miller (1984))

To investigate further the role of culture in dispositional attributions, Joan Miller (1984) compared middle-class North Americans and Indian Hindus from each of four age groups (adults, and 15-, 11- and 8-year-olds). Participants narrated prosocial and antisocial behaviour and gave their own spontaneous explanations of the causes of this behaviour. Miller coded responses to identify the proportion of dispositional and contextual attributions that participants made. Among the youngest children there was little cross-cultural difference (see Figure 9.9). As age increased, however, the two groups diverged, mainly because the Americans increasingly adopted dispositional attributions. For context attributions the results were reversed.

The important lesson this study teaches us is that cultural factors have a significant impact on attribution and social explanation.[E]

Structure and function of attitudes

A short history of attitudes

Attitude is a word that is part of our commonsense language. Many years ago, the social psychologist Gordon Allport referred to attitude as social psychology's most indispensable concept. In the 1935 *Handbook of social psychology*, which was highly influential at the time, he wrote:

> *The concept of attitudes is probably the most distinctive and indispensable concept in contemporary American social psychology. No other term appears more frequently in the experimental and theoretical literature.* (Allport, 1935, p. 798)

Attitude
(a) A relatively enduring organisation of beliefs, feelings and behavioural tendencies towards socially significant objects, groups, events or symbols. (b) A general feeling or evaluation—positive or negative—about some person, object or issue.

In the historical context in which Allport was writing, his view is not remarkable. Others, such as Thomas and Znaniecki (1918) and Watson (1930), had previously equated social psychology and attitude research—actually defining social psychology as the scientific study of attitudes! The early 1930s also witnessed the first generation of questionnaire-based scales to measure attitudes. According to Allport, an attitude is:

> *a mental and neural state of readiness, organised through experience, exerting a directive or dynamic influence upon the individual's response to all objects and situations with which it is related.* (Allport, 1935, p. 810)

Allport was not to know that such a fashionable concept would become the centre of much controversy in the decades ahead. For example, a radical behavioural view would emerge to argue that an attitude is merely a figment of the imagination—people invent attitudes to explain behaviour that has already occurred.

In charting the history of attitude research in social psychology, Bill McGuire (1986) identified three main phases separated by periods of waning interest:

1. a concentration on attitude measurement and how these measurements related to behaviour (1920s and 1930s)
2. a focus on the dynamics of change in an individual's attitudes (1950s and 1960s)
3. a focus on the cognitive and social structure and function of attitudes and attitude systems (1980s and 1990s).

The word 'attitude' is derived from the Latin *aptus*, which means 'fit and ready for action'. This ancient meaning refers to something that is directly observable, such as a boxer in a boxing ring. Today, however, attitude researchers view 'attitude' as a construct that, although not directly observable, precedes behaviour and guides our choices and decisions for action.

Attitude research in psychology and the social sciences has generated enormous interest and many hundreds, probably thousands, of studies covering almost every conceivable topic about which attitudes might be expressed. During the 1960s and 1970s attitude research entered a period of pessimism and decline. To some extent, this was a reaction to concern about the apparent lack of relationship between expressed attitudes and overt behaviour.

However, during the 1980s attitudes again became a centre of attention for social psychologists, stimulated by cognitive psychology's impact on social psychology (see reviews

[E]Vaughan, M. G., & Hogg, M. A. (2014). Social cognition and social thinking. In *Social psychology* (7th ed., pp. 80–99). Frenchs Forest, NSW: Pearson Australia.

by Olson & Zanna, 1993; Tesser & Shaffer, 1990). This resurgence included a significant focus on how information processing and memory, and affect and feelings might affect attitude formation and change (Haddock & Zanna, 1999; Lieberman, 2000; Murphy, Monahan & Zajonc, 1995). There has also been extensive research on attitude strength and accessibility, on how attitudes relate to behaviour (Ajzen, 2001), and on implicit measures of attitude (Crano & Prislin, 2006; Fazio & Olson, 2003b). Most recently, there has been a focus on biochemical dimensions of attitude phenomena (Blascovich & Mendes, 2010) and on neural activity associated with attitudes (Stanley, Phelps & Banaji, 2008).

We take the view that attitudes are basic to, and pervasive, in human life. In doing this, we will not take McGuire's evolutionary sequence too literally, as the three foci he refers to have always been, and continue to be, of interest to social psychologists. Without having attitudes, people would have difficulty in construing and reacting to events, in trying to make decisions and in making sense of their relationships with other people in everyday life. Attitudes continue to fascinate researchers and remain a key, if sometimes controversial, part of social psychology.

Let us now look at the anatomy of an attitude.

Attitude structure

One of the most fundamental psychological questions that can be asked about attitudes is whether they are a unitary construct or whether they have a number of different components.

One component

One-component attitude model
An attitude consists of affect towards or evaluation of the object.

Thurstone preferred a **one-component attitude model**, defining an attitude as "the affect for or against a psychological object" (1931, p. 261). A later text focusing on how one constructs scales to measure attitudes reiterated this view: an attitude is "the degree of positive or negative affect associated with some psychological object" (Edwards, 1957, p. 2). How simple can you get—do you like the object or not? With hindsight, it can be argued that the dominant feature of affect became the basis of a more sophisticated sociocognitive model proposed by Pratkanis and Greenwald (1989).

Two components

Two-component attitude model
An attitude consists of a mental readiness to act. It also guides evaluative (judgemental) responses.

Allport (1935) favoured a **two-component attitude model**. To Thurstone's 'affect' Allport added a second component—a state of mental readiness. Mental readiness is a predisposition which has a relatively consistent influence on how we decide what is good or bad, desirable or undesirable, and so on. An attitude is therefore a private event. Its existence is unobservable externally and can only be inferred, perhaps by examining our own mental processes introspectively. As we see later, we might also make inferences by examining what we say and what we do. You cannot see, touch or physically examine an attitude; it is a hypothetical construct.

Three components

Three-component attitude model
An attitude consists of cognitive, affective and behavioural components. This threefold division has an ancient heritage, stressing thought, feeling and action as basic to human experience.

A third view is the **three-component attitude model**, which has its roots in ancient philosophy:

> *The trichotomy of human experience into thought, feeling, and action, although not logically compelling, is so pervasive in Indo-European thought (being found in Hellenic, Zoroastrian and Hindu philosophy) as to suggest that it corresponds to something basic in our way of conceptualisation, perhaps ... reflecting the three evolutionary layers of the brain, cerebral cortex, limbic system, and old brain.* (McGuire, 1989, p. 40)

The three-component model of attitude was particularly popular in the 1960s (e.g. Krech, Crutchfield & Ballachey, 1962; Rosenberg & Hovland, 1960). It was also represented in the later work of Himmelfarb and Eagly (1974), who described an attitude as a relatively enduring organisation of beliefs about, and feelings and behavioural tendencies towards, socially significant objects, groups, events or symbols. Note that this definition not only included the three components but also emphasised that attitudes are:

- *relatively permanent*: that is, they persist across time and situations—a momentary feeling is not an attitude
- limited to *socially significant* events or objects
- *generalisable*, with at least some degree of abstraction. If you drop a book on your toe and find that it hurts, this is not enough to form an attitude, because it is a single event in one place and at one time. But if the experience makes you dislike books or libraries, or clumsiness in general, then that dislike is an attitude.

Each attitude, then, is made up of thoughts and ideas, a cluster of feelings, likes and dislikes, and behavioural intentions. Other theorists who have favoured the three-component model include Thomas Ostrom (1968) and Steven Breckler (1984).

Despite the appeal of the 'trinity', this model presents a problem by prejudging a link between attitude and behaviour (Zanna & Rempel, 1988), itself a thorny and complex issue that is dealt with in detail later. Suffice to say that most modern definitions of attitude involve both belief and feeling structures and are much concerned with how, if each can indeed be measured, the resulting data may help predict people's actions. (Based on what you have read so far, try to answer the first focus question.)

Attitude functions

Presumably attitudes exist because they are useful—they serve a purpose, they have a function. The approaches we have considered so far make at least an implicit assumption of purpose. Some writers have been more explicit. Daniel Katz (1960), for example, proposed that there are various kinds of attitude, each serving a different function, such as:

- knowledge
- instrumentality (means to an end or goal)
- ego defence (protecting one's self-esteem)
- value expressiveness (allowing people to display those values that uniquely identify and define them).

An attitude saves cognitive energy, as we do not have to figure out 'from scratch' how we should relate to the object or situation in question (Smith, Bruner & White, 1956), a function that parallels the utility of a **schema** and fits the cognitive miser or motivated tactician models of contemporary social cognition, and of a **stereotype** (e.g. Fiske & Taylor, 2008).

Russell Fazio (1989) later argued that the main function of any kind of attitude is a utilitarian one: that of object appraisal. This should hold regardless of whether the attitude has a positive or negative valence (i.e. whether our feelings about the object are good or bad). Merely possessing an attitude is useful because of the orientation towards the object that it provides for the person. For example, having a negative attitude towards snakes (believing they are dangerous) is useful if we cannot differentiate between safe and deadly varieties. However, for an attitude truly to fulfil this function it must be accessible. We develop this aspect of Fazio's thinking about attitude function when we deal with the link between attitude and behaviour.

Schema
Cognitive structure that represents knowledge about a concept or type of stimulus, including its attributes and the relations among those attributes.

Stereotype
Widely shared and simplified evaluative image of a social group and its members.

Cognitive consistency

Cognitive consistency theories A group of attitude theories stressing that people try to maintain internal consistency, order and agreement among their various cognitions.

Cognition The knowledge, beliefs, thoughts and ideas that people have about themselves and their environment. May also refer to mental processes through which knowledge is acquired, including perception, memory and thinking.

Sociocognitive model Attitude theory highlighting an evaluative component. Knowledge of an object is represented in memory along with a summary of how to appraise it.

In the late 1950s and 1960s cognitive consistency theories came to dominate social psychology, and their emphasis on cognition dealt a fatal blow to simplistic reinforcement explanations (e.g. by learning theorists such as Thorndike, Hull and Skinner) in social psychology (Greenwald et al. 2002). The best known of these theories was cognitive dissonance theory (Cooper, 2007; Festinger, 1957).

As well as specifying that beliefs are the building blocks of attitude structure, this family of theories focused on inconsistencies among people's beliefs. Consistency theories differ in how they define consistency and inconsistency, but they all assume that people find inconsistent beliefs aversive. Two thoughts are inconsistent if one seems to contradict the other, and such a state of mind is bothersome. This disharmony is known as *dissonance*. Consistency theories argue that people are motivated to change one or more contradictory beliefs so that the belief system as a whole is in harmony. The outcome is restoration of consistency.

Cognition and evaluation

We noted above the existence of a one-component view of attitudes—initially one in which affect reigned supreme (Thurstone, 1931), but subsequently focusing on evaluation as the core component (e.g. Osgood, Suci & Tannenbaum, 1957). This simple idea resurfaces in a more complicated guise in Anthony Pratkanis and Tony Greenwald's sociocognitive model, where an attitude is defined as 'a person's evaluation of an object of thought' (1989, p. 247). An attitude object (see Figure 9.10) is represented in memory by:

- an object label and the rules for applying that label
- an evaluative summary of that object
- a knowledge structure supporting that evaluation.

For example, the attitude object we know as a 'shark' may be represented in memory as a really big fish with very sharp teeth (*label*); that lives in the sea and eats other fish and sometimes people (*rules*); is scary and best avoided while swimming (*evaluative summary*); and is a scientifically and fictionally well-documented threat to our physical wellbeing (*knowledge structure*). However, despite the cognitive emphasis, it was the evaluative component that Pratkanis and Greenwald highlighted.

The evaluative dimension of attitudes is, of course, a central focus of research on prejudice where the key problem is that members of one group harbour negative attitudes towards members of another group (Dovidio, Glick & Rudman, 2005; Jones, 1996). In

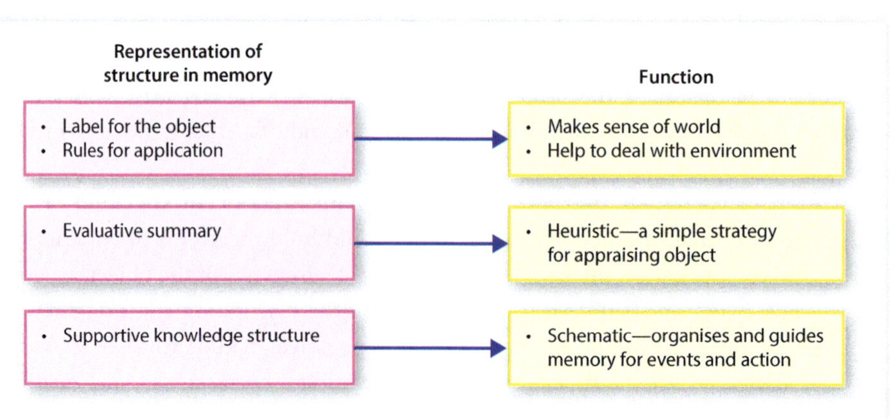

Figure 9.10 The sociocognitive model of attitude structure and function

This theory draws on research in social cognition and studies of memory. Just as physical objects or even people can be represented in memory, so too can an attitude object

(**Source:** based on Pratkanis & Greenwald (1989))

the attitude literature, various terms have been used almost interchangeably in denoting this evaluative component, such as 'affect', 'evaluation', 'emotion' and 'feeling', suggesting an urgent need for the terminology to be tidied up and standardised (Breckler & Wiggins (1989a, 1989b). Recent research on affect and emotion has helped sort some of this out by theorising about the role of cognitive appraisals of stimuli in people's experience of affect and emotion (e.g. Blascovich 2008; Lazarus, 1991; see Keltner & Lerner, 2010). When we apply this knowledge to the study of an attitude, we can distinguish between *affect* (an emotional reaction to an attitude object) and *evaluation* (particular kinds of thought, belief and judgement about the object).

Decision making and attitudes

Do we perform cognitive algebra?

Information processing approaches emphasise how complex it is to acquire knowledge and to form and change our attitudes. According to **information integration theory** (Anderson, 1971, 1981), we use **cognitive algebra** to construct our attitudes from information we receive about attitude objects. People are sophisticated problem solvers and vigilant evaluators of new information. How we receive and combine this information provides the basis for attitude structure. The salience of some items and the order in which they are received become important determinants of the way in which they are processed. As new information arrives, people evaluate it and combine it with existing information stored in memory. For example, a warning from health authorities that a certain brand of food may cause serious illness may lead people to re-evaluate their attitude, change their behaviour and not eat that brand again.

In Norman Anderson's approach, we acquire and re-evaluate attitudes by using cognitive algebra. We 'mentally' average out the values attached to discrete bits of information that are collated and stored in memory about an attitude object. Ordinary people habitually use such mathematics: for example, if you think a friend is shy, energetic and compassionate, your overall attitude is an average of the evaluations you attach to those traits. You would calculate a different average for another friend who was outgoing, energetic and charismatic.

Information processing
The evaluation of information; in relation to attitudes, the means by which people acquire knowledge and form and change attitudes.

Information integration theory
The idea that a person's attitude can be estimated by averaging across the positive and negative ratings of the object.

Cognitive algebra
Approach to the study of impression formation that focuses on how people combine attributes that have valence into an overall positive or negative impression.

Attitudes and automatic judgements

As a challenge to classical attitude theory, Patricia Devine (1989) suggested that people's attitudes are underpinned by implicit and automatic judgements of which they are unaware. Because these judgements are automatic and unconscious, they are less influenced by *social desirability bias* (i.e. how others might react). As such, they should therefore be a more reliable measure of a person's 'true' attitudes.

According to Norbert Schwarz (2000), a model of attitude as an implicit construct could help us better understand the relationship between people's attitudes and their behaviour (see below). Others are more cautious. For example, implicit measures (again, see below) may be as dependent on context as explicit measures (attitudes), but in different ways (Glaser & Banaji, 1999). Implicit measures correlate only weakly with both explicit self-reports and overt behaviour (Hilton & Karpinski, 2000), and correlations between implicit and explicit measures of intergroup attitudes are generally low (Dovidio, Kawakami & Beach, 2001). In considering developments in attitude theory, van der Pligt and de Vries (2000) proposed a decision-making strategy continuum, which ranges from intuition at one end to controlled information processing (e.g. Anderson, 1971) at the other.

Dispute over the best way to characterise attitudes continues and shows little sign of abating. Is an attitude a directive and organised state of readiness (Allport), an outcome of algebraic calculation (Anderson) or an automatic judgement (Devine)?

Can attitudes predict behaviour?

Why study attitudes if scientists disagree about how best to define them? One answer is that attitudes may be useful for predicting what people will do—maybe if we change people's attitudes, we might be able to change their behaviour. Perhaps with tongue in cheek, Crano and Prislin have written in a recent review: 'Because attitudes predict behavior, they are considered the crown jewel of social psychology' (2006, p. 360). As we shall see, a number of behavioural scientists have questioned this assumption.

For instance, Gregson and Stacey (1981) found only a small positive correlation between attitudes and self-reported alcohol consumption. Furthermore, there was no evidence of any benefits in focusing on attitude change rather than on economic incentives to control alcohol use (e.g. avoiding fines, increasing taxes). This sort of finding has caused some critics to question the utility of the concept of attitude: if attitude measures bear no relation to what people actually do, then what is the use of the concept? It is interesting that an early study of ethnic attitudes by LaPiere (1934) revealed a glaring inconsistency between what people do and what they say.

Following LaPiere's study, which vividly called into question the predictive utility of questionnaires, researchers have used more sophisticated methods to study the attitude–behaviour relationship, but still mainly found relatively low correspondence between questionnaire measures of attitudes and measures of actual behaviour. After reviewing this research, Wicker (1969) concluded that the correlation between attitudes and behaviour is seldom as high as 0.30 (which, when squared, indicates that only 9 percent of the variability in a behaviour is accounted for by an attitude). In fact, Wicker found that the average correlation between attitudes and behaviour was only 0.15. This view was seized upon during the 1970s as damning evidence—the attitude concept is not worth a fig, since it has little predictive power. A sense of despair settled on the field (Abelson, 1972). Nevertheless, attitudes are still being researched (Banaji & Heiphetz, 2010; Fazio & Olson, 2003a).

What gradually emerged was that attitudes and overt behaviour are not related in a one-to-one fashion. There are conditions that promote or disrupt the correspondence between having an attitude and behaving (Doll & Ajzen, 1992; Smith & Stasson, 2000). For example, attitude–behaviour consistency can vary according to whether:

- an attitude is more rather than less accessible (see below)
- an attitude is expressed publicly, say in a group, or privately, such as when responding to a questionnaire
- an individual identifies strongly or weakly with a group for which the attitude is normative.

Not all classes of social behaviour can be predicted accurately from verbally

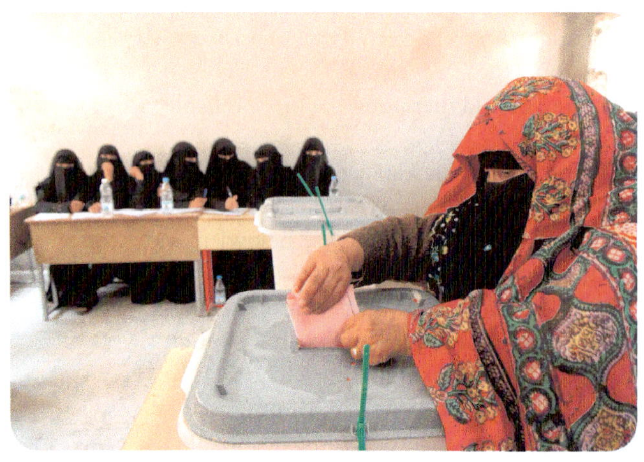

Attitudes and behaviour This voter is under surveillance. Will her selection reflect her own view, or might it be constrained by a prevailing norm? (**Source:** © AFP.)

expressed attitudes. We look now at research that has explored why attitude–behaviour correspondence is often weak, and what factors may strengthen the correspondence.

Beliefs, intentions and behaviour

According to Martin Fishbein (1967a, 1967b, 1971), the basic ingredient of an attitude is affect, a position that reflects Thurstone's (1931) early definition. However, an attitude measure based entirely on a unidimensional, bipolar evaluative scale (such as good/bad) does not predict reliably how a person will later behave. Better prediction depends on an account of the interaction between attitudes, beliefs and behavioural intentions, and the connections of all of these with subsequent actions.

In this equation, we need to establish both how strong and how valuable are a person's beliefs: some beliefs will carry more weight than others in relation to the final act. For example, the strength or weakness of a person's religious convictions may be pivotal in their decision-making processes regarding moral behaviour—moral norms may play a very important role in attitude–behaviour relations (Manstead, 2000). Without this information, trying to predict an outcome for a given individual must inevitably be a hit-or-miss affair.

Consider the example in Table 9.1. A young, heterosexually active man might believe, strongly or not, that certain things are true about two forms of contraception, the pill and the condom. *Belief strength* (or expectancy) has a probability estimate, ranging from 0 to 1, regarding the truth; for example, he may hold a very strong belief (0.90) that the pill is a highly reliable method of birth control. Reliability of a contraceptive is a 'good' thing, so his *evaluation* (or value) of the pill is +2, say, on a five-point scale ranging from –2 to +2. Belief strength and evaluation interact, producing a final rating of +1.80. (Like Anderson, Fishbein's view incorporates the idea that people are able to perform cognitive algebra.)

Next, the young man might be fairly sure (0.70) that the condom is less reliable (–1), a rating of –0.70. Likewise, he thinks that using a condom is potentially embarrassing in a sexual encounter. His further belief that using a condom has no known side effects is not sufficient to offset the effects of the other two beliefs. Check the hypothetical algebra in Table 9.1. Consequently, the young man's intention to use a condom, should he possess one, may be quite low (perhaps he hopes that the women who cross his path use the pill!). Only by having all of this information could we be fairly confident about predicting his future behaviour.

This approach to prediction also offers a method of measurement, the expectancy–value technique. In subsequent work with his colleague Icek Ajzen, Fishbein developed the *theory of reasoned action* to link beliefs to intentions to behaviour (Ajzen & Fishbein, 1980; Fishbein & Ajzen, 1974). We return to this model later. Fishbein and Ajzen's work was a significant advance in understanding issues that had previously complicated the overall relationship

Table 9.1 A young man's hypothetical attitude towards contraceptive use: the strength and value of his beliefs

	Man's belief about woman using pill					Man's belief about man using condom				
Attribute	**Strength of belief**		**Value of belief**		**Result**	**Strength of belief**		**Value of belief**		**Result**
Reliability	0.90	×	+2	=	+1.80	0.70	×	–1	=	–0.70
Embarrassment	1.00	×	+2	=	+2.00	0.80	×	–2	=	–1.60
Side effects	0.10	×	–1	=	–0.10	1.00	×	+2	=	+2.00
Outcome					+3.70					–0.30

The strength of a belief, in this example, is the probability (from 0 to 1) that a person thinks that the belief is true. The value of a belief is an evaluation on a bipolar scale (in this case, ranging from +2 to –2).

between attitudes and behaviour. Predictions can be clarified when the inherent links are brought to the surface. Furthermore, behavioural predictions can be much improved if the measures of attitudes are specific rather than general.

Specific attitudes

Ajzen and Fishbein believed that success in predicting the way we behave is determined by asking whether we would perform a given act or series of acts. The key lies in asking questions that are quite specific rather than ones that deal with generalities.

Ajzen and Fishbein argued that much previous attitude research had suffered from either trying to predict specific behaviours from general attitudes or vice versa, so that low correlations were to be expected. This is, in essence, what LaPiere did. An example of a specific attitude predicting specific behaviour would be a student's attitude towards a psychology exam predicting how diligently he or she would study for that exam. In contrast, an example of a general attitude predicting a general class of behaviour would be attitudes towards psychology as a whole predicting the behaviour generally relevant to learning more about psychology, such as reading magazine articles or talking with your tutor. How interested you are in psychology generally is not likely to be predictive of how well you prepare for a specific psychology exam.

In a two-year longitudinal study by Davidson and Jacard (1979), women's attitudes towards birth control were measured at different levels of specificity and used as predictors of their actual use of the contraceptive pill. The measures, ranging from very general to very specific, were correlated as follows with actual pill use (correlations in parentheses): 'Attitude towards birth control' (0.08); 'Attitude towards birth control pills' (0.32); 'Attitude towards using birth control pills' (0.53); and 'Attitude towards using birth control pills during the next two years' (0.57). Thus, this last measure was the most highly correlated with actual use of the contraceptive pill. It indicates quite clearly that the closer the question is to the actual behaviour, the more accurately the behaviour is predicted. (See Kraus, 1995, for a meta-analysis of attitudes as predictors of behaviour.)

Meta-analysis
Statistical procedure that combines data from different studies to measure the overall reliability and strength of specific effects.

Multiple-act criterion
Term for a general behavioural index based on an average or combination of several specific behaviours.

General attitudes

Fishbein and Ajzen (1975) also argued that we can predict behaviour from more general attitudes, but only if we adopt a multiple-act criterion. This criterion is a general behavioural index based on an average or combination of various specific behaviours. General attitudes usually predict multiple-act criteria much better than they predict single acts, because single acts are usually affected by many factors. For example, the specific behaviour of participating in a paper-recycling program on a given day is a function of many factors, even the weather. Yet a person engaging in such behaviour may claim to be 'environmentally conscious', a general attitude. Environmental attitudes are no doubt one determinant of this behaviour, but they are not the only, or even perhaps the major, one.

Theory of reasoned action
Fishbein and Ajzen's model of the links between attitude and behaviour. A major feature is the proposition that the best way to predict a behaviour is to ask whether the person intends to do it.

Reasoned action

The ideas outlined so far were integrated into a general model of the links between attitude and behaviour—the theory of reasoned action (Ajzen & Fishbein, 1980; Fishbein & Ajzen, 1974). The model encapsulated three processes of beliefs, intention and action, and included the following components:

- *Subjective norm*—a product of what the person thinks others believe. Significant others provide direct or indirect information about 'what is the proper thing to do'.
- *Attitude towards the behaviour*—a product of the person's beliefs about the target behaviour and how these beliefs are evaluated (refer back to the cognitive algebra in Table 5.1).

Note that this is an attitude towards behaviour (such as taking a birth control pill in Davidson and Jacard's study), not towards the object (such as the pill itself).

- *Behavioural intention*—an internal declaration to act.
- *Behaviour*—the action performed.

Usually, an action will be performed if (1) the person's attitude is favourable; and (2) the social norm is also favourable. In early tests of the theory, Fishbein and his colleagues (Fishbein & Feldman, 1963; Fishbein & Coombs, 1974) gave participants a series of statements about the attributes of various attitude objects: for example, political candidates. The participants estimated *expectancies*—that is, how likely it was that the object (candidate) possessed the various attributes—and gave the attributes a *value*. These expectancies and values were then used to predict the participants' feelings towards the attitude object, assessed by asking the participants how much they liked or disliked that object. The correlation between the scores and the participants' feelings was high, pointing to some promise for the model.

Other research reported that, when people's voting intentions were later compared with how they actually voted, the correlations were:

- 0.80 in the 1976 American presidential election (Fishbein, Ajzen & Hinkle, 1980)
- 0.89 in a referendum on nuclear power (Fishbein, Bowman, Thomas, Jacard & Ajzen, 1980).

Overall, if you know someone's very specific behavioural intentions, then you are effectively almost there in terms of predicting what they will actually do—their behaviour. Meta-analyses of relevant research suggest this is the case but that some hurdles remain regarding, for example, behavioural opportunities (Gollwitzer & Sheeran, 2006; Webb & Sheeran, 2006).

Planned behaviour: the role of volition

The theory of reasoned action (TRA) emphasises not only the rationality of human behaviour but also the belief that the behaviour is under the person's conscious control: for example, 'I know I can stop smoking if I really want to'. However, some actions are less under people's control than others.

Consequently, the basic model was extended by Ajzen (1989) to emphasise the role of volition. Perceived behavioural control is the extent to which the person believes it is easy or difficult to perform an act. The process of coming to such a decision includes consideration of past experiences, as well as present obstacles that the person may envisage. For example, Ajzen and Madden (1986) found that students, not surprisingly, want to get A-grades in their courses: A-grades are highly valued by the students (attitude), and they are the grades that their family and friends want them to get (subjective norm). However, prediction of actually getting an A will be unreliable unless the students' perceptions of their own abilities are taken into account.

Ajzen argued that perceived behavioural control can act on either the behavioural intention or directly on the behaviour itself. He referred to this modified model as the **theory of planned behaviour** (TPB). In a subsequent meta-analysis, Richard Cooke and Paschal Sheeran (2004) have referred to TPB as 'probably the dominant account of the relationship between cognitions and behaviour in social psychology' (2004, p. 159; also see Ajzen & Fishbein, 2005). The two theories, TRA and TPB, are not in conflict. The concepts and the way in which they are linked in each theory are shown in Figure 9.11.

Theory of planned behaviour
Modification by Ajzen of the theory of reasoned action. It suggests that predicting a behaviour from an attitude measure is improved if people believe they have control over that behaviour.

In one study, Beck and Ajzen (1991) started with students' self-reports of the extent to which they had been dishonest in the past. The behaviour sampled included exam cheating, shoplifting and telling lies to avoid completing written assignments, actions that were quite often reported. They found that measuring the perception of control that students thought they had over these actions improved the accuracy of prediction of future actions and, to some extent, the actual performance of the act. This was most successful in the case of cheating, which may well be planned in a more deliberate way than shoplifting or lying.

In another study, Madden, Ellen and Ajzen (1992) measured students' perceptions of control in relation to nine behaviours. These ranged from 'getting a good night's sleep' (quite hard to control) to 'taking vitamin supplements' (quite easy to control). The results were calculated to compare predictive power by squaring the correlation coefficient (i.e. r^2) between each of the two predictors (sleep and vitamins) and each of the outcomes (intentions and actions). Perceived control improved the prediction accuracy for both intentions and actions, and this improvement was substantially effective in predicting the action itself. These effects are evident in the steep gradient of the two lower lines in Figure 9.12, an outcome that has been confirmed in an independent study using a wide range of 30 behaviours (Sheeran, Trafimow, Finlay & Norman, 2002).

Features of both models have been used to understand people's attitudes towards their health. Debbie Terry and her colleagues (Terry, Gallois & McCamish, 1993) have shown how Fishbein and Ajzen's concepts can be applied to the study of safe-sex behaviour as a response to the threat of contracting HIV (see Box 9.5). Specifically, the target behaviour included monogamous relationships, non-penetrative sex and the use of condoms. All of the variables shown in Figure 9.11 can be applied in this setting. In the context of practising safe sex, the particular variable of perceived behavioural control needs to be accounted for, particularly where neither of the sex partners may be fully confident of controlling the wishes of the other person. A practical question that may need to be examined is the degree of control that a woman might perceive she has about whether a condom will be used in her next sexual encounter.

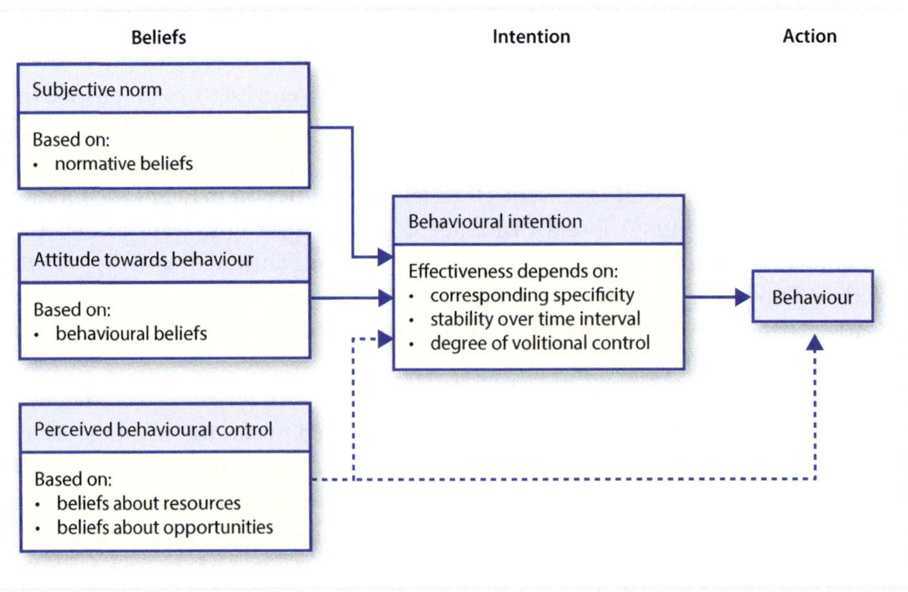

Figure 9.11 A comparison of the theory of reasoned action (TRA) and the theory of planned behaviour (TPB)

The solid lines show the concepts and links in the original theory of reasoned action; the dotted lines show an addition introduced in the theory of planned behaviour (**Source:** based on Ajzen & Fishbein (1980); Madden, Ellen & Ajzen (1992))

Research and applications 9.5

Reasoned action, planned behaviour and safe sex

TRA and TPB have proved useful in understanding and promoting responsible sexual behaviour

Social psychologists have increasingly turned their attention to promoting health practices such as avoiding the abuse of alcohol, tobacco and other substances; promoting dental hygiene; vaccinating against infectious diseases; participating in cervical smear tests; and using sunscreen products.

Another sphere of application has been the promotion of contraceptive practices to avoid unwanted pregnancies. Health professionals have also been concerned about the spread of HIV and contraction of AIDS.

In this context, social psychologists have mounted a concerted campaign of research promoting condom use, safe sex and monogamous relationships. Several researchers have explicitly recognised Fishbein and Ajzen's (Fishbein & Ajzen, 1974; Ajzen & Fishbein, 1980) theory of reasoned action as a model that helps to account for variability in people's willingness to practise safe sex (see Terry, Gallois & McCamish, 1993). One feature of this work has been to focus on establishing how much people feel they can actually exert control over their health. A woman with this sense of control is more likely to wear a seat belt, examine her breasts, use a contraceptive, have sex in an exclusive relationship, and discuss her partner's sexual and intravenous drug-use history.

Apart from a sense of control, other factors such as perceptions of condom proposers (those who initiate condom use) and the expectations and experience of safe sex are implicated in initiating safe sex (Hodges, Klaaren & Wheatley, 2000). Coupled with these factors, cultural background also plays a role in the gender and sexuality equation. For example, Conley, Collins and Garcia (2000) found that Chinese Americans reacted more negatively than European Americans to the female condom proposer. Furthermore, Japanese Americans perceived the female condom proposer to be less sexually attractive than did the Chinese or European Americans.

A problem with practising safe sex with one's partner is that it is not a behaviour that comes completely under one individual's *volitional control*, whereas going for a run usually is. The theory of reasoned action, together with its extension, the theory of planned behaviour (see Figure 9.11), provides a framework for psychologists and other health professionals to target particular variables that have the potential to encourage safe sex, as well as other health behaviour.

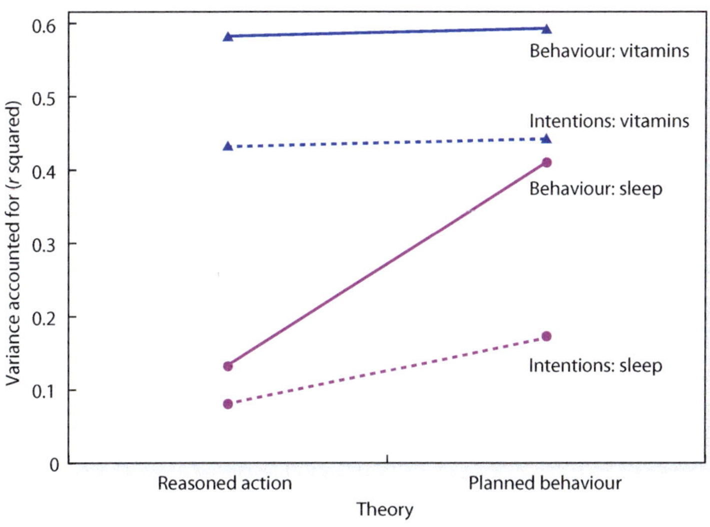

Figure 9.12 Theories of reasoned action and planned behaviour compared: the effect of including perceived behavioural control as a variable
(**Source:** based on data from Madden, Ellen & Ajzen (1992))

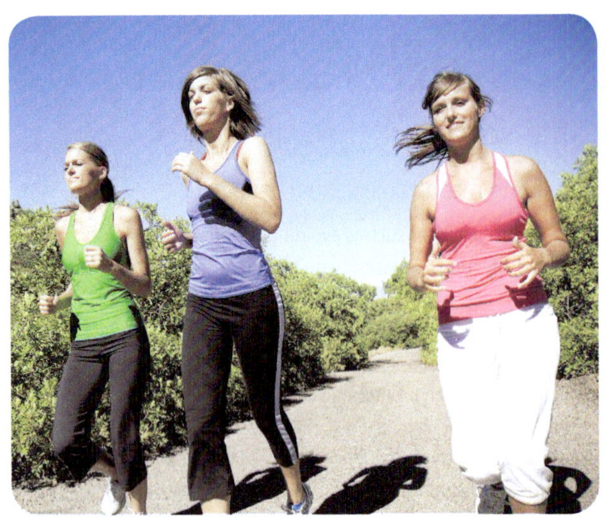

Perceived behavioural control The search for physical fitness includes the belief that 'I can do this!' Having company adds a supportive social norm (**Source:** © Yobro10/ Dreamstime.com.)

In critically evaluating both TRA and TPB, Tony Manstead and Dianne Parker (1995) argued that the inclusion of 'perceived behavioural control' in TPB is an improvement on the original theory. In a meta-analysis by Armitage and Conner (2001), perceived behavioural control emerged as a significant variable and could account for up to 20 percent of prospective actual behaviour.

TPB has also been applied to the prediction of driver behaviour in Britain (e.g. Parker, Manstead & Stradling, 1995; Conner et al., 2007). Studies have measured both the intentions of drivers and their behaviours, such as speeding, cutting in, weaving recklessly and illegal overtaking on the inside lanes of a motorway. The study by Conner and his colleagues introduced actual behaviour measures—one a driving simulator, and the other real on-road driving caught on a discreet camera. Their results suggest that the TPB can provide a basis for developing interventions designed to reduce speeding on the roads. The tendency to speed is based partly upon a driver's intentions to speed and partly on the absence of a moral norm not to speed.

Aside from the usual variable associated with the TRA and TPB models, some researchers have pointed to the role of people's *moral values* in determining action (e.g. Gorsuch & Ortbergh, 1983; Manstead, 2000; Pagel & Davidson, 1984; Schwartz, 1977). For example, if someone wanted to find out whether we would donate money to charity, they would do well to find out whether acting charitably is a priority in our lives. In this specific context, Greg Maio and Jim Olson (1995) found that general altruistic values predicted charitable behaviour (donating to cancer research), but only where the context emphasised the *expression* of one's values. Where the context emphasised rewards and punishments (i.e. a utilitarian emphasis), values did not predict donating.

Habit is also a predictor of future behaviour in that an action can become relatively automatic (discussed in a later section), and can operate independently of processes underlying TPB. David Trafimow (2000) found that male and female students who were in the habit of using condoms reported that they would continue to do so on the next occasion. In effect, habitual condom users do not 'need' to use reasoned decisions, such as thinking about what their attitudes are or about what norms are appropriate. In a TPB study of binge drinking (Norman & Conner, 2006), the way that students viewed their drinking history could predict their future behaviour. For example, if Bill believes he is a binge drinker, he will attend less to his attitude towards alcohol abuse and will also feel that he has less control over how much he drinks.

Both the TRA and TPB models have implications for how we can strive for a healthy lifestyle (Conner, Norman & Bell, 2002; Stroebe, 2011). Likewise, in health psychology, **protection motivation theory** focuses on how people can make a start to protect their health, maintain better practices and avoid risky behaviour (see Box 9.6 and Figure 9.13).

Protection motivation theory Adopting a healthy behaviour requires cognitive balancing between the perceived threat of illness and one's capacity to cope with the health regimen.

Various issues to which these models have been applied include HIV prevention (Smith & Stasson, 2000), condom use and safer sex behaviour (Sheeran & Taylor, 1999), alcohol consumption (Conner, Warren, Close & Sparks, 1999), smoking (Godin, Valois, Lepage & Desharnais, 1992) and healthy eating (Conner, Norman & Bell, 2002). However, the models are not restricted to the health domain. For example, Fox-Cardamone, Hinkle and Hogue (2000) used TPB to examine antinuclear behaviour. Antinuclear attitudes emerged as significant predictors of either antinuclear intentions or behaviour. All three theories share

Research and applications 9.6

Can we protect ourselves against major diseases?

According to statistics from the US Center for Disease Control and Prevention, cardiovascular disease and cancer were by far the leading causes of death in the United States in 2009; a statistic that prevails in most Western nations. It is well known that preventive behaviour for both diseases includes routine medical examinations, regular blood pressure readings, exercising aerobically for at least 20 minutes three times per week, eating a well-balanced diet that is low in salt and fat, maintaining a healthy weight and not smoking. It is a major challenge for health psychologists to find a model of health promotion that is robust enough to encourage people to engage in these preventive behaviours.

According to Floyd, Prentice-Dunn and Rogers (2000), protection motivation theory has emerged as just such a model. The model was developed initially to explain the effects of fear-arousing appeals on maladaptive health attitudes and behaviour, and was derived from Fishbein's theories of expectancy–value and reasoned action. Other components built into protection motivation theory included the effects of intrinsic and extrinsic reward (related to social learning theory) and Bandura's (1986, 1992) concept of self-efficacy, which in turn is closely related to that of *perceived behavioural control* in TPB (Ajzen, 1998).

From their meta-analysis of research based on 65 studies and more than 20 health issues, Floyd, Prentice-Dunn and Rogers argue that adaptive intentions and behaviour are facilitated by:

- an increase in the perceived severity of a health threat
- the vulnerability of the individual to that threat
- the perceived effectiveness of taking protective action
- self-efficacy.

In considering why Joe, for example, might either continue to smoke or decide to quit, protection motivation theory specifies two mediating cognitive processes:

1. *Threat appraisal*—smoking has intrinsic rewards (e.g. taste in mouth, nicotine effect) and extrinsic rewards (e.g. his friends think it's cool). These are weighed up against the extent to which Joe thinks there is a severe risk to his health (e.g. after reading the latest brochure in his doctor's waiting room) and that he is vulnerable (e.g. because a close relative who smoked died of lung cancer).
2. *Coping appraisal*—Joe takes into account response efficacy (whether nicotine replacement therapy might work) and self-efficacy (whether he thinks he can adhere to the regimen).

The trade-off when Joe compares his appraisals of threat and coping would be his level of protection motivation and whether he decides to quit smoking (see Figure 5.5).

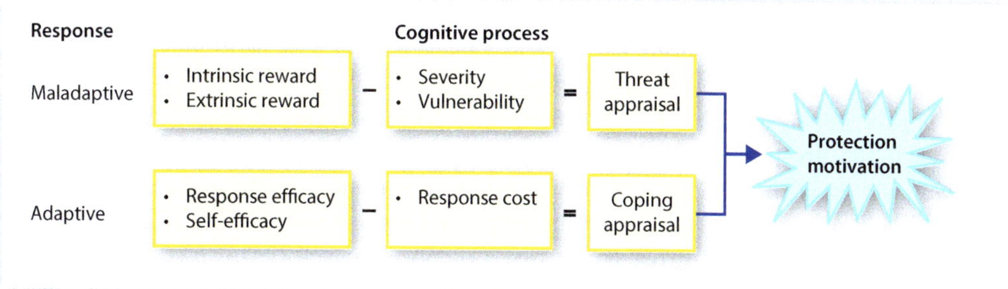

Figure 9.13 Mediating cognitive processes in protection motivation theory

This theory grew from psychological research into health promotion. Adopting a healthy practice will depend on several cognitive processes that balance perceived threat against the capacity to cope with a health regimen
(**Source:** based on Floyd, Prentice-Dunn & Rogers (2000))

the idea that motivation towards protection results from a perceived threat and the desire to avoid potential negative outcomes (Floyd, Prentice-Dunn & Rogers, 2000).

There is a reservation about TRA and TPB—it is assumed that attitudes are rational and socially significant behaviour is intentional, reasoned and planned. This may not always be true. How would you apply these theories to answer the second focus question?

Self-efficacy Expectations that we have about our capacity to succeed in particular tasks.

Attitude accessibility

Most models of attitude feature a cognitive component, in that beliefs are the building blocks of the more general concept of attitude, and even approaches that emphasise an evaluative component agree on one matter: attitudes are represented in memory (Olson & Zanna, 1993).

Accessible attitudes are those that can be recalled from memory more easily and can therefore be expressed more quickly (Eagly & Chaiken, 1998). They can exert a strong influence on behaviour (Fazio, 1986) and are associated with greater attitude–behaviour consistency (Doll & Ajzen, 1992). They are also more stable, more selective in judging relevant information and more resistant to change (Fazio, 1995). There is some evidence that affective evaluations are faster than cognitive evaluations, suggesting more evaluative attitudes are more accessible in memory (Verplanken & Aarts, 1999; Verplanken, Hofstee & Janssen, 1998).

Most studies of attitude accessibility have focused on highly accessible attitudes, drawing on Fazio's (1995) model of attitudes as an association in memory between an object and an evaluation. The rationale behind Fazio's model is that the extent to which an attitude is 'handy' or functional and useful for the individual depends on the extent to which the attitude can be automatically activated in memory. The likelihood of automatic activation depends on the strength of the association between the object and the evaluation (Bargh, Chaiken, Govender & Pratto, 1992). Strong object–evaluation associations should therefore be highly functional because they help us make decisions.

Although the ideas behind attitude accessibility are intuitively appealing and supported by some research (e.g. Fazio, Ledbetter & Towles-Schwen, 2000), there is also some evidence that implicit measures (as object–evaluation associations) correlate only weakly with explicit self-reports—what people actually say (Hilton & Karpinski, 2000). We return to this topic later when we examine how attitudes are measured.

As well as facilitating decision making, accessible attitudes orient visual attention and categorisation processes (Roskos-Ewoldsen & Fazio, 1992; Smith, Fazio & Cejka, 1996), and free up resources for coping with stress (Fazio & Powell, 1997). How might accessible attitudes affect the way we categorise? Smith, Fazio and Cejka (1996) showed that, when choosing from a number of possible categories to describe an object, we are more likely to select an accessible one. For example, when participants rehearsed their attitudes towards dairy products, yoghurt was more likely to cue as a *dairy product*. On the other hand, when attitudes towards health food were experimentally enhanced, and therefore made more accessible in memory, yoghurt was more likely to cue as a *health food* (Eagly & Chaiken, 1998).

Fazio's studies confirmed earlier findings that perceptions of stimuli will probably be biased in the direction of an individual's attitude (Lambert, Solomon & Watson, 1949; Zanna, 1993). However, he also showed that costs are associated with highly accessible attitudes. Recall that accessible attitudes are stable over time. Thus, if the object of an attitude changes, accessible attitudes toward that object may function less well (Fazio, Ledbetter & Towles-Schwen, 2000). Accessibility can produce insensitivity to change—we have become set in our ways. Consequently, someone who feels negative about a particular attitude object may not be able to detect if the 'object' has changed for better or perhaps worse (see Box 9.7).

Accessibility can also be conceptualised in the language of connectionism (Van Overwalle & Siebler, 2005). An accessible attitude is a cognitive node in the mind that is well connected to other cognitive nodes (through learning and perhaps conditioning), so that the focal attitude can be activated in different ways and along different cognitive paths:

> *This allows a view of the mind as an adaptive learning mechanism that develops accurate mental representations of the world. Learning is modeled as a process of online adaptation of existing knowledge to novel information ... the network changes the weights of the connections with the attitude object so as to better represent the accumulated history of co-occurrences between objects and their attributes and evaluations.* (Van Overwalle & Siebler, 2005, p. 232)

Research and applications 9.7

Accessible attitudes can be costly

There may be costs associated with highly accessible attitudes. Russell Fazio and his colleagues tested this idea in several experiments using computer-based morphing (Fazio, Ledbetter & Towles-Schwen, 2000): 24 same-sex digital facial photographs were paired so that one image in each pair was relatively attractive and one was not, based on earlier data. Five morphs (composites) of the images of each pair were created that varied in attractiveness determined by the percentage (e.g. 67/33, 50/50, 13/87) that each image contributed to a morph.

In part 1 of an experimental sequence, participants 'formed' attitudes that were either highly accessible (HA) or less accessible (LA). HA participants verbally rated how attractive each morph was, whereas LA participants verbally estimated the morph's probable physical height. Part 2 involved the detection of change in an image. Participants were told that they would see more faces, some of which were different photographs of people they had already seen, and they were to choose both quickly and accurately whether each image was the same or different from those seen earlier. HA participants were slower to respond than LA participants and also made more errors than LA participants. In an experimental variation, they also noticed less change in a morphed image.

All attitudes are functional, and accessible attitudes even more so, since they usually deal with objects, events and people that are stable. However, if the attitude object changes over time, then a highly accessible attitude may become dysfunctional—it is stuck in time.

Van Overwalle and Siebler suggest that a connectionist approach is consistent with: (1) dual-process models of attitude change, and (2) the notion of algebraic weights placed on beliefs, introduced by Fishbein (see the example in Table 9.1).

Attitude strength and direct experience

Do strong attitudes guide behaviour? The results of a study of attitudes towards Greenpeace suggest they do (Holland, Verplanken & Van Knippenberg, 2002). People with very positive attitudes towards Greenpeace were much more likely to make a donation to the cause than those with weak positive attitudes.

Almost by definition, strong attitudes must be highly accessible. They come to mind more readily and exert more influence over behaviour than weak attitudes. Fazio argued that attitudes are evaluative associations with objects, which makes his approach a one-component model. Associations can vary in strength from 'no link' (i.e. a non-attitude), to a weak link, to a strong link. Only an association that is strong allows the **automatic activation** of an attitude (Fazio, 1995; Fazio, Blascovich & Driscoll, 1992; Fazio & Powell, 1997; Fazio, Sanbonmatsu, Powell & Kardes, 1986; see Figure 9.14). As we go about our daily activities: 'we seamlessly and spontaneously evaluate the stimuli in our paths, including physical objects, people, words, pictures, faces, letters, and even odors' (Ferguson, 2007, p. 596).

Automatic activation
According to Fazio, attitudes that have a strong evaluative link to situational cues are more likely to come automatically to mind from memory.

Direct experience of an object and having a vested interest in it (i.e. something with a strong effect on your life) make the attitude more accessible and strengthen its effect on behaviour. For example, people who have had a nuclear reactor built in their neighbourhood will have stronger and more clearly defined attitudes regarding the safety of nuclear reactors. These people will be more motivated by their attitudes—they may be more involved in protests or more likely to move house.

As another example, consider attitudes towards doctor-assisted suicide (Haddock, Rothman, Reber & Schwarz, 1999). As subjective experience with this form of dying increased—its certainty, intensity and importance—the corresponding attitude about doctor-assisted suicide became stronger. It became more certain, intense and important.

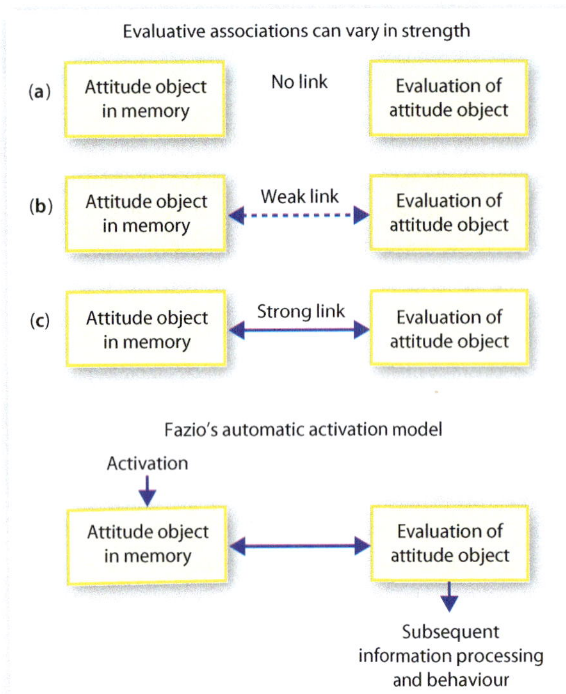

Figure 9.14 When is an attitude accessible?

A stronger attitude is more accessible than a weaker attitude. It can be automatically activated and will exert more influence over behaviour

The more often you *think* about an attitude, the more likely it is to resurface and influence your behaviour through easier decision making (Fazio, Blascovich & Driscoll, 1992). Powell and Fazio (1984) were able to make an attitude more accessible simply by asking on six different occasions what people's attitudes were as opposed to asking them only once. Accessing general attitudes can affect behaviour in specific situations. If the general attitude is never accessed, it cannot affect behaviour. Therefore, the activation step of Fazio's model is critical, since only activated attitudes can guide subsequent information processing and behaviour. Think of a sports coach priming a team by asking the question 'Which is the greatest team?' demanding a shouted response of 'We are!' and repeating this scenario a number of times before the match begins.

In addition to the role of strength, an attitude becomes more accessible as direct experience with the attitude object increases. Attitudes formed through actual experience are more consistently related to behaviour (Regan & Fazio, 1977; Doll & Ajzen, 1992). Suppose Mary has participated in several psychology experiments but William has only read about them. We can predict Mary's willingness to participate in the future more accurately than William's (Fazio & Zanna, 1978). Another example: your attitude to UFOs is far less likely to predict how you will act should you encounter one (!) than your attitude to lecturers is likely to predict your lecture room behaviour. Likewise, it would be reassuring to think that those people who have been caught driving with excessive blood alcohol levels would be less likely to drink and drive in the future. Unfortunately, this is not always the case.

Therefore, although direct experience seems appealing as an influence on attitude accessibility, establishing its actual effectiveness is a difficult task. We consider the role of direct experience again in the context of attitude formation in a later section.

Apart from attitude accessibility and direct experience with the attitude object, issues such as attitude salience, ambivalence, consistency between affect and cognition, attitude extremity, affective intensity, certainty, importance, latitudes of rejection and non-commitment are common themes in attitude research that fall under the general rubric of 'attitude strength'. Not surprisingly, attitude strength may consist of many related constructs rather than just one (Krosnick, Boninger, Chuang, Berent & Carnot, 1993). Although some dimensions of attitude strength are strongly related, most are not.

Reflecting on the attitude–behaviour link

Let us take stock of what research tells us (Glassman & Albarracín, 2006). As attitudes are being *formed*, they correlate more strongly with a future behaviour when:

- the attitudes are *accessible* (easy to recall)
- the attitudes are *stable over time*
- people have had *direct experience* with the attitude object
- people *frequently report* their attitudes.

The attitude–behaviour link is stronger when relevant information—such as persuasive arguments—is pertinent to the actual behaviour, one-sided and supportive of the attitude object, rather than two-sided. We deal with the topic of attitude formation below, and the role of persuasive arguments is part of our treatment of attitude change.

Moderator variables

Although it is difficult to predict single acts from general attitudes, prediction can be improved by the addition of a **moderator variable** that specifies conditions under which the attitude–behaviour relationship is stronger or weaker. Moderators include the situation, personality, habit, sense of control and direct experience. The attitude itself can also act as a moderator—for example, an attitude that functions to emphasise a person's self-concept and central values has stronger attitude–behaviour correspondence than one that simply maximises rewards and minimises punishments (Maio & Olson, 1994; Verplanken & Holland, 2002). Ironically, moderator variables may turn out to be more powerful predictors of an action than the more general underlying attitude. We consider two cases.

Moderator variable A variable that qualifies an otherwise simple hypothesis with a view to improving its predictive power (e.g. A causes B, but only when C (the moderator) is present).

Situational variables

Aspects of the situation, or context, can cause people to act in a way that is inconsistent with their attitudes (Calder & Ross, 1973). Weak attitudes are particularly susceptible to context (Lavine, Huff, Wagner & Sweeney, 1998), and in many cases what tends to happen is that social norms that are contextually salient overwhelm people's underlying attitudes. For instance, if university students expect each other to dress in jeans and casual clothes, these expectations represent a powerful norm for how students dress on campus.

Norms have always been considered important in attitude–behaviour relations, but they have generally been separated from attitudes: attitudes are 'in here' (private, internalised cognitive constructs), norms are 'out there' (public, external pressures representing the cumulative expectations of others). This view of norms has been challenged by social identity theory, which sees no such distinction—attitudes can be personal and idiosyncratic but much more typically they are a normative property of a group, and group identification causes one to internalise the group's normative properties, including its attitudes, as an aspect of self (e.g. Abrams & Hogg, 1990a; Hogg & Smith, 2007; Turner, 1991).

This idea has been applied to attitude–behaviour relations to argue that attitudes are more likely to express themselves as behaviour if the attitudes and associated behaviour are normative properties of a contextually salient social group with which people identify (Hogg & Smith, 2007; Terry & Hogg, 1996; Terry, Hogg & White, 2000). To test this, Terry and Hogg (1996) conducted two longitudinal questionnaire studies of students' intentions to take regular exercise and to protect themselves from the sun. These intentions were stronger when participants identified strongly with a self-relevant student peer group whom participants believed took regular exercise or habitually protected themselves from the sun (Figure 9.15).

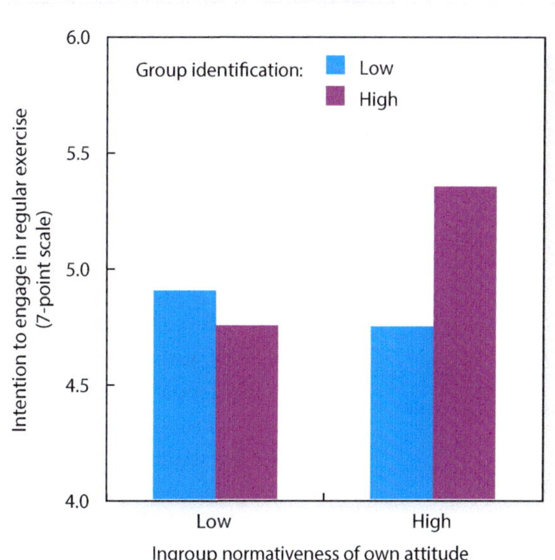

Figure 9.15 The role of norms and group identification in attitude–behaviour consistency

Students expressed a stronger intention to engage in regular exercise when they felt their attitudes towards exercise were normative of a student peer group with which they identified strongly
(**Source:** based on data by Terry & Hogg (1996))

Individual differences

Social psychologists tend to be divided into two camps—those who prefer situational explanations of social behaviour and those who prefer personality and individual difference explanations (Ross & Nisbett, 1991). Although this distinction has become less stark in recent years (Funder & Fast, 2010), it nevertheless has impacted attitude research. For example, Walter Mischel (1968) argued that situational characteristics were more reliable predictors of behaviour than were personality traits. Whereas Bem and Allen (1974) and Vaughan (1977) have shown that people who were consistent in their *answers* on a personality scale were more likely to be consistent in their *behaviour* across a variety of relevant situations than people who gave variable answers. For example, a high scorer on an extroversion–introversion scale would be more likely to behave in an extroverted manner and a low scorer in an introverted manner, across different social settings. On the other hand, those who were variable (mid-range scorers) in their answers on the scale would not behave consistently.

It is therefore useful to know how people's behavioural *habits* are related to their *degree of control* over the behaviour (Langer, 1975; Petty & Cacioppo, 1981; Triandis, 1980; Verplanken, Aarts, van Knippenberg & Moonen, 1998)—the study of habits has experienced a recent revival (see Neal, Wood, Labrecque & Lally, 2012; Wood & Neal, 2007). Harry Triandis (1977) proposed a model similar to Fishbein and Ajzen's, which included a habit factor to reflect the number of times a person had performed a particular action in the past. Smoking, for instance, is habitual for many people and is often partly due to a physiological and/or psychological dependency. Thus, the behaviour of smokers may bear little relationship to their attitudes towards cigarettes. Stuart Oskamp (1984) reported that about 70 percent of smokers agreed that 'smoking is one of the causes of lung cancer' and that 'cigarette smoking causes disease and death'.

In a review of research on 'habit', Bas Verplanken and Henk Aarts (1999) concluded that the relationship between attitudes and behaviour and between intentions and behaviour were near zero when habits were strong but sizeable when habits were weak. However, psychologists are fiercely vigilant in protecting their theories! In this instance, Ajzen (2002) does not see an inconsistency between habitual behaviour and planned behaviour:

> *The theory of planned behavior [and of reasoned action] does not propose that individuals review their behavioral, normative, and control beliefs prior to every enactment of a frequently performed behavior. Instead, attitudes and intentions—once formed and well-established—are assumed to be activated automatically and to guide behavior without the necessity of conscious supervision.* (Ajzen, 2002, p. 108)

Mood as a moderator variable may be considered both a situational and a personality variable. Carolyn Semmler and Neil Brewer (2002) examined the effects of trial-induced mood on how jurors processed information and made decisions. They found that being sad did not affect a juror's judgement, despite an increase in irrelevant thought. However, angry jurors actually reported more irrelevant thoughts, detected fewer inconsistencies in the witness's testimony and judged the defendant more harshly.

If we replace 'mood' with terms like 'affect' and 'emotion', we invoke part of the three-component model of attitude structure discussed earlier. In this wider context, there has been considerable research into affect-based evaluations of an attitude object (e.g. 'I hate broccoli, but I love ice cream') especially in the context of persuasion and advertising.

Cognitive biases, one of which is self–other discrepancy, are also moderators of attitude–behaviour correspondence. Angela Paglia and Robin Room (1999) studied what more than 800 people expected to happen when they drank alcohol and also how readily available they thought alcohol should be. They found that support for tighter control over alcohol availability stems partly from what people expect to happen, both from their own drinking and from the drinking of others. There was a distinct self–other discrepancy: people expect alcohol to affect others more adversely than themselves! Furthermore, the greater the bias, the greater the support for alcohol restriction.

Finally, some people are more focused than others on what has been called their *self-identity*—their sense of who they are as defined by the roles they occupy in society; although similar to social identity, self-identity is more focused on roles than group membership (Terry, Hogg & White, 1999). Self-identity has been viewed as an influence on people's intentions to act, which is a component of the theory of planned behaviour, discussed above (Hagger & Chatzisarantis, 2006). In one study, people were more likely to express an intention to donate blood if being a blood donor was an important part of their self-identity (Charng, Piliavin & Callero, 1988).

Forming attitudes

Attitudes are learned as part of the socialisation process (Fishbein & Ajzen, 1975; McGuire, 1969; Oskamp, 1977). They may develop through direct experiences or vicariously through interactions with others, or be a product of cognitive processes and thought. Generally, social psychologists have confined their work to understanding the basic psychological processes that underlie **attitude formation** rather than exploring how particular classes of attitude develop. The study of these processes usually involves laboratory experiments rather than survey or public opinion research.[F]

Attitude formation
The process of forming our attitudes, mainly from our own experiences, the influences of others and our emotional reactions.

Concepts related to attitudes

Values

We have treated attitudes as a relatively high-level concept involving affect as a central dimension, with many theorists arguing that beliefs constitute an additional dimension. If we accept both views, an attitude is a set of integrated beliefs with an affective loading. From such an approach springs a further level of analysis, and another term, **values** (e.g. Bernard, Maio & Olson, 2003; Maio, 2010; Rohan, 2000).

Values
A higher order concept thought to provide a structure for organising attitudes.

Values and attitudes are usually measured differently. Attitudes are measured to reflect varying degrees of favourability towards an object, whereas values are rated for their importance as guiding principles in life. An early emphasis on the global concept of values was the basis for a psychological test (Allport & Vernon, 1931) designed to measure the relative importance to a person of six broad classes of value orientation:

1 *theoretical*—an interest in problem solving, the basis of how things work
2 *economic*—an interest in economic matters, finance and money affairs
3 *aesthetic*—an interest in the arts, theatre, music, etc.
4 *social*—a concern for one's colleagues, a social welfare orientation
5 *political*—an interest in political structures and power arrangements
6 *religious*—a concern with theology, the afterlife and morals.

Milton Rokeach (1973) later suggested that values should be conceived less in terms of interests or activities and more as preferred goals (end-states). He distinguished between *terminal values* (e.g. equality and freedom) and *instrumental values* (e.g. honesty and ambition). A terminal value, such as equality, could have significant effects on the way someone might

[F]Vaughan, M. G., & Hogg, M. A. (2014). Social cognition and social thinking. In *Social psychology* (7th ed., pp. 136-155). Frenchs Forest, NSW: Pearson Australia.

feel about racial issues, which is just what Rokeach found. From this viewpoint, a value is a higher order concept, having broad control over an individual's more specific attitudes. For example, measuring values can help to predict people's attitudes to the unemployed (Heaven, 1990), to industrial action (Feather, 2002), and to beliefs in a just world (Feather, 1991). When values are primed, we are more likely to make choices consistent with our values. For example, if information enhances our thoughts about the environment, we are more likely to behave in an environmentally friendly way (Verplanken & Holland, 2002).

Hilde Himmelweit and her colleagues conducted a longitudinal study, spanning almost a quarter of a century, of social psychological influences on voting in Britain (Himmelweit, Humphreys & Jaeger, 1985). They found that specific attitudes were usually poor predictors, while broader sociopolitical values and party identifications were much better predictors. In another large-scale study by Miles Hewstone (1986), this time of attitudes of French, Italian, German and British students towards European integration, general value orientation changes were seen to have some influence on changed attitudes towards integration.

According to Norm Feather (1994), values are general beliefs about desirable behaviour and goals, with an 'oughtness' quality about them. They both transcend attitudes and influence the form that attitudes take. Values offer standards for evaluating actions, justifying opinions and conduct, planning behaviour, deciding between different alternatives, engaging in social influence and presenting the self to others. Within the person, they are organised into hierarchies, and their relative importance may alter during a lifetime. Value systems vary across individuals, groups and cultures.

Feather (2002) tested some of these principles among a group of third-party participants in a study of an ongoing major industrial dispute. Judgements about the quality of the behaviour (e.g. procedural fairness) of both the employer and the union were based on values such as authority, wealth, power, equality and being prosocial. Geert Hofstede (1980) and Shalom Schwartz (1992), among others, have also explored the way that entire cultures can be characterised and differentiated by their underlying value systems.

Can values predict behaviour? If the target behaviour is a specific act, it is very unlikely, given that a value is an even more general concept than an attitude. Although Bardi and Schwartz (2003) found correlations between some values and self-reported congruent behaviour (e.g. traditionalism and observing traditional holiday customs), they did not collect actual behavioural data.

Ideology

Ideology
A systematically interrelated set of beliefs whose primary function is explanation. It circumscribes thinking, making it difficult for the holder to escape from its mould.

Ideology overlaps to some extent with the term 'value'. It connotes an integrated and widely shared system of beliefs, usually with a social or political reference, that serves an explanatory function (Thompson, 1990). Most familiar to us are the religious and sociopolitical ideologies that serve as rallying points for many of the world's most intransigent intergroup conflicts. Ideologies have a tendency to make the state of things as they are seem quite natural (the naturalistic fallacy), to justify or legitimise the status quo (Jost & van der Toorn, 2012; Jost & Hunyadi, 2002; Major, Quinton & McCoy, 2002), and to enhance hierarchical social relations (e.g. Sidanius, Levin, Federico & Pratto, 2001; Sidanius & Pratto, 1999). Ideologies also frame more specific values, attitudes and behavioural intentions (e.g. Crandall, 1994).

Philip Tetlock (1989) has proposed that terminal values, such as those described by Rokeach (1973), underlie many *political ideologies*. For example, Machiavellianism as an ideology, named after Machiavelli (a 16th-century Florentine diplomat considered by some to have been the first social scientist), is the notion that craft and deceit are justified in pursuing and maintaining power in the political world (Saucier, 2000). Ideologies can vary as a function of two characteristics:

1 They may assign different priorities to particular values: traditionally, we might expect liberals and conservatives to rank 'individual freedom' and 'national security' in opposite ways.
2 Some ideologies are pluralistic and others monistic. A pluralistic ideology can tolerate a conflict of values: for example, neoliberalism as a pluralistic ideology emphasises economic growth and also a concern with social justice. A monistic ideology will be quite intolerant of conflict, seeing issues in starkly simplistic terms. An example of a monistic ideology is Manicheism—the notion that the world is divided between good and evil principles.

Mick Billig (1991) has suggested that much of our everyday thinking arises from what he calls ideological dilemmas. Teachers, for example, face the dilemma of being an authority and yet encouraging equality between teacher and student. When conflict between values arises, it can trigger a clash of attitudes between groups. For example, Katz and Hass (1988) reported a polarisation of ethnic attitudes in a community when values such as communalism and individualism clashed.

Ideology, in the guise of ideological orthodoxy, has also been implicated in societal extremism. Ideology, because of its all-embracing explanatory function, provides an immensely comforting buffer against uncertainty: uncertainty about what to think, what to do, who one is, and ultimately the nature of existence (Hogg, 2007b, 2012; Solomon, Greenberg, Pyszczynski & Pryzbylinski, 1995; Van den Bos, 2009). It is only a short step to recognise that people will go to great lengths to protect their ideology and the group that defines it. One reason why religious ideologies are so powerful and enduring, and why religious fundamentalism arises, is precisely because organised religions are uncertainty-reducing groups that have sophisticated ideologies that define one's self and identity and normatively regulate both secular and existential aspects of life (Hogg, Adelman & Blagg, 2010).

According to **terror management theory** (e.g. Greenberg, Solomon, & Pyszczynski, 1997; Pyszczynski, Greenberg & Solomon, 1999; Solomon, Greenberg & Pyszczynski, 1991), people may also subscribe to an ideology and defend their world view as a way to buffer themselves against paralysing terror over the inevitability of their own death. Numerous studies have shown that making a person's own death salient leads to world-view defence.

Terror management theory
The notion that the most fundamental human motivation is to reduce the terror of the inevitability of death. Self-esteem may be centrally implicated in effective terror management.

Social representations

Researchers who work in a **social representations** tradition have a somewhat different perspective on attitudes. First introduced by Serge Moscovici (1961) and based on earlier work by the French sociologist Emile Durkheim (1912/1995) on 'collective representations', social representations refer to the way that people elaborate simplified and shared understandings of their world through social interaction (Deaux & Philogene, 2001; Farr & Moscovici, 1984; Lorenzi-Cioldi & Clémence, 2001; Moscovici, 1981, 1988, 2000; Purkhardt, 1995).

Social representations
Collectively elaborated explanations of unfamiliar and complex phenomena that transform them into a familiar and simple form.

Moscovici maintained that people's beliefs are socially constructed; they are shaped by what other people believe and say and they are shared with other members of one's community:

> *Our reactions to events, our responses to stimuli, are related to a given definition, common to all the members of the community to which we belong.* (Moscovici, 1983, p. 5)

From an attitudinal perspective, the important point is that specific attitudes are framed by, and embedded within, wider representational structures, which are in turn grounded in social groups. In this sense, attitudes tend to reflect the society or groups in which people live their lives.

This type of perspective on attitudes reflects a broader 'top–down' perspective on social behaviour, which has been a hallmark of European social psychology. It prompted the American social psychologist William McGuire (1986) to observe that 'the two movements serve mutually supplementary uses', in that the European concept of collective representations highlights how *alike* group members are, while the American individualist tradition highlights how *different* they are (see also Tajfel, 1972).

Social representations may influence the evaluative tone of attitudes 'nested' within them. For example, Pascal Moliner and Eric Tafani (1997) have argued that attitudes towards objects are based on the evaluative components of the representation of those objects, and that a change in attitudes towards an object may be accompanied by changes in the evaluative dimension of its representation.

Umbereen Rafiq and her colleagues studied how Muslim and Christian students in the United Kingdom represented the second Iraq war. They focused on causal networks used by each group as explanations of the conflict (Rafiq, Jobanuptra & Muncer, 2006). Muslims and Christians agreed that there were causal links (sometimes bi-directional) between racism, religious prejudice and the history of conflict in the Middle East; however, Christians were more likely than Muslims to believe that the war was connected with a hunt for terrorist cells in Iraq—a reason consistently emphasised by then US President G. W. Bush. Ironically, God's Will did not feature in either the Muslim or the Christian causal network!

Measuring attitudes

Attitude scales

How should we measure attitudes; explicitly or implicitly? Some forms of attitude measurement can be completely explicit: people are simply asked to agree or disagree with various statements about their beliefs. Particularly in the early days of attitude research, in the 1930s, it was assumed that explicit measures would get at people's real beliefs and opinions. There was intense US media interest in predicting election results based on opinion polling (in particular, the Gallup Poll), and in establishing what election candidates believed and how they might act. The result was frenzied development of attitude questionnaires targeting a host of social issues.

In addition to scales based on adding scores across items, other researchers tried to get a better fit between a single item and a specific behaviour. We might ask: can this fit be improved if an attitude measure includes both an evaluative and a belief component? To this end, Fishbein and Ajzen (1974) developed the **expectancy-value model**, in which each contributing belief underlying an attitude domain is weighted by the strength of its relationship to the attitude object. The main elements of this model were described earlier (see also Table 9.1). Despite some criticisms (see Eagly & Chaiken, 1993), this technique has had predictive success in a variety of settings—in marketing and consumer research (Assael, 1981), politics (Bowman & Fishbein, 1978), family planning (Vinokur-Kaplan, 1978), classroom attendance (Fredericks & Dossett, 1983), seat-belt wearing (Budd, North & Spencer, 1984), preventing HIV infection (Terry, Gallois & McCamish, 1993), and how mothers feed their infants (Manstead, Proffitt & Smart, 1983).[G]

Expectancy-value model
Direct experience with an attitude object informs a person how much that object should be liked or disliked in the future.

[G]Vaughan, M. G., & Hogg, M. A. (2014). Social cognition and social thinking. In *Social psychology* (7th ed., pp. 159–163). Frenchs Forest, NSW: Pearson Australia.

Attitudes, arguments and behaviour

Attitudes do not readily predict behaviour, and the attitude–behaviour relationship can be so weak that some researchers have, in frustration, even suggested abandoning the attitude concept entirely. We will now focus on how attitudes can change over time, concentrating our attention on what kinds of intervention might bring about such change, and on the nature of the processes involved. This entails a focus on the cognitive dynamics of attitude change and on how individuals can change other individuals' attitudes, rather than on how attitudes are part of group norms and how group processes are involved in norm change, and in attitude change through conformity to norms.

We trust you will conclude that much of the reservation about the usefulness of the concept of attitude is misguided. In particular, we hope to show that discrepancies between attitudes and behaviour, rather than being an embarrassment to attitude theory, actually engage the very processes through which **attitude change** can occur.

The persuasion and attitude change literature is enormous (Albarracín & Vargas, 2010; Maio & Haddock, 2010; Visser & Cooper, 2007)—there are thousands of studies and a daunting variety of theories and perspectives. In our coverage we have focused on two general orientations. The first concentrates on people's use of arguments to convince others that a change of mind, and perhaps of behaviour, is needed. Research in this area has focused on the nature of the message—that is, the persuasive communication that will be effective—and considers a large number of variables that may determine what will do the job in changing another person's point of view. Obvious areas of application relate to political propaganda and advertising.

The second orientation focuses on the active participation of the person. By getting people to carry out certain activities, we may actually be trying to change their underlying attitudes. This path to attitude change is the focus of **cognitive dissonance**, one of the consistency theories of attitude. Whereas the first orientation starts from the premise that you reason with people to change how they think and act, the second orientation eliminates reasoning: simply persuade others to act differently, even if you have to use trickery; later they may come to *think* differently (i.e. change their attitude) and should then continue acting the way you want.

Attitude change
Any significant modification of an individual's attitude. In the persuasion process, this involves the communicator, the communication, the medium used, and the characteristics of the audience. Attitude change can also occur by inducing someone to perform an act that runs counter to an existing attitude.

Cognitive dissonance
State of psychological tension, produced by simultaneously having two opposing cognitions. People are motivated to reduce the tension, often by changing or rejecting one of the cognitions. Festinger proposed that we seek harmony in our attitudes, beliefs and behaviours, and try to reduce tension from inconsistency among these elements.

Persuasive communication

> *The receptive powers of the masses are very restricted, and their understanding is feeble. On the other hand, they quickly forget. Such being the case, all effective propaganda must be confined to a few bare essentials and those must be expressed as far as possible in stereotyped formulas. These slogans should be persistently repeated until the very last individual has come to grasp the idea that has been put forward. If this principle be forgotten and if an attempt be made to be abstract and general, the propaganda will turn out ineffective; for the public will not be able to digest or retain what is offered to them in this way. Therefore, the greater the scope of the message that has to be presented, the more necessary it is for the propaganda to discover that plan of action which is psychologically the most efficient.* (Hitler, *Mein Kampf*, 1933)

Has there ever been a more dramatic, mesmerising and chilling communicator than Adolf Hitler? His massive audiences at the Nazi rallies of the 1930s and 1940s might not have been so impressed had they known what he thought of them. The extreme case of Hitler, but also of other demagogues, allows us to connect the study of persuasive communication to leadership, rhetoric (e.g. Billig, 1991, 1996), and social mobilisation and crowd behaviour.

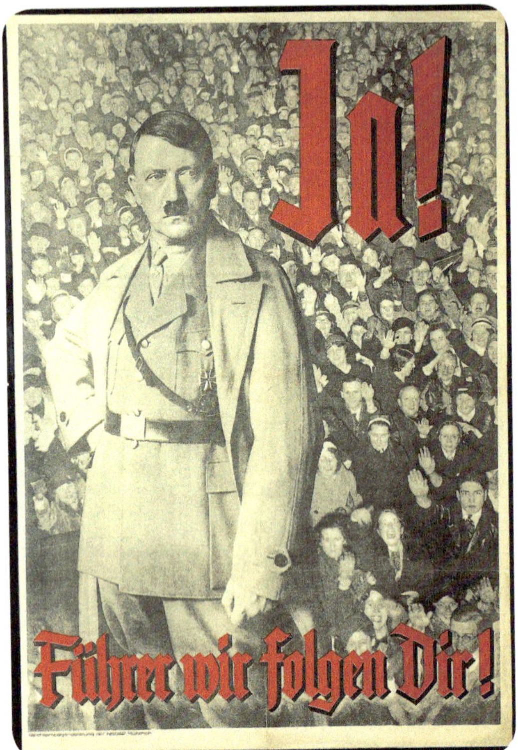

Persuading the masses Hitler felt that the content of an effective public message needed to be simple. Slogans were a key ingredient of Nazi propaganda
(**Source:** Imperial War Museum/Dorling Kindersley.)

Research on the relationship between **persuasive communication** and attitude change is, however, generally more narrowly focused, and has been most thoroughly applied to advertising and marketing (Johnson, Pham & Johar, 2007). According to Schwerin and Newell (1981, p. 7), behavioural change 'obviously cannot occur without [attitude change] having taken place'. For a long time, social psychologists have been interested in the nature of successful versus unsuccessful persuasion. Yet, despite the large part that persuasive messages play in influencing behaviour, only in the past 50 or so years have social scientists studied what makes persuasive messages effective.

Systematic investigation began towards the end of the Second World War, at a time when President Roosevelt was concerned that Americans, after being victorious in Europe, would lose the will to fight on against Japan. Carl Hovland was contracted by the US War Department to investigate how propaganda could be used to rally support for the American war effort—as it already had for the German cause by Hitler and the Nazi party. After the war, Hovland continued this work at Yale University in what was the first coordinated research program focusing on the social psychology of persuasion. Research funding was again politically motivated, this time by the Cold War—the United States' perception of threat from the Soviet Union, and its 'wish to justify its ways to the classes and win the hearts and minds of the masses' (McGuire, 1986, p. 99). The main features of this pioneering work were outlined in the research team's book, *Communication and persuasion* (Hovland, Janis & Kelley, 1953). They suggested that the key to understanding why people attend to, understand, remember and accept a persuasive message is to study the characteristics of the person presenting the message, the content of the message, and the characteristics of the receiver of the message.

Persuasive communication
Message intended to change an attitude and related behaviours of an audience.

The general model of the Yale approach, shown in Figure 9.16, is still employed as the basis of contemporary *communications theory* in marketing and advertising (see Belch & Belch, 2012). Hovland, Janis and Kelley asked, 'Who says what to whom and with what effect?' and studied three general variables involved in persuasion:

1. the communicator, or the source (who)
2. the communication, or message (what)
3. the audience (to whom).

Hovland and his colleagues identified four distinct steps in the persuasion process: attention, comprehension, acceptance, and retention. This research program spanned nearly three decades and produced a vast amount of data.

Not all findings from the early Yale research program have endured. For example, people with high self-esteem are just as easily persuaded as those with low self-esteem, but they do not want to admit it (Baumeister & Covington, 1985). And when persuasion does occur, people may even deny it—when people do succumb to persuasion they may conveniently fail to recall their original opinion (Bem & McConnell, 1970)!

Most contemporary social psychologists view the persuasion process as a series of steps. They do not always agree about what the important steps are, but they do agree that the audience has at least to pay attention to the communicator's message, understand the content and think about what was said (Eagly & Chaiken, 1984). The audience's thoughts are critical

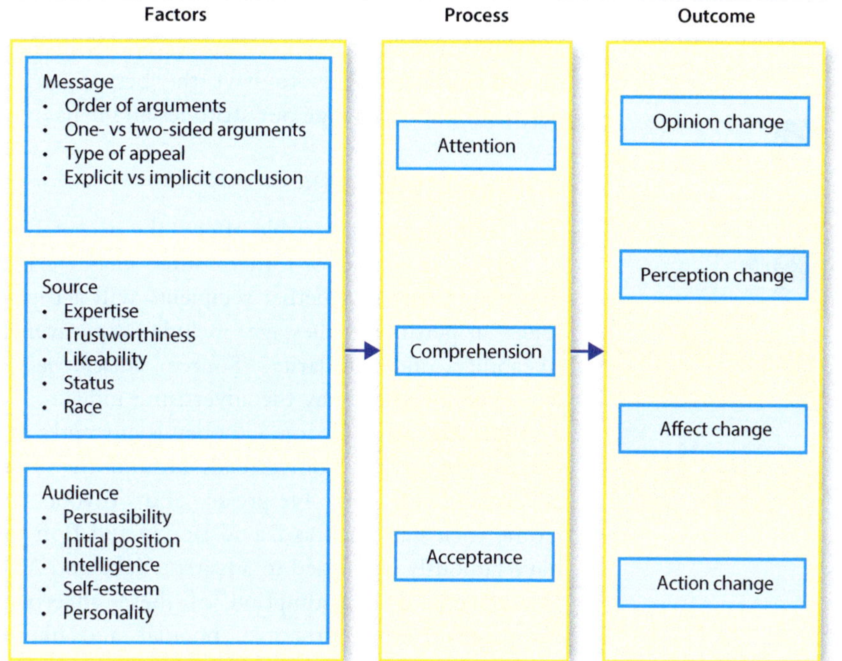

Figure 9.16 The Yale approach to communication and persuasion

In this classic research, various message, source and audience factors were found to affect the extent that people can be persuaded. See Box 9.11 for details of such message factors
(**Source:** based on Janis & Hovland (1959))

in this process (Petty & Cacioppo, 1981); the message will ultimately be accepted if it arouses favourable thoughts, whereas it will be rejected if the recipients argue strongly against it in their minds.

People are not oblivious to persuasion attempts. We can hardly avoid commercial advertising, public education programs and political propaganda. Interestingly, most people consider that they are less likely to be influenced than others by advertisements. This has been called the **third-person effect** ('You and I are not influenced, but they are'). For example, if we see a mundane product being advertised by using attractive models in an exotic setting, we assume that we (and those like us) are wiser than others to the tricks of the advertising industry. In reality, we are just as susceptible.

Third-person effect
Most people think that they are less influenced than others by advertisements.

Julie Duck and her colleagues have conducted a series of studies of the third-person effect, demonstrating its application to political advertising and AIDS prevention (see Duck, Hogg & Terry, 2000).

In the next three sections, we look at each of the three links in the persuasion chain: the communicator, the message and the audience. However, in any given context all three are of course operative. Some of the studies noted below do indeed analyse more than one of these three variables at a time, and they often interact: for example, whether an argument should present a one-sided or a two-sided case can depend on how intelligent the audience is.

The communicator

The Yale communication program showed early on that there is a group of variables relating to characteristics of the source (communicator) that can have significant effects on how acceptable we find a message. Great expertise, good physical looks and extensive interpersonal and verbal skills make a communicator more effective. Harry Triandis (1971) has argued that a communicator who is an expert, with knowledge, ability and skill, demands more of our respect. Furthermore, people we feel familiar with, close and attracted to are able to influence us more than others. In addition, people who have power have some control

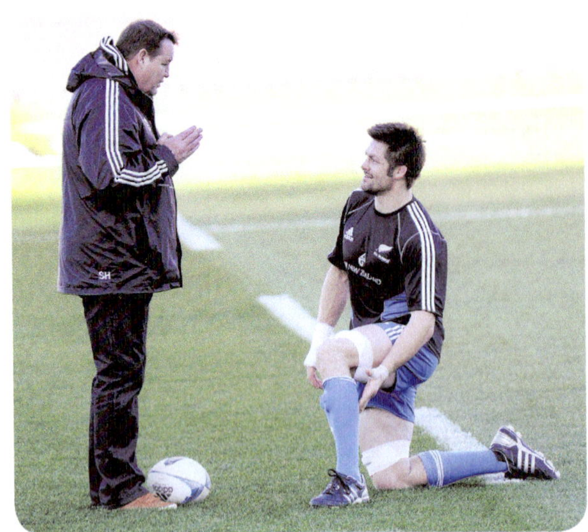

Source credibility The All Blacks captain is not kneeling in awe, but he is listening carefully to his coach's advice about the game plan (**Source:** SNPA/Ross Setford.)

over the kinds of reinforcement we might receive, and are thus influential. In all of these cases, such sources of influence are likely to have the best chance of persuading us to change our attitudes and behaviour.

Source credibility

The communicator variable affects the acceptability of persuasive messages. Other source characteristics that play a part in whether recipients will accept or reject a persuasive message include attractiveness, likeability and similarity. Source *attractiveness* is exploited mercilessly by the advertising industry. For example, the actor George Clooney is currently used extensively in TV commercials around the world advertising Martini, Nespresso and Toyota, and iconic rock stars such as David Bowie and Bon Jovi have famously been used to advertise Sake and Advil respectively. The assumption of these advertising campaigns is that attractive, popular and likeable spokespersons are persuasive, and thus are instrumental in enhancing consumer demand for a product. Attitude research generally supports this logic (Chaiken, 1979, 1983).

With regard to *similarity*, because we tend to like people who are similar to us we are more persuaded by similar than dissimilar sources: for example, a member of your peer group should be more persuasive than a stranger. However, it is not quite this simple (Petty & Cacioppo, 1981). When the issue concerns a matter of taste or judgement (e.g. who was Italy's greatest football player of all time?), similar sources are accepted more readily than dissimilar sources. But when the issue concerns a matter of fact (e.g. at which Olympic Games did your country win its greatest number of gold medals?), dissimilar sources do better (Goethals & Nelson, 1973).

We have already noted that no single communication variable can be treated in isolation, and that what works best in the persuasion process is an interaction of three categories of variables ('communication language' terms are given in parentheses):

1 **source** (sender)—from whom does the communication come?
2 **message** (signal)—what medium is used, and what kinds of argument are involved?
3 **audience** (receiver)—who is the target?

Source
The point of origin of a persuasive communication.

Message
Communication from a source directed to an audience.

Audience
Intended target of a persuasive communication.

Many experiments have focused on a single variable; others on two variables, one from each of two categories. An example of the latter kind was a study by Steve Bochner and Chester Insko (1966), which dealt with source *credibility* in combination with the discrepancy between the opinion of the target and that of the source. With respect to credibility, Bochner and Insko expected that an audience would pay more attention to the opinion of the communicator who was thought to be more believable. They predicted that there would be more room for attitude change when the target's opinion was more discrepant from that of the source.

Bochner and Insko's participants were students who were initially asked how much sleep was required to maintain one's health. Most said eight hours. They were then exposed to two sources of opinion that varied in expertise and therefore credibility. One was a Nobel Prize-winning physiologist with expertise in sleep research (higher credibility) and the other a YMCA instructor (lower credibility). Discrepancy was manipulated in terms of the amount of variation between student opinion and that of the source. If the source said that five hours was enough, the discrepancy was three hours with respect to the typical view of

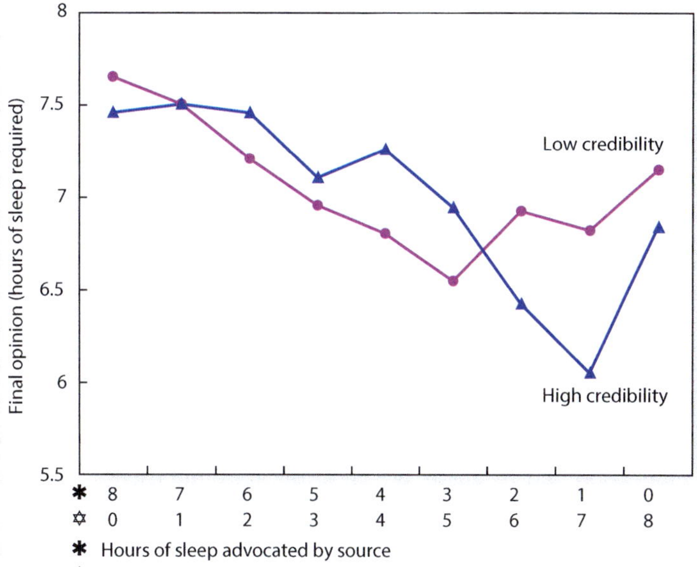

Figure 9.17 The effect of communicator credibility and position discrepancy on opinion change

As a position adopted in a message becomes increasingly discrepant from what most people would accept, a more credible communicator becomes very effective in inducing opinion change
(**Source:** based on data from Bochner & Insko (1966))

eight hours: the pressure to shift should be higher than if the discrepancy was only one hour. However, what would happen if the source said that two hours was sufficient? Look at the results in Figure 9.17.

In terms of the discrepancy variable, more opinion change occurred at moderate levels of difference between the students and the source. It seems that extreme discrepancy is not a good tactic in influencing a target. The audience will resist if the difference is too great and may look for ways of discrediting the communicator ('They don't know what they are talking about!'). However, this effect interacted with the variable of credibility. It was the expert who induced the greatest amount of change, and this took place when discrepancy was marked. In Bochner and Insko's study, the change was greatest when the highly credible source advocated one hour of sleep and students had suggested eight hours, a discrepancy of seven hours.

Interaction effects in research point to nuances in the way that one or more variables can determine a given outcome, and one example of this relates to source credibility. When a message is simple, that is, it does not require much elaboration or thought processing, source credibility acts as a heuristic: 'this person is famous, so what they say must be true'. However, a more complex message requires more elaboration or thought processing. In this context, Zakary Tormala and his associates have found that source credibility has more than one role and its capacity to persuade is 'all in the timing'. People's thinking became more confident when the identity of the source followed the message, but their thinking became more favourable when the identity of the source preceded the message (Tormala, Briñol & Petty, 2007).

The message

An important idea not communicated persuasively is like having no idea at all. (Bernbach, 2002)

Several message variables have been intensively investigated for their relative power to induce attitude change. When, for example, should we present both sides of an argument rather than just our own? This variable seems to interact quite strongly with characteristics of the audience. If the audience is against the argument but is also fairly intelligent, it is more effective to present both sides. However, it is better to present only one side if a less intelligent audience is already favourably disposed towards the argument (Lumsdaine & Janis, 1953; McGinnies, 1966).

Comparative advertising, in which a rival product is presented as inferior to a target product, is a common instance of using two-sided messages. When a consumer is not very motivated to buy the target product, comparative advertising can work, as this type of advertising is geared simply to making a product appear better (Pechmann & Esteban, 1994). An attentive and interested consumer, on the other hand, is likely to process message information quite carefully. If loyalty to a rival brand is high, comparative advertising of a new target brand is not very effective (Nye, Roth & Shimp, 2008). Explanations of how messages are handled in terms of dual-processing models of attitude change are dealt with below.

Effects of repetition

In the advertising industry, it is a maxim that a message needs to be repeated over and over again in order to be both understood and recalled. We all know how intensely irritating this can be, and a sceptic might conclude that this maxim is self-interested—it justifies more advertising and thus boom times for advertising agencies. If we believe the advertising industry, however, this is not a major motive. According to Ray (1988), the main goal is to strive for repetition minimisation: that is, to have the maximum impact with the minimum exposure and therefore the most cost-effective expenditure. It seems that television advertising exposure reinforces preferences more than it motivates brand choices, and that the optimum rate is two to three times per week (Tellis, 1987).

In general, the issue of message repetition invites, as we shall see below, examination of the way in which information is processed and of how memory works. Somewhat more startling is a finding that simple repetition of a statement gives it the *ring of truth* (Arkes, Boehm & Xu, 1991; Moons, Mackie & Garcia-Marques, 2009)! Repeated exposure to an object clearly increases familiarity with that object. Repetition of a name can make that name seem famous (Jacoby, Kelly, Brown & Jasechko, 1989). (Note also that an increase in familiarity between people can increase interpersonal liking.) There is a catch to the use of repetition, identified in a study of TV and internet advertising: it may not work very well with a totally new product, and may even become decreasingly effective. Even a little brand familiarity helps (Campbell & Keller, 2003).

Another variable that has received substantial attention, because of the way in which it has been used by the media to induce people to obey the law or to care for their health, is the use of fear.

Does fear work?

Fear-arousing messages may enhance persuasion—but how fearful can a message become and still be effective? Many agencies in our community persist with forms of advertising that are intended to frighten us into complying with their advice or admonitions. Health workers may visit the local school to lecture children on how 'smoking is dangerous to your health'. To drive the point home, they might show pictures of a diseased lung. Television advertising may remind you that 'if you drink, don't drive', and perhaps try to reinforce this message with graphic scenes of carnage on the roads. In the late 1980s a legendary advertising campaign associated the Grim Reaper with unsafe sexual practices and the likelihood of contracting HIV. Does fear work? The answer is a mixed one.

In an early study by Janis and Feshbach (1953), there were three different experimental conditions under which participants were encouraged to take better care of their teeth. In a low-fear condition, they were told of the painful outcomes of diseased teeth and gums, and suggestions were made about how to maintain good oral health. In a moderate-fear condition, the warning about oral disease was more explicit. In a high-fear condition, they were told that the disease could spread to other parts of their body, and very unpleasant visual slides were used showing decayed teeth and diseased gums. The participants reported on their current dental habits and were followed up one week later. Janis and Feshbach found an inverse relationship between degree of (presumed) fear arousal and change in dental hygiene practices. The low-fear participants were taking the best care of their teeth after one week, followed by the moderate-fear group and then the high-fear group.

Leventhal, Watts and Pagano (1967) reported a conflicting result from a study of how a fearful communication might aid in persuading people to stop smoking. The participants were volunteers who wished to give up smoking. In a moderate-fear condition, the participants listened to a talk with charts illustrating the link between death from lung cancer and the rate at which cigarettes were used. In a high-fear condition, they also saw a graphic film about an operation on a patient with lung cancer. Their results showed a greater willingness to stop smoking among people in the high-fear condition.

How do we explain the discrepancy between these results? Both Janis (1967) and McGuire (1969) suggested that an inverted U-curve hypothesis might be applied to the conflicting results (see Figure 9.18). McGuire's analysis distinguishes two parameters that could control the way we respond to a persuasive message, one involving comprehension and the other involving the degree to which we yield to change. The more we can understand what is being presented to us and can conceive of ways to put this into effect, the more likely we are to go along with a particular message.

In line with dual-process models of information processing, when fear is at a very low level an audience may be little motivated to attend to the message because the message does not spell out sufficiently the harmful consequences of an act (Keller & Block, 1995). As fear increases, so does arousal, interest and attention to what is going on. However, a very frightening presentation of an idea may arouse so much anxiety, even a state of panic, that we become distracted, miss some of the factual content of the message and are unable to process the information properly or know what to do.

What we do not know is whether the high-fear condition in the Janis and Feshbach study aroused more fear than the one in the Leventhal, Watts and Pagano study. If it did, then a curvilinear fit might be appropriate for the data. Therefore, there may be a limit to the effectiveness of fear-arousing messages. Disturbing TV images, for example, may distract people from the intended message or, even if the message is attended to, may so upset people that the entire episode is avoided.

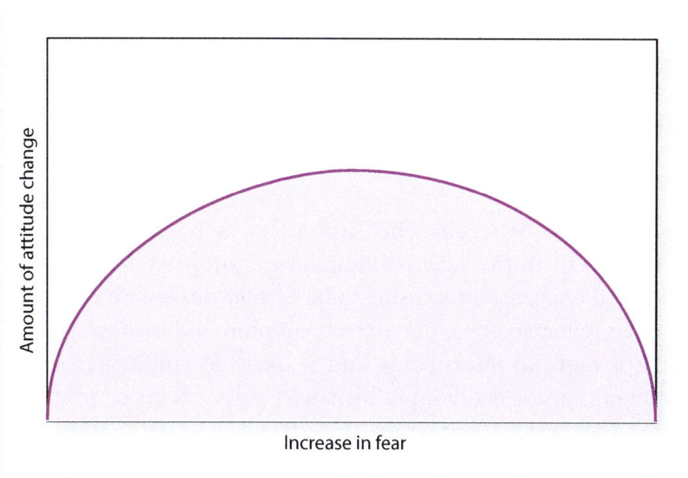

Figure 9.18 The inverted U-curve relationship between fear and attitude change

The amount of attitude change increases as a function of fear up to a medium level of arousal. At high levels of fear, however, there is a fall-off in attitude change. This could be due to lack of attention to the stimulus, or to the disruptive effects of intense emotion, or both

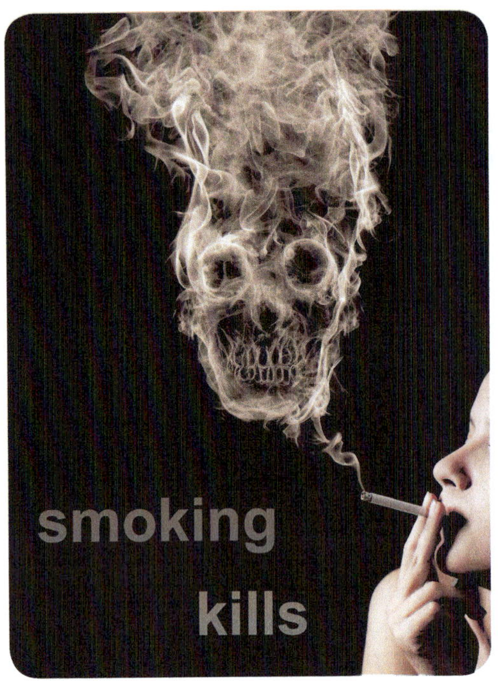

Does fear work? New fear campaigns to quit smoking now are relentless. Whether fear alone as a factor actually works Box 6.1 remains unproven
(**Source:** Kamenetskiy Konstantin/Shutterstock.)

According to *protection motivation theory* fear appeals should work to eliminate dangerous health practices if they include an effective presentation of how to cope with the danger (see Wood, 2000, for a review). Kim Witte and her colleagues, for example, combined a fear appeal with the promotion of self-protective behaviours in a campaign to reduce the spread of genital warts (Witte, Berkowitz, Cameron & McKeon, 1998).

These approaches to the study of the differential effects of scary messages do not directly address the inverted U-curve hypothesis. Whether a message achieves its goals is probably determined by a trade-off between the perception of danger (*threat appraisal*) and whether people believe they can carry out the corrective behaviour (*coping appraisal*). The underlying idea here is consistent with Blascovich's bio-psychosocial model of challenge and threat (Blascovich 2008, Blascovich & Tomaka, 1996)—a demand can be perceived as a threat if one feels one does not have the resources to cope, and as a challenge if one feels one does have the resources to cope.

The nature of threat appraisal was examined in a German study of stress-related illness. Enny Das and her colleagues reason that ordinary people in a health-risk setting ask themselves two questions:

1. How vulnerable am I?
2. How severe is the risk?

In this study (Das, de Wit & Stroebe, 2003), risk following long-term stress could range from fairly mild (e.g. fever or cold hands and feet) to very severe (e.g. stomach ulcers or heart disease). Once it was accepted there was even a mild risk (the second question), people were more likely to follow a health recommendation provided they believed they were very vulnerable to a threat (the first question). This therefore suggests that impactful messages about risky health practices should pinpoint the matter of *vulnerability* to a greater degree than simply severity.

There is an additional conceptual twist in understanding the effect of fearful messages. If the fear is so extreme that it makes us aware of our own death and mortality, then terror management processes may come into play. According to **terror management theory** (Greenberg, Solomon & Pyszczynski, 1997; Pyszczynski, Greenberg & Solomon, 1999) thoughts of our own death create 'paralyzing terror'. This makes us seek symbolic immortality, which we achieve by identifying with and psychologically defending cultural institutions and ideologies that we subscribe to. Thus, fear-laden messages may lead to ideological conviction and zealous identification with groups, rather than to attitude and behaviour change related to the focus of the message. However, there are other methods being used to encourage people to quit smoking (see Box 9.10).

Terror management theory
The notion that the most fundamental human motivation is to reduce the terror of the inevitability of death. Self-esteem may be centrally implicated in effective terror management.

Facts versus feelings

That a distinction is commonly drawn between belief and affect as components of an attitude (e.g. Haddock & Zanna, 1999). In the advertising industry, a related distinction is sometimes made between *factual* and *evaluative* advertising. The former deals with claims of fact and is thought to be objective, whereas the latter reflects opinion and is subjective. A factually oriented advertisement is high on information and is likely to emphasise one or more attributes among the following: price, quality, performance, components or contents, availability, special offer, taste, packaging, guarantees or warranties, safety, nutrition, independent research, company-sponsored research or new ideas. However, the simple recall of facts from an advertisement does not guarantee a change in the brand purchased. Furthermore, if there is factual content in a message, it is important for people to be able to assimilate and understand the general conclusion of the message (Albion & Faris, 1979; Beattie & Mitchell, 1985).

Even if a distinction is made between beliefs and feelings, evaluating an object (say, judging whether it is good or bad) is not identical to experiencing affect or an emotion. From this point of view, we can repeat the argument that attitudes are fundamentally evaluations, which is where Thurstone (1928) started out. Applying this to an advertising context, evaluation means that instead of conveying facts or objective claims, the message is couched in such a way that it makes the consumer feel generally 'good' about the product. A common method in evaluative advertising is to capitalise on the *transfer of affect*, which itself is based on learning by association.

The distinction between facts and feelings does not imply that a given advertisement contains only factual or only evaluative material. On the contrary, modern marketing strategy favours using both approaches in all advertisements. A consumer can be led to *feel* that one product is superior to another by subtle associations with music or colour, or through the use of attractive models. The same consumer can be led to *believe* that the product is a better buy because it is better value for money.

Social psychologists debate whether the kind of appeal should fit the basis on which an attitude is held (Petty & Wegener, 1998). According to Edwards (1990), if the underlying attitude is emotional (affect-based), then the appeal should be as well, but if the attitude is centred on beliefs (cognition-based), then a factual appeal should work better. Millar and Millar (1990) argue for a mismatch: for example, using a factual appeal when the attitude is emotional. However, the attitude objects used by Edwards (e.g. photographs of strangers, a fictitious insecticide) were unknown to the participants, whereas Millar and Millar tapped established attitudes (a list of drinks actually generated by the participants), so participants could counter with effective arguments.

The medium and the message

Shelly Chaiken and Alice Eagly (1983) compared the relative effects on an audience of presenting messages in video, audio and written forms. This has obvious implications for advertising. Which has more impact on the consumer: television, radio or print media? It depends. If the message is simple, as much advertising is, the probable answer is: video > audio > written. A moderating variable in this context is the relative ease or difficulty of comprehension required of the audience. If the points of a message require considerable processing by the target, a written medium is likely to be best. Readers have the chance to go back at will, mull over what is being said and then read on. If the material is quite complex, then newspapers and magazines can come into their own. However, there is an interesting interaction with the difficulty of the message. Look at the difference in effectiveness between various media in Figure 9.19. When the message was easy to comprehend, Chaiken and Eagly found that a videotaped presentation brought about most opinion change. When the message was difficult, however, opinion change was greatest when the material was written. Only recently has research included a focus on computer-mediated attitude change (e.g. Sassenberg & Boos, 2003).

Framing a message

The way in which a message is framed or slanted can have subtle effects on its meaning, and therefore on whether it is accepted. For example, if the issue of 'affirmative action' is presented as 'equal opportunity' rather than 'reverse discrimination', people will view it more favourably (Bosveld, Koomen & Vogelaar, 1997). In their review of how to promote health-

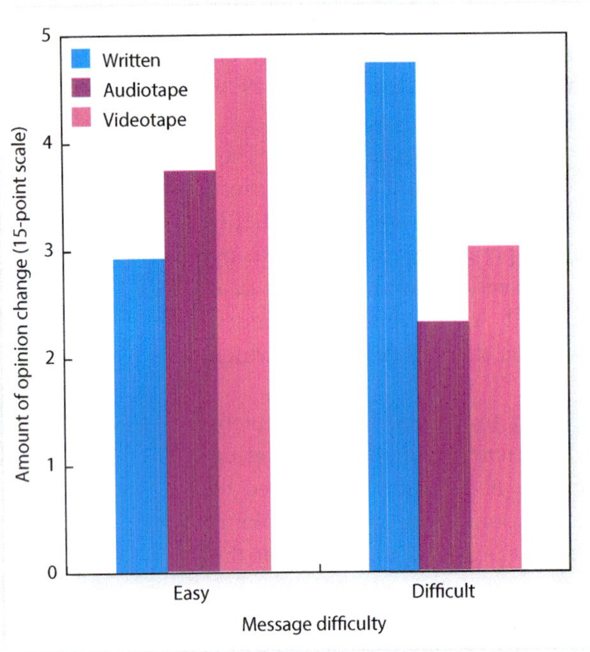

Figure 9.19 The effects of source modality and message difficulty on opinion change

Using sound or a visual image rather than the printed word makes an easily understood message more acceptable. However, a difficult message profits from using a verbal document
(**Source:** based on Chaiken & Eagly (1983))

related behaviour, Alexander Rothman and Peter Salovey (1997) found that message framing plays an important role. If the behaviour relates to detecting an illness, such as breast self-examination, the message should be framed in terms of preventing loss; but if the behaviour leads to a positive outcome, such as taking regular exercise, the message should be framed in terms of gain.

The sleeper effect

A persuasive message should have its greatest impact just after it is presented. It is counter-intuitive to think that its power might increase with the passage of time, and yet this is precisely what the **sleeper effect** suggests (Kelman & Hovland, 1953). An early finding in the Yale attitude change program (Hovland, Lumsdaine & Sheffield, 1949) was that films promoting more positive attitudes among American soldiers towards their British allies in the Second World War became more effective well after they had been viewed. Kelman and Hovland reasoned that we initially associate the conclusion of a message with: (1) the quality of its argument, and (2) other cues, such as the credibility of its source. Of these, memory of the argument becomes more enduring as time goes by. Take the part played by source credibility as it interacts with our views on how much sleep we need each night, discussed earlier (see Figure 9.17). Were we to take a measure of the impact of an extreme message about a month later, the sleeper effect predicts that the less credible source would probably be as persuasive as the more credible source: the message survives but the source does not.

Sleeper effect
The impact of a persuasive message can increase over time when a discounting cue, such as an invalid source, can no longer be recalled.

Bill Crano and Radmila Prislin (2006) have described the sleeper effect, usually associated with studies in mass communication, as an 'old chestnut'. Its reliability has long been questioned (e.g. Gillig & Greenwald, 1974), but it has been replicated under quite strict conditions (e.g. Pratkanis, Greenwald, Leippe & Baumgardner, 1988). More recently, a meta-analysis by Kumkale and Albarracín (2004) has detailed the particular circumstances where it is robust and points to a reawakened interest in the literature.

The sleeper effect may have some passing resemblance to the phenomena of latent influence and conversion in the minority influence literature (Moscovici, 1980; for a review see Martin & Hewstone, 1998). Groups that hold a minority view can, if they adopt the right behavioural style (Mugny, 1982) and are not outright rejected as an outgroup (Crano & Seyranian, 2009), be quite effective in changing the attitudes of the majority; but typically there is initial resistance and the attitude change comes later in the form of a sudden conversion.

The audience

Self-esteem

In their 1950s studies, Hovland and his colleagues had noted that a distracted audience is more easily persuaded than one that is paying full attention, provided that the message is simple; and that people with low self-esteem are more susceptible than those with high self-esteem. Bill McGuire (1968) suggested that the relationship between persuasibility and self-esteem is actually curvilinear: that is, it follows an inverted U-curve of the kind shown in Figure 9.17 (substituting 'self-esteem' for 'fear'). This curve suggests that people with either low or high self-esteem are less persuasible than those with moderate self-esteem. He reasoned that those with low self-esteem would be either less attentive or else more anxious when processing a message, whereas those with high self-esteem would be less susceptible to influence, presumably because they are generally more self-assured. According to a review by Nancy Rhodes and Wendy Wood (1992), research generally confirms this curvilinear relationship. As an aside, McGuire has also proposed a similar curvilinear relationship between intelligence and persuasibility.

Men and women

Another consistent, but more controversial, finding is that women are more easily persuaded than men (Cooper, 1979; Eagly, 1978). Crutchfield (1955) was the first to report this effect when he found that women were more conforming and susceptible to social influence than men. Some researchers proposed that this difference exists because women are socialised to be cooperative and non-assertive and are therefore less resistant than men to attempts to influence them (Eagly, Wood & Fishbaugh, 1981). Sistrunk and McDavid (1971) favoured another explanation—women are more easily influenced than men, but only when the subject discussed is one with which men are more familiar. When the topic is female-oriented, men are more influenced than women.

This finding led to the proposition that the consistent difference found in persuasibility had been due to a methodological bias. The persuasive messages used in attitude research had typically dealt with male-oriented topics, and the researchers were usually male. If the topics had not been gender-biased, the male–female differences would not have been found. Because more recent studies are more sophisticated in both design and execution (e.g. Eagly & Carli, 1981), the conclusion they support is now widely accepted.

Linda Carli (1990) investigated male–female differences in both the audience and the source. Participants heard a recorded message read by either a man or a woman, who spoke either tentatively or assertively. When the reader was female and tentative rather than assertive, male listeners were more easily persuaded than female listeners. In contrast, male readers were equally influential in each condition. This suggests that gender-related persuasiveness is a complex interaction of who is speaking, who is listening and whether the message is delivered in a gender-stereotyped way.

Katherine Covell and her colleagues investigated the effectiveness of tobacco and alcohol advertising as a function of gender and generation (Covell, Dion & Dion, 1994). The participants were male and female adolescents and their mothers and fathers. They rated the image and the quality of the advertised products and showed a preference for image-oriented over quality-oriented advertising. A gender difference was restricted to the adolescents, among whom females showed an even higher preference for image-oriented advertising. Covell, Dion and Dion suggested that, when advertisements target adolescents and feature alcohol and tobacco, young women might be particularly attentive to image-oriented messages and judge drinking and smoking to be more desirable.

In general, studies of gender differences in attitude change mirror those of social influence in small groups (see the review by Carli, 2001).

Individual differences

Research into individual differences in persuasibility has focused on individual differences in *need for cognition* (Haugtvedt & Petty, 1992), *need for closure* (Kruglanski & Webster, 1996; Kruglanski, Webster & Klem, 1993), *need to evaluate* (Jarvis & Petty, 1995) and *preference for consistency* (Cialdini, Trost & Newsom, 1995). Individual differences have also been found in *attitude importance* (Zuwerink & Devine, 1996). In these studies, people who scored high on these various needs were less likely to be persuaded than those who scored low. However, the relationship between personality variables and persuasion is not simple. The role of the **moderator variable** is important. For instance, in almost all cases, social contextual factors influence the personality–persuasibility relationship.

Moderator variable
A variable that qualifies an otherwise simple hypothesis with a view to improving its predictive power (e.g. A causes B, but only when C (the moderator) is present).

Age

Penny Visser and Jon Krosnick (1998) and Tom Tyler and Regina Schuller (1991) have suggested up to five plausible hypotheses about a relationship between age and susceptibility to attitude change:

1. *Increasing persistence*—susceptibility to attitude change is high in early adulthood but decreases gradually across the lifespan; attitudes reflect the accumulation of relevant experiences (a negative linear line).
2. *Impressionable years*—core attitudes, values and beliefs are crystallised during a period of great plasticity in early adulthood (an S-curve).
3. *Life stages*—there is a high susceptibility during early adulthood and later life, but a lower susceptibility throughout middle adulthood (a U-curve).
4. *Lifelong openness*—individuals are to some extent susceptible to attitude change throughout their lives.
5. *Persistence*—most of an individual's fundamental orientations are established firmly during pre-adult socialisation; susceptibility to attitude change thereafter is low.

These hypotheses are derived as much from developmental psychology as from social psychology. Which has the greatest explanatory power remains an open question. Tyler and Schuller's (1991) field study of attitudes towards the government supports the *lifelong openness* hypothesis: that is, age is generally irrelevant to attitude change. On the other hand, Visser and Krosnick's (1998) laboratory experiments support the *life stages* hypothesis. Rutland's (1999) research on the development of prejudice shows that negative attitudes towards ethnic and national outgroups only crystallise in later childhood (around age 10).

Disconfirmation bias
The tendency to notice, refute and regard as weak, arguments that contradict our prior beliefs.

Other variables

There are at least two other audience variables that relate to the persuasion process.

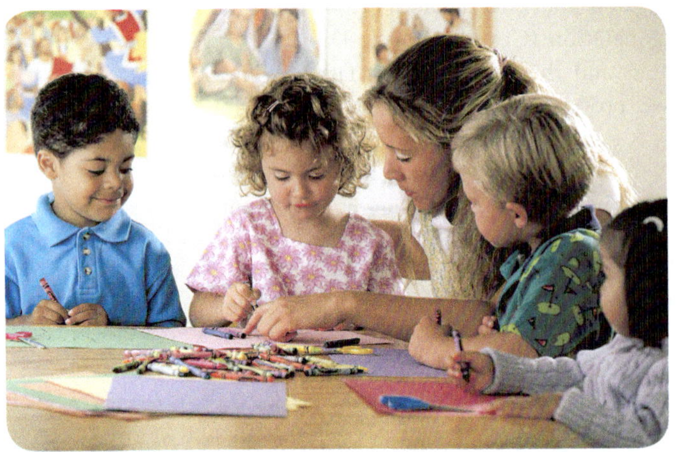

The impressionable years Respected adults, such as this teacher, are enormously influential in the development of young children's attitudes
(**Source:** Pearson Australia Pty Ltd.)

1 *Prior beliefs* affect persuasibility. There is evidence for a **disconfirmation bias** in argument evaluation. Arguments that are incompatible with prior beliefs are scrutinised longer, subjected to more extensive refutational analyses and are judged weaker than arguments compatible with prior beliefs. Furthermore, the magnitude and form of a disconfirmation bias is higher if prior beliefs are accompanied by emotional conviction (Edwards & Smith, 1996). Even if arguments contain only facts, prior beliefs affect whether factual information is considered at all. In a political controversy over the stranding of a Soviet submarine near a Swedish naval base in 1981, the contending sides were most unwilling to accept facts introduced by each other into the debate, querying whether they

were relevant and reliable (Lindstrom, 1997). The disconfirmation bias is evident daily in media political discussions. For example, the disaster of the *Kursk,* a Russian submarine that sank in the Barents Sea in 2000, and the refusal of Western help in the rescue mission, sparked a similar debate to that in 1981.

2 *Cognitive biases* are important in both attitude formation and change. For example, Duck, Hogg and Terry (1999) demonstrated the *third-person effect* in media persuasion (discussed earlier). According to this bias, people believe that they are less influenced than others by persuasion attempts. Students' perceptions of the impact of AIDS advertisements on themselves, students (ingroup), non-students (outgroup) and people in general were examined. Results showed that perceived self–other differences varied with how strongly students identified with being students. Those who did not identify strongly as students (low identifiers) exhibited the third-person effect, while those who did identify strongly as students (high identifiers) were more willing to acknowledge impact on themselves and the student ingroup.

In closing, we stress that the three major categories of variables dealt with—source, message and audience—interact in practice. For example, whether one would choose to employ an expert source to deliver a message can depend on the target group:

> *A guiding principle in both marketing research and in persuasion theory is to 'know your audience' … marketers realize that a key to capturing a significant portion of the market share is to target one's product to those who are most likely to want or need it.* (Jacks & Cameron, 2003, p. 145)

In the next section we examine how the persuasion process works.

Dual-process models of persuasion

Much time and energy has been spent studying how we respond to the content of a message. Although different approaches have been taken by Petty and Cacioppo (e.g. Petty & Cacioppo, 1986a, 1986b) and by Chaiken (e.g. Chaiken, 1987; Chaiken, Liberman & Eagly, 1989), there are elements in common. Each approach postulates two processes and draws on developments in research on memory from cognitive psychology. Both theories deal with persuasion cues. Sometimes it may not be the quality and type of the persuasion cues that matter but rather the quantity of message processing that underlies attitude change (Mackie, Worth & Asuncion, 1990). After more than 20 years of research, are these theories still relevant?

> *Without question, the dual-process models remain today's most influential persuasion paradigms, as they have been since their inception. In these models, source and message may play distinct roles that, in concert with motivation and ability to process information, determine the outcomes of persuasive interactions.* (Crano & Prislin, 2006, p. 348)

Elaboration-likelihood model

According to Richard Petty and John Cacioppo's **elaboration-likelihood model** (ELM), when people receive a persuasive message they think about the arguments it makes. However, they do not necessarily think deeply or carefully, because to do so requires considerable cognitive effort. People are cognitive tacticians who are motivated to expend valuable cognitive capital only on issues that are important to them. Persuasion follows two routes, depending on whether people expend a great deal or very little cognitive effort on the message.

Elaboration-likelihood model
Petty and Cacioppo's model of attitude change: when people attend to a message carefully, they use a central route to process it; otherwise they use a peripheral route. This model competes with the heuristic–systematic model.

If the arguments of the message are followed closely, a *central route* is used. We digest the arguments in a message, extract a point that meets our needs and even indulge mentally in counter-arguments if we disagree with some of them. If the central route to persuasion is to be used, the points in the message need to be put convincingly, as we will be required to expend considerable cognitive effort—that is, to work hard—on them. For example, suppose that your doctor told you that you needed major surgery. The chances are that you would take

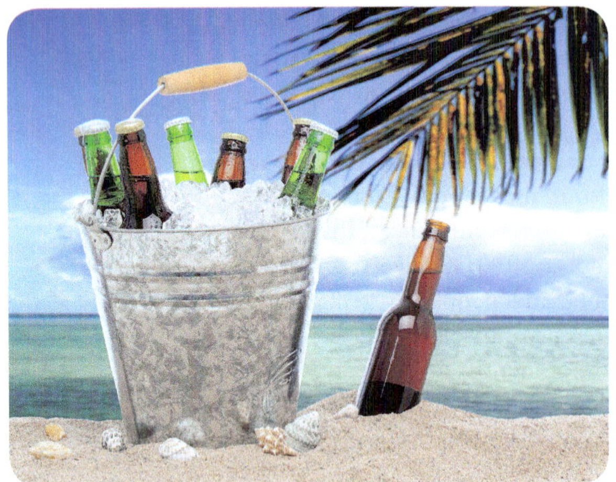

Peripheral cues in advertising Feeling hot and thirsty? Fancy a cold beer?
(**Source:** Steve Cukrov/Shutterstock)

a considerable amount of convincing, that you would listen carefully to what the doctor says, read what you could about the matter and even seek a second medical opinion. On the other hand, when arguments are not well attended to a *peripheral route* is followed. By using peripheral cues we act in a less diligent fashion, preferring a consumer product on a superficial whim, such as an advertisement in which the product is used by an attractive model. The alternative routes available according to the elaboration–likelihood model are shown in Figure 9.20.

Heuristic-systematic model

Heuristic-systematic model Chaiken's model of attitude change: when people attend to a message carefully, they use systematic processing; otherwise they process information by using heuristics, or 'mental shortcuts'. This model competes with the elaboration–likelihood model.

Shelley Chaiken's **heuristic-systematic model** (HSM) deals with the same phenomena using slightly different concepts, distinguishing between *systematic* processing and *heuristic* processing. Systematic processing occurs when people scan and consider available arguments. In the case of heuristic processing, we do not indulge in careful reasoning but instead use cognitive heuristics, such as thinking that longer arguments are stronger. Persuasive messages are not always processed systematically. Chaiken has suggested that people sometimes employ cognitive heuristics to simplify the task of handling information.

You will recall that heuristics are simple decision rules or 'mental shortcuts', the tools that cognitive misers and motivated tacticians use. So, when we are judging the reliability of a message, we may resort to such truisms as 'statistics don't lie' or 'you can't trust a politician' as an easy way of making up our minds. As previously discussed, this feature of judgement is actively exploited by advertising companies when they seek to influence consumers by portraying their products as supported by scientific research or expert opinion. For instance, washing detergents are often advertised in laboratory settings, showing technical equipment and authoritative-looking people in white coats.

At what point would we switch from heuristic to systematic processing? According to Petty (Petty & Wegener, 1998), people have a *sufficiency threshold*: heuristics will be used as long as they satisfy our need to be confident in the attitude that we adopt.

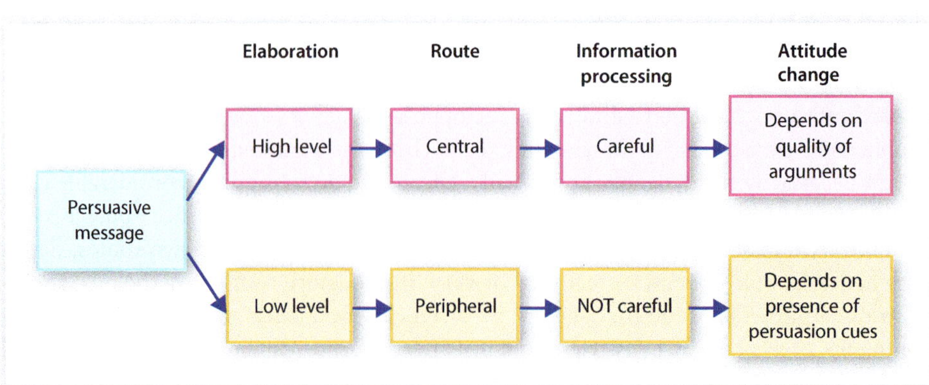

Figure 9.20 The elaboration–likelihood model of persuasion
(**Source:** based on Petty & Cacioppo (1986b))

When we lack sufficient confidence, we resort to the more effortful systematic mode of processing.

The role of cognition is fundamental in handling a persuasive message, but how well we concentrate on the content of a message can be subtly affected by something as transient as our *mood*. Diane Mackie, for example, has shown that merely being in a good mood changes the way we attend to information (Mackie & Worth, 1989; see also Petty, Schuman, Richman & Stratham, 1993). Using background music is a widely used advertising ploy to engender a mellow feeling. There is a sneaky reason behind this—feeling 'good' makes it difficult for us to process a message systematically. When time is limited, which is typical of TV advertising, feeling really good leads us to flick on to autopilot, i.e. to use a peripheral route (ELM) or heuristic processing (HSM).

Think again about how advertisers present everyday merchandise: cues like feel-good background music have an additional and longer term 'benefit' (Gorn, 1982). Marketing strategists George and Michael Belch (2012) noted that, through classical conditioning, a product repeatedly associated with a good mood can become evaluated positively—in time—in the absence of music or other positive contextual cues.

However, Duane Wegener demonstrated that people who are already happy do not always scrutinise messages superficially. If the message content is in line with our attitudes (therefore congruent with our already good mood), then being happy as well leads to more extensive processing (Wegener, Petty & Smith, 1995). What is involved here is an interaction between two of the three major persuasion factors noted in the Yale program: a supportive message and a happy audience.

In addition, feeling 'good' makes it difficult to process a message systematically. When time is limited, such as when we watch a TV advertisement, feeling really good can make us more susceptible to peripheral heuristic processing. Bohner, Chaiken and Hunyadi (1994) induced either a happy or a sad mood in students who then heard arguments that were strong, weak or ambiguous. All arguments were attributed to a highly credible source. When the message was unambiguous, sad participants were more easily influenced when they used heuristic processing. The effects of a sad mood have also been studied in a mock court setting (Semmler & Brewer, 2002). When jurors feel sad, their accuracy (i.e. systematic processing) in detecting witness inconsistencies and their perceptions of witness reliability and a defendant's culpability are improved.

How emotional the content of a message is can influence our 'choice' between processing methods according to its level of fear. Information tended to be processed centrally for low-fear messages and peripherally for high-fear messages (Hale, Lemieux & Mongeau, 1995).

Contrary to the common view that happy people scrutinise messages superficially, sometimes being happy leads to more extensive processing. Happy people may actually be more attentive because the message seems more relevant to their happy mood (the *hedonic contingency* hypothesis—Wegener, Petty & Smith, 1995).

As a reminder that social processes can be complex, consider a study by Chaiken and Maheswaran (1994): systematic processing can be eroded when certain variables interact (see Box 9.8).

In summary, when people are motivated to attend to a message and to deal with it *thoughtfully*, they use a central route to process it according to the ELM (Petty & Cacioppo) or process it systematically according to the HSM (Chaiken). When attention is reduced so that people become cognitively *lazy*, they use a peripheral route (Petty & Cacioppo) or resort to heuristics—simple decision rules (Chaiken).

Research and applications 9.8

Systematic processing can be undermined

This study dealt with complex interactions between source and message variables, as well as task importance, in relation to whether people use heuristic or systematic processing. In New York, students were asked to rate a new telephone-answering machine in an experiment with three independent variables:

1. *Task importance*. Some students believed that their opinion would weigh heavily, since sample size was small, in whether the machine would be distributed throughout New York; other students thought that their opinion would merely contribute to a much larger sample of New Yorkers and would not alter the outcome very much.
2. *Source credibility*. The product description was supposedly written by either a high-credibility source (Consumer Reports) or a low-credibility source (the sales staff of Kmart).
3. *Message type*. A pretest established eight product features, four of which were important (e.g. could take different cassette types, screening of incoming calls) and four unimportant (e.g. colour range, special bolts for a wall). The important-to-unimportant ratio of these features was varied to create messages that were strong (4:2), ambiguous (3:3) or weak (2:4).

The findings for the students showed that:

- For the unimportant task (their opinion did not count for much), the machine was rated in terms of the credibility of the source—heuristic processing was used—regardless of whether the message was strong, ambiguous or weak.
- For the important task (their opinion really counted), the machine was rated in terms of message content—systematic processing was used—provided the message was clearly strong or clearly weak. Source credibility did not affect these ratings.
- However, source credibility did play a role when the task was important but the message was ambiguous. Both systematic and heuristic processing were used.

Source: Chaiken & Maheswaran (1994)

Compliance

Compliance
Superficial, public and transitory change in behaviour and expressed attitudes in response to requests, coercion or group pressure.

The literature on social influence sometimes uses the term **compliance** interchangeably with conformity. This can happen when 'conformity' is broadly defined to include a change in behaviour, as well as beliefs, as a consequence of group pressure. In this section, compliance refers to a surface *behavioural* response to a *request by another individual*; whereas conformity, refers to the influence of a group upon an individual that usually produces more enduring internalised changes in one's attitudes and beliefs (see Hogg, 2010). Because compliance is more closely associated with behaviour, and conformity with attitudes, the compliance–conformity distinction engages with the attitude–behaviour relationship (see Sheeran, 2002). Compliance is also more closely associated with individuals having some form of power over you (French & Raven, 1959—see Fiske & Berdahl, 2007).

We are confronted daily with demands and requests. Often they are put to us in a straightforward and clear manner, such as when a friend asks you to dinner, and nothing more is requested. At other times, requests have a 'hidden agenda': for example, an acquaintance invites you to dinner to get you into the right mood to ask you to finance a new business venture. The result is often the same—we comply.

What are the factors and situations that make us more compliant, and why is it that we are more influenced on some occasions than others? Generally, people influence us when they use effective tactics or have powerful attributes.

Tactics for enhancing compliance

Persuading people to comply with requests to buy certain products has been the cornerstone of many economies. It is not surprising, therefore, that over the years many different tactics have been devised to enhance compliance. Salespeople, especially, have designed and refined many indirect procedures for inducing compliance, as their livelihood depends on it. We have all come across these tactics.

These tactics typically involve strategic self-presentation designed to elicit different emotions to compel others to comply. Ned Jones and Thane Pittman (1982) describe five such strategies and emotions: *intimidation* is an attempt to elicit fear by getting others to think you are dangerous; *exemplification* is an attempt to elicit guilt by getting others to regard you as a morally respectable individual; *supplication* is an attempt to elicit pity by getting others to believe you are helpless and needy; *self-promotion* is an attempt to elicit respect and confidence by persuading others that you are competent; and *ingratiation* is simply an attempt to get others to like you in order to secure compliance with a subsequent request. These last two, self-promotion and ingratiation, service two of the most common goals of social interaction: to get people to think you are competent and to get people to like you (Leary, 1995)—competence and warmth are the two most basic dimensions on which we evaluate people (Fiske, Cuddy & Glick, 2007).

Ingratiation

Ingratiation (Jones, 1964) is a particularly common tactic. A person attempts to influence others by first agreeing with them and getting them to like him/her. Next, various requests are made. You would be using ingratiation if you agreed with other people to appear similar to them or to make them feel good, made yourself look attractive, paid compliments, dropped names of those held in high esteem or physically touched them. However, ingratiation that is transparent can backfire, leading to the 'ingratiator's dilemma': the more obvious it is that an ingratiator will profit by impressing the target person, the less likely it is that the tactic will succeed (see Gordon, 1996, for a meta-analysis).

Using the **reciprocity principle** is another tactic, based on the social norm that 'we should treat others the way they treat us'. If we do others a favour, they feel obliged to reciprocate. Judith Regan (1971) showed that greater compliance was obtained from people who had previously received a favour than from those who had received none. Similarly, *guilt arousal* produces more compliance. People who are induced to feel guilty are more likely to comply with a later request to behave altruistically: for example, to make a phone call to save native trees, to agree to donate blood, or at a university to participate in an experiment (Carlsmith & Gross, 1969; Darlington & Macker, 1966; Freedman, Wallington & Bless, 1967).

Have you had your car windscreen washed while waiting at traffic lights? If the cleaner washes it before you can refuse, there is subtle pressure on you to pay for the service. In some cities (e.g. in Portugal), people might guide you into parking spaces that one could have easily located and then ask for money. These are real-life examples of persuasion to give money that involves activation of the reciprocity principle.

Multiple requests

A very effective tactic is the use of **multiple requests**. Instead of a single request, a two-step procedure is used, with the first request functioning as a set-up or softener for the second, real request. Three classic variations are the foot-in-the-door, the door-in-the-face and low-balling tactics (see Figure 9.21; for a recent review, see Cialdini & Goldstein, 2004).

According to the **foot-in-the-door tactic**, if someone agrees to a small request, they will be more willing to comply with a later, large request. Some salespeople use this approach,

Ingratiation
Strategic attempt to get someone to like you in order to obtain compliance with a request.

Reciprocity principle
The law of 'doing unto others as they do to you'. It can refer to an attempt to gain compliance by first doing someone a favour, or to mutual aggression or mutual attraction.

Multiple requests
Tactics for gaining compliance using a two-step procedure: the first request functions as a set-up for the second, real request.

Foot-in-the-door tactic
Multiple-request technique to gain compliance, in which the focal request is preceded by a smaller request that is bound to be accepted.

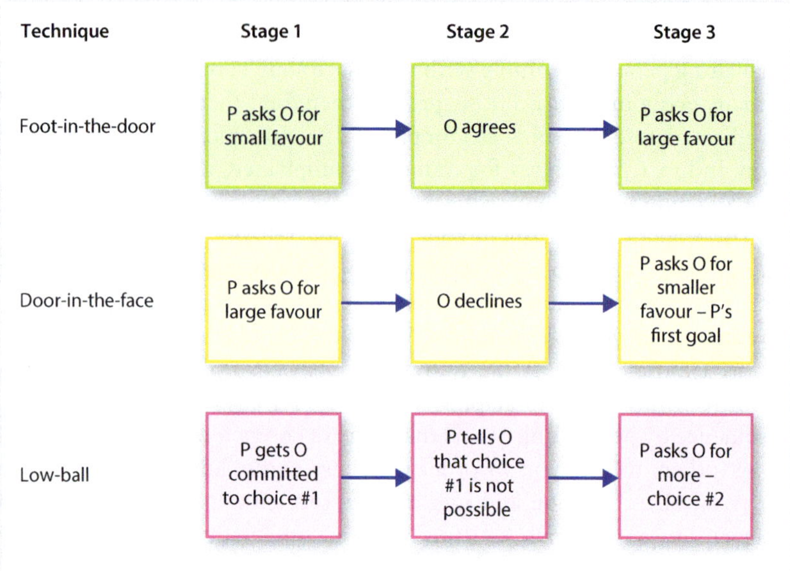

Figure 9.21 Three classic techniques for inducing compliance

and it underlies the saying 'if you give them an inch, they'll take a mile'. At first they might telephone you to ask just a few questions 'for a small survey that we are doing' and then entice you to join 'the hundreds of others in your area' who subscribe to their product.

In a study by Jonathan Freedman and Scott Fraser (1966), people were first contacted in their home to answer a few simple questions about the kind of soap they used at home. Later, they were more willing to comply with the larger request of allowing six people to make a thorough inventory of all the household items present. Only 22 percent complied when they received the larger request 'cold', but 53 percent complied when they had been softened up by the initial questions about soap.

The foot-in-the-door tactic may not always work. If the initial request appears too small or the second too large the link between the requests breaks down (Foss & Dempsey, 1979; Zuckerman, Lazzaro & Waldgeir, 1979). Nevertheless, a review by Saks (1978) suggested that, if the technique is tuned carefully, people can even be induced to act as donors for organ and tissue transplants (Saks, 1978).

In a refinement of the tactic, people agreed to a series of graded requests rather than jumping from a small to a large request. They were presented with two preliminary requests, increasingly demanding, prior to an ultimate request (Goldman, Creason & McCall, 1981; Dolinski, 2000). This proved more effective than the classic foot-in-the-door technique. Think of this, perhaps, as the 'two-feet-in-the-door technique'! Graded requests occur often when someone asks someone out on a 'date'. At first, a prospective partner might not agree to go out with you, but might well agree to go with you to study in the library. Your next tactic is to request another meeting, and eventually a proper date.

In a Polish field experiment, Darius Dolinski (2000) arranged for a young man to ask people in the city of Wroclaw for directions to Zubrzyckiego Street. There is no such street. Most said they did not know, although a few gave precise directions! Further down the street, the same people were then asked by a young woman to look after a huge bag for five minutes while she went up to the fifth floor in an apartment building to see a friend. A control group was asked to look after the bag, but not for the street directions. Compliance with the second, more demanding request was higher in the experimental group (see Figure 9.22).

Since there is reasonable evidence across a variety of studies that the foot-in-the-door technique actually works, what psychological process could account for it? A likely candidate for an explanation is Daryl Bem's (1967) self-perception theory (DeJong (1979). By complying with a small request, people become committed to their behaviour and develop a picture of themselves as 'giving'. The subsequent large request compels them to appear consistent. Dolinski explained his results in the same way. In trying to help a stranger, although unsuccessfully, his participants would have inferred that they were altruistic. They were therefore more susceptible to a later influence—even if that request was more demanding.

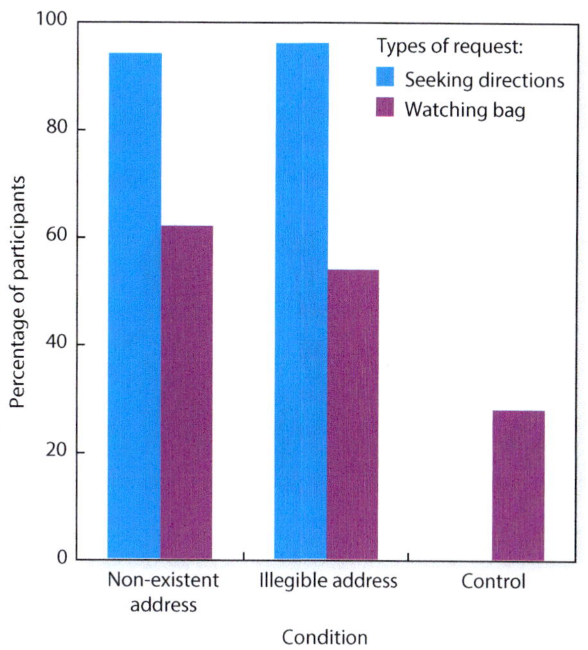

Figure 9.22 The foot-in-the-door technique: compliance with an impossible request followed by a possible request

Percentage of participants who answered 'I do not know' when asked about a non-existent or illegible address and of those who then complied with the request to keep an eye on the confederate's bag
(**Source:** based on data from Dolinski (2000), Experiment 2)

Similarly, Bob Cialdini and Melanie Trost (1998) explain the effect in terms of the principle of *self-consistency*. We try to manage our self-concept in such a way that, if we are charitable on one occasion, then we should be charitable again on the second occasion. Donald Gorassini and James Olson (1995), however, are sceptical that something as dramatic as self-conceptual change mediates the effect. Instead, they proposed an explanation with fewer assumptions. The foot-in-the-door tactic alters people's interpretation of situations that activate attitudes enhancing compliance. The self is left out of the loop.

What happens if an attempt to get a foot in the door fails? Commonsense suggests that this should reduce the likelihood of future compliance. Surprisingly, the opposite strategy, the **door-in-the-face tactic**, can prove successful (Cialdini et al., 1975; Patch, 1986). Here, a person is asked a large favour first and a small request second. Politicians especially are masters of this art. To illustrate, say that the government warns the media that student fees will need to go up 30 percent. Will you be angry? Later, however, it announces officially that the increase will 'only' be 10 percent—the actual figure planned. You probably feel relieved and think 'that's not so bad', and consequently are more accepting.

Door-in-the-face tactic
Multiple-request technique to gain compliance, in which the focal request is preceded by a larger request that is bound to be refused.

Cialdini et al. (1975) tested this tactic by approaching students with a huge request: 'Would you serve as a voluntary counsellor at a youth offenders' centre two hours a week for the next two years?' Virtually no one agreed. However, when the researchers then asked for a considerably smaller request, 'Would you chaperone a group of these offenders on a two-hour trip to the zoo?', 50 percent agreed. When the second request was presented alone, less than 17 percent complied. For the tactic to be effective, the researchers noted that the final request should come from the same person who made the initial request. According to them, participants perceived the scaled-down request as a concession by the influencer, and consequently they felt pressure to reciprocate. If some other person were to make the second request, reciprocation would not be necessary.

According to Cialdini, the door-in-the-face technique may well capitalise on a contrast effect: just as lukewarm water feels cool when you have just had your hand in hot water, a second request seems more reasonable and acceptable when it is contrasted with a larger request. This procedure is prevalent in sales settings. Suppose you tell an estate agent that

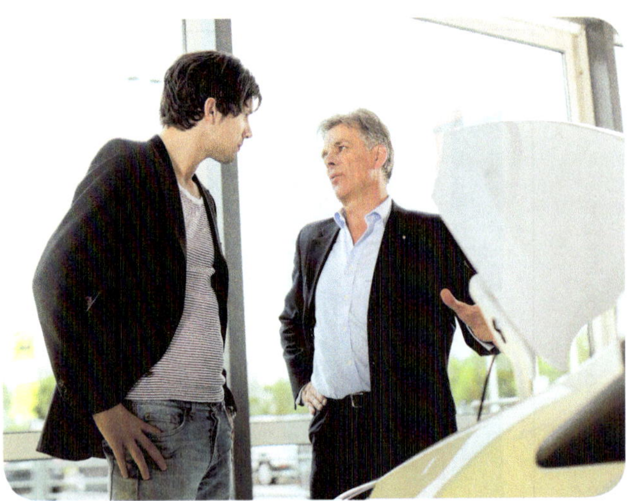

Low ball After 'consulting' with his boss, a salesman will tell a keen buyer that the quoted price for a new car no longer includes certain attractive extras
(**Source:** Kzenon/Shutterstock.)

you would like to spend quite a lot of hard-earned money on a small flat and she shows you a few rundown and overpriced examples. Then the higher-priced flats (the ones she really wants to show you!) look like extremely good bargains. In doing this, the estate agent has used the door-in-the-face tactic.

The other multiple-request technique used in similar situations is the **low-ball tactic** (check the first focus question). Here, the influencer changes the rules halfway and manages to get away with it. Its effectiveness depends on inducing the customer to agree to a request before revealing certain hidden costs. It is based on the principle that once people are committed to an action, they are more likely to accept a slight increase in the cost of that action. This tendency for people to stick with decisions is also captured in the notion of *sunk costs* (Fox & Hoffman, 2002), where once a course of action is decided on, people will continue to invest in it even if the costs increase dramatically.

Low-ball tactic
Technique for inducing compliance in which a person who agrees to a request still feels committed after finding that there are hidden costs.

Suppose you shop around for a car and are confronted with the following chain of events. The car salesperson makes you a very attractive offer—a high trade-in price for your old car—and then suggests a reduction on the marked purchase price for the car you have set your heart on. You decide to buy it and are ready to sign the papers. The salesperson then goes off to check the agreement with the boss, comes back, looks very disappointed and informs you that the boss will not sanction it because they would lose too much money on the deal. You can still have the car, but at the marked price. What should you do? Surprisingly, many customers still go ahead with the deal. It seems that, once you are committed, you are hooked and reluctant to back out. A commonplace example of low-balling is when someone asks 'Could you do me a favour?' and you agree before actually knowing what will be expected of you.

Just how effective low-balling can be was demonstrated by Cialdini, Cacioppo, Bassett and Miller (1978). They asked half their participants to be in an experiment that began at 7 a.m. The other half were asked first to commit to participating in an experiment and then were informed that it would start at 7 am. The latter group had been low-balled and complied more often (56 percent) than the control group (31 percent) and also tended to keep their appointments.

These studies show us the circumstances in which compliance is likely to occur. Sometimes our decision to comply may be rational: we weigh the pros and cons of our action. However, often we act before we think. According to Ellen Langer and her colleagues, much compliance is due to **mindlessness**: we agree without giving it a thought. Langer conducted experiments in which people were asked to comply with requests with little or no justification. In their study, a person about to use a photocopier was interrupted by an experimenter, who requested priority use for: (1) no reason, (2) a non-informative reason ('I have to make copies'), or (3) a justified reason ('I'm in a rush'). They found that, as long as the request was small, people were likely to agree, even for a spurious reason. There was lower compliance when there was no reason (Langer, Blank & Chanowitz, 1978).

Mindlessness
The act of agreeing to a request without giving it a thought. A small request is likely to be agreed to, even if a spurious reason is provided.

Though being mindless may be a deciding factor in compliant behaviour, studies of power strategies indicate that this compliance often depends on the sources of power used.

Action research

At about the time that Hovland and his associates were studying attitude change in the US Army, the expatriate German psychologist Kurt Lewin was undertaking another piece of practical wartime research on the home front for a civilian government agency. With the aim of conserving supplies at a time of food shortages and rationing, he tried to convince American housewives to feed their families unusual but highly nutritious foods, such as beef hearts and kidneys, rather than steak or roast beef.

Lewin considered that attitude change could best be achieved if the recipients were somehow actively engaged in the change process rather than just being passive recipients. He referred to this involvement of the participants in the actual research process, and its outcome, as **action research**. Lewin demonstrated that an active discussion among 'housewives' about how best to present beef hearts and other similar foods to their families was much more effective than merely giving them a persuasive lecture presentation. His data showed that 32 percent of the women in the discussion group went on to serve the new food, compared with only 3 percent in the lecture group (Lewin, 1943).

Action research
The simultaneous activities of undertaking social science research, involving participants in the process, and addressing a social problem.

The emphasis on action by participants fitted in with parts of the attitude change program of Hovland and his associates. For instance, Irving Janis and Bert King (1954) investigated the effects of role playing by their participants. They found that those who gave a speech arguing against something that they believed in (i.e. acted out a role) experienced more attitude change than when they listened passively to a speech arguing against their position.

This early study of counter-attitudinal behaviour foreshadowed research into cognitive dissonance (discussed in the next section). One of Lewin's students was Leon Festinger, who believed that humans are active processors and organisers of the information they receive from the world around them and of the cognitions (attitudes, beliefs, ideas, opinions) they have about the world. He accepted the consistency principle and argued that people will even change their ideas to make them consistent with what they are feeling or with how they are acting (Festinger, 1980). This would be the basis of the theory of cognitive dissonance.

In recent years, action research has been used increasingly by social psychologists to address community health issues relating to smoking, sun exposure and risky sexual practices. For example, prompted by the fact that Australia has one of the highest rates of melanoma in the world, David Hill and his colleagues (Hill, White, Marks & Borland, 1993) conducted a three-year study dedicated to changing attitudes and behaviour related to sun exposure, called the SunSmart health promotion program. This campaign was called SLIP! SLOP! SLAP! ('slip on a shirt, slop on some sunscreen, slap on a hat'), and was conducted via an array of media over three successive summers throughout the state of Victoria in southern Australia. Hill and associates found a significant change among 4500 participants in sun-related behaviour over this period. There was:

- a drop in those reporting sunburn—11 to 7 percent
- an increase in hat wearing—19 to 29 percent
- an increase in sunscreen use—12 to 21 percent
- an increase in body area covered by clothing—67 to 71 percent.

Check the ongoing work of the Cancer Council Victoria at www.cancervic.org.au.

An important correlate of these behavioural changes was attitude change. Agreement declined with items such as 'A suntanned person is more healthy' and 'There is little chance I'll get skin cancer'. Action research methods have also been used to reduce smoking (see Box 9.10).

More recently, there have been media campaigns focusing on nearly 1400 patients living with HIV or AIDS in France (Peretti-Watel, Obadia, Dray-Spira, Lert & Moatti, 2005). The respondents reported that information provided in the mass media helped them to manage their sexual life by using condoms and avoiding secondary infection.

Cognitive dissonance and attitude change

People are allowed to change their minds and, as we all know, they do. In this section we deal with the theory of cognitive dissonance. Its major premise is that cognitive dissonance is an unpleasant state of psychological tension generated when a person has two or more cognitions (bits of information) that are inconsistent or clash. Cognitions are thoughts, attitudes, beliefs or states of awareness of behaviour. For example, if a woman believes that monogamy is an important feature of her marriage and yet is having an extramarital affair, she may experience a measure of guilt and discomfort (dissonance). One of a family of **cognitive consistency theories**, it was developed by Leon Festinger (1957) and became the most studied topic in social psychology during the 1960s (see Cooper, 2007).

Cognitive consistency theories
A group of attitude theories stressing that people try to maintain internal consistency, order and agreement among their various cognitions.

Festinger proposed that we seek harmony in our attitudes, beliefs and behaviour, and try to reduce tension from inconsistency between these elements. The theory holds that people will try to reduce dissonance by changing one or more of the inconsistent cognitions (e.g. in the case of the unfaithful wife, 'what's wrong with a little fun if no one finds out?'), by looking for additional evidence to bolster one side or the other ('my husband doesn't understand me'), or by derogating the source of one of the cognitions ('fidelity is a construct of religious indoctrination'). The maxim appears to be: *The greater the dissonance, the stronger the attempts to reduce it.* Experiencing dissonance leads people to feel physiologically 'on edge'—as evidenced by changes in the electrical conductivity of the skin that can be detected by a polygraph.

Selective exposure hypothesis
People tend to avoid potentially dissonant information.

For dissonance to lead to attitude change, it is necessary that two sets of attitudes are in contradiction (see Box 9.9). Because dissonance is unpleasant, people will tend to avoid exposure to ideas that bring it about. According to the **selective exposure hypothesis**, people are remarkably choosy when potentially dissonant information is on the horizon. Exceptions are when their attitude is either: (1) very strong, and they can integrate or argue against contrary information, or (2) very weak, and it seems better to discover the truth now and then make appropriate attitudinal and behavioural changes (Frey, 1986; Frey & Rosch, 1984).

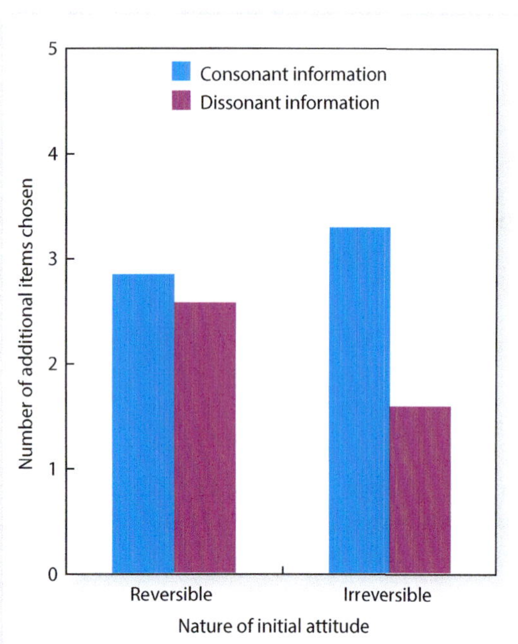

Figure 9.23 Selection of consonant and dissonant information as a function of attitude irreversibility
(**Source:** based on data from Frey & Rosch (1984))

For example, Dieter Frey and Marita Rosch (1984) gave German high-school students written profiles on the basis of which they had to form an attitude about whether to terminate or continue the employment of a 'manager'. Half the participants were told that their attitude was reversible (they could change their mind later on) and half that their attitude was irreversible. Then they selected as many bits of additional information as they wished from a pool containing five items of consonant information (in support of their attitude) and five items of dissonant information (in opposition to their attitude). Participants chose more consonant than dissonant information, and the effect was greatly magnified in the irreversible condition (see Figure 9.23).

A virtue of cognitive dissonance theory is that it is stated in a broad and general way. It is applicable in many situations, particularly those involving attitude or behaviour change. For instance, it has been applied to understanding:

Research and applications 9.9

The impact of student exchange on national stereotypes

Student exchanges provide a wonderful opportunity for sojourners to confront stereotypic attitudes about other nations with new information gleaned from personal experience in a foreign country. From a cognitive dissonance perspective, one would expect (or hope) that pleasant personal experiences would conflict with ingrained negative attitudes towards a foreign nation, and would arouse cognitive dissonance which, under the circumstances, could only be resolved by changing the initial attitude.

A study by Wolfgang Stroebe and his colleagues of American students on one-year exchanges in Germany and France illustrates this idea. They found that in the case of sojourners in Germany, reality matched existing attitudes and consequently there was no dissonance and no attitude change. Sojourners in France, however, found that realities were less pleasant than pre-existing attitudes had led them to believe. There was dissonance, and consequently they departed from France with changed attitudes—unfortunately changed for the worse (Stroebe, Lenkert & Jonas, 1988). These findings are consistent with other research into sojourners' attitudes (e.g. Klineberg & Hull, 1979), and they foreshadow the complexity of studying the way that stereotypes may change after direct contact with an outgroup.

- people's feelings of regret and changes of attitude after making a decision
- their patterns of exposing themselves to and searching for new information
- reasons that people seek social support for their beliefs
- attitude change in situations where lack of support from fellow ingroup members acted as a dissonant cognition
- attitude change in situations where a person has said or done something contrary to their customary beliefs or practice
- attitude change to rationalise hypocritical behaviour (Stone & Fernandez, 2008; Stone, Wiegand, Cooper & Aronson, 1997).

Dissonance theory is often grouped with balance theory as one of a family of models assuming that people try to be consistent in thought and action. A particularly appealing feature of dissonance theory is that it can generate non-obvious predictions about how people make choices when faced with conflicting attitudes and behaviours (Insko, 1967). Dissonance research falls largely into one of three research paradigms (Worchel, Cooper & Goethals, 1988): effort justification, induced compliance, and free choice. Let us see how these differ.

Effort justification

Now here is a surprise. The moment you choose between alternatives, you invite a state of dissonance. Suppose you need some takeaway food tonight. You make the momentous decision to go to the hamburger joint rather than the Chinese takeaway. You keep mulling over the alternatives even after making your choice. Tonight's the night for a hamburger—you can taste it in your mouth already! The hamburger will be evaluated more favourably, or perhaps the Chinese will become less attractive, or maybe both—and tomorrow is another day. The way the **effort justification** paradigm works is shown in Figure 9.24.

Effort justification A special case of cognitive dissonance: inconsistency is experienced when a person makes a considerable effort to achieve a modest goal.

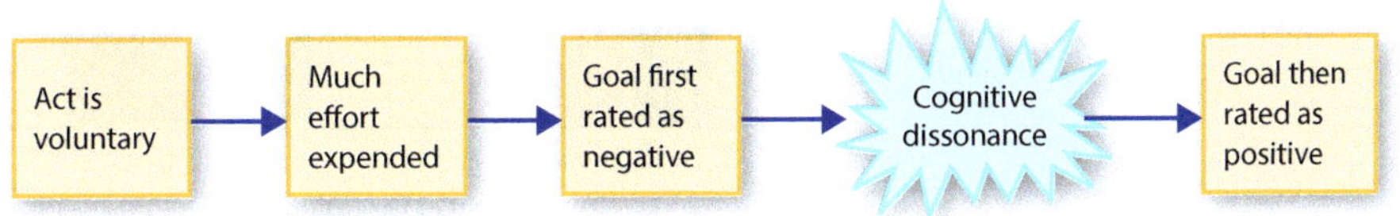

Figure 9.24 The general model of the effort justification paradigm

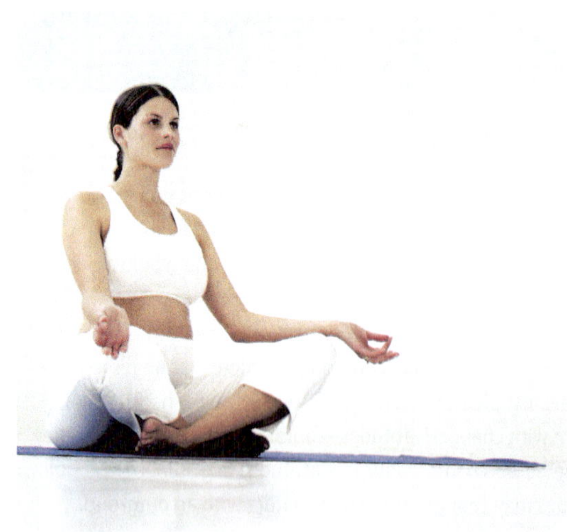

Effort justification She looks incredibly serene. All that dedication to yoga has paid off and, she believes, will ease the birth of her baby
(**Source:** Pearson Australia Pty Ltd.)

An often quoted early study by Elliott Aronson and Judson Mills (1959) explored what effort justification means. Female students volunteered to take part in a group discussion about sex, but were told that, before they could join a group, they must first pass a screening test for their capacity to speak frankly. Those who agreed were assigned to one of two conditions. In the severe condition, they were given a list of obscene words and explicit sexual descriptions to read aloud; in the mild condition, they were to read words that included some such as 'petting' and 'prostitution'.

After being initiated, they listened over headphones to a discussion held by a group with a view to joining in during the following week. What they heard was tame—far short of embarrassing. The discussion was in fact a recording in which the participants had been primed to mumble, be incoherent and plain boring. As well as the severe and mild initiation conditions, there was a control condition in which the participants did not undergo the screening experience.

The hypothesis was that the severe condition would cause some suffering to the participants, but yet they had volunteered to participate. The act of volunteering for embarrassment should cause dissonance. The predicted outcome would be increased liking for the chosen option (to participate in the discussion group), because the choice had entailed suffering. To make this sequence consonant would require the participant to rate the group discussion as more interesting than it really was. The hypothesis was confirmed. Those who went through the severe initiation thought that both the group discussion and the other group members were much more interesting than did those in the mild or control conditions (see Figure 9.25).

Later studies have shown that effort justification is a useful device to induce important behavioural changes relating to phobias and alcohol abuse. An interesting example is a study by Joel Cooper and Danny Axsom (1982). The participants were women who felt they needed help to lose weight and were willing to try a 'new experimental procedure'. They were required to come to a laboratory, where they were weighed and the procedure was explained to them.

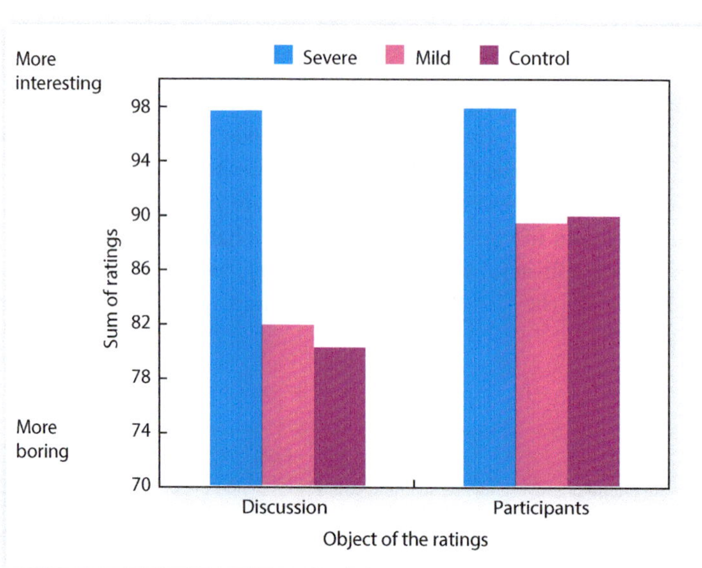

Figure 9.25 Interest in a group discussion in relation to the severity of the initiation procedure

Some degree of 'suffering' makes a voluntary activity seem more attractive
(**Source:** based on data from Aronson & Mills (1959))

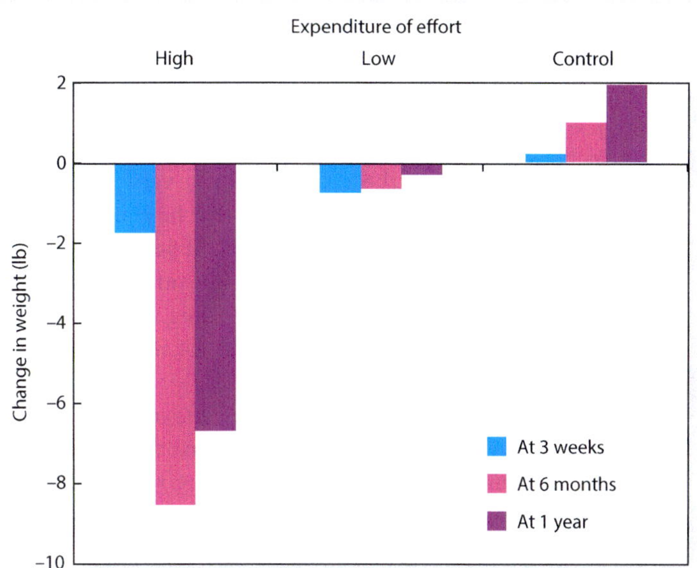

Figure 9.26 Change in weight among overweight women after expending psychological effort

You may think that physical effort should reduce weight. This study suggests that mental effort is an important ingredient in a program's effectiveness
(**Source:** based on data from Cooper & Axsom (1982))

In a high-effort condition, some were told that they needed to participate in a variety of time-consuming and effortful tasks, including reading tongue twisters aloud for a session lasting 40 minutes. These tasks required psychological effort rather than physical exercise. When the effort was low, the tasks were shorter and easier; and in a control condition, the volunteers did not participate in any tasks at all but were simply weighed and asked to report again at a later date. The high-effort and low-effort groups came to the laboratory for five sessions over a period of three weeks, at which point they were weighed again. The results are shown in Figure 9.26.

Cooper and Axsom were encouraged to find that the weight loss in the high-effort group was not just an artefact of the interest shown in the women during the time of the five-week study. The participants were contacted again after six months and after one year and agreed to be weighed again. The weight loss was much more marked after time had elapsed. After six months, a remarkable 94 percent of the high-effort group had lost some weight, while only 39 percent of the low-effort group had managed to do so.

Induced compliance

Sometimes people are induced to act in a way that is inconsistent with their attitudes. An important aspect of the induced compliance paradigm is that the inducement should not be so strong that people feel they have been forced against their will. Festinger and Carlsmith (1959) carried out a seminal experiment in which students who had volunteered to participate in a psychology experiment were asked to perform an extremely boring task for an hour, believing that they were contributing to research on 'measures of performance'.

Induced compliance
A special case of cognitive dissonance: inconsistency is experienced when a person is persuaded to behave in a way that is contrary to an attitude.

Imagine that you are the volunteer and that in front of you is a board, on which there are several rows of square pegs, each one sitting in a square hole. You are asked to turn each peg a quarter of a turn to the left and then a quarter of a turn back to the right. When you have finished turning all the pegs, you are instructed to start all over again, repeating the sequence over and over for 20 minutes. (This was not designed to be fun!) When the 20 minutes are up, the experimenter tells you that you have finished the first part, and you can now start on the second part, this time taking spools of thread off another peg board and placing them all back on again, and again, and again. Finally, the mind-numbing jobs are over.

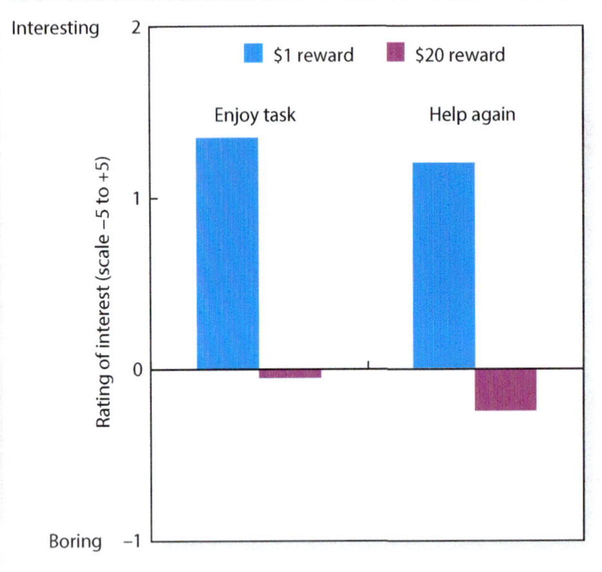

Figure 9.27 The effect of incentives on evaluating a boring task in an induced-compliance context

One of social psychology's counter-intuitive findings: commitment to return to repeat a boring task is maximised, as is dissonance, by offering a minimal reward (**Source:** based on data from Festinger & Carlsmith (1959))

At this point, the experimenter lets you in on a secret: you were a control participant, but you can now be of 'real' help. It seems that a confederate of the experimenter has failed to show up. Could you fill in? All you have to do is tell the next person that the tasks are really very interesting. The experimenter explains that he is interested in the effects of preconceptions on people's work on a task. Later, the experimenter offers a monetary incentive if you would be willing to be on call to help again at some time in the future. Luckily, you are never called.

In the Festinger and Carlsmith study, participants in one condition were paid the princely sum of $1 for agreeing to cooperate in this way, while others in a second condition were paid $20 for agreeing to help. The experimental design also included a control group of participants who were not asked to tell anyone how interesting the truly boring experience had been, and they were paid no incentive. On a later occasion, all were asked to rate how interesting or otherwise this task had been.

According to the induced compliance paradigm, dissonance follows from the fact that you have agreed to say things about what you have experienced when you know that the opposite is true. You have been induced to behave in a *counter-attitudinal* way.

The variation in levels of incentive adds an interesting twist. Participants who were paid $20 could explain their lie to themselves with the thought, 'I did it for the $20. It must have been a lousy task, indeed'—$20 was a tidy sum in the mid-1950s. In other words, dissonance would probably not exist in this condition. On the other hand, those who told the lie and were paid only $1 were confronted with a dilemma: 'I have done a really boring task, then told someone else that it was interesting, and finally even agreed to come back and do this again for a measly $1!' Herein lies the dissonance. One way of reducing the continuing arousal would be for these participants to convince themselves that the experiment was really quite interesting after all. The results of this now classic study are shown in Figure 9.27.

The interest ratings of the two reward groups confirmed the main predictions. The $1 group rated the task as fairly interesting, whereas the $20 group found it slightly boring (while control participants found it even more so). The $1 participants were also more willing to take part in similar experiments in the future. The main thrust of this experiment, which was to use a smaller reward to bring about a larger attitude change, has been replicated several times. To modify an old saying: 'If you are going to lead a donkey on, use a carrot, but make it a small one if you want the donkey to enjoy the trip.'

Talking of carrots brings us to consider eating fried grasshoppers. An intriguing experiment carried out in a military setting by Philip Zimbardo and his colleagues (Zimbardo, Weisenberg, Firestone & Levy, 1965) tackled this culinary question. The participants were asked to comply with the aversive request to eat grasshoppers by an authority figure whose interpersonal style was either positive (warm) or negative (cold). According to the induced compliance variation of cognitive dissonance, **post-decisional conflict** (and consequent attitude change) should be greater when the communicator is negative—how else could one justify behaving voluntarily in a counter-attitudinal way? Read what happened in this study in Box 9.9, and check the results in Figure 9.28.

Post-decisional conflict
The dissonance associated with behaving in a counter-attitudinal way. Dissonance can be reduced by bringing the attitude into line with the behaviour.

Research classic 9.9

To know grasshoppers is to love them

Attitude change following induced compliance

Let us consider a scenario, involving young military cadets, was actually researched by Phil Zimbardo and his colleagues (Zimbardo, Ebbesen & Maslach, 1977). They arranged for an officer in command to suggest to the cadets that they might eat a few fried grasshoppers, and mild social pressure was put on them to comply. By administering a questionnaire about food habits earlier, they had ascertained that all the cadets thought there were limits to what they should be expected to eat, and that a meal of fried grasshoppers was one such limit. However, the officer gave them a talk indicating that modern soldiers in combat conditions should be mobile and, among other things, be ready literally to eat off the land. After his talk, the cadets were each given a plate with five fried grasshoppers and invited to try them out.

A critical feature of the experiment was the way in which the request was made. For half the cadets the officer was cheerful, informal and permissive. For the other half, he was cool, official and stiff. There was also a control group who gave two sets of food ratings but were never induced, or had the chance, to eat grasshoppers. The social pressure on the experimental participants had to be subtle enough for them to feel they had freely chosen whether or not to eat the grasshoppers. Indeed, an order to eat would not arouse dissonance, because a cadet could then justify his compliance by saying 'He made me do it'. Furthermore, the cadets who listened to the positive officer might justify complying by thinking 'I did it as a favour for this nice guy'. However, those who might eat the grasshoppers for the negative officer could not justify their behaviour in this way. The resulting experience should be dissonance, and the easy way of reducing this would be to change their feelings about grasshoppers as a source of food.

As it turned out, about 50 percent of the cadets actually ate some grasshoppers. Those who complied ate, on average, two of the five hoppers sitting on their plate. The results in Figure 9.28 show the percentage of participants who changed their ratings of liking or disliking grasshoppers as food. It is interesting to note that, in both the negative and positive officer conditions, eaters were more favourable and non-eaters less favourable. This suggests that a degree of self-justification was required to account for an act that was voluntary but aversive. However, the most interesting result concerned the negative officer condition. This is the case in which dissonance should be maximal and, in line with the theory, it was here that the biggest change towards liking the little beasties was recorded.

Source: based on Zimbardo, Ebbesen & Maslach (1977); Zimbardo, Weisenberg, Firestone & Levy (1965)

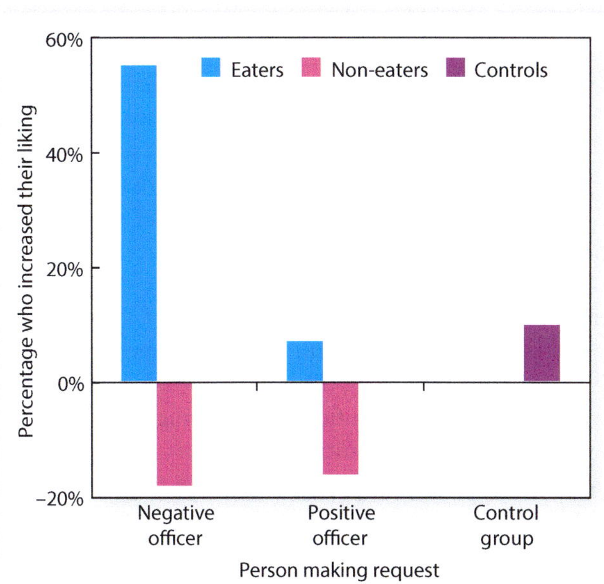

Figure 9.28 Degree of liking fried grasshoppers as food by military cadets in relation to the interpersonal style of an officer

As with Figure 6.12, here is another counter-intuitive outcome: complying with an unpleasant request can seem more attractive when the person making the request is less attractive
(**Source:** based on data from Zimbardo, Weisenberg, Firestone & Levy (1965))

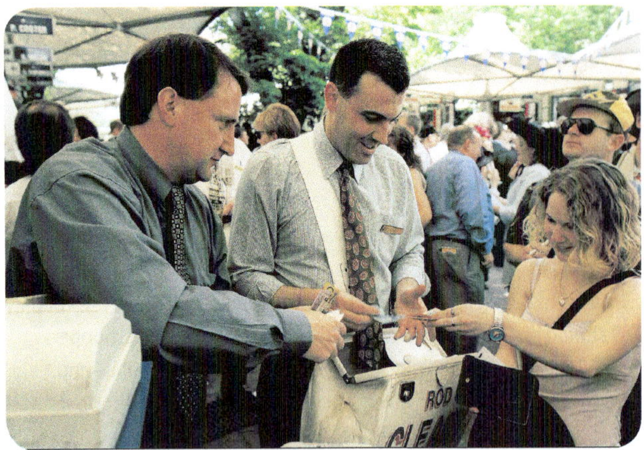

Free choice Sometimes dissonance is self-induced. Simply making a bet on the Melbourne Cup can convince us that our horse is more likely to win!
(**Source:** AAP Image/Philip Quirk/Wildlight.)

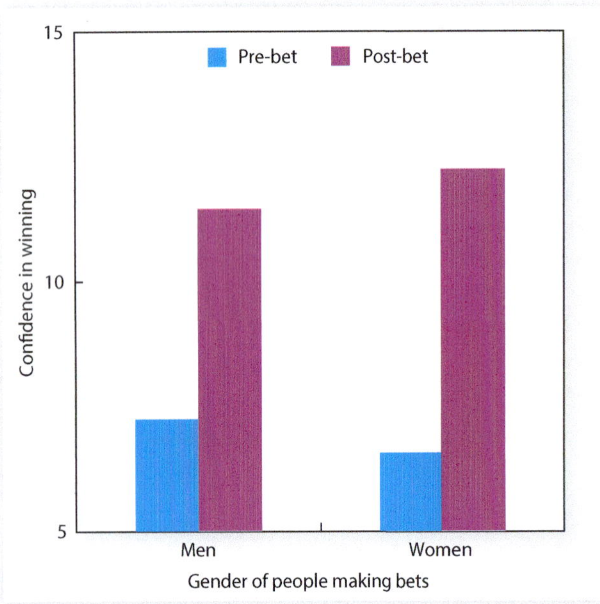

Figure 9.29 Degree of confidence in winning before and after making a bet

Making a commitment reduces dissonance. When we make a bet we 'had better believe' we have just increased our chances of winning!
(**Source:** based on data from Younger, Walker & Arrowood (1977))

Inducing people to act inconsistently with their attitudes is not easy and often requires a subtle approach. Counter-attitudinal actions with foreseeable negative consequences, such as being quoted in a newspaper saying that smoking is not harmful, requires an intricate inducement; whereas actions with less serious or negative consequences, such as voting anonymously that smoking is harmless, may be less difficult to bring about. However, once people have been induced to act counter-attitudinally, the theory predicts that dissonance will be strong and that they will seek to justify their action (Riess, Kalle & Tedeschi, 1981).

Free choice

Suppose that your choices between alternative courses of action are fairly evenly balanced, and that you are committed to making some kind of decision. This applies to numerous situations in our everyday lives: whether to buy this product or that; go to this tourist spot or another for a holiday; take this job offer or some other one. Based on Festinger's (1964) blueprint of the process of conflict in decision making, the pre-decision period is marked by uncertainty and dissonance, and the post-decision period by relative calm and confidence.

Free-choice dissonance reduction is likely to be a feature of bets laid on the outcome of sporting events, horse racing, gambling and so on. Once a person has made a choice between decision alternatives, dissonance theory predicts that the person making a bet will become more confident about a successful outcome. Jonathan Younger and his colleagues interviewed people at a Canadian national exposition who were either about to bet or had just placed their bets on games such as bingo and wheel of fortune, and asked them to rate their confidence in winning. They found that people who had already made their bet were more confident of winning (Younger, Walker & Arrowood 1977; see Figure 9.29).

However, dissonance theory is not the only contender that might account for results in the free-choice paradigm. There is a line of studies that contrasts people's preference for intuitive rather than rational predictions of outcomes using the **representativeness heuristic** (Kahneman & Tversky, 1973). For example, we are less confident of winning a lottery if we opt to exchange our purchased ticket for a new ticket. Intuitively, it doesn't feel right—the cognitive load of assessing the competing choice probabilities is excessive. We sometimes even 'refrain from changing checkout lines at the grocery store or from switching answers on multiple-choice tests' (Risen & Gilovich, 2007, p. 21)!

Representativeness heuristic
A cognitive shortcut in which instances are assigned to categories or types on the basis of overall similarity or resemblance to the category.

The role of self

According to Elliot Aronson (e.g. 1999) *self-consistency* is central to dissonance. People strive for a view of themselves as moral and competent human beings (Merritt et al. 2012). Counter-attitudinal behaviour is inconsistent with this view, and is thus distressing and motivates change, particularly among people who think relatively highly of themselves (i.e. they have higher self-esteem).

This idea that self-consistency is crucial for dissonance is taken up in a slightly different guise by **self-affirmation theory** (Steele, 1988; Steele, Spencer & Lynch, 1993; also see Sherman & Cohen, 2006). The key idea is that, if your self-concept is evaluatively challenged in one domain, then you can rectify the problem by publicly making positive statements about yourself in another domain. For example, if my competence as a scholar is challenged, I might emphasise (affirm) that I am a wonderful cook and a great athlete. From a dissonance perspective, negative behaviours are particularly threatening to one's sense of self. People who have high self-esteem can respond via self-affirmation—they experience no dissonance. However, people who have low self-esteem and are therefore less able to self-affirm, do experience dissonance. Here, there is a conflict: Aronson (self-consistency) predicts greater dissonance under high self-esteem, whereas Steele (self-affirmation) predicts greater dissonance under low self-esteem (see Tesser, 2000).

Self-affirmation theory
The theory that people reduce the impact of threat to their self-concept by focusing on and affirming their competence in some other area.

Jeff Stone (2003) has suggested that these contradictions involving self-esteem can be accounted for by recasting an explanation in terms of *self-standards*. When we evaluate our actions to judge if they are good or sensible rather than bad or foolish, we use our personal (individualised) standards or normative (group, or cultural) standards as yardsticks. The standards operating at a point in time are those that are readily or chronically accessible in memory. If we believe we have acted foolishly, dissonance will probably occur; but self-esteem will not enter the equation unless a personal standard has been brought to mind.

Overall, dissonance research involving the self, self-concept and self-esteem remains fluid, though this much seems agreed:

> *contemporary views of the self in dissonance have at least one common bond—they all make important assumptions about how people assess the meaning and significance of their behavior.*
> (Stone & Cooper, 2001, p. 241)

Vicarious dissonance

There is some intriguing evidence that people can experience dissonance vicariously (Cooper & Hogg, 2007; Norton, Monin, Cooper & Hogg, 2003). When two people share a strong bond, such as identifying strongly with the same group, dissonance experienced by one person may be felt by the other. This implies that a community advertisement could induce dissonance in viewers who watch someone 'like them' engaging in counter-attitudinal behaviour. The viewer does not actually have to behave counter-attitudinally. If the viewer also engages in counter-attitudinal behaviour, there may be a rebound effect because the common category member being observed provides social support for the viewer's dissonance.

Research conducted in Australia by Blake McKimmie and his colleagues found that ingroup social support for counter-attitudinal behaviour reduces dissonance (McKimmie et al., 2003). Other researchers found that endorsement of ingroup normative attitudes to do with pro-environmental behaviours strengthened when participants had observed an ingroup member acting hypocritically and when an outgroup member remarked negatively on the hypocrisy—endorsement was weakest when an outgroup member did not appear to notice the hypocrisy (Gaffney, Hogg, Cooper & Stone, 2012).

Alternative views to dissonance

Cognitive dissonance theory has had a chequered history in social psychology (see Visser & Cooper, 2003). Festinger's original ideas have been refined and sharpened. Dissonance was not as easy to create as Festinger originally believed, and in some cases other theories (e.g. self-perception theory, discussed next) may provide a better explanation of attitude change than cognitive dissonance. Despite this, cognitive dissonance theory remains one of the most widely accepted explanations of attitude change and much other social behaviour. It has generated well over 1000 empirical studies and will probably continue to be an integral part of social psychological theory for many years (Beauvois & Joule, 1996; Cooper, 2007; Cooper & Croyle, 1984; Joule & Beauvois, 1998).

Self-perception theory

Self-perception theory
Bem's idea that we gain knowledge of ourselves only by making self-attributions: for example, we infer our own attitudes from our own behaviour.

Some of the results of the dissonance experiments can be explained by **self-perception theory** (Bem, 1972). Some have suggested that attitude change does not occur according to the basic mechanisms proposed by dissonance theory and there have been several experimental attempts to compare the two. Both theories have been shown to be helpful in understanding behaviour (Fazio, Zanna & Cooper, 1977).

To understand the uses of each theory, imagine that attitudes fall on a continuum, spread over a range of acceptable choices. The idea that there are latitudes of acceptance and rejection around attitudes forms the basis of social judgement theory (Sherif & Sherif, 1967). If you are in favour of keeping the drinking age at 18, you might also agree to 17 or 19. There is a latitude of acceptance around your position. Alternatively, there is also a latitude of rejection: you might definitely be against a legal drinking age of either 15 or 21. Mostly we act within our own latitudes of acceptance. Sometimes we may go outside them: for instance, when we pay twice the amount for a dinner at a restaurant than we planned. If you feel you chose freely, you will experience dissonance.

A view that integrates self-perception and dissonance theories suggests that, when your actions fall within your range of acceptance, self-perception theory best accounts for your response. So, if you had been willing to pay up to 25 percent more than your original budget, there would be no real conflict: 'I suppose I was willing to pay that little bit more.' However, when you find yourself acting outside your previous range of acceptance, dissonance theory gives a better account of your response. We reduce our dissonance only by changing our attitude: 'I paid twice what I had budgeted, but that's okay because I thought the food was fantastic' (Fazio, Zanna & Cooper, 1977). Thus attitudes may be changed either through a self-attributional process such as self-perception or through attempts to reduce the feeling of cognitive dissonance.

A new look at cognitive dissonance

Joel Cooper and Russell Fazio (1984), in their *new look* model, countered some of the objections to cognitive dissonance theory. One controversy was how to retain and defend the concept of attitude when a person's observed behaviour and beliefs are in contradiction. According to Cooper and Fazio, when behaviour is counter-attitudinal we try to figure out what the consequences might be. If these are thought to be negative and fairly serious, we must then check to see if our action was voluntary. If it was, we then accept responsibility, experience arousal from the state of dissonance that follows and bring the relevant attitude into line, so reducing dissonance. This revision, shown in Figure 9.30, also includes attributional processes, in terms both of whether we acted according to our free will and of whether external influences were more or less important.

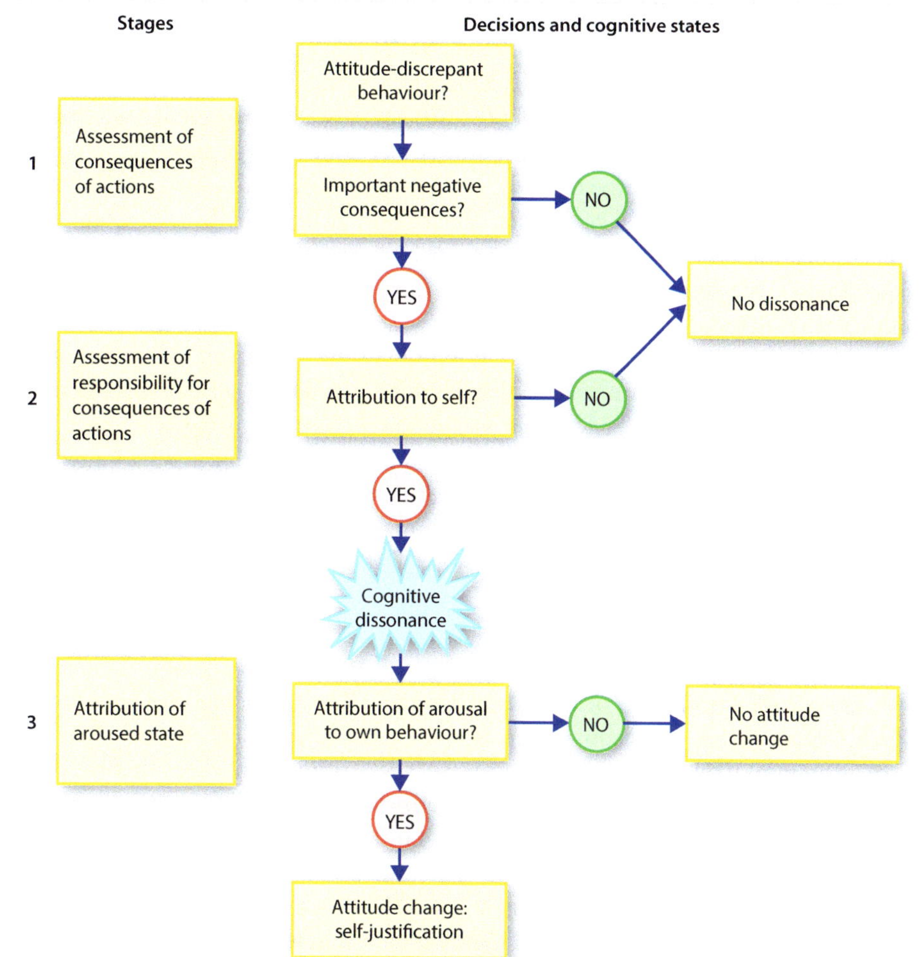

Figure 9.30
A revised cognitive dissonance model of attitude-discrepant behaviour
(**Source:** based on Cooper & Fazio (1984))

The new look model is supported by considerable evidence (Cooper, 1999), but so is the traditional cognitive dissonance theory that focuses on inconsistency rather than behavioural consequences (e.g. Harmon-Jones, 2000).

Resistance to persuasion

When we feel strongly about an issue we can be quite stubborn in resisting attempts to change our position (Zuwerink & Devine, 1996). However, much of the material presented in this section highlights factors that are conducive to our altering our attitudes, very often beyond a level of direct awareness. Yet far more attempts at persuasion fail than ever succeed. Researchers have identified three major reasons: reactance, forewarning, and inoculation.

Reactance

We are more easily persuaded if we think the message is not deliberately intended to be persuasive. Where a deliberate persuasion attempt is suspected, a process of **reactance** can be triggered. Think back to an occasion when someone obviously tried to change your

Reactance
Brehm's theory that people try to protect their freedom to act. When they perceive that this freedom has been curtailed, they will act to regain it.

attitudes. You might recall having an unpleasant reaction, and even hardening your existing attitude—perhaps becoming even more opposed to the other person's position.

Jack Brehm (1966) coined the term 'reactance' to describe this process—a psychological state that we experience when someone tries to limit our personal freedom. Research suggests that, when we feel this way, we can engage in covert counter-argument and attempts to undermine source credibility (Silvia, 2006), and go on to shift more overtly in the opposite direction, an effect known as *negative attitude change*. The treatment a doctor recommends to a patient is sometimes responded to in this way (Rhodewalt & Strube, 1985).

Some of you may be familiar with the biblical story set in the Garden of Eden. God said, 'I forbid you to eat that apple.' Eve (egged on by the serpent) thought 'Right! Let's see how it tastes.' Brad Bushman and Angela Stack (1996) tested this idea in an interesting study of warning labels for television films with violent content. Two kinds of labels were compared: (a) *tainted fruit* labels, in which a warning was relatively low-key, suggesting that a film's content could have harmful effects; (b) *forbidden fruit* labels, in which the warning was more overt and seemed like censorship—the very thing that a network could be anxious to avoid. Perhaps you will not be surprised that strong warnings increase interest in the violent films and viewers in this study responded in kind.

Forewarning

Forewarning
Advance knowledge that one is to be the target of a persuasion attempt. Forewarning often produces resistance to persuasion.

Forewarning is prior knowledge of persuasive intent—telling someone that you are going to influence them. When we know this in advance, persuasion is less effective (Cialdini & Petty, 1979; Johnson, 1994), especially with respect to attitudes and issues that we consider important (Petty & Cacioppo, 1979). When people are forewarned, they have time to rehearse counter-arguments that can be used as a defence. From this point of view, forewarning can be thought of as a special case of inoculation. A meta-analysis of research on forewarning by Wendy Wood and Jeffrey Quinn (2003) concluded that forewarning produces resistance (a boomerang effect) among people who are highly involved in the issue, but slight agreement with the persuasive message among those who are less involved.

Inoculation

> *The Chinese Communists have developed a peculiar brand of soul surgery which they practice with impressive skill—the process of 'thought reform'. They first demonstrated this to the American public during the Korean conflict ... And more recently we have seen ... Western civilians released from Chinese prisons, repeating their false confessions, insisting upon their guilt, praising the 'justice' and 'leniency' which they have received, and expounding the 'truth' and 'righteousness' of all Communist doctrine.* (R. J. Lifton, 1956; cited in Bernard, Maio & Olson, 2003, p. 63)

Inoculation
A way of making people resistant to persuasion. By providing them with a diluted counter-argument, they can build up effective refutations to a later, stronger argument.

As the term suggests, **inoculation** is a form of protection. In biology, we can inject a weakened or inert form of disease-producing germs into the patient to build up resistance to a more powerful form. In social psychology, we might seek an analogous method of providing a defence against persuasive ideas (McGuire, 1964). The technique of inoculation, described as 'the grandparent theory of resistance of attitude change' (Eagly & Chaiken, 1993, p. 561), is initiated by exposing a person to a weakened counter-attitudinal argument.

Bill McGuire and his associates (e.g. McGuire & Papageorgis, 1961; Anderson & McGuire, 1965) became interested in the technique following reports of 'brainwashing' of American soldiers imprisoned by Chinese forces during the Korean War of the early 1950s. Some of these made public statements denouncing the American government and saying they wanted to remain in China when the war ended. McGuire reasoned that these soldiers were mostly inexperienced young men who had not previously been exposed to attacks on the American way of life and were not forearmed with a defence against the Marxist logic.

McGuire applied the biological analogy to the field of persuasive communications, distinguishing two kinds of defence:

1. *The supportive defence*—based on attitude bolstering. Resistance could be strengthened by providing additional arguments that back up the original beliefs.
2. *The inoculation defence*—employs counter-arguments, and may be more effective. A person learns what the opposition's arguments are and then hears them demolished.

Inoculation at the outset poses some degree of threat, since a counter-argument is an attack on one's attitude (Insko, 1967). Note that the inoculation defence picks up on the advantage of a two-sided presentation, discussed earlier in relation to characteristics of a persuasive message. In general terms, this defence starts with a weak attack on the person's position, as a strong one might be fatal! The person can then be told that the weak argument is not too strong and should be easy to rebut, or else an argument is to be provided that deals directly with the weak attack. Increased resistance to persuasion may come about because we become motivated to defend our beliefs, and we acquire some skill in doing this.

Bill McGuire and Demetrios Papageorgis (1961) put both forms of defence to the test. Students were asked to indicate their agreement on a 15-point scale with a series of truisms relating to health beliefs, such as:

- It's a good idea to brush your teeth after every meal if at all possible.
- The effects of penicillin have been, almost without exception, of great benefit to mankind.
- Everyone should get a yearly chest X-ray to detect any signs of TB at an early stage.
- Mental illness is not contagious.

Before the experiment began, many of the students very thoroughly endorsed these propositions by scoring 15 on the 15-point response scale. The main variables of interest were the effects of introducing defences and attacks on these health beliefs in the form of essays offering arguments for or against the truisms. Students who were in the defence groups were in either (a) a *supportive* defence group (the students received support for their position), or (b) an *inoculation* defence group (their position was subjected to a weak attack, which was then refuted). There were also two control groups, one in which the students were neither attacked nor defended, and another that read essays that strongly attacked the truisms but none defending them.

Not surprisingly, control participants who had been neither attacked nor defended continued to show the highest level of acceptance of the truisms. The crucial findings shown in Figure 9.31 were:

- Students equipped with a supportive defence were a little more resistant to an attack when compared with the control group who had been attacked without any defence (compare the data in columns 2 and 4).
- Students who had been inoculated were substantially strengthened in their defence against a strong attack compared with the same control group (compare the data in columns 1 and 4).

Inoculation is clearly a strong defence against persuasion (also see Jacks & Cameron, 2003). However, McGuire (1964) has noted that the weaker supportive defence should not be ignored, although it is most effective when attacks upon one's position are well understood, so that established and rehearsed supportive arguments can be called up. For example, try persuading committed visitors to your door that they are in error when they are intent on telling you about the wonders of their religion. The chances are that they have heard your counter-arguments before. McGuire favoured the inoculation defence when the audience is to be exposed to a new argument. By having to deal with a mild earlier

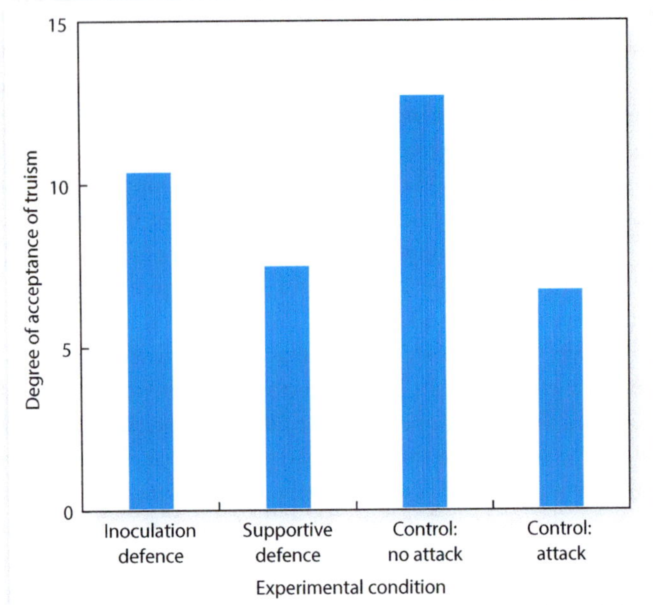

Figure 9.31 Degree of acceptance of health truisms in modes of reading and writing as a function of supportive and inoculation defences

One of the best forms of defence against counter-arguments is to be exposed to small doses of these arguments
(**Source:** based on data from McGuire & Papageorgis (1961))

attack on their position, they will be better equipped to innovate when a stronger one is mounted.

Inoculation has been used in some kinds of advertising. An example is issue/advocacy advertising in which a company protects consumer loyalty from 'attitude slippage' by issuing media releases on controversial issues (see Burgoon, Pfau & Birk, 1995). For example, a chemical company may issue a statement about environmental pollution in order to inoculate its consumers against allegations of environmental misconduct from competing companies, or from other 'enemies' such as a local green party. This practice is now widespread: an alcohol company may fund alcohol research and alcohol-moderation campaigns, and a fashion company may support the protection of wildlife.

Attitude accessibility and strength

Attitude *accessibility* and attitude *strength* are among other variables connected to people's resistance to persuasion:

- Accessible attitudes come to mind more easily and are likely to be stronger. When applied to the study of resistance, Michael Pfau and his colleagues confirmed what we might expect. An attitude that is accessible and strong is more resistant to persuasion (Pfau, Compton, Parker, et al., 2004; Pfau, Roskos-Ewoldsen, Wood, et al., 2003). In the case of inoculation, the initial threat to one's attitude makes the attitude more accessible, and even more so if we form counter-arguments.
- On a different tack, Zakary Tormala and Richard Petty (2002) have shown that success in resisting persuasion can rebound on the persuader by strengthening the target person's initial attitude. This effect held up even when the message was strong (Tormala & Petty, 2004a) or came from an expert source (Tormala & Petty, 2004b).

To be effective, a persuasive message must account for the kinds of real-life decisions that people later make—their *post-message behaviour*. Consider the varied campaigns directed at risky behaviour, such as trying to dissuade young people from drinking alcohol. Dolores Albarracín and her colleagues found that warnings about health and injury were not effective in promoting abstinence. A message such as 'just say no' to offers of alcohol may not stand much chance at the next teenage party. Young people who indulge in a 'trial' drink will immediately be in conflict—experience dissonance—between their behaviour and the content of the message. One outcome could be a weakening of the very attitude that the message was designed to support (Albarracín, Cohen & Kumkale, 2003).

Research on resistance to persuasion has expanded during the last decade and been applied to a wide range of persuasion domains (see Knowles & Linn, 2004). However, let us close this section with an irony. McGuire's original work was triggered by the dramatic events surrounding wartime brainwashing in the 1950s. Those real-world events were actually deep-reaching attempts to induce value conversion rather than more surface-level attitude change, and resonate today with the strategies of religious cults that are determined to undermine people's cherished values (Bernard, Maio & Olson, 2003). For this reason, more research attention to strategies for defending values against psychological attacks would be timely.[H]

Types of social influence

Social psychology was defined by Gordon Allport as 'an attempt to understand and explain how the thoughts, feelings, and behaviours of individuals are influenced by the actual, imagined, or implied presence of others' (1954a, p. 5). This widely accepted and often quoted definition of social psychology identifies a potential problem for the study of **social influence**—how does the study of social influence differ from the study of social psychology as a whole? There is no straightforward answer. Instead, we will look at the kinds of issues that are researched by social psychologists who claim to be studying social influence.

Social influence
Process whereby attitudes and behaviour are influenced by the real or implied presence of other people.

Social life is characterised by argument, conflict and controversy in which individuals or groups try to change the thoughts, feelings and behaviour of others by persuasion, argument, example, command, propaganda or force. People can be quite aware of influence attempts and can form impressions of how affected they and other people are by different types of influence.

Social life is also characterised by **norms**: that is, by attitudinal and behavioural uniformities among people, or what Turner has called 'normative social similarities and differences between people' (1991, p. 2). One of the most interesting sets of issues in social influence, perhaps even in social psychology, is how people construct norms, how they conform to or are regulated by those norms, and how those norms change.

Norms
Attitudinal and behavioural uniformities that define group membership and differentiate between groups.

Leaders play a key a role in the construction of norms and, more broadly, in processes of influence and persuasion. Leadership is thus an influence process (Hogg, 2010), but it is also a group process because norms are emergent properties of groups, and where there are leaders there are followers.

Compliance, obedience, conformity

We are all familiar with the difference between yielding to direct or indirect pressure from a group or an individual, and being genuinely persuaded. For example, you may simply agree publicly with other people's attitudes, comply with their requests or go along with their behaviour, yet privately not feel persuaded at all. On other occasions, you may privately change your innermost beliefs in line with their views or their behaviour. This has not gone unnoticed by social psychologists, who find it useful to distinguish between coercive **compliance** on the one hand and persuasive influence on the other.

Compliance
Superficial, public and transitory change in behaviour and expressed attitudes in response to requests, coercion or group pressure.

[H]Vaughan, M. G., & Hogg, M. A. (2014). Social cognition and social thinking. In *Social psychology* (7th ed., pp. 174–209). Frenchs Forest, NSW: Pearson Australia.

Some forms of social influence produce public compliance—an outward change in behaviour and expressed attitudes in response to a request from another person, or as a consequence of persuasion or coercion. As compliance does not reflect internal change, it usually persists only while behaviour is under surveillance. For example, children may obey parental directives to keep their room tidy, but only if they know that their parents are watching! An important prerequisite for coercive compulsion and compliance is that the source of social influence is perceived by the target of influence to have power; power is the basis of compliance (Moscovici, 1976).

However, because evidence for internal mental states is gleaned from observed behaviour, it can be difficult to know whether compliant behaviour does or does not reflect internalisation (Allen, 1965)—although some recent neuroscience studies have begun to chart brain activity differences associated with compliant behaviour versus more deep-seated cognitive changes (cf. Berns et al., 2005). People's strategic control over their behaviour for self-presentation and communication purposes can amplify this difficulty. Research into compliance with direct requests has generally been conducted within an attitude-change and persuasion framework.

In contrast to compliance, other forms of social influence produce private acceptance and internalisation. There is subjective acceptance and conversion (Moscovici, 1976), which produces true internal change that persists in the absence of surveillance. Conformity is not based on power but rather on the subjective validity of social norms (Festinger, 1950): that is, a feeling of confidence and certainty that the beliefs and actions described by the norm are correct, appropriate, valid and socially desirable. Under these circumstances, the norm becomes an internalised standard for behaviour, and thus surveillance is unnecessary. However, in making determinations about the validity and self-relevance of group norms, we often turn to leaders we trust as members of our group—and this can cause us to perceive them as having charisma (e.g. Platow, van Knippenberg, Haslam, van Knippenberg & Spears, 2006) and power (Turner, 2005).

Reference group
Kelley's term for a group that is psychologically significant for our behaviour and attitudes.

Membership group
Kelley's term for a group to which we belong by some objective external criterion.

Hal Kelley (1952) has made a valuable distinction between reference group and membership group. **Reference groups** are groups that are psychologically significant for people's attitudes and behaviour, either in the positive sense that we seek to behave in accordance with their norms, or in the negative sense that we seek to behave in opposition to their norms. **Membership groups** are groups to which we belong (which we are *in*) by some objective criterion, external designation or social consensus. A positive reference group is a source of conformity (which will be socially validated if that group also happens to be our membership group), while a negative reference group that is also our membership group has enormous coercive power to produce compliance. For example, if I am a student but I despise all the attributes of being a student, and if I would much rather be a lecturer because I value lecturer norms so much more, then 'student' is my membership group and is also a negative reference group, while 'lecturer' is a positive reference group but not my membership group. I will comply with student norms but conform to lecturer norms.

Dual-process dependency model
General model of social influence in which two separate processes operate—dependency on others for social approval and for information about reality.

The general distinction between coercive compliance and persuasive influence is a theme that surfaces repeatedly in different guises in social influence research. The distinction maps on to a general view in social psychology that two quite separate processes are responsible for social influence phenomena. Thus John Turner and his colleagues refer to traditional perspectives on social influence as representing a **dual-process dependency model** (e.g. Turner, 1991). This dual-process approach is currently perhaps most obvious in Richard Petty and John Cacioppo's (1986b) elaboration–likelihood model and Shelley Chaiken's (Bohner, Moskowitz & Chaiken, 1995) heuristic–systematic model of attitude change (Eagly & Chaiken, 1993).

Power and influence

We have noted that compliance tends to be associated with power relations, whereas conformity is not. Compliance is affected not only by the persuasive tactics that people use to make requests but also by how much power they are perceived to have. **Power** can be interpreted as the capacity or ability to exert influence; and influence is power in action. For example, John French and Bert Raven (1959) identified five bases of social power, and later Raven (1965, 1993) expanded this to six: reward power, coercive power, informational power, expert power, legitimate power and referent power (see Figure 9.32).

Power
Capacity to influence others while resisting their attempts to influence.

Because it is almost a truism in psychology that the power to administer reinforcements or punishments should influence behaviour, there have been virtually no attempts to demonstrate reward and coercive power (Collins & Raven, 1969). One general problem is that reinforcement formulations, particularly of complex social behaviour, tend to strike enormous difficulty in specifying in advance what are rewards and what are punishments, yet find it very easy to do so after the event. Thus reinforcement formulations tend to be unfalsifiable, and it may be more useful to focus on the cognitive and social processes that cause specific individuals in certain contexts to treat some things as reinforcement and others as punishment.

While information may have the power to influence, it is clearly not true that all information has such power. If we were earnestly to tell you that we had knowledge that pigs really do fly, it is very unlikely that you would be persuaded. For you to be persuaded, other influence processes would also have to be operating: for instance, the information might have to be perceived to be consistent with normative expectations, or coercive or reward power might have to operate.

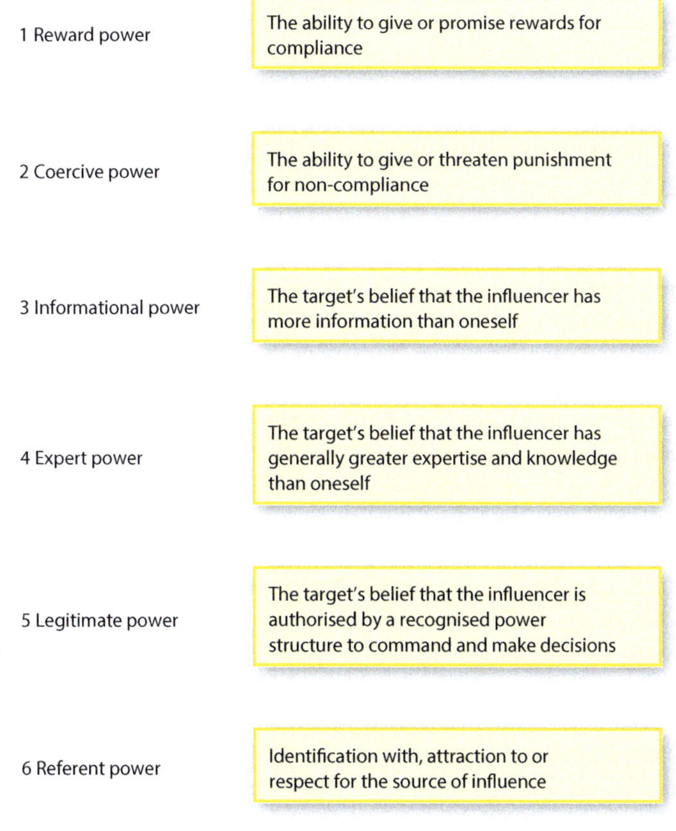

Figure 9.32 There are many different sources of power that people can access to persuade others
Source: based on Raven (1965)

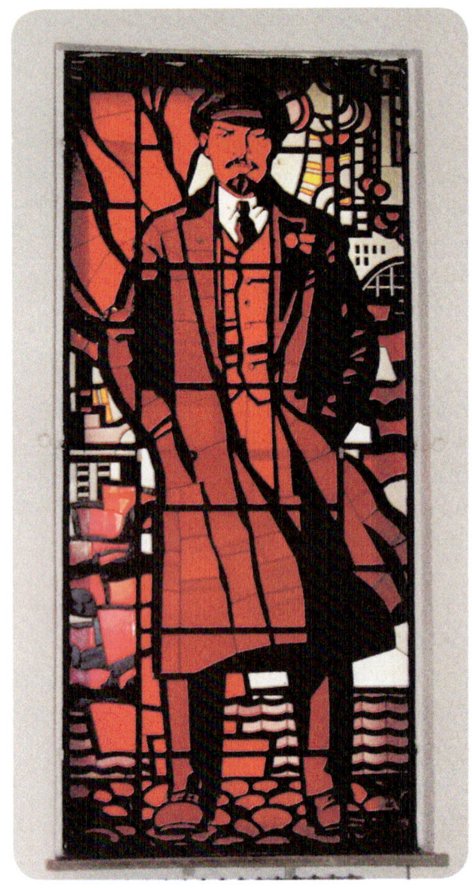

Legitimate power A Bolshevik revolutionary, Lenin became a powerful figure and was ultimately authorised by a power structure in Russia to command and make decisions (**Source:** Graham M. Vaughan.)

However, information can be influential when it originates from an expert source. Steve Bochner and Chester Insko (1966) provided a nice illustration of expert power. They found that participants more readily accepted information that people did not need much sleep when the information was attributed to a Nobel Prize-winning physiologist than to a less prestigious source. The information lost the power to influence only when it became intrinsically implausible—stating that almost no sleep was needed (see Figure 9.17).

Legitimate power is based in authority and is probably best illustrated by a consideration of obedience (see below). Referent power may operate through a range of processes (see also Collins & Raven, 1969), including consensual validation, social approval and group identification (all of which are discussed below in the section on conformity). Focusing on legitimacy and power, Adam Galinsky and his colleagues have pursued a line of research showing, among other things, that people who believe they have legitimate power are more likely to take action to pursue goals—they feel empowered (Galinsky, Gruenfeld & Magee, 2003), and that people who do not feel their power is legitimate or associated with status can be extremely destructive (Fast, Halevy & Galinsky, 2012).

In addition to power as the ability to influence, there are other perspectives on social power (Fiske & Berdahl, 2007; Keltner, Gruenfeld & Anderson, 2003; Ng, 1996). For example, Fiske (1993b; Fiske & Dépret, 1996; Goodwin, Gubin, Fiske & Yzerbyt, 2000) presents a social cognitive and attributional analysis of power imbalance within a group. Serge Moscovici (1976) actually contrasts power with influence, treating them as two different processes. Power is the control of behaviour through domination that produces compliance and submission: if people have power, in this sense, they do not need influence; and if they can influence effectively, they need not resort to power. There is also a significant literature on intergroup power relations (e.g. Hornsey, Spears, Cremers & Hogg, 2003; Jost & Major, 2001).

Power can also be considered as a role within a group that is defined by effective influence over followers: that is, as a leadership position. However, the relationship between power and leadership is not clear-cut. Some leaders certainly do influence by the exercise of power through coercion—they are the all-too-familiar autocratic or dictatorial leaders who may cajole and use ideological methods to keep their power elite in line, but most certainly exercise raw power over the masses (e.g. Moghaddam, in press). However, most leaders influence by persuasion and by instilling their vision in the rest of the group. Groups tend to permit their leaders to be idiosyncratic and innovative (Abrams, Randsley de Moura, Marques & Hutchison, 2008; Hollander, 1985), and they see their leaders as being charismatic (Avolio & Yammarino, 2003) and, in many cases, as having legitimate authority (Tyler, 1997).

Generally, leadership researchers distinguish leadership from power (e.g. Chemers, 2001; Lord, Brown & Harvey, 2001). Leadership is a process of influence that enlists and mobilises others in the attainment of collective goals; it imbues people with the group's attitudes and goals, and inspires them to work towards achieving them. Leadership is not a process that requires people to exercise power over others in order to gain compliance or, more extremely, in order to coerce or force people. Leadership may actually be more closely associated with conformity processes than power processes and power may be a social construct rather than a cause of effective leadership (Hogg, 2010; Hogg & van Knippenberg, 2003; Hogg, van Knippenberg & Rast, 2012; Reid & Ng, 1999).

John Turner (2005) has critiqued traditional perspectives on power and influence. The traditional perspective is that power rests on control of resources, and that power is the basis of influence that psychologically attaches people to groups. In contrast, Turner argues that attachment to and identification with a group is the basis of influence processes. Those who are influential are invested with power, and power allows control of resources. Turner's approach is a social identity analysis. It invokes social identity theory's conceptualisation of influence in groups (e.g. Turner, 1981b; see below) and of leadership in groups (e.g. Hogg & van Knippenberg, 2003).

Obedience to authority

In 1951 Solomon Asch published the results of a now classic experiment on conformity, in which student participants conformed to erroneous judgements of line lengths made by a numerical majority (see later in this section for details). Some critics were simply unimpressed by this study: the task, judging line length, was trivial, and there were no significant consequences for self and others of conforming or resisting.

Stanley Milgram (1974, 1992) was one of these critics; in the early 1960s he tried to replicate Asch's study, but with a task that had important consequences attached to the decision to conform or remain independent. He decided to have experimental confederates apparently administer electric shocks to another person to see whether the true participant, who was not a confederate, would conform. Before being able to start the study, Milgram needed to run a control group to obtain a base rate for people's willingness to shock someone *without* social pressure from confederates. For Milgram, this almost immediately became a crucial question in its own right. In fact, he never actually went ahead with his original conformity study, and the control group became the basis of one of social psychology's most dramatic research programs.

A wider social issue influenced Milgram. Adolf Eichmann was the Nazi official most directly responsible for the logistics of Hitler's 'Final Solution', in which six million Jews were systematically annihilated. Hannah Arendt (1963) reported his trial in her book *Eichmann in Jerusalem*, bearing the riveting subtitle *A report on the banality of evil*. This captures a disturbing finding, one that applied to Eichmann and later to other war criminals who have been brought to trial. These 'monsters' may not have been monsters at all. They were often mild-mannered, softly spoken, courteous people who repeatedly and politely explained that they did what they did not because they hated Jews (or Muslims, etc.) but because they were ordered to do it—they were simply obeying orders. Looks can, of course, be deceiving. Peter Malkin, the Israeli agent who captured Adolf Eichmann in 1960, discovered that Eichmann knew some Hebrew words, and he asked:

> *'Perhaps you're familiar with some other words,' I said.* 'Aba. Ima. *Do those ring a bell?'*
>
> 'Aba, Ima,' *he mused, trying hard to recall. 'I don't really remember. What do they mean?'*
>
> *'Daddy, Mommy. It's what Jewish children scream when they're torn from their parents' arms.' I paused, almost unable to contain myself. 'My sister's boy, my favorite playmate, he was just your son's age. Also blond and blue-eyed, just like your son. And you killed him.'*
>
> *Genuinely perplexed by the observation, he actually waited a moment to see if I would clarify it. 'Yes,' he said finally, 'but he was Jewish, wasn't he?'* (Malkin & Stein, 1990, p. 110)

Milgram brought these strands together in a series of experiments with the underlying feature that people are socialised to respect the authority of the state (Milgram, 1963, 1974; see Blass, 2004). If we enter an **agentic state**, we can absolve ourselves of responsibility for what happens next. Participants in Milgram's experiments were recruited from the community by advertisement and reported to a laboratory at Yale University to participate in a study of the effect of punishment on human learning. They arrived in pairs and drew lots to determine their roles in the study (one was the 'learner', the other the 'teacher'). See Box 9.10 for a description of what happened next, and check how the shock generator looked in Figure 9.33.

Agentic state
A frame of mind thought by Milgram to characterise unquestioning obedience, in which people as agents transfer personal responsibility to the person giving orders.

Research classic | 9.10

Milgram's procedure in an early study of obedience to authority

Together with the experimenter in the Yale laboratory, there was a teacher (the real participant) and a learner (actually, a confederate).

The learner's role was to learn a list of paired associates, and the teacher's role was to administer an electric shock to the learner every time the learner gave a wrong associate to the cue word. The teacher saw the learner being strapped to a chair and having electrode paste and electrodes attached to his arm. The teacher overheard the experimenter explain that the paste was to prevent blistering and burning, and overheard the learner telling the experimenter that he had a slight heart condition. The experimenter also explained that, although the shocks might be painful, they would cause no permanent tissue damage.

The teacher was now taken into a separate room housing a shock generator (see Figure 9.33). He was told to administer progressively larger shocks to the learner every time the learner made a mistake—15 volts (V) for the first mistake, 30 V for the next mistake, 45 V for the next, and so on. An important feature of the shock generator was the descriptive labels attached to the scale of increasing voltage. The teacher was given a sample shock of 45 V, and then the experiment commenced.

The learner got some pairs correct but also made some errors, and very soon the teacher had reached 75 V, at which point the learner grunted in pain. At 120 V the learner shouted out to the experimenter that the shocks were becoming painful. At 150 V the learner, or now more accurately the 'victim', demanded to be released from the experiment, and at 180 V he cried out that he could stand it no longer. The victim continued to cry out in pain at each shock, rising to an 'agonised scream' at 250 V. At 300 V the victim ceased responding to the cue words; the teacher was told to treat this as a 'wrong answer'.

Throughout the experiment, the teacher was agitated and tense, and often asked to break off. To such requests, the experimenter responded with an ordered sequence of replies proceeding from a mild 'please continue', through 'the experiment requires that you continue' and 'it is absolutely essential that you continue', to the ultimate 'you have no other choice, you must go on'.

A panel of 110 experts on human behaviour, including 39 psychiatrists, were asked to predict how far a normal, psychologically balanced human being would go in this experiment. These experts believed that only about 10 percent would exceed 180 V, and no one would obey to the end. These predictions, together with the actual and the remarkably different behaviour of the participants, are shown schematically in Figure 9.34. Compare these with the actual behaviour of the participants (Figure 9.34).

In a slight variant of the procedure described above, in which the victim could not be seen or heard but pounded on the wall at 300 V and 315 V and then went silent, almost everyone continued to 255 V, and 65 percent continued to the very end—administering massive electric shocks to someone who was not responding and who had previously reported having a heart complaint!

The participants in this experiment were quite normal people—forty 20–50-year-old men from a range of occupations. Unknown to them, however, the entire experiment involved an elaborate deception in which they were always the teacher, and the learner/victim was actually an experimental stooge (an avuncular-looking middle-aged man) who had been carefully briefed on how to react. No electric shocks were actually administered apart from the 45 V sample shock to the teacher.

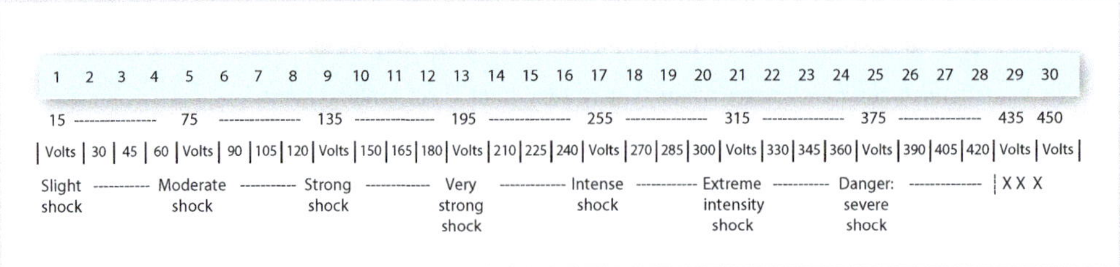

1 2 3 4 5 6 7 8 9 10 11 12 13 14 15 16 17 18 19 20 21 22 23 24 25 26 27 28 29 30
15 --------------- 75 --------------- 135 --------------- 195 --------------- 255 --------------- 315 --------------- 375 --------------- 435 450
| Volts | 30 | 45 | 60 | Volts | 90 | 105 | 120 | Volts | 150 | 165 | 180 | Volts | 210 | 225 | 240 | Volts | 270 | 285 | 300 | Volts | 330 | 345 | 360 | Volts | 390 | 405 | 420 | Volts | Volts |
Slight shock ---------- Moderate shock ---------- Strong shock ---------- Very strong shock ---------- Intense shock ---------- Extreme intensity shock ---------- Danger: severe shock ---------- | X X X

Figure 9.33 Milgram's shock generator

Participants in Milgram's obedience studies were confronted with a 15–450 volt shock generator that had different descriptive labels, including the frighteningly evocative 'XXX', attached to the more impersonal voltage values
(**Source:** Milgram (1963, 1974))

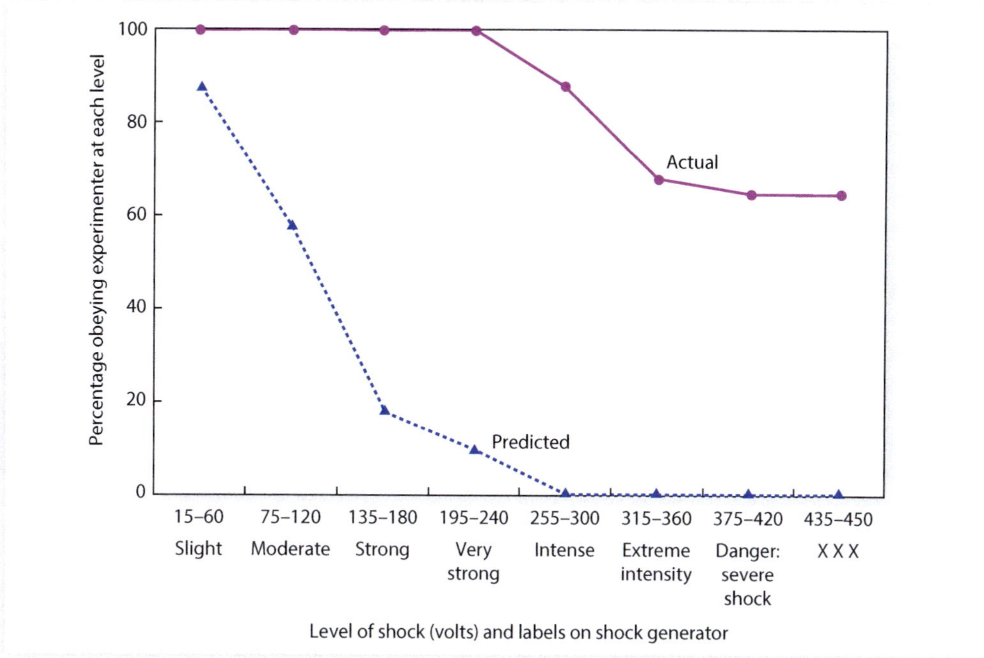

Figure 9.34 Predicted versus actual levels of shock given to a victim in Milgram's obedience-to-authority experiment

'Experts' on human behaviour predicted that very few normal, psychologically balanced people would obey orders to administer more than a 'strong' electric shock to the 'incompetent' learner in Milgram's experiment—in actual fact, 65 percent of people were obedient right to the very end, going beyond 'danger: severe shock', into a zone labelled 'XXX'

(**Source:** based on data from Milgram (1974))

Note: See extracts from Milgram's work at www.panarchy.org/milgram/obedience.html.

Factors influencing obedience

Milgram (1974) conducted 18 experiments, in which he varied different parameters to investigate factors influencing obedience. In all but one experiment the participants were 20–50-year-old males, not attending university, from a range of occupations and socioeconomic levels. In one study in which women were the participants, exactly the same level of obedience was obtained as with male participants. In an attempt to see if 21st-century Americans would be obedient like their 1970s counterparts, Jerry Burger (2009) conducted a partial replication of the original Milgram studies (a full replication was not possible due to research ethics concerns—see below). Burger discovered only slightly lower levels of obedience than in the original 1970s studies.

Milgram's experiment has been replicated in Italy, Germany, Australia, Britain, Jordan, Spain, Austria and the Netherlands (Smith, Bond & Kağitçibaşi, 2006). Complete obedience ranged from over 90 percent in Spain and the Netherlands (Meeus & Raaijmakers, 1986), through over 80 percent in Italy, Germany and Austria (Mantell, 1971), to a low of 40 percent among Australian men and only 16 percent among Australian women (Kilham & Mann, 1974). Some studies have also used modified settings: for example, Wim Meeus and Quinten Raaijmakers (1986) used an administrative obedience setting in which an 'interviewer' was required to harass a 'job applicant'.

One reason that people continue to administer electric shocks may be that the experiment starts very innocuously with quite trivial shocks, and once they have committed themselves to a course of action (i.e. to give shocks), it can be difficult subsequently to change their

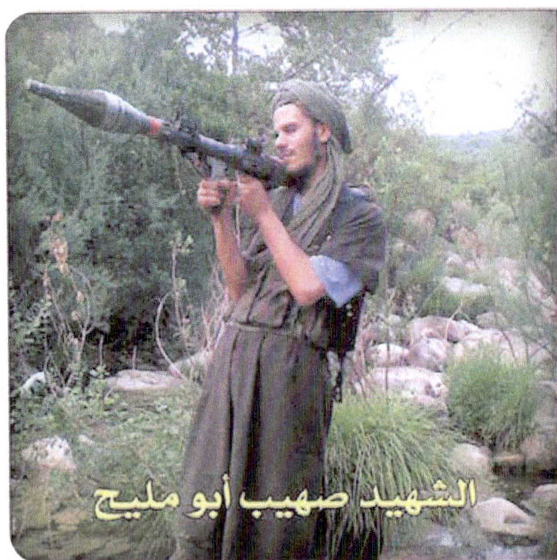

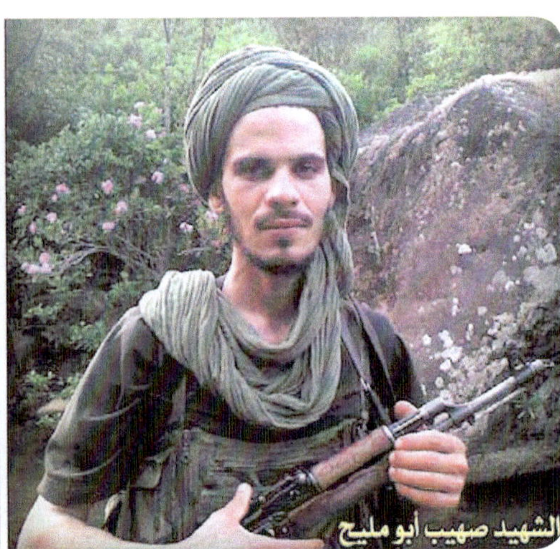

Obedience to authority This young man symbolises complete unquestioning obedience and reportedly made the ultimate sacrifice (**Source:** AFP PHOTO/ SITE.)

mind. The process, which reflects the psychology of sunk costs in which once committed to a course of action people will continue their commitment even if the costs increase dramatically (Fox & Hoffman, 2002), may be similar to that involved in the foot-in-the-door technique of persuasion (Freedman & Fraser, 1966).

An important factor in obedience is *immediacy of the victim*—how close or obvious the victim is to the participant. Milgram (1974) varied the level of immediacy across a number of experiments. We have seen above that 65 percent of people 'shocked to the limit' of 450 V when the victim was unseen and unheard except for pounding on the wall. In an even less immediate condition in which the victim was neither seen nor heard at all, 100 percent of people went to the end. The baseline condition (the one described in detail above) yielded 62.5 percent obedience. As immediacy increased from this baseline, obedience decreased: when the victim was visible in the same room, 40 percent obeyed to the limit; and when the teacher actually had to hold the victim's hand down on to the electrode to receive the shock, obedience dropped to a still frighteningly high 30 percent.

Immediacy may prevent dehumanisation of the victim (cf. Haslam, 2006; Haslam, Loughnan & Kashima, 2008), making it easier to view a victim as a living and breathing person like oneself and thus to empathise with their thoughts and feelings. Hence, pregnant women express greater commitment to their pregnancy after having seen an ultrasound scan that clearly reveals body parts (Lydon & Dunkel-Schetter, 1994); and it is easier to press a button to wipe out an entire village from 12 000 metres or from deep under the ocean in a submarine than it is to shoot an individual enemy from close range.

Another important factor is *immediacy of the authority figure*. Obedience was reduced to 20.5 percent when the experimenter was absent from the room and relayed directions by telephone. When the experimenter gave no orders at all, and the participant was entirely free to choose when to stop, 2.5 percent still persisted to the end. Perhaps the most dramatic influence on obedience is group pressure. The presence of two disobedient peers (i.e. others who appeared to revolt and refused to continue after giving shocks in the 150–210 V range) reduced complete obedience to 10 percent, while two obedient peers raised complete obedience to 92.5 percent.

Group pressure probably has its effects because the actions of others help to confirm that it is either legitimate or illegitimate to continue administering the shocks. Another important factor is the legitimacy of the authority figure, which allows people to abdicate personal responsibility for their actions. For example, Brad Bushman (1984, 1988) had confederates, dressed in uniform, neat attire or a shabby outfit stand next to someone fumbling for change for a parking meter. The confederate stopped passers-by and 'ordered' them to give the person change for the meter. Over 70 percent obeyed the uniformed confederate (giving 'because they had been told to' as the reason) and about 50 percent obeyed a confederate who was either neatly attired or shabbily dressed (generally giving altruism as a reason). These studies suggest that mere emblems of authority can create unquestioning obedience.

Milgram's original experiments were conducted by lab-coated scientists at prestigious Yale University, and the purpose of the research was quite clearly the pursuit of scientific knowledge. What would happen if these trappings of legitimate authority were removed? Milgram ran one experiment in a rundown inner-city office building. The research was ostensibly sponsored by a private commercial research firm. Obedience dropped, but to a still remarkably high 48 percent.

Milgram's research addresses one of humanity's great failings—the tendency for people to obey orders without first thinking about (1) what they are being asked to do, and (2) the consequences of their obedience for other living beings. However, obedience can sometimes be beneficial: for example, many organisations would grind to a halt or would be catastrophically dysfunctional if their members continually painstakingly negotiated orders (think about an emergency surgery team, a flight crew, a commando unit). (Now consider the first focus question.) However, the pitfalls of blind obedience, contingent on immediacy, group pressure, group norms and legitimacy, are also many. For example, American research has shown that medication errors in hospitals can be attributed to the fact that nurses overwhelmingly defer to doctors' orders, even when metaphorical alarm bells are ringing (Lesar, Briceland & Stein, 1977).

In another study focusing on organisational obedience, 77 percent of participants who were playing the role of board members of a pharmaceutical company advocated continued marketing of a hazardous drug merely because they felt that the chair of the board favoured this decision (Brief, Dukerich & Doran, 1991).

Before closing this section to deal next with ethical concerns about Milgram's experiments, we should note that reservations have been raised about their logic. The connection between destructive obedience as Milgram conceived it on one hand, and the holocaust itself on the other, has been questioned. In Bob Cialdini and Noah Goldstein's (2004) review of social influence research, they pointed out that:

- Milgram's participants were troubled by the orders they were given, whereas many of the perpetrators of Holocaust atrocities obeyed orders willingly and sometimes sadistically.
- Although the Nazi chain of command and the experimenter in Milgram's studies had apparent legitimate authority, the experimenter had expert authority as well.

The ethical legacy of Milgram's experiments

One enduring legacy of Milgram's experiments is the heated debate that it stirred up over research ethics (Baumrind, 1964; Rosnow, 1981). Recall that Milgram's participants really believed they were administering severe electric shocks that were causing extreme pain to another human being. Milgram was careful to interview and, with the assistance of a psychiatrist, to follow up the more than 1000 participants in his experiments. There was no evidence of psychopathology, and 83.7 percent of those who had taken part indicated that they were glad, or very glad, to have been in the experiment (Milgram, 1992, p. 186). Only 1.3 percent were sorry or very sorry to have participated.

The ethical issues really revolve around three questions concerning the ethics of subjecting experimental participants to short-term stress:

1 Is the research important? If not, then such stress is unjustifiable. However, it can be difficult to assess the 'importance' of research objectively.
2 Is the participant free to terminate the experiment at any time? How free were Milgram's participants? In one sense they were free to do whatever they wanted, but it was never made explicit to them that they could terminate whenever they wished—in fact, the very purpose of the study was to persuade them to remain!
3 Did the participant freely consent to being in the experiment in the first place? In Milgram's experiments the participants did not give fully informed consent: they

volunteered to take part, but the true nature of the experiment was not fully explained to them.

This raises the issue of deception in social psychology research. Herbert Kelman (1967) distinguishes two reasons for deceiving people: the first is to induce them to take part in an otherwise unpleasant experiment. This is, ethically, a highly dubious practice. The second reason is that in order to study the automatic operation of psychological processes, participants need to be naive regarding the hypotheses, and this often involves some deception concerning the true purpose of the study and the procedures used.

The fallout from this debate has been a code of ethics to guide psychologists in conducting research. The principal components of the code are:

- participation must be based on fully informed consent
- participants must be explicitly informed that they can withdraw, without penalty, at any stage of the study
- participants must be fully and honestly debriefed at the end of the study.

Modern university ethics committees would be unlikely to approve the impressively brazen deceptions that produced many of social psychology's classic research programs of the 1950s, 1960s and early 1970s. What is more likely to be endorsed is the use of minor and harmless procedural deceptions enshrined in clever cover stories that are considered essential to preserve the scientific rigour of much experimental social psychology. See the American Psychological Association's Code of Ethics (2002) at www.apa.org/ethics/code2002.html.

Conformity

The formation and influence of norms

Conformity Deep-seated, private and enduring change in behaviour and attitudes due to group pressure.

Although much social influence is reflected in compliance with direct requests and obedience to authority, social influence can also operate in a less direct manner through **conformity** to social or group norms. For example, Floyd Allport (1924) observed that people in groups gave less extreme and more conservative judgements of odours and weights than when they were alone. It seemed as if, in the absence of direct pressure, the group could cause members to converge and thus become more similar to one another.

Muzafer Sherif (1936) explicitly linked this convergence effect to the development of *group norms*. Proceeding from the premise that people need to be certain and confident that what they are doing, thinking or feeling is correct and appropriate, Sherif argued that people use the behaviour of others to establish the range of possible behaviour: we can call this the **frame of reference**, or relevant *social comparative context*. Average, central or middle positions in such frames of reference are typically perceived to be more correct than fringe positions, thus people tend to adopt them. Sherif believed that this explained the origins of social norms and the concomitant convergence that accentuates consensus within groups.

Frame of reference Complete range of subjectively conceivable positions that relevant people can occupy in a particular context on some attitudinal or behavioural dimension.

Autokinesis Optical illusion in which a pinpoint of light shining in complete darkness appears to move about.

To test this idea, he conducted his classic studies using **autokinesis** (see Box 9.16 and Figure 9.35 for details), in which small groups making estimates of physical movement quickly converged over a series of trials on the mean of the group's estimates and remained influenced by this norm even when they later made estimates alone.

It is worth emphasising that normative pressure is one of the most effective ways to change people's behaviour. For example, we noted that Kurt Lewin (1947) tried to encourage American housewives to change the eating habits of their families—specifically to eat more offal (beef hearts and kidneys). Three groups of 13 to 17 housewives attended an interesting factual lecture that, among other things, stressed how valuable such a change in eating habits would be to the war effort (it was 1943). Another three groups were given information but were also encouraged to talk among themselves and arrive at some kind of consensus (i.e. establish a norm) about buying the food.

A follow-up survey revealed that the norm was far more effective than the abstract information in causing some change in behaviour: only 3 percent of the information group had changed their behaviour, compared with 32 percent of the norm group. Subsequent research confirmed that it was the norm not the attendant discussion that was the crucial factor (Bennett, 1955).

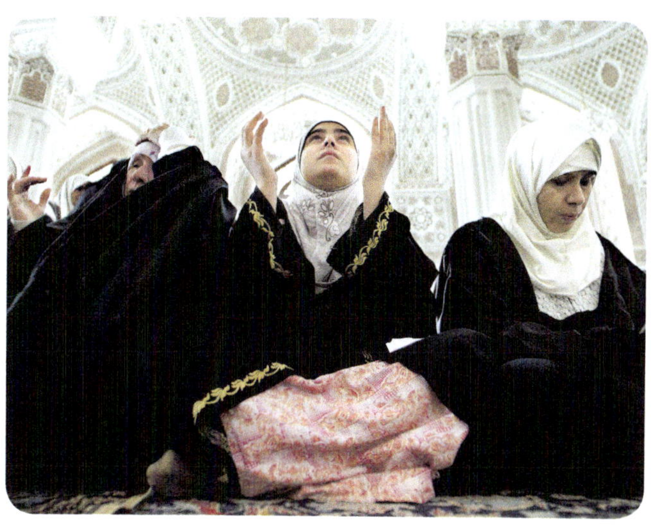

Conformity and group acceptance
All groups have norms
(**Source:** AFP PHOTO/ Henghameh FAHIMI.)

Yielding to majority group pressure

Like Sherif, Solomon Asch (1952) believed that conformity reflects a relatively rational process in which people construct a norm from other people's behaviour in order to determine correct and appropriate behaviour for themselves. Clearly, if you are already confident and certain about what is appropriate and correct, then others' behaviour will be largely irrelevant and thus not influential. In Sherif's study, the object of judgement was ambiguous: participants were uncertain, so a norm arose rapidly and was highly effective in guiding behaviour. Asch argued that if the object of judgement was entirely unambiguous (i.e. one would expect no disagreement between judges), then disagreement, or alternative perceptions, would have no effect on behaviour: people would remain entirely independent of group influence.

To test this idea, Asch (1951, 1956) created a classic experimental paradigm. Students, participating in what they thought was a visual discrimination task, seated themselves around a table in groups of seven to nine. They took turns in a fixed order to call out publicly which of three comparison lines was the same length as a standard line (see Figure 9.35). There were 18 trials. In reality, only one person was a true naive participant, and he answered second to last. The others were experimental confederates instructed to give erroneous responses on 12 focal trials: on 6 trials they picked a line that was too long and on 6 a line that was too short. There was a control condition in which participants performed the task privately with no group influence; as less than 1 percent of the control participants' responses were errors, it can be assumed that the task was unambiguous.

The experimental results were intriguing. There were large individual differences, with about 25 percent of participants remaining steadfastly independent throughout, about 50 percent conforming to the erroneous majority on 6 or more focal trials, and 5 percent conforming on all 12 focal trials. The average conformity rate was 33 percent: computed as the total number of instances of conformity across the experiment, divided by the product of the number of participants in the experiment and the number of focal trials in the sequence.

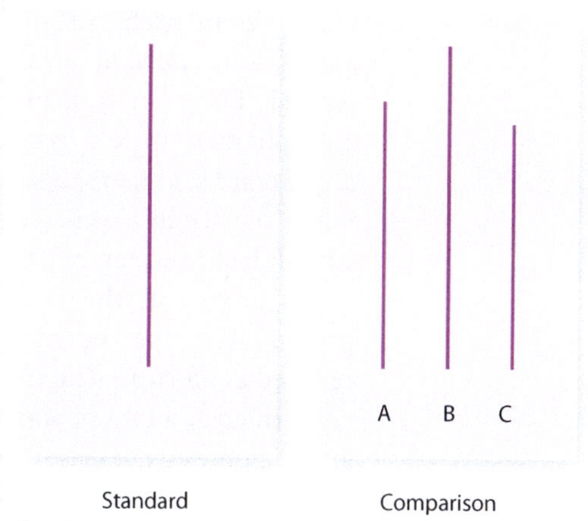

Figure 9.35 Sample lines used in conformity experiment

Participants in Asch's conformity studies had simply to say which one of the three comparison lines was the same length as the standard line
(**Source:** based on Asch (1951))

After the experiment, Asch asked his participants why they conformed. They all said they had initially experienced uncertainty and self-doubt because of the disagreement between themselves and the group, and that this gradually evolved into self-consciousness, fear of disapproval, and feelings of anxiety and even loneliness. Different reasons were given for yielding. Most participants knew they saw things differently from the group but felt that their perceptions may have been inaccurate and that the group was actually correct. Others did not believe that the group was correct but simply went along with the group in order not to stand out. (Consider how this might apply to Tom's self-doubts in the second focus question.) A small minority reported that they actually saw the lines as the group did. Independents were either entirely confident in the accuracy of their own judgements or were emotionally affected but guided by a belief in individualism or in doing the task as directed (i.e. being accurate and correct).

These subjective accounts should be treated cautiously—perhaps the participants were merely trying to verbally justify their behaviour and engage in self-presentation. For instance, an fMRI study by Berns and his colleagues found that those who conformed may actually have experienced changed perception, and that those who did not conform showed brain activity in the amygdale associated with elevated emotions—a cost of nonconformity may be accentuated by emotions and anxiety (Berns et al., 2005).

Nevertheless, the subjective accounts suggest, perhaps in line with the fMRI evidence, that one reason why people conform, even when the stimulus is completely unambiguous, may be to avoid censure, ridicule and social disapproval. This is a real fear. In another version of his experiment, Asch (1951) had 16 naive participants confronting one confederate who gave incorrect answers. The participants found the confederate's behaviour ludicrous and openly ridiculed and laughed at him. Even the experimenter found the situation so bizarre that he could not contain his mirth and also ended up laughing at the poor confederate!

Perhaps, then, if participants were not worried about social disapproval, there would be no subjective pressure to conform. To test this idea, Asch conducted another variation of the experiment, in which the incorrect majority called out their judgements publicly but the single naive participant wrote his down privately. Conformity dropped to 12.5 percent.

Morton Deutsch and Harold Gerard (1955) extended this modification. They wondered whether they could entirely eradicate pressure to conform if: (a) the task was unambiguous; (b) the participant was anonymous and responded privately; and (c) the participant was not under any sort of surveillance by the group. Why should you conform to an erroneous majority when there is an obvious, unambiguous and objectively correct answer, and the group has no way of knowing what you are doing?

To test this idea, Deutsch and Gerard confronted a naive participant face to face with three confederates, who made unanimously incorrect judgements of lines on focal trials, exactly as in Asch's original experiment. In another condition, the naive participant was anonymous, isolated in a cubicle and allowed to respond privately—no group pressure existed. There was a third condition in which participants responded face to face, but with an explicit group goal to be as accurate as possible—group pressure was maximised. Deutsch and Gerard also manipulated subjective uncertainty by having half the participants respond while the stimuli were present (the procedure used by Asch) and half respond after the stimuli had been removed (there would be scope for feeling uncertain).

As predicted, the results showed that decreasing uncertainty and decreasing group pressure (i.e. the motivation and ability of the group to censure lack of conformity) reduced conformity (Figure 9.36). Perhaps the most interesting finding was that people still conformed at a rate of about 23 percent even when uncertainty was low (stimulus present) and responses were private and anonymous.

The discovery that participants still conformed when isolated in cubicles greatly facilitated the systematic investigation of factors influencing conformity. Richard Crutchfield (1955) devised an apparatus in which participants in cubicles believed they were communicating with one another by pressing buttons on a console that illuminated responses, when in reality the cubicles were not interconnected and the experimenter was the source of all communication. In this way, many participants could be run simultaneously and yet all

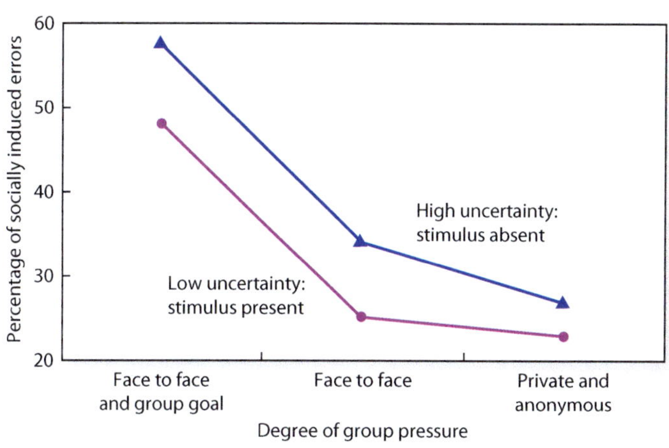

Figure 9.36 Conformity as a function of uncertainty and perceived group pressure

- The length of lines was estimated either (a) when they were present (low uncertainty) or (b) after they had been removed (high uncertainty)
- Participants were confronted with the judgements of an incorrect and unanimous majority
- Influence (percentage of errors) was stronger in the high uncertainty condition
- Influence was weaker when accuracy was stressed as an important group goal
- Influence was further weakened when judgements were private and anonymous

(**Source:** based on data from Deutsch & Gerard (1955))

would believe they were being exposed to a unanimous group. The time-consuming, costly and risky practice of using confederates was no longer necessary, and data could now be collected much more quickly under more controlled and varied experimental conditions (Allen, 1965, 1975). Nowadays, one can, of course, use a much more efficient computerised variant of Crutchfield's methodology.

Who conforms? Individual and group characteristics

The existence of significant individual differences in conformity led to a search for personality attributes that predispose some people to conform more than others. Those who conform tend to have low self-esteem, a high need for social support or approval, a need for self-control, low IQ, high anxiety, feelings of self-blame and insecurity in the group, feelings of inferiority, feelings of relatively low status in the group, and a generally authoritarian personality (Costanzo, 1970; Crutchfield, 1955; Elms & Milgram, 1966; Raven & French, 1958; Stang, 1972). However, contradictory findings, and evidence that people who conform in one situation do not conform in another, suggest that situational factors may be more important than personality in conformity (Barocas & Gorlow, 1967; Barron, 1953; McGuire, 1968; Vaughan, 1964).

Alice Eagly drew a similar conclusion about gender differences in conformity. Women have been shown to conform slightly more than men in some conformity studies. This can be explained in terms of the tasks used in some of these studies—tasks with which women had less familiarity and expertise. Women were therefore more uncertain and thus more influenced than men (Eagly, 1978, 1983; Eagly & Carli, 1981).

A good example of this was a study by Frank Sistrunk and John McDavid (1971), in which males and females were exposed to group pressure in identifying various stimuli. For some, the stimuli were traditionally masculine items (e.g. identifying a special type of wrench), for some, traditionally feminine items (e.g. identifying types of needlework), and for others the stimuli were neutral (e.g. identifying rock stars). As expected, women conformed more on masculine items, men more on feminine items, and both groups equally on neutral (non gender-stereotypical) items—see Figure 9.37.

Women do, however, tend to conform a little more than men in public interactive settings like that involved in the Asch paradigm. One explanation is that it reflects women's greater concern with maintaining group harmony (Eagly, 1978). However, a later study put the emphasis on men's behaviour; women conformed equally in public and private contexts whereas it was men who were particularly resistant to influence in public settings (Eagly, Wood, & Fishbaugh, 1981).

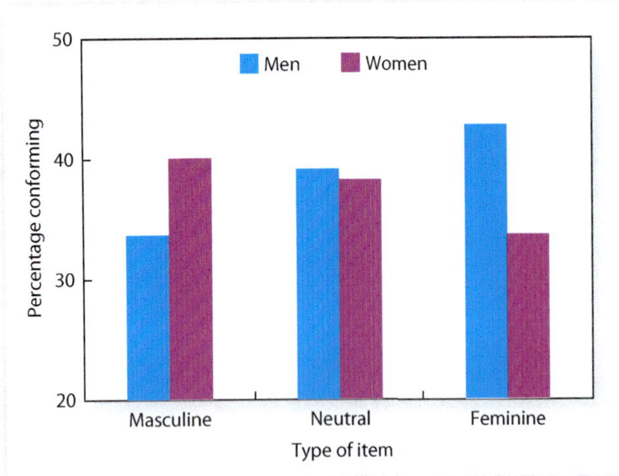

Figure 9.37 Conformity as a function of gender of participant and gender-stereotypicality of task

When a task is male-stereotypical, more women conform. When the task is female-stereotypical, more men conform
(**Source:** based on data from Sistrunk & McDavid (1971))

Cultural norms

Do cultural norms affect conformity? Peter Smith and his colleagues surveyed conformity studies that used Asch's paradigm or a variant thereof (Smith, Bond & Kağitçibaşi (2006). They found significant intercultural variation. The level of conformity (i.e. percentage of incorrect responses) ranged from a low of 14 percent among Belgian students (Doms, 1983) to a high of 58 percent among Indian teachers in Fiji (Chandra, 1973), with an overall average of 31.2 percent. Conformity was lower among participants from individualist cultures in North America and north-western Europe (25.3 percent) than among participants from collectivist or interdependent cultures in Africa, Asia, Oceania and South America (37.1 percent).

A meta-analysis of studies using the Asch paradigm in 17 countries (R. Bond & Smith, 1996) confirmed that people who score high on Geert Hofstede's (1980) collectivism scale conform more than people who score low. For example, Norwegians, who have a reputation for social unity and responsibility, were more conformist than the French, who value critical judgement, diverse opinions and dissent (Milgram, 1961); and the Bantu of Zimbabwe, who have strong sanctions against nonconformity, were highly conformist (Whittaker & Meade, 1967).

The higher level of conformity in collectivist or interdependent cultures arises because conformity is viewed favourably, as a form of social glue (Markus & Kitayama, 1991). What is perhaps more surprising is that, although conformity is lower in individualist Western societies, it is still remarkably high; even when conformity has negative overtones, people find it difficult to resist conforming to a group norm.

Situational factors in conformity

The two situational factors in conformity that have been most exhaustively researched are group size and group unanimity (Allen, 1965, 1975).

Group size

Solomon Asch (1952) found that as the unanimous group increased from 1 person to 2 to 3, and on up to 15, the conformity rate increased and then decreased slightly: 3, 13, 33, 35 and down to 31 percent. Although some research reports a linear relationship between size and conformity (e.g. Mann, 1977), the most robust finding is that conformity reaches its full strength with a 3–5 person majority, and additional members have little effect (e.g. Stang, 1976).

Group size may have a different effect depending on the type of judgement being made and the motivation of the individual (Campbell & Fairey, 1989). With matters of taste, where there is no objectively correct answer (e.g. musical preferences), and where you are concerned about 'fitting in', group size will have a relatively linear effect: the larger the majority, the more you will be swayed. When there is a correct response and you are concerned about being correct, then the views of one or two others will usually be sufficient: the views of additional others will be largely redundant.

Finally, David Wilder (1977) observed that size may not refer to the actual number of physically separate people in the group but to the number of seemingly *independent* sources of influence in the group. For instance, a majority of three individuals who are perceived to be independent will be more influential than a majority of, say, five who are perceived to be in collusion and thus represent a single information source. In fact, people may actually find it difficult to represent more than four or five different pieces of information. Instead, they usually assimilate additional group members into one or other of these initial sources of information—hence the relative lack of effect of group size above three to five members.

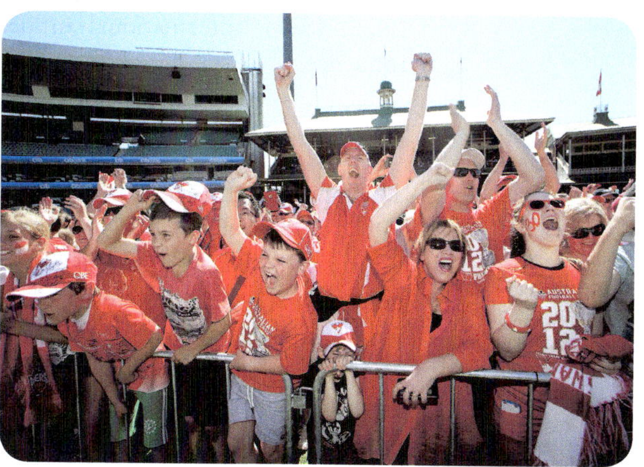

Group size and conformity This might be an occasion to go along with the happy throng!
(**Source:** AAP Image/Warren Clarke.)

Group unanimity

In Asch's original experiment, the erroneous majority was unanimous and the conformity rate was 33 percent. Subsequent experiments have shown that conformity is significantly reduced if the majority is not unanimous (Allen, 1975). Asch himself found that a correct supporter (i.e. a member of the majority who always gave the correct answer, and thus agreed with and supported the true participant) reduced conformity from 33 to 5.5 percent.

It seems that support for remaining independent is not the crucial factor in reducing conformity. Rather, any sort of lack of unanimity among the majority seems to be effective. For example, Asch found that a dissenter who was even more wildly incorrect than the majority was equally effective. Vernon Allen and John Levine (1971) conducted an experiment in which participants who were asked to make visual judgements were provided either with a supporter who had normal vision or a supporter who wore such thick glasses as to raise serious doubts about his ability to see anything at all, let alone judge lines accurately. In the absence of any support, participants conformed 97 percent of the time. The 'competent' supporter reduced conformity to 36 percent, but most surprising was the fact that the 'incompetent' supporter reduced conformity as well, to 64 percent (see Figure 9.38).

Supporters, dissenters and deviates may be effective in reducing conformity because they shatter the unanimity of the majority and thus raise or legitimise the possibility of alternative ways of responding or behaving. For example, Charlan Nemeth and Cynthia Chiles (1988) confronted participants with four confederates who either all correctly identified blue slides as 'blue', or among whom one consistently called the blue slide 'green'. Participants were then exposed to another group that unanimously called red slides 'orange'. The participants who had previously been exposed to the consistent dissenter were more likely to correctly call the red slides 'red'.

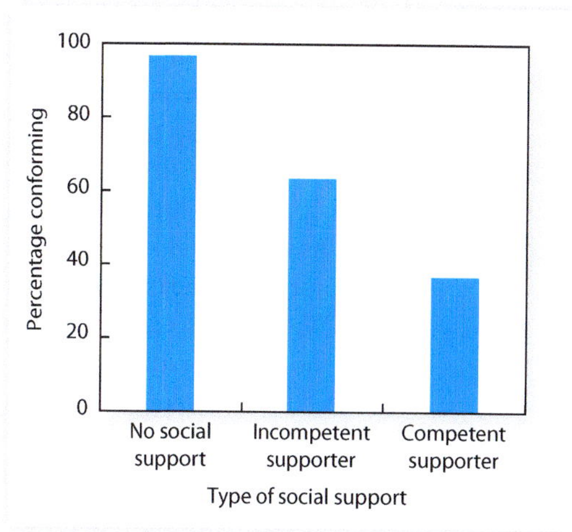

Figure 9.38 Conformity as a function of presence or absence of support, and of competence of supporter

Social support on a line judgement task reduced conformity, even when the supporter was patently unable to make accurate judgements because he was visually impaired
(**Source:** based on data from Allen & Levine (1971))

Processes of conformity

Social psychologists have proposed three main processes of social influence to account specifically for conformity

(Nail, 1986): informational influence, normative influence, and referent informational influence.

Informational and normative influence

Informational influence
An influence to accept information from another as evidence about reality.

The most enduring distinction is between informational influence and normative influence (Deutsch & Gerard, 1955; Kelley, 1952). **Informational influence** is an influence to accept information from another as *evidence* about reality. We need to feel confident that our perceptions, beliefs and feelings are correct. Informational influence comes into play when we are uncertain, either because stimuli are intrinsically ambiguous or because there is social disagreement. When this happens, we initially make objective tests against reality; otherwise, we make social comparisons, as Festinger and others have pointed out (Festinger, 1950, 1954; Suls & Wheeler, 2000). Effective informational influence causes true cognitive change.

Informational influence was probably partially responsible for the convergence effects in Sherif's (1936) study that we have already discussed. Reality was ambiguous, and participants used other people's estimates as information to remove the ambiguity and resolve subjective uncertainty. In that kind of experimental setting, when participants were told that the apparent movement was in fact an illusion, they did not conform (e.g. Alexander, Zucker & Brody, 1970); presumably, since reality itself was uncertain, their own subjective uncertainty was interpreted as a correct and valid representation of reality, and thus informational influence did not operate. On the other hand, Asch's (1952) stimuli were designed to be unambiguous in order to exclude informational influence. However, Asch did note that conformity increased as the comparison lines were made more similar to one another and the judgement task thus became more difficult. The moral? Informational influence rules in moments of certainty, not times of doubt.

Normative influence
An influence to conform with the positive expectation of others, to gain social approval or to avoid social disapproval.

Normative influence is an influence to conform to the positive expectations of others. People have a need for social approval and acceptance, which causes them to 'go along with' the group for instrumental reasons—to cultivate approval and acceptance, avoid censure or disapproval, or to achieve specific goals. Normative influence comes into play when we believe the group has the power and ability to reward or punish us according to what we do. For this to be effective we need to believe we are under surveillance by the group. Effective normative influence creates surface compliance in public settings rather than true, enduring cognitive change. There is considerable evidence that people often conform to a majority in public but do not necessarily internalise this as it does not carry over to private settings or endure over time (Nail, 1986).

There is little doubt that normative influence was the principal cause of conformity in the Asch paradigm—the lines being judged were unambiguous (informational influence would not be operating), but participants' behaviour was under direct surveillance by the group. We have also seen that privacy, anonymity and lack of surveillance reduced conformity in the Asch paradigm, presumably because normative influence was weakened.

In reflecting on Deutsch and Gerard's (1955) study we can note that, even under conditions in which neither informational nor normative influence would be expected to operate, they found residual conformity at a remarkably high rate of about 23 percent. Perhaps social influence in groups needs to be explained in a different way.

Referent informational influence

The distinction between informational and normative influence is only one among many different terminologies that have been used in social psychology to distinguish between two types of social influence. It represents what John Turner and his colleagues call a dual-process dependency model of social influence (Abrams & Hogg, 1990a; Hogg & Turner, 1987a; Turner, 1991). People are influenced by others because they are dependent on them either for information that removes ambiguity and thus establishes subjective validity, or for reasons of social approval and acceptance.

This dual-process perspective has been challenged on the grounds that as an explanation of conformity it underemphasises the role of group belongingness. After all, an important feature of conformity is that we are influenced because we feel we belong, psychologically, to the group, and therefore the norms of the group are relevant standards for our own behaviour. The dual-process model has drifted away from group norms and group belongingness and focused on *interpersonal* dependency, which could just as well occur between individuals as among group members.

This challenge has come from **social identity theory** (Tajfel & Turner, 1979; also Abrams & Hogg, 2010; Hogg, 2006), which proposes a separate social influence process responsible for conformity to group norms, called **referent informational influence** (Hogg & Turner, 1987a; Turner, 1981b; also Hogg, in press).

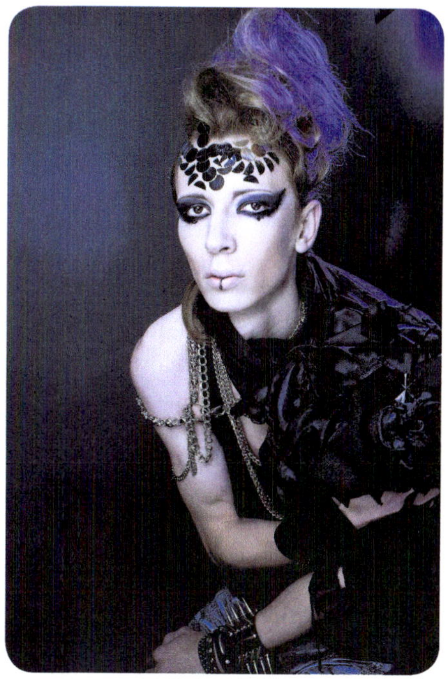

Marching to a different drum An independent spirit? No. This young Goth is conforming to a subgroup norm
(**Source:** Photocreative/Shutterstock.)

When our membership in a group becomes psychologically salient, several things happen. We feel a sense of belonging; we define ourselves in terms of the group. We also recruit from memory and use information available in the social context to determine the relevant attributes that are based on our group's norms. We can glean information from the way that outgroup members, or even unrelated individuals, behave. But the most immediate source is the behaviour of fellow ingroup members, particularly those we consider to be generally reliable sources of the information we need. The ingroup norm that fits the context captures and accentuates both similarities among ingroup members and differences between our group and the relevant outgroup—it obeys the **metacontrast principle**.

Social identity theory
Theory of group membership and intergroup relations based on self-categorisation, social comparison and the construction of a shared self-definition in terms of ingroup-defining properties.

Referent informational influence
Pressure to conform with a group norm that defines oneself as a group member.

Metacontrast principle
The prototype of a group is that position within the group that has the largest ratio of 'differences to ingroup positions' to 'differences to outgroup positions'.

The process of *self-categorisation* associated with social identity processes, group belongingness and group behaviour (Turner et al., 1987) brings us to see ourselves through the lens of our group. We assimilate our thoughts, feelings and behaviour to the group norm and act accordingly. To the extent that members of the group construct a similar group norm, self-categorisation produces intragroup convergence on that norm and increases uniformity within the group—the typical conformity effect.

Referent informational influence differs from normative and informational influence in a number of important ways. People conform because they are group members, not to validate physical reality or to avoid social disapproval. People do not conform to other people but to a norm: other people act as a source of information about the appropriate ingroup norm. Because the norm is an internalised representation, people can conform to it without the surveillance of group members, or for that matter anybody else.

Referent informational influence has direct support from a series of four conformity experiments by Hogg and Turner (1987a). For example, under conditions of private responding (i.e. no normative influence), participants conformed to a non-unanimous majority containing a correct supporter (i.e. no informational influence) only if it was the participant's explicit or implicit ingroup (see also Abrams, Wetherell, Cochrane, Hogg & Turner, 1990). Other support for referent informational influence comes from research into group polarisation (e.g. Turner, Wetherell, & Hogg, 1989), crowd behaviour (e.g. Reicher, 1984), and social identity and stereotyping (e.g. Oakes, Haslam, & Turner, 1994).

Minority influence and social change

Our discussion of social influence, particularly conformity, has dealt with how individuals yield to direct or indirect social influence, most often from a numerical majority. Dissenters, deviates or independents have mainly been of interest indirectly, either as a means of investigating the effects of different types of majority or to investigate conformist personality attributes. However, we are all familiar with a very different, and very common, type of influence that can occur in a group: an individual or a numerical minority can sometimes change the views of the majority. Often such influence is based (in the case of individuals) on leadership or (in the case of subgroups) legitimate power.

However, minorities are typically at an influence disadvantage relative to majorities. Often, they are less numerous, and in the eyes of the majority, they have less legitimate power and are less worthy of serious consideration. Asch (1952), as we saw above, found that a single deviate (who was a confederate) from a correct majority (true participants) was ridiculed and laughed at. Sometimes, however, a minority that has little or no legitimate power can be influential and ultimately sway the majority to its own viewpoint. For example, in a variant of the single deviate study, Asch (1952) found a quite different response. When a correct majority of 11 true participants was confronted by a deviant/incorrect minority of 9 confederates, the majority remained independent (i.e. continued responding correctly) but took the minority's responses far more seriously—no one laughed. Clearly, the minority had some influence over the majority, albeit not enough in this experiment to produce manifest conformity.

History illustrates the power of minorities. Think of it this way: if the only form of social influence was majority influence, then social homogeneity would have been reached tens of thousands of years ago, individuals and groups always being swayed to adopt the views and practices of the growing numerical majority. Minorities, particularly those that are active and organised, introduce innovations that ultimately produce social change: without **minority influence**, social change would be very difficult to explain.

Minority influence
Social influence processes whereby numerical or power minorities change the attitudes of the majority.

For example, American anti-war rallies during the 1960s had an effect on majority attitudes that hastened withdrawal from Vietnam. Similarly, the suffragettes of the 1920s gradually changed public opinion so that women were granted the vote, and the Campaign for Nuclear Disarmament rallies in Western Europe in the early 1980s gradually shifted public opinion away from the 'benefits' of nuclear proliferation. Most recently, the 2011 popular uprisings across North Africa and the Middle East, dubbed the 'Arab Spring', have to varying degrees changed majority attitudes regarding governance in those countries. An excellent example of an active minority is Greenpeace: the group is numerically small (in terms of 'activist' members) but has important influence on public opinion through the high profile of some of its members and the wide publicity of its views.

The sorts of question that are important here are whether minorities and majorities gain influence via different social practices and, more fundamentally, whether the underlying psychology is different. There have been several recent overviews of minority influence research and theory (Hogg, 2010; Martin & Hewstone, 2003, 2008, 2010; Martin, Hewstone, Martin & Gardikiotis, 2008), and an earlier meta-analysis of research findings (Wood, Lundgren, Ouellette, Busceme & Blackstone, 1994).

Beyond conformity

Social influence research has generally adopted a perspective in which people conform to majorities because they are dependent on them for normative and informational reasons. Moscovici and his colleagues mounted a systematic critique of this perspective (Moscovici, 1976; Moscovici & Faucheux, 1972). They argued that there had been a **conformity bias**

Conformity bias
Tendency for social psychology to treat group influence as a one-way process in which individuals or minorities always conform to majorities.

underpinned by a functionalist assumption in the literature on social influence. Nearly all research focused on how individuals or minorities yield to majority influence and conform to the majority, and assumed that social influence satisfies an adaptive requirement of human life, to align with the status quo and thus produce uniformity, perpetuate stability and sustain the status quo. In this sense, social influence *is* conformity. Clearly, conformity is an important need for individuals, groups and society. However, innovation and normative *change* are sometimes required to adapt to altered circumstances. Such change is difficult to understand from a conformity perspective, because it requires an understanding of the dynamics of active minorities.

Moscovici and Faucheux (1972) also famously 'turned Asch on his head'. They cleverly suggested that Asch's studies had actually been studies of minority influence, not majority influence. The Asch paradigm appears to pit a lone individual (true participant) against an erroneous majority (confederates) on an unambiguous physical perception task. Clearly, a case of majority influence in the absence of subjective uncertainty? Perhaps not.

The certainty with which we hold views lies in the amount of agreement we encounter for those views: ambiguity and uncertainty are not properties of objects 'out there' but of other people's disagreement with us. This point is just as valid for matters of taste (if everyone disagrees with your taste in music, your taste is likely to change) as for matters of physical perception (if everyone disagrees with your perception of length, your perception is likely to change) (Moscovici, 1976, 1985a; Tajfel, 1969; Turner, 1985).

This sense of uncertainty would be particularly acute when an obviously correct perception is challenged. Asch's lines were *not* 'unambiguous'; there was disagreement between confederates and participants over the length of the lines. In reality, Asch's lone participant was a member of a large majority (those people outside the experiment who would call the lines 'correctly': that is, the rest of humanity) confronted by a small minority (the confederates who called the lines 'incorrectly'). Asch's participants were influenced by a minority: participants who remained 'independent' can be considered to be the conformists! 'Independence' in this sense is nicely described by the American writer Henry Thoreau in his famous quote from *Walden* (1854): 'If a man does not keep pace with his companions, perhaps it is because he hears a different drummer.'

In contrast to traditional conformity research, Moscovici (1976, 1985a) believed that there is disagreement and conflict within groups, and that there are three *social influence modalities* that define how people respond to such social conflict:

1 *Conformity*—majority influence in which the majority persuades the minority or deviates to adopt the majority viewpoint
2 *Normalisation*—mutual compromise leading to convergence
3 *Innovation*—a minority creates and accentuates conflict in order to persuade the majority to adopt the minority viewpoint[1]

Groupthink

Groupthink
A mode of thinking in highly cohesive groups in which the desire to reach unanimous agreement overrides the motivation to adopt proper rational decision-making procedures.

Groups sometimes employ deficient decision-making procedures that produce poor decisions. The consequences of such decisions can be disastrous. Irving Janis (1972) used an archival method, relying on retrospective accounts and content analysis, to compare a number of American foreign policy decisions that had unfavourable outcomes (e.g. the 1961 Bay of Pigs fiasco, the 1941 defence of Pearl Harbor) with others that had favourable outcomes (e.g. the 1962 Cuban missile crisis). Janis coined the term **groupthink** to describe the group decision-making process that produced the poor decisions. Groupthink was

[1]Vaughan, M. G., & Hogg, M. A. (2014). Social cognition and social thinking. In *Social psychology* (7th ed., pp. 214–233). Frenchs Forest, NSW: Pearson Australia.

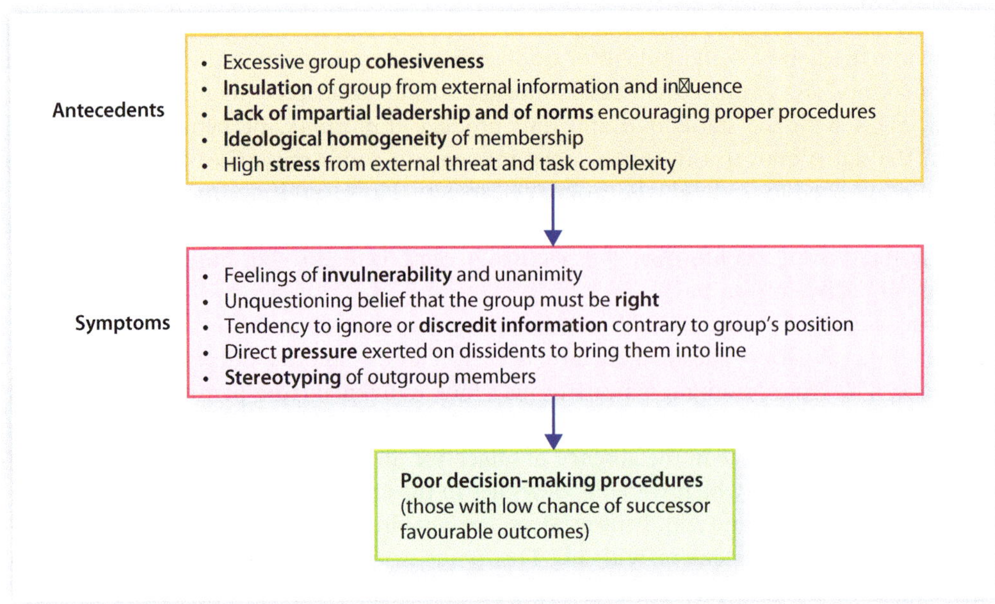

Figure 9.39 Antecedents, symptoms and consequences of groupthink
(**Source:** Janis & Mann (1977))

defined as a mode of thinking in which the desire to reach unanimous agreement overrides the motivation to adopt proper rational decision-making procedures (Janis, 1982; Janis & Mann, 1977).

The antecedents, symptoms and consequences of groupthink are displayed in Figure 9.39. The principal cause of groupthink is excessive group cohesiveness, but there are other antecedents that relate to basic structural faults in the group and to the immediate decision-making context. Together, these factors generate a range of symptoms that are associated with defective decision-making procedures: for example, there is inadequate and biased discussion and consideration of objectives and alternative solutions, and a failure to seek the advice of experts outside the group (see the third and fourth focus questions).

Descriptive studies of groupthink (e.g. Hart, 1990; Hensley & Griffin, 1986; Tetlock, 1979) largely support the general model (but see Tetlock, Peterson, McGuire, Chang & Feld, 1992), whereas experimental studies tend to find mixed or little support for the role of cohesiveness. Experiments establish background conditions for groupthink in four-person laboratory or quasi-naturalistic groups, and then manipulate cohesiveness (usually as friends versus strangers), and either a leadership variable (directiveness or need-for-power) or procedural directions for effective decision making.

Some have found no relationship between cohesiveness and groupthink (Flowers, 1977; Fodor & Smith, 1982), some have found a positive relationship only under certain conditions (Callaway & Esser, 1984; Courtright, 1978; Turner, Pratkanis, Probasco & Leve, 1992), and some a negative relationship (Leana, 1985).

Group polarisation The grounding of the entire QANTAS Airlines fleet in 2011 astounded the Pilots Association. A spokesman described the board's action as 'nothing short of crazy' and said that the CEO (pictured) 'was completely mad'
(**Source:** Sam Ruttyn/Newspix © Newspix/ News Ltd/3rd Party Managed Reproduction & Supply Rights.)

These problems have led people to suggest other ways to approach the explanation of groupthink (Aldag & Fuller, 1993; Hogg, 1993). For example, group cohesiveness may need to be more precisely defined before its relationship to groupthink can be specified (Longley & Pruitt, 1980; McCauley, 1989); at present, it ranges from close friendship to group-based liking. Hogg and Hains (1998) conducted a laboratory study of four-person discussion groups involving 472 participants to find that symptoms of groupthink were associated with cohesiveness, but only where cohesion represented group-based liking, not friendship or interpersonal attraction.

It has also been suggested that groupthink is merely a specific instance of 'risky shift': a group that already tends towards making a risky decision polarises through discussion to an even more risky decision (Myers & Lamm, 1975; see below). Others have suggested that groupthink may not really be a group process at all but just an aggregation of coping responses adopted by individuals to combat excessive stress (Callaway, Marriott & Esser, 1985). Group members are under decision-making stress and thus adopt defensive coping strategies that involve suboptimal decision-making procedures, which are symptomatic of groupthink. This behaviour is mutually reinforced by members of the group and thus produces defective group decisions.[J]

Behavioural style and the genetic model

Building on this critique, Moscovici (1976) proposed a genetic model of social influence. He called it a 'genetic' model because it focused on the way in which the dynamics of social conflict can generate (are genetic of) social change. He believed that, in order to create change, active minorities actually go out of their way to create, draw attention to and accentuate conflict. The core premise was that all attempts at influence create conflict based on disagreement between the source and the target of influence. Because people generally do not like conflict, they try to avoid or resolve it. In the case of disagreement with a minority, an easy and common resolution is to simply dismiss, discredit or even pathologise the minority (Papastamou, 1986).

However, it is difficult to dismiss a minority if it 'stands up to' the majority and adopts a behavioural style that conveys uncompromising certainty about and commitment to its position, and a genuine belief that the majority ought to change to adopt its position. Under these circumstances, the majority takes the minority seriously, reconsidering its own beliefs and considering the minority's position as a viable alternative.

The most effective behavioural style a minority can adopt to prevail over the majority is one in which, among other things, the minority promulgates a message that is consistent across time and context, shows *investment* in its position by making significant personal and material sacrifices, and evinces *autonomy* by acting out of principle rather than from ulterior or instrumental motives. *Consistency* is the most important behavioural style for effective minority influence, as it speaks directly to the existence of an alternative norm and identity rather than merely an alternative opinion. Specifically, it:

- disrupts the majority norm and produces uncertainty and doubt
- draws attention to the minority as an entity (e.g. Hamilton & Sherman, 1996)
- conveys the clear impression that there is an alternative coherent point of view
- demonstrates certainty and an unshakable commitment to this point of view
- shows that (and how) the only solution to the conflict is espousal of the minority's viewpoint.

From an attribution theory perspective such as Kelley's (1967), this form of consistent and distinctive behaviour cannot be discounted—it demands to be explained. Furthermore, the

[J]Vaughan, M. G., & Hogg, M. A. (2014). Social cognition and social thinking. In *Social psychology* (7th ed., pp. 312–313). Frenchs Forest, NSW: Pearson Australia.

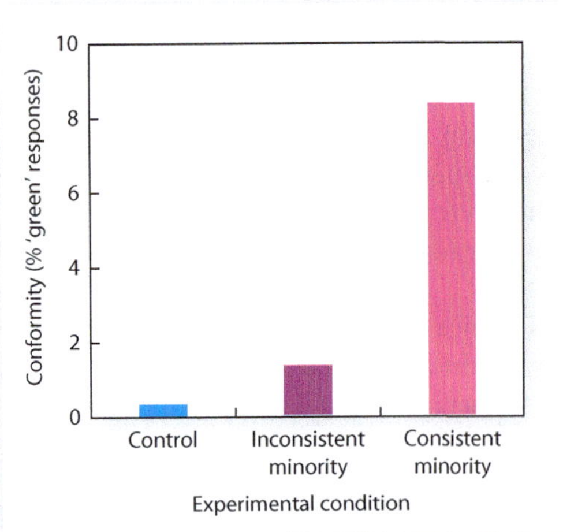

Figure 9.40 Conformity to a minority as a function of minority consistency

Although not as effective as a consistent majority, a consistent two-person minority in a six-person group was more influential than an inconsistent minority; that four people were influenced by two is quite remarkable
(**Source:** based on data from Moscovici, Lage & Naffrechoux (1969))

behaviour is likely to be internally attributed by an observer to invariant and perhaps essentialist (e.g. Haslam, Rothschild, & Ernst, 1998) properties of the minority rather than to transient or situational factors.

All of this makes the minority even more of a force to be reckoned with and a focus of deliberation by the majority. Overall, a minority that is consistent raises uncertainty. It begs the question: if this minority espouses its viewpoint time and time again, is it the obvious and most viable resolution? (Considering these points, might Aleksei and Ivan have a chance against the system in the fourth focus question?)

Moscovici and his colleagues demonstrated the role of consistency in a series of ingenious experiments, referred to as the 'blue–green' studies (Maass & Clark, 1984). In a modified version of the Asch paradigm, Moscovici, Lage and Naffrechoux (1969) had four participants confront two confederates in a colour perception task involving blue slides that varied only in intensity. The confederates were either consistent, always calling the slides 'green', or inconsistent, calling the slides 'green' two-thirds of the time and 'blue' one-third of the time. There was also a control condition with no confederates, just six true participants. Figure 9.40 shows that the consistent minority were more influential than the inconsistent minority (9 percent versus 2 percent). We might say that the reported rate of 9 percent for the consistent minority is not that high when compared with a consistent majority (recall that Asch reported an average conformity rate of 33 percent). Nevertheless, this simple experiment highlighted the fact that a minority of two could influence a majority of four.

There are two other notable results from an extension of this experiment, in which participants' real colour thresholds were tested privately after the social influence stage: (1) both experimental groups showed a lower threshold for 'green' than the control group—that is, they erred towards seeing ambiguous green–blue slides as 'green'; and (2) this effect was greater among experimental participants who were resistant to the minority—that is, participants who did not publicly call the blue slides 'green'.

Serge Moscovici and Elisabeth Lage (1976) employed the same colour perception task to compare consistent and inconsistent minorities with consistent and inconsistent majorities. There was also a control condition. As before, the only minority to produce conformity was the consistent minority (10 percent conformity). Although this does not compare well with the rate of conformity to the consistent majority (40 percent), it is comparable with the rate of conformity to the inconsistent majority (12 percent). However, the most important finding was that the *only* participants in the entire experiment who actually changed their blue–green thresholds were those in the consistent minority condition. Other studies have shown that the most important aspects of consistency are synchronic consistency (i.e. consensus) among members of the minority (Nemeth, Wachtler &

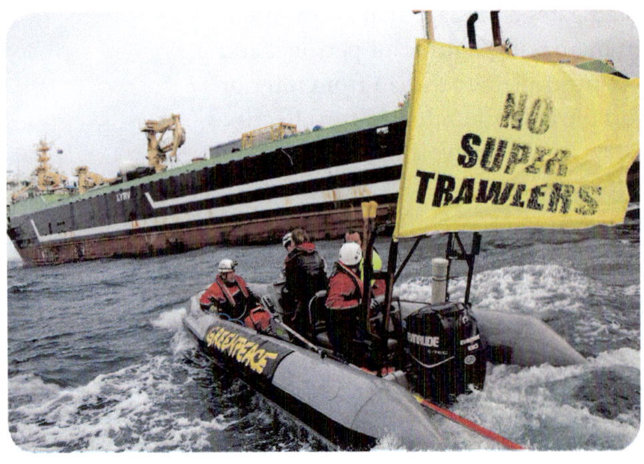

An active minority with style Greenpeace activists try to intercept a huge fishing trawler bound for Port Lincoln, South Australia
(**Source:** EPA/GREENPEACE/HANDOUT.)

Endicott, 1977) and perceived consistency, not merely objective repetition (Nemeth, Swedlund & Kanki, 1974).

Moscovici's (1976) focus on the importance of behavioural style was extended by Gabriel Mugny (1982) who focused on the strategic use of behavioural styles by real, active minorities struggling to change societal practices. Because minorities are typically powerless, they must negotiate with the majority rather than unilaterally adopt a behavioural style. Mugny distinguished between rigid and flexible negotiating styles, arguing that a rigid minority that refuses to compromise on any issues risks being rejected as dogmatic, and a minority that is too flexible, shifting its ground and compromising, risks being rejected as inconsistent (the classic case of 'flip-flopping'). There is a fine line to tread, but some flexibility is more effective than total rigidity. A minority should continue to be consistent with regard to its core position but should adopt a relatively open-minded and reasonable negotiating style on less core issues (e.g. Mugny & Papastamou, 1981).

Conversion theory

In 1980 Moscovici supplemented his earlier account of social influence based on behavioural style with his conversion theory (Moscovici, 1980, 1985a), and this remains the dominant explanation of minority influence. His earlier approach focused largely on how a minority's behavioural style (in particular, attributions based on the minority's consistent behaviour) could enhance its influence over a majority. Conversion theory is a more cognitive account of how a member of the majority processes the minority's message.

Moscovici argued that majorities and minorities exert influence through different processes:

1. *Majority influence* produces direct public compliance for reasons of normative or informational dependence. People engage in a *comparison process*, in which they concentrate attention on what others say to know how to fit in with them. Majority views are accepted passively without much thought. The outcome is public compliance with majority views with little or no private attitude change.
2. *Minority influence* produces indirect, often latent, private change in opinion due to the cognitive conflict and restructuring that deviant ideas produce. People engage in a *validation process* in which they carefully examine and cogitate over the validity of their beliefs. The outcome is little or no overt public agreement with the minority, for fear of being viewed as a member of the minority, but a degree of private internal attitude change that may only surface later on. Minorities produce a **conversion effect** as a consequence of active consideration of the minority point of view.

Conversion effect
When minority influence brings about a sudden and dramatic internal and private change in the attitudes of a majority.

Moscovici's dual-process model of influence embodies a distinction that is very similar to that discussed earlier between normative and informational influence (cf. Deutsch & Gerard, 1967), and is related to Petty and Cacioppo's (1986a) distinction between peripheral and central processing, and Chaiken's (Bohner, Moskowitz & Chaiken, 1995) distinction between heuristic and systematic processing Eagly & Chaiken, 1993).

Empirical evidence for conversion theory can be organised around three testable hypotheses (Martin & Hewstone, 2003): direction-of-attention, content-of-thinking, differential-influence. There is support for the *direction-of-attention hypothesis*—majority influence causes people to focus on their relationship to the majority (interpersonal focus), whereas minority influence causes people to focus on the minority message itself (message focus) (e.g. Campbell, Tesser & Fairey, 1986). There is also support for the *content-of-thinking hypothesis*—majority influence leads to superficial examination of arguments, whereas minority influence leads to detailed evaluation of arguments (e.g. Maass & Clark, 1983; Martin, 1996; Mucchi-Faina, Maass & Volpato, 1991).

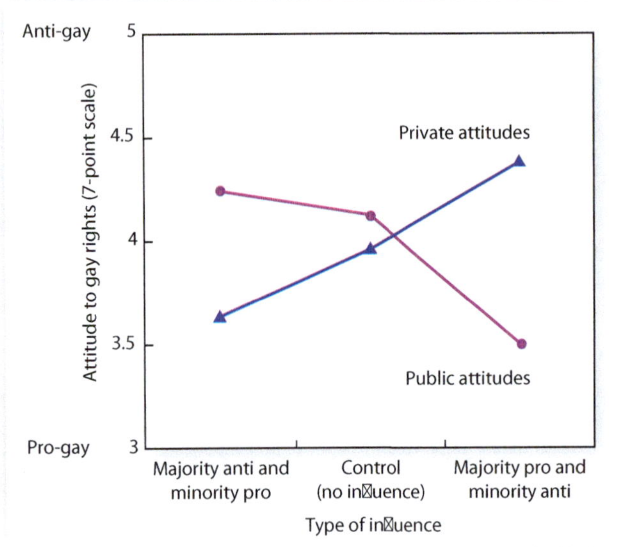

Figure 9.41 Public and private attitude change in response to majority and minority influence

Relative to a no-influence control condition, heterosexual *public* attitudes towards gay rights closely reflected the pro- or anti-gay attitudes of the majority. However, *private* attitudes reflected the pro- or anti-gay attitudes of the minority (**Source:** based on data from Maass & Clark (1983))

The *differential-influence hypothesis*—that majority influence produces more public/direct influence than private/indirect influence, whereas minority influence produces the opposite—has received most research attention and support (see Wood, Lundgren, Ouellette, Busceme & Blackstone, 1994). For example, the studies described above by Moscovici, Lage and Naffrechoux (1969) and Moscovici and Lage (1976) found, as would be expected from conversion theory, that conversion through minority influence took longer to manifest itself than compliance through majority influence: there was evidence for private change in colour thresholds (i.e. conversion) among participants exposed to a consistent minority, although they did not behave (or had not yet behaved) publicly in line with this change.

Another series of studies, by Anne Maass and Russell Clark (1983, 1986), report three experiments investigating people's public and private reactions to majority and minority influence regarding the issue of gay rights. In one of these experiments, Maass & Clark (1983) found that publicly expressed attitudes conformed to the expressed views of the majority (i.e. if the majority was pro-gay, then so were the participants), while privately expressed attitudes shifted towards the position espoused by the minority (see Figure 9.41).

Perhaps the most intriguing support for the *differential-influence hypothesis* comes from a series of fascinating experiments by Moscovici and Personnaz (1980, 1986), who employed the blue–green paradigm described above. Individual participants, judging the colour of obviously blue slides that varied only in intensity, were exposed to a single confederate who always called the blue slides 'green'. They were led to believe that most people (82 percent) would respond as the confederate did, or that only very few people (18 percent) would. In this way, the confederate was a source of majority or minority influence. Participants publicly called out the colour of the slide and then (and this is the ingenious twist introduced by Moscovici and Personnaz) the slide was removed and participants wrote down privately the colour of the after-image. Unknown to most people, including the participants, the after-image is always the complementary colour. So, for blue slides the after-image would be yellow, and for green slides it would be purple.

There were three phases to the experiment: an influence phase, where participants were exposed to the confederate, preceded and followed by phases where the confederate was absent and there was thus no influence. The results were remarkable (see Figure 9.42). Majority influence hardly affected the chromatic after-image: it remained yellow, indicating that participants had seen a blue slide. Minority influence, however, shifted the after-image towards purple, indicating that participants had actually 'seen' a green slide! The effect persisted even when the minority confederate was absent.

This controversial finding clearly supports the idea that minority influence produces indirect, latent internal change, while majority influence produces direct, immediate behavioural compliance. Moscovici and Personnaz have been able to replicate it, but others have been less successful. For example, in a direct replication Machteld Doms and Eddy van Avermaet (1980) found after-image changes after both minority and majority influence, while Richard Sorrentino and his colleagues found no after-image shift after minority influence, except among participants who were suspicious of the experiment (Sorrentino, King & Leo, 1980).

To try to resolve the contradictory findings, Robin Martin conducted a series of five careful replications of Moscovici and Personnaz's paradigm (Martin, 1998). His pattern of findings revealed that participants tended to show a degree of after-image shift only if they paid close attention to the blue slides—this occurred among participants who were either suspicious of the experiment or who were exposed to many, rather than a few, slides.

The key point is that circumstances that made people attend more closely to the blue slides caused them actually to see more green in the slides and thus to report an after-image that was shifted towards the after-image of green. These findings suggest that Moscovici and his colleagues' intriguing after-image findings may not reflect distinct minority/majority influence processes but may be a methodological artefact. This does not mean that conversion theory is wrong, but it does question the status of the blue–green studies as evidence for conversion theory. Martin (1998) comes to the relatively cautious conclusion that the findings may at least partially be an artefact of the amount of attention participants were paying to the slides: the greater the attention, the greater the after-image shift.

Convergent-divergent theory

Charlan Nemeth (1986, 1995) offered a slightly different account of majority/minority differences in influence. Because people expect to share attitudes with the majority, the discovery through majority influence that their attitudes are in fact in disagreement with those of the majority is surprising and stressful. It leads to a self-protective narrowing of focus of attention. This produces convergent thinking that inhibits consideration of alternative views. In contrast, because people do not expect to share attitudes with a minority, the discovery of disagreement associated with minority influence is unsurprising and not stressful and does not narrow focus of attention. It allows divergent thinking that involves consideration of a range of alternative views, even those not proposed by the minority.

In this way, Nemeth believes that exposure to minority views can stimulate innovation and creativity, generate more and better ideas, and lead to superior decision making in groups. The key

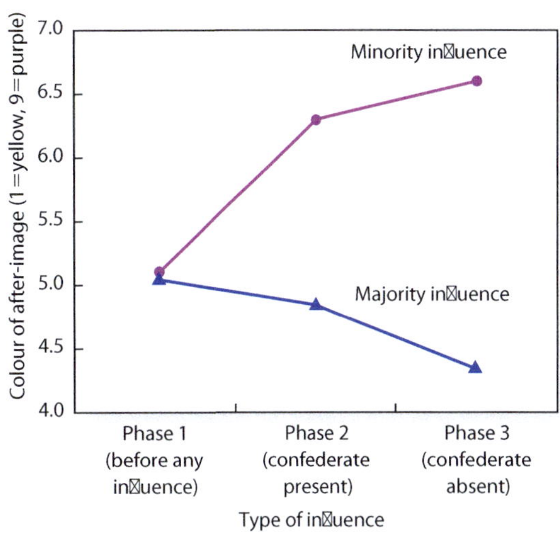

Figure 9.42 Reported colour of chromatic after-image as a result of majority and minority influence

Participants exposed to a majority member who wrongly identified blue slides as 'green' did not change their perception: their after-images did not alter. However, participants exposed to a minority member who called the blue slides 'green' did change their perception: their after-images changed and continued to change even after influence had ceased
(**Source:** based on data from Moscovici & Personnaz (1980))

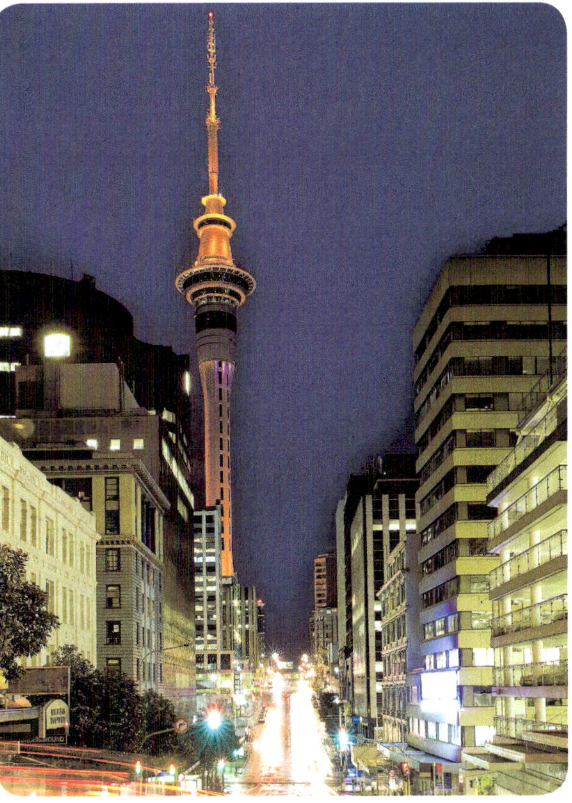

Conversion If you and your friends repeatedly and consistently told your friend Pierre that this was the Eiffel Tower, would he eventually believe you?
(**Source:** EPA/GREENPEACE/HANDOUT.)

difference between Nemeth's (1986) convergent–divergent theory and Moscovici's (1980) conversion theory hinges on the relationship between 'stress' and message processing: for Nemeth, majority-induced stress restricts message processing; for Moscovici, minority-induced stress elaborates message processing.

Convergent–divergent theory is supported by research using relatively straightforward cognitive tasks. Minority influence improves performance relative to majority influence on tasks that benefit from divergent thinking (e.g. Martin & Hewstone, 1999; Nemeth & Wachtler, 1983); majority influence improves performance relative to minority influence on tasks that benefit from convergent thinking (e.g. Peterson & Nemeth, 1996); and minority influence leads to the generation of more creative and novel judgements than does majority influence (e.g. Mucchi-Faina, Maass & Volpato, 1991; Nemeth & Wachtler, 1983).

For example, the Nemeth studies (Nemeth, 1986; Nemeth & Wachtler, 1983) employed Asch-type and blue–green paradigms in which participants exposed to majority or minority influence converged, with little thought, on majority responses; but minorities stimulated divergent, novel, creative thinking, and more active information processing, which increased the probability of correct answers. Angelica Mucchi-Faina and her colleagues used a different paradigm to find that students at the University of Perugia generated more original and creative ideas for promoting the international image of the city of Perugia when they had been exposed to a conventional majority and a creative minority than vice versa, or where the majority and the minority were both original or both conventional (Mucchi-Faina, Maass & Volpato, 1991).

Research on convergent–divergent theory also shows that minority influence leads people to explore different strategies for problem solving whereas majority influence restricts people to the majority-endorsed strategy (e.g. Butera, Mugny, Legrenzi & Pérez, 1996; Peterson & Nemeth, 1996), and that minority influence encourages issue-relevant thinking whereas majority influence encourages message-relevant thinking (e.g. De Dreu, De Vries, Gordijn & Schuurman, 1999).

Social identity and self-categorisation

We already saw above that the social identity theory of influence in groups, referent informational influence theory (e.g. Abrams & Hogg, 1990a; Hogg & Turner, 1987a; Turner & Oakes, 1989), views prototypical ingroup members as the most reliable source of information about what is normative for the group—the attitudes and behaviours that define and characterise the group. Through the process of self-categorisation, group members perceive themselves and behave in line with the norm.

From this perspective, minorities should be extremely ineffective sources of influence. Groups in society that promulgate minority viewpoints are generally widely stigmatised by the majority as social outgroups, or are 'psychologised' as deviant individuals. Their views are, at best, rejected as irrelevant, but they are often ridiculed and trivialised in an attempt to discredit the minority (e.g. the treatment of gays, environmentalists, intellectuals). All this resistance on the part of the majority makes it very difficult for minorities to have effective influence.

So, from a social identity perspective, how can a minority within one's group be influential? The problem for ingroup minorities is that the majority group makes intragroup social comparisons that highlight and accentuate the minority's otherness, essentially concretising a majority-versus-minority intergroup contrast within the group (David & Turner, 2001).

The key to effective minority influence is for the minority to somehow make the majority shift its level of social comparison to focus on intergroup comparisons with a genuine shared outgroup. This process automatically transcends intragroup divisions and focuses attention on the minority's ingroup credentials. The minority is now viewed as part of the ingroup, and there is indirect attitude change that may not be manifested overtly. For example, a radical faction within Islam will have more influence within Islam if Muslims make intergroup comparisons between Islam and the West than if they dwell on intra-Islam comparisons between majority and minority factions.

Research confirms that minorities do indeed exert more influence if they are perceived by the majority as an ingroup (Maass, Clark & Haberkorn, 1982; Martin, 1988; Mugny & Papastamou, 1982); and studies by David and Turner (1996, 1999) show that ingroup minorities produced more indirect attitude change (i.e. conversion) than did outgroup minorities, and majorities produced surface compliance. However, other research has found that an outgroup minority has just as much indirect influence as an ingroup minority (see review by Pérez & Mugny, 1998) and, according to Martin and Hewstone (2003), more research is needed to confirm that conversion is generated by the process of self-categorisation.

Vested interest and the leniency contract

Overall minorities are more influential if they can avoid being categorised by the majority as a despised outgroup and can be considered by the majority as part of the ingroup. The challenge for a minority is to be able to achieve this at the same time as promulgating an unwaveringly consistent alternative viewpoint that differs from the majority position. How can minorities successfully have it both ways—be thought of as an ingroup *and* hold an unwavering outgroup position?

The trick psychologically is to establish one's legitimate ingroup credentials before drawing undue critical attention to one's distinct minority viewpoint. Bill Crano's context–comparison model of minority influence describes how this may happen (e.g. Crano, 2001; Crano & Alvaro, 1998; Crano & Chen, 1998; Crano & Seyranian, 2009). When a minority's message involves weak or unvested attitudes (i.e. attitudes that are relatively flexible, not fixed or absolute), an ingroup minority can be quite persuasive—the message is more likely to be distinctive and attract attention and elaboration, and, by virtue of the message being unvested and the minority a clear ingroup, there is little threat of derogation or rejection of the minority. An outgroup minority is likely to be derogated and have no influence.

When the message involves strong or vested (i.e. fixed, inflexible and absolute) attitudes, it is more difficult for the minority to prevail. The message is not only highly distinctive but speaks to core group attributes. The inclination is to reject the message and the minority outright. However, the fact that the minority is actually part of the ingroup makes members reluctant to do so—to derogate people who are, after all, ingroup members. One way out of this dilemma is to establish with the minority what Crano calls a leniency contract. Essentially, the majority assumes that, because the minority is an ingroup minority, it is unlikely to want to destroy the majority's core attributes, and in turn the majority is lenient towards the minority and its views. This enables the majority to elaborate open-mindedly on the ingroup minority's message, without defensiveness or hostility and without derogating the minority. This leniency toward an ingroup minority leads to indirect attitude change. An outgroup minority does not invite leniency and is therefore likely to be strongly derogated as a threat to core group attitudes.

The logic behind this analysis is that disagreement between people who define themselves as members of the same group is both unexpected and unnerving—it raises subjective uncertainty about themselves and their attributes, and motivates uncertainty reduction (Hogg, 2007b, 2012). Where common ingroup membership is important and 'inescapable', there will be a degree of redefinition of group attributes in line with the minority: that is, the minority has been effective. Where common ingroup membership is unimportant and easily denied, there will be no redefinition of ingroup attributes in line with the minority: that is, the minority will be ineffective.

Attribution and social impact

Attribution
The process of assigning a cause to our own behaviour, and that of others.

Many aspects of minority influence suggest an underlying **attribution** process (Hewstone, 1989; Kelley, 1967). Effective minorities are consistent and consensual, distinct from the majority, unmotivated by self-interest or external pressures, and flexible in style. This combination of factors encourages a perception that the minority has chosen its position freely. It is therefore difficult to explain away its position in terms of idiosyncrasies of individuals (although this is, as we saw above, a strategy that is attempted), or in terms of external inducements or threats. Perhaps, then, there is actually some intrinsic merit to its position. This encourages people to take the minority seriously (although, again, social forces work against this) and at least consider its position; such cognitive work is an important precondition for subsequent attitude change.

Although majorities and minorities can be defined in terms of power, they also of course refer to numbers of people. Although 'minorities' are often both less powerful and less numerous (e.g. people from Somalia living in Australia or New Zealand), they can be less powerful but more numerous (e.g. Tibetans versus Chinese in Tibet). Perhaps not surprisingly, an attempt has been made to explain minority influence purely in terms of social influence consequences of relative numerosity.

Social impact
The effect that other people have on our attitudes and behaviour, usually as a consequence of factors such as group size, and temporal and physical immediacy.

Bibb Latané drew on **social impact** theory to argue that, as a source of influence increases in size (number), it has more influence (Latané, 1981; Latané & Wolf, 1981). However, as the cumulative source of influence gets larger, the impact of each additional source is reduced—a single source has enormous impact, the addition of a second source increases impact but not by as much as the first, a third even less, and so on. A good analogy is switching on a single light in a dark room—the impact is huge. A second light improves things, but only a little. If you have 10 lights on, the impact of an eleventh is negligible. Evidence does support this idea: the more numerous the source of influence, the more impact it has, with incremental changes due to additional sources decreasing with increasing size (e.g. Mullen, 1983; Tanford & Penrod, 1984).

But how does this account for the fact that minorities can actually have influence? One explanation is that the effect of a large majority on an individual majority member has reached a plateau: additional members or 'bits' of majority influence have relatively little impact. Although a minority viewpoint has relatively little impact, it has not yet attained a plateau: additional members or 'bits' of minority influence have a relatively large impact. In this way, exposure to minority positions can, paradoxically, have greater impact than exposure to majority viewpoints.[K]

[K]Vaughan, M. G., & Hogg, M. A. (2014). Social influence. In *Social psychology* (7th ed.,pp. 233–241). Frenchs Forest, NSW: Pearson Australia.

Summary

- Social cognition refers to cognitive processes and structures that affect and are affected by social context. It is assumed that people have a limited capacity to process information and are cognitive misers who take all sorts of cognitive shortcuts; or they are motivated tacticians who choose, on the basis of their goals, motives and needs, among an array of cognitive strategies.
- The overall impressions we form of other people are dominated by stereotypes, unfavourable information, first impressions and idiosyncratic personal constructs. Research suggests that in forming impressions of other people we weight components and then average them in complex ways; or certain components may influence the interpretation and meaning of all other components and dominate the resulting impression.
- Schemas are cognitive structures that represent knowledge about people, events, roles, the self and the general processing of information. Once invoked, schemas bias all aspects of information processing and inference in such a way that the schema remains unassailed.
- The encoding of information is heavily influenced by the salience of stimuli and by the cognitive accessibility of existing schemas.
- We tend to remember people mainly in terms of their traits but also in terms of their behaviour and appearance. They can be stored as individual people, or as category members.
- The processes we use to make inferences fall far short of ideal. Our schemas dominate us, we disregard regression effects and base-rate information, and we perceive illusory correlations. We rely on cognitive shortcuts (heuristics) such as representativeness, availability, and anchoring and adjustment, rather than on more optimal information-processing techniques.
- Affect and emotion are cognitively underpinned by appraisals of accountability, and our needs, goals and capacity to deal with a demand in a particular situation. In turn, affect influences social cognition—it infuses social cognition only where people process information in an open and constructive manner that involves active elaboration of stimulus details and information from memory.
- Social cognition has been criticised for being too cognitive and for not properly relating cognitive processes and structures to language, social interaction and social structure, consequently failing to address many topics of central concern to social psychology. This situation has improved in recent years; however, social neuroscience may fall prey to these limitations in an even bigger way.
- People are naive psychologists seeking to understand the causes of their own and other people's behaviour.
- Much like scientists, people take account of consensus, consistency and distinctiveness information in deciding whether to attribute behaviour internally to personality traits and dispositions, or externally to situational factors.
- People are actually poor scientists when it comes to making attributions. They are biased in many different ways, the most significant of which is a tendency to attribute others' behaviour dispositionally and their own behaviour externally, and a tendency to protect the self-concept by externally attributing their own failures and internally attributing their successes.
- Attributions for the behaviour of people as ingroup or outgroup members are ethnocentric and based on stereotypes. However, this bias is affected by the real or perceived nature of intergroup relations.
- Stereotypes may originate in a need for groups to attribute the cause of large-scale distressing events to outgroups that have (stereotypical) properties that are causally linked to the events.
- People resort to causal attributions only when there is no readily available social knowledge (e.g. scripts, causal schemata, social representations, cultural beliefs) to explain things automatically.
- Social representations are simplified causal theories of complex phenomena that are socially constructed through communication contextualised by intergroup relations. Rumour may play a key role in social representations.

- Conspiracy theories are one particularly bizarre but sadly prevalent type of causal theory that often persists in the face of overwhelming evidence that the theory is wrong.
- Attitudes have been a major interest of social psychologists for many years. They have been described as the most important concept in social psychology.
- Theories of attitude structure generally agree that attitudes are lasting general evaluations of socially significant objects (including people and issues). Some emphasise that attitudes are relatively enduring organisations of beliefs and behavioural tendencies towards social objects.
- Attitude structure has been studied mostly from a cognitive viewpoint. Balance theory and the theory of cognitive dissonance suggested that people strive to be internally consistent in their attitudes and beliefs.
- A strong attitude has a powerful evaluative association with the attitude object. It is more accessible in memory and more likely to be activated and the related behaviour performed. A more accessible attitude can involve a cost; high accessibility can lead to insensitivity to change in the attitude object.
- Attitudes that are accessible are more likely to be acted on.
- A value is a higher order concept that can play a guiding and organising role in relation to attitudes. Ideology and social representations are other related concepts.
- Measuring attitudes is both important and difficult. Traditional attitude scales of the 1930s are less frequently used today. While the response format of many modern measures is still based on the old Likert scale, the data is analysed by sophisticated statistical programs.
- A variety of physiological and behavioural indexes, both explicit and implicit, have been used to measure attitudes. The implicit association test has proved particularly popular and has gained traction when a more valid measure of a socially sensitive topic is required. Brain imaging technology is also being used to record neural processes correlated with implicit attitudes.
- The Yale research program was a major approach to the study of communication and persuasion. It focused on three kinds of factors: the source of a message (*who* factors), the message itself (*what* factors), and the audience (*to whom* factors).
- A communicator variable that has been studied in some depth is source credibility. A well-researched message variable is an appeal based on fear. There has been renewed interest in the sleeper effect, according to which some messages gain impact after the passage of time.
- Two important areas of our lives that employ relevant principles from social-psychological research are advertising and political propaganda.
- Two models dealing with how a persuasive message is learned draw heavily on social cognition. Petty and Cacioppo's elaboration–likelihood model proposes that, when people attend to a message carefully, they use a central route to process it; otherwise they use a peripheral route. Chaiken's heuristic–systematic model suggests that people use systematic processing when they attend to a message carefully; otherwise they use heuristic processing. The models are not in conflict.
- A variety of techniques that deal with ways of inducing another person to comply with our requests have been intensively studied: these include ingratiation, reciprocity and guilt arousal. There are also multiple-request techniques (foot-in-the-door, door-in-the-face and low-balling), in which a first request functions as a set-up for the second, real request.
- Festinger's cognitive dissonance theory is a major approach to the topic of attitude change. It addresses not only conflict between a person's beliefs but also discrepancy between behaviour and underlying attitudes, and behaviour and self-conception. It includes three variations on the way in which dissonance is brought about: effort justification, induced compliance, and free choice.
- Reactance is an increase in resistance to persuasion when the communicator's efforts to persuade are obvious. Techniques for building up resistance include forewarning and the inoculation defence. In recent years, manufacturing companies have used inoculating media releases to shore up consumer loyalty.
- Social influence can produce surface behavioural compliance with requests, obedience of commands, internalised conformity to group norms and deep-seated attitude change.

- People tend to be more readily influenced by reference groups, because they are psychologically significant for our attitudes and behaviour, than by membership groups, as they are simply groups to which we belong by some external criterion.
- Given the right circumstances, we all have the potential to obey commands blindly, even if the consequences of such obedience include harm to others.
- Obedience is affected by the proximity and legitimacy of authority, by the proximity of the victim, and by the degree of social support for obedience or disobedience.
- Group norms are enormously powerful sources of conformity: we all tend to yield to the majority.
- Conformity can be reduced if the task is unambiguous and we are not under surveillance, although even under these circumstances there is often residual conformity. Lack of unanimity among the majority is particularly effective in reducing conformity.
- People may conform in order to feel sure about the objective validity of their perceptions and opinions, to obtain social approval and avoid social disapproval, or to express or validate their social identity as members of a specific group.

Review questions

A. Fill in the missing words to complete the following statements.

1. According to Asch (1946) you are more likely to remember information presented first as a result of the ____________________. Whereas, remembering information presented last in a list refers to the ____________________.
2. Social inference involves the ____________ process to identify, sample and combine information to form ______________ and make ______________.
3. Anchoring and adjustment is a __________ often used by professionals as a selling technique. It describes the process in which a person uses a specific value or target number as a starting point, known as an __________, and subsequently __________ that information until an acceptable value is reached.
4. ______________ attribution refers to the process of assigning or labeling the behaviour of others behaviour based on individual characteristics, as opposed to ______________ that stem from the environment or culture.
5. The ____________________explains how as humans we pay particular attention to intentional behaviour that underlies various dispositions. For example, we infer that a friendly comment made by someone is due to an ____________________ to be friendly.
6. The self-serving bias is the tendency to attribute positive outcomes or behaviours to ____________________(otherwise known as a self-enhancing bias) and negative outcomes or behaviours to ____________________ (known as the self-protecting bias)

B. Please select one statement that best answers each of the following questions.

7. According to Asch (1964) which of the following statements is most accurate?
   a) a negative first impression is more resistant to change than a positive one
   b) first impressions last
   c) first impressions mean very little
   d) both a) and b)
8. A schema is defined as:
   a) a mental script or mental concept about a situation or event that helps us organise and interpret information.
   b) thoughts, beliefs or attitudes that allows us to make sense of a situation, person or event by filling in missing information that is stored in memory as a result of life experiences
   c) schemas can contribute to stereotypes and make it difficult to retain new information that does not conform to our established ideas about the world
   d) all of the above
9. Anna is 4 years old. She knows that a horse is large, has hair, four legs, and a tail. When Anna encounters a cow for the first time, she initially called it a horse. This is an example of:
   a) stereotype
   b) social judgeability
   c) schema
   d) negativity

10. Social encoding refers to the process of seeking information from an external social environment and representing it in the mind. Which of the following represents the four key stages of social encoding.

a) pre-attentive analysis, focal attention, comprehension, elaborative reasoning
b) pre-attentive analysis, comprehension, focal attention, elaborative reasoning
c) focal attention, pre-attentive analysis , comprehension, elaborative reasoning
d) focal attention, comprehension, pre-attentive analysis, elaborative reasoning

11. Social inference relies on which of the following mechanisms:

a) a top-down deductive approach related to general schemas
b) a bottom-up inductive approach that relies on specific instances
c) both a) and b)
d) none of the above

12. The theory of how people explain our own or others' behavior is called:

a) cognitive theory
b) impression theory
c) communication theory
d) attribution theory

13. The tendency for people to place an emphasis on internal characteristics rather than external factors, in explaining another person's behavior is called:

a) correspondent inferences error
b) cognitive bias error
c) fundamental attribution error
d) inferential analysis error

14. You notice a car behind you is driving erratically for a few kilometers and the driver soon cuts you off while driving through a busy intersection. Your immediate thought is "that person is a jerk!". However, this is the first time his driving has been erratic as his pregnant wife is in labour and he is desperate to get to the hospital. Your initial thought was an example of a:

a) correspondent inferences error
b) cognitive bias error
c) fundamental attribution error
d) inferential analysis error

15. Persuasive communication relies on which of the following:

a) expertise, popularity and attractiveness, rapid speech, perceived manipulation, linguistic power and fear
b) expertise, popularity and attractiveness, slow speech, perceived manipulation, linguistic power and fear
c) it depends on the person and the chosen audience
d) none of the above

16. The foot-in the door, door-in-the-face and low-ball are all types of what?

a) diseases
b) attitudes
c) tactics for requests
d) motivation strategies

17. Which of the following are NOT examples of various forms of cognitive dissonances:

a) induced compliance
b) effort justification
c) selective exposure hypothesis
d) all of the above

18. A psychological frame of mind whereby an individual allows others to direct their actions and behaviours and pass responsibility for the consequences of the behaviour on the authority figure relates to which obedience term?

a) dual-process dependency model

b) compliance

c) legitimate power

d) agentic state

C. Fill in the missing words to complete the following table.

19. There are three common types of schemas: Fill in the blanks.

Types of Schemas	Definition	Example
Script		20 years later, I remember going to the 1996 footy grand final
	Schemas about individuals or specific knowledge about someone	My sister is very creative but a poor athlete
	Schemas about various occupations or roles	

CHAPTER 10

Communication

The content in this section has been compiled from:
Drench Chapter 5

Drench, M.E., Noonan, A.C., Sharby, N., & Ventura, S.H. (2012). Motivation, adherence and collaborative treatment planning. In *Pyschosocial aspects of health care* (3rd ed., pp. 77-113). Upper Saddle River, N.J: Pearson Education.

CHAPTER 10

Communication

Communication involves the interpretation of meaning from interpersonal interactions, elements of body language and expressions. In health care settings, effective communication can dramatically effect therapeutic outcomes. For example, if communication breaks down it can become a barrier to a patient's capacity to follow through with medical recommendations and/or adhere to a treatment plan. In this chapter, evidence-based components of effective communication are explored to provide foundational learning that can be practised to enhance client and/or patient interviews.

After studying this chapter you should be able to:

- Describe the core elements of communication
- Describe effective techniques of verbal communication
- Describe effective techniques of non-verbal communication
- Describe barriers to effective communication
- Identify levels and sources of conflict in communication.

Patrick was late again! In frustration, I asked the nurse why he was never down in physical therapy (PT) for his scheduled appointments. She said, "He's the most impossible amputee I've ever worked with. Come with me, and you'll understand." As we approached his room, she shouted, "Patrick, get out of bed!" and threw up the shade. Depressed and angry, he shouted obscenities at the nurse and pulled the covers over his head.

I was absolutely appalled at her lack of sensitivity and compassion. No wonder he refused to have PT that day. I determined another strategy was in order. The following morning, I entered his room, smiled, and said, "Patrick, it's time to get up for PT. Your appointment is in 30 minutes. Will that work for you?" He nodded, and I left. One-half hour later, on the dot, he wheeled his chair into the clinic.

—*From the journal of Lindsay Cushing, physical therapist student*

"Communication is the interpretation of meaning from interpersonal interactions and extends far beyond verbal information to include elements of body movement, expressions, and subconscious mechanisms" (Davis, 2009, p. 78). Health care providers are required to communicate on a daily basis with clients, clients' families and friends, third-party payers, equipment vendors, and other health care professionals. Effective and timely communication is key to providing successful client- and family-centred health care and achieving optimal health outcomes. It enables providers to understand individual needs, helps clarify complicated issues, and promotes client adherence to complex treatment regimens. It is especially important when working with clients who have limited or no English proficiency skills, those with limited health literacy, and clients whose cultural backgrounds are not well understood by providers (Saha, Beach, & Cooper, 2008).

First and foremost, communication is the means by which we establish a therapeutic relationship with each client. There is strong support for including core communication studies and other professional behaviours, such as caring and empathy, in health care curricula and continuing education programs to better prepare client- and family-centred practitioners (Ang, 2002; Bonvicini et al., 2008; Greenfield, Anderson, Cox, & Tanner, 2008; Henkin, Dee, & Beatus, 2000; Raica, 2009; Taylor, Wook Lee, Kielhofner, & Ketkar, 2009). Learning experiences that promote the use of open-ended inquiries, active listening, reflective practice, empathy, and other caring behaviours can better prepare novice clinicians for the transition from the classroom to the clinic (Greenfield et al., 2008).

Although clients consider a provider's demonstration of caring and empathy to be extremely important to them, such demonstrations are often lacking in many medical encounters (Bonvicini et al., 2008). Unless providers are able to display these qualities to clients, interventions may be ineffective, regardless of the providers' clinical skills (Charon, 2001). Empathy is the ability to identify with and understand someone's situation, feelings, and emotions and recognise that the client is someone's mother, daughter, wife, or sibling. This includes imagining what it feels like to "be in the clients' shoes," to actually see things through their eyes, to not only hear what they are saying but to absorb their verbal and nonverbal cues (Davis, 2009; Fox et al., 2009).

In a study of general practitioners who had been patients, participants stated, "You never really appreciate what it's like being a patient until you are a patient . . . suddenly you realize that you feel very small and that you don't have much of a voice and you don't feel very powerful . . . you feel very vulnerable and you can get very emotional, and you cannot be very rational about things" (Fox et al., 2009, p. 1582). Other participants indicated feelings of anxiety, shock, and loss of control. Waiting for a medical procedure, one participant indicated that being an "insider" in the health care system gave her the ability to be seen more quickly than other patients who lacked such power. While she still felt anxious and some sense of disempowerment, she recognised that her feelings were tempered because of her professional medical status. Respondents indicated that, as a result of their experiences, they developed a better understanding of and enhanced emotional connection with future patients. Recognising their own disempowering feelings, they worked harder to empathise with patients, to recognise their emotions, and to empower them in clinical decision making.

Studies show that an empathetic approach to client care leads to improvements in the quality of client–provider relationships, enhanced treatment outcomes, and enrichment of practitioners' own lives (Davis, 2009; Greenfield et al., 2008). The first step in developing empathy is to practice effective communication skills. Good communication skills allow health care providers to focus on the person, not the disease; to build a therapeutic alliance that improves both the client's and provider's perspectives; and to achieve more appropriate therapeutic goals (Saha et al., 2008; Teal & Street, 2009).

Health care professionals agree that they must possess effective communication skills to motivate clients, promote adherence with treatment protocols, and ensure appropriate, cost-efficient outcomes (Pettrey, 2003; Vanderhoff, 2005). Studies show that poor communication often results in negative consequences. If information is not relayed adequately, inaccurate diagnoses can result (Sutcliffe, Lewton, & Rosenthal, 2004). Clients may grow dissatisfied and frustrated with health care providers, become nonadherent with treatment plans, or seek alternative care, resulting in higher medical costs. In addition, practitioners can also become frustrated and develop symptoms of burnout. To prevent the latter, it is helpful for providers to recognise their own limitations, know that they cannot *cure* everyone, and practice stress management strategies to help balance work and family life (Greenfield et al., 2008).

Although individuals may believe they are clearly conveying messages to others, receivers may not always hear the message senders thought they were conveying. The opening journal entry in this chapter provides a good example. The nurse thought she was helping Patrick prepare for therapy, but he responded to her approach as an unwelcome interruption to his sleep. In addition, her behaviour suggested disapproval and judgement. In contrast, Lindsay reframed the situation, giving Patrick the opportunity to take control and "save face." As a result, she was successful in motivating him. A health professional's role is to provide clients with factual information that helps them formulate their own decisions, not offer value judgements. In this chapter, we discuss the components of effective communication and their importance in conducting a client-centred patient interview.

Elements of effective communication

Communication begins when the sender expresses an idea, either verbally or nonverbally. Verbal messages are influenced by paralanguage cues, such as tone of voice, pitch, volume, and speed. Nonverbal messages may be sent intentionally or unintentionally. They include facial expression, touch, proxemics, and behaviour. The receiver interprets the message within a context that is mediated by these influencing factors. The receiver's understanding of the meaning of the message is further affected by what he or she perceives and feels. People's perceptions may vary depending on social role, literacy level, cultural background, personal needs, age, and prior life experiences. The physical context in which a discussion takes place, the time of day, the individual's mental status, and other factors occurring in one or more of the participants' lives may also influence the communication process (Barringer & Glod, 1998).

Communication between health care providers and clients differs from day-to-day social interactions with friends or family members. Individuals choose their friends but not necessarily their clients. Social relationships are based on enjoyment and mutual satisfaction, whereas professional affiliations exist for the benefit of the client. A health professional may elect to end a friendship based on another individual's unacceptable social responses but may be obligated to continue treating a client who behaves similarly. During social interactions, individuals share problems and experiences, whereas in therapeutic situations, the focus is solely on the client's concerns. In social surroundings, people often speak without thinking beforehand about what they are going to say or how it will influence others. In health care settings, communication should be planned in advance, whenever possible, to help facilitate accurate communication. To ensure that messages are being correctly interpreted by both sender and receiver, health care professionals need to continuously observe and analyse their interactions with others (Vanderhoff, 2005). Providing feedback and paraphrasing messages may help ensure clarification.

Levels of communication

Communication occurs at four levels. It starts at the *intrapersonal level,* as we absorb information from our environment and begin to develop and formulate our thoughts and ideas. Once we decide to send a message to another person, we start to communicate at the *interpersonal level.* Here, the opportunity for misinterpretation begins. A higher level of communication takes place when we participate in a *small group discussion* with more than one other individual. This frequently occurs at team and family meetings. People enter with differing goals, objectives, and backgrounds, and the chances of misinterpretation or conflict increase. Finally, *organisational communication* takes place when *several groups* within a facility meet to discuss problems or establish policies. Egos, personal agendas, and professional differences may all interfere with the exchange. Everyone needs to strive to keep the channels of communication open and effective (Davis, 2006).

Developing client-practitioner rapport

As health care professionals, we might neglect to think about the culture shock that clients experience when they encounter the health care setting. Clients enter with their own concerns, anxieties, and value systems. They have their personal routine and may be accustomed to privacy. In an inpatient setting, they may have an unknown and unwanted roommate. We socialise them into *our* world. We often require them to wear particular attire and eat at preset times. They select what they are eating from limited menus. In addition to coping with their illness, disease, or disability, we expect them to value our expertise and follow our instructions. Is it any wonder why clients may feel dependent, vulnerable, or afraid?

Studies confirm that practitioners who adopt a friendly and reassuring manner are more effective than those who do not. In fact, in one study of empathy and its relationship to the common cold, researchers found that clinician empathy, as perceived by patients, significantly decreased illness duration and severity associated with immune system changes (Rakel et al., 2009). The adage that a picture is worth a thousand words may seem almost too basic to mention, but a perceived inhospitable health care environment can damage an impression before the provider even begins to speak. Facial expressions and postures may be the first "picture" or impression the client receives, depending on his or her learning style, cultural context, and other factors. Explaining who you are and why you are there can establish a therapeutic foundation, and a smile can be very comforting. Pulling up a chair to sit at eye level with a client who is seated or reclining can make the health professional seem open to communication and collaboration rather than authoritative and distant. Taken together, these simple measures demonstrate a willingness to spend the time needed for clients and providers to get to know each other. Evidence shows that when providers use these techniques, clients' psychological well-being and their ability to recall information at a later date both improve (Stiefel et al., 2010).

Prior to entering a client's room or greeting a client in the clinic or home setting, providers should clear their thoughts in order to be mindful and focused on the person they are about to meet. By taking time to practice this simple strategy, practitioners make themselves ready to be truly present in each and every experience. The process involves practitioners becoming aware of their thoughts and reflecting on their biases and expectations, which enables them to remain nonjudgemental and ready to listen intently to what the client has to say (Epstein, 1999; Hutchinson, 2005). Therapists who are aware of their own thoughts and feelings and who are oriented toward the interpersonal aspects of client interactions achieve more effective therapeutic relationships and better outcomes. In occupational therapy, this concept is referred to as "use of self." It involves the therapist's use of his or her own personality, perceptions, and judgements as part of the therapeutic process (Taylor et al., 2009).

Health care professionals often work with very distressed people, whose emotional strain can affect their ability to communicate. Our attempts to deal with difficult situations can affect our own ability to communicate and be compassionate (Halstead, 2001). In a busy health care setting, providers are frequently under stress. It may be easy to fall into the habit of concentrating on the illness, disease, or injury rather than on the client as a person. Although this may be an appropriate response in the emergency department, it is not appropriate in most other cases. Before we can effectively treat a client, we must develop a good relationship or rapport (Schneider, Kaplan, Greenfield, Li, & Wilson, 2004).

In our efforts to be empathetic and compassionate, though, we need to be genuine and not offer false reassurances. "I know how you feel" is not authentic—we do not know how they feel. Instead, we might say, "This must be difficult for you," "Tell me how this is affecting you," or "How are you feeling?" Similarly, we may not be able to tell them that "everything will be all right." Clients have a right, and often a need, to express their emotions regarding their illness or disability. The provider's role is to listen and be empathetic (Halstead, 2001).

It is important for providers to ask clients about their health practices. Do they eat a balanced diet? Do they exercise regularly? Do they use seat belts? Do they consume drugs or alcohol? As clients talk, providers can practice active listening skills by leaning toward the client, nodding, and asking clarifying questions. Keep in mind that some clients find touch comforting; others do not. It may be appropriate for providers to touch a client's arm or shoulder to demonstrate caring. If the client withdraws or appears uncomfortable, responsive providers will withdraw their touch and avoid unnecessary touch in the future.

Before beginning to examine or treat clients, providers can let clients know what to expect to help build a sense of trust and respect and allay anxiety. The extra minutes it takes to develop this sense of rapport is well worth the effort as the treatment program progresses. Consider the case of Donnie, a physical therapist student completing an internship in a skilled nursing facility. On his way to meet a new client who was admitted following a stroke, he stopped by the nurses' station to review her medical record. A staff member said, "Good luck with Mrs. Benson. She is in a bad mood today and refuses to do anything." Donnie approached the room with trepidation. As he entered, he took time to note the pictures and personal items on the bedside table. He introduced himself to the client and said, "From your pictures, I see that you like to dance." She responded, "I was quite a dancer in my day." As Donnie developed a therapeutic relationship with her, she allowed him to proceed. Following an evaluation, he asked her if she would like to dance with him. A few minutes later, the staff was amazed as they saw Donnie and Mrs. Benson smiling and *waltzing* down the corridor.

As health care professionals, we need to develop an awareness and ability to reflect on our own attitudes, styles, and approaches to clients. Rather than assuming that a client is "difficult," it is important to question our own attitudes and develop more effective strategies. Taking the time to view clients as the "experts" in *their individual situations* and allowing time for them to express their desires, values, and emotions may improve therapeutic relationships and lead to better client outcomes (Beach & Inui, 2006; Greenfield et al., 2008). This is especially important in a health care environment in which clients are quickly discharged. In addition to treating the client, the health care provider must play the roles of educator and facilitator, helping clients become independent in their own care as quickly as possible (Vanderhoff, 2005).

Client-sensitive language

As Martin (1999) noted, "language shapes thought" (p. 44). Thinking about clients as their illness or disability reinforces emotional detachment. For some, the person *becomes* the diagnosis, which frames the context in how we connect. Focusing on the individual enables us to see his or her abilities, needs, desires, and goals rather than the impairments. For example, the common expression of "confined to a wheelchair" promotes a negative connotation of being limited, even imprisoned. The wheelchair, in fact, is just the opposite. It is liberating, providing a means of mobility, of accessing the world. Refer to Table 10.1 for other examples of diminishing and empowering language.

In addition to empowering clients, we show respect by using "people-first" language. The terminology we use reflects how we think about clients (Martin, 1999). Consider how the nurse in Lindsay's journal referred to Patrick as "the most impossible amputee." Patrick is not the amputation. He is a person who has undergone a surgical amputation of his lower limb. We often hear health care workers using terminology such as "that CVA," "the shoulder," or "the arthritic client." People are not their impairments, functional limitations, or disabilities, but rather the person with a stroke, the woman with a shoulder problem, the client with arthritis. Acknowledging their individuality and totality is part of a therapeutic outcome. Providers need to be aware of this and encourage others to avoid referring to clients by their diagnoses or body parts.

Table 10.1 Examples of Diminishing and Empowering Terminology

Diminishing Terminology	Empowering Terminology
• Stroke victim	• Person who has had a stroke
• Stricken with polio	• Person who has polio
• Afflicted with cerebral palsy	• Person with cerebral palsy; diagnosed with cerebral palsy
• Suffers from Parkinson's disease	• Person who has Parkinson's disease
• Mute; dumb	• Person who is unable to speak
• Confined to a wheelchair	• Uses a wheelchair
• The handicapped; impaired; disabled; crippled; deformed	• Person with a disability or impairment
• Normal (as though a person with a disability is not normal)	• Person without a disability
• The blind	• Person who is visually impaired; person who is blind
• Epileptic	• Person with epilepsy; person with a seizure disorder
• Schizophrenic	• Person with schizophrenia
• Alcoholic	• Person with alcoholism
• Fits	• Seizures
• Victim of ...	• Survivor of ...
• Suffering from	• Diagnosed with

Similarly, choice of words, tone, and volume can communicate certain messages, even when they are unintended. For example, by referring to older clients as "honey" or "dear," health providers may inadvertently transmit messages of dependence or incompetence to older adults by infantilising them, using what has become known as *elderspeak* (Williams, Kemper, & Hummert, 2004, p. 17).

Mindfulness: being present in the moment

> Today, I had an experience that made me very sad. I've been on my rotation at the hospital for three months, and my supervisor seems very pleased with my skills. I have a lot of independence and am responsible for my own caseload. A therapist was out sick with the flu today, and I was asked to pick up two of her clients on top of my own. Boy was I overwhelmed! I only had time to skim the charts and then rush in and do the best treatment I could with very little time.
>
> Later, I was scheduled to examine Ms. Jones, a newly admitted client. She's a 23-year-old woman who was in a car accident that caused a fracture-dislocation at the lumbar 4-5 level of the spinal cord. At this time, she has paraplegia, with no sensation in her lower extremities. I was feeling so rushed that I just barged into her room and quickly introduced myself before I started bombarding her with questions about her past medical history and current status. Then I began running through the items on the evaluation form as quickly as I could. She started crying and then shouted, "You're just like all the others! I'm a person." I felt so terrible. I realized I was not treating her as a client, but as an object. I quickly apologized and fled the room. I immediately recognized my mistake. I had let my frustration take over, and as a result, I failed to be there for her when she needed me.
>
> —*From the journal of Mark Smart, occupational therapy student*

Today, the need to be highly productive places significant demands on health care practitioners. The ability to simultaneously perform multiple tasks is expected. While running from client to client, it is easy to forget that each person is a unique human being. What messages does this behaviour convey? When providers work with one client but are preoccupied with others, they risk giving the client the impression that he or she is "in the way" and "unimportant." To avoid this, providers should practice mindfulness. This requires that we fully attend to each task (Epstein, 1999; Epstein & Street, 2007; Hutchinson, 2005; Kabat-Zinn, 1994; Kearney, Weininger, Vachon, Harrison, & Mount, 2009; Mead & Bower, 2002; Mentgen, 2001; Teal & Street, 2009).

How do providers become mindful in the midst of a chaotic health care environment? Studies show that mindful practitioners develop self-awareness, clearing their minds of mental clutter, so that they are able to focus on the present moment. Mindfulness involves self-assessment, the ability to be aware of one's own opinions, prejudices, and expectations. Practitioners must understand and respect what the client is feeling and distinguish the client's feelings from their own. The mindful practitioner welcomes uncertainty, and difficult patients become interesting (Epstein & Street, 2007; Hutchinson, 2005; Kabat-Zinn, 1994; Kearney et al., 2009; Mead & Bower, 2002; Mentgen, 2001). Whereas all practitioners rely on academic knowledge, the mindful practitioner also relies on knowledge of the self and client. Barriers to mindfulness include emphasis on explicit rather than tacit knowledge, time constraints, and the desire to maintain emotional distance from clients. To develop mindfulness, practitioners learn to actively listen to their clients and observe and learn from mentors in clinical settings. In addition, practitioners may want to practice meditation (Epstein, 1999) or maintain a personal journal of their client encounters to reflect on and learn from their actions in practice (Epstein, 1999; Schon, 1983; Wainwright, Shepard, Harman, & Stephens, 2010).

It only takes a minute to focus and give complete attention to the client. This small intervention can greatly enhance the effectiveness of the treatment. Clients are aware of the state of mind we bring to the interaction. Had Mark, the occupational therapy student, been able to eliminate the distractions and fully attend to Ms. Jones, he might have developed a rapport with her and been more successful in eliciting information. She might have become a partner in her care and been spared feeling like a "victim" of *his* distress.

Verbal communication

Vocabulary

It is important to match your chosen communication technique as closely as possible to the preferred style of the client, which may mean adjusting your typical approach. For example, you may need to speak more slowly or more loudly, consider how you make eye contact, and, perhaps, not ask too many questions of a client who comes from a culture that uses indirect language skills. This is information that may not be readily apparent and can only be identified by carefully observing a client's response to you.

As stated earlier, communication involves sending a message to a receiver (an audience). When sending a message, it is important for the sender to keep in mind the needs of the audience. First, consider the importance of vocabulary. When talking to another health care professional who shares our common language, providers should use medical terminology. However, when speaking with a client, providers need to use words that the client understands; for example, you would use a different language with an adult who has undergone a heart transplant than with a child who has a developmental delay. Sometimes, clients nod and smile, apparently signaling that they understand, even when they do not. Checking with clients to determine what they have heard helps avoid misunderstandings. Providers can ask them to repeat the information or ask questions to determine clarity of understanding.

Using medical terminology may unknowingly frighten clients. For example, suggesting that a client go to a short-term care facility for rehabilitation following surgery may be routine to the provider, but the client may hear, "I am being sent to a nursing home and will never go home again." To avoid such miscommunication, observe clients' nonverbal responses. If they appear upset by something said, ask questions to clarify misconceptions or concerns prior to moving on to new topics or activities. Whatever vocabulary providers choose, it is essential to speak with clients at their level of understanding (Vanderhoff, 2005). Words are building blocks, but they are only a part of verbal communication.

Paralanguage

Paralanguage, an important component of verbal communication, includes pitch, tone, speed, volume, emotional quality, stress, and accent (Purtilo & Haddad, 2007). The phrase "It's not what you say but how you say it that counts" illustrates the idea that what one says can be interpreted many different ways. Sometimes, especially when we are stressed, busy, or impatient, what we planned to say comes out sounding all wrong.

When we are in a hurry, we tend to talk faster. When we are excited or angry, we talk louder. If we are nervous, the listener may detect a higher pitch or tone. Accents may be difficult for some to understand. When communicating with clients, it is important to appear calm and concerned. Maintain an appropriate tone and volume to convey a sense of trust and interest. Take time to emphasise key words so the listener "hears" them and recognises their importance. Volume should vary depending on the size of the room and the hearing capabilities of the audience.

Active listening

Active listening is an essential evaluation tool (Jensen, Gwyer, Shepard, & Hack, 2000). The onus falls on the health care provider to intently listen to clients' stories, understand their needs within the context of their lives, create a plan of care in collaboration with clients and significant others, and teach clients and significant others the skills they need to carry out the plan of care (Vanderhoff, 2005). Although hearing implies the ability to perceive sound, *active listening* involves being alert and receptive to both verbal and nonverbal communication cues. Whenever possible, eliminate the physical and mental distractions that may hinder communication. Strive to appear relaxed and interested in what clients have to say. Listen to their stories. This is not the time to spend reviewing the medical record and previous documentation. Although making some notes may be appropriate, ignoring the client while taking copious notes is not effective (Davis, 2009).

Florence Nightingale is reported to have said, "We must not talk to them [clients], not at them, but with them" (Attewell, 1998). Active listening shows clients that you are fully present in the moment, grasping the meaning of what they are saying. One difference noted between "expert" and "novice" physical therapists (Jensen et al., 2000) relates to the importance of listening. Skilled clinicians claim that they "got much more information from listening than from structuring questions" and that "if you go in and listen to the clients, they will tell you" (p. 33). It is very powerful for the client to feel your complete presence.

Active listening skills are also relevant in other situations and can clarify miscommunication and de-escalate conflict. Consider this scenario: A busy phlebotomist enters a client's room to draw blood and discovers the speech-language pathologist in the midst of treatment. Knowing how many clients he still needs to see, he demands emotionally, "You'll have to stop for a minute. I need to draw blood immediately. I'm in a hurry." Although the therapist may have the urge to respond in kind, anger will not resolve the situation and may even inflame it. The potential conflict may be diffused by a process of active listening, which includes a three-step framework: restatement, reflection, and clarification (Davis, 2006). Through this process, listeners let speakers know they were heard and understood: "I understand that you're in a hurry and want to see this client immediately." Listeners then describe how they think the speaker feels and gives him or her the opportunity to clarify feelings: "It sounds like you're having a hectic day and are upset." Finally, the listener summarises the situation and asks for a potential solution: "We can stop for a moment or two and let you draw some blood" or "We'll be done in about fifteen minutes, if you want to come back." Either response would reduce conflict and allow both health care providers to proceed with client care, always a primary concern. Ask yourself: What are the medical priorities? What would most benefit the client at this time? Active listening is a challenging skill to develop and requires practice. When used effectively, it can improve therapeutic interactions as well as diffuse angry situations, leading to effective solutions.

It is not always easy for providers to be "therapeutic" in their approach, especially when they are the target of disappointment, frustration, and blame. Expert clinicians do not judge or categorise clients as difficult or nonadherent. Instead, they evaluate the challenge and accept the responsibility of developing alternate communication solutions (Jensen et al.,

2000). Consider Joyce, a woman with multiple sclerosis, who bellowed at the occupational therapist, "When I came here, they told me that I would be able to dress myself within a week. Well, I can't. It's all your fault! If I had a better therapist, I would be home by now." Although the therapist might reflexively respond defensively, it is therapeutically beneficial to take a different approach. In this case, the occupational therapist could say, "I understand that when you first came to this hospital, you thought you'd be able to take care of yourself. You now see that this will take more time and be more involved than you anticipated. You sound frustrated. Unfortunately, there are no quick solutions. We have to work on your balance and strength so that you're able to be more independent."

How will you react the next time you are confronted by an angry client or colleague? Keep in mind that clients sometimes just need to talk to express their fear, anger, or frustration with their illness, injury, or disability. Providers may be called on to listen therapeutically, without responding, to affirm that what clients are experiencing is normal and understandable, even if the clients need to repeat the story multiple times to everyone with whom they come in contact (Halstead, 2001).

Clinicians should be aware that when they are under stress they may be tempted to respond inappropriately. When emotionally upset, providers should recognise their feelings, take responsibility for their actions, and not blame others. Not all situations will work out the way we would like, even for expert clinicians. People are emotional; they may become angry and frustrated and verbally "strike out" when they feel they cannot control a situation. Providers must do their best to maintain a level head and respond appropriately to clients, family members, and other health care professionals. If, however, a health care professional says something inappropriate, a well-timed apology is in order. These strategies not only improve communication capabilities but also allow health care professionals to provide more effective client care.

On occasion, professional caregivers may feel anger or resentment toward their clients. Recognise that this is a normal reaction. To be compassionate with our clients, we need to recognise and respond to our own feelings and needs (Halstead, 2001). Studies have shown that health providers who practice meditation, mindfulness, and/or participate in reflective writing are less likely to lose perspective or experience burnout on the job. They are also more likely to be engaged with their clients and coworkers, be less judgemental of themselves and others, be more empathetic, have a greater sense of self-actualisation, and be better appreciated by their clients (Kearney et al., 2009).

Nonverbal communication

Although verbal communication is important, people also convey messages without saying a word. It is imperative to "tune in" to the nonverbal cues we give and receive. If we are unaware of the nonverbal signals we send to clients, we may inadvertently jeopardise our therapeutic relationships. Open to ambiguous interpretation and not always easy to understand, nonverbal communication strongly influences the perceived meaning of messages. For example, a provider enters a client's room and finds him in tears. Should the clinician immediately assume the client is depressed about his condition? Should the health care provider leave and avoid interacting? Instead, he opens a dialogue and discovers that these are tears of joy over news of a new grandchild. This information may motivate him to achieve the goal of returning home. It is important to verify assumptions and not accept seemingly pat conclusions. By reading body language, tone of voice, pacing of speech, and other forms of paralanguage, we can better hear the message and "read between the lines" (Coulehan & Block, 2001).

Facial expressions

Facial expressions are important because they convey emotions. Following a biopsy, a frightened client is alert to the expression on the doctor's face as she walks into the room to announce the diagnosis. Is the news good or bad? Afraid and lacking information, we attempt to learn what we can by watching people. Research shows that fear, sadness, and anger are identified by looking at one's eyes, whereas happiness and disgust are best identified by looking at an individual's mouth (Ekman, 1999). What do the health care providers' facial expressions convey to clients? What do clients' expressions convey to the health care provider?

When treating a client, it is important to be aware of the expression on the person's face. Consider the adage, "The eyes are the mirror of the soul." Is the person in pain? Does he or she wince when moved from the bed to the chair? Some clients will report when they feel pain; others are stoic and silent. Observing facial expressions and nonverbal language and communicating with clients assists providers in better understanding what clients may be thinking and feeling.

Touch

Touch is another form of nonverbal communication. In health care settings, providers touch clients to examine, evaluate, treat, and comfort them. In fact, as health care professionals, we often have intimate contact with clients that otherwise would be restricted to their significant others.

There are several forms of touch. *Procedural* or *instrumental* touch occurs when our hands come in contact with clients, as we carry out interventions, such as moving a client into bed, performing range-of-motion exercises, or drawing blood. *Expressive* or *caring* touch involves contact that is meant to convey emotional support. This may include resting a hand on a client's arm or shoulder (Barringer & Glod, 1998; Routasalo, 1999). Although expressive or caring touch may be "therapeutic," it should not be confused with the complementary/alternative approach known as *therapeutic touch*. This is a technique in which a health care practitioner combines mindfulness, intent, and hand movements to promote healing by balancing energy fields. Hands may be placed directly on the skin, over clothing, or several inches above the client's body (Hayes & Cox, 1999; Herdtner, 2000; Monroe, 2009; Umbreit, 2000).

Health professionals' touching style is influenced by their cultural backgrounds, previous experience, and education. Although many studies show that touch has a calming and comforting effect on clients, individual responses to touch vary, depending on age, gender, parts of the body being touched, physical environment, cultural heritage, prior experience, and personal interpretation of the meaning of the touch (Monroe, 2009; Routasalo, 1999).

Like verbal communication, the true meaning of a touch may be misinterpreted by either a client or health care provider. Touch that is intended to be comforting may be perceived as controlling or as a sexual advance (Schacher, Stalker, & Teram, 1999). Therefore, it is important to inform clients about what you are going to do and the reason for it. Touch should be firm enough to let the client feel safe and secure but should not be so firm as to cause unnecessary discomfort. We constantly need to assess how clients are responding to our touch. Do they withdraw? Do they appear physically or emotionally uncomfortable? If so, clarify the response with them. Keep the lines of communication open.

Spatial distances/proxemics

Spatial distances also convey nonverbal information. Sitting down to speak with someone seated in a wheelchair puts you at the same level as the client and conveys equality and respect. Standing over clients and talking down to them may convey a message of superiority. Standing in a doorway to talk to clients may imply that you are too busy to interact with them or do not really care what they have to say. Moving closer to clients sends a positive message that, as a health care provider, you are interested.

The concept of *proxemics* represents another aspect of spatial distances. Proxemics identifies the distances we maintain while communicating with others. These distances may vary depending on culture. However, according to Davis (2009), proxemics generally involves four different zones of space: intimate, personal, social, and public. Interactions within different spaces may evoke different meanings for clients, varying from feelings of comfort to those of discomfort, depending on the individual's previous experiences and the relationships with health care providers. When providing health care interventions, we frequently enter intimate or personal zones, and this should be done with great sensitivity. For example, one could say, "May I please hold your arm so that I can obtain your blood pressure?"

Distracting behaviours

Constantly checking your watch, answering telephone calls, responding to pagers, or talking with others while you are with clients conveys a message that you are really too busy to be with them, have other things to do, or are disinterested. Clients may become uncomfortable and feel unimportant. They may fail to relay valuable information because they do not want to "hold you up" or think you do not care. Although there are times when clinicians need to respond to outside distractions, these need to be prioritised and limited.

It is important to remember that clients and families do not always share the perspective or priorities of health care providers (Woltersdorf, 1998). Whereas the latter are usually goal centred, clients and family members tend to be emotionally centred. Through listening, observing, and avoiding distracting behaviours before speaking, providers can learn about clients' emotional needs and discover how best to help them.

Written communication

Written communication is extremely important in the health care setting. For example, letters are written to doctors to describe client progress, to third-party payers to justify treatments and request equipment, and to other health care professionals who are collaborating in client care. In addition, information is recorded in the medical record, and written instructions are given to clients to assist them in following recommended suggestions and home care programs.

One advantage of written over verbal communication is that printed material is more permanent (Vanderhoff, 2005). Providers can refer to notes to review client progress. Clients can refer to the written word to remind them, for example, about what medications to take and when. They can review the information at their own pace, as often as necessary. However, when preparing written information, the target readers must be kept in mind. Many studies have identified incongruities in the reading levels of written health care materials and the literacy skills of the intended audience (McCray, 2005). Write to your audience; use appropriate, culturally sensitive terminology; and ensure that the information is accurate, clear, concise, understandable, and legible.

Electronic communication

The media is a significant shaper of values and attitudes. It is becoming increasingly more common for health care professionals and clients to provide and/or access information via television and radio broadcasts and Internet websites rather than through print media such as newspapers, magazines, and bulletins. Electronic communication is transforming the way health care professionals and clients gather information and interact with one another. Clinical decision-making software and online sources of medical information that clients explore are two examples. Rapid Internet access and inexpensive web cameras have made videoconferencing possible, and that same technology allows professionals to assess situations, such as the status of a wound, without additional clinic visits (Jadad & Delamothe, 2004).

An important consideration for using electronic forms of communication is that transmissions can be intercepted by unintended audiences, thereby making confidentiality a paramount concern. In addition, clients may obtain information from websites that present inaccurate data. You can provide an important professional service by instructing clients about the best ways to assess the quality and reliability of medically related websites.

Many clients and practitioners now prefer to communicate by electronic mail (e-mail), a trend that is becoming more prevalent because it allows individuals to ask or answer questions any time of the day or night (Kummervold, Trondsen, Andreassen, Gammon, & Hjortdahl, 2004). Because there is no opportunity to read nonverbal cues through e-mail, it is important to ensure that messages are as clear as possible. Utilise professional communication skills with formal salutations and closings, appropriate terminology, correct punctuation, and dictionary spelling for all words. Read your message prior to sending, and correct any errors or potential sources of misinterpretation. Remember that e-mail communications become an official part of clients' medical records as well as an important indication of your professionalism and clinical abilities.

Electronic communication can be a detriment or boon for people with disabilities and those who are ageing. Not everyone is computer literate or has access. Helping clients to gain access to electronic aids such as print magnifiers, talking computers, and other forms of assistive technology can provide flexibility and improve access to information that can be used to improve health and wellness.

Using humour to communicate

Many strategies are used to assist in developing relationships with clients. When used appropriately, humour can be one of them. It may open the lines of communication, decrease stress, and establish a sense of camaraderie. Humour has been shown to be an effective coping strategy for clients and their family members, as well as health care providers. In addition, it has been shown to increase job productivity (Wanzer, Booth-Butterfield, & Booth-Butterfield, 2005) and decrease the number of malpractice claims filed (Levinson, Roter, Mullooly, Dull, & Frankel, 1997). Effective use of humour has also been shown to lead to more positive perceived or actual outcomes (Cann, Zapata, & Davis, 2009). Although humour does not *solve* problems, it can diminish their impact.

Laughter involves every major system in the body. When you laugh, you enjoy yourself, blissfully unaware of the release of catecholamine, which will boost your alertness and enhance your ability to solve problems. You probably are not focusing on how your dilated blood vessels, increased heart rate, and circulation are spreading a high-density lipoprotein throughout your body, which may lower your risk of heart disease. Your lungs expand, bringing in more oxygen and expelling more carbon dioxide than you did before you laughed. Your muscular tension is released, as you exercise your diaphragm, facial, upper extremity, thoracic, and abdominal muscles, and stress hormones are lowered (Hassed, 2001).

Schmitt's (1990) research indicated that most clients welcome laughter. The majority of clients in her survey strongly agreed with its benefits, stating, "Laughing helps me get through difficult times," "Sometimes, laughing works as well as a pain pill," "When I laugh, I feel better," "I appreciate an opportunity to laugh when I feel sad," and "Rehabilitation hospitals should encourage laughter to help clients feel better about their stay" (p. 145). Clients perceive that nurses who laugh with them are being therapeutic.

When used inappropriately, however, humour may interfere with communication or offend others (Cann et al., 2009). At its extreme, it may even cause psychological harm. Struggling to maintain his sitting balance, a 25-year-old man with a traumatic brain injury wildly threw a ball, which landed far from the desired target. The recreation therapist responded, "Well, we won't be picking *you* to pitch on the centre's team." Although she was trying to lighten his mood, the client, a former semiprofessional baseball player, took this message to heart and became quite depressed. He refused to "try again," thus setting back his progress.

Inappropriate humour may antagonise and alienate people. Once this has occurred, it can be difficult or impossible to reestablish a therapeutic relationship. Make sure you know and understand your client prior to injecting humour into your conversation. If a client appears offended by something you said, apologise, assure the client that you meant no disrespect, and be sure to avoid such topics in the future. Attempt to reestablish a sense of rapport and mutual respect with the client. If, over time, you believe that is impossible, the client may benefit by having his or her care transferred to someone else.

Think about the potential impact of humour. Try to put yourself in the position of the client, friend, or family member. Does the humour have the same effect on you as it did before? Clients are in a vulnerable position when they come to you. Although humour can be an excellent communication tool when used in a therapeutic manner, it can also have undesirable effects. You may be unaware of where sensitive areas lie. Avoid jokes related to gender, politics, religion, culture, or sexual orientation. When integrating humour into health care interactions, it is wise to proceed with caution.

Barriers to effective communication

Role uncertainty

Communication can be negatively affected by a number of factors, including role uncertainty. Clients may not know what we expect of them and not know what to expect from us. For example, older clients may expect health professionals to be somewhat paternalistic and willingly hand over the responsibility for their health and well-being to their health care providers. More commonly, clients and health professionals expect to work collaboratively in treatment planning. This may be uncomfortable for older clients, who want to be told what to do and may be reluctant to ask questions. They may appear passive to a younger generation of clinicians. It is important to encourage them to assume a more active role in their health care.

In an inpatient setting, clients often have contact with many different professionals during the course of a day. Team members may have different expectations for them, providing them with conflicting information, further contributing to their role uncertainty. Another complicating factor is that everyone is in a hurry, which may confuse clients, who may hesitate to ask questions or discuss physical or psychosocial concerns because they do not want to bother their providers (Northouse & Northouse, 1998).

Sensory overload

Sensory overload may adversely affect both receptive and expressive communication (Purtilo & Haddad, 2007). Are directions understandable, amidst a frightening environment of intravenous poles and buzzing machines? Institutional smells, distracting visual stimuli, and unfamiliar touch can bombard clients' senses. As a result, they may become unable to organise their thoughts to effectively communicate and may leave a health care provider's office not really understanding what the provider said or knowing what they are expected to do next. People process information at varying rates. Instructions to a client may seem abundantly clear to us, but they may not be easy for others to fathom. Providers can help diminish sensory overload by meeting clients one on one in a quiet room and eliminating distractions.

Voice and word choice

It is important to give clear, simple instructions using a tone and volume that are easy to hear and comprehend. Whenever possible, provide clients with written instructions, including pictures, if this enhances understanding. Providers may ask the client to repeat directions or demonstrate a task. If the instructions are for home use, ask, "Can you picture yourself doing this on your own at home?" If the client says no, ask why not. This creates an opportunity to promote understanding and allow clients to voice questions or concerns in a safe environment. Whenever possible, give clients a period of time to think about the instructions. Review them at the next session and ask for a demonstration to determine whether the client truly understands or has any questions.

Physical appearance

Consider the saying "First impressions are lasting." People often judge others based on their appearance, which may include height, weight, hairstyle, clothing, skin colour, piercings, tattoos, accessories, and physical attractiveness. We tend to gravitate to individuals who are similar to ourselves and may have overt or covert biases against those who differ from us. Providers need to recognise that seeing the client as being "similar to" or "different from" themselves may affect their emotional and cognitive responses to a situation (Garden, 2008). Health care professionals need to be aware of their own biases and refrain from making judgements about clients based on physical appearances. Conversely, providers should realise that their first impression of clients may affect relationships. Uniforms, stethoscopes, and other tools of the trade convey messages. Although a professional appearance may help inspire trust and confidence in clients and allay a measure of anxiety, it may create a barrier for others.

Sometimes health providers misinterpret the functional impact of apparent physical limitations. One study examined people who were blind or visually impaired to determine barriers to effective health care (O'Day, Killeen, & Iezzoni, 2004). The two barriers the researchers identified were (1) the assumption made by health providers that clients who are blind or visually impaired would not be able to fully participate in their own care, and (2) the failure of providers to have written materials available in alternative formats, including Braille, large print, or audiotape. Failure to accommodate different abilities in health care, such as providing wheelchair-accessible examination rooms and alternative forms of communication, demonstrates a bias toward "ableism," which can cause people with disabilities to feel unwelcome. Conversely, developing universally accessible services demonstrates respect for differences and facilitates access and participation for all clients.

Gender differences

Differences in communication styles between men and women can lead to misinterpretation of messages (James & Cinelli, 2003). In general, women like to talk to others when they have a problem or need to make a decision, whereas men like to keep their problems to themselves. Women tend to be relationship oriented and want to connect with others more so than men do. To men, status and dominance are often more important than relationship building. Women tend to ask questions to build rapport, whereas men like to tell others what to do and provide information rather than asking questions. When women are involved in disagreements, there is great potential for disruption of the relationship that exists between the opposing parties. When men disagree, they tend to express their disagreement, move on to other topics, and forget about it. Disagreements rarely impact other aspects of their relationships. As listeners, women tend to nod their heads to indicate they are listening, whereas men only nod their heads when they agree with the speaker (Lieberman, 2010).

Loscalzo (1999) studied the communication styles of men and women who were being treated for cancer. He found that women tend to be better communicators than men, who tend to compartmentalise their lives. During times of stress, women want to talk about what is happening, while men would rather not. What seems to help men is to have a plan for solving problems and getting on with life. Whereas most women enjoy communicating about problems and joining support groups, men want health care providers to help them identify problems and come up with solutions. Loscalzo also found that women generally cope with a cancer diagnosis better than men, both as clients and as caregivers. Men are frequently unwilling to join support groups, and when they do, they use the group for educational purposes only. Conversely, women use support groups to share experiences and encourage one another.

Although certain characteristics of communication are attributable to men and others to women, it is important to realise that most people are able to adapt communication styles to fit specific needs. Very few people use one style all of the time. This concept is demonstrated in health care through the practice of *safety culture*. Safety culture refers to a set of professional behaviours designed to deliberately avoid the influence of status, gender, and other social or cultural norms in favor of "best practices" for communication in health care (Carney, West, Neily, Mills, & Bagian, 2010).

Students and health care professionals will most likely find differences in communication styles between men and women, as well as between those of different professions. Recognising your own communication style and adapting it to meet the existing circumstances are of utmost importance to ensure positive client outcomes. Whereas women may be more comfortable making decisions via consensus, and men may be more comfortable giving orders, each may need to move out of his or her comfort zone and communicate using a less familiar style to ensure effective communication. Table 10.2 provides an overview of male versus female communication styles.

Table 10.2 Gender differences in communication

Male communication style	Female communication style
Give information/report	Collect information/gain rapport
Talk about things (sports, business)	Talk about people
Focus on facts, reason, and logic	Focus on feelings, senses, and meaning
Thrive on competition	Thrive on harmony and relating
"Know" by analysing and figuring things out	"Know" by intuition
Assertive	Cooperative
Seek intellectual understanding	
Focused, specific, and logical	Holistic—"wise angled"
Comfortable with rules, order, structure	Comfortable with fluidity
Want to think	Want to feel

Source: Simon & Pedersen (2005).

Cultural barriers

As stated earlier, individuals are usually more comfortable with people from a similar culture. They may even inadvertently be biased and treat people from other cultures differently. In fact, a review of the literature on cultural differences in medical communication revealed that during doctor/patient encounters, White doctors behaved less effectively when interacting with patients from minority groups than with those who were White, and patients from minority groups were less expressive or assertive during the medical encounter than their White counterparts (Schouten & Meeuwesen, 2006).

In today's multicultural environment, language barriers affect one's ability to communicate effectively. If a client speaks a different language, it is important to provide a professional interpreter to assist with the communication process. Family members are usually not the most appropriate resource. Clients do not always want to discuss their concerns in front of family. In certain cultures, for example, men prefer not to reveal their problems to their wives or children. In addition, well-intentioned family members may edit or misinterpret messages being translated (Misra-Hebert, 2003).

Beyond language, other cultural influences affect communication, including differences in values, beliefs, emotions, and nonverbal cues. People from some cultures are encouraged to cry when they feel pain; individuals from other cultures are discouraged from doing so and may, in fact, hide their pain. This could certainly affect treatment interventions. In cross-cultural encounters, providers need to understand the client's interpretation of authority figures, the use of physical contact, communication style, and the role of gender, sexuality, and the family in decision making. Failure to appropriately interpret this information can adversely affect health outcomes (Misra-Hebert, 2003).

Ideally, administrators should recruit and hire health professionals who share languages and cultures with the people who live in the communities being served. However, this may not be feasible due to lower representation of minority cultures in health care professions. Therefore, health providers are advised to learn as much as possible about the cultures and languages of the communities they serve. In all settings, the use of clear, culturally appropriate written instructions, complete with pictures or videotapes/DVDs and available in various languages, greatly enhances communication between clients and providers (Thompson et al., 2007).

Improving the cultural competence of health care providers is one way of responding to the demographic changes in the United States and decreasing health disparities (Teal & Street, 2009). Research has shown that culturally competent communication skills can be taught and, when implemented in the clinical setting, improve patient care (Misra-Hebert, 2003). It has also been suggested that courses on communication skills training, which include role-playing and facilitation by experienced trainers, should be required in all health professional education programs (Stiefel et al., 2010).

Conflict

Health care providers interact daily with clients, families, colleagues, insurance providers, and others. Everyone brings his or her background, culture, beliefs, and goals into the workplace, and viewpoints vary. Even when people share similar goals, they may have different perspectives and priorities regarding those goals. Conflict becomes inevitable (Xu & Davidhizar, 2004). Although some people seem to thrive on conflict, many are uncomfortable with it and either try to avoid it or handle it poorly. To manage conflict effectively, we need to change our own behaviour or alter the situation.

Despite the negative connotations of conflict, it has both positive and negative elements. Managed appropriately, conflict can lead to positive changes, such as decreased stress levels, improved staff cohesiveness, job satisfaction, and creative problem solving. Ignored, avoided, or poorly managed conflict negatively affects all people involved. It can permeate an organisation, group, or relationship, decreasing everyone's ability to work effectively (Lipcamon & Mainwaring, 2004). Sometimes, coworkers are able to adequately resolve their issues independently. At other times, the assistance of managers, supervisors, or neutral third parties is required.

Conflict involves tension or disagreement between two or more opposing forces. It is a process in which one party perceives that its interests are being opposed or negatively affected by another. Once that occurs, people need to decide how to deal with the situation, even if their choice is to do nothing. If they respond emotionally, actions will lead to reactions and conflict is under way.

In the health care system, individuals work both independently and interdependently. Opinions about the most appropriate form of care may differ. In one study of clinical decision making in intensive care units, physicians and nurses identified conflict during patient management discussions (Coombs, 2003). In another study with more than 200 patients in intensive care, doctors and nurses documented 248 conflicts concerning vital matters of patient care, as well as disputes between teams and families, among team members, and among family members (Studdert et al., 2003). Time constraints and limited resources influence decision making. As health professionals work together to provide client-centred care, roles may overlap and lines of authority for ultimate decision making may blur. Conflict is often a by-product. Consider the conflict described in this case:

> My supervisor reprimanded me this morning in front of a client and his daughter. I was so embarrassed! I became so nervous that my hands were shaking as I tried to continue with the treatment. I knew Mr. Chen had lost all confidence in my abilities. He looked as if he feared I was going to hurt him. His daughter asked me if I was sure I knew what I was doing. Finally, my supervisor suggested I leave and finish up some paperwork while he completed the treatment. I left the room and ran to the ladies' room in tears to compose myself. Later in the day, my supervisor acted as if nothing had happened. We continued to treat other patients. I was anxious and afraid I would make another mistake, but I didn't say anything to him.
>
> Tonight, I talked with my roommate. She told me that I should meet with my supervisor first thing in the morning and discuss the situation. I know she's right. I can accept constructive criticism, but I think he handled it inappropriately. He could have directed me to correct my error and then talked to me later in the staff room, away from the client and his daughter. The client's safety wasn't at risk. As much as I hate confrontation and would like to pretend this never happened, I know my roommate is right. If I don't say something, I'll always be afraid that he'll do this to me again, and my ability to learn will be in jeopardy. He probably doesn't even know how he made me feel.
>
> —*From the journal of Shannon Sullivan, nursing student*

Although Shannon would have preferred to ignore this situation, she realised that strategy would not solve her problem and could negatively affect her educational experience and her ability to treat clients effectively. If she is able to discuss her feelings and situation with her supervisor, she may be able to develop a better working relationship with him. Together, they could develop learning objectives and discuss appropriate feedback mechanisms. Shannon might be more at ease treating clients in the presence of her supervisor, and she could learn how to improve her nursing skills from him.

Levels of conflict

Conflict can occur at personal, interpersonal, intragroup, or intergroup levels, as discussed in the following sections.

Personal conflict

At the personal level, conflict occurs within an individual (Dove, 1998). He or she may receive pressure from colleagues to do something that is not in accordance with his or her personal value system. For example, a supervisor may suggest that an occupational therapist delegate portions of a client's treatment to an occupational therapy assistant in order to increase productivity. The occupational therapist may believe that the client requires the attention and skills of a therapist and that it is inappropriate to delegate this part of the care. As a result, the occupational therapist may feel internal personal conflict and have to decide whether to adhere to the supervisor's suggestion or confront the supervisor to discuss the situation. The ultimate decision will be influenced by how strongly the occupational therapist feels about the level of care needed, the experience of both the occupational therapist and the assistant, and the conflict-management style the occupational therapist uses in this situation.

An individual may also experience interrole conflicts at a personal level. Consider Tim Gallagher, a nurse in the intensive care unit in a large urban hospital. Toward the end of his shift, Tim hurries to complete paperwork, ignoring the patients' call buttons buzzing around him. Other nurses leave their documentation to respond to the patients' needs. While Tim always leaves on time, the other nurses work overtime to complete their duties. Although they do not confront Tim, they vent their anger among themselves. When one of the nurses finally tells him how much the others resent his behaviour, he informs her that he is a single parent, caring for two preschool-age children. If he does not pick the children up at the day care centre at the appointed time, he is charged a penalty for each minute he is late. He cannot afford to be late. Torn between his parental role of needing to get his children on time and his professional role of being a team player and attending to client care and documentation, Tim may be experiencing personal conflict of an interrole nature. This conflict is causing internal stress for him and creating an interpersonal conflict between Tim and the other nurses.

Interpersonal conflict

Conflict develops at the interpersonal level when two or more individuals exhibit conflicting values or beliefs (Dove, 1998). For example, interpersonal conflicts frequently occur between nursing home staff members and residents' family members (Nelson & Cox, 2003; Pillemer, Hegeman, Albright, & Henderson, 1998). Nursing homes are structured organisations with rules and regulations. Sometimes they appear to provide impersonal client care. Family members, however, may provide more personal, albeit infrequent, care. Discrepancies about what is best for the client may arise. While staff members focus on the technical aspects of care, families may perceive that the emotional components are lacking and that their experiences are undervalued. Similarly, staff members might feel unappreciated by families. Because many nursing home residents, especially those with cognitive impairments, are unable to provide accurate information about their experiences, well-intentioned families may misinterpret what they see. Interpersonal conflict may ensue. If time restrictions further limit communication between staff and families, minor interpersonal conflicts can escalate into larger problems (Pillemer et al., 1998).

Intragroup conflict

Intragroup conflict exists when members within a group disagree with each other as to what course of action should be taken (Dove, 1998). Consider the Minelli family. For more than 10 years, Mr. Minelli has been caring for his wife at home. As her Alzheimer's disease has progressed, she has started to wander and is becoming combative. Mr. Minelli is seeking advice from his children. Of the six adult children in the family, three of them work in health care. Only the youngest daughter lives nearby.

The local daughter is the mother of five young children and has a husband who frequently travels for business. Experiencing interrole conflict between her roles as a mother, wife, and daughter, she cares for her nuclear family, while cleaning her parents' house and doing their laundry and shopping. Exhausted and frustrated, she suggested to her father that he consider placing her mother in a nursing home. The oldest son, who is a pediatrician, disagrees and has offered to pay for daytime respite care. The oldest daughter, who is a nurse, agrees with her younger sister. She believes her mother would receive excellent care in a long-term facility and that her father would be relieved of the burden. The youngest son, who is a pharmacist, thinks that everyone should "chip in" to build an apartment for the parents at his sister's house, making it easier for her to assist them. His sister's husband does not support this idea.

This family is experiencing intragroup conflict, and it is tearing them apart. Mr. Minelli wants to do whatever is best for his wife, but he does not know what that is. He loves his children and does not want to hurt their feelings, yet he is unable to make a decision. Siblings have heated arguments over the telephone and by e-mail correspondence. Alliances and counteralliances have developed. If the conflict remains unresolved, the family may be further torn apart. The Minelli family may need a neutral party, such as a social worker, to mediate the situation.

Intergroup conflict

Intergroup conflict arises between two or more groups of people, departments, or organisations that have conflicting beliefs or needs (Dove, 1998). Consider Carmen Garcia, a 94-year-old woman recovering from a motor vehicle accident in which she sustained multiple fractures and internal injuries. She was in both the intensive care and medical/surgical units for several weeks and is now ready to be discharged from the acute care hospital. The health care team recommended that she go to a transitional care unit, where she will receive nursing care and therapy to increase her strength and endurance. In contrast, Mrs. Garcia and her family want her to go home. Her children and grandchildren believe that their cultural values oblige them to care for her at home, out of respect for her position in the family and their love.

Members of the health care team are quite concerned about the family's ability to care for Mrs. Garcia at home because she is weak and cannot bear weight on her casted right leg. She also has a fracture of her left humerus. Hospital staff members fear that either she will be further injured at home or that a family member will get hurt trying to help her.

The meeting between the two groups was confrontational. Even though a social worker attempted to mediate the situation, members of both groups refused to change their positions. Christmas was fast approaching, and both Mrs. Garcia and her family believed that this would be her last one at home. They wanted to spend it together in a family environment, not in the cafeteria of a health facility. The family ultimately brought Mrs. Garcia home, discharged against medical advice.

Sources of conflict

Conflicts include content, psychological, and procedural components (Moore, 1996). *Content issues* are related to specific factors, such as time and money. In the managed health care environment, a primary care physician may be in conflict with an insurance provider over how long a client may be able to stay in an acute care hospital following surgery. A physical therapist and a parent may be in conflict over the appropriate care of a child.

> I visited my client and her family today. It was time to discuss the possibility of ordering a wheelchair for Brenda. Her mother became extremely insistent that Brenda's stroller was just fine for getting her around and that the use of a wheelchair would make her appear much more disabled. By using a trial wheelchair and some accessories I had available, I was able to demonstrate to Brenda's mother that Brenda could be significantly more functional and less disabled if her posture was improved. To my surprise, the demonstration proved convincing!
>
> —*From the journal of Ron Johansen, physical therapist student*

By reframing the above situation, Ron was able to suggest an alternate perspective. The wheelchair became a symbol of independence rather than disability.

Psychological elements of conflict are multidimensional and include trust, respect, and the desire for inclusion (Moore, 1996). Involving clients, families, and appropriate care providers in decision making, introducing change slowly, and encouraging feedback can help reduce conflict (Davidhizar, Giger, & Poole, 1997). Using active listening techniques can also improve communication and diminish conflict. Listening to concerns and ideas attentively, eliminating unnecessary interruptions, and ensuring confidentiality will help cultivate a sense of trust. Providing adequate information and showing respect for everyone increases the probability that all involved will be able to manage conflict without the need for outside interventions (Purtilo & Haddad, 2007).

Procedural components of conflict involve policies, the chain of command, and decision-making responsibility. When policies are unclear, individuals may interpret them differently, resulting in conflicting views as to the appropriate course of action. Because content, psychological, and procedural components are interrelated, a conflict cannot be completely resolved until all three elements in this "satisfaction triangle" have been addressed (Moore, 1996).

Conflict can emanate from many sources. As discussed earlier, differing personal beliefs, goals, interests, and values may lead to conflict. Possible incompatibilities, based on temperaments, race, religion, culture, or other biases, may also result in conflict. Members of different cultures view conflict in different ways, a factor that must be taken into consideration when dealing with both clients and colleagues (Nibler & Harris, 2003; Xu & Davidhizar, 2004).

There is much ambiguity in health care. Individuals interpret available information in different ways, depending on their backgrounds and life experiences. Clients may be uncertain about options and potential outcomes. Decisions are complex, because many individuals are involved at different levels, which can result in competition for power, prestige, and status.

Lack of communication and unclear expectations are also sources of conflict. For example, in health care settings, clients may receive conflicting information from different staff members. Consider Nancy, a new mother who is having difficulty breast-feeding. Nurses on each of three successive shifts have offered her different and conflicting strategies. She is frustrated, confused, and anxious.

E-mail communication may also be a source of conflict. E-mail interactions lack both the verbal and nonverbal cues of face-to-face communication, leaving room for misinterpretation. In addition, people may be tempted to respond instantaneously to e-mail messages, rather than taking the time to consider what they are going to say. To prevent unnecessary conflict, it is important to follow-up on e-mail messages with telephone calls and face-to-face meetings to clarify questions or concerns (Umiker, 1997; Zweibel & Goldstein, 2001).

Life circumstances may also create conflict (Northouse & Northouse, 1998). For example, in contemporary society, family members often live long distances from each other, creating a geographic barrier when adult children attempt to assist parents with medical problems. Older adults sometimes fail to ask pertinent questions of their health care providers and, therefore, clients may not receive the services they need. Consider Ramona, a medical assistant working in southern California. Her elderly parents were both ill and living on the east coast. Ramona's mother had heart problems and required dialysis treatments twice a week. Her father had difficulty walking after having bilateral total hip replacements. In addition, he had a long history of smoking and emphysema.

Ramona became very frustrated when her attempts to contact her parents' primary care physician by e-mail were unsuccessful. She believed that the physician was not doing everything he could to help her parents. She made arrangements to fly home to accompany them to their next appointment. After Ramona described how much difficulty her parents were having, the physician immediately recommended a homemaker to assist with routine housekeeping and a company to provide meals. The doctor apologised profusely, stating that he was unaware of the difficulties Ramona's parents were having at home. In the end, enhanced communication made it possible for appropriate resources to be put into place.

Lack of advance directives from a legally incompetent client may be another source of conflict. Questions may exist about what is the "right" or "best" thing to do. Health care providers and clients' medical care surrogates do not always agree about the most appropriate care for a client who is unable to express his or her own wishes. Alpers and Lo (1999) describe a client who no longer had decision-making capabilities and had not left a clear advance directive. The family claimed that the client believed in the sanctity of life. Despite no hope for recovery, family members wanted the health care providers to prolong his life as long as possible. The health care professionals thought that the client was enduring unnecessary pain and suffering while life support systems kept him alive. Although his wife agreed with the health care team in principle, she would not go against the wishes of her children. This case illustrates the stress that family surrogates may experience and the need to provide them with the support and information required to help them make wise decisions.

Strategies to manage conflict

Four elements affect the outcome of conflict: the issues at hand, cooperation among involved parties, the power bases of the participants, and the effectiveness of their communication skills (Miller, 1998). When conflict concerns relatively minor issues, cooperation and resolution may be fast and easy. At other times, conflict is related to substantive issues, where individuals or groups interpret facts differently, have opposing goals, or disagree on acceptable methods. When conflicting parties disagree on principles, cooperation may be nonexistent and resolution more difficult to achieve.

Although many health care professionals consider clinical skills as being most important for competent practice, they sometimes fail to recognise that communication and the ability to manage conflict successfully are of primary importance in ensuring effective health care outcomes (Pettrey, 2003). This is especially true in today's health care environment where there is an emphasis on interdisciplinary care. There is a tendency for individuals to "band together" in a "us" against "them" mentality. This can result in intragroup and intergroup conflict. Teams that work together to openly discuss differences and solve problems are much more effective than those that set up competitive goals (Alper, Tjosvold, & Law, 1998).

The ability to communicate effectively greatly assists people and groups in resolving conflicts. It is imperative to focus on the pertinent issues and avoid blaming and name-calling. When participants lose focus, the number of issues involved tends to expand, and the emphasis shifts toward winning rather than compromising. People begin to attack each other rather than the issues. Power tactics, including coercion and deception, are often employed.

Unfortunately, in today's society, violent behaviour is becoming more prevalent. This may occur in the inpatient, outpatient, or home care settings and may involve coworkers, clients, or clients' family members. Organisations need to update staff members so they have the necessary skills to manage violent conflict in the workplace while continuing to deliver quality patient care. Educational programs are also needed to help providers recognise the warning signs of violence and understand the appropriate use of de-escalation and other interpersonal skills to contain and manage such situations (Young & Turner, 2009).

Thomas and Kilmann (1974) identified five styles of managing conflict—*avoidance, accommodation, competition, compromise,* and *collaboration*—that continue to be studied today (Lipcamon & Mainwaring, 2004). Most authors agree that no one single strategy is best. Rather, each situation needs to be evaluated to determine which strategy would be the most effective (Eason & Brown, 1999; Henrikson, 1998; Northouse & Northouse, 1998; Umiker, 1997). Although we have the ability to utilise each of the strategies in a given situation, each of us has our own preferred style of managing conflict. Understanding the strengths and weaknesses of each strategy and learning to identify our own as well as our colleagues' and clients' preferred styles will help us become better communicators and more effective health care providers. The following section describes the strengths and liabilities of each of these styles of managing conflict.

Avoidance

Avoidance is an unassertive and uncooperative conflict management strategy in which individuals simply ignore or evade the fact that a conflict exists (Eason & Brown, 1999; Northouse & Northouse, 1998; Umiker, 1997). People who are passive and uncomfortable addressing conflict frequently use this style. Avoidance can be counterproductive, often prolonging, rather than resolving, issues and increasing stress levels. Consider a staff therapist who works in a large medical centre. As clients are referred to the department, their names are posted on the bulletin board, and therapists select them. Most of the staff members add clients to their caseloads as the names become available, but one therapist purposely avoids "difficult" clients, leaving colleagues to care for those who have more complicated needs. Other staff members recognise this but do not address the situation with him. As a result, nothing changes—the problem continues, the rest of the staff remains frustrated, and staff morale decreases.

There are times when avoidance is a positive and necessary strategy. If individuals are angry, avoidance allows for a cooling-off period. It provides people with time to gain composure and gather additional information prior to addressing the issues. If a problem is perceived to be trivial, people may prefer to ignore it rather than deal with it. In addition, some problems resolve themselves over time. In those cases, it may not be worth the time and energy needed to confront them. When a problem is out of a provider's control, he or she may want to avoid becoming involved. In health care, minor conflicts might need to be set aside to ensure effective client care.

Accommodation

Accommodation is an unassertive but cooperative approach to conflict management. A person neglects his or her own needs to meet the needs of others. Those who seek constant approval frequently use this strategy (Eason & Brown, 1999; Henrikson, 1998; Northouse & Northouse, 1998; Umiker, 1997). Although this approach may appear to promote harmony and solve conflicts quickly, it may also be superficial and temporary. People who constantly accommodate may feel angry and frustrated because they failed to seize the opportunity to express their own thoughts, opinions, and feelings. For example, Shelley, a respiratory therapist, initially volunteered to work on major holidays so that her colleagues, whose extended families live out of state, could have the time off. What began as "team player behaviour" became expected by the staff. Now, harboring feelings of frustration, she would like to have a holiday off but continues to accommodate colleagues' expectations. A better resolution may have emerged if Shelley had expressed her feelings, and the group had taken the time to consider alternative solutions.

Accommodation is an appropriate strategy to use when one realises that the other party is right or when there is little chance of "winning." It can also be used when one party has little interest in the situation or when the outcome does not particularly affect him or her. In health care settings, accommodation may sometimes be useful to promote harmony and maintain good interpersonal relationships among staff members or interdisciplinary teams.

Competition

Competition is an aggressive, uncompromising approach to managing conflict. It is power driven and frequently used by assertive individuals interested in pursuing their own goals, even at the expense of others (Eason & Brown, 1999; Henrikson, 1998; Northouse & Northouse, 1998; Umiker, 1997). Think of a situation in which a student proposes an alternative evidence-based treatment approach rather than one an experienced practitioner has been using for many years. The supervisor refuses to consider the students' proposal or listen to the rationale, insisting that it be done her way. This style may result in quick, short-term agreements. However, the results are based upon an "I win, you lose" strategy, which may be counterproductive over time and negatively affect client outcomes.

Compromise

Compromise is a strategy midway between competition and accommodation. It includes an element of assertiveness, as well as a component of cooperation (Eason & Brown, 1999; Henrikson, 1998; Northouse & Northouse, 1998; Umiker, 1997). People who compromise use a "give-and-take" strategy. They are concerned with their own needs, as well as the needs and concerns of others, and realise that neither side can win completely. Although both parties may agree to the final outcome, neither side is perfectly satisfied with the results. Whereas this method may result in faster resolution of problems, more innovative and satisfying results may be achieved if the parties continue to negotiate.

Compromise can be an effective means of settling conflict. Consider Melissa, a 15-year-old girl with juvenile rheumatoid arthritis. Her medication made her drowsy and impaired her ability to think clearly, affecting her schoolwork. Her physician compromised and prescribed another medication that was not as effective but had fewer side effects.

Collaboration

Collaboration involves both assertiveness and cooperation. It is a problem-solving approach in which all parties want to fully address the concerns of everyone. It is designed to promote a "win–win" solution, with everyone committed to the final outcome. Participants believe that the achievement of mutual goals is more important than individual objectives (Eason & Brown, 1999; Henrikson, 1998; Northouse & Northouse, 1998; Umiker, 1997). Imagine a situation in which a manager enlists input from the entire staff to address how they might change the hours and staffing patterns of their operation. Although most authors agree that this is the preferred approach to managing conflict, it is the most difficult and often the most time consuming to achieve and, therefore, may not be appropriate in all situations.

People need to explore differences, identify commonalities, and work together to develop problem-solving strategies and initiate solutions acceptable to all involved. This requires everyone's dedication and hard work. As a result of the time and energy expended, innovative, cost-effective solutions usually result. Because both sides "win," everyone tends to feel satisfied. This helps build stronger relationships, promote trust, improve morale, decrease stress, and set the stage for more positive conflict resolution in the future.

It is important to note that the five styles of managing conflict just discussed may be used to varying degrees or in combination with one another, depending on the circumstances in each situation. A good communicator expresses his or her own viewpoints, listens carefully to the opinions of others, and works collaboratively to develop cooperative problem-solving strategies that lead to solutions acceptable to all parties (Miller, 1998; Umiker, 1997).

Mediation

Sometimes, individuals or groups may be unable to resolve conflict, and it escalates. Members of each side may try to convert otherwise neutral parties to their points of view. Stress levels increase while productivity decreases. At such junctures, mediation may be required (Fraser, 2001). A neutral third party is invited to facilitate the process. The mediator begins by developing a rapport with the parties in conflict. Once the conflict has been defined, alternative solutions are generated, with each possible solution considered until an agreement can be reached (Fraser, 2001; Rotarius & Liberman, 2000).

To be successful, individuals cannot blame one another. They must carefully listen to and understand all issues in the disagreement. For mediation to be successful, everyone has to agree from the outset to accept and implement the final decision, even if they do not agree with it.

The client interview

The first section of this chapter described the components and importance of communication. This section provides information and suggestions for putting communication skills into practice. Client-interview models and the explanatory model of care are described. Skilled health care providers can efficiently and effectively develop a client-centred plan of care when they take the time to utilise effective communication techniques and listen to their client's stories during the interview process.

I don't think that I did a very good job with my client evaluation today. It was the first time I did one on my own, so of course, I was kind of nervous. Before I got started, my supervisor and I went over the chart, the diagnosis, and the kinds of symptoms to look for. Last night, I made a careful list to make sure that I didn't leave anything out.

Somehow, even though I asked all the right questions, I did not feel like things went very well. As I read down the list of questions, she answered briefly, using just a few words each time. She seemed sort of bored and did not offer any extra information. Although there was enough data to get started on the treatment, I didn't feel like I knew much about her or what she would like to get out of our sessions. Worse still, I am not sure how to motivate her to follow through on the home exercises.

—*From the journal of Jackie Marsh, occupational therapy student*

It has been said that there are three T's in TreaTmenT. The first "T" represents the *theory* that provides the scientific and philosophical basis for what we do. The second "T" stands for *technique*, which informs us what to do and how to do it—the so-called "tools of the trade." The final "T" is for *therapeutic* alliance, which allows us to apply our theories and techniques in a collaborative way with our clients to promote effective outcomes.

Developing relationships with clients is the most essential skill that we bring to the treatment setting. It is the foundation on which we build trust, understand each client's needs, and develop individualised treatment plans (Haidet & Paterniti, 2003; Smith & Hoppe, 1991). We begin to forge these alliances as soon as we meet and greet each new client. In this chapter, we discussed the importance of communication skills. You should also consider collaborative treatment planning as a tool to support motivation and adherence. These skills provide the basis for all interactions within the health care setting and are an essential component of the client interview.

"The client interview is at the core of clinical interaction and the clinician's most important and intimate professional activity" (Kern et al., 2005, p. 65). In essence, the clinical interview is where the science of medicine joins the art of client care (Coulehan & Block, 2001; Epstein, 1999). The nature of the ideal interview is dynamic rather than static and it consists of more than just reviewing a checklist of symptoms to trigger information about clients' perceptions of their complaints. A good interviewer establishes a climate of safety in which clients feel they can discuss personal and psychosocial factors that contribute to the impact and meaning of various somatic symptoms. This information is crucial to effective client interventions. In this section, we describe the elements of a good client interview and explain how to perform one successfully.

Types of interviews

The biomedical model interview

The biomedical model of health care is founded on the premise that anatomy, physiology, pathology and other biological forces are responsible for health and illness, function and dysfunction. Therefore, the biomedical client interview was designed to identify disease or dysfunction and to determine an appropriate medical intervention (Donnelly, 1996); or, to phrase it more casually, it was concerned only with the "two Fs"—to find it and fix it (Tongue, Epps, & Forese, 2005).

Using the traditional biomedical model, health professionals have been taught to start the client interview by taking a history. They are instructed to ask open-ended questions that elicit client concerns and complaints. This is followed by the use of close-ended questions to gather specific diagnostic information. The intent is to allow the client to describe what has prompted the need for the visit and to provide increasingly specific information to determine a diagnosis and plan of care. However, this often does not proceed optimally. Studies have shown that, on average, practitioners who utilise this interviewing style interrupt clients after less than 20 seconds! Following this interruption, the provider takes control of the interview, and the client rarely has an opportunity to redirect it toward his or her concerns (Beckwith & Frankel, 1984; Lipkin, Frankel, Beckman, Charon, & Fein,1995). "The biomedical approach to medicine all too often overrides concern about patients' psychological and social experiences of illness" (Garden, 2008, p. 122).

Studies examining the biomedical interview model show that significant diagnostic information is never communicated by the client to the provider (Haidet & Paterniti, 2003; Smith & Hoppe, 1991). In part, this happens because the interviewer assumes that the first problem mentioned by the client is the most important one, and the focus quickly narrows to that issue. However, this is often not the primary problem or even the real reason that caused the client to seek medical attention (Roter & Hall, 1992). When this approach is taken, the care that is provided does not rise to the standard of evidence-based practice. Focusing only on symptoms or problems that the provider identifies as important generates biased and incomplete information, leading to inaccurate diagnoses and plans of care (Lipkin et al., 1995; Smith & Hoppe, 1991).

The biomedical interview is also designed to include social issues, sometimes known as a social history. This is where psychosocial information is usually requested. However, because the collection of information is typically provider driven within this model, questions are directed away from personal factors toward biomedical concerns (Smith & Hoppe, 1991). This lack of attention or acknowledgment of client concerns is prevalent, even in such emotionally laden settings as cancer care (Stacey, Henderson, MacArthur, & Dohan, 2009).

Consider the case of Mr. Mansur, who left an appointment with his orthopedist feeling very confused and upset. He went to the doctor because he was having pain in his knees that made walking difficult. The doctor conducted a very thorough exam, and in the process, determined that Mr. Mansur also had severe carpal tunnel syndrome. She spent the remainder of the visit discussing the importance of having surgical correction of his carpal tunnel syndrome. Because the physician judged the client's carpal tunnel syndrome to be a more serious problem than his knee pain, she lost sight of the reason why Mr. Mansur had sought medical advice and assistance in the first place. The client left the office determined to change health care professionals because this one did not understand his needs.

The client-centred interview

"True patient-centred care places increased emphasis on the therapeutic encounter between the patient and the provider" (Tripicchio, Bykerk, & Wegner, 2009, p. 55). It abolishes the power differential that can exist in the client–provider relationship and creates an equal and collaborative partnership. Each client is viewed as the expert on his or her health and is given the opportunity to be heard and respected (Roter & Hall, 1992). This paradigm necessitates shared decision making, which considers the clients' beliefs and concerns as highly as those of the care provider (Tongue et al., 2005). Thus, there is shared knowledge, control, and decision making. The client-centred interview produces significantly better results as seen by improved outcomes, including trust, adherence, and empowerment, as well as client and provider satisfaction (Garden, 2008; Haidet & Paterniti, 2003; Kleinman, Eisenberg, & Good, 1978; Platt & Platt, 2003; Smith & Hoppe, 1991; Tongue et al., 2005).

A cornerstone of client-centred care is hearing clients' stories and learning what their symptoms and discomforts mean to them (Roter & Hall, 1992). Key questions that need to be answered include these: "Who is this person?" "What does she want from our encounter?" and "How does the client perceive or understand his health?" (Coulehan et al., 2001; Epstein, 1999). A provider who facilitates client storytelling will learn information about the client, as well as the problem that motivated him or her to come to the appointment. This approach enables the provider to obtain a more accurate medical history and provides a solid foundation, allowing the client and provider to develop a more effective relationship (Platt et al., 2001). Client-centred interviewing allows clients to set the direction of the exchange. It is the responsibility of the health provider to follow up on the client's lead by asking clarifying questions and offering reflections and information. A sample of questions providers might ask during the interview is found in Boxes 10.1 and 10.2.

It is important to assess whether the client has mental or spiritual distress along with physical changes or pain (Donnelly, 1996). Stress is prevalent in today's world and affects each of us differently, depending on an individual's available levels of support and his or her resilience in managing these issues. The client-centred model of care allows us to elicit

Box 10.1 Sample open-ended questions

- Tell me about yourself.
- I'd like to know about you as a person.
- What brings you here today?
- Tell me more about that.
- How are things going for you?
- Is anything bothering you?
- How does that affect you?
- How do you feel about that?
- What do you think is going on?
- What are your concerns?
- What are your expectations?
- What do you think can be changed?
- What are your thoughts about your treatment plan?
- How can I help you?
- Is there anything else bothering you?
- Is there anything else that you would like to tell me?

information about the challenges our clients are facing, as well as the strategies and supports they find helpful. We can ask simple questions as described in Box 10.2 to obtain information. When we know what underlying factors may be contributing to the client's distress, we can collaborate to strengthen their support systems or help them find new resources if needed.

A problem that is frequently noted by health care providers is that clients bring up questions just as the care provider is leaving the room. Often, these are very important issues and may even be the primary reasons the client made the appointment. By providing clients time and comfort in which to express all their concerns, the client-centred interview makes it possible to avoid "doorknob" questions. Statements such as "Is there anything more you can tell me?" or "Is there anything else you would like me to know?" will allow this information to surface at an appropriate time and be included in the diagnostic process.

Explanatory model of care

Arthur Kleinman is a psychiatrist and anthropologist who has done ground-breaking work on the interface between culture and medical care. In his approach to care, client interviews generate mini-ethnographies that help to explain how clients perceive their own problems. He calls the belief system that each person uses to understand his or her health and medical issues the *explanatory model*. It is important to keep in mind that health providers also have explanatory models that may substantially differ from or even conflict with the client's model (Kleinman et al., 1978). The importance of understanding the explanatory models of both the health care provider and the client is widely accepted as an important component of client-centred interviews (Coulehan & Block, 2001; Coulehan et al., 2001; Donnelly, 1996;

Box 10.2 Sample psychosocial questions (social history)

- Tell me about your living situation.
- What is your job like?
- Tell me about your family.
- What kinds of stress do you feel?
- What do you do to manage your stress?
- Who helps you with that?
- How does that affect your health?
- What are your social supports?
- What are you feeling?
- How far did you go in school? Do you ever have trouble understanding the things people tell you or give you to read? (health literacy)

Haidet & Paterniti, 2003; Platt et al., 2001; Smith & Hoppe, 1991; Stacey et al., 2009). What is most challenging about this paradigm is the need for providers to remain nonjudgemental and to respect the client's model as highly as the biomedical factors when designing a plan of care.

Each client is unique and has his or her own story to tell. Medical concerns do not occur in a vacuum, but as a component of everything the client is experiencing, as well as the cultural context and beliefs that shape the client's expectations. It is important to get the whole story. In other words, we can do a good physical exam, but can still miss important information if we do not incorporate the meaning of the problem to the client. Further, we may not be able to provide clients with care they will be willing to agree to if we do not ask what is acceptable to them. Eliciting each client's "explanation" provides the information needed to uncover clients' belief systems and understanding of their circumstances. This approach ties in nicely with the health belief model of behaviour change.

Effective implementation of Kleinman's explanatory model requires that clients be guided through the process of providing this information. In turn, the provider helps the client to understand his or her explanatory model of health care and to place client concerns within that context. Together, client and provider can develop a collaborative plan of action to address client concerns by utilise the client's own resources and those available through the health care system. The most important step in this process is for providers to present themselves as client allies, ready to negotiate therapeutic plans that make sense to both the health care professional and the client. The latter is the most important aspect of this model, because it helps develop client trust and adherence (Kleinman, 1988; Kleinman et al., 1978).

Using the explanatory model requires breaking down the power differential that traditionally has existed between clients and providers. Eliciting clients' explanatory models of their medical conditions requires skills that are new to some health care providers. Examples of questions that may be helpful are included in Box 10.3. One should be flexible when asking questions and use words or phrases that seem most appropriate for each individual. The key questions to ask are these: "What do you think is wrong?" "What caused it?" and "What do you want me to do?" (Kleinman, 1988, p. 239). This will allow the health care provider to understand the meaning the client has attached to his or her condition, as well as open the opportunity for a dialogue on how to proceed with treatment.

Box 10.3 Questions to Elicit Clients' Explanatory Models

- Tell me what brings you here today? What do you call your problem?
- What do you think has caused your problem?
- Why do you think it started when it did?
- Tell me your ideas about how the problem will change over time.
- What do you think your sickness does to you? How does it work?
- How severe is your illness? How long will it last?
- Tell me about the difficulties that your problem causes for you.
- How has this problem affected your life?
- What do you think is the best plan of care for you?
- What do you think is the best thing I can do for you?
- What kind of treatment do you think you should receive?
- What worries you most about your illness?
- Tell me what you are most afraid of.

Sources: Kleinman (1988), Kleinman et al. (1978), and Johnson, Hardt, & Kleinman (1995).

Invite, listen, summarise

Boyle and associates (2005) have developed a simple system that guides practitioners in performing a client-centred interview. They call this strategy *invite, listen, and summarise.* It provides a helpful mnemonic device to help interviewers recall the necessary steps. At the beginning of the interview, health professionals briefly identify themselves and make a remark such as "You and I have never met before, and I would like to know something about you as a person before we begin our examination." This allows the clinician to see the client as a person first and to understand his or her story. It also provides a powerful message to clients: that the clinician wants to know them as people and is interested in their opinions. Other phrases that can be used to *invite* the client to provide important information include "Tell me a little about yourself" or "Tell me what brings you here today" (Boyle et al., 2005, p. 30).

Professionals actively *listen* to the client's story and use appropriate communication skills to show that they are engaged. As clinicians listen, they process and reflect on what they are hearing, while providing cues to the client to continue. During this stage, they request more information or provide confirmation that they are listening, by using statements such as "Tell me more," "Anything else you can tell me?" "What do you think about this?" "How do you feel about that?" (Boyle et al., 2005, p. 30). The clinician does not interrupt the flow of information or take control of the interview to pursue areas that might be important for diagnosis or treatment.

At this point, clinicians *summarise* what they have heard, using statements such as "You have been having chest pain for several weeks that does not seem related to exercise; did I hear that correctly?" "It sounds like there is a lot going on in your family, and I would like to know a little more about that" or "In the past, you have not been satisfied with your medical care because it did not fit with what you believe to be the best route to follow." This process of summarising ensures that the client has been correctly heard and understood, which is important to all involved parties.

Once you have heard the client's story and elicited the symptoms, impact on life, and his or her understanding of the problem, you can move on to more close-ended questions and perform tests to narrow the diagnosis and treatment options. This is also the time to present your understanding and knowledge of the client's difficulties. You can describe how the symptoms reflect or affect physical or emotional functioning and what kinds of interventions you believe are most effective. There is often more than one solution to the client's difficulties, and you can present several viable options, while explaining which ones you feel will be most effective. Finally, the provider must be willing to negotiate with clients about the best course of treatment.

In the beginning

Entire books have been written on how to perform a good client interview. It is beyond the scope of this chapter to cover all potential encounters in different practice settings. However, this section provides basic information for organising, structuring, and conducting the interview.

Planning for the client interview begins before the client even arrives in the office or clinic. It is assumed that the clinician will be knowledgeable, professional, and have well-developed communication skills. Before actually beginning the interview, it is important to prepare the room, the area, and yourself. Remember that it is not just the provider who interacts with the client but the office staff, receptionist, aides, students, and others, such as food service staff and cleaning personnel.

In any setting, the entire staff must help make the visit successful. It is important to realise that clients may be feeling a number of unpleasant emotions, including nervousness, embarrassment, worry, or anxiety. By providing a welcoming and respectful environment, clients will feel reassured that they are in good hands. For example, clients should be received into an area that ensures private interactions with friendly receptionists and that waiting areas are neat, clean, and pleasant. It is important to consider the furnishings and decorations that are used. Because many clients come from cultures other than Anglo American, artwork or other decorations that represent other cultures may help to indicate that this facility is welcoming to all.

The interview space should be private, quiet, and nondistracting, preferably with a door that closes. Clients can be distracted by a bustling clinic with ringing telephones, people walking in and out of the area, and perhaps an open clinic space where clients can see or hear each other. This will impair the client's ability to focus on the interview and provide answers with the depth and clarity that is needed. For this reason, it is also a good idea to separate clients from those who accompanied them to the appointment so that they can freely answer all questions and disclose their concerns. This, of course, would not be appropriate if clients need to have someone help provide a detailed medical history for them or to assist with communication due to hearing loss, literacy issues, and or other communication concerns. In addition, during an initial assessment, a client may need to be examined more fully than in later treatments, so concerns about physical privacy may exist.

Many students are anxious or uncertain about how to best communicate with clients. This is both understandable and positive. It indicates that students recognise and care about the psychosocial needs of their clients and understand the role of client–provider interactions. It is reassuring to know that while words are important, the caring, attentive, nonjudgemental attitude of the provider also speaks volumes. In the next section, we will emphasise that what you say is not nearly as important as how well you listen. Truly hearing the client is one of the most crucial skills we can bring to the encounter.

Asking and listening

As stated earlier, the successful client interview depends on skillful communication techniques. It permits us to hear each client's story, while gathering information about both the diagnosis and the type of care that will be acceptable to him or her. It also requires proficiency at organising the structure and flow of the interview, pacing the questions and response times, using both open-ended and close-ended questions, and, of course, listening carefully to hear what the client is telling us. Perhaps the most essential skill in the client interview is silence, which allows the client time to tell us everything that we need to know (Smith & Hoppe, 1991). Research has confirmed that if the client is allowed to speak uninterrupted at the beginning of the interview, he or she is able to relay 80 percent of all relevant information in 2 to 3 minutes (Beckwith & Frankel, 1984; Lipkin et al., 1995; Tongue et al., 2005). One foundational belief of the client-centred interview is that the client has all the information the health care provider needs. Therefore, you must learn to listen attentively and wait for the client to give you that information (Shepard, 2007; Smith & Hoppe, 1991). It is very important to hear the clients' whole story if you are going to be asking them to incorporate changes, such as new medications, diet, or activity levels, into their lifestyles.

The interview typically begins with a simple greeting and an introduction, if the client is new to the provider: "Hello, my name is Jan, and I am going to be your nurse today." The introduction can quickly establish the relationship between the client and provider. A general rule is that the way providers introduce themselves should match the terms in which the client is addressed. If providers use formal terms for themselves, then the client must also be addressed using formal language, such as Mr., Mrs., Ms., or Dr. Some uncertainty exists about whether it is better to use formal or informal names, but the typical suggestion is that usage start out on a formal level and progress to an informal level as the relationship develops (Lipkin et al., 1995). Another way to handle this is to ask clients what they would like to be called.

In a busy health practice, confusion can arise over the roles of the many types of providers the client may encounter. It is not only rude, but very disconcerting, to interact with professionals who have not identified their roles on the team. Are you the nurse, the social worker, the doctor, or the medical technician? It is also helpful to briefly describe your role and what you will be doing, even if it is something as basic as taking vital signs.

After the initial greeting, the provider can make a remark about a neutral subject, such as the weather or the traffic. Avoid starting by casually asking, "How are you doing today?" because clients may reflexively answer "Fine," when in fact, they are not fine at all (Tongue et al., 2005). Once the client and provider are comfortably settled, the provider can ask an open-ended question, such as "Tell me how you are doing" or "Tell me what brought you here today." Remember that it is important to be patient and listen without interrupting; if we allow clients a few minutes to speak, they will tell us almost everything we need to know. Rather than being silent or immobile, we should nod, smile, and make statements such as "MmHm," "I see," "Tell me more about that," and "What was that like for you?"

Johnson, Hardt, and Kleinman (1995) suggest several skills that are necessary as part of the conversation to elicit the client's explanatory model. During this conversational portion of the interview, providers need to give their full attention to the client and be nonjudgemental about the information that is provided. This takes practice, because it involves not only words but body language. The questions provided in Box 10.1 are examples of the kind of information you will need to acquire and can be used as a guide. Remember to be flexible and authentic in your interview so that you are not stiff or stilted. Use words or phrases that are comfortable to you and the clients and be sensitive about how many questions to ask. You may need to interpret the reason for client reluctance to answer certain questions: Are they embarrassed by the question? Do they understand what you are trying to ask? Demonstrating interest and openness to what the client is and is not saying will generally provide sufficient information to reveal client concerns.

A mistake many providers make is asking too many questions, especially those that require only a yes/no or one-word answer. For example, rather than asking "How many servings of fruits and vegetables do you eat on a typical day?" "Do you have more pain in the morning or the evening?" or "Is your pain sharp, dull, or throbbing?" you can say "Tell me about your diet" or "Describe your pain to me." This can be followed up by asking the client to tell you more or by restating what you have heard and asking if you have correctly understood. It is important to ask how the condition affects the client, what he or she has done to try to deal with the problem, and what preferences, if any, the client has for care. Remember, before leaving this portion of the interview, it is important to ask if clients have anything else they think is important for you to know about their health or well-being.

Finally, health literacy is a factor that must be considered in all client interviews. It is particularly relevant when the client is a non-native English speaker and has limited English proficiency. For the purposes of a client-centred interview, the provider should avoid making any assumptions about literacy and should find a way for clients to demonstrate their understanding of information provided in medical encounters (Coulehan & Block, 2001). One technique is to ask clients to explain or describe in their own words what they have just heard you say. We can also ask if they have different words to explain the same thing.

[A]Drench, M.E., Noonan, A.C., Sharby, N., & Ventura, S.H. (2012). Motivation, adherence and collaborative treatment planning. In *Pyschosocial aspects of health care* (3rd ed., pp. 77–113). Upper Saddle River, NJ: Pearson Education.

Summary

This chapter described the importance of communication and its relevance to health care. It is imperative to develop a rapport with a client in order to provide quality care. We reviewed the components of communication, which include being present in the moment, practicing mindfulness, using and appropriately interpreting verbal and nonverbal communication, the importance of active listening and understanding what the client is saying, and the use of client-sensitive language.

Appropriate and inappropriate humour in communication was described. Used effectively, humour can decrease tension and assist health care professionals in developing relationships with clients. Used inappropriately, humour can damage relationships, negatively effect adherence to treatment programs, and damage outcomes. Barriers to effective communication, such as role uncertainty, sensory overload, voice and word choice, physical appearance, and gender and cross-cultural differences were discussed.

This chapter also defined and presented an overview of conflict. Sources of conflict were identified, and elements of conflict resolution were explored. The advantages and disadvantages of common approaches to managing conflict were discussed. Methods of alternative conflict resolution were introduced.

Performing a good client interview is one of the most essential functions of the health provider. It allows us to develop relationships with clients, listen and hear their stories, and learn about how health concerns affect their lives. By using the concept of client-centred care, we are able to convey our willingness to understand and respond empathetically to those concerns. This is also the most effective and efficient way to obtain important diagnostic information. Students and novice health care professionals are often concerned about saying and doing the right thing. Rest assured that the practices of active listening, reflecting, and asking follow-up questions will provide you with the foundation needed to establish an effective plan of care that integrates client concerns with evidence-based practice.[A]

Review questions

A. Fill in the missing words to complete the following statements.

1. Facial expression, ____________, ______________distances, and distracting behaviours are some examples of non-verbal communication.
2. There are four levels of conflict which can occur at _________, __________________, __________________, or ____________ levels.

B. Read the following statements and answer with the most correct definition.

3. The four levels of communication are known as:
   - **a)** intrapersonal, interpersonal, large group discussion, organisational communication
   - **b)** intrapersonal, interpersonal, small group discussion, organisational communication
   - **c)** intergenerational, interpersonal, large group discussion, organisational communication
   - **d)** intergenerational, interpersonal, small group discussion, organisational communication
4. In effective communication, developing rapport with clients involves:
   - **a)** clinician empathy, validation and collaboration
   - **b)** awareness of both practitioner and client's non-verbal and verbal behaviour (e.g. body language and using client-sensitive language)
   - **c)** clinician awareness of the setting/environment (e.g. seating arrangements)
   - **d)** all of the above
5. Paralanguage refers to which of the following?
   - **a)** it is an important component of nonverbal communication and includes, pitch, tone, speed, volume, emotional quality, stress and accent.
   - **b)** it is an important component of verbal communication and includes, pitch, tone, speed, volume, emotional quality, stress and accent.
   - **c)** it involves being aware and receptive of both verbal and nonverbal communication cues
   - **d)** none of the above
6. Which of the following are barriers to communication?
   - **a)** sensory overload
   - **b)** role uncertainty
   - **c)** gender differences
   - **d)** all of the above
7. Which of the following statements best describes intragroup conflict?
   - **a)** conflict within individuals (two or more) that may be related to differences in values or beliefs
   - **b)** conflict within two or more groups of people or organisations that have differences in values or beliefs
   - **c)** conflict related to when members within a family, group or community do not agree with each other
   - **d)** conflict that occurs at an individual level where a person may be living incongruently with their values of beliefs

8. Strategies to manage conflict include:
   a) collaboration, avoidance, accommodation, competition, compromise, and mediation
   b) collaboration, avoidance, rebelling, competition, compromise, and mediation
   c) avoidance, accommodation, rebelling, competition , compromise, and mediation
   d) avoidance, accommodation, competition, compromise, and mediation

9. Which of the following best describes the client-centred interview?
   a) exploring the client's history through the use of closed and open-ended questions to develop a specific diagnosis and treatment plan
   b) hearing client's stories and learning what their symptoms and distress mean to them by taking the clients lead, asking clarifying questions, offering reflections and validation to ensure a strong therapeutic relationship is developed and maintained.
   c) is about developing mini-ethnographies to help the client develop a deeper understanding of their difficulties
   d) all of the above

CHAPTER 11

Personality

The content in this section has been compiled from:
Maltby, Day, & Macaskill, Chapter 4

Maltby, J., Day, L., & Macaskill, A. (2013). Theories and measurement of intelligence. In J. Maltby, L. Day, & A. Macaskill (Eds.), *Personality, individual differences and intelligence* (3rd ed., pp. 77–88). Harlow, Essex: Pearson Education.

Maltby, Day, & Macaskill, Chapter 6

Maltby, J., Day, L., & Macaskill, A. (2013). Theories and measurement of intelligence. In J. Maltby, L. Day, & A. Macaskill (Eds.), *Personality, individual differences and intelligence* (3rd ed., pp. 124–147). Harlow, Essex: Pearson Education.

Maltby, Day, & Macaskill, Chapter 7

Maltby, J., Day, L., & Macaskill, A. (2013). Theories and measurement of intelligence. In J. Maltby, L. Day, & A. Macaskill (Eds.), *Personality, individual differences and intelligence* (3rd ed., pp. 152–171). Harlow, Essex: Pearson Education.

CHAPTER 11

Personality

Personality is regarded as an individual's typical way of thinking, feeling, and behaving. In chapter nine we learnt how our social context can influence behaviour, though we aren't exclusively a product of the social environment. Personality – consisting of traits – can in part account for one's behaviour. In health care, understanding the structure of personality can allow us to predict how individuals may respond in certain situations, which can facilitate positive therapeutic outcomes. In this chapter we examine key theories on personality, including both humanistic and trait models, and examine how individual differences in personality can influence how a person functions.

After studying this chapter you should be able to:

- Identify learning theorists and describe how their application of concepts derived from learning theory apply to personality
- Describe humanistic personality theories: Maslow and Rogers
- Define personality traits
- Identify and describe core trait theories of personality:
  - Sheldon (1970)
  - early lexical approaches
  - Allport (1961)
  - Cattell (1965)
  - Eysenck (1947)
  - five-factor model (Costa & McCrae, 1992).

Attempts to apply learning theory approaches to personality

The theorists that we will explore now all made serious attempts to apply concepts derived from learning theory to personality. John Dollard and Neal Miller, two of the earliest of these theorists, both worked at Yale University. They are somewhat unique in that their aim was to try to integrate learning theory principles with Freud's psychoanalytic approach. Both Dollard and Miller had trained as Freudian analysts, Dollard at the Berlin Institute and Miller at the Vienna Institute. By background, Dollard was a social scientist, teaching anthropology, sociology and psychology and only specialising in psychology later in his career. Miller had trained as an academic psychologist before his analytic training. Both men were impressed with the work of the learning theorists while also influenced by Freud's theory. They sought to develop a synthesis of the two concepts to create a theory of personality.

Dollard and Miller collaborated on animal laboratory studies, mainly using rats, sharing Skinner's view that animal learning could be generalised to humans. However, unlike Skinner, they allowed for inner causation in behaviour. They believed that, because of the higher mental processes of humans, our behaviour does not consist merely of responding to stimuli in our environment; instead, we can also respond to inner stimuli, and thoughts can be reinforcing for us. This is the first attempt to allow cognitive processing within a primarily learning theory model. The principles of learning demonstrated in lower species in the laboratory still applied to human learning but, because of their superior mental processes, humans were capable of more complexity. Thoughts and memories could cue behaviour within their model. This also allowed humans to plan ahead and anticipate events. There was even a role for the unconscious.

Dollard and Miller acknowledged the importance of unconscious processes in human behaviour, but their definition of the unconscious is different from Freud's—who saw the unconscious as comprising the sex and death instincts, which were inherited from birth. Dollard and Miller suggest that we are unaware of some processes because we acquired our drives and the cues before we learnt to talk and consequently they are not labelled. Examples might be some of our secondary drives for social contact, love and so on that we learnt as infants from our initial contacts with our parents. We have learnt to associate a particular smell, perhaps with the good feeling of being fed, but are unconscious of it. In future when we are exposed to the smell, it will affect our behaviour at an unconscious level. Other cues may be unconscious, as they are not labelled in our society. For example, in Japanese society to lose face (to be embarrassed or humiliated, especially publicly) is an important concept, and there is a richer vocabulary in Japanese for labelling the experience than is the case in English, where the concept is not so important. Whether labels are readily available also affects how we perceive cues. The well-known example always cited here is that of the Inuit people (people who live on the arctic coasts, including Siberia, Alaska and Greenland) and their wealth of labels for different types of snow. Consequently, they make discriminations between types of snow that English speakers would find difficult or even impossible to do. This then accounts for material being in the unconscious because it is **unlabelled**.

Unlabelled
In learning theory, this term accounts for material being in the unconscious.

Cues may also be unconscious because they have been repressed. Dollard and Miller suggest that the defence mechanism of repression is a learned response, like the rest of our behaviour. When we discussed repression previously, as a Freudian defence mechanism, we saw that it involves suppressing inconvenient or disagreeable feelings or thoughts. If we cannot remember something, it cannot upset us. For Dollard and Miller, repression is about a failure to label the upsetting thoughts or memories so that they are not easy to recall and making a decision not to think about it. When you recall unpleasant events, this reinforces the negative experience you originally had. Repression avoids this, and not labelling the feelings makes it harder for them to be recalled to conscious thought. Dollard and Miller accepted the importance of the effects of unconscious motivation and Freudian defence mechanism on behaviour, but they expressed defence mechanisms in learning theory terminology. The interested reader can find a very readable account in their book, *Personality and Psychotherapy*, published in 1950.

The stimulus-response model of personality of Dollard and Miller

As expected in a stimulus–response (S–R) theory, the emphasis was on how behaviour is learnt. From Hull, another early American learning theory researcher, Dollard and Miller borrowed the term **habit** to label the association between stimulus and response. Within their model, personality is composed largely of learned habits, and they go on to explain how these habits are acquired and maintained.

Habit
The label describing the association between the stimulus and the response.

Primary drives
Innate physiological drives associated with ensuring survival for the individual. They include hunger, thirst, the need for sleep and the avoidance of pain

Primary reinforcers
This refers to something that is naturally reinforcing without any learning having to occur. It is sometimes called an unconditioned response.

Secondary reinforcers
Items or events that were originally neutral but have acquired a value as a reinforcer through being associated with primary drive reduction.

They agreed with Freud that the infant is born with some innate drives, which they termed **primary drives**, but disagreed with Freud about the nature of these drives. These innate primitive drives are physiological drives associated with ensuring survival for the individual. They include hunger, thirst, the need for sleep and the avoidance of pain. Reduction of these drives provides the most powerful reinforcement for the individual. Dollard and Miller (1950) claim that this reinforcement occurs automatically and unconsciously, and, to be maximally effective, it should immediately follow the response. Like many other personality theorists with a clinical background, Dollard and Miller focus mainly on psychopathology in the development of their theory and then extrapolate from this to normal development. For example, if an infant is left to become extremely hungry (primary drive), then it cries very loudly for attention (response). If the mother then feeds the infant, what the infant is said to have learnt is that making a fuss is rewarded. Such a child might then go on to make an excessive fuss every time they have a drive that requires satisfaction. In this terminology, making a fuss has become a habit. The baby whose primary drive of hunger was quickly met would not have this habit of over-reacting and would develop normal levels of response, in this case distress. In most western societies, primary drives are rarely directly observed, apart from in infant feeding, as societies have developed means of reducing them before they become pressing. The process for doing this involves the acquisition of what Dollard and Miller termed **secondary drives**. These secondary drives are learned mainly to help us cope with our primary drives. An example would be of setting regular mealtimes so that you are motivated to eat at particular times before the primary drive of hunger becomes overwhelming and therefore distressing. Associated with these primary and secondary drives are different types of reinforcement. For the innate primary drives, **primary reinforcers** are food, water, sleep and so on. Secondary drives similarly have **secondary reinforcers**. These secondary reinforcers are items or events that were originally neutral but have acquired a value as a reinforcer through being associated with primary drive reduction. A mother smiling at her child is a secondary reinforcer as it is associated with physical well-being. Money is also a secondary reinforcer as it is associated with being able to buy food, provide shelter and so on.

Dollard and Miller describe the learning of habits as being composed of four constituent parts: the initial drive, the cue to act, the response and reinforcement of the response. As discussed earlier, the drive stimulates the person to act. It does not guide them how to act but simply lets the person know that they want something. A drive might be hunger. Cues provide guidance about how to act or respond in S–R terminology. You notice a billboard advertising a new Chinese takeaway. This might be the cue for you to respond, by taking a detour past the takeaway to get something to eat. If you then pick up a delicious meal that you enjoy hugely, you will no longer be hungry; your drive will have been satisfied. In this situation, the Chinese meal constitutes reinforcement. Reinforcement refers to the effect that a response has. As the meal was good, it reinforced your action of going to get it; next time you are in a similar position, hungry when walking home, you may be tempted to repeat the experience. In S–R terms, a habit has been formed. If, on the other hand, the meal was disgusting and the portions were tiny, the experience of visiting the takeaway would not have been reinforcing and you are unlikely to visit it again. In S–R terms, if the response does not satisfy the drive, it will undergo extinction. It does not mean that you will never again visit the takeaway, but you are less likely to do so. Remember that habits can be both positive and negative. They are simply associations between stimuli and responses.

Dollard and Miller (1941, 1950) were particularly interested in what happened when we became frustrated in our attempts to satisfy our drives. They described four types of conflict situations that we could face. The conflict is caused by our tendencies to wish to obtain (termed 'approach') certain goals or objects. They developed a simple diagrammatic system to illustrate these conflicts, as they felt that this helped them to understand exactly what was going on in any situation (see Figure 11.1).

- **Approach-approach conflict** – This describes the situation where there are two equally desirable goals, but they are incompatible. This could be when you are asked to choose between two equally desirable objects to have as a gift. You really want both but can only have one. Both goals are positive but incompatible.
- **Avoidance-avoidance conflict** – This is the situation where you are faced with what you perceive as two equally undesirable alternatives. You have a spare hour, and your partner asks you to go jogging, which you hate; or you could offer to do the ironing as an excuse not to go jogging, but you equally hate ironing. Here, for you, both goals are undesirable and incompatible in terms of having neither the wish nor the time to do both.
- **Approach-avoidance conflict** – Here there is one goal, but while an element of it is attractive, an aspect of it is equally unattractive. For example, you are offered a place in what seems an ideal house; however, one of your housemates would be someone you really do not like.
- **Double approach-avoidance conflict** – Here there may be multiple goals, some desirable and some undesirable. This is more like most situations, where there are a variety of factors, positives and negatives, to take into consideration before being able to make a decision.

Although we have used human examples to illustrate the analysis of conflict situations, Dollard and Miller used laboratory animals rather than humans to demonstrate that this system was accurate at predicting behaviour.

For Dollard and Miller, therefore, behaviour is motivated by the need to reduce our primary or

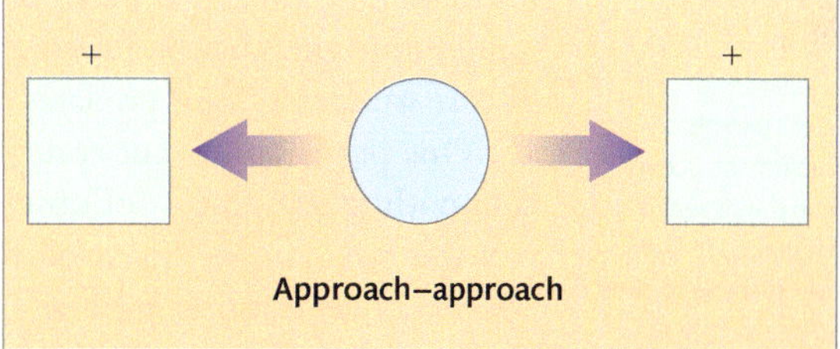

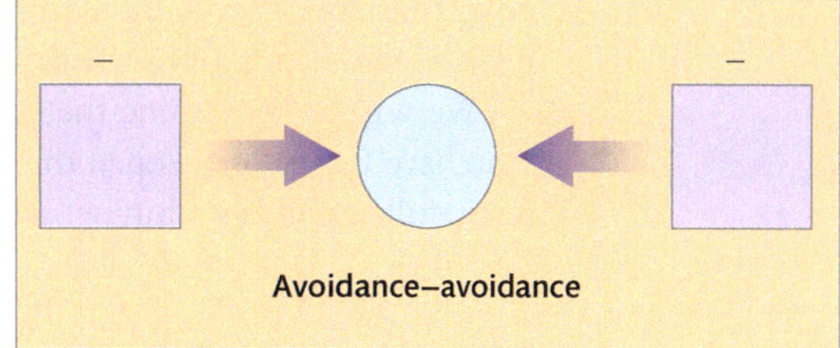

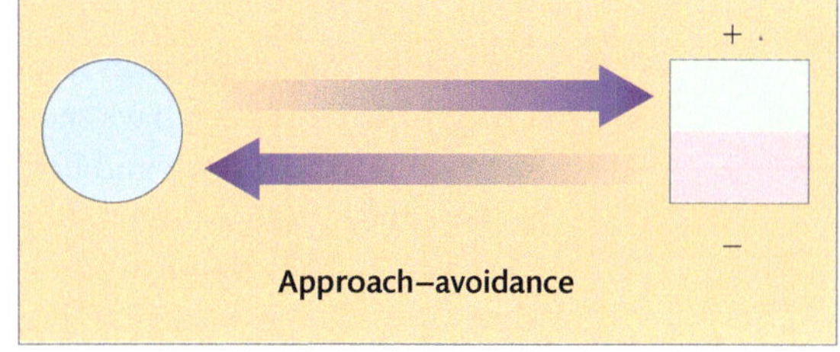

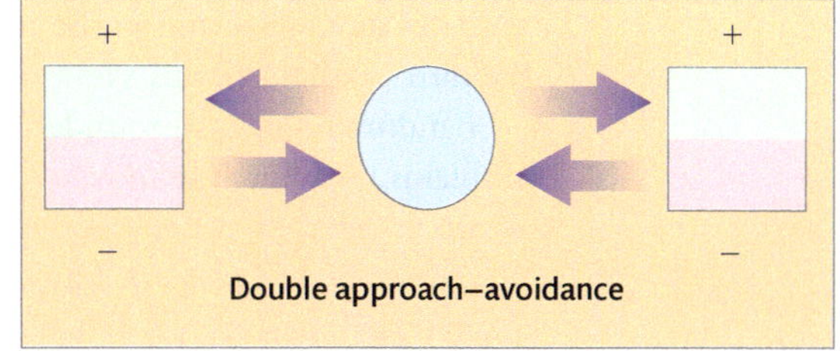

Figure 11.1 The Dollard and Miller system for analysing conflicts.

secondary drives, and we learn new behaviours in the process. It is a deterministic account of human development. It is more complex than the early learning theory models as it allows for the inner influence of human cognitive processes; making it a forerunner of cognitive models of personality.

One aspect of Dollard and Miller's model that is subject to criticism from behaviourists as not being radical enough is their approach to the treatment of mental disorder. For them, as with the other learning theorists, psychopathology consists of learned, unproductive, unhelpful habits or responses. In their integrative approach, they suggested that some of these habits might be unconscious because of the reasons we have discussed earlier and that this factor added to the complexity. The aim of treatment is to remove these ineffective habits and replace them with new, more effective habits. Unlike the earlier behaviourists, Dollard and Miller did not adopt a purely deconditioning approach to treatment; they maintain significant elements of psychotherapy, the 'talking cure', in their approach. There are two phases to their treatment: first is a **talking phase**, where the problem habits are identified, explored and labelled. In the second phase, the patient is encouraged to learn more adaptive habits and apply them in their life. They call this phase the **performance phase**. They departed from their Freudian psychoanalytic training in not attending to the problems that patients had experienced in the past. They felt that past emotional issues do not have to be relived in therapy for them to be resolved. The past is only helpful sometimes in helping patients understand the source of their problems. Their focus was on current problems in living and future strategies. This predates the current treatment practice in cognitive therapy.

Talking phase
In Dollard and Miller's two phases of treatment, this phase occurs when problem habits are identified, explored and labelled.

Performance phase
In Dollard and Miller's two phases of treatment, occurs when the patient is encouraged to learn more adaptive habits and apply them in their life.

One other significant contribution made by Dollard and Miller (1941) was to recognise and outline the process of observational learning. They demonstrated how performance on a novel task can be improved by seeing someone else perform the task. This increases the speed of the learning process. They suggested that observational learning is important in development as children learn from observing adults and other children in situations that are novel to them. They stressed that observational learning could explain how both adaptive and maladaptive habits are learned.

We will now examine the contributions of theorists Albert Bandura and Michael Rotter, who have further developed this concept of social and observational learning in ways that can be usefully applied within personality theorising.

Albert Bandura and social learning theory

One of the major questions in personality theorising is whether inner or outer forces control our behaviour. As we have seen, the psychoanalysts would have us believe that inner forces determine who we are and how we behave. The learning theorists that we have examined so far conceptualise human beings as being at the mercy of outer forces. The environment determines your opportunities for learning new behaviour, the interests you are likely to develop and your history of learning. Dollard and Miller allowed for some inner influence from the higher cognitive functioning possessed by humans but said that principles of reinforcement external to the individual are thought mainly to control human behaviour. Bandura challenges this view, as we shall see.

Bandura's work is grounded in the learning theory tradition, but his focus is on human problems in living. He moved from animal studies to focusing on purely human behaviour, although he kept the methodology of undertaking mainly laboratory-based research. His laboratory techniques are much more sophisticated, emphasising observation in situations designed to simulate real-life experiences. He is interested in developing theory and applying it to behavioural problems to facilitate positive change in individuals and groups.

The model of the individual in his approach is of an active player responding both to inner stimuli and the external environment and moving back and forward in a dynamic system. Individuals are seen to be influential in determining their own motivation, development and behaviour. Bandura (1978; 1989) uses the term **reciprocal determinism** to label the processes that drive behaviour. He sees an individual as being influenced by personal factors, behaviour and environmental factors. All three factors interact with one another to influence how individuals behave. The direction of these interactions is displayed in Figure 11.2.

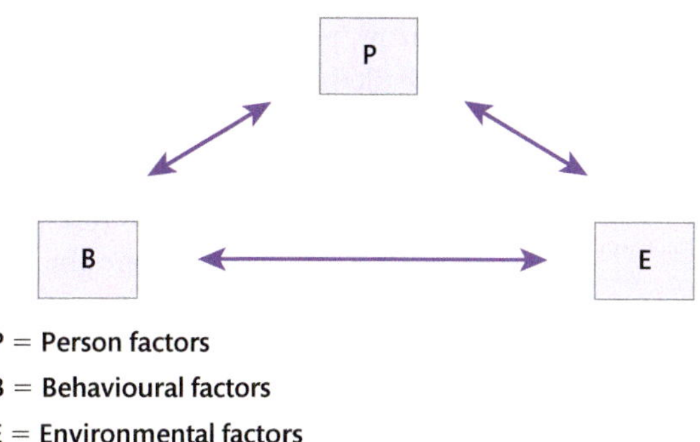

P = Person factors
B = Behavioural factors
E = Environmental factors

Figure 11.2 The interacting factors in reciprocal determinism.

Personal factors include the individual's cognitions, emotions and biological variables that contribute to their inner state. This is a major break from the traditional learning theory approaches that we have examined previously. These personal factors can impact on both an individual's behaviour and on their environment. If you truly think you will fail at a task in a specific setting, Bandura (1995) has shown that this greatly increases the likelihood of failure, as you approach the task differently. Your cognitions are affecting your behaviour. If you do not like opera, then you are unlikely to choose to go to an opera. Here your cognitions are influencing the environments you experience. Similarly, if you hate smoking, you may avoid bars that you know will be smoky. Here, environmental factors and personal cognitions are impacting on your behaviour.

Reciprocal determinism The belief that cognitive and environmental events interact to motivate behaviour.

Personal factors Include the individual's cognitions, emotions and biological variables that contribute to their inner state.

Behavioural factors Aspects of an individual's behaviour.

Environmental factors Aspects of the environment.

Reciprocal causation A term introduced by Albert Bandura to refer to the mutual influence between sets of factors.

Bandura also suggests that **behavioural factors** can affect the individual's cognitions, feelings and emotions. Supposing you go skiing for the first time with some friends, and you prove to be good at it. You get your balance quickly, and the instructor is complimentary. You now have the cognition that 'This is something I can do.' Your feelings may also change from apprehension about whether you could do it, to feeling positive about skiing. The converse might also be true if your initial experience of skiing was awful. Your behaviour with regard to the skiing experience has influenced your cognitions and your feelings, and both are likely to influence whether you choose to ski in future. If you take up skiing, you may even become an expert and your body will develop neurological networks reflecting your expertise. In this way, Bandura (2001) demonstrated how our behaviour affects our cognitions, feelings, emotions and even our neurobiology in some instances.

With regard to the environment, we have seen from the earlier examples how **environmental factors** like polluted environments may affect our behavioural choices. The hole in the ozone layer is another good example that has resulted in us having to take more care to avoid burning when it is sunny. We may have to spend time and money buying sunscreens or we may avoid sunbathing (behavioural factors). In addition, we may also worry about sunburn and plan ways to avoid it (personal factors). We hope that these examples give you an idea of Bandura's model of **reciprocal causation** in action. You surely can think of other examples. Doing this makes you aware of the complexity of learned behaviour that, unlike the earlier models, Bandura's model can handle.

Unlike Skinner, Bandura (1995; 1998) believes that individuals do possess free will and are not at the mercy of their drives and reinforcement schedules in their learning environment. For Bandura, our cognitive processes allow us some control in selecting the situations we operate in and in creating or transforming situations. We may have to work, but we can choose what we do in our leisure; or we may work towards changing a work

Personal agency
The belief that you can change things to make them better for yourself or others.

Proxy agency
Occurs when the individual enlists other people to help change some of the factors impacting on their life.

Collectove agency
Describes the situation where a group of individuals come together believing that they can make a difference to their own and/or others' life circumstances.

situation to make it more amenable to us. We can start businesses or interest groups or throw parties to provide the experiences and environments that we need. Bandura has labelled this personal agency: the belief that you can change things to make them better for yourself or others. Bandura (1999) has extended the concept to include proxy agency, where the individual enlists other people to help change some of the factors impacting on their life. They may ask a family member to look after their child so that they can get a job, or so that they can change their life in some other way. Bandura points out that there can be a downside to proxy agency in that people may in the process surrender their power to the other, who may not have their best interests at heart, and/or they may become subservient and give up control of their lives. He prefers the idea of collective agency, which is where a group of individuals come together believing that they can make a difference to their own and/or others' life circumstances. An example might be the recent emergence of farmers' markets. Here, like-minded people, who wish to earn a sustainable income from the produce they farm, organise markets to sell their produce directly to the public for a fair price.

Learning within Bandura's model

Within Bandura's model, personality development is about how we learn to become the person we are, and this then explains why we behave as we do. Bandura (1977) suggests that, for learning to be effective, individuals have to be aware of the consequences of their behaviour. He demonstrated that people think about the consequences of their behaviour in learning situations. We think beyond the immediate situation and anticipate possible outcomes with an eye to the future. Being aware of the consequences of our behaviour also allows us forethought, in that we can anticipate what possible outcomes may follow our behaviour, and this knowledge can affect how we choose to behave and what we learn in the situation. Bandura (1995; 1999) sees awareness of the consequences of our behaviour and foresight as being human attributes as we possess language and symbolic thought which make it easier to record the consequences of our actions.

One of the most well-known aspects of Bandura's work is observational learning. As discussed in chapter one, learning occurs by watching and following what other people do and imitating their behaviour that occurs by classical or operant conditioning. What happens is that an individual watches someone perform a novel behaviour, and, when they are required to perform the same behaviour, they copy what they have previously seen. This is termed modelling by Bandura.

You may recall from your earlier readings that Bandura and Walters (1963) undertook a series of famous studies with a doll (Bobo). To summarise, nursery school children were divided into two groups. One group, the experimental group, watched an adult playing aggressively with a plastic doll called 'Bobo'. The adult hit and kicked the doll, shouting things like 'Throw him in the air.' The second group of children, the control group, did not see the aggressive play. Later, both groups of children were allowed to play with the doll. Children in the experimental group displayed twice as much aggression towards the doll as did those in the control group.

Forethought
Deliberation, consideration or planning beforehand.

Observational learning
Learning by watching and analysing the behaviour of another.

Characteristics of the model
Main features of the approach.

From variations of this study, Bandura (1977) concluded that three factors are important in modelling. Firstly, the characteristics of the model influence how likely we are to imitate them. The more similar to ourselves the model is, the more likely we are to imitate them. Models undertaking simple behaviour are more likely to be copied than they are if the behaviour is complex. The type of behaviour being modelled also has an effect, with hostile and aggressive behaviour more likely to be modelled. Secondly, the **attributes of the observer** exert an influence. Less confident individuals and those with low self-esteem or those who feel incompetent in the situation are more likely to imitate the model. Individuals with a learning history of being rewarded for conforming behaviour or who are highly dependent also imitate models more. Finally, Bandura showed that the **consequences of imitating a behaviour** are the most influential factor. If individuals believe that imitating a behaviour will bring positive results, then they are more likely to do so.

While we have talked about modelling using the term 'imitation', Bandura is insistent that modelling involves more than passive imitation. It is an active process of learning through observation, where the observer makes judgements and constructs symbolic representations of the behaviours observed. These symbolic representations may be verbal descriptions or visual images, and they are used to guide the individuals' future behaviour in similar situations. Bandura has studied the factors that may influence these processes in great detail; interested readers can refer to the further reading provided at the end of the discussion. Here we will restrict ourselves to a more aerial view of his theory as it relates to aspects of personality and its development. It is sufficient for us to be aware that modelling is not a passive process of observation, but an active process where the observer reviews what they have learnt and makes judgements about it and may decide to keep or discard parts of the behaviour. A distinction is also made between what we have learned (knowledge acquired) and what we can do (performance). Performance is seen to involve trial and error as we gradually shape our behaviour into the desired format. We may also acquire knowledge that we do not use, like learning about ways to murder someone from watching television; fortunately, few of us ever put this knowledge to use.

While reinforcement is crucial for learning in classical and operant conditioning, Bandura demonstrates that it is not always necessary in observational learning. You notice vivid billboard adverts, or loud noises, because they command your attention. You may not think about the information at the time; however, when faced with an array of soap powder at the supermarket, you recognise the one from the billboard. Bandura also demonstrates that we can, and frequently do, reinforce our own behaviour. This **self-reinforcement** is where we evaluate our own behaviour; we may stop doing something we are getting no pleasure from, or that we judge as harming us in some way, while continuing to do things that bring positive reinforcement. The other crucial element for learning that Bandura identifies is an **incentive** so that we are motivated to learn. Here, **forethought** plays an important part, as well as the more traditional cues for learning. Forethought can allow us to anticipate reinforcements and thus motivate our behaviour. He suggests that motivation is crucial with observational learning, as it requires practice for the skills to be perfected. Motivation and reinforcement are much more dynamic complex processes in this model.

Bandura (2002) is keen to encourage the application of his social learning theory to address global problems such as the AIDS pandemic, population growth and gender inequalities. He sees social modelling and observational learning as being core components of behavioural change. The modelling principles in his famous Bobo study were incorporated into serial dramas and soap operas by a well-known writer (Sabido, 1981; 2002). These dramas incorporate positive role models demonstrating beneficial lifestyles, negative role models displaying detrimental lifestyles and individuals who are making the transition from negative to more positive life roles. Bandura (2002) reports that these dramas provide individuals with positive role models. They also provide the inspiration for viewers to make positive changes in their own lives. To assist in the change process, supporting resources on linked websites or in post-programme information slots are made available to the viewers. These dramas are tailored for different cultures and are delivered in Africa, Asia and Latin

Attributes of the observer
Key characteristics of the person observing the behaviour.

Consequences of imitating a behaviour
The results or outcomes of reproducing or copying behaviour.

Self-reinforcement
Occurs when we evaluate our own behaviour; we may stop doing something we are getting no pleasure from, or that we judge as harming us in some way, while continuing to do things that bring positive reinforcement.

Incentive
Something that provides the motivation to learn.

Forethought
Deliberation, consideration or planning beforehand.

America (Bandura, 2000; Brown and Cody, 1991; Singhal and Rogers, 1989; Vaughan *et al.*, 1995). You see examples of post-programme information slots closer to home, with helpline details being provided after popular soap operas when particular social issues are included in the programme.

Personality development in social learning theory

It is this emphasis on observational learning that has led to the term 'social' being included in the theory, to stress that it is about how people learn from other individuals. In terms of how children develop their personalities, it is a learning process where parents, peers and others provide role models for children to learn from through observational learning mainly. The children learn to model their behaviour on successful models in their environment. This might be a sibling who manages to avoid trouble in one situation and a friend who gets on well in another and so on. Unfortunately, parents and others are not always consistent in their reinforcement, as we have seen, so the picture is more complicated than it might seem at first. Role models will be more or less effective, as will individual children's learning. Children will be exposed to different experiences, different environments and different cultures, and all of these influences help account for the observed diversity of human beings. The child is at the centre of these learning experiences and actively shaping the process. It is a truly dynamic, complex process.

Identifying goals to achieve is a crucial part of this process, and obtaining external feedback from relevant others on progress made towards achieving these goals plays an important part in maintaining motivation and ultimate success (Bandura, 1991). Bandura also demonstrated that goal achievement depends heavily on self-regulatory processes (Bandura, 1990; 1991; 1994; 1999; 2002). These **internal self-regulatory processes** include self-criticism, self-praise, valuation of own personal standards, re-evaluation of own personal standards if necessary, self-persuasion, evaluation of attainment and acceptance of challenges. Bandura (1990) describes these processes as being attempts at self-influence, and he has shown that the more of these factors involved in achieving a goal, the higher the levels of motivation to succeed. He identified self-efficacy as one of the most powerful of the self-regulatory processes, and we shall examine it next.

Internal self-regulatory processes
Bandura describes these processes as being attempts at self-influence that include self-criticism, self-praise; valuation of own personal standards; re-evaluation of own personal standards if necessary; self-persuasion, evaluation of attainment, acceptance of challenges.

Self-efficacy as a self-regulatory process

Self-efficacy is defined as being your belief that if you perform some behaviour, it will get you a desired positive outcome (Bandura, 1989; 1994). It has become a really hot topic in psychology during the past 10 or so years and has stimulated a great deal of research, especially in health. Individuals have been shown to vary greatly in their levels of self-efficacy related to specific tasks. If we take smokers who wish to stop smoking as an example, they will vary greatly in whether they believe that they can achieve their goal. It is a special kind of confidence in your ability to perform. In the smoking example, it might be that the smoker felt that not smoking at home and at work was achievable (high self-efficacy) but that not smoking when out with friends would be more difficult (low self-efficacy). Their overall judgement would depend on the relative amount of time they spent in each activity, and perhaps on their past experiences of similar success in a relevant area and so on. Bandura (1997) has shown that high self-efficacy significantly increases the likelihood of achieving success. Self-efficacy will influence whether a task will be attempted as well as the effort put into it and the persistence with which it is pursued in the face of difficulties or apparent lack of progress. For example, one recent study of the factors that affected the likelihood of relapse in a smoking cessation programme found that low levels of self-efficacy in individuals were a significant predictor (Segan *et al.*, 2006). Another study looked at factors that predicted heavy drinking in anxiety-provoking social situations for a student population in the United States (Gilles *et al.*, 2006). The students most likely to drink heavily in these situations had low self-efficacy for avoiding heavy drinking in social situations and a correspondingly high belief that alcohol facilitated social interactions. Halkitis *et al.*, (2005) looked at adherence with HIV antiretroviral treatment in 300 HIV-positive men. They found that poorer adherence was associated with low self-efficacy towards adherence, amongst other factors. Having confidence in your ability to succeed at something is consistently shown to be a significant factor in a wide range of scenarios (Bandura, 1997).

An example will help to clarify the application of self-efficacy. Let us compare two students, Dan and Stuart, who have to give assessed seminar presentations.

One student, Dan, is quite looking forward to his presentation. He knows that if he does well he will get a good mark, and he really wants to do well this year to get a good degree. He knows from experience that, although he will be anxious initially, once he gets started he likes public speaking and will enjoy it. He is interested in the topic, and he is already quite well informed about it. He knows that he can organise his work effectively as he has received good marks previously when he has given himself sufficient time to undertake the preparatory work well. Not surprisingly then, his self-efficacy is high with regard to the seminar presentation; he feels confident about all the component parts that go into producing a good seminar presentation, and he has some positive experiences to reinforce this. The one proviso he has is about ensuring that he has enough time to complete the task. As his motivation to succeed is high and his self-efficacy is high, he is more likely to devote the time to the work. The chances of Dan succeeding in delivering a good presentation are also correspondingly high.

Stuart dreads the event. He hates public speaking, and he has no confidence in his ability to master the constituent parts of the task. He knows that he has to do it, but his self-efficacy in relation to the task is low. As a result, thinking about it makes him anxious. He tries to put it out of his mind, and he avoids cues that remind him about it, like going to the library to prepare and so on. He indulges in ostrich-like behaviour and, consequently, his chances of success are reduced. His initial low self-efficacy rating has resulted in him not being motivated to perform the task. Self-efficacy has been shown to be an important variable in predicting educational achievement. Lane and Lane (2001) showed that self-efficacy was a good predictor of British students' achievement on sports science courses. Hoy and Davis (2006) demonstrated that, in school situations, teachers' ratings of their own self-efficacy in teaching are associated with the levels of achievement attained by their pupils.

Increasing self-efficacy ratings

The good news is that Bandura (1997) has demonstrated that self-efficacy can be modified by several different methods. Bandura (1999) has shown that the most straightforward way to improve self-efficacy is to get the person to 'perform the dreaded task'. If someone can be encouraged and supported to do something they fear, it has a dramatic effect on their self-efficacy. If the level of their performance is an issue, then further self-regulatory processes may be called into play so that the individual sees it as a gradual process. The first goal will be to perform, and subsequent goals may be about making improvements to their performance. **Vicarious experience** has also been shown to have an effect (Bandura, 1994). This is where the individual sees someone, whom they know shares the same fears as theirs, actually performing the task. Their cognitions become more positive, and they may say something like, 'If they can learn to do it, then so can I.' This then changes their self-efficacy directly. The final method is termed **participant modelling**. In this method, the person with low self-efficacy shadows a person who is successfully completing the task. Even this imitative behaviour has been shown to lower anxiety.

Vicarious experience
Occurs when the individual sees a person that they know shares the same fears as them actually performing the task they dread doing. This has a positive effect on the observer's self-efficacy.

Participant modelling
Occurs when the low self-efficacy person shadows a high-efficacy person in a new or dreaded task.

Returning to the student seminar example discussed earlier, Bandura's model outlines three possible courses of action for the student low in self-efficacy. He would suggest that observing another anxious student perform successfully and discussing how they prepared for the seminar would be very helpful in raising self-efficacy. Taking this action allows the student to change their cognitions, to see that they can learn to deliver a good presentation as well. Another technique would be to pair up the anxious student with someone less anxious. The anxious student would follow the confident student through the preparation and performance. Any possibility for feedback in the process would increase the chances of success by increasing the anxious student's confidence that they were progressing in the right direction. So, obtaining feedback on the content is valuable, as is rehearsing the presentation with a friendly audience of family or friends. Once this rehearsal has been achieved, it again increases confidence. Any steps to improve confidence will improve the chances of a successful outcome.

Self-efficacy and the other self-regulatory processes help us to maintain our motivation and to be resilient even when faced with setbacks to our progress. Bandura (1990) quotes interesting examples of such resilience, including that displayed by the author James Joyce, whose book *Dubliners* was rejected by 22 publishers before becoming a success. Similarly, the artist Van Gogh died a pauper, having only ever sold one of his many paintings that are now worth a fortune. There are many more examples of amazing resilience shown by individuals in the face of rejection and apparent failure. Bandura sees the self-regulatory processes such as self-efficacy as being important in helping us to survive hard knocks and continue to strive to achieve our goals. Benight and Bandura (2004) published an extensive review of research undertaken on the role of self-efficacy in helping individuals recover from traumatic experiences. They looked at natural disasters, war, terrorist attacks, loss of a spouse and other interpersonal traumas. They concluded that individuals who believe that they can overcome their difficulties (high in self-efficacy) are consistently shown, in all the studies they examined, to make a better recovery.

Measuring self-efficacy

There are psychometric tests that have developed to measure General Self-Efficacy: Sherer *et al.*'s (1982) General Self-Efficacy Scale, Schwarzer and Jerusalem's (1995) General Perceived Self-Efficacy Scale, and Chen *et al.*'s (2001) New General Self-Efficacy Scale. Sherer *et al.*'s General Self-Efficacy Scale aims to measure self-efficacy via items that measure a general set of expectations that the respondent brings into new situations that they face. An example item from this scale is 'If I can't do a job the first time, I keep trying until I can'. Schwarzer and Jerusalem's General Perceived Self-Efficacy Scale is designed to measure general self-efficacy by examining the participant's beliefs around their own capability to handle new and difficult tasks in a variety of different domains. An example item from this measure is 'I can handle whatever comes my way'. Chen *et al.*'s New General Self-Efficacy Scale is designed to measure the respondent's belief in their overall competence at being able to produce a necessary performance across a variety of possible 'achievement' situations. An example item from this scale is 'I will be able to achieve most of the goals that I have set for myself'.

However, Bandura is critical of attempts to measure self-efficacy with global scales. He points out that few people are confident about every aspect of their lives and the tasks they have to perform. Hence, self-efficacy is measured in relation to specific tasks. It demands confidence judgements to be made about the constituent skills or knowledge elements that make up a task. Researchers need to undertake this analysis systematically to ensure that all the relevant components are assessed. Bandura (2006) provides detailed guidance on measuring self-efficacy. Consequently, Bandura suggests that new and separate scales need

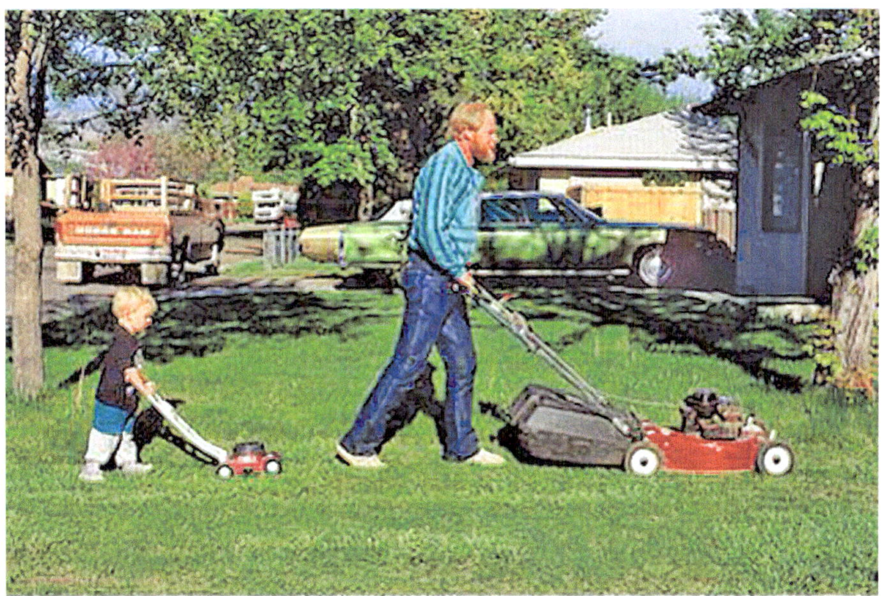

Children copy adults' behaviour in many different and subtle ways.
Source: Alamy Images/David R. Frazier Photolibrary, Inc.

to be developed for each self-efficacy domain. So, for example, Bandura (2006) suggests the following.

- **Children's Self-Efficacy Scale**, which measures children's self-efficacy around a number of learning situations that students may experience at school, e.g. Self-Efficacy for Academic Achievement ('Learn reading, writing and language skills'), Self-Efficacy for Self-Regulated Learning ('Organise my schoolwork') and Social Self-Efficacy ('Carry on conversations with others').
- **Teacher Self-Efficacy Scale**, which measures teachers' self-efficacy around a number of teaching situations in which teachers may face challenges, e.g. Efficacy to Influence Decision-Making ('Get the instructional materials and equipment I need'), Disciplinary Self-Efficacy ('Get children to follow classroom rules') and Efficacy to Create a Positive School Climate ('Make students enjoy coming to school').
- **Parental Self-Efficacy**, which measure parents' self-efficacy around a number of situations in which parents may face challenges, e.g. Efficacy in Setting Limits, Monitoring Activities and Influencing Peer Affiliations ('Keep track of what your children are doing when they are outside the home'), Efficacy to Exercise Control over High-Risk Behaviour ('Prevent your children from doing things you do not want them to do outside the home') and Resiliency of Self-Efficacy ('Keep up your spirits when you suffer hardships').

Julian Rotter and locus of control

We now want to introduce you to an important concept, **locus of control**, that has been and is still used extensively in research in personality and individual differences. This concept was first described by Julian Rotter (1966), another American learning theory researcher, who carried out most of his research at the University of Connecticut, where he still works. We will begin by examining the theoretical background to the concept of locus of control before going on to explore how locus of control is measured. There is a wealth of research on locus of control, as it has been and continues to be as popular a research tool as are measures

Locus of control
Theory developed by Julian Rotter; describes how people tend to ascribe their chances of future successes or failures either to internal or external causes.

of self-efficacy. For this reason, we present only a brief taste of some of the research findings here, with an indication of the areas of research where it has been applied.

Like Bandura, Rotter felt that animal studies were too simplistic to address the complexity of human behaviour. Rotter was interested in how you might predict how individuals would respond in particular situations. Supposing someone makes a nasty remark about you in front of other people. You could respond angrily; you could mock them for doing it; you could get upset; you could go quiet; or you could walk away. There are a variety of possibilities. Rotter (1966) aimed to predict which option an individual might choose in a particular situation. He termed this the **behaviour potential**; that is, the likelihood of a specific behaviour occurring in a particular situation. The response that you choose will be the one with the strongest behaviour potential in that situation. However, the crucial question is, how is the strength of the behaviour potential determined? Rotter developed a formula to answer this question:

Behaviour potential
The likelihood of a specific behaviour occurring in a particular situation.

Expectancy
Our subjective estimate of the likely outcome of a course of behaviour.

Reinforcement value
Refers to our preferences amongst the possible reinforcements available to us.

Generalised expectancies
Explains the process whereby individuals come to believe, based on their learning experiences, either that reinforcements are controlled by outside forces or that their behaviour controls reinforcements.

Behaviour potential = Reinforcement value × Expectancy

In this formula, **expectancy** is our subjective estimate of the likely outcome of a course of behaviour. It is what we *expect* will happen. In learning theory terminology, it is our estimate of probability of our behaviour receiving a particular reinforcement in that situation. This is generally based on our experience of the same or similar situations. In the nasty insult example, it is your estimate of what you expect will happen if, for example, you mock the person. You may estimate that they will blush and feel ashamed of having made the nasty remark. Each option will have a different expectancy associated with it. This expectancy influences how you choose to behave in that situation. The final variable that contributes to predicting our behaviour is **reinforcement value**. This refers to our preferences amongst the possible reinforcements available. You may be more inclined to help someone move some furniture if you know they will buy you a drink as a thank you.

To summarise, Rotter suggests that to predict behaviour in a particular situation, we need to know what the options are and what the individual sees as being the possible outcomes for each option. The individual then assesses the likely outcome of each option (expectancy). Next, they assess how much they value this outcome. The behaviour that is likely to occur (behaviour potential) will be the behaviour that gets the highest rating. A summary of this decision-making process for our hypothetical example is shown in Table 11.1.

In novel situations, where by definition we have no experience to guide us, Rotter (1966) suggests that we rely on what he calls **generalised expectancies**. What he showed to be important about this concept is that individuals come to believe on the basis of their other learning experiences that either reinforcement is controlled by outside forces or that their behaviour controls reinforcement (Rotter, 1966). The question he was interested in was whether it makes a difference if people believe that the reinforcement they receive is linked to how they perform, compared to individuals who believe that the reinforcement they receive is unrelated to their own behaviour. He labelled individuals who believe that reinforcement depends on external forces as externals. The external forces may include powerful others in

Table 11.1 Application of Rotter's equation for predicting behaviour to an insult. **Stimulus:** Someone you know, Angela, makes a nasty remark about you in front of other people.

Behavioural option	Possible outcome	Rating of expectancy of outcome	Value of the outcome to the individual	Behaviour potential (probability that option will occur)
Angry reply	Argument	High	Low	Low
Mocking comment	Angela is embarrassed	High	High	High
Get upset	Angela feels remorse	Low	High	Low
Say nothing	Feel silly	High	Low	Low
Walk away	Feel silly	High	Low	Low

the person's world, luck, God, fate, the State and so on. What is crucial is that externals believe that the locus of control is external to them. What they do does not influence the outcomes. Individuals who believe that their behaviour does make a difference to the outcome are labelled internals. Rotter (1966) demonstrated that locus of control is a relatively stable personality characteristic and developed a scale to assess it, the IE Scale. It is assessed via a 30-item forced-choice scale. Scores are on a continuum of I–E, and Rotter does not suggest a cut-off point to separate externals from internals. He has published normative scores for particular groups to allow comparisons to be made. Although other assessment tools to measure locus of control have been developed since Rotter's scale was published, his IE Scale is still the most widely used in research. Some sample items from the scale are shown in Figure 11.3.

The impact of locus of control on behaviour

Rotter (1982) demonstrated that people with an internal locus of control are more likely to feel in control of their lives and to feel empowered to try to change things in their environment. Individuals with an external locus of control are more likely to feel powerless and helpless to change things and to be dependent on others. Research has shown that internality increases with age. Children become more internal as they develop into adulthood. Internality becomes stable in middle age and does not decrease in old age. Warm, supportive parents who encourage independence in their offspring have been shown to foster the development of internality in their children (de Mann *et al.*, 1992).

Locus of control scores tend to correlate with anxiety, and there tend be more externals than internals among people with mental health problems (Lefcourt, 1992). A major review of studies on depression and locus of control concluded that external scores correlate positively with higher levels of depression (Benassi *et al*, 1988). This link with externality and depression is still reported currently, and it also links with suicidal behaviour. Cvengros *et al.* (2005) examined relationships between locus of control and levels of depression in patients suffering chronic kidney disease. They compared patient scores on health, locus of control, depression and progression of the illness over a 22-month period. Results

Respondents are asked to circle either of the two statements to indicate which statement they agree with.

Item 2

- Many of the unhappy things in people's lives are partly due to bad luck. (external locus of control)
- People's misfortunes result from the mistakes they make. (internal locus of control)

Item 9

- I have often found that what is going to happen will happen. (external locus of control)
- Trusting to fate has never turned out as well for me as making a decision to take a definite course of action. (internal locus of control)

Item 29

- What happens to me is my own doing. (internal locus of control)
- Sometimes I feel that I don't have enough control over the direction my life is taking. (external locus of control)

Figure 11.3 Sample items from Rotter's locus of control scale.
Source: Rotter (1966).

demonstrated that patients who experienced an increase in their locus of control scores, demonstrating that they felt that they had more control over aspects of their condition, were less likely to be depressed. Liu *et al.* (2005) surveyed 1,362 adolescents in five schools in rural China and examined the relationships between locus of control, suicidal behaviours, life stressors, depression and family characteristics. They reported that high scores on the external locus of control were a risk factor for suicidal ideation and suicide attempts, along with high life stress, increasing age and depression.

A similar pattern is found for physical health, with internals becoming better informed about their illness and coping better with physical illness. Externals are more likely to adopt a passive patient role, while internals are more likely to get involved in their treatment by adopting healthier behaviour (Powell, 1992). Internal locus of control has been shown to be associated with improved quality of life in patients undergoing treatment for HIV (Préau and the APROCO study group, 2005). The study assessed quality of life, locus of control and demographic and health factors in 309 HIV-infected patients at the start of their treatment programme and then monitored the sample over 44 months of treatment. After 44 months of treatment, internal locus of control was a determinant of higher quality of both physical and mental health. Similar results, demonstrating better quality of life for internals, have been reported for individuals suffering from chronic illnesses such as epilepsy (Amir *et al.*, 1999), diabetes (Aalto *et al.*, 1997) and migraines (Allen *et al.*, 2000).

Locus of control has also been shown to impact on behaviour in many other situations. Lerner *et al.* (2005) carried out a study examining risk and protective factors in psychological distress experienced by 6,000 immigrants who had come to Israel from Russia. In a survey taken 5 years after the immigration, the researchers showed that psychological distress levels in the participants were linked with having an external locus of control as well as with other negative health and social factors. Locus of control is also applied in organisational research. For example, Allen *et al.* (2005) looked at the role of locus of control among other variables in predicting whether employees acted on their intention to change jobs, or whether they simply talked about it. They found that individuals with an internal locus of control were more likely to translate their intention to change jobs into action and change their job.

Locus of control has also been applied in educational contexts. Martinez (1994) showed that internals tend to achieve greater academic success than externals do. It is suggested that when internals do well in examinations or essays, they tend to attribute their success to their own abilities or to having worked hard. Externals, on the other hand, are more likely to put their success down to luck or an easy test. These differences in causal attribution will affect the confidence with which internals and externals approach academic assessment. Bender (1995) has suggested that the experience of continued failure despite trying at school leads to the development of an external locus of control in schoolchildren. They see that trying hard brings no reward, so they give up and may come to see failure as their destiny. Anderman and Midgley (1997) suggest that in the circumstances of repeated failure, having an external locus of control protects the individual's self-esteem. It is then not their fault that they fail. Internals, on the other hand, will be more confident and have higher expectations of themselves, both of which increase their probability of success. With very few exceptions, it appears that internals are more successful than externals in most situations. However, remember that the IE Scale is a continuum, and scores tend to cluster around the middle of the scale with few very extreme scores.[A]

[A]Maltby, J., Day, L., & Macaskill, A. (2013). Theories and measurement of intelligence. In *Personality, Individual Differences and Intelligence* (3rd ed., pp. 77–88). Harlow, Essex: Pearson Education Limited.

Humanistic theories applied to school education

What was your school like? Were you allowed to construct your timetable, decide which subjects to study, have no obligatory assessment? Were the teachers concerned that you had enough time to play and enjoy yourself? This was probably not your experience of school. It is most likely to have had a set curriculum, obligatory coursework, tests and examinations. The theorists that we examine here suggest that such educational conformity frequently stifles our individuality and creativity as human beings and encourages competition rather than cooperation. There is one school in England that defies this educational conformity. Summerhill was set up by the famous educationalist A. S. Neil in 1923, in Lyme Regis. In 1927 the school was moved to Suffolk, where it still operates today, run by Neil's son.

Neil believed that children must live their own lives, not the lives that their parents or school teachers think they should live. Neil believed that our aim in life is to find happiness. By living different experiences, Neil felt, we will find things that interest us; and this will make us happy and provide us with the motivation to work at these things. He strongly believed that traditional education stifles creativity in most children, and that they lose their love of learning and exploring new ideas. He established Summerhill to provide the ideal learning environment, giving children freedom to choose their interests and to develop their personalities freely within a democratically run community. The Summerhill philosophy exemplifies many of the ideas expounded by the personality theorists who are discussed here. There are scheduled lessons at Summerhill; however, each child is given a blank timetable, and they are free to attend lessons as they choose. Many new pupils say they have no intention of ever going to lessons again, but such is the culture of the school that they are drawn to participate in learning because the experiences are fun. The basic belief in Summerhill, shared by the theorists who we discuss here, is that as a species we are inquisitive and want to learn – and that if we are given the freedom to learn, then we will learn. There is no compulsory coursework; there are no tests or examinations. Neil believed that education must be a preparation for life and that children will learn what they want to learn and be happier as a result. He felt that only by giving children the freedom to develop as they choose will their true personalities develop. He believed that assessment, examinations and prizes sidetrack proper personality development. Children in conventional education, he claimed, are socialised into developing in ways that meet the expectations of others, such as parents and teachers, and the children's true selves can often be lost in the process.

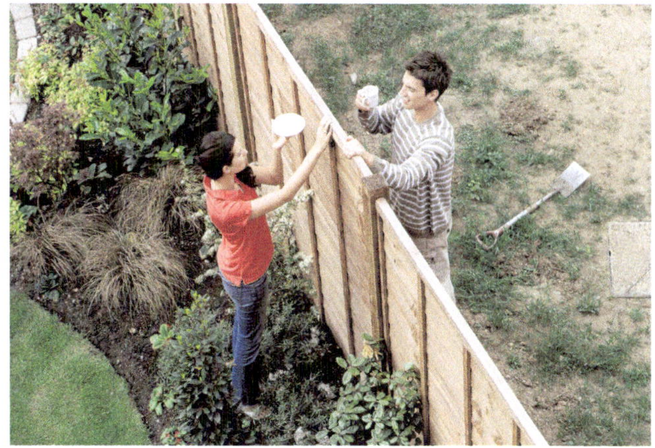

Source: Alamy Images/Image Source Black

This is obviously a very contentious stance and one that you may want to discuss further with your fellow students. Do you think it would have been a good experience for you? In 1999 the school received an unfavourable Office for Standards in Education (Ofsted) report from the government school inspectors. The school was in danger of being closed, but it took the government to court and actually won the case. From the site you can access the Ofsted report and details of the court case. Summerhill is of interest to us as it practises many of the principles outlined by Abraham Maslow and Carl Rogers, the two personality theorists presented here, and we will return to it later.

Both Maslow and Rogers were American psychologists, but European psychology and philosophy heavily influenced their ideas. In this discussion, we will examine the historical roots of the approach that influenced both theorists and helped define the key principles. Each theorist is presented in turn and then the overall approach is evaluated.

Historical roots and key elements of the humanistic approach

In early twentieth-century American psychology, the two main influences were the psychoanalytic tradition and the learning theory approaches that we have covered previously. Maslow and Rogers were initially educated in the psychoanalytic tradition, and the dominant learning theory approaches played a significant part in their early education as psychologists. However, as neither theorist was comfortable with these approaches, they developed alternative approaches. These approaches drew on the European tradition of existential philosophy, epitomised in the writings of Friedrich Nietzsche, Søren Kierkegaard and Jean-Paul Sartre. There is no one agreed-upon definition of existential philosophy. It addresses what is called ontology, defined as 'the science of being'. Existential philosophers are concerned with how we find meaning for our existence, what motivates us to keep on living. They emphasise the uniqueness of human beings and focus on issues of free will and human responsibility. These existential themes are incorporated into the work of both Maslow and Rogers.

Maslow and Rogers' theories are often described as humanistic personality theories. Several characteristics define humanistic approaches. There is always an emphasis on *personal growth*. Human beings are seen to be motivated by a need to grow and develop in a positive way. Human nature is conceptualised as being positive, unlike the Freudian conception of human nature as innately aggressive and destructive. The focus in humanistic theories is on the here and now. Individuals are discouraged from focusing on the past. While the past may have helped to shape the person you are, you are seen as being able to change. Within humanistic approaches, individuals are encouraged to savour the moment without worrying overly about the past or the future. There is also an emphasis on personal responsibility. Borrowing from the existential philosophers, there is an emphasis on human beings having free will in terms of the choices they make in their lives; and consequently, they are responsible for these choices. Sometimes we assume that we do not have a choice, but the humanists would suggest that this is because we find the alternatives too hard to undertake. Examples of this include Albert Ellis' rational-emotive behaviour therapy. Ellis' theory, although classified as a cognitive theory, also shares this humanistic bent.

The final defining feature of humanistic theories is an emphasis on the phenomenology of the individual person. Phenomenological approaches focus on trying to understand individual experience and consciousness. The concept of the uniqueness of each individual and their experience is stressed. Individuals are conceptualised as being the experts on themselves, and humanistic therapists aim merely to help their clients understand what their problems are and not to provide solutions.

Abraham Maslow and self-actualisation

We looked earlier at Maslow's hierarchy of needs. Here we will concentrate on his view of human nature and human motivation.

Human nature and human motivation

Maslow wanted to move from the early focus of psychology on clinical populations and the related psychopathology to explore how to make the average human being happier and healthier. He began with the assumption that human nature is basically good, as opposed to the negative conceptualisation of humans provided by Freud. Maslow described human beings as having innate tendencies towards healthy growth and development that he labelled **instinctoid tendencies** (Maslow, 1954). These positive instinctoid tendencies were conceptualised by Maslow as being weak and easily overcome by negative environmental influences. If the instinctoid tendencies in children are fostered, they will have the capacity to display honesty, trust, kindness, love and generosity and will develop constructively into healthy individuals. Conversely, if children grow up in an unhealthy environment they can easily lose their positive instinctoid tendencies and grow up to become destructive, aggressive and unloving individuals, engaging in self-destructive and self-defeating behaviour (Maslow, 1954; 1965; 1968; 1970). Maslow suggests that such individuals feature among Freud's case studies, and he acknowledges that psychoanalytic theories and therapies provide useful tools for psychologists having to deal with this disturbed population. However, his wish was to focus on the positive possibilities in human development; he felt that this approach, alongside the work of the psychoanalysts, would then provide a complete theory of human personality (Maslow, 1968).

Maslow's interest was in trying to understand what motivates us to go about our lives and make the choices that we do. As we saw previously, this is a fundamental area for personality theories to address. In his early doctoral studies, Maslow had become interested in the needs that animals display, and he demonstrated that it was possible to organise these needs into a hierarchy. The needs lower in the hierarchy must be satisfied before we address higher-level needs. From his observations, he suggested that a similar system existed for human beings. He described two distinct types of human motivations. The first are **deficiency motives**; that is, basic needs that we are driven to fulfil. These include drives like hunger, thirst and the need for safety and to be loved by someone. Maslow conceptualises these needs as representing something that we lack and are motivated to get. If we are hungry, once we have obtained sufficient food, this need is met. The need then ceases to be a motivator. Maslow gave examples of the economic depression in America in the 1930s, when thousands of people lost their jobs. Feeding their family became the dominant need for many people, so they were happy to get any job that would allow them to achieve their goal. He compares this situation with economically affluent times and suggests that, when people are wealthier, their motivational needs change. Hunger is no longer a threat, so they are motivated to get a better house or car, or a more interesting job and so on.

The second type of needs Maslow outlines are **growth motives**, sometimes called **being motives** or **B-motives**. These needs are unique to each individual and are conceptualised as gaining intensity as they are met. He suggests that these needs are about developing the individual's potential. They include things like giving love unselfishly; increases in drive, like curiosity and the thirst for knowledge; developing skills and having new experiences. Maslow felt that the personal growth involved in these B-motives was exciting and rewarding for the individuals and served to stimulate them further. This is a crucial difference between deficiency motives and growth motives. Deficiency motives create a negative motivational

Instinctoid tendencies
Maslow's description of human beings as having innate tendencies towards healthy growth and development.

Deficiency motives
Some basic needs that we lack and are motivated to get. They include drives like hunger, thirst, the need for safety and the need to be loved. They are the basic motives that ensure human survival. Deficiency motives create a negative motivational state that can only be changed by satisfying the need.

Growth motives
Sometimes called being motives or B-motives, these needs are unique to each individual and are responsible for the development of the individual to their full potential. Growth motives represent a higher level of functioning. They differ from deficiency motives in that they create a positive motivational state that continues to develop.

state that can be changed only by satisfying the need; in contrast, growth motives can be enjoyable, and satisfying these needs can act as further motivation to achieve personal goals and ambitions. In this way, deficiency motives are seen to ensure our survival, while growth needs represent a higher level of functioning that can result in us becoming happier, healthier and more fulfilled as individuals. Maslow suggested that the psychoanalysts had overemphasised drive reduction as a motivator for human behaviour because this tended to be true of the clinical populations that were their focus. He acknowledged that human motives were complex and that behaviour could be motivated by several needs. For example, an apparently simple behaviour like eating might be motivated by hunger, the need to be with others or by the need for emotional comfort when a love affair goes wrong; we are sure you can think of other motives. If we ate only to fulfil our hunger needs, obesity would not be such a health problem in western societies.

Hierarchy of needs

Maslow (1970) felt that it would be difficult to produce lists of human needs given the complexity of human motivation and the way that behaviour could be motivated by several needs. However, he argued that needs vary significantly in terms of their importance for ensuring our survival. To this end, he developed what has become his famous hierarchy of needs. Some needs have to be met before other needs are acknowledged and begin to motivate our behaviour. We saw this earlier in the economic depression example. Maslow's hierarchy of needs is displayed in Figure 11.4. It begins with lower-level or survival needs, which have to be satisfied first before we seek gratification of our higher-order needs.

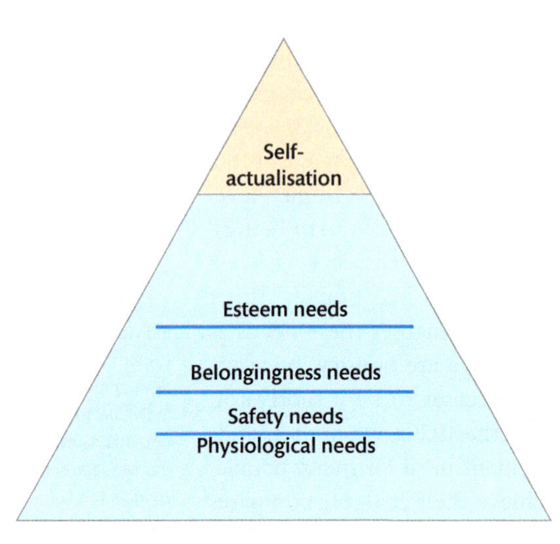

Figure 11.4 Maslow's hierarchy of needs.

Our physiological needs include hunger, thirst, sleep, oxygen, the elimination of bodily waste and sex. Most of these are deficiency needs, and once they are satisfied, the motivation to pursue the activity ceases. If we are thirsty we have a drink of water, and the need is satisfied. The exceptions are sexual drive, the need for elimination and sleep; these are considered to be growth needs (Maslow, 1968). Sexual needs, for example, do not decrease with gratification but frequently increase. Rarely in western cultures are individuals in the position of being motivated only by their physiological needs; however, we can imagine that if you were starving, food would be your number one priority and all your other needs for respect, love and the like would be of little importance. Once our physiological needs are satisfied, we then turn our attention to the next level of needs as a source of motivation.

The safety needs

Needs at the next level of Maslow's hierarchy include needs for security, safe circumstances to live within, self-protection, law-abiding communities and a sense of order. Although Maslow tended to focus on the positive aspects of these drives, what emerges at this level are your fears and anxieties about your own safety – and these motivate your behaviour. If you live in a large estate where violence and crime are rife, you can imagine being motivated to work either at getting a house in a safer place or at changing the environment to make it safer. Which you would choose is likely to be influenced by other personality factors, such as your levels of altruism and political and situational factors. For others, the choice might be getting securer locks on their doors or altering their behaviour to minimise the risk of being harmed. All of these behaviours Maslow would conceptualise as being motivated by our need for security.

Maslow (1970) pointed out that the safety needs can be clearly observed in infants and young children where they are upset by loud unexplained noises, rough handling or major changes in their daily routine. He strongly believed that children need routines, consistently enforced rules and limits imposed on their behaviour to meet their safety needs. The absence of this safe, relatively predictable environment would impact badly on a child's development, although Maslow did not specify the specific negative effects likely to occur.

His contention was that we all prefer to live in stable societies, where we feel safe and are not continually at risk of being robbed or mugged or our homes burgled. This may be one of the reasons that, in general elections, voters always seem to be interested in issues of law and order. Maslow would say that such prospective voters are being motivated by their safety needs to take an interest in such things. Our safety needs also motivate us to buy insurance and save for a pension or a rainy day, and they may motivate us to train for a secure job where we feel our skills will always be in demand and we are unlikely to be made redundant. Maslow (1968) pointed out that the downside of safety needs is that they can stifle our growth by encouraging us always to opt for the safe choice and thereby minimise risk in our life.

Belongingness and love needs

Once our physiological and safety needs are largely taken care of, Maslow states that our needs for belongingness and love become more important motivators of our behaviour. He is saying that we all need to feel that we are needed and accepted by others. Human beings are conceptualised as social beings, and we need to feel that we are rooted in communities, with ties to family and friends. Our need for belongingness motivates us to make friends, to join clubs and other organisations where we can meet people and socialise. Once our more basic needs have been met, we become more aware of our loneliness, absence of companions and friends, and we become motivated to do something about it. Maslow defined two distinct types of love that were based on different needs, D-love and B-love. The first is **D-love**, which is based on a deficiency need, hence the label. It is the love that we seek to meet the emptiness inside ourselves. We want it for ourselves; the loved one is there to meet our needs. In this way, it is a relatively selfish deficiency need. Maslow defines this love as consisting of individual yearning for affection, tenderness, feelings of elation and sexual arousal. It does not always bring out the best in individuals, as they may display all sorts of manipulative behaviour to try to get the attention of the person they desire. It can sometimes be observed in the young child competing for their mother's attention with their younger sibling. Maslow contrasts this need for love and belongingness for ourselves with the ability we have to love others. He calls this latter type of love **B-love** and suggests that, once our basic needs for D-love have been met, we become capable of attaining B-love. B-love or Being-love is about being able to love others in a non-possessive, unconditional way, simply loving them for being. It involves showing respect for the other, accepting their individuality, putting their needs before your own on occasion and valuing them. B-love is a growth need, and Maslow sees it as representing an emotionally mature type of love. It is possible only when the basic needs have been sufficiently gratified. At this stage, Maslow (1970) considers that the person is moving towards **self-actualisation**. Maslow was concerned about the high numbers of individuals living alone in western cultures and felt that, while this lifestyle is valued by some individuals, for most it creates loneliness as belongingness and love needs may not be met sufficiently.

D-love
Defined by Maslow as consisting of individual yearning for affection, tenderness, feelings of elation and sexual arousal. It is a deficiency need and can result in selfish, manipulative behaviour.

B-love
Involves being able to love others in a non-possessive, unconditional way. It is simply loving them for being. It is a growth need, and Maslow sees it as representing an emotionally mature type of love.

Self-actualisation
The sole motivator in Rogers' model. It is an innate, positive drive to develop and realise our potential.

The esteem needs

Esteem needs are the last of our basic needs. Maslow (1970) divided these into two types of needs. The first type of esteem need is based on our need to see ourselves as competent, achieving individuals. Secondly, there is the need for esteem based on the evaluation of others. He claimed that we have a need for respect and admiration from other people but advises that this must be deserved. He suggests that the incompetent individual who lies, cheats or buys their way into a position of authority will still feel inferior and will not enjoy their position, as their real esteem needs – especially their need to see themselves as competent and achieving – are not being met (Maslow, 1970).

The need for self-actualisation

The highest level of need is for self-actualisation. Maslow (1968; 1970) argues that once our basic needs have been met, we start to focus on what we want from life. Individuals may be very successful financially and have enough power and success that all their lower-level needs are being met, but they may still not be happy and contented. They are still searching for something. This restlessness comes from their need for self-actualisation. Self-actualisation demands that individuals develop themselves so that they achieve their full potential. It is about maximising their talents and finding meaning in life, so that they are at peace with themselves. Maslow is eager to stress that this process will be different for everyone depending on the individual's talents and interests. It is a growth need that emerges only after the other basic needs have been addressed. For this reason, Maslow (1968; 1970) describes it as coming to prominence only in older people. This idea is similar to Jung's concept of individuation. Young adults are seen as being taken up with addressing their basic needs, such as getting an education and finding work, somewhere to live, love and relationships. Maslow (1964) is clear that not all individuals achieve self-actualisation, although many strive to do so. Self-actualised individuals are thought to be rare. He suggests that the model of motivation we have just described does not fit these self-actualised individuals. He suggests that the needs of self-actualisers are qualitatively different; he describes them as **metaneeds**. The foci of metaneeds are very different, being concerned with higher aesthetic and moral values such as beauty, truth, justice and ethics. We shall be looking in some more detail shortly at the qualities of self-actualised individuals after we have concluded the discussion of Maslow's model of motivation.

Metaneeds
The needs of self-actualising individuals. These are higher-level needs that are qualitatively different, being concerned with concepts such as beauty, truth, justice and ethics.

Discussion of basic needs

Maslow's model appears very neat and simple at one level, but he stressed that his hierarchical model is an oversimplification of the actual relationship between needs and behaviour. The reality is that, while the order makes sense for most people, there will be individual exceptions. The priority of our needs will vary depending on our personal circumstances across time, so that it is not a static model. At any level, a need does not have to be totally gratified for us to be motivated by higher-order needs. Maslow estimated some average figures for need fulfilment in the average American, suggesting that on average around 85 percent of individual physical needs are met, 70 percent of safety needs, 50 percent of belongingness and love, 40 percent of self-esteem needs and 10 percent of self-actualisation needs. Thinking about percentage need in this way helps to get across Maslow's idea that the degree to which a need is unfulfilled will influence the impact it has on the individual's behaviour. For example, if a long-term relationship ends, the belongingness and love needs are likely to be much less satisfied than they were previously. This results in the individual becoming more motivated to seek solace with others, and the person will derive some comfort from being with friends and other relatives as this helps increase their sense of belonging.

Maslow (1968; 1970) claimed that his model had universal applicability, but that the means of gratification might change within cultures. He felt that we share many of the basic needs, such as physiological and safety needs, with other animals, but the higher-order needs are distinctly human. The higher apes display a need for love and belongingness, but Maslow felt that self-actualisation is a uniquely human pursuit.

He stressed that the motivation for behaviour is frequently immensely complex and that many behaviours are motivated by a variety of needs. Using the example of sexual behaviour, Maslow pointed out that it can be motivated by a physiological need for sexual release, or it can be a need for love and affection, a wish to feel masculine or feminine or to express a sense of mastery in a situation and so on. Thus, the activities we engage in may also satisfy more than one set of needs at any one time. Maslow (1970) also acknowledges the importance of unconscious motivation. He perceives the instinctoid tendencies as being quite weak and easily overcome by situational factors, and consequently we may often not be consciously aware of how they affect our motivation. However, unlike Freud, who claims that unconscious motives originating in our past experiences cause our behaviour and also determine our goals, Maslow sees human beings as being future-oriented. For Maslow, our ultimate goal is self-actualisation driven on by our motivational needs. It is the instinctoid needs that he conceptualises as frequently influencing us unconsciously. There is some inconsistency in Maslow's theorising here as he also accepts the validity of the Freudian defence mechanisms. He accepted that they play a crucial role in preventing individuals knowing themselves and yet the individual is unconscious of their effect. So, here we have further evidence of unconscious motivation based on past experiences influencing behaviour. In Maslow's defence, he wanted his focus to be on healthy individuals. He was clear that the psychologically healthy individual needs to use defence mechanisms much less, and therefore the role of unconscious motivation based on past experiences is also less.

Characteristics of self-actualisers

Maslow wanted his theory to be about human aspirations and abilities. He did not want to focus on clinical populations and their psychopathology, as is the case with so many other personality theories. To meet this aim, he undertook interview studies of individuals who appeared to him to be self-actualised; he also conducted studies of famous historical figures, using any documents about them that he could find. Among those he studied were Albert Einstein, Eleanor Roosevelt, William James, Thomas Jefferson, Albert Schweitzer, Jane Addams and Baruch Spinoza (Maslow, 1968). He described this research as undertaking a holistic analysis, the aim of which was to understand individuals in some depth. From this study, he outlined the characteristics of self-actualising individuals. At the outset we need to acknowledge, as Maslow (1970) did, that this data was impressionistic and did not meet conventional scientific standards in terms of reliability and validity. However, Maslow published these studies as he felt that the topic was so important.

Every healthy person studied was described by Maslow as being creative. The creativity of the self-actualised was a way of approaching life. It did not necessarily mean that they painted pictures or produced poetry and so on, which is how we tend to think conventionally about creativity. Rather, they approached everyday tasks in novel ways. They might be a conventionally creative person as well, but an example he gave was of a woman who expressed her creativity in producing very interesting meals and presenting them beautifully in quite novel ways. Self-actualisers found little everyday things interesting, and Maslow compares them with young children who take such pleasure from small discoveries. Self-actualisers have not lost their awe of the world and their interest in the minutiae.

Being cognition
The different style of thinking adopted by self-actualisers. It is non-judgemental and involves feelings of being at one with the world. It is a transient state experienced at times of self-actualisation.

Peak experiences
The different style of thinking adopted by self-actualisers. It is non-judgemental and involves feelings of being at one with the world. It is a transient state experienced at times of self-actualisation.

Deficiency cognition
The term Maslow used to describe the thoughts we have when we are making judgements about how well our experiences are meeting our deficiency needs.

Self-actualisers also think differently, according to Maslow (1962). He claimed that self-actualisers engage more often in what he termed **being cognition (B-cognition)**. This is a non-judgemental form of thought. It is about accepting oneself and the world and just being and feeling at one with the world. Maslow referred to B-cognition occurring at moments of experiencing self-actualisation in what he termed **peak experiences**; and obviously, self-actualisers have more of these peak experiences. More recently, Csikszentmihalyi (1999) has defined this concept of peak experiences in some detail, although he has renamed them optimal experiences. The characteristics that Csikszentmihalyi describes as defining such experiences are summarised in Table 11.2. This list will give you a much better understanding of Maslow's concept of peak experience.

B-cognition is contrasted with the more normally occurring **deficiency cognition (D-cognition)**. D-cognition is judgemental, and in it we see ourselves as distinct from the world around us. It is about making judgements about how well our experiences are meeting our deficiency needs. Maslow (1962) stresses that B-cognition states are transient even for self-actualisers. He points out that it is dangerous to exist continually in a passive, non-judgemental, non-intervening state.

In terms of their personal characteristics, self-actualisers tend to have higher levels of self-acceptance. They also accept others more easily, being less judgemental and more tolerant of others. Maslow also claimed that they perceive reality more accurately with fewer distortions. This is linked to them being more in touch with themselves and being less psychologically defended. The use of a defence mechanism tends to distort reality. For example, if you failed to get a job you really wanted, the defended individual might say that the process was unfair, or deny that they wanted the job, while the self-actualiser is more likely to be truthful.

Self-actualisers tend to have well-developed ethical and moral standards and are more likely to accept responsibility for their actions. They have greater self-knowledge and tend to follow their codes of ethics. They also have a strong wish to help others and are concerned about the welfare of the communities in which they live. This quality is the same as Adler's concept of social interest, and Maslow acknowledges a debt to Adler for this concept. Self-actualisers are good at focusing on problems and seeing them through to resolution. They are often more interested in the big picture than the minor details. In their working lives, they are more likely to be motivated by a desire to fulfil their inner potential than by promises of more wealth or other trappings of success. They do things because they want to rather than it being a way to get on at work. In this way, they are more independent and less influenced by cultural norms and much more likely to make up their own minds about issues and act accordingly.

In their personalities, self-actualisers tend to have deeper personal relationships, preferring to have a few close friends rather than a wide circle of acquaintances. Maslow also claimed

Table 11.2 The characteristics of peak experiences

1	The individual's attention is totally absorbed by the activity.
2	The activity has clear objectives so that the person has a clear goal to work towards.
3	It is a challenging activity that requires the person's full attention but is not so difficult that they cannot make meaningful progress.
4	The person is able to concentrate fully on the task at hand, and other parts of their life do not impinge on what they are doing.
5	The individual feels in control of the activity.
6	The activity is so personally engrossing that the individual does not think about themselves while engaging in it.
7	All sense of time is lost while the person is engaged. Most commonly, time passes very quickly.
8	The activity tends to be one where feedback is clearly available, so that the person is aware of making progress even though it may be based on only a personal evaluation.

that they are more likely to demonstrate the non-possessive B-love. Their sense of humour is also different. They find jokes based on superiority or aggressive hostility offensive and prefer more philosophically based humour.

Maslow's description of self-actualising individuals makes them sound like absolute paragons of virtue. However, as Maslow (1968; 1970) points out, this is far from the case. No one is a self-actualising individual all the time in all their activities. Similarly, peak experiences come and go. At times, self-actualising individuals can be as annoying and irritating as anyone. Like Albert Ellis, Maslow strongly believed that there are no perfect human beings, but some are happier than others.

Personality development

Maslow did not provide a great deal of detailed information about personality development; rather, he outlined some core principles. Firstly, he conceptualised children as having an innate drive to develop. This is a positive drive fuelled by the motivational needs outlined in his hierarchy of needs. Maslow felt that, as children become socialised, there is a crucial time for their development. This is when they decide whether they are going to listen to what he terms 'their inner voice' and develop according to their own instinctoid needs or whether they are going to follow their parental dictates. Maslow concluded that parental expectations and cultural expectations influence most children, but this is because children are seldom given real choices. If you cast your mind back to the material you read about Summerhill School in the introduction to this discussion, Summerhill exemplifies the sort of learning experience that Maslow felt was the ideal for creating happy, fulfilled individuals. Children are not coerced but are given choices, and Maslow assumed that their natural desire to grow will direct them towards engaging in learning experiences. This is the reported Summerhill experience. There are rules – indeed, quite a large number of them – but they are formulated with the pupils and enforced by the whole community. Maslow is clear that children need rules and limits to meet their safety needs. Like Adler, he felt that pampering is very bad for children and that having some rules to come up against is beneficial. Children need to be given considerable freedom of choice but they also need to be given responsibilities. In this way, they are encouraged always to take responsibility for their behaviour. The satisfaction of a child's needs, as specified in Maslow's hierarchy, is the best way to encourage healthy development; as long as this is done in a disciplined way and the child is not pampered.

Mental illness and its treatment in Maslow's approach

For Maslow (1970) there was one underlying cause for all mental illness and psychological disturbance, and that was the failure to satisfy the individual's fundamental needs as outlined in the hierarchy. He felt the lower the level of need that is not being satisfied, the more profound the disturbance. For example, someone who has failed to find any place in the world and in relationships that make them feel safe is more disturbed than someone who is still searching for love and respect. In this conceptualisation, it is clear that the basic needs have a psychological aspect to them and are not merely physical needs. Safety is not just about a safe environment, although it is part of it. If you feel unsafe where you live, you are more likely to be anxious and it will impact your psychological health. Similarly, if you do not have any family or close relationships that you feel secure in, you are going to be very anxious and upset as your needs are not being met.

In terms of treatment, Maslow adopted an eclectic approach. He was against all diagnostic labels and the medical model that they implied. To improve their health, individuals needed to be assisted towards self-actualisation. Maslow was a trained psychoanalyst, and he used psychoanalysis on occasion for severe problems. For less disturbed individuals, he would use briefer therapies, including behaviour therapy. He was also a fan of group therapy and encounter groups for healthy individuals to help them to self-actualise further. We will discuss encounter groups in more detail later in the discussion, when we look at the work of Carl Rogers. Thus Maslow is seen as adopting an eclectic approach to therapy – even utilising psychoanalysis, which is somewhat at odds with his rejection of the medical model and his conceptualisation of the causes of psychological disturbance. This inconsistency did not appear to concern him.

Evaluation of Maslow's theory

We will now evaluate Maslow's theory using eight criteria: description, explanation, empirical validity, testable concepts, comprehensiveness, parsimony, heuristic value and applied value.

Description

Maslow provides a reasonable, if somewhat simplified, description of human behaviour. The theory therefore is high on face validity. However, he does present an extremely positive and almost simplistic view of human nature and human beings. This is somewhat at odds with his acceptance of many Freudian defence mechanisms, as we have discussed earlier in this discussion. Defence mechanisms refer to the complexity of human motivation and the difficulties in explaining behaviour even to ourselves. Maslow does not acknowledge these inconsistencies in his theorising.

It seems somewhat simplistic to claim that blocks to self-actualisation are at the root of all human behavioural problems. There is no mention of genetic susceptibilities to mental illness and sociopathic conditions, for example. To put so much emphasis on environmental influences is untenable, as biological evidence shows.

Explanation

While Maslow's theory seems to present a neat, rational explanation of human motivation, it does appear to suggest that motivation is more clear-cut than it generally is, and that the link between our needs and our behaviour is obvious. The reality is that behaviour is frequently the result of many different motivators. For example, if you take the case of someone doing a menial job that is poorly paid, the assumption from Maslow is that they are working to earn money to meet their physiological and safety needs. The job itself is not inherently satisfying; however, they may work with a good set of colleagues, and this may meet their belongingness needs and compensate for the nature of the work, so they are not motivated to seek more conducive or better paid work. An example of this might be where a member of a company cleaning staff shows a marked reluctance to become a supervisor even though it paid more. Although the job might bring extra money and be physically easier, they might not consider this compensation for the loss of comradeship from the other cleaners. Maslow has provided useful insights into human motivational needs, but perhaps not the whole picture.

Maslow's work on defining types of needs and types of love is interesting. It was a new, very creative approach to these topics. In his work on general needs and types of love, he presents a less positive perspective on human beings, seeing us as capable of being manipulative, disrespectful of others and very demanding in the way that we treat others. This is somewhat at odds with his generally positive view of human beings, but he does not really acknowledge these inconsistencies in his theory.

Empirical validity

While self-actualisation is at the core of Maslow's theory, the research on which it is based is dubious. He selected a very small sample of participants to investigate the concept. These were not randomly selected; rather, Maslow chose to examine individuals whom he believed to be self-actualisers. He did not use any objective measures to assess these individuals, and there was a lack of consistency in assessment between individuals. In all, it was an extremely subjective process, more descriptive than evaluative.

Testable concepts

Many of Maslow's other concepts are also difficult to define precisely and therefore difficult to test empirically. Examples include peak experiences where it is unclear exactly what is meant. Self-actualisers are thought to be rare individuals, yet researchers such as Leiby (1997) report that drug-induced peak experiences are common. This raises the issue of whether and how these artificially induced experiences relate to self-actualisation. Ravizza (1977) reported that many athletes report peak experiences but are not self-actualisers in any other aspects of their lives. Thus, questions are raised about the relationship between peak experiences and self-actualisation.

The basis for Maslow's selection of the five basic needs is also unclear. He does not provide a rationale for their selection, and many other human needs can be identified. His theorising embraces many assumptions about human behaviour that are stated authoritatively, but the supporting evidence is either absent or weak. He did argue against the empiricism of existing psychological methodologies, but this does not excuse his lack of attention to providing objective support for this theory (Maslow, 1970).

Most of the concepts in Maslow's theory are imprecisely defined, so they are difficult to research. There have been more systematic attempts to measure self-actualisation. Shostrum (1966) developed a measure called the personal orientation inventory (POI). It is a self-report questionnaire with 150 items that are answered positively or negatively. It measures the degree to which individuals are inner-directed on one major scale and whether they use their time effectively on the second major scale, both of which are thought to relate to self-actualisation, as we have seen. There are 10 subscales measuring self-actualising values, feeling reactivity, existentiality, self-regard, spontaneity, self-acceptance, nature of humankind, synergy, acceptance of aggression and capacity for intimate contact. While the validity and the usefulness of the measure was established using several samples (Dosamantes-Alperson and Merrill, 1980; Knapp, 1976), there are problems with it. Participants do not like the forced-choice response mode, feeling that it does not give an accurate reflection of their views, and other researchers have reported that it correlates poorly with other related measures such as the purpose in life test (PIL) devised by Crumbaugh and Maholick (1969). Mittleman (1991) reviews much of this work on self-actualisation and concludes that self-actualisation is difficult to measure, but the most reliable aspect of it relates only to possessing openness to experience.

Comprehensiveness

Maslow's theory is really focused on positive growth and, as such, it is not a comprehensive theory. His approach was new and creative, making a welcome change to the previous theories with their emphasis on psychopathology. He did attempt some discussion of psychopathology and adopted aspects of Freud's model, but this was not done in a systematic or comprehensive fashion. The explanation of human motivation is also limited. There is much more emphasis on self-actualisation, but even here the precise detail is missing.

Maslow does not spell out exactly how self-actualisation can be achieved. Similarly, he talks only in very general terms about the development of personality.

Parsimony

Maslow's theory is very concise for a theory of human personality. We have already discussed how his concept of motivation is limited and how the selection of five basic needs is somewhat arbitrary. The description of personality development is lacking in detail. We have also discussed the limitations of Maslow's treatment of psychopathology and how the adoption of Freudian concepts such as defence mechanisms is inconsistent with the rest of his theory. As a general theory, the conclusion must be that it is too parsimonious.

Heuristic value

Although Maslow's theory has many limitations, it undoubtedly has had a major impact on many researchers, both in psychology and other disciplines. He was one of the first theorists to focus on the healthy side of human psychological development. His focus on human achievement and human values introduced new foci for psychologists. By vehemently questioning the dominant laboratory study approach to psychology, he caused psychologists to review their research methodologies (Maslow, 1970). He stressed the need to ask meaningful questions rather than pursue more trivial research that could easily be addressed by the existing laboratory-based practices. He wanted researchers to think creatively about developing methodologies that could address important real-life issues, although it might mean losing some control of the laboratory-based studies. He also influenced subsequent theorists such as Rogers, as we shall see.

Applied value

The area where Maslow's work has had most impact is in business. His theory of motivation became and is still popular with managers. It led to an increasing emphasis on the need to offer development opportunities to employees. Maslow stressed the importance of consulting with employees and fostering a sense of belonging within companies, and this concept has been embraced by generations of business managers (Maslow, 1967). His influence also extended to counselling and healthcare professional training, as it provided a neat system for examining human motivational needs. Maslow's work also had a major impact on educational programmes. He emphasised the importance of student-centred learning, suggesting that individuals want to learn and that the role of educators is to provide the environment to facilitate such learning. As discussed in the introduction, he saw schools like Summerhill as offering this learning environment.

Carl Rogers and person-centred therapy

In our review of Carl Rogers' theory, we are first going to outline the basic principles underlying the theory.

Basic principles underlying the theory

Carl Rogers, like most of the personality theorists we have studied, based his theory on disturbed clinical populations. His initial work was based mainly on his experience of working with disturbed adolescents, as detailed in the Profile box. Many of the therapists that Rogers worked with initially at the American equivalent of the National Society for the Prevention of Cruelty to Children (NSPCC) were psychoanalytically trained, but he increasingly felt uncomfortable working psychoanalytically. His personality theory grew out of his theory of therapy. He acknowledged that experience plays an important part in personality development, but he could not accept the Freudian notion that the early years largely dictate adult development. He felt that individuals can play an active role in shaping their own lives. He, like Maslow, saw human beings as being future-oriented and believed that our future goals influence our current behaviour. In this way, he saw individuals as having the power to shape their own lives.

This focus on the power of the individual to change their lives is reflected in the title of his approach. He first named it client-centred therapy. The term 'patient' was the norm at the time among therapists and is very much associated with the medical model of illness where the doctor/therapist is the expert who provides treatment and hopefully a cure to the patient. In this relationship, the therapist is the expert and the patient is less powerful and receives the expert's knowledge. Therefore the medical model has traditionally assigned a relatively passive role to the patient. Adopting an existential humanistic stance, as we discussed in the introduction, Rogers (1951) felt that individuals are the best experts on themselves, not the therapist. He selected the term 'client' to suggest a more equal role, similar to that of customer and provider. The term 'client-centred' reflects Rogers' view that clients are the experts on themselves and that the role of the therapist is to help the client to better recognise their problems and formulate their issues. In this way, the therapist acts more as a facilitator. Once clients understood what the problem was, Rogers felt that they would know how to solve it in a way that suited their particular life situation. Later he changed the term to 'person-centred', feeling that the term 'person' is more power-neutral than the word 'client'.

Rogers adopted a phenomenological position about the nature of reality. He stressed that we all function within a perceptual or subjective frame of reference (Rogers, 1956). He denied the possibility of an objective reality that we all share. Instead, we all perceive our own reality. Sometimes students have a problem with this idea, as you may be having. However, if you think about the unreliability of eyewitness testimony, something that social psychologists have spent some time studying (Kassin *et at.*, 1989; Loftus, 1979), the meaning will become clearer. We know that even in experimental situations, there are significant individual differences in terms of the interpretation of events and the details seen

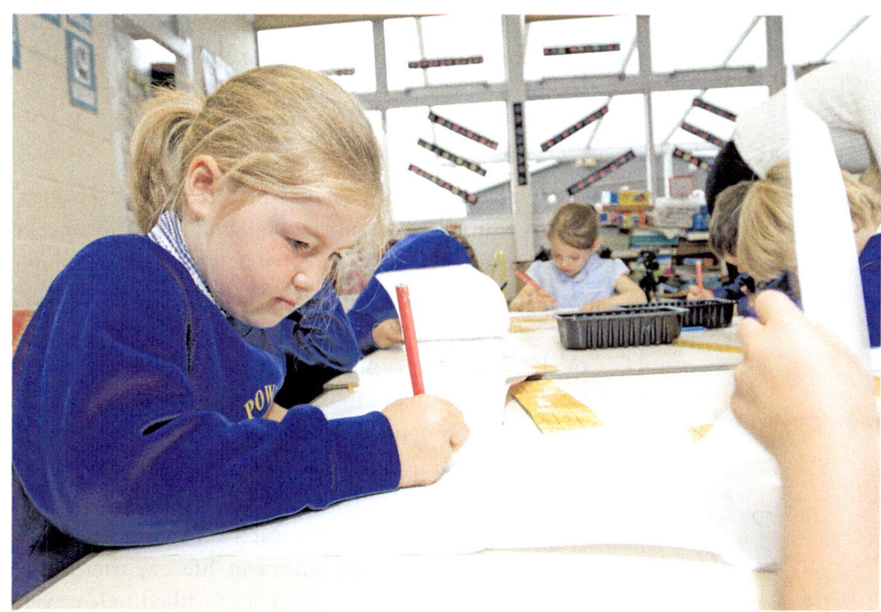

Rogers believed that we are the best experts on ourselves and that people are capable of working out their own solutions to their own problems.
Source: Pearson Education Ltd. Jules Selmes

by different observers. Rogers points out that how we perceive a situation depends on our mood, the type of person we are, our beliefs, our past experiences and so on. This relates to the ABC model, used in rational-emotive behaviour therapy, to conceptualise our perceptual processes. Rogers, like Ellis, accepts that everyone perceives situations differently; therefore, to understand an individual, you have to try to understand how they see the world. We will return to this later when we discuss Rogers' approach to counselling and therapy.

Self-actualisation

Self-actualisation The sole motivator in Rogers' model. It is an innate, positive drive to develop and realise our potential.

Rogers (1961) stressed the uniqueness of each individual. He felt that clients are the best experts on themselves and that people are capable of working out their own solutions to their own problems. He believed that each person has a natural tendency towards growth and self-actualisation. His definition of **self-actualisation** is the same as Maslow's, discussed earlier: it is an innate, positive drive to develop and realise our potential. Individuals are described as having an innate actualising tendency. It is our single basic motivating drive, and it is a positive drive towards growth. From birth, Rogers suggested we all have a drive towards actualising our potential, to become what we are capable of becoming.

Rogers (1959; 1977) claimed that we can all cope with our lives and remain psychologically healthy as long as our actualising potential is not blocked. Blocks in our actualising tendency are the cause of all psychological problems. This role for the actualising tendency differs from Maslow's conception. You will recall that, for Maslow, psychological problems result from an individual's needs not being met, and he is specific about these needs. The role that Rogers ascribed to self-actualisation is less specific. It is a general positive motivator; indeed, our only motivator. There are two aspects to it. The biological aspect includes the *drive for satisfaction* of our basic needs such as food, water, sleep, safety and sexual reproduction. The psychological aspect involves the development of our potential and the qualities that make us more worthwhile human beings (Rogers, 1959). Rogers paid most attention to the psychological aspect, self-actualisation, as he conceptualised it as being crucial for our psychological health. It is a positive drive towards growth for Rogers, just as it was for Maslow. Rogers (1977) suggested that we develop our capacity for self-destructive, aggressive and harmful behaviour only under perverse circumstances, such as growing up in a difficult environment with few opportunities for self-actualisation or not being given the freedom to develop according to our true nature. In these circumstances, our self-actualisation is blocked and problems occur. Individuals may become psychologically distressed and/or demonstrate antisocial behaviour.

Effect of society on self-actualisation

To understand fully the process of self-actualisation, we need to examine Rogers' conception of the self. Rogers made a distinction between our real self and our self-concept (see Figure 11.5). The real self is defined as being our underlying organismic self. This is, if you like, the genetic blueprint for the person we are capable of becoming if our development occurs within totally favourable circumstances. If we had these ideal developmental experiences, Rogers suggested, our behavioural choices would be guided purely by our actualising tendency. Self-actualisation would then be within everyone's reach once you had lived long enough to accrue sufficient life experiences to discover what truly made you fulfilled. However,

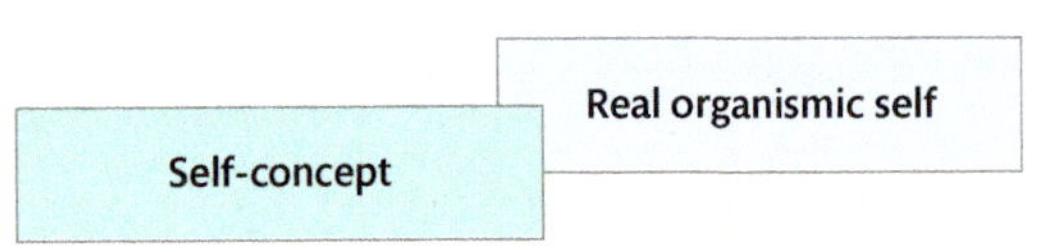

Figure 11.5 Rogers' two aspects of the self.

Rogers argued that this is rarely, if ever, the case. The explanation for this is quite complex, and we will go through it in stages.

He asserted that human beings as a species are social animals. We all need to be liked/loved by other people. Rogers was very clear about the nature of the emotional experience that is necessary for optimum development, and he termed it **unconditional positive regard**. He preferred this to the term 'love' as he asserted that love is seldom truly unconditional. Unconditional positive regard means accepting someone for who they are and valuing them just for being. The term 'regard' means seeing oneself as making a positive difference in someone else's life. It is about knowing that someone would truly miss you were you to die tomorrow. They would feel that they had a gap in their life that would always be there. It is an unselfish love, like Maslow's Being-love (B-love). You want what is best for the other above what is best for you. However, Rogers suggested that unconditional positive regard is rare and that mostly what we experience is conditional positive regard. As part of the socialisation process, we learn that we are loved/liked more when we do what others want us to do. When we behave in ways that please our parents, for example, they reward us with praise and this makes us feel good. We have obtained positive regard from them. For the most part, the positive regard we experience is not unconditional. When we misbehave, or fail an examination or refuse to do something that our parents desperately want us to do, we are likely to have experienced a sense of having disappointed our parents and being less loved and loveable as a result. These experiences help us to learn what we need to do to get positive regard from other people.

Unconditional positive regard
Non-judgemental valuing of an individual. It is the term Rogers preferred over 'love', as he felt that most of what is termed love is not unconditional.

Conditions of worth
The criteria we use to judge the adequacy of our own behaviour. They are based on other people's judgements about what is desirable behaviour.

Self-concept
The term used to refer to our perception of who we are. It is based largely on the evaluations that other people have made of us during our development.

Even more crucially, we develop what Rogers called **conditions of worth** related to these experiences. We learn that we are loved more when we do things that make our parents or other people in our social world happy. This need for positive regard leads to us acquiring conditions of worth, which we use to evaluate the impact that our behaviour is likely to have on others. What is important about conditions of worth is that they can distort the natural direction of our actualising tendency. For example, if one of my conditions of worth is that I am loved more when I am helpful and agree to do things that my friends want, I am going to find it difficult to say no to these friends when they ask for my help. I may well find myself doing lots of things that I do not really want to do. This is often the case with individuals who lack assertiveness, for example. They always agree to do things for others because their condition of worth dictates that, by doing so, they will be liked and that, conversely, if they refuse, they will be disliked. Conditions of worth are important as they can keep us doing things that do not meet our real needs, and this makes it difficult for us ever to achieve self-actualisation.

We began this section by referring to two aspects of the self: the real organismic self and the self-concept. Conditions of worth, as we shall now see, impact on our self-concept. As children grow and become socialised, they develop a sense of who they are as people. Rogers termed this their **self-concept**. It is our perception of who we are based largely on how other people have described us and evaluated us. You may have been told in your family that you are the clever one or the good-looking one, and you will have internalised this description as part of who you are. The easiest way to access your self-concept is to answer the question, 'Who am I?' Most of us find it relatively easy to produce a list of adjectives to describe ourselves, and this is our self-concept. We use the conditions of worth that we have acquired as our self-concept has developed, to evaluate our own behaviour and to help us make choices in our lives. We are conscious of the contents of our self-concept, whereas our real organismic self may have become obscured as a result of our developmental experiences of socialisation. As we saw in our discussion of conditions of worth, we may end up making choices that make other people happy but do not meet the needs of our real self. In the longer term, we are unlikely to be able to self-actualise; if this is the case, we will experience feelings of being discontented at least and perhaps even psychological illnesses such as depression.

The conditions of worth linked to our self-concept can be problematic as they keep us doing things that do not meet our real needs. We also tend to perceive things so that they fit our self-concept. For example, suppose you do not think you are a very able student and then, in an assignment, you get an A-grade. You are unlikely to say, 'I did that piece of work well and I deserved that mark'. Instead, you are more likely to explain your mark to your friends by saying that you were lucky or that the instructor was a soft marker and so on. This is because getting an A-grade does not fit with your concept of yourself as a poor student academically. In this way, our self-concept can serve to lower our own levels of self-regard.

You may ask, why do we maintain a self-concept if aspects of it are ineffective? There are several reasons, as follows. Firstly, we use it and our related conditions of worth to judge our own personal adequacy. This is potentially problematic, as our self-concept will contain conditions of worth that were applicable to us at an earlier age. These conditions of worth are very deeply embedded and are therefore more resistant to change. As you will know from learning theory, knowledge that we acquire early is more resistant to change. Say, for example, you met an eminent businessman who, from a modest start, had become wealthy and successful. All the evidence is that he is an able man and obviously very bright to have achieved all that he had achieved. On learning that you were at university, he comments that he has always been 'thick'. He tells you that he failed the grammar school entrance examination and was always useless at learning. He goes on to say that this was a great disappointment to his parents. Obviously, he had learnt a great deal to be as successful as he was, but still he judged himself according to a condition of worth he had acquired as a child. Rogers felt that conditions of worth have the effect of lowering our sense of worth and make it less likely that we will have the confidence to attempt change. If we believe that we are uncoordinated, for example, then we are unlikely to enrol for a dancing class or take up gymnastics. In these ways, our self-concept and conditions of worth are important; they dictate the way in which we interact with people to meet our own needs, and they influence the choices we make in our lives.

Thus we can see that our self-concept is socially constructed. To summarise, we tend to judge ourselves according to what others think of us rather than on what we ourselves feel. We behave this way because of our high need for positive regard. This may result in us relying more on other people's judgements about our personal worth than on our own views. Rogers (1959) suggested that, because of our high need for positive regard, our organismic valuing processes may be overwhelmed. We are out of touch with our real needs. Only if we are raised with sufficient unconditional positive regard is there likely to be congruence between the self and the self-concept, and the better the match between the two, the more psychologically healthy we will be as adults. Rogers believed that parents and educational establishments can create helpful environments. These are environments that foster creativity, with democratic rules that enable us to be curious, self-reliant and respectful of others and ourselves within safe limits. This is very much the environment that is provided at Summerhill, the school we discussed in the introduction. Harrington, Block and Block (1987) used data from a longitudinal study, set up by Block and Block in 1968 at the University of California, to show that children raised in such environments were more creative in later life than were children in a matched control group that did not experience a creative environment. This is a major study documenting around 100 young people from age 3. The longitudinal study concluded after the retirement of the main researcher, but an overview of 30 years of research on the participants has been published (Block and Block, 2006). We have included the web address at the end of the discussion for anyone wanting to know more about this research.

Developmental impact on the child of their parents' self-concept

For Rogers, one important way that parents impacted on their children related to the adequacy of the parents' self-concepts. In his model, the healthy individual has experienced significant amounts of unconditional positive regard and consequently has relatively few conditions of worth. Here two points are worth noting. Firstly, Rogers did not specify precisely how much unconditional positive regard qualifies as a significant amount. He is always very vague about this, but the assumption is that none of us get enough. Secondly, as a consequence, we all have some conditions of worth. Individuals with fewer conditions of worth are classified as high-functioning adults, while those with more conditions of worth are classified as low-functioning. High-functioning adults are more accepting of themselves and of others and therefore impose fewer conditions of worth on their children, for example. Low-functioning individuals have many more conditions of worth, are consequently less accepting and more judgemental, and impose more conditions of worth on their children. The ways that the adequacy of parents' self-concept affects how they relate to their own children are summarised in Figure 11.6.

From this discussion, you can see that having conditions of worth makes us judgemental of both others and ourselves. Being self-accepting means that you are less judgemental of yourself and others. In psychological terms, self-accepting individuals are less psychologically defended, so that Rogers claimed they perceive the world more accurately and have less need to distort situations to fit with their self-concept. Take the example of someone who is interviewed for a job that they really want. Although they prepared well and thought that they performed well at interview, they did not get the job. In Rogers' view, the self-

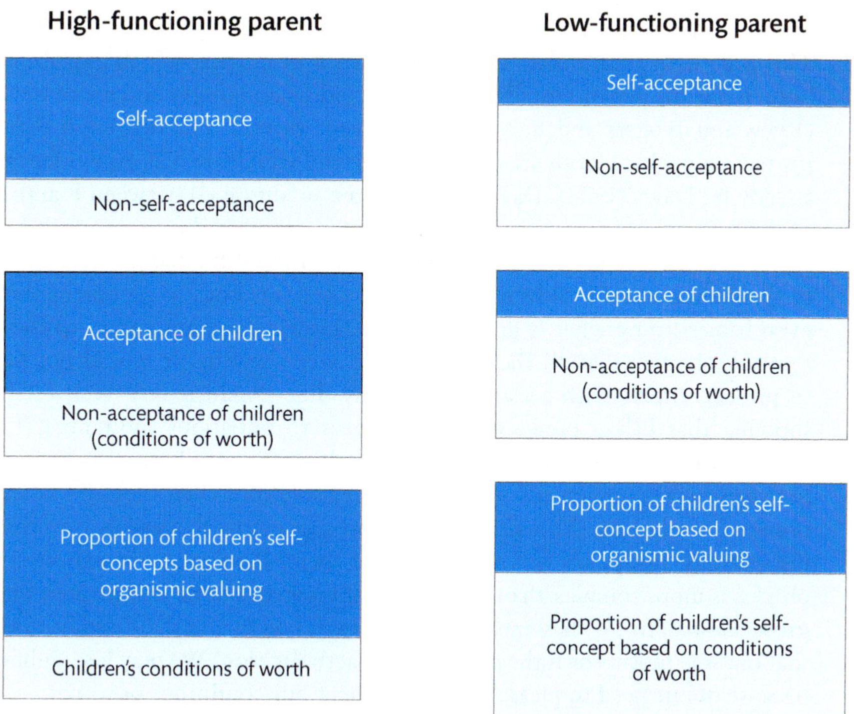

Figure 11.6 Degree of self-acceptance of parents in relation to their acceptance of their children, and the extent of conditions of worth imposed on their children.

accepting person will accept that they were not right for the position in some way. On the other hand, the individual with low self-acceptance will defend their self-esteem by asserting that they really did not want the job and had only applied for the experience of being interviewed or something similar. This exemplifies what Rogers meant by distorting their perception of reality.

Rogers was keen that his ideas were tested, and Wylie (1979) and Swann (1984) found some support among students for this idea, although it is not completely clear how well the measures they used actually assessed perceptual distortions. They asked individuals to report how they would react to various scenarios involving failure and then asked a friend of the participant to assess how honest they thought the person's judgement was. Perceptual distortions of this type are notoriously difficult to measure. The model of Freudian defence mechanisms suggest that distorting our perception so that we rationalise our failures is a psychologically adaptive response, as it serves to protect our self-esteem. It is problematic only if it is taken to extreme in the Freudian model.

Given Rogers' emphasis on the importance of the subjective worldview, it is quite strange to find him discussing individual perceptual distortions of reality. His emphasis in therapy, as we shall see, was to accept the individual's perceptions – distorted or otherwise. The point he made was that the healthy individual has fewer distortions, and they are more accepting of themselves. In the course of therapy, Rogers would expect perceptual distortions to decrease as the individual became more in touch with their organismic values that can lead to self-actualisation. We will return to this in more detail when we discuss Rogers' approach to therapy.

The role of the actualising tendency in development

Organismic valuing
An ongoing process whereby experiences are symbolised and valued according to optimal enhancement of the organism and self.

From infancy, Rogers claimed, we interact with the world in terms of our self-actualising tendency. Towards this end, infants are seen as engaging in an organismic valuing process. This is defined as an innate bodily process for evaluating which experiences are 'right' or 'wrong' for the person. Infants will value food when hungry and reject it when full. Rogers (1959) and Rogers and Stevens (1967) went further and suggested that infants 'know' instinctively which foods are good for them and which are bad. As evidence, Rogers quoted a study by Davis (1928). Davis studied three infants aged between 8 and 10 months. Two of the babies were on a particular diet for 6 months, and one was on it for 1 year. Nurses interpreted the babies pointing to various foods, and the babies were given this food. All the babies remained healthy, and Rogers quoted this study as supporting his hypothesis that even babies know what is good for them. However, examination of the choices of food available showed that all the food choices were healthy. It would not have been ethical to present infants with a totally unhealthy diet. There is now well-established evidence showing that babies prefer sweet substances to nutritious substances (Lipsitt, 1977). In Lipsitt's study, infants under 4 months were shown to suck longer and to have shorter pauses between sucking when fed sugar-and-water solutions then they did when fed nutritious, non-sweet solutions. This finding lends no support to Rogers' notion that human beings instinctively always know what is good for them. Rogers (1980) admitted that the valuing process is more complex than he initially envisaged; but he still insisted that if adults are to grow constructively, they must trust their own bodies and their own intuitions. The idea is that our sole motivator is the drive for self-actualisation. We may lose sight of our real needs because of our need to please others and meet our conditions of worth.

For Rogers (1961), as we have seen, parents play a significant role in determining how in touch the child ultimately is with their self-actualising tendency. To maximise the chances of self-actualisation, the child needs to grow up with relatively few conditions of worth. Rogers (1977) saw schools and the wider society as having a crucial role to play here also, as we have seen (Rogers, 1951; 1969; 1983; Rogers and Freiberg, 1993). He advocated student-centred teaching, where the role of the educational establishment is to provide the conditions that facilitate the child's learning. As we have previously discussed, educational establishments such as Summerhill meet Rogers' principles. These schools do not encourage competition and are relatively non-judgemental. The rules that are enforced are democratically agreed ones that ensure the children are in a safe, humane environment. Rogers felt that if conditions of trust develop, it is easier for individuals to work towards self-actualisation guided by their actualising tendency (Rogers and Freiberg, 1993). In a trusting, non-judgemental environment, it is easier for children to evaluate their experiences and have the confidence to select those that they enjoy and find worthwhile. Rogers stated that such children will be more in touch with their true selves and, as such, will instinctively know which experiences are good for them. Traditional schooling, in Rogers' view, encouraged the development of conditions of worth in the child and stifled creativity. Children need to be respected and to have freedom to make choices in their lives. This freedom also brings with it responsibilities, and Rogers suggested that children must also respect others and acknowledge that others too have the right to make their own decisions. This position is very similar to the rights and responsibilities that Albert Ellis saw as the corollary of human free will.

There are no stages in the development of self-actualisation in Rogers' theory. The emphasis is on providing the right environment for optimum growth to occur. Rogers was keen to promote the development of what he termed person-centred families, where his principles would be applied, as well as person-centred educational establishments. Personality development can be a lifelong process, Rogers felt. Unlike Freud and many of the other psychoanalysts that we have studied, Rogers does not see childhood as determining the adult personality. Individuals are always open to change in his model, and personality growth can occur at any age.

The endpoint of self-actualisation for Rogers was what he called the **fully functioning person**. Such an individual is described as being very open to experience and high in self-acceptance, with few, if any, conditions of worth. As a result, they have a positive self-concept and high self-esteem. Their organismic valuing process guides the choices they make in life, and other people's expectations and judgements of them do not influence them. If they make mistakes, they are able to acknowledge them openly and learn from them. Rogers suggested that such individuals are true to their inner selves. He gave examples of artists like El Greco, who painted in a style that was not accepted at the time; even so, he did not deviate from it to gain social acceptance or to make money, being convinced that it was right for him and it was art. A summary of the attributes of the fully functioning person is given in Table 11.3. Rogers saw individuals as continually growing, and he suggested that we have a concept of how we wish to grow; this description is also included in Table 11.3.

Fully functioning person
The person who has achieved self-actualisation. Such individuals have few conditions of worth. They are high in self-acceptance and in touch with their organismic valuing processes.

In terms of personal relationships, the fully functioning individual respects the rights of others and cares deeply for them. Such individuals display high levels of unconditional positive regard for the other people in their lives and are capable of forming deep relationships. Self-actualisation is not conceptualised as the endpoint of development but rather as a journey that the individual is on. It is a process that the individual is continually engaged in, seeking out satisfying experiences and discarding unsatisfying ones whenever possible or compensating for them in other ways. For example, the individual who undertakes a job that they find dull and boring may continue to do the job as no other option is readily available and they need money to live, but they may experience self-actualisation in other ways. Such an individual may find activities such as gardening or other hobbies, or voluntary work in the community

Table 11.3 Rogers' goals for counselling and for living

Overall goal	**Overall goals for development throughout life**
The fully functioning (mature) person	What Rogers terms the person of tomorrow
Personal qualities	**Personal qualities**
• Open to experience and able to perceive realistically	• Openness to the world, both inner and outer
• Rational and not defensive	• Desire for authenticity
• Engaged in existential process of living	• Scepticism regarding science and technology
• Trusts in their own organismic valuing process	• Desire for wholeness as a human being
• Construes experience in an existential manner	• The wish for intimacy
• Accepts responsibility for being different from others	• Accepts other people as they are
• Accepts responsibility for own behaviour	• Cares for others
• Relates creatively towards the environment	• Attitude of closeness towards nature
• Accepts others as unique individuals	• Anti-institutional in approach
• Prizes herself or himself	• Trusts their own internal authority
• Prizes others	• Material things are unimportant
• Relates openly and freely on the basis of immediate experiencing	• A yearning for spiritual values and experiences
• Communicates rich self-awareness when desired	

or close relationships within their family that fulfil their needs for self-actualisation. The self-actualising individual is described as being *congruent* with the totality of their lives. They feel satisfied with their life and believe that they fit within it. From this it is clear that self-actualisation is about an attitude to life, to oneself and to others. It is part of an ongoing process of living.

Rogers' conceptualisation of psychological problems

The fully functioning person, as we have seen, is the ideal and is rarely achieved as most of us have conditions of worth associated with our self-concept. The greater the conditions of worth associated with an individual's self-concept, the less psychologically healthy they are in Rogers' model. The individual is alienated from their true self, and this situation is expressed either in feelings of discontent, symptoms of psychological illness or antisocial behaviour or combinations of all three. Rogers avoided using diagnostic labels to describe his clients as he felt that using labels served to stress the expertise of the therapist and consequently disempowered the client. We discussed this approach in some detail, you will remember, in the introduction when we covered Rogers' objections to the medical model of illness and treatment. Clients simply need to be provided with an empowering environment that will allow them to get in touch with their true selves. This will then provide the guidance necessary for them to make helpful changes in the way that they run their lives. This environment is provided through an empowering relationship with the therapist, and we shall examine this concept next.

The principles of Rogerian counselling

Rogers' theory of personality originated in his clinical work with disturbed clients. His aim was to develop a more effective method of helping individuals, and through this his conceptualisation of what human beings are like emerged. He believed that human nature is positive and that we are motivated towards positive growth and continual development. The disturbed individual has deviated from this positive path, as they have not had sufficiently growth-enhancing relationships, experiences and environments. The aim of therapy is to provide the client with the experience of a good relationship in a safe environment. This focus becomes even more apparent when we examine Rogers' goals for counselling in Table 11.3 and see that the goals for counselling are identical to his goals for living. The aim in counselling is to provide a safe environment and experience of a good relationship as Rogers believed that this will be sufficient to allow the individual to get in touch with their true organismic self and rediscover their way to self-actualisation. It is about finding their true selves. This may sound like 'hippie' sentiments, and Rogerian counselling and derivatives of it were very popular in the 1960s and 1970s with the general public, especially the young. Group sessions based on Rogerian principles were common and led to what became known as the encounter group experience. These were groups set up to allow people to explore aspects of themselves in a psychologically safe environment. Through these encounters with themselves and others, they would find their true selves (Rogers, 1970). We will now examine in more detail Rogers' approach to therapy and the provision of a psychologically safe, empowering environment.

The aim of therapy was to facilitate a reintegration of the self-concept. To understand what this means, we need to return to conditions of worth and what they imply. If you have many conditions of worth, you are very aware of having imperfections as you have an image of the ideal person that you should be. If you were this ideal, then you would be more loveable and more admired than you currently are. It might involve being smarter, kinder, more organised, healthier or whatever. This would be our **ideal self**. We use this ideal self to judge ourselves. When we do not meet the criteria in our ideal self, our self-esteem is lowered, making us feel even worse about ourselves. To put it simply, the individual with few conditions of worth accepts themselves as they are, and the gap between their ideal self and real self is a narrow one. The person with many conditions of worth has a much wider perceptual gap between how they see themselves and how they would like to be; their ideal self. The existence of this gap leads to unhappiness and discontent and, in extreme conditions, depression. The aim of therapy is to reduce this gap and to reintegrate the self-concept with the real self. The individual then becomes more accepting of who they are and are happier consequently. At this point, many students then ask, 'But what if the client appears to be a thoroughly rotten

Ideal self
The image that individuals have of the person that they would like to be. Individuals use their concept of their ideal self to judge themselves.

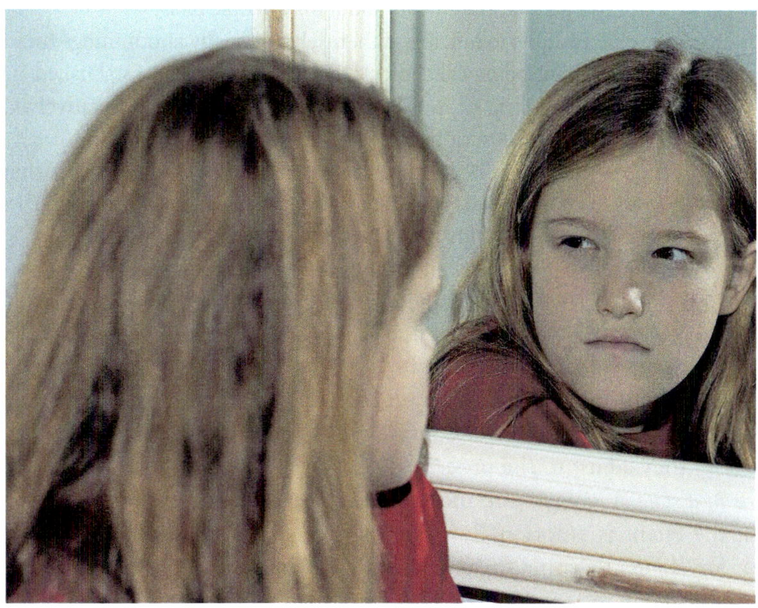

Ideas of how we see and reflect on ourselves are very important in Rogers' theory.
Source: Pearson Education Ltd. Tudor Photography

individual? Does Rogerian therapy still involve helping the person feel good about themselves?' The answer to this question lies in Rogers' conception of human nature and the source of human motivation. If you recall from earlier in the discussion, Rogers asserted that human nature is basically benign. As a species, we want to do good things, and our actualising tendency, the sole source of motivational energy, is a positive drive towards growth. So, to return to the question posed, Rogers did not accept the idea that individuals are rotten. The apparently rotten individual had their actualising tendency blocked at some point because of poor relationship and/or environmental experiences. Counselling aims to allow the individual to rediscover their actualising tendency, and, in doing so, they will be able to solve their problems and choose a more constructive way forward. This will then maximise their chances of happiness. Rogers, like Ellis, saw human beings as a hedonistic species, with happiness/contentment as our ultimate goal.

To achieve successful counselling, Rogers emphasised that the relationship between client and therapist is crucial. The clients have the ability to change within themselves, and the counsellor's role is to facilitate the process. To achieve a successful outcome, the counsellor needs to possess certain qualities and the client needs to be in a certain psychological state so that a relationship that facilitates growth in the client is created. These conditions have come to be labelled the **core conditions of counselling** and will now be described in turn. None of the conditions are considered more important than the others; Rogers (1959) stated that all need to be present.

The core conditions of counselling which facilitate personal growth

a Both the *client and the therapist must be in psychological contact*. By this condition, Rogers meant that counselling is about more than simply chatting to someone. It is not about exchanging pleasantries, although counsellors may do so initially to help put clients at their ease. It is about discussing inner feelings focused on the self. Rogers (1961) suggested that clients frequently go through stages in their conversations with their therapist before they are making true deep psychological contact (Figure 11.7). These stages are described as follows:

- **Stage 1** – The client's talk is about other people mostly, not themselves. Clients may make general statements or discuss their children or work colleagues and so on.
- **Stage 2** – Although the client begins to talk about feelings, they do not refer these feelings to themselves. They are still general statements about how people feel.
- **Stage 3** – Now the client begins to talk about themselves, usually about things they have done in the past. At this point, psychological contact is becoming properly established.
- **Stage 4** – Here the client begins to express how they feel now, but very tentatively. Clients still express their feelings at a fairly descriptive level.
- **Stage 5** – At this point, the client begins to live their feelings within the counselling session. Emotions are expressed spontaneously, and the client is focused on the present. They may still be a little tentative in recognising fully how they feel.
- **Stage 6** – Now the client can accept their feelings fully and explores them freely.
- **Stage 7** – This is the final stage, where the client has come to accept their own feelings and is also more open to the feelings of others. The person is in touch with themself psychologically and can also relate to others in the same way.

Obviously, there will be individual differences in how long this process takes. Some individuals may establish psychological contact within the first session, while for others it will take longer as they adjust to the process.

b *The client is in a state of incongruence* and feels anxious about it. By this condition, Rogers meant that the client is emotionally upset. It is this emotional upset that provides the motivation for clients to come for counselling. If you are happy and your life is going well, you are unlikely to feel the need to seek out a counsellor.

c *The counsellor is congruent in the relationship.* Rogers said that the counsellor must be genuine and not simply role-playing. Counsellors must be aware of their own feelings and be at ease with them. They must also be able to communicate their feelings if this is appropriate. To facilitate this congruence, most schools of counselling now require trainee counsellors to undertake personal counselling or therapy as part of their training. Counsellors are also required to have their work supervised regularly by another trained counsellor. This is a further check that they are dealing honestly with any feelings that the clients may provoke in them.

d The therapist experiences **unconditional positive regard** for the client. This is one of the crucial qualities required by counsellors, according to Rogers (1951; 1961). Experiencing unconditional positive regard requires the therapist not to judge the client, but to value them as another human being. They have worth simply because they exist within Rogers' humanistic perspective, and all human beings should be treated with respect and dignity.

e The therapist experiences an **empathic understanding** of the client's internal frame of reference. This condition is about accepting that there is no external reality, but that we all have a subjective view of the world. We discussed taking this phenomenological perspective in the introduction to humanistic theories at the start of the discussion. The role of the therapist is to try to understand the client's view of the world, so that they can better understand why the client feels as they do. Empathy is a concept that is often

Unconditional positive regard
Non-judgemental valuing of an individual. It is the term Rogers preferred over 'love', as he felt that most of what is termed love is not unconditional.

Empathic understanding
Within Rogers' theory of counselling, refers to the therapist understanding the client's internal frame of reference. This is about accepting that there is no external reality, but that we all have a subjective view of the world.

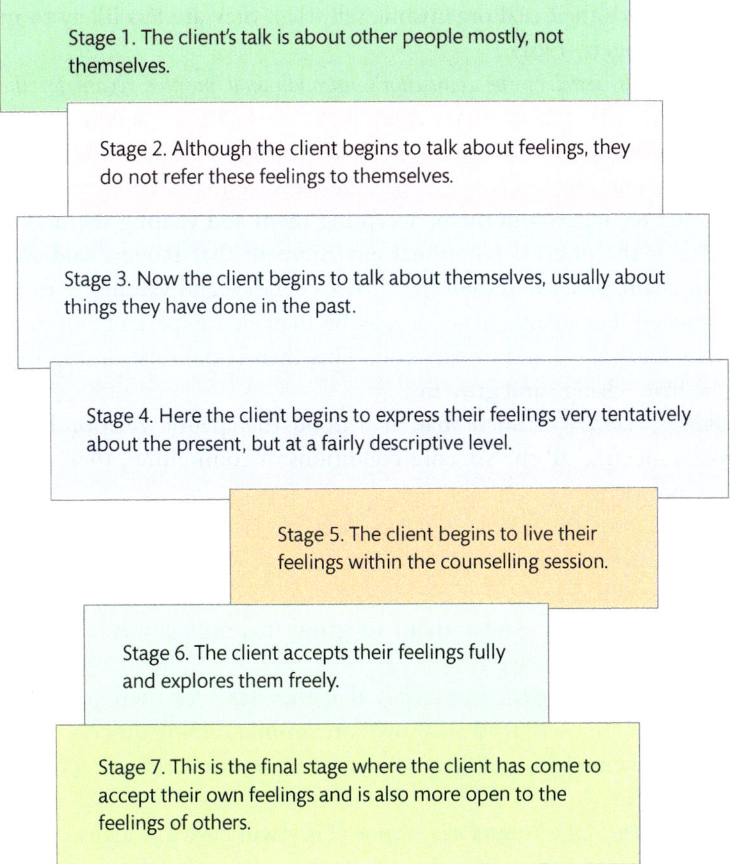

Figure 11.7 The seven stages that clients frequently go through before they make true deep psychological contact with their therapist.

misunderstood and is frequently confused with sympathy. Comparing the two concepts is a useful way of increasing our understanding of them. Sympathy is what we usually give to our friends when they are having problems. We agree that what has happened to them is awful, and we say that we understand how they are feeling. What we are actually doing is saying that we know what they are going through, yet Rogers would say that we can never truly understand what someone else is going through. Further, when expressing sympathy we are agreeing with the individual's negative interpretation of the event. We are reinforcing their perception of the event as awful. However, the role of the counsellor is to help the client feel better about what has happened, so reinforcing the client's negative worldview of the event is not a good starting point. To be empathic, the counsellor is required simply to try to understand what the client is experiencing and feeling and not to judge or evaluate the experience. The counsellor, by listening carefully and asking questions to help them really understand what has happened, also helps the client to become clearer in their own mind about their situation. In this way, the counsellor is facilitating the client's understanding of their situation.

By not judging the client, the therapist also introduces the client to the idea of not judging themselves. Rogers believes that continually judging oneself is unhelpful. It implies that you are comparing yourself with an ideal self, as we have already discussed. Self-acceptance is the goal for counselling and for living in Rogers' model. It is accepted that, as human beings, we will make mistakes, but the aim is to help people learn from their mistakes. This position is very similar to that advocated by Albert Ellis in his rational-emotive behaviour therapy. Rogers went further in that he felt that, if individuals are in touch with their real organismic self, then they are less likely to make mistakes in their lives (Rogers, 1961).

f The *client perceives the counsellor's unconditional positive regard for them and the counsellor's empathic understanding of their difficulties.* Rogers (1959) emphasised that it is crucial for the counsellor to be able to convey their empathy and unconditional positive regard to the client. The client needs to experience this feeling of being valued and of someone really trying to understand them, accepting them and valuing them as another human being. This is the positive emotional environment that Rogers said we all need to optimise our chances of self-actualising. It is acceptance and valuing with no conditions of worth attached. For many clients, it may be their first experience of such a relationship where they feel valued and understood. This then is the relationship that Roger claimed will facilitate change and growth.

Rogers (1959) claimed that, if a good therapeutic relationship is established, which involves meeting all the six core conditions of counselling, then clients will change in the following ways:

- Clients will have *more realistic perceptions of their world.* They will also be more open to new experiences.
- Clients will *behave more rationally.* They will be more in touch with their actualising tendency, which guides them to grow in positive ways. They will engage more in developing themselves.
- The level of *personal responsibility* that they take for their own behavioural choices will increase. They will trust their own organismic valuing process. They will have learnt how to help themselves, and they will have a clearer understanding of the nature of the choices they make.
- Clients' *levels of self-regard will increase.* They will have lost many of their conditions of worth and have a much higher degree of unconditional self-acceptance. Their feelings about themselves are now based on their own values rather than on the praise and needs of others in their lives. Fundamentally, they will know that as people they are sound although sometimes

they may behave in mistaken ways. This is similar to the distinction Ellis made between judging behaviour, but not the person.

- Clients will also have an *increased capacity for good personal relations*. If you are self-accepting, as we saw earlier in the discussion of conditions of worth and parenting, then you are more likely to accept others without conditions of worth attached. Rogers (1959) clearly defined what he meant by good personal relationships. He felt that such relationships involve accepting others as unique individuals, prizing them, relating openly and freely to them, communicating appropriately and being genuine in your feelings.
- Rogers believed that self-actualisation resulted in the individual *living ethically*. The individual is seen as a trustworthy person who does not infringe on the rights of others and can distinguish between good and evil. Rogers suggested that the following qualities within the individual contribute to this change:
  - They trust in their own internal feelings rather than relying on external authority to do what is right. This is based on Rogers' positive view of human nature and human motivation.
  - Their value system will focus more on people and relationships, and they will be fairly indifferent to material things.
  - They will develop more of a closeness and a reverence for nature. They will feel more at one with the world.
  - Rogers suggests that they will also have a yearning for values to guide their lives and for spiritual experiences.

These were very substantial claims to make about the benefits of Rogerian counselling, and Rogers was keen to provide research to assess its validity. Much of his early research involved the case study approach, where he would provide a detailed account of a client's progress (Rogers, 1954). To improve on the evaluation of the effects of counselling, Rogers adopted the Q-sort to measure clients' self-concepts.

At the start of counselling, the correlation between the client's current self-concept and ideal self is low. What this means is that the individual does not accept themselves as they are; they may wish to be cleverer, more reliable or whatever. After counselling, the correlation between the self and the ideal self tends to be much higher. What this means in practice is that individuals are selecting the same items to describe how they are and how they would like to be. Rogers and his colleagues carried out ambitious research projects to assess the effectiveness of client-centred therapy. Truax and Carkhuff (1967) provide a detailed review of this work. The studies quoted provide some support for the effectiveness of Rogerian counselling, but not all the studies are unproblematic. Many of the measures of improvement are not objectively based; rather, they are self-report ratings completed by the client and/or therapist. Obviously, if clients and therapists have invested significant amounts of time and perhaps money on therapy, they are unlikely to rate the experience as having been worthless. More objective measures of changes in the client's behaviour would be preferable for measuring the effectiveness of therapy. There is also a lack of long-term follow-up studies to assess how lasting any changes obtained are.

Evaluation of Rogers' theory

We will now evaluate Rogers' theory using the eight criteria identified previously: description, explanation, empirical validity, testable concepts, comprehensiveness, parsimony, heuristic value and applied value.

Description

Rogers, like Maslow, is criticised for his overly optimistic conceptualisation of human beings. As a total description of human behaviour, Rogers' theory is limited. His initial focus is on abnormal development and psychopathology and its treatment. However, his concept of conditions of worth provides a very valuable way of describing the mechanisms that we use to evaluate our own behaviour. His description of how the self is construed is innovative, and his comparison of self and ideal self is valuable. Intuitively, these concepts seem to provide useful descriptions and are therefore high in face validity.

His phenomenological approach represents a real attempt to engage with the world as individuals experience it. However, such an approach, with its focus on conscious experience, excludes what many will conceptualise as the rich world of the unconscious. Another danger of Rogers' approach is that it may rely so much on individual observations that objective measurement is ignored and no knowledge is generated that is applicable to the wider science of psychology. Rogers was very aware of this, and his utilisation of measures such as the Q-sort was his attempt to overcome this shortcoming.

Explanation

Rogers attempted to explain a vast range of human behaviour, ranging from what we require for optimum individual development to the nature of the society that would promote psychological health. However, he used the same principles that he developed for counselling troubled individuals to propose solutions for societies and indeed for the world's problems. This ignores the social, historical and political factors that play a crucial role in developing and maintaining these problems and leads to his explanations being limited in scope and somewhat reductionist in nature. His underlying thesis was that, if individuals communicated better, then society's problems would be solved. While good communication is helpful, it is unrealistic and overly optimistic to see it as the solution to what are very complex problems.

Empirical validity

Rogers was very aware of the need to provide empirical evidence to validate his theory. There is a lot of research on his therapy in particular. The results are generally positive, but all of this research is heavily reliant on self-report measures. Clients self-assess their progress, but this is hardly objective evidence given that they have invested considerable time and frequently money in their treatment, so are unlikely to evaluate it as a negative undertaking. Similarly, therapists provide reports of clients' progress, and here the tendency must surely be to provide a positive assessment. There is a need for more objective measures of therapeutic progress using standardised instruments and/or involving significant others of the client in the assessment of progress.

As we saw earlier, Rogers' idea about human beings knowing intuitively what is good for them received little research support. We know from work on the relationship between attitudes and behaviour that knowing some behaviour is harmful is not a good predictor of whether we practise that behaviour. If this were not so, we would not currently be having problems with binge drinking, obesity, smoking and many other health issues in our society.

Testable concepts

As mentioned already, Rogers was keen to construct a testable theory, and he did encourage research on his concepts. Despite this, some of his concepts are not easy to define. The concept of empathy has been researched, and reliable measures are available. However, concepts like unconditional positive regard and genuineness are more difficult to define and have proved difficult to measure. Rogers does need to be commended for his attempts to produce a testable theory and a therapy that can be evaluated. Traditionally, his counselling approach has been described as being non-directive, in that the therapist does not claim to know what is best for the client. Clients produce their own solutions. This idea that Rogerian therapists are somehow less directive than other therapists is contentious. As videos of his therapy sessions show, Rogers himself made considerable use of non-verbal signals when interacting with his clients. In this way he is likely to have influenced clients. This claim of non-directiveness can thus be seen to be difficult to assess objectively.

Comprehensiveness

Most of Rogers' work focuses on understanding psychopathology and developing an intervention that could be used as an effective treatment. This meant that his early work was not very comprehensive. Later in his life, he expanded his interests to look in more detail at development, education and the effect of culture and society's institutions on mental health. In this way, his approach became more comprehensive. His work on social and political structures, while interesting, is very speculative.

Parsimony

Rogers has chosen to take a broad approach to human behaviour; despite this, his theory utilises very few concepts. He fails the parsimony criteria by using too few concepts and assumptions. This results in imprecision, as his concepts are applied very widely to explain very different phenomena. A good example is his explanation of psychopathology. This is too simplistic to explain the full range of psychopathologies that have been documented and results in a reductionist approach.

Heuristic value

Rogers' work has provoked a great deal of controversy within psychology and continues to provoke debate. This in itself is a valuable contribution to make to a science. His humanistic and phenomenological stance has led to a re-evaluation of the importance of the individual and their subjective worldview. His emphasis on the concepts of self and ideal self also led to more attention being paid to these concepts and significant amounts of research being undertaken. His ideas about the core conditions of counselling also led therapy and counselling trainers to reflect on the educational training of counsellors, and useful debates ensued.

Applied value

Rogers' theory has been applied widely. This is certainly one of its strengths. His views of therapy have helped define the training of most counsellors. The recent trend, to encourage counselling psychologists to be trained in several schools of counselling, generally results in trainee counsellors beginning their education with Rogerian therapy. This means that most counsellors are familiar with the core conditions and develop active listening skills and empathy for their clients.

Rogers was also extremely influential in the development of group approaches to psychological treatments. The development of encounter groups in the 1960s and 1970s was attributable to Rogers' influence. These were group experiences designed to help individuals explore their true inner selves and thereby set them on the road to self-actualisation.

Final comments

Now you should understand what is meant by humanistic theories in psychology and how they evolved. You should be familiar with the developmental experiences that influenced the theorising of Maslow and Rogers and appreciate Maslow and Rogers' conceptualisations of human nature. You should also be familiar with Maslow's hierarchy of needs and the motives related to it, understand the principles of personality development and the causes of mental illness as described by Maslow and Rogers, be familiar with Rogers' conceptualisation of self-actualisation and its importance in development and understand the principles of Rogerian counselling, including the importance of the core conditions of counselling.[B]

Introduction

Easygoing, intelligent, funny, caring, professional man, aged 44, **good in a crisis,** seeks **warm, friendly, intelligent** woman of a similar age. Enjoys good food, wine, cinema and theatre.

Vibrant, charismatic, passionate, energetic sportswoman, aged 32, **loves all outdoor activities, foreign travel,** cooking, reading and gardening, seeks country-dwelling male with similar interests.

At this point, you may be wondering what lonely-hearts advertisements are doing in a textbook on personality. However, we want you to think about the image of the individuals that these advertisements convey. Most of us are good at doing this; from a short description of an individual, we can build up a mental picture of them and make decisions about which individuals we are attracted to and might like to meet and which hold no appeal for us. What we are doing is using our knowledge of personality traits to build up an image of the person from their description. We have highlighted the words that label personality traits in the advertisements above, and it is worth taking a moment to reflect on what you understand by each of them and how you value them. Is the picture of a vibrant, charismatic, passionate, energetic woman - one you value positively - or one you find unappealing?

Nomoethic
An approach to personality based on the assumption that a finite set of variables exists that can be used to describe human personality. The aim is to identify these personality variables or traits that occur consistently across groups of people.

What these types of adverts suggest is that from a few personality traits and statements about interests, we may be able to build up an image of the individual. This in effect is what trait personality theorists aim to do, but in a more rigorous, scientific way. Trait theorists employ the nomothetic approach to personality. The aim is to identify those personality variables or traits that occur consistently across groups of people. Each individual can then be located within this set of variables. The aim is to identify the main traits that usefully distinguish between types of people. In achieving this, they hope to uncover the basic structure of personality. This is one of the major aims of studying human personality. It is a major undertaking, and we will now explore the progress that has been made, starting with the Ancient Greeks.

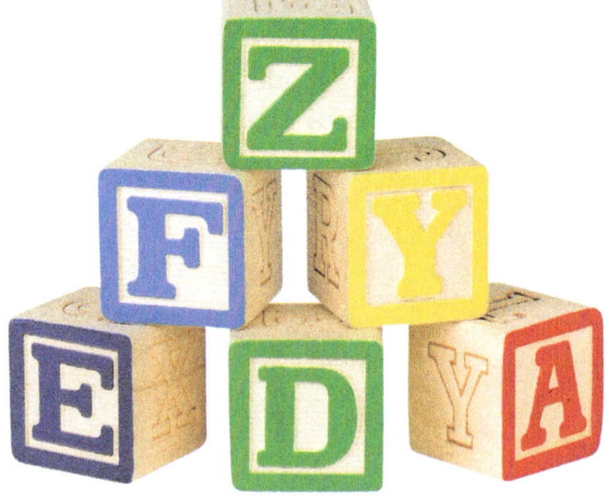

Source: Getty Images/Photodisc

Emergence of personality traits

The Ancient Greek philosopher, Aristotle (384–322 BC), provides the first written description of personality traits, or dispositions, as he preferred to call them. He described individual differences in traits such as modesty, bravery and vanity, seeing them as important determinants of whether a person behaved ethically. One of his students, Theophrastus (371–287 BC), published an account of 30 personality

[B] Maltby, J., Day, L., & Macaskill, A. (2013). Theories and measurement of intelligence. In J. Maltby, L. Day, & A. Macaskill (Eds.), *Personality, individual differences and intelligence* (3rd ed., pp. 124–147). Harlow, Essex: Pearson Education.

characters or types. These were early attempts to describe the commonly acknowledged differences between individuals and to identify individuals with similar dispositions. The task can be thought of as putting some order or structure into our everyday observations so that they are easier to conceptualise and discuss.

Another Ancient Greek philosopher, Hippocrates (460–377 BC), described physical illness as being caused by the balance of bodily fluids, or humours, as he labelled them. These fluids included blood, black bile, yellow bile and phlegm. Another Ancient Greek, a physician named Galen (AD 130–200), expanded on Hippocrates' theory of the humours and applied it to describe human temperament or personality (Stelmack and Stalikas, 1991). When the humours were in balance, an equitable temperament was the result. If the humours were out of balance, then physical illness and mental disturbance occurred. The terms Galen used to describe these mental disturbances are still part of the English language. An excess of black bile resulted in a **melancholic temperament**, associated with depressed mood and feelings of anxiety. Strong activity in the body fluids resulted in an individual with strong emotions described as being of **choleric temperament**, meaning that they had a tendency to become angry easily. Individuals of **phlegmatic temperament** were calm, as there was low humorous activity, while individuals of **sanguine temperament** were confident and optimistic.

Melancholic temperament Associated with depressed mood and feelings of anxiety.

Choleric temperament Describing an individual who has a tendency to be easily angered

Phlegmatic temperament Describes an individual who is calm.

Sanguine temperament Describes an individual who is confident and optimistic.

In the Middle Ages the German philosopher Immanuel Kant (1724–1804) revisited the humoural temperaments and produced a description of four personality types. These were based on the strength of the individual's feelings and how active the person was. Melancholic individuals had weak feelings, while sanguine individuals had strong feelings. Phlegmatic individuals had low levels of activity, while choleric individuals had much higher levels of activity.

These early writers all described types of personality rather than personality traits. This is an important distinction. Personality types describe discrete categories into which individuals can be placed. Personality traits are continuous dimensions, and individuals can be positioned along the dimension depending on how much of the trait they possess.

It was Wilhelm Wundt, the founding father of modern-day psychology, who changed the categorical types of personality into trait dimensions. He revisited the humoural terms in his description of personality, reclassifying the old types in two dimensions based on their mood stability and the strength of their emotions. Individuals could then be placed along the dimensions of mood stability and strength of emotions rather than being simply placed in one category. Wundt's classification system is displayed in Figure 11.8.

It is true to say that little progress was made in terms of classifying personality traits from the time of the Ancient Greeks to the middle of the nineteenth century, when the clinical theories emerged. The reason for the delay in the emergence of trait theories is easily understandable. There are a huge number of terms in all languages to describe personality traits. For trait approaches to personality to develop scientifically, some systematic way of structuring these terms and identifying the common dimensions underlying them was necessary. It was the invention of statistical techniques such as correlation and factor analysis that made this possible, as we shall see.

Defining personality traits

Up until now, we have used the term 'trait' to describe personality. We are sure you have understood what we have been saying, but we should begin this section with a definition of exactly what psychologists mean by a personality trait. Frequently, terms that have a very specific meaning in psychology are also part of our everyday language. This can result in some confusion about the precise meaning of terms; hence psychology's obsession with defining the terms that we use. According to Burger (1997), 'A trait is a dimension of personality used to categorise people according to the degree to which they manifest a particular characteristic.'

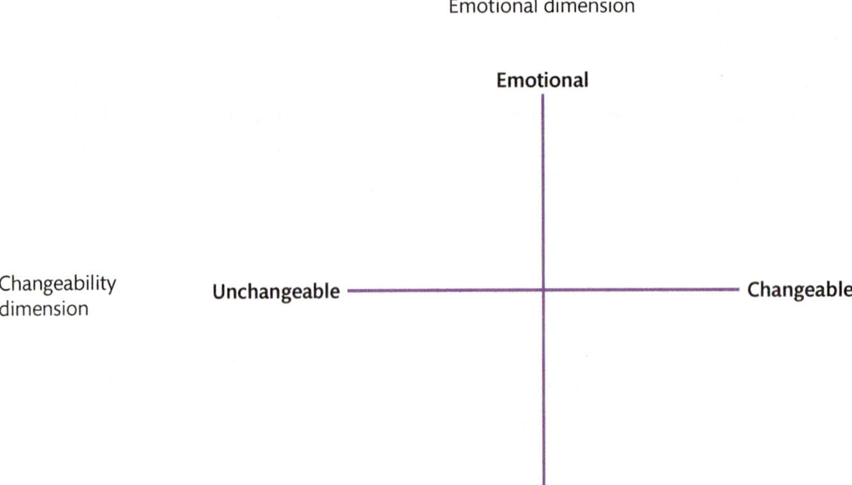

Figure 11.8 Wundt's emotionality and changeability dimensions of personality.

Two assumptions underlie trait theory. The first assumption is that personality characteristics are relatively stable over time; the second is that traits show stability across situations. A person's behaviour may alter on different occasions, but the assumption is that there is some internal consistency in the ways that individuals behave. For example, someone who is described as an extravert may be very outgoing and chatty at a party but less so in a psychology seminar. In both situations, this person is likely to be more sociable than an introverted individual. We also assume that personality traits influence behaviour. The person is outgoing and chatty because they are an extravert. These are somewhat circular arguments, and the psychologist has to move beyond them. Trait theorists have to be able to make a distinction between the internal qualities of the individual and the way they behave. The causal relationship between the two then has to be explained if we are to avoid circular arguments. To say that individuals become angry easily because they have an angry disposition does not get us very far. We need to know where their angry disposition has come from and how it influences their day-to-day behaviour.

It follows logically from the trait approach that trait theorists are more interested in general descriptions of behaviour than in understanding the individual and making predictions about individual behaviour. They take the trait continuum and provide descriptions of how groups of people at different points on the continuum might be expected to behave. For example, they might compare a group high in aggression with a group with low scores on the same trait and observe how they behave in a debate. They are interested in typical group behaviour. It is frequently a descriptive rather than an explanatory approach. Some trait theorists are more interested in describing personality and predicting behaviour than in identifying what caused the behaviour. This can lead to circular reasoning. An individual is said to behave in a certain way because they are an anxious person. When asked to explain why an individual is anxious, the response is that they are anxious because they have behaved in a certain way.

Increasingly, however, the identification processes are only the first stage. Trait theorists are becoming more interested in providing explanations for behaviour. Trait approaches make it relatively easy to make comparisons among people; individuals can be placed on a continuum relative to others, and groups can also be compared. However, trait theorists have little to say about personality change. The theorists with an interest in personality change have come from a clinical background, while trait theorists are more likely to be academic psychologists.

To recap, within psychology, traits are considered the fundamental units of personality. They represent dispositions to respond in certain ways. For a long time, there were arguments about how much the situation influenced the individual's behaviour and how much was down to their personality traits. It is now generally accepted that, while situational factors will affect behaviour, dispositional effects on that behaviour will still be observable. Mischel (1999) has produced an elegant definition of a personality trait that incorporates this. He suggests that a trait is the 'conditional probability of a category of behaviours in a category of contexts'. Hence, if a person is an extravert, then degrees of extraverted behaviour will be observable from that person in a variety of situations.

The development of trait theories within psychology

During the rest of this discussion we are going to take you through the development and establishment of the core trait theories of personality in psychology. These include the work of:

- Sheldon
- early lexical approaches
- Allport
- Cattell
- Eysenck
- the five-factor model.

Endomorphy
A term used by Sheldon to link the digestive system of the body to a temperament of love of relaxation and comfort.

Mesomorphy
A term used by Sheldon to link the musculature and the circulatory system of the body to a temperament of being physically assertive and competitive.

Ectomorphy
A term used by Sheldon to link the nervous system and the brain system of the body to a temperament of need for privacy, restraint and inhibition.

Sheldon and somatotypes

Although the psychoanalyst Jung introduced the terms 'extraversion' and 'introversion', the real founding figure of trait psychology is considered to be an American psychologist, William Sheldon (1899–1977). He outlined what came to be a very well-known description of personality called somatotypes, which is based on physique and temperament. From his surveys of thousands of individuals, he concluded that there are three basic types of physique: **endomorphy**, **mesomorphy** and **ectomorphy** (Sheldon, 1970). Using correlational techniques, he demonstrated that each body type was associated with a particular temperament. A summary of his theory is displayed in Table 11.4

While accepting that everyone had the same internal organs, Sheldon felt that individuals were different in terms of which organs were most prominent in their bodies and thus where

Table 11.4 Sheldon's theory of physique and temperament

	Physique		Temperament	
	Focus on part of body	**Physique**	**Temperament**	**Description**
Ectomorph	Nervous system and the brain	Light-boned with a slight musculature	**Cerebrotonia**	A need for privacy, restrained, inhibited
Mesomorph	Musculature and the circulatory system	Large, bony with well-defined muscles	**Somatotonia**	Physically assertive, competitive, keen on physical activity
Endomorph	Digestive system, particularly the stomach	Rounded body tending towards fatness	**Viscerotonia**	Associated with a love of relaxation and comfort; like food and are sociable

Table 11.5 Evidence for the lexical hypothesis

Personality descriptor	Synonyms	Number
honest	trustworthy, truthful, veracious, trusty, honourable, creditable, decent, law-abiding, uncorrupted, uncorrupt, incorruptible, ethical, moral, virtuous, principled, upright, high-minded, dependable, reliable, reputable, above-board, straight, square-dealing, fair, just, candid, frank, sincere, direct, ingenuous, sound	31
warm	amiable, friendly, cheerful, cordial, affable, pleasant, genial, kindly, hospitable, hearty, affectionate, mellow, loving	13
pedantic	perfectionistic, scrupulous, finicky, fussy, punctilious, fastidious, meticulous, exact, quibbling	9
aberrant – meaning odd or peculiar	not included	

Source: Oxford Concise Thesaurus, Oxford, UK: Oxford University Press, 2007.

their body's focus lay. Table 11.4 represents the extremes of each type, but Sheldon produced a detailed atlas of male body types where bodies were matched against these extremes using a seven-point grading scale. He planned a similar female body atlas, but this was never produced. You may still come across descriptions of Sheldon's body types in popular texts. In terms of personality theorising, Sheldon's work was important as it marked the start of the utilisation of psychometric approaches to the study of personality. He carried out extensive surveys of large populations, collected different measures from individuals using questionnaires and applied statistical techniques to the analysis of his data.

Early lexical approaches to personality and the lexical hypothesis

Several of the early researchers used dictionaries or *Roget's Thesaurus* to try to identify and count the number of words that describe personality traits. Sir Francis Galton (1822–1911) was an Englishman who is best known for his early studies on genetic influences on intelligence, but he was also interested in the relationships between language and personality. He suggested that the most meaningful personality descriptors will tend to become encoded in language as single words. Galton (1884) provides the first documented source of a dictionary and/or thesaurus being used to elicit words describing personality.

This approach has come to be known as the lexical hypothesis. It suggests that it is the individual differences between people that are important that become encoded as single terms. This appears to be a sensible assumption. Two additional criteria are included in the lexical hypothesis. First, frequency of use is also assumed to correspond with importance. Again, it seems logical that the words we use most to describe personality will be labelling the aspects of personality that we think are most important. Secondly, the number of words in a language that refer to each trait will be related to how important that trait is in describing human personality. An example from a thesaurus is included in Table 11.5 to help clarify what we mean. From the table, you can see that the personality descriptor 'honest' has 31 synonyms listed, suggesting that it is a more important descriptor of personality than the word 'aberrant', which is not listed in the *Oxford Concise Thesaurus* (2007). Similarly, the word 'warm' describes a more useful descriptor of personality than 'pedantic' does.

While most of the early work was conducted on the English language, it is assumed that, if the lexical hypothesis is a valid theory, then it should apply cross-culturally (Norman, 1963). This is the final assumption of the lexical hypothesis. We will return to the cross-cultural question later in the discussion. To summarise, it states that, if individual differences between people are important, there will be words to describe them; the more frequently a personality descriptor is used, the more important the personality characteristic; finally, the more synonyms of the word there are, the more important the difference.

Gordon Allport

Initially, lexical researchers were limited to counting the terms used, identifying synonyms and producing lists of these words. One of the first psychologists to produce such a list was the American Gordon Allport (1897–1967). With a colleague, he identified 18,000 words, of which 4,500 described personality traits (Allport and Odbert, 1936). Allport published the first psychology text on personality traits, *Personality Traits: Their Classification and Measurement* (1921), and he is believed to have taught the first course on personality in the United States in 1924. While promoting the concept of personality traits, Allport (1961) was quite clear about the limitations of the trait approach. He felt that it was almost impossible to use an individual's personality traits to predict how they will behave in a specific situation. He acknowledged that there is variability in everyone's behaviour, but that there is also some constancy. Personality traits constitute this constant portion of behaviour. He suggested that personality traits have a physical presence in our nervous systems. He suggested that advances in technology would one day enable psychologists to identify personality traits from inspection of the nervous system.

Although interested in traits, Allport adopted a unified approach to personality, suggesting that it is the way that the component traits come together that is important. It is how the traits come together that produces the uniqueness of all individuals, which he was keen to stress. Together, these traits produce a unified personality that is capable of constant evolution and change. Allport felt that change is a component part of the personality system that is necessary to allow us to adapt to new situations and grow to cope with them. He adopted a very positive conceptualisation of human nature. He suggested that human beings are normally rational, creative, active and self-reliant. This was a very different view of human nature from the Freudian one that was dominant at the time.

Allport made the distinction between nomothetic and idiographic approaches to the study of personality. Allport felt that both approaches bring unique insights into our understanding of personality. He felt that the nomothetic approach allows the identification of **common personality traits** (Allport, 1961). He saw these common traits as ways of classifying groups of individuals, with one group being classified as being more dominant, happier or whatever than another comparable group. He felt that such comparisons based on common traits are not particularly useful. Of more use is what he termed the **personal disposition** of the individual. The personal disposition represents the unique characteristics of the individual. This approach emphasises the uniqueness of each person, and Allport (1961) felt that this was potentially a more fruitful approach towards developing a real understanding of personality.

Personality traits were further classified into cardinal, central and secondary traits. **Cardinal traits** are single traits that may dominate an individual's personality and heavily influence their behaviour. These may be thought of as obsessions or ruling passions that produce a need that demands to be fulfilled. For example, someone may have a cardinal trait of competitiveness that permeates virtually every aspect of their behaviour. They strive to be best at everything they do. **Central traits** are the five to ten traits that Allport felt best describe an individual's personality. **Secondary traits** are more concerned with an individual's preferences and are not a core constituent of their personality. Secondary traits may only become apparent in particular situations – unlike central traits, which have a more general applicability.

Common traits
Ways of classifying groups of individuals, with one group being classified as being more dominant, happier or whatever than another comparable group.

Personal dispositions
Represent the unique characteristics of the individual. This approach emphasises the uniqueness of each person.

Central traits
The five to ten traits that Allport felt best describe an individual's personality. They are generally applicable to that person regardless of situational factors.

Secondary traits
Traits that are more concerned with an individual's preferences and are not a core constituent of their personality. Secondary traits may become apparent only in particular situations

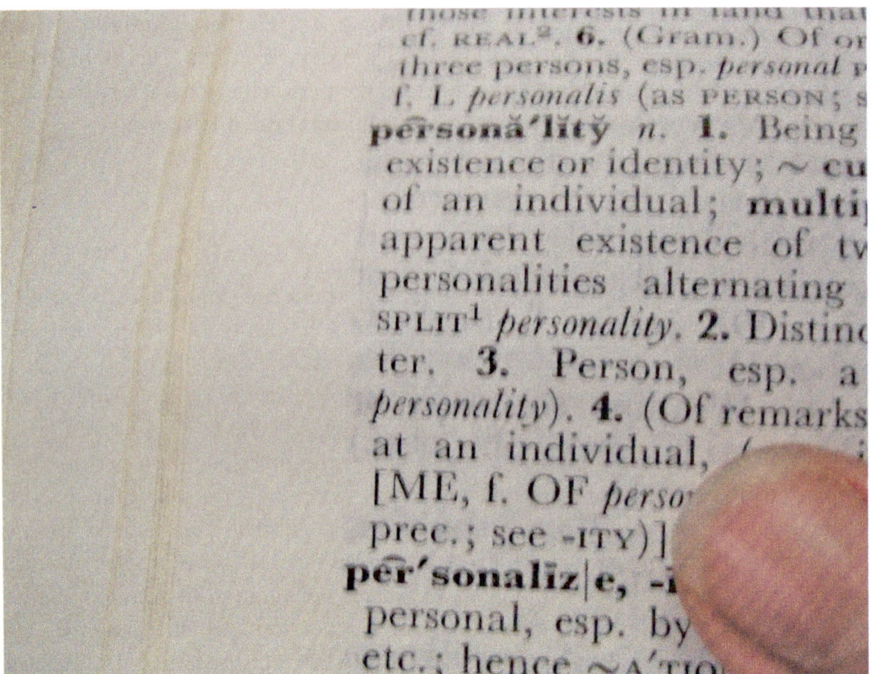

The aim of lexical approaches is to find underlying dimensions to the many ways we describe our personality.
Source: Pearson Education Ltd

The other major contribution that Allport made to personality theorising relates to the concept of self. He emphasised the importance of the concept to any theory of personality as he felt it is crucial to the development of identity and individuality. He hypothesised that children are not born with a concept of self, but that it gradually develops. He felt that it is a lifelong process of development. The child first becomes aware of the separateness of themselves from others in their environment and from this comes their sense of self-identity. As a result of their experiences while becoming integrated into their family and wider society, they develop self-esteem. Allport felt that the concept of self presented a challenge to psychologists as it is difficult to define precisely, consisting as it does of several component parts. He used the term **proprium** as a synonym for the self, suggesting that the term represented all the constituent parts that go to make up the concept of self.

Proprium
A synonym for the self, used by Allport. The term represents all the constituent parts that go to make up the concept of self.

Allport's major impact on personality theory was in terms of stressing the limitations of the trait approaches as they were currently adopted. He raised the issue about the relative influence of personality and situation in determining behaviour, something still of concern to psychologists. His inclusion of the concept of self as a legitimate and central concern of personality theorists was also important in the trait tradition of personality research. His distinction between nomothetic and idiographic approaches to the study of personality is an important one. He did not develop any standardised measures of personality traits as such; this was left to other theorists, as we shall see. His list of 4,500 personality traits is too long to be of much practical use in assessing personality.

Raymond Cattell and the emergence of the factor analytic approach

The real advances in trait approaches were only possible after the invention of the technique of factor analysis. Allport did not engage with factor analysis; however, the next theorist that we examine, Raymond Cattell, made full use of the technique, having been instructed in it by Spearman, the inventor of factor analysis. Following from this early scientific training, Cattell was keen to apply empirical methods to discover the basic structure of personality. From the lists of personality traits, he noted that many traits are very similar, and he argued that the existing lists could be reduced to a much smaller number of traits. This smaller number of traits would represent the basic components of personality. Cattell's work thus marks the beginning of the search for the structure of personality using factor analysis. Put simply, the procedure involves identifying lists of the most frequently used sets of words that seem to describe aspects of personality; large samples of individuals are then asked to rate the degree to which the attributes apply to them. This data set is then factor-analysed to identify which attributes cluster together. Clusters are composed of items that correlate with each other. So, for example, you might have the variables 'determined', 'persistent', 'productive' and 'goal-directed' that turn out to be highly correlated with each other and thus form a cluster or factor that you could perhaps call achievement-oriented. What this method gives you is a general measure of some ability – in this instance, achievement orientation – that you obtain by measuring the individual's ratings of their determination, persistence, productivity and goal-directedness.

Types of traits

Cattell (1965) defined personality as being the characteristics of the individual that allow prediction of how they will behave in a given situation. His approach to personality was a broad one, and he identified a range of traits, as we shall see. Later in his career, he became interested in the ways that personality traits and situational variables interact to affect the way that individuals behave. Traits are conceptualised as being relatively stable, long-lasting building blocks of personality.

Cattell makes distinctions between types of traits. The first distinction relates to whether traits are genetically determined or the result of environmental experiences. The genetically determined traits are called **constitutional traits** while the environmentally induced traits are called **environmental-mold traits**. This distinction represents the nature versus nurture debate that occurs repeatedly in every area of psychology. In this application, it asks whether individual differences are caused by inherited aspects of our personality, or are they explained by how we have been treated and the environmental experiences we have had? Cattell (1982) was keen to try to establish the relative contribution of genetics and environment to various personality traits. He developed a statistical procedure called **multiple abstract variance analysis (MAVA)** to accomplish this. He administered personality tests to assess a particular trait in relation to complex samples consisting of family members raised together, family members raised apart, identical twins raised together, identical twins raised apart, unrelated children raised together and unrelated children raised apart. Using complex statistical procedures, the test allows the researcher to calculate the precise degree of influence that genetic and environmental factors have in the development of a particular personality trait.

Next, Cattell defines three different types of traits: ability, temperament and dynamic traits. **Ability traits** determine how well you deal with a particular situation and how well you reach whatever your goal is in that situation. For example, the various aspects of intelligence are good examples of ability traits. He also identifies individual differences in the styles that people adopt when they are pursuing their goals. These are labelled **temperament traits**. Some people may be laidback and easygoing, or irritable, or anxious and so on, in the way that they typically approach life. These then are examples of temperament traits.

Constitutional traits
The genetically determined personality traits in Cattell's system.

Environmental-mold traits
The environmentally induced traits in Cattell's system.

Multiple abstract variance analysis (MAVA)
A statistical technique developed by Cattell that allows the researcher to establish the relative contribution of genetics and environment to various personality traits.

Ability traits
Traits that determine how well you deal with a particular situation and how well you reach whatever your goal is in that situation.

Temperament traits
The individual differences in the styles that people adopt when they are pursuing their goals.

Dynamic traits
The traits that motivate us and energise our behaviour.

Attitudes
One of three dynamic traits in Cattell's theory of personality. Attitudes represent a specific trait and help to predict how we will behave in a particular situation.

Sentiments
One of three dynamic traits in Cattell's theory of personality. Sentiments are complex attitudes that include our opinions and interests that help determine how we feel about people or situations.

Dynamic lattice
A term to describe Cattell's dynamic traits of attitudes, sentiments and ergs are organised in very complex and interrelated ways.

Common traits
Ways of classifying groups of individuals, with one group being classified as being more dominant, happier or whatever than another comparable group.

Unique traits
Rarer traits that tend to be unique to individuals.

Surface traits
Collections of traits that cluster together in many individuals; that is, the scores on these traits are correlated with each other. Factor analysis uncovers a single underlying

Source trait
The common trait revealed by factor

Cattell, like many of the other theorists we have examined, was interested in what motivates human behaviour. This is a core area for personality theories to explain. He suggested that we have **dynamic traits** that motivate us and energise our behaviour (Cattell, 1965). For example, an individual may be motivated to succeed and be very competitive, or they may be ambitious, or driven to care for others, be artistic and so on. As Cattell (1965) considered the question of motivation to be at the heart of personality theorising, the dynamic traits were heavily researched. He concluded that there are three types of dynamic traits: **attitudes**, **sentiments** and **ergs**. Attitudes are defined as hypothetical constructs that express our particular interests in people or objects in specific situations. Attitudes help to predict how we will behave in a particular situation. Cattell (1950) defined sentiments as complex attitudes that include our opinions and interests that help determine how we feel about people or situations. Cattell (1979) considered ergs to be innate motivators. He suggested that ergs are innate drives. They cause us to recognise and attend to some stimuli more readily than others, and to seek satisfaction of our drives.

Cattell suggests that all these types of dynamic traits are organised in very complex and interrelated ways to produce the **dynamic lattice**. The aim is to explain how we have to acquire particular traits to achieve our goals. For example, if your goal is learning to ski, you need to learn to copy the instructor. You have to demonstrate patience and perseverance in practising. You have to tolerate being a figure of fun when you fall over, and you may have to conquer fear to go on the drag lift and so on. How others react to you will also affect the lattice as will your attitudes towards others and the mood you are in. This then gives a hint of the complexity involved. It is fair to say that this system certainly does not simplify the explanation of behaviour in any real way, and other psychologists have not followed up this work.

A further distinction is between **common traits** and **unique traits**. Common traits are those shared by many people. They would include intelligence, sociability, dependency and so on. Unique traits are rarer and specific to individuals. A unique trait might be an interest in collecting fishing reels by a particular maker or an interest in a particular entertainer or the like. They are specialised interests, if you like, that motivate individuals to pursue certain related activities. While Cattell's work is concerned almost exclusively with common traits, he includes the concept of unique traits to emphasise the uniqueness of human beings. He also stressed that the uniqueness of individuals is also because of the unique ways that common traits come together in different individuals. Different individuals will have different mixtures of common traits making up their personalities, thus making them unique.

Cattell (1950) suggested an important distinction between **surface traits** and **source traits**. Surface traits are collections of traits descriptors that cluster together in many individuals and situations. For example, individuals who are sociable also tend to be carefree, hopeful and contented. These are all surface traits; when you measure individuals on each of these surface traits, you find that their scores on each one are correlated with all the others. That is, if an individual scores highly on sociability, they also score highly on the carefree trait, the hopefulness trait and the contentedness trait. The technique of factor analysis suggests that there is an underlying trait, what Cattell calls a **source trait**, that is responsible for the observed variance in the surface traits. In this case, it is the source trait of extraversion. Extraversion is measured by the scores of the surface traits of sociability, carefreeness, hopefulness and contentedness. The surface traits relate to the overt behaviours that individuals display. The source trait, on the other hand, is the major difference in personality that is responsible for all these related differences in observed behaviour. In simple terms, being high in the source trait of extraversion causes you to display behaviour that is more sociable, to have more hopeful attitudes and so on.

The source traits are identified using the statistical technique of factor analysis, as we have previously discussed. Source traits are important as they represent the actual underlying structure of personality. If psychologists can identify the basic structure of personality, then they will be better able to predict behaviour. This has become the main quest for trait theorists. As we have seen, there are an enormous number of personality traits; identifying the source traits will reduce this number. By using a smaller number of source traits, psychologists can then construct personality tests that include only measures of surface traits that relate to the source traits. Personality tests produced in this way will provide better measures of individual differences in personality.

Cattell (1957) makes it clear that it is necessary to use a broad range of personality descriptors to ensure that the appropriate source traits are discovered. He began his quest for the underlying structure of personality with the list of 4,500 trait names as identified by Allport and Odbert (1936). Firstly, using teams of raters, Cattell removed all the synonyms. This left him with a list of 171 trait names. By getting raters to assess individuals on these traits, he reduced the list further to produce 36 surface traits. Ten other surface traits were identified in further studies on personality assessment and from a review of the psychiatric literature. Thus, Cattell concluded that 46 surface traits are sufficient to describe individual differences in personality (Cattell and Kline, 1977).

Beginning with these 46 surface traits, Cattell used a variety of approaches to uncover the source traits of personality. The aim was to factor-analyse measures of all the 46 surface traits collected from large samples of individuals. If you look at factor analysis, you will see that large numbers of participants are required for factor analysis. Cattell used different data collection procedures to obtain his data sets. One source of data he called **L-data**, short for 'life record data'. These are measurements of behaviour taken from the person's actual life. Ideally it might be things like the A-level grades the person got, the degree they were awarded, the number of car accidents they had and so on. Such data could be difficult to obtain, so Cattell settled for ratings of the individual's behaviour by individuals who knew them well in a particular situation. In a school setting it might be teacher's ratings of aspects of the individual's ability, sociability, conscientiousness, and/or fellow students' ratings. In a work setting, it might be ratings by colleagues or managers, for example. These individuals would rate aspects of their target colleague's behaviour using a 10-point Likert Scale.

A second type of data collection involved using personality questionnaires. Cattell called this **Q-data**. This is the paper-and-pencil questionnaire that is widely used as an assessment tool in psychology.

Cattell's final method of generating data involved getting participants to complete tests under standardised testing conditions, but the tests are such that the responses cannot be faked. He called the data collected **T-data** and claimed that it represents truly objective test data. In normal questionnaires, respondents may lie about some of their answers to create a good impression, for example. However, participants completing the objective tests that produce T-data do not know what is being measured, so they cannot distort their answers. Cattell (1965) gives the Rorschach inkblot test as an example of such a test. Participants are presented with a series of different inkblots and have to report what they see. Clinical psychologists then interpret this information.

From the factor analyses of huge data sets gathered using these different procedures, Cattell identified 16 major source factors (Cattell, 1971; Cattell and Kline, 1977). Further research identified another 7 factors; however, his best-known measure of personality, the Sixteen Personality Factor (16PF) questionnaire uses the original 16 factors as they are the most robust measures. Cattell and his co-researchers have identified these 16 source traits as representing the basic structure of personality. He also ranked the traits in terms of how important they were in predicting an individual's behaviour. In the following list, we will present the 16 factors in this order, so that the most predictive items come first. Each factor represents a continuum along which individuals are ranked. At one end, individuals possess

L-data
Short for 'life record data'. These are measurements of behaviour taken from the person's actual life or observations on the individual from individuals who know them well.

Q-data
Refers to pen-and-paper, self-assessed personality questionnaires.

T-data
Produced when participants are asked to complete tests where they do not know what the test is measuring so that they cannot fake or distort their answers.

extremely high levels of the factor; at the other end, their levels are extremely low. Cattell (1965) was at pains to point out that almost all of the source traits have positive and negative aspects at each end of the continuum. We will highlight an example as we go through the trait descriptions. In labelling the source traits, we will use the factor letters that Cattell used to describe each factor, followed by what the scales measure (which has come to be the popular name for each of the scales) and then by the technical labels that Cattell has assigned to each factor (in parentheses). By doing this, we want to ensure that you will recognise the traits in other texts, where any of these names may be used.

- **Factor A, Outgoing–Reserved (affectothymia–schizothymia).** This factor measures whether individuals are outgoing or reserved. It is the largest factor. The technical labels Cattell chose for the endpoints of this factor, affectothymia (outgoing) and schizothymia (reserved), reflect the history of the employment of this trait in psychiatry. The outgoing–reserved dimension was shown to be important in determining which individuals were hospitalised for mental illness (Cattell, 1965).
- **Factor B, Intelligence (High '8'–Low '8').** Cattell was the first to include intelligence as an ability trait. He rated it as the second best predictor of behaviour in his initial analysis of the factors that best predict actual behaviour.
- **Factor C, Stable–Emotional (high ego strength–low ego strength).** This source trait measures emotional stability and the ability an individual has to control their impulses and solve problems effectively (Cattell, 1965). At the positive end, individuals are rated as being stable individuals who cope well in their lives and are realistic in their approach to life. At the negative end, individuals are emotionally labile. They are more neurotic and highly anxious.
- **Factor E, Assertive–Humble (dominance–submissiveness).** At the dominant end individuals display the surface traits of boastfulness, aggression, self-assertiveness, conceit, forcefulness, wilfulness, egotism and vigour. Humble or submissive individuals are seen to be modest, unsure, quiet, obedient, meek and retiring. This trait is the first to display a mixture of positive and negative attributes at each end of the scale. Dominant individuals have positive qualities of vigour and forcefulness but are boastful and egotistical.
- **Factor F, Happy-go-lucky–Sober (surgency–desurgency).** When discussing this term, Cattell defended his creation of new terms like surgency to describe his source traits. He suggests that the common names for traits often do not accurately represent what psychologists mean, so it is better to use a technical term that can be defined more precisely. High surgency individuals are cheerful, sociable, responsive, joyous, witty, humorous, talkative and energetic. He suggests that this is more than simply happy-go-lucky, the popular name for the term. Desurgent individuals are pessimistic, inclined to depression, reclusive, introspective, given to worrying, retiring and subdued. Cattell (1980) stated that this is the most important single predictive factor in children's personalities. He explored the influence of genetic factors on this trait and suggested that 55 percent of the variance on this trait is due to heredity.
- **Factor G, Conscientious–Expedient (high superego–low superego).** Cattell (1965) compares this factor to Freud's concept of the superego. Individuals high in conscientiousness are persistent and reliable and exercise good self-control. At the other end of the continuum, expedient individuals tend to take the line of least resistance rather than be guided by their principles.
- **Factor H, Venturesome–Shy (parmia–threctia).** Here Cattell contrasts the bold, genial, adventurous, gregarious, individual (venturesome) with the shy, aloof, self-contained, timid individual (shy). Cattell's technical labels for these terms are not as obscure as they seem at first sight. The terms relate to the autonomic nervous system, specifically the sympathetic and parasympathetic systems. The sympathetic nervous system produces the body's fight-or-flight response in the presence of a stressor of some

sort. Put simply, the parasympathetic system is involved in maintaining more normal, relaxed functioning. *Parmia* is an abbreviation of 'parasympathetic immunity', meaning that the individual remains calm under potentially threatening circumstances. They are immune to the effects of the sympathetic system. Similarly, *threctia* stands for 'threat reactivity' and hence is used to label an individual who has a reactive sympathetic system. Cattell (1982) undertook studies on the heritability of this trait and concluded that the genetic factor accounted for approximately 40 percent of the variance.

- **Factor I, Tender-minded–Tough-minded (premsia–harria).** The popular name describes this trait well. Tough-minded individuals are mature, independent-minded, self-sufficient and realistic. Tender-minded individuals are gentle, imaginative, anxious, impatient, demanding, immature, creative, neurotic and sentimental. The technical terms are derived from the phrases 'protected emotional sensitivity' (*premsia*) and 'hard realism' (*harria*).
- **Factor L, Suspicious–Trusting (protension–alaxia).** Individuals high in factor L are at the suspicious end of the continuum and, as well as being suspicious, are jealous and withdrawn from others. Those scoring low on factor L are trusting, composed and understanding. Cattell (1957) explains that the technical term *protension* is derived from the words 'projection' and 'tension'. *Alaxia* is from the term 'relaxation'.
- **Factor M, Imaginative–Practical (autia–praxernia).** The individual high in factor M is unconventional, intellectual and imaginative. They may often be unconcerned with the practicalities of life. The technical term *autia* comes from the word 'autistic'. *Praxernia* is derived from 'practical and concerned'. Such individuals are conventional, practical, logical, with a tendency to worry, and conscientious.
- **Factor N, Shrewd–Forthright (shrewdness–artlessness).** Here the descriptors fit the labels well. The shrewd individual is astute, worldly, smart and insightful (Cattell and Kline, 1977). The forthright individual is spontaneous, unpretentious and somewhat naïve.
- **Factor O, Apprehensive–Placid (guilt-proneness–assurance).** High levels of guilt-proneness are conceptualised as a purely negative trait by Cattell and Kline (1977). It is seen to be typical of criminals, alcoholics, other drug abusers and individuals suffering from manic depression. Individuals low in factor O are placid, resilient and self-confident (Cattell and Kline, 1977).

As the factors are presented in their order of importance in explaining individual differences in behaviour, the remaining four Q factors are therefore not particularly good predictors of behaviour; however, some of them have been researched extensively.

- **Factor Q_1, Experimenting–Conservative (radicalism– conservatism).** It is suggested that conservatives have a general fear of uncertainty and thus opt for the known and the well established. Radicals, on the other hand, prefer the non-conventional and conform less to the rules of society than conservatives do (Cattell, 1957).
- **Factor Q_2, Self-sufficiency–Group-tied (self-sufficiency–group adherence).** This factor is self-explanatory. It describes the individual's preference to go it alone or their need to be part of a group.
- **Factor Q_3, Controlled–Casual (high self-concept–low integration).** Individuals high in factor Q_3 are compulsive individuals. They crave a controlled environment that is highly predictable. Individuals low in factor Q_3 are undisciplined, lax individuals who have a preference for disorganisation in their surroundings.
- **Factor Q_4, Tense–Relaxed (high ergic tension–low ergic tension).** Again, this factor is largely self-explanatory. Those high in factor Q_4 are tense, driven individuals, while at the other end of the continuum, individuals are relaxed and easygoing (Cattell, 1973).

Contribution of Cattell

As we have seen, Cattell was keen to develop a comprehensive, empirically based trait theory of personality. He acknowledged the complexity of factors that all contribute to explain human behaviour, including genetics and environmental factors as well as ability and personality characteristics. Cattell (1965, 1980) was adamant that the test of any good personality theory was its ability to predict behaviour; he even produced an extremely complex mathematical equation that he suggested could do this. He wrote about the effect of learning on personality development and even turned his attention to classifying abnormal behaviour. While he produced vast amounts of empirically based work and attempted to develop a truly comprehensive theory of personality, he is best known in psychology for the 16PF (Cattell *et al.*, 1970).

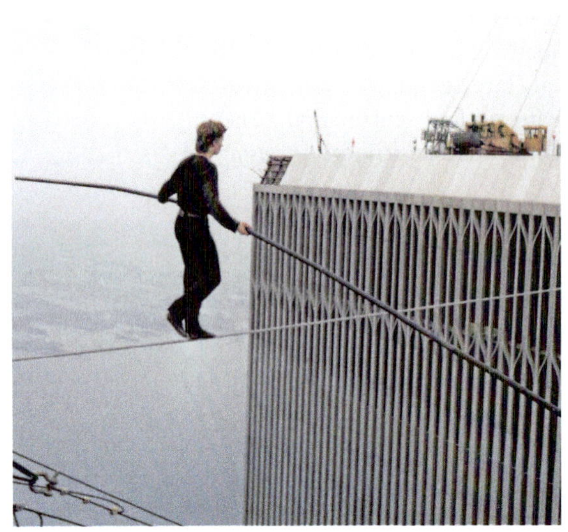

Which one of Cattell's 16 personality factors might describe this man: outgoing–reserved, stable–emotional, happy-go-lucky–sober, venturesome–shy, apprehensive–placid, experimenting–conservative?
Source: The Kobal Collection/Discover Films/BBC

The Sixteen Personality Factor (16PF) questionnaire has become a standard measure of personality and has been used consistently since its publication. However, the internal consistencies of some of the scales were quite low, and it has been revised and improved (Conn and Rieke, 1994). To do this, the questionnaire has been changed substantially, with over 50 percent of the items being new or significantly modified.

Although these revisions have produced a better measure psychometrically, it does mean that studies using the 16PF cannot be directly compared with the work that uses the earlier measure. The earlier measure had good predictability. Studies were undertaken that linked participation in church activities to differences in personality characteristics (Cattell, 1973; Cattell and Child, 1975). Other researchers demonstrated that the 16PF was a good predictor of success in different school subjects (Barton *et al.*, 1971).

Given the amount that Cattell published, it is perhaps surprising that this work has not had more impact. Part of the reason for this is that much of his work is difficult to understand. His use of obscure labels for his factors and the complex systems that he postulated are not reader-friendly. He put great emphasis on the objectivity of his approach and did not acknowledge the inherent subjectivity involved in factor analysis, linked to the initial selection of traits the researcher chooses to measure and the explanatory labels they select for their underlying factors. Trait approaches generally will be evaluated at the end of the discussion so are not repeated here. What we need to remember at this point is that Cattell suggested that the underlying structure of personality consists of 16 factors.

Hans Eysenck's trait theory of personality

When Hans Eysenck began to work in the area of personality, he observed that there were two schools within psychology. The first consisted of personality theorists whose main focus was on the development of theories, with little, if any, emphasis on evaluating these theories with empirical evidence. The second group was made up of experimental psychologists who had little interest in individual differences. Eysenck (1947) stressed the need for an integration of these two approaches. He outlined his goals as being to identify the main dimensions of personality, devise means of measuring them and test them using experimental, quantitative procedures. He felt that these steps would lead to the development of sound personality theory.

Eysenck (1947; 1952) accepted the conventional wisdom that assumed that children inherit personality characteristics from their parents and other members of their family. At the time he was writing, the main theoretical slant in psychology was that babies were relatively blank slates and that, while development was limited by differences in intelligence or physical skills, it was environmental experiences, particularly parenting styles, that largely influenced the development of personality. This was a legacy from the strong tradition of behaviourism. Over 50 years ago, Eysenck was stressing the importance of genetic inheritance, a view that has gained ground within psychology. We know from physiology that there are differences in physiological functioning between individuals and that these biological differences often translate into different behaviour. Eysenck's early claim that there is a large biological determinant to personality was originally met with scepticism, but, it has become accepted as supporting evidence has emerged from biological research.

Eysenck began by examining historical approaches to personality, including the work of Hippocrates and Galen that we covered earlier. His aim was to uncover the underlying structure of personality. The historical evidence suggested to him that there are different personality types, and the definition of personality that he adopted incorporates this concept. Eysenck (1970) defines personality as being the way that an individual's character, temperament, intelligence, physique and nervous system are organised. He suggests that this organisation is relatively stable and long-lasting. Traits are the relatively stable, long-lasting characteristics of the individual. In common with other trait researchers, Eysenck utilised factor analysis. He collected measurements of personality traits from large samples of individuals and factor-analysed them. After many years of research, he concluded that there are three basic personality dimensions, which he called types, and that all traits can be subsumed within these three types. Before we examine the three types, we need to become familiar with Eysenck's model of personality.

Eysenck's structure of personality

Beginning with observations of individual behaviour that he calls **specific responses**, Eysenck developed a hierarchical typology. An example of the methodology he used will make this clearer. For example, you would watch someone talking with their friends one evening and carefully observe their specific responses. If this person spends a great deal of their time talking with friends, you can begin to observe some of what Eysenck calls their **habitual responses**. Thus, habitual responses are the ways that individuals typically behave in a situation. From continued observations of the same individual, you might observe that this person seeks out occasions to interact with others and really enjoys social events. The conclusion would be that this person is very sociable or, in personality terms, they possess the trait of sociability. This structure of personality is shown in Figure 11.9. From the figure, you can see that specific responses that are found together in the individual make up habitual responses, and collections of habitual responses that the individual produces make up the next level of personality traits. Using factor analyses, Eysenck argued that traits such as sociability, liveliness, activity, assertiveness and sensation-seeking are highly correlated. This means that an individual's scores on each of these traits are likely to be very similar. This collection of traits then forms a **supertrait** or **personality type**. Each supertrait represents a continuum along which individuals can be placed, depending on the degree of the attribute they possess.

Supertrait
A term used by Eysenck to describe a collection of traits.

Personality type
A term used by Eysenck to describe a collection of traits.

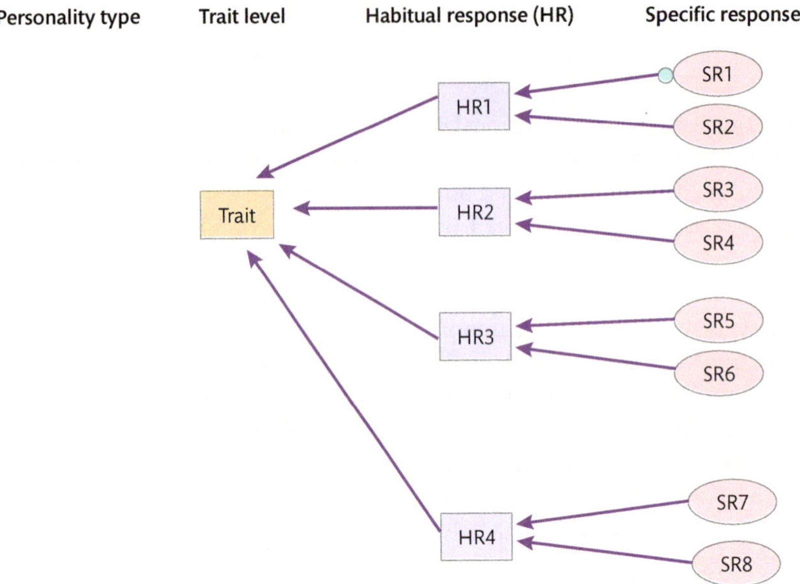

Figure 11.9 Eysenck's hierarchical model of personality.
Source: Adapted from Eysenck, H. J. (1967). *The Biological Basis of Personality*. Springfield, IL: Charles C. Thomas, p. 36. Reprinted courtesy of Charles C. Thomas Publisher, Ltd.

Extraversion
Sociable, talkative, active, spontaneous, adventurous, enthusiastic, person-oriented, assertive personality traits.

Introversion
Within Jungian theory, reflects a hesitant, reflective,quiet and retiring nature.

Extraverts
This term describes individuals who are very sociable, energetic, optimistic, friendly and assertive

Introverts
This term describes individuals who are reserved, independent rather than followers socially, even-paced rather than sluggish in terms of their pace of work.

Neuroticism
Tense, anxious, emotional, moody traits

Eysenck originally suggested that there are two supertraits. The first is a measure of sociability with **extraversion** at one end of the continuum and **introversion** at the other. **Extraverts** are sociable and impulsive people who like excitement and whose orientation is towards external reality. **Introverts** are quiet, introspective individuals who are oriented towards inner reality and who prefer a well-ordered life. The personality traits that make up extraversion are shown in Figure 11.10.

The second personality type or supertrait is **neuroticism**. Individuals can be placed on this dimension according to the degree of neuroticism they possess. Eysenck (1965b) defines neurotics as emotionally unstable individuals. He describes several types of neurotic behaviour. Some individuals high in neuroticism may have unreasonable fears (phobias) of certain objects, places, animals or people. Others may have obsessional or impulsive symptoms. The distinguishing feature of neurotic behaviour is that the individual displays an anxiety or fear level that is disproportionate to the realities of the situation. The traits that make up neuroticism are shown in Figure 11.11. Eysenck does separate out one group of neurotics who are free from anxiety and fear, and he labels this group **psychopaths**. These are individuals who behave in an antisocial manner and seem unable to appreciate the consequences of their actions despite any punishment meted out (Eysenck, 1965b). Such individuals are described as acting as if they have no conscience and showing no remorse for things they have done. Psychopathic personalities are likely to be found within the prison population.

The recognition of this group of psychopaths by Eysenck led to the identification of a third personality factor. As the two personality types (extraversion and neuroticism) did not adequately explain all of Eysenck's data, he added a third type, **psychoticism**. It is the severity of the disorder that differentiates psychotics from neurotics. Psychotics display the most severe type of psychopathology, frequently being insensitive to others, hostile, cruel and inhumane with a strong need to ridicule and upset others. The traits that come together to form psychoticism are shown in Figure 11.12.

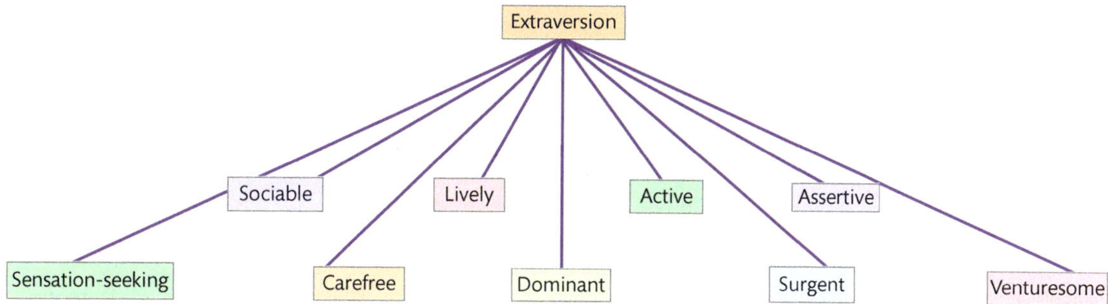

Figure 11.10 Traits that make up extraversion.
Source: Based on Eysenck and Eysenck (1985a).

Eysenck and Eysenck (1985a) stated that, despite having all these undesirable traits, psychotics still tend to be creative individuals. Eysenck quoted several sources of evidence to support his hypothesis. First, he provided historical examples of individuals he felt were geniuses and who had all displayed personality traits typical of psychoticism. He defined geniuses as being extremely creative individuals, and he suggested that many of the traits associated with psychoticism could be perceived as aiding a creative career. Traits such as being egocentric, so you always put yourself first; being tough-minded, so that you pursue your own goals regardless of others or circumstances; being unempathic, so that you are not affected by other people's emotions and problems. Psychological studies of great individuals have demonstrated that they have needed to be self-centred and persistent to overcome the obstacles that they faced in their lives and that they also possess the ability to think in unusual, almost bizarre, ways (Simonton, 1994). Eysenck (1995) cited evidence that psychotic individuals perform well on tests of creativity that require divergent thinking. By divergent thinking, he meant the ability to produce novel ideas that are different from those that most people produce. He claimed that psychotics and geniuses have an overinclusive cognitive style that allows them to consider divergent solutions to problems. These views of Eysenck's are not universally accepted. As Simonton (1994) points out, humanistic psychologists such as Maslow and Rogers asserted that creativity is the result of optimum mental health, which implies balanced personalities. Eysenck (1995) did admit that more research is required in this area.

Psychopaths
There are individuals that behave an antisocial manner and seem unable to appreciate the consequences of their actions despite any punishment meted out.

Psychoticism
Impulsive, antisocial, egocentric personality traits.

Eysenck (1967) claimed that these three types or supertraits make up the basic structure of personality, and he developed an instrument to measure the three types and their supporting

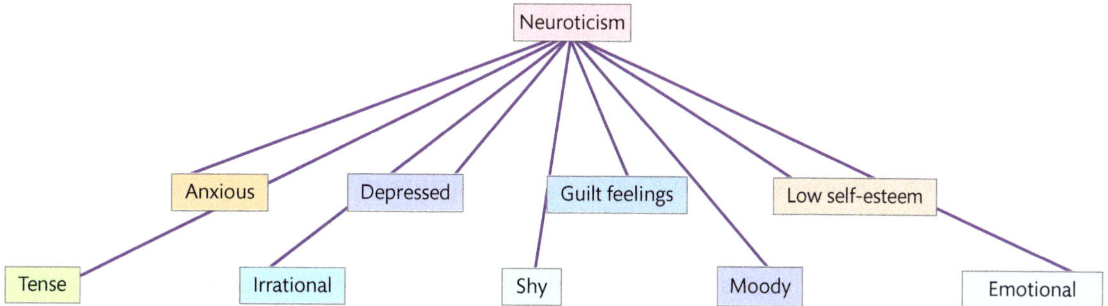

Figure 11.11 Traits that make up neuroticism.
Source: Based on Eysenck and Eysenck (1985a).

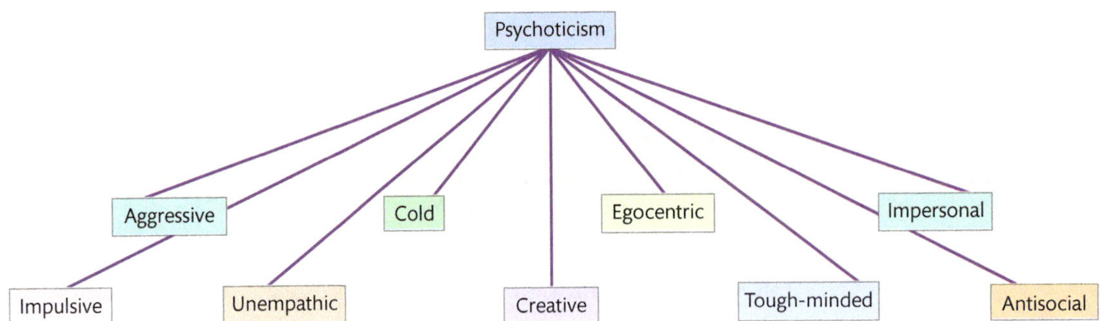

Figure 11.12 Traits that make up psychoticism.
Source: Based on Eysenck and Eysenck (1985a).

traits. This is called the Eysenck Personality Questionnaire (EPQ; H. Eysenck and S. Eysenck, 1975). He suggested that there is a link between the clinical conditions of neurosis and psychoses and his scales of neuroticism and psychoticism. Individuals who score highly on neuroticism or psychoticism are not necessarily neurotic or psychotic, but he argued that they are at risk of developing these disorders. High scores indicate a predisposition, which may develop under adverse circumstances.

Eysenck's next task was to explain why individuals who differed along the supertrait dimensions should behave differently. His theoretical exposition, while not ignoring environmental influences, was heavily biological. Indeed, Eysenck (1982a) claimed that about two-thirds of the variance in personality development can be attributed to biological factors. Environment plays a part, particularly in influencing how traits are expressed, but Eysenck would argue that biology has imposed limits on how much an individual personality can change.

Research evidence for Eysenck's types

Many predictions have been made from this theory, and there is a high level of support over a period of 40 years. For example, Eysenck (1965b) reported that extraverts compared with introverts prefer to socialise. They like louder music and brighter colours, and they are more likely to smoke, drink more alcohol and engage in more varied sexual activities. These differences generally continue to be reported in the literature. Amirkham *et al.* (1995) found that extraverts are more likely than introverts to attract and maintain networks of friends and to approach others for help when they are undergoing a crisis. Eysenck and Eysenck (1975) reported that extraverts, because of their need for variety in their lives, have more career changes or job changes. Extraverts are also more likely to change relationship partners more frequently. Campbell and Hawley (1982) looked at the study habits and the preferred location for studying of students and found that introverts prefer to study in quiet areas, while extraverts study in areas where there are other people and opportunities to socialise. Extraverts also took more study breaks than introverts did, indicating that they have a higher need for change in their activities and environment. Davies and Parasuraman (1992) reported that extraverts tire more easily than introverts on tasks requiring vigilance and are more likely to make errors. While there continues to be a significant amount of research utilising versions of the EPQ (H. Eysenck and S. Eysenck, 1975; 1991), the neuroticism and the extraversion scales have proved to be good reliable measures psychometrically; the psychoticism scale is more problematic, with much lower internal reliability statistics. Eysenck (1967) admitted that this scale is less robust and did refine it somewhat (Eysenck, 1992) but, despite this, it remains the weakest measure.

If the three-factor solution represents the basic structure of personality, it should be found cross-culturally. Eysenck and Eysenck undertook a considerable programme of cross-cultural research to explore whether the theory held. His EPQ was carefully translated into many different languages. This research is summarised in Eysenck and Eysenck (1982). He reported that the primary factors were found in at least 24 nations in both males and females. His sample included African, Asian, North American and many European cultures. From this data and from twin studies, Eysenck concluded that the three-factor structure has a genetic basis and represents the basic structure of personality.

Sybil Eysenck produced a child's version of the EPQ, called the Junior Eysenck Personality Questionnaire (S. Eysenck, 1965). It was also translated into many languages, and again the cross-cultural evidence was consistent. Studies of children found the same three factors cross-culturally. This provided additional evidence for the theory. H. Eysenck followed up this research with longitudinal studies to demonstrate that the structure was stable across time (H. Eysenck, 1967, 1982a, 1990b, 1993; S. Eysenck *et al.*, 1993; 1994). S. Eysenck concluded that all this research provided confirmatory evidence that there is a genetic basis for the primary personality types. They are all found cross-culturally, despite social pressures within different cultures to develop in specific ways. The same structures are found in children as in adults. Reviews of studies of identical and fraternal twins, raised together and raised apart, found the same structures and personality similarities between individual biological relatives and lend considerable support for a significant genetic component to personality. As mentioned previously, details of genetic studies of personality are included later.

Eysenck (1990b) does still see a role for the environment in the development of personality. He suggested that, while individuals' genes provide a strong tendency to become a certain type of person, some modification is possible. He suggested that the way that children are socialised was crucial here. However, he did not provide a detailed developmental theory to explain how the environment might intervene in development or to specify the environment that would promote healthy development.

Psychopathology and Eysenck's therapeutic approach

Eysenck was a behaviourist, and therefore he placed a lot of emphasis on how learned behaviour was acquired. Thus, healthy and abnormal behaviour is the result of the way that individuals respond to the stimuli in their environment. Some individuals are more susceptible to developing psychopathology because of their inherited vulnerabilities. For example, Eysenck suggested that individuals who score highly on the personality trait neurosis are more likely to develop clinical neuroses than are those with low scores.

Eysenck's approach to treatment involved behaviour therapy. He was extremely hostile to all other therapies but particularly targeted psychoanalytic approaches. Indeed, Eysenck (1965a) claimed that the only effective therapy was behaviour therapy. As mentioned in the Profile box, Eysenck developed clinical psychology training in the United Kingdom and was an active clinician as well as a personality researcher for much of his life.

Eysenck's contribution to trait theorising

Eysenck's theorising is fairly comprehensive, although not all aspects of it are equally well developed. This is particularly true of the developmental aspects and the biological basis. He also focuses heavily on genetic factors and pays much less attention to the social context within which much behaviour occurs and that may affect personality and behaviour in particular situations. He would argue that personality determines to some degree the situations that individuals choose to be in, but that is debatable to some extent. In terms of heuristic value, Eysenck has been very influential. His critique of all therapies, apart from behaviour therapy, stimulated therapists to evaluate their work and led to a large increase in evaluative research on therapies. His work also has significant applied value. He demonstrated a rigorous approach to personality theorising. He moved beyond many personality trait researchers in that he tried to provide not merely a description of personality structure but also an explanation of what caused differences in personality, with his genetic studies and his biological theory. He also provided a fairly robust measure of personality. His work has stimulated an enormous amount of research. Eysenck founded the journal *Personality and Individual Differences*, and its continued growth and development attests to his influence over many years.

In one other aspect, his theory can perhaps be criticised for being too parsimonious, having only three factors. Do three factors really represent the basic structure of personality? This question of the number of factors necessary to describe personality structure is what we shall discuss next. There has been considerable debate in the psychological literature about the number of factors required for an adequate description of personality and, as we shall see, before his death Eysenck contributed to this discussion (Eysenck, 1991).

The five-factor model

Psychologists increasingly agree that five supertraits may adequately describe the structure of personality. The evidence to support this contention has come from several sources. There is still some debate, as we shall see, about how to label these factors; but this is perhaps unsurprising given that assigning labels is the most subjective aspect of factor analysis. Researchers are likely to have different opinions about which words best describe the constituent traits that make up a supertrait. We shall begin by examining the evidence for five factors, and then we will look at where this leaves Eysenck's three-factor model and Cattell's 16-factor model. Finally, we will evaluate the trait approach to personality.

Evidential sources for the five-factor model

There are three evidential sources for the five-factor model:

- the lexical approach;
- factor analysis evidence for the five-factor model;
- other evidence in support of the five-factor model of personality.

The lexical approach

You will recall that earlier in this discussion, we discussed the lexical hypothesis. This is the hypothesis that it is the differences in personality that are important for social interaction, and human societies have labelled these differences as single terms. Several detailed accounts of the lexical approach and its history are available if you want to explore this theory further (De Raad, 2000; Saucier and Goldberg, 2001).

You will recall that Cattell's 16PF came from the factor analysis of the list of 4,500 trait names identified by Allport and Odbert (1936). Cattell produced a 16-factor solution. Fiske (1949) reanalysed the same data but could not reproduce the 16 factors; he published instead a five-factor solution. This work was ignored for a long time. Tupes and Christal (1961/1992) reported five factors from analyses of trait words in eight different samples. Norman (1963) revisited the earlier research and reproduced the same five-factor structure using personality ratings of individuals given by their peers. Digman and Takemoto-Chock (1981) carried out further analyses and confirmed Norman's five-factor solution. Goldberg (1981) reviewed all the research and made a convincing argument for the Big Five. Since then, Goldberg and his team have carried out an extensive research programme investigating personality traits, and

Goldberg (1990) concluded that in the English language trait descriptors are versions of five major features of personality: love, work, affect, power and intellect. Since then, the research has spread to other languages. Saucier and Ostendorf (1999) used a set of 500 personality traits and found a five-factor structure in the German language, for example.

Saucier and Goldberg (2001) have described the lexical approach to investigating whether the five-factor structure is universally applicable as an emic approach to research. Basically, what the researchers do is to use the personality terms that are found in the native language of the country. They contrast this with what they call the etic approach, which uses personality questionnaires translated from another language that in practice tends to be English. Saucier and Goldberg (2001) report that etic approaches tend to replicate the five-factor structure while there is more variability reported in studies using emic approaches. Perugini and Di-Blas (2002) discuss this issue further in relation to emic and etic data that they collected on Italian samples. They point out that in the etic approach, the questionnaires being translated are based on five-factor structures found in the original language. Goldberg and his research team make a case for the necessity of further study of cultural differences in personality trait use that are being found using emic approaches as a core part of the search for the universal structure of personality. Goldberg's research team has made available copyrighted free adjective scales that can be used to measure the five factors and personality scales for measuring them. These can be accessed from his website and the address is included at the end of the discussion.

Emic approach
A lexical approach to personality research using the personality terms that are found in the native language of the country

Etic approach
Uses personality questionnaires translated from another language, which in practice tends to be English.

Factor analysis evidence for the five-factor model of personality

This is the second source of evidence for the existence of a structure of five factors. Costa and McCrae (1985; 1989; 1992; 1997) are arguably the most influential researchers in this area, and their factor solution has come to be called the Big Five model. This approach requires large samples of participants to complete at least two personality questionnaires. The resultant data set is then factor-analysed to uncover clusters of traits. The consistent finding is the emergence of five factors or dimensions of personality.

It is important to stress that it is the analysis of data that has produced the factors, not exploration of a theory about the number of factors necessary in a model. This is not the usual approach in psychology. Usually researchers begin with a theoretically based hypothesis about some aspect of behaviour. They then collect their data, and their results either support or refute their original theory-driven hypothesis. In contrast, with the five-factor research, the hypothesis that five factors represent the basic structure of personality has come from the data that was collected. In other words, the Big Five model is a data-derived hypothesis as opposed to a theoretically based one.

These are the factors described by the American personality researchers Costa and McCrae (1992), who measured personality with their well-known Neuroticism, Extraversion, Openness Personality Inventory (NEO-PI-R). The Big Five factors are Openness, Conscientiousness, Extraversion, Agreeableness and Neuroticism. You can use the acronym OCEAN to help you remember what the factors are called. More detailed descriptions of each factor are now provided. Each factor represents a continuum along which individuals can be placed according to their scores.

- **Openness** – This factor refers to the individual having an openness to new experiences. It includes the characteristics of showing intellectual curiosity, divergent thinking and a willingness to consider new ideas and an active imagination. Individuals scoring highly on openness are unconventional and independent thinkers. Individuals with low scores are more conventional and prefer the familiar to the new.
- **Conscientiousness** – This factor describes our degree of self-discipline and control. Individuals with high scores on this factor are determined, organised and plan for events

OCEAN
This is an acronym that refers to the factors of the Big Five trait theory of personality factors. The letters refer to the super traits of Openness, Conscientiousness, Extraversion, Agreeableness and Neuroticism.

in their lives. Individuals with low scores tend to be careless, easily distracted from their goals or the tasks that they are undertaking and undependable. If you look closely at the trait descriptors included in conscientiousness, you will see that they are all attributes likely to become apparent in work situations. For this reason, they are sometimes referred to as the will to achieve or work dimension.

- **Extraversion** – This factor is a measure of the individual's sociability. It is the same factor as described by Eysenck earlier in this discussion and by the psychoanalyst Jung. Individuals who score highly on extraversion are very sociable, energetic, optimistic, friendly and assertive. Individuals with high scores are labelled extraverts. As with the Eysenck and Jung descriptions, individuals with low scores are labelled introverts. Introverts are described as being reserved and independent rather than followers socially and even-paced rather than sluggish in terms of their pace of work.
- **Agreeableness** – This factor relates very much to characteristics of the individual that are relevent for social interaction. Individuals with high scores are trusting, helpful, soft-hearted and sympathetic. Those with low scores are suspicious, antagonistic, unhelpful, sceptical and uncooperative.
- **Neuroticism** – This factor measures an individual's emotional stability and personal adjustment. Costa and McCrae (1992) suggest that, although a range of emotions exists, individuals who score highly on one also rate highly on others. In psychological terms, the various emotional states are highly correlated. Thus, the individual who scores highly on neuroticism experiences wide swings in their mood and they are volatile in their emotions. Individuals with low scores on the neuroticism factor are calm, well adjusted and not prone to extreme maladaptive emotional states. (Indeed, in some five-factor models of personality, this dimension is referred to as emotional stability.)

These are the five main dimensions popularly known as the Big Five. Within each of the main dimensions there are more specific personality attributes that cluster together, and all contribute to the category score. These subordinate traits are sometimes called facets (Costa and McCrae, 1992). The Big Five model is a hierarchical model similar in concept to Eysenck's model. Each of the Big Five factors consists of six facets or subordinate traits. The facets included in the NEO-PI-R (Costa and McCrae, 1992) are shown in Table 11.6. Thus, an individual's scores on the traits of fantasy, aesthetics, feelings, actions, ideas and values combine to produce their scores on the openness factor. The NEO-PI-R then allows measurement at a general factor level or on more specific factors. Obviously, the more specific the measure, the greater the likelihood of using it to actually predict behaviour.

Other evidence in support of the Big Five

There is too much research supporting the Big Five for us to review it all here. Instead, we will cite some examples from the main areas. In terms of how well this model fits with other measures of personality, the evidence is largely positive. McCrae and Costa (1989) factor-analysed scores on the Myers–Briggs Type Inventory and found that it supports a five-factor structure. Boyle (1989) reported that the five-factor model is also broadly compatible with Cattell's fourteen-factor measure and Eysenck's three-factor measure. The latest measure of the 16PFI allows scoring on the Big Five (Conn and Rieke, 1994). Goldberg (1993) compared the five-factor model with Eysenck's three-factor model and concluded that two of the factors – extraversion and neuroticism – are very similar, and that psychoticism can be subsumed under agreeableness and conscientiousness.

The NEO-PI-R has also been translated into several other languages, and the same factor structure has been replicated (McCrae and Costa, 1997; McCrae *et al.*, 1998; 2000). If you recall, this evidence is not uncontentious, based as it is on the etic approach to personality

Table 11.6 The constituent facets of the Big Five factors

Openness	Conscientiousness	Extraversion	Agreeableness	Neuroticism
Fantasy	Competence	Warmth	Trust	Anxiety
Aesthetics	Order	Gregariousness	Straightforwardness	Angry hostility
Feelings	Dutifulness	Assertiveness	Altruism	Depressions
Actions	Achievement-striving	Activity	Compliance	Self-consciousness
Ideas	Self-discipline	Excitement-seeking	Modesty	Impulsiveness
Values	Deliberation	Positive emotions	Tender-mindedness	Vulnerability

Source: Based on Costa and McCrae (1985).

research that we discussed earlier. These researchers (McCrae and Costa, 1997; McCrae *et al.*, 1998; 2000) have also demonstrated that the observed personality differences are stable over time and have a genetic basis. To summarise, Costa and McCrae (1992) claim that the five factors represent the universal structure of personality based on all the evidence we have discussed. The factors are found in different languages, ages of people and races.

Evaluation of the Big Five and trait approaches

Can we conclude then that the Big Five represent the structure of personality? Unfortunately, it is premature to say that there is total consensus on the model. Increasingly, there is debate about a six-factor model and the existence of higher order factors. Among researchers who agree that there are five factors, there is still some level of disagreement about the exact nature of each of the five factors. Indeed, Saucier and Goldberg (1998) and Saucier (1995) argue that research should look for solutions beyond the current five-factor models. This is the scientific approach – to search for contradictory evidence instead of purely focusing on searching for confirmation, as the present research does.

There is some debate about how the factors should be labelled. Labelling factors depends on the researcher's judgement about the best descriptor for the cluster of correlated traits. For example, the agreeableness factor has also been labelled conformity (Fiske, 1949) and likeability (Norman, 1963). The same debate applies for all the other factors.

Peabody and Goldberg (1989) have also demonstrated that the measures that are included in a questionnaire crucially affect the final factors produced. If a questionnaire does not have many items that measure openness, for example, then the description of openness that is produced will be narrower. There is still some argument about the number of traits, with studies reporting different numbers between Eysenck's three and seven (Ashton and Lee, 2001, 2007; Briggs, 1989; Church and Burke, 1994; Zuckerman *et al.*, 1993). McCrae and Costa (1995) suggest that the number depends on the nature of the trait measures that are included. They point out that five-factor models tend not to include evaluative traits like moral/immoral. If evaluative traits are included, Almagor *et al.*, (1995) have suggested that a seven-factor solution emerges.

There has been some debate about what exactly some of the factors mean (Digman 1990). Are they perhaps linguistic categories that do not actually represent the underlying structure of personality? Is it that the five factors represent our ability to describe personality traits in language and are nothing to do with underlying structures? There is no easy answer to this question, although the accumulating weight of research evidence would seem to negate it. Is it perhaps that our cognitive abilities only allow for a five-factor structure but the reality is more complex and subtle?

Briggs (1989) has criticised the model for being atheoretical. As we have discussed earlier, the model is data-driven and was not derived from a theoretical base. There are currently some attempts to address this with genetic studies and the search for a physiological basis for the observed differences. This criticism applies more generally to the trait approach, although theorists such as Eysenck saw theory building as being crucial within his approach.

One of the more general criticisms of trait approaches to personality is related to how the various measures are interpreted and used. For example, Mischel (1968; 1983a; 1990) has pointed out that many of these measures are largely descriptive and do not predict behaviour particularly well. Despite this claim, many of these measures are widely used to make important decisions about individuals' lives, and in workplace situations are often blindly interpreted by people who are not psychologists. Mischel (1968) demonstrates that, on average, personality trait measures statistically account for only around 10 percent of the variance observed in behaviour. In other words, 90 percent of the variance in behaviour is down to something other than the effect of personality. However, Kraus (1995) has shown that the variance figure is not insignificant and is similar to that found in studies measuring the relationship between attitudes and behaviour. Mischel's criticism of the overreliance on trait measures to assess individuals has had beneficial effects in work settings. The practice currently is to use multiple measures of personality assessment in work settings. Psychometric assessments, individual and group tasks and interviews are frequently used together as an assessment package, and this prevents overreliance on the psychometric tool.

Final comments

In summary, we have described the nomothetic approach to personality research. You should now appreciate the long history of attempts to describe and explain differences in personality. You should understand what is meant by the lexical hypothesis and be familiar with the approach to data analysis employed by trait theorists. You should also be aware of the contributions of Allport, Cattell and Eysenck to understanding personality, as well as the approaches that have resulted in the identification of the Big Five personality traits.[C]

[C]Maltby, J., Day, L., & Macaskill, A. (2013). Theories and measurement of intelligence. In J. Maltby, L. Day, & A. Macaskill (Eds.), *Personality, individual differences and intelligence* (3rd ed., pp. 152–171). Harlow, Essex: Pearson Education.

Summary

- Dollard and Miller made the first attempt to allow for cognitive processing in learning theory. They allow for unconscious influences on motivation but strictly define what they mean by the unconscious.
- Dollard and Miller outlined a stimulus–response (S–R) theory of learning. This includes the consideration of primary drives and secondary drives.
- Dollard and Miller demonstrated that observational learning played an important role in learning. Role models are observed, and their performance is imitated.
- Bandura was the first learning theorist to allocate a significant role in learning to inner cognitive processes. Bandura uses the term reciprocal determinism to label the processes that drive behaviour. He sees an individual as being influenced by three interacting factors: personal factors, behaviour and environmental factors.
- Bandura further develops Dollard and Miller's concept of observational learning and has demonstrated its importance in the acquisition of aggressive behaviour, in particular with the Bobo doll study. He demonstrated that the characteristics of the model, attributes of the observer and the consequences of imitating behaviour are all influential factors in the learning process.
- For Bandura, modelling behaviour was an active process of learning through observation where the observer makes judgements and constructs symbolic representations.
- Bandura demonstrated that humans use self-reinforcement to control our behaviour via internal self-regulatory processes.
- Self-efficacy is identified as one of the most powerful of the self-regulatory processes.
- Rotter demonstrated that the likelihood of a behaviour occurring, termed behaviour potential, is predicted by our expectancy and reinforcement value.
- Rotter termed our generalised expectancies in new situations as locus of control.
- Two assumptions underlie trait theory. The first is that personality characteristics are relatively stable over time. The second is that traits show stability across situations.
- Trait theorists are aiming to find the basic structure of personality and to produce reliable ways of measuring personality differences.
- William Sheldon outlined a description of personality, called somatotypes, based on physique and temperament. He described three basic types of physique – endomorphy, mesomorphy and ectomorphy – and demonstrated that each body type was associated with a particular temperament.
- The lexical hypothesis was first put forth by Sir Francis Galton. It suggests that it is the important individual differences between people that come to be encoded as single word terms (trait descriptors). The lexical hypothesis led to attempts to categorise the important personality traits. With the advent of factor analysis, these trait lists were analysed to try to uncover the underlying structure.
- Gordon Allport identified 18,000 words, of which 4,500 described personality traits.
- Allport conceptualised human nature as normally being rational, creative, active and self-reliant. He used the idiographic approach to discover personal dispositions. He described three types of personality traits: cardinal, central and secondary.
- Allport emphasised the importance of the concept of self to any theory of personality. He hypothesised that children were not born with a concept of self but that it gradually developed, and it was a lifelong process. Allport was a pioneer in trait theory, and one of his important contributions was to alert psychologists to the limitations of trait approaches.
- Cattell's work marks the beginning of the search for the structure of personality using factor analysis. He made a distinction between traits that are genetically determined and those that are the result of environmental experiences. He defined three different types of traits: ability, temperament and dynamic. He subdivided dynamic traits into three types: attributes, sentiments and ergs. All these types of dynamic

traits are organised in complex and interrelated ways to produce a dynamic lattice. He makes a further distinction between common traits and unique traits. The latter account for the uniqueness of human beings.

- Cattell made an important distinction between surface traits and source traits. Surface traits are collections of trait descriptors that cluster together in many individuals and situations. Using factor analysis, he uncovered underlying traits that he called source traits. These are responsible for the observed variance in the surface traits.
- Cattell used a variety of approaches to uncover the source traits of personality. He finally produced 16 factors and claimed that they represent the basic structure of personality. He developed the 16PF as a measurement tool.
- Eysenck's goals were to identify the main dimensions of personality, devise means of measuring them and test them using experimental, quantitative procedures. He defined personality as being the way that an individual's character, temperament, intelligence, physique and nervous system are organised. Traits are the relatively stable, long-lasting characteristics of the individual.
- Eysenck developed a hierarchical model of personality types. At the bottom level are specific behavioural responses called habitual responses. These come together to make up personality traits. Clusters of traits come together to make up personality types. Using factor analysis, Eysenck identified three types or supertraits that he hypothesised made up the basic structure of personality. He developed the Eysenck Personality Questionnaire (EPQ) to measure these three types and their underlying traits.
- Eysenck claimed that about two-thirds of the variance in personality development can be attributed to biological factors. Environment influences how traits are expressed, but Eysenck argues that biology has imposed limits on how much an individual personality can change.
- There is good support for neuroticism and extraversion, including cross-cultural, developmental and longitudinal stability data. Psychoticism is the least reliable dimension.
- Eysenck provided not merely a description of personality structure but also an explanation of what causes differences in personality, with his genetic studies and his biological theory. His work has stimulated an enormous amount of research.
- There is a growing consensus that five supertraits make up the basic structure of personality. While there are arguments about the names accorded to these factors, those chosen by Costa and McCrae are the most popular. The Big Five factors are Openness, Conscientiousness, Extraversion, Agreeableness and Neuroticism (OCEAN).
- There are several sources of evidence underpinning the Big Five structure of personality. The first of these uses the lexical approach to uncover the structures. The second approach uses the factor analysis of personality questionnaires.
- The Big Five model is hierarchical, similar in concept to Eysenck's model. Each of the Big Five factors consists of six facets or subordinate traits. Costa and Macrae's NEO-PI-R measures both the subordinate traits and the supertraits.
- There is increasing agreement that there are five factors, but there is still some level of disagreement about the exact nature of each of the five factors. Debate continues about how the factors should be labelled.
- The lack of an underpinning theory is problematic for some psychologists. This trait approach is data-driven, not theoretically driven, although theoretical support is now developing.

Review questions

A. A Fill in the missing words to complete the following statements.

1. Carl Rogers believed that unconditional positive regard, ___________ understanding and ___________ are necessary and sufficient conditions for therapy.
2. William Sheldon outlined various descriptions of personality known as somatotypes which are based on __________ and ______________.
3. Gordon Allport organised traits into a hierarchy of three levels that include __________ traits, ________ traits and ________ traits.

B. Please select one statement that best answers each of the following questions.

4. Which of the following learning theorists contributed to personality theory?
   a) Abraham Maslow and Carl Rogers
   b) Albert Bandura and Julian Rotter
   c) Sigmund Freud and Carl Jung
   d) all of the above
5. Which of the following statements accurately defines the humanistic approach to personality?
   a) there is an emphasis on personal growth rather than deficits
   b) human nature is considered to be a positive, present-focused process with an emphasis on phenomenology of the individual persons conscious experience
   c) free will and responsibility are core concepts of the humanistic approach
   d) all of the above
6. According to Maslow's Hierarchy of Needs, what is the first need that must be met?
   a) safety
   b) belonging
   c) esteem
   d) physiological
7. Which of the following statements best describes the process of self-actualisation?
   a) Is when a person is very social but lacks autonomy
   b) Is a common presentation in society
   c) occurs when an individual's actual self and ideal self are congruent with each other
   d) all of the above
8. Temperament as defined by Galen includes which of the following characteristics:
   a) openness, extraversion, conscientiousness, agreeableness and neuroticism
   b) cerebrotonia, somatotonia and viscerotonia
   c) melancholic, phlegmatic, choleric and sanguine
   d) none of the above
9. Sheldon describes a mesomorph as which of the following characteristics in terms of physique?
   a) light-boned with a slight musculature
   b) big-boned with well-defined muscles
   c) rounded body tending towards fatness
   d) none of the above

10. True or False? Using a statistical process known as a factor analysis, Raymond Cattell generated sixteen dimensions of personality known as the 16PF that were derived from a list of 4,500 traits.

11. Hans Eysenck's theory of personality is based on which of the following dimensions?

a) openness, extraversion, conscientiousness, agreeableness and neuroticism

b) openness, extraversion, conscientiousness, agreeableness and psychosis

c) introversion versus extraversion, neuroticism versus stability and psychoticism versus socialisation

d) introversion versus extraversion, neuroticism versus instability and psychosis versus socialisation

12. Anna is described as a positive, warm, assertive and outgoing person. Based on Costa and McCrea's Big-Five facets, Anna is most likely to be classified as showing which of the following dimensions?

a) openness

b) conscientiousness

c) agreeableness

d) extraversion

CHAPTER 12

Pain

The content in this section has been compiled from:
Morrison, chapter 16

Morrison, V., & Bennett, P. (2009). Pain. In V. Morrison & P. Bennett (Eds.), *An introduction to health psychology* (2nd ed., pp. 479–510). Harlow, Essex: Pearson Education.

CHAPTER 12

Pain

Pain is defined as an unpleasant sensory and emotional experience associated with actual or potential tissue damage, or described in terms of such damage. Pain can alter an individual's functional, psychological and social life, while also indirectly influencing interactions and therapeutic outcomes in health care settings (e.g., adherence to treatment). In this chapter, we examine how pain influences behaviour, emphasising key theories of pain and providing pain management strategies.

After studying this chapter you should be able to:

- Describe different types of pain: acute and chronic
- Identify and describe biological models of pain
- Describe the psychobiological theory of pain: Melzack and Wall
- Describe how people can be helped to cope with pain.

The experience of pain

Pain occurs in a variety of medical conditions, and sometimes in the absence of any physical problems. So prevalent is this experience that we have taken an entire chapter to examine its aetiology and treatment. This chapter examines a number of physiological and psychological explanations for our differing experiences of pain. It first examines the experience of pain: how various types of pain are defined, how prevalent they are, and how we respond to acute and chronic pain. It then considers the role of emotion, cognitions and attention in mediating the experience of pain. The next section describes the gate theory of pain developed by Melzack and Wall, which explains how both biological and psychological factors combine to create our experience of pain. Finally, the chapter goes on to consider a number of psychological interventions used in the treatment of both acute and chronic pain.

Pain is a familiar sensation for most of us. It is functional. It is unpleasant, and it warns us of potential damage to the body. A reflex action when we feel pain is to pull away from its cause or to try to reduce it in some way. Pain may also signal the onset of disease—and is the symptom most likely to lead an individual to seeking medical help. The value of pain as a warning indicator is shown by the disadvantages experienced by those who feel no pain. People with a condition known as congenital universal insensitivity to pain (CUIP) usually die at a young age because they fail to respond to illnesses of which the main symptom is pain (such as appendicitis) or to avoid situations that risk their health (Nagasako *et al.* 2003). They could, for example, receive extensive burns by sitting too close to a hot fire without experiencing the warning signs that most of us take for granted.

Despite its survival benefits, when pain lasts for a long time, it feels destructive and problematic. It can be so difficult to ignore that it takes over our lives. Chronic pain may be the result of long-term conditions such as rheumatoid arthritis. It may endure long after the time of physical damage, or even be experienced in areas of the body that no longer exist. Many people who have had an arm or leg amputated go on to experience **phantom limb pain**, in which they feel pain in their non-existent limb – sometimes for many years. Accordingly, pain can also be maladaptive and contribute to long-term problems for an affected individual.

Phantom limb pain
A phenomenon that occurs following amputation of a limb, in which the individual feels like they still have their limb, and the limb is in pain.

Migraine
A headache with symptoms including nausea, vomiting or sensitivity to light. Associated with changes in vascular flow within the brain.

Trigeminal neuralgia
A painful inflammation of the trigeminal nerve that causes sharp and severe facial pain.

Types of pain

Medical definitions have categorised various types of pain, including:

- *Acute pain*: despite most people's experience of acute pain as lasting only a few minutes, acute pain is defined as pain lasting less than three to six months. Some episodes of acute pain, usually involving some form of injury, may occur only once, and generally the pain disappears once the damaged tissue has healed. Examples include toothache and childbirth. However, acute pain may be recurrent. Conditions such as **migraine**, headaches or **trigeminal neuralgia** may involve repeated episodes of pain, each one of which can be defined as 'acute' but which are also part of a longer-term condition.
- *Chronic pain*: this is pain that continues for more than three to six months. Chronic pain generally begins with an episode of acute pain that fails to improve over time. In this category, there are two broad types of pain: (1) pain with an identifiable cause such as rheumatoid arthritis or a back injury, and (2) pain with no identifiable cause. The latter is not unusual—85 percent of cases of back pain have no known physical cause (Deyo 1991). Chronic pain can, itself, be divided into two types:
  1. *Chronic benign pain*: in which long-term pain is experienced to a similar degree over time. An example of this may be lower back pain.
  2. *Chronic progressive pain*: here, the pain becomes progressively worse over time due to the progression of a disease such as rheumatoid arthritis.

Another way of thinking about types of pain is to think about the nature of the pain. Here, three dimensions of experience are frequently used:

1. *the type of pain*: including stabbing, shooting, throbbing, aching, piercing, sharp and hot;
2. *the severity of pain*: from mild discomfort to excruciating;
3. *the pattern of pain*: including brief, continuous and intermittent.

The prevalence of pain

It would be difficult to find many people who had not experienced some degree of acute pain in the last month or so, but chronic pain is also remarkably common. Blyth *et al.* (2003) found that 21 percent of a large community sample reported some degree of chronic pain. The most frequently reported causes were injury (38 percent), sports injury (13 percent) and a 'health problem' (29 percent). Nearly 80 percent of those who reported having chronic pain had consulted a doctor about it in the six months before the survey. Eriksen *et al.* (2003) reported similar prevalence levels: 19 percent of their community sample had some degree of chronic pain. Older people were more likely to report pain than younger people. Divorced or separated people were more likely to report having pain than married people. Not surprisingly, perhaps, people with jobs that involved 'high physical strain' were more likely to report chronic pain than those in more sedentary jobs. These high levels of pain appear to be a universal finding. Across Africa, 50 percent of adults are likely to complain of lower back pain in any one year (Louw *et al.* 2007). Perhaps more alarming is the large numbers of young people that experience some degree of debilitating pain. Skoffer (2007) for example, examined a sample of Danish schoolchildren aged between 15 and 16 years. More than half their sample reported pain or discomfort in their lower back; a quarter experienced a decreased function as a consequence of this pain. The pain appears to have been caused mainly by carrying a heavy satchel over one shoulder. Another way of looking at the prevalence of pain is to examine the use of analgesics within the general population. A Finnish study gives us some relevant data. Turunen *et al.* (2005) found that in a population sample of people aged 15–74 years old, 8.5 percent used over-the-counter analgesics daily, and 13.6 percent used analgesics at least several times a week.

Pain is a primary reason for visiting a doctor. For example, Mantyselka et al. (2001) reported that 40 percent of primary care visits were the result of pain; '21 percent of their sample who attended their doctor with a primary symptom of pain had experienced pain for more than six months, and 80 percent reported limited physical function as a consequence of their pain. The most common areas of pain were in the lower back, abdomen and head. Among particular patient groups, levels of pain can be even higher. Potter *et al.* (2003), for example, reported that 64 percent of people receiving care from a hospice, the majority of whom had a diagnosis of terminal cancer, reported pain as one of their primary symptoms. The cost of pain is not only physical and psychological, but also economic. Maniadakis and Gray (2000) estimated the direct costs to the British health service of treating back pain in 1998 to be £1,632 million. The *indirect* costs of back pain to the economy in terms of days off sick, production losses in industry, the costs of 'informal' care of people with back pain, and so on, were even greater – an estimated £10,668 million.

Living with pain

To say that chronic pain is unpleasant is understating its potential effects. Pain can have a profound effect on an affected individual and those close to them, so much so that many people with chronic pain organise their day around their pain. They may be prevented from engaging in physical, social and even work activities. Some may even find looking after themselves on a day-to-day basis difficult. It may affect social and marital relationships, resulting in conflict between couples – which may itself exacerbate the pain (Lang *et al.* 1996). It may also affect an individual's financial situation, as they may lose their job because of pain-related disability. It is noteworthy that people who have physically demanding jobs are more likely to experience pain than those in sedentary jobs – and most likely to lose them due to any physical limitations caused by pain (Eriksen et al. 2003)' to 'As noted earlier, people who have physically demanding jobs are more likely to experience pain than those in sedentary jobs – and most likely to lose them due to any physical limitations caused by pain (Eriksen et al. 2003)

Not surprisingly, levels of depression are high among people with chronic pain (Lépine and Briley 2004). However, the direction of association between depression and pain is not always clear. It is possible that some people who are depressed focus on bodily symptoms or minor aches and pains and are more likely to perceive them as painful 'symptoms' of disease than people who are not depressed. That is, depression may lead to high levels of reporting of pain symptoms. In other cases, the strain of living with pain and the restrictions on life that it imposes may lead to depression. There may indeed be a *reciprocal* relationship between depression and pain. People who are depressed may feel unable to cope with their pain and thus limit their activity to minimise any pain they experience. This lack of activity may lead to a stiffening of joints and muscles, which results in increased pain when they do attempt activities. This, in turn, may restrict their activity further and increase their depression. And so the cycle continues. The case of Mrs B provides an example of this.

I have a headache all the time. Some days are worse than others. When it's bad, its pounding and I cannot escape it. When I have a good day, I can feel it, but it is not so dominating. When I have a bad day, I don't want to do anything. I struggle to go to work as I do not want to lose my job. But I take 10 hours to do 5 hours' work. I can't concentrate, everything feels bad. I just want to lie down and not move. I don't want to do things at the weekend, but I know I must. But it really gets me down. I do things, but I'm not really all there . . . I don't enjoy them really. So, even when I do things I should enjoy I don't enjoy them like I used to . . . and knowing this makes me feel depressed, as I cannot see an end to the pain . . .

A further factor that may influence how people respond to pain comes from their interactions with their social environment. Pain brings a number of costs – it may also bring a number of (often unconscious) benefits to both the person in pain and those around them. Bokan *et al.* (1981) identified three kinds of 'gain' or reward associated with pain:

1. *primary (intrapersonal) gain*: occurs when expressions of pain (wincing, clutching painful areas, and so on) results in the cessation or reduction of an aversive consequence – for example, someone taking over a household chore that causes pain;
2. *secondary (interpersonal) gain*: occurs when pain behaviour results in a positive outcome, such as expressions of sympathy or care;
3. *tertiary gain*: involves feelings of pleasure or satisfaction that someone other than the individual in pain may experience when they help them.

A further type of gain may stem from an individual's beliefs about their pain. If they believe that when they do certain things the pain they experience indicates they are causing themselves physical harm, the relief gained from avoiding that activity may also reinforce inaction and lack of activity.

These various reward systems can lead to considerable problems. If an individual in pain experiences an environment in which their expressions of pain are rewarded by outcomes that they desire and that those around them gain satisfaction from providing, this may result in them doing less and less to help themselves, leading to increasing inactivity, muscle stiffness and wastage, which exacerbate any problems they may have.

Take the case of Mr Jones, who had chronic backache for a number of months. Over this time, he found that certain activities increased his pain. Activities such as standing while raising his hands and lifting proved particularly difficult. Unfortunately, these activities corresponded to those involved in washing the dishes following a meal. Because of this, he worried that any pain he expe-

rienced was because of the position he was adopting while washing up. As a result, although he did not complain about doing the washing-up, he showed his pain through winces and an awkward stance at the sink. His wife, alert to his non-verbal behaviour and not wishing her husband to be in pain, offered to do the washing-up for him on a couple of occasions, and soon he stopped doing it altogether. As a result, Mr Jones felt better because he was avoiding his worries and a boring task, and Mrs Jones felt better because she cared about her husband and wanted to do the best she could for him. It seems like a win–win situation. However, both parties may eventually lose as a result of this process: Mr Jones because his increasing inactivity will lead to further back problems; Mrs Jones because she will potentially become overburdened and resentful of her role as a 'carer'.

Brena and Chapman (1983) described the so-called 'five Ds' that may result from such an environment:

1. dramatisation of complaints;
2. disuse through inactivity;
3. drug misuse as a result of over-medication in response to pain behaviour;
4. dependency on others due to learned helplessness and impaired use of personal coping skills;
5. disability due to inactivity.

Real world 12.1

Ethnicity and pain

An anaesthetist who had worked in a variety of countries was describing the amount of anaesthetic he had to give to people having the same operation in different countries across Europe and the USA. He suggested that if the UK acted as a sort of 'baseline' against which to compare other countries, then people in the USA liked to be knocked out completely and not to experience any pain at all – so they needed more anaesthetic than people in the UK. By contrast, he suggested that people from Scandinavian countries expected to experience a reasonable amount of pain following surgery, so they needed less anaesthetic than people from the UK. Whether his story is true or not, it raises issues about whether there are differences in pain expectations and tolerance across countries and cultures.

A number of studies have examined similar issues, studying ethnic differences in the experience of both acute and chronic pain in the USA. Sheffield *et al.* (2000), for example, found that African American participants in their study rated a series of thermal stimuli as more unpleasant and showed a tendency to rate their pain as more intense than whites. Incidentally, women also showed a tendency to rate the stimuli as more unpleasant and more intense than men. Similarly, Riley *et al.* (2002) found that African American patients experiencing chronic pain reported significantly higher levels of pain unpleasantness, emotional response to pain and pain behaviour, but not pain intensity, than their white counterparts. In a similar study, Green *et al.* (2003) reported that African Americans with chronic pain reported more pain, sleep disturbance and depression than their white counterparts.

These data evoke a number of questions. The first question that has to be asked is why are we interested in this type of issue? Why should we expect such differences, and what if anything do they tell us? Are any differences biological or genetic? Are they the result of socio-cultural factors? Are they cognitively mediated? Are they the results of biased reporting of results – are there studies out there that have found no differences in pain experiences and responses between different social and ethnic groups that do not get reported? The data tell us very little about the origins of any between-group differences – and lead to dangers of negative stereotyping.

Ironically, these emerging stereotypes conflict with at least some health professionals' beliefs about ethnic differences in pain thresholds. What evidence there is suggests that African Americans are likely to be offered less analgesic than their white counterparts, at least in some US hospitals. But stereotypes do seem to influence our expectations of different social groups and how they are treated. Morris (1999), for example, noted that the least powerful groups within any culture are the most likely to experience disregard for their pain – and the most powerful are likely to have access to good pain relief should it be required. He cited historical examples of the disregard of pain among insane people in the eighteenth century, and black American women in the nineteenth century. One interesting belief noted by Morris, was that in the eighteenth and nineteenth century labourers were thought to have 'coarse' nerves that freed them from pain while undertaking hard manual work, while upper-class men and women were thought to have 'refined' nervous systems that would not allow them to engage in such labour without harm. Care should be taken not to establish more racial or ethnic stereotypes.

By contrast, many people cope well with chronic pain for significant periods of time without encountering such problems, and many environments will encourage activity and minimise the pain experience. Evers *et al.* (2003), for example, found that patients with rheumatoid arthritis who had good social support reported less pain and better physical functioning than those who were less well supported. This may be the result of a number of factors. People who are well supported may be encouraged by friends to take part in activities which maintain function and prevent joint stiffening and other factors that contribute to pain. The emotional support that such people provide may also influence the experience of pain. Interestingly, patients with pain express similar levels of satisfaction with their partners whether they are too supportive or encourage independence and more positive coping strategies (Holtzman *et al.* 2004).

Biological models of pain

Perhaps the simplest biological theory of pain is that there are 'pain receptors' in the skin and elsewhere in the body that when activated transmit information to a centre in the brain that processes pain-related information. Once activated, this 'pain centre' produces the sensory experience of pain. This type of theory, known as a specificity theory, was first proposed in the third century BC by Epicurus and was taken up later by Descartes and others in the seventeenth century. Von Frey (1894; see Norrsell *et al.* 1999) added to this theory by suggesting that our skin includes three different types of nerve, each of which responds to touch, warmth or pain. These theories were further elaborated by Goldscheider (1884; see Norrsell *et al.* 1999), whose pattern theory of pain suggested that pain sensations occurred only when the degree of nerve stimulation crossed a certain threshold. These basic biological models of pain, with some elaboration, remained dominant until the 1960s. They were supported by the identification of nerves that were sensitive to different types of pain, and nerve tracts that led from the skin to the spine, where they linked with other nerves before leading to the brain (see below).

These theories have one common tenet: that the sensation of pain is a direct representation of the degree of physical damage or sensation sustained by the individual. This tenet has the benefit of simplicity. Unfortunately, it can easily be shown to be wrong. We have already hinted at a number of factors that influence our experience of pain. Three other sets of evidence have been used to challenge these simple biological theories of pain:

1. pain in the absence of pain receptors;
2. 'pain receptors' that do not transmit pain;
3. the influence of psychological factors on the experience of pain.

Pain in the absence of pain receptors

Perhaps the most obvious evidence to counter these simple biological models is the evidence that many people experience pain in the absence of any nerve pain receptors. The most dramatic example of this phenomenon is known as 'phantom limb pain', which involves sensations, sometimes extremely painful, that feel located in a patient's missing limb following amputation. Up to 70 percent of amputees report phantom limb pain a week after amputation, and over half of these people continue to experience phantom limb pain for many months or even years after their surgery (Dijkstra *et al.* 2002). Two years following amputation, nearly a third of patients who initially experienced phantom limb pain still experience significant pain despite using strong opiate medication (Mishra *et al.* 2007). Interestingly, people who have their upper limb amputated are far less likely to experience phantom limb pain than those who have had a leg amputated. Similar experiences are reported by people with spinal cord injuries and paralysis. Unfortunately, phantom limb pain is difficult to treat and can have a significant negative impact on those with the condition.

'Pain receptors' that do not transmit pain

A second physical phenomenon that presents problems for these early theories stems from the experiences of people with CUIP referred to above. Individuals with this condition may experience painless bone fractures and ulceration to their hands and feet, which may go unnoticed. They may also fail to identify pain as a symptom of severe disease and sustain dramatic injuries as a result of a failure to respond to danger signals. Some people with CUIP may even experience ulceration of the cornea of the eye as they fail to protect against strong sunlight (Nagasako *et al.* 2003). Individuals with CUIP appear to have intact pain pathways, so they present the opposite problem to that posed by phantom limbs: a failure to perceive pain in the presence of an apparently intact pain pathway.

Psychological influences on pain

A number of psychological factors have been found to influence the experience of pain. Three of the key ones are:

1. *Mood*: anxiety and depression reduce pain tolerance and increase the reporting of pain.
2. *Attention*: focusing on pain increases the experience of pain.
3. *Cognitions*: expectations of increases or reductions in pain can be self-fulfilling.

Mood and pain

Mood influences the perception of pain—and pain influences mood. Evidence of the influence of mood on the experience of pain can be found in studies in which participants are asked to rate or tolerate pain until their discomfort is too great to tolerate it any further. These have shown that depressed or anxious participants report the equivalent pain stimulus as more painful than people without any mood disorder (e.g. Mel'nikova 1993) and tolerate pain for significantly less time (Pinerua-Shuhaibar *et al.* 1999).

Short-term mood states may also affect the experience of pain. Fisher and Johnston (1996b), for example, gave patients with lower back pain a simple mood induction procedure in which they were asked either about upsetting aspects of their condition or to report more positive aspects of their condition and how they were coping with it. Before and after this procedure, participants were given a plastic bag into which were placed as many packets of rice as they felt able to tolerate and then held the bag until it felt uncomfortable. In comparison with their performance at baseline, participants who reported the upsetting issues (and were therefore assumed to be more depressed) performed less well. By contrast, those whose mood was improved were able to hold the same weights for a longer period than baseline. This was an important study, as it used real patients faced with a task similar to their everyday activities.

Evidence of a reciprocal relationship between pain and mood has also been reported in a number of studies. Magni *et al.* (1994), for example, followed over two thousand participants for a period of eight years. They found that participants who reported chronic pain at the beginning of the study were nearly three times more likely to become depressed over the follow-up period than those without this problem. By contrast, another group of people who were depressed and free of pain at the beginning of the study were over twice as likely to report having had a significant period of pain over the follow-up period. The authors speculated that depression may predict some 'pain conditions' while some 'pain conditions' may predict depression, although the nature of these two conditions was not clear. Suffice it to say that there is an interaction between pain and mood that can operate in both directions.

Attention and pain

One of the ways that mood may influence our perception of pain is by influencing the attention we pay to any pain sensations. Depressed or anxious people may pay more attention to pain sensations than other people, and this focus may significantly influence their experience of pain. Focusing on pain seems to increase its impact: focusing on other things seems to reduce it. Many people who experience injuries while playing sports requiring effort and concentration, for example, do not notice the extent of any injuries until after the game has finished. Less anecdotally, there is evidence that fewer people experience pain following physical trauma at times of intense stress, such as being on the battlefield, than when similar levels of injury are sustained in less stressful situations (Beecher 1946). This may be because of attentional factors – in the battlefield there are many important distractions from one's own pain. However, other factors may also have been involved. It is possible, for example, that the soldiers were simply pleased to be alive following battle and thought that their injury would result in them being sent away from the battlefield. Civilians would be more likely to view their injuries as unwelcome and likely to interfere with their day-to-day activities. The issue here, therefore, may be the meaning ascribed to the injury and pain as much as the degree of attention paid to it.

Despite these alternative explanations, more controlled evaluations of the relationship between attention and pain have shown that the use of distraction can reduce pain, while experimental manipulations that increase attention to painful stimuli result in increased reporting of pain. James and Hardardottir (2002), for example, asked patients to place their lower arm in freezing cold water (an excruciatingly painful procedure known as the **cold pressor test**) and to either concentrate on a computer-based task or the pain sensations. Those who focused on the pain were least able to tolerate it and pulled their arm out of the water significantly earlier than those in the distraction task.

Cold pressor test Procedure in which participants place their arm in a mixture of water and ice maintaining the water temperature at between 0 and 3°C.

Attentional bias may also explain why some people with acute pain go on to develop chronic pain, while others do not. Vlaeyen *et al.* (1995) suggested that people who develop chronic pain in the absence of any clear physical injury or inflammation may respond to acute pain with a degree of fear, worry about its consequences and begin to check themselves for any pain sensations. Because they are now paying attention to a variety of aches and pains that may pass unnoticed in other people, they label their pain as symptomatic of an underlying problem. They may also stop engaging in activities that could trigger an episode of pain. In an experimental study that relates to this process, Nouwen *et al.* (2006) asked patients with chronic pain and individuals with no such problem to focus on the pain experienced during a cold pressor task (and therefore not related to the medical cause of their pain). Patients with chronic pain reported more pain and withdrew their hand from the water earlier than those in the control group. Further evidence of this process is provided by Dehghani *et al.* (2003). Their study, which used the dot probe task to explore attentional bias towards pain-related stimuli, found that people with chronic pain were more attentive to words describing the sensory experience of pain than neutral words or words describing its emotional or behavioural consequences. Their results also indicated that people with high levels of fear of pain both attended to relevant words more quickly and then had difficulty in focusing their attention away from them. Both results support the attentional hypothesis of chronic pain.

Cognition and pain

Mood may influence pain by influencing our thoughts about the nature and consequences of any pain. The types of thought that may influence the pain experience include:

- attributions concerning the cause of pain;
- beliefs about the ability to tolerate pain;

- beliefs about the ability to control pain;
- expectations of pain relief – the placebo effect.

A simple example of how attributions concerning the cause of pain may influence the pain experience was described by Cassell (1982) in a case report in which one patient's pain was easily controlled with codeine when they attributed it to **sciatica** but required strong opiate analgesia when they attributed the same pain to having cancer. Walsh and Radcliffe (2002) found that the beliefs of people with chronic back pain influenced their willingness to take part in an exercise programme. Those people who believed their pain was the result of physical damage to their spine were more reluctant to engage in exercise than those who attributed it to 'psychological' factors – because they were afraid that exercise would exacerbate their damaged back and increase their pain. Similarly, Murphy *et al.* (1997) found that the activities of people with lower back pain were more restricted by their expectations of pain than by the actual pain they experienced. They were most restricted when the pain they experienced exceeded the level of pain they expected – presumably because they considered this additional pain to indicate some physical damage as a result of their exercise. One particular cognitive response to pain, known as catastrophising (e.g. 'This pain means something is seriously wrong!') is consistently associated with poor outcomes in relation to pain, including reports of pre-operative pain (Roth *et al.* 2007), pain following physiotherapy (Hill *et al.* 2007), and restrictions in activity as a consequence of pain (Voerman *et al.* 2007).

Sciatica
Pain down the leg, which is caused by irritation of the main nerve into the leg, the sciatic nerve. This pain tends to be caused where the nerves pass through and emerge from the lower bones of the spine (lumbar vertebrae).

People who feel able to tolerate or manage their pain are less restricted by their pain. Maly *et al.* (2007) found that patients with osteoarthritis of the knee with high levels of belief in their ability to manage their pain walked more than those with less strong beliefs. Similarly, fit cyclists who believed in their ability to control or manage their pain allowed themselves to experience more painful exercise than those with lower control beliefs (Motl *et al.* 2007). Individuals with high control beliefs may also experience less pain. Jensen *et al.* (2001), for example, found that among a group of patients with chronic pain involved in a pain management programme, increased perceptions of control over pain accompanied reductions in reported pain. Experimental studies also provide support. In one such study, van den Hout *et al.* (2000) randomly assigned healthy participants to one of three preparatory conditions before they were given a cold pressor task. The preparatory conditions involved a task during which participants were given feedback indicating high levels of control over the task, low levels of control, or no feedback. Despite the fact that the initial task was not pain-related, it seemed to have some carry-over to the cold pressor task. In this, participants who received the high control feedback tolerated the cold pressor task for significantly longer than those who received low control feedback. Perceived control may also influence pain-related behaviour in patient populations. In a partial replication of their study of the effect of mood on pain behaviour described above, Fisher and Johnston (1996) allocated patients with chronic pain to conditions in which their perceptions of control over their pain were experimentally increased or decreased. Control was increased by asking patients to talk about times when they had been in control of their pain and decreased by asking them to recount periods when their control was low. Patients in the increased control condition performed their lifting task for longer than those in the decreased control condition.

Expectations of pain relief: the placebo response

One of the most fascinating phenomena associated with pain is known as the placebo response. If you were to give an inert tablet with no biochemical effects to people experiencing some degree of pain, *tell* them that it will have no effect, a percentage of those individuals (and probably quite a significant percentage) would report some relief from pain as a result of being given the 'tablet'. Red 'tablets' are more effective than blue 'tablets' in this context (Huskisson 1974). There appears to be some benefit to simply being given what appears to be treatment, whether this is a tablet, injection or more culturally diverse form of treatment. This phenomenon is known as the placebo effect.

A placebo (from the Latin, 'I please') is an inert preparation that has no pharmacological effects. Two of hundreds of studies provide examples of its impact. Verdugo and Ochoa (1994) examined the placebo response to an injection of saline (salt water) close to the area of maximum pain in patients with neuropathic pain – that is, pain that seems to be generated by the nerves themselves – which can be difficult to treat with conventional analgesia. Following this simple intervention, nearly two-thirds of the patients reported a 50 percent or greater reduction in pain. In a similar study, Fine *et al.* (1994) tested a placebo injected into patients with chronic lower back pain. All participants in the study reported significant reductions in pain beginning between fifteen minutes and one hour after the injection and lasting up to several days. These are not unusual findings. Across a range of studies, the percentage of individuals to report at least a 50 percent reduction in pain following being given a placebo ranges from a lowly 7 percent to nearly 50 percent across a variety of conditions and periods of time (McQuay and Moore 2005). Its effect is not limited to pain. The placebo effect can be found in inflammation, the speed of wound healing, immune responses to infection, and the treatment of conditions as diverse as angina, asthma and depression (Humphrey 2002). If a placebo is given following treatment with an active drug, the patient may not only show the degree of benefit in symptom reduction experienced during the active treatment, they may also experience the same side-effects as they did while on the active drug (Suchman and Ader 1992).

Two key mechanisms through which placebo is assumed to work have been posited. The first involves a classical conditioned response, which has been implicated in immune and respiratory responses. A second process, particularly relevant to pain, involves our expectations of pain or pain relief (Price *et al.* 2008). We experience a reduction in pain because we expect a reduction in pain. The logic of this theory (and consistent with explanations of pain experiences described earlier in the chapter), is that if we can somehow change expectations about the efficacy or otherwise of a particular placebo treatment, then the effectiveness of that placebo treatment will also vary. In one of the few studies to attempt this, Fedele *et al.* (1989) found that repeated use of a placebo over several menstrual cycles in women suffering from painful periods resulted in a lowering of the placebo's success in controlling pain. Although they did not directly measure the beliefs and expectations of these women, such a finding is consistent with a gradual change of expectations in the effectiveness of the treatment leading to a reduction in placebo response. Of course, just as positive expectations can lead to a reduction in pain, negative expectations can lead to increases in pain – the nocebo response. Patients recently diagnosed as having a serious illness or patients who distrust their therapy, for example, are likely to report more pain than others (Benedetti *et al.* 2007).

On a slightly tangential note, the placebo effect is considered so important and pervasive that the best trials of the effectiveness of a new intervention involve a comparison with a placebo version of the intervention, for which trial participants have an equal expectation of effectiveness. To simply compare an intervention with no-treatment condition is no longer considered a good test of the effectiveness of an intervention. It must fare significantly better than a placebo to be considered an effective treatment. Medical placebos are relatively easy to construct – usually a tablet or injection identical to the real intervention. Psychological placebos are more difficult to construct, but typically involve as a minimum the same amount of time spent with the participants in some apparently 'psychological' act (e.g. a non-specific discussion of a problem) as the active therapy.

A psycho-biological theory of pain

Gate control theory of pain
A theory of pain developed by Melzack and Wall in which a 'gate' is used as a metaphor for the chemicals, including endorphins, that mitigate the experience of pain.

The evidence considered previously suggests that two sets of processes are involved in the experience of pain: one involving sensory information from the site of the painful stimulation, the other involving emotional and cognitive processes. The **gate control theory of pain** proposed by Melzack and Wall (e.g. 1965) takes both processes into account and is generally recognised as the best theoretical account of pain we now have. Melzack and Wall used the analogy of a gate to explain the pain experience. The essence of their gate control theory of pain is that the degree of pain we experience is the result of two sets of processes:

1. Pain receptors in the skin and organs transmit information about physical damage to a series of 'gates' in the spinal column (see Figure 12.1). Within the gates, these nerves link to other nerves along the spinal column that transmit information up to pain centres in the brain.
2. At the same time as we experience physical damage, we also experience related cognitions and emotions – fear, alarm, and so on. This information results in the activation of nerve fibres taking information from the brain down the spinal column to the gate at which the incoming pain signals enter the spinal column.

The degree of pain we experience is a result of differing levels of activation in these two systems. Activation of the sensory nerves from the site of the pain to the spinal column 'opens' the gate. This activates the nerves leading to the pain centres and is recognised as pain – that is the essence of the biological theories of pain described above. However, the downward pathways activated by emotional and cognitive factors can also influence the position of the gate. Anxious thoughts or focusing attention on pain 'open' the gate and increase our experience of pain; calming or distracting thoughts 'close' the gate. This, in effect, prevents neural impulses travelling up through the spinal cord to the brain and reduces the experience of pain. The intensity of pain we experience at any time will be a function of these two sometimes competing and sometimes complementary processes.

Pain sensations are transmitted from the site of an injury to the spinal gate by nerves known as nociceptors, three types of which have been identified:

- A delta fibres (types I and II):
  - respond to light touch, mechanical and thermal stimuli. Carry information about brief sharp pain;
  - very strong noxious stimuli related to potential or actual damage to tissues. The experience is short-lasting.
- C polymodal fibres:
  - slow conducting; carry information about dull, throbbing, pain – which is experienced for a longer period than that from the A delta fibres.

Perhaps the most important characteristic of these different fibres is that they transmit information at different speeds. As a result, our response to injury usually involves two phases:

1. The first, mediated by A delta fibres, involves the experience of sharp pain.
2. This is followed by a more chronic throbbing pain mediated by the C polymodal fibres.

A second set of nerves, known as A beta fibres, also transmit tactile information, particularly related to gentle touch. These fibres can work to our advantage as they provide information that competes with the A delta and C fibres at the spinal column. When we receive an injury, activation of the A delta fibres is initiated and sends 'pain signals' via the spinal column to the brain. The first instinct we have following such an injury is to rub the site of the injury. This simple act reduces the amount of pain we experience. This occurs because rubbing the site of injury activates A beta fibres. Because they transmit information more quickly than C fibres, this information also reaches the brain more quickly and reduces the degree of activation that would have been triggered by the C fibres alone. Thus, in the terms of

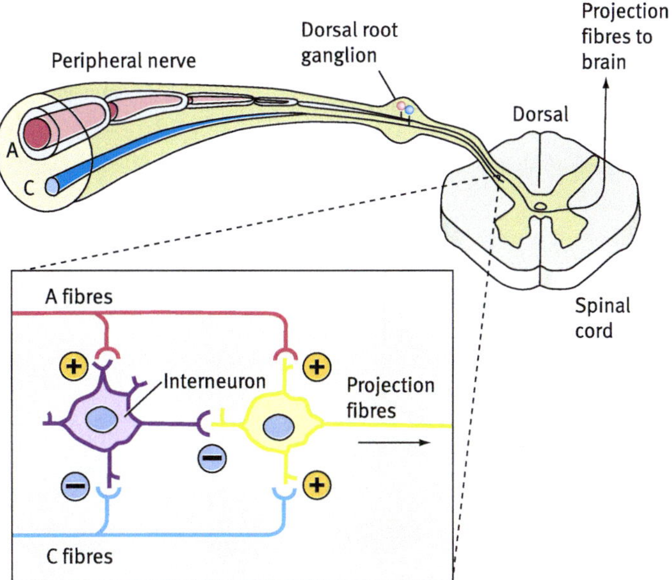

Figure 12.1 The transmission of information along the A and C fibres to the gelatinosa substantia in the spinal cord and upwards to the brain.
Source: adapted from Rosenzweig, Leiman and Breedlove (1996: 272)

Melzack and Wall, activation of A beta fibres to touch and gentle stimuli can close the pain gate. Activation of A delta and C fibres to painful stimuli opens the gate.

The A and C fibres transmit information to areas in the spinal cord known as the substantia gelatinosa. These lie within the dorsal horn of each part of the spinal column (see Figure 12.1). Nerve impulses here trigger the release of a chemical known as substance P into the substantia gelatinosa. This, in turn, activates nerve fibres known as T(ransmitter) fibres, which transmit the sensation of pain to the brain:

- Information from A fibres is taken to the **thalamus** and on to the cortex, where the individual can plan and initiate action to remove them from the source of the pain.
- Information from the C fibres follows a pathway to the **limbic system**, **hypothalamus** and autonomic nervous system. Activity within the limbic system adds an emotional content, such as fear or alarm, to the experience of pain. The hypothalamus controls activity within the autonomic nervous system, which allows us to respond quickly to remove ourselves from harm.

Thalamus
Area of the brain that links the basic functions of the hindbrain and midbrain with the higher centres of processing, the cerebral cortex. Regulates attention and contributes to memory functions. The portion that enters the limbic system is involved in the experience of emotions.

Limbic system
A series of structures in the brain, often referred to as the 'emotional computer' because of its role in coordinating emotions. It links sensory information to emotionally relevant behaviour, in particular responses to fear and anger.

Hypothalamus
Area of the brain that regulates appetite, sexual arousal and thirst. Also appears to have some control over emotions.

What do YOU Think?

We have already identified a number of factors that influence our experience of pain. Think how *you* react to pain. Do these factors reflect your own experience of pain? And how do we come to respond to pain in the way we do? Do you rub yourself if you are bruised to ease the pain? If so, why? Did you learn to do it as a response to previous pain experiences – or were you told to do so by a parent or friend? Are you stoic in the face of pain? If so, is this a result of how others have expected you to respond? 'Big boys don't cry': cultural and childhood experiences may encourage different ways of expressing both emotional and physical pain in men and women. Do they affect how you respond to pain? Or do you respond in ways determined by your personality? People who are generally anxious may be more prone to respond to pain with catastrophic thinking, anxiety and high levels of physiological arousal – resulting in a relatively high experience of pain (and other labelling of bodily sensations as 'symptoms' of disease). People who are more relaxed and optimistic may have a less emotional response to pain and experience relatively less pain. Is this the case for you?

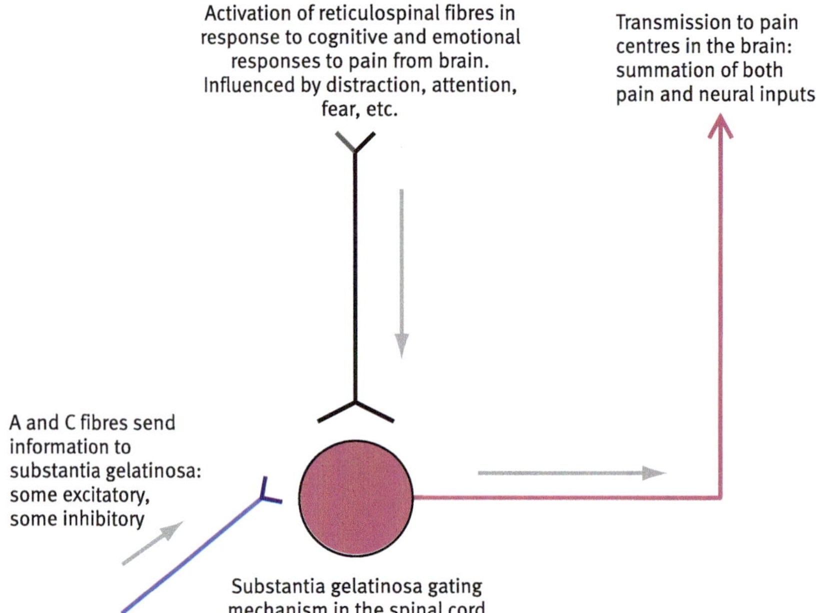

Figure 12.2 A schematic view of the gate control mechanism postulated by Melzack and Wall.

The results of this neural activity are transmitted *down* the spinal column through nerve pathways known as reticulospinal fibres to the spinal gate mechanism (see Figure 12.2). These may trigger the release of a variety of chemicals into the 'soup' of chemicals in the substantia gelatinosa (and brain), the most important of which are naturally occurring opiate-like substances called **endorphins**. These 'close' the gate and moderate the degree of pain experienced. Activity in this system is mediated by a number of factors, each of which influences the release of endorphins. These include:

- *Focusing on the pain*: worrying, or **catastrophising**, reduces the amount of endorphins released and opens the gate.
- *Emotional and cognitive factors*: feeling optimistic and unconcerned about the 'meaning' of the pain increases endorphin release and closes the gate – anxiety, worry, anger or depression opens the gate.
- *Physical factors*: relaxation increases endorphin release and lessens the experience of pain.

Pain medication will also 'close' the pain gate.

Endorphins
Naturally occurring opiate-like chemicals released in the brain and spinal cord. They reduce the experience of pain and can induce feelings of relaxation or pleasure. Associated with the so-called 'runner's high'.

Catastrophising
The act of constructing catastrophic thoughts.

Future understandings of pain: the neuromatrix

Despite the success of the gate theory of pain, it has still struggled to account for one important type of pain – phantom limb pain. The theory cannot account for pain in the absence of stimulation by the A and C fibres. In response to these limitations, Melzack (2005) has developed a more complex theory of the mechanisms of pain that attempts to explain this mysterious phenomenon. His model has three key assumptions:

1. The same neural processes that are involved in pain perception in the intact body are involved in pain perception in the phantom limb.
2. All the qualities that we normally feel from the body, including pain, can be felt in the absence of inputs from the body.

3. The body is perceived as a unity and is identified as the 'self', distinct from other people and the surrounding world.

Melzack contended that the anatomical substrate of the 'body-self' is a large, widespread network of neurons linking the thalamus, cortex and limbic system in the brain. He termed this system the 'neuromatrix'. We process and integrate pain-related information within the neuromatrix. Related information about a pain experience (physical elements of the injury, emotional reactions to the injury, and so on) combine to form a 'neurosignature' or network of information about the nature and emotional reaction to a pain stimulus. Neurosignatures have two components:

1. *the body-self matrix*: processes and integrates incoming sensory and emotional information;
2. *the action neuromatrix*: develops behavioural responses in response to these networks.

Behavioural responses to pain can only occur after information about the nature of the pain, its cause, and physical and emotional consequences have been, at least, partially processed and integrated. We do not move away from a hot object, for example, until we realise that it is the cause of pain and that continuing to be near it will cause further pain and potential injury. We only become consciously aware of pain after this integrated network of information is then projected to what Melzack terms the 'sentient neural hub': the seat of consciousness. Here, the stream of nerve impulses is converted into a continually changing stream of awareness.

So far, Melzack's new theory does not explain the experience of phantom limb pain. This moves us from an explanation of how we feel pain from external sources to one explaining how we feel pain generated by the body itself. Melzack suggested that the neuromatrix is pre-wired to 'assume' that the limbs can move. Accordingly, in people who have had limbs removed, the body still sends signals to try to move them. When they do not move in response to these signals, stronger and more frequent messages may be sent to the muscles, and these are perceived as pain. Melzack's theory of pain is still relatively new and has only recently been subjected to empirical research. However, what data there are provide broad support for the existence of a neuromatrix, but we have yet to locate it within any particular brain area (Derbyshire 2000).

Helping people to cope with pain

The first-line treatment for *acute* pain is generally some form of pharmacological treatment – varying in strength from aspirin to some form of opium derivative such as pethidine. Psychological interventions generally form a second-level intervention. The American Agency for Health Care Policy (1992), for example, suggested that these should be used for those who find this type of intervention 'appealing', where patients may benefit from reducing or avoiding pharmacological treatment, have high levels of anxiety, would need prolonged pain relief and/or who have incomplete pain relief following pharmacological intervention. By contrast, increasing numbers of patients with *chronic* pain resulting from conditions as varied as rheumatoid arthritis and lower back pain are being taught to manage their pain using psychological approaches in order to minimise the amount of painkilling medication they need to take and to maintain or improve their quality of life. It is important that the effectiveness of these interventions is evaluated as part of the day-to-day care of patients as well as in research studies. So, before we look at some of the approaches used to treat both acute and chronic pain, we examine some simple, and not so simple, ways of measuring pain.

Measuring pain

The simplest measure of pain involves the use of a simple linear visual analogue or numerical rating scales – typically varying from a score of 0, registering no pain, to 100, rating the most pain you could imagine. This type of measure is quick to administer and score and is frequently used in clinical settings. A limitation of the approach is that patients often find it quite difficult to consider pain in numerical terms. Another simple approach involves patients rating their pain on a series of adjectives denoting increasing pain: mild, distressing, excruciating, and so on. This has the advantage of being more easily comprehensible to patients than numeric scales – it uses concepts patients are more familiar with. However, this approach has its disadvantages, as many patients tend to rate themselves somewhere in the middle of such scales, making them less sensitive to subtle differences in pain than analogue scales.

One important limitation of these measures is that they simply measure the sensation of pain. However, we have already noted that the experience of pain is multidimensional. It involves emotional, cognitive and behavioural responses as well as sensory experiences. A number of measures have tried to address these inadequacies. Perhaps the best known of these is the McGill pain questionnaire (e.g. Melzack 1975). This is more complicated to administer and interpret than the simple scales described above. However, it provides a multidimensional understanding of the nature of the pain that an individual is experiencing. In its various forms, it measures:

- *the type of pain*: including throbbing, shooting, stabbing, cramping, gnawing, hot and tender, using a four-point scale from 'none' to 'severe';
- *the emotional response to the pain*: including tiring, exhausting, fearful and punishing;
- *the intensity of the pain*: on a scale from 'no pain' to 'worst possible pain';
- *the timing of pain*: whether it is brief, continuous or intermittent.

While this measure extends our assessment of pain, it does not address all the responses to it. It does not, for example, measure pain in relation to movement or measure an individual's behavioural response to pain. How much does it restrict their daily life? Can they walk up stairs, or lift heavy weights? These may all have to be measured separately. Turk and Okifuji (1999) suggested that one can also measure the pain behaviour in which an individual engages. They suggested measuring:

- *verbal/vocalisations*: sighs, moans, complaints
- *motor behaviour*: facial grimacing, distorted gait (limping), rigid or unstable posture, excessively slow or laboured movement, seek help/pain reducing behaviour
- *treatment behaviours*: taking medication, use of protective device (e.g. cane, cervical collar), visit doctor
- *functional limitations*: resting, reduced activity.

Each of these may become a target for some of the interventions discussed below.

Acute pain

A number of approaches have been used to help people to cope with acute pain. Any procedures used need to be relatively easy to learn and use. Accordingly, most approaches to acute pain control have focused on:

- increasing patients' sense of control over the pain experience and medical procedures that may be causing the pain;
- teaching coping skills, including distraction techniques and relaxation;
- hypnosis.

Some of these are discussed further in the context of preparing people for the experience of surgery in Chapter 10. Here, we address other ways of achieving these goals.

Increasing control: patient-controlled anaesthesia

The experience of pain following trauma or surgical operations can be made worse by patients' fears that they cannot control their pain. They may be frightened that when they are in significant pain the nurses may be too busy to give them painkillers, that the pain will be so bad that it will not be controlled by the type of painkiller they will be given, and so on. To alleviate such fears, patients may exaggerate reports of pain or pester health-care professionals to give them painkillers in order to avoid periods of inadequate analgesia. This may result in them experiencing unnecessary anxiety and using more medication than necessary.

One way that each of these issues can be addressed is through the use of **patient-controlled analgesia** (PCA). Using this method, the patient controls how much analgesic drug they receive through an intravenous drip – albeit with some controls built into the delivery system so they cannot exceed a specified dosage. It is assumed that because patients can control the timing of their pain relief, they will be less anxious about the control of their pain, be more satisfied with their analgesia and use less analgesic. Systematic reviews of this approach, summarised in *Bandolier* (2003), suggest that this is the case. The majority of studies that have compared levels of satisfaction with PCA against health-care professional-controlled analgesia have found higher levels of satisfaction with PCA. There is also consistent evidence that PCA may result in less use of analgesics than when health professionals have control over pain control. Van der Vyver *et al.* (2002), for example, reported a systematic review of the use of analgesia and pain control during childbirth. In all cases of comparison between PCA and doctor-controlled analgesia, they found that women used less analgesia. Children can also use PCA systems. Birmingham *et al.* (2003) reported data from over a hundred children for whom PCA was used for acute post-operative pain control. Satisfactory analgesia was obtained in 90 percent of cases, with no evidence of toxicity or serious adverse effects. It therefore seems a safe, beneficial form of treatment for a wide range of people.

Patient-controlled analgesia (PCA)
A technique through which small doses of analgesic drugs, usually opioids, are administered (usually by an intravenous drip and controlled by a pump) by patients themselves. It is mostly used for the control of post-operative pain.

Teaching coping skills

DISTRACTION. We have already noted in the chapter that focusing on pain tends to increase the experience of pain, while distraction decreases it. Given the apparent simplicity of teaching distraction techniques, these would seem to be sensible strategies to teach patients who are in acute pain or who have to undergo painful procedures. The procedure seems to work. Callaghan and Li (2002), for example, taught women undergoing a hysterectomy to distract themselves from worrisome thoughts prior to their operation. Compared with women only given information about the procedure, they reported less pain and evidenced less distress after the operation. Fauerbach *et al.* (2002) also reported success after teaching distraction skills – but only if patients actively focused on something other than the pain experience rather than simply trying not to think of the pain. Their study involved a comparison of an intervention designed to reduce the negative emotional aspects of a painful procedure and one designed to distract completely from the procedure – both of which should reduce the intensity of any pain (see above). In their study, patients receiving regular, extremely painful, dressing changes to burns were randomly assigned to an emotional control or distraction condition. In the first condition, participants were asked to focus on the sensory experience of their dressing change 'while noticing subtle variations in the sensory experience and the ebb and flow of pain sensations', to focus on the present and not to anticipate or dwell on future and past pain, limiting thoughts to those about the sensory experience and not its implications or other potentially **catastrophic thoughts**. In the distraction condition, participants were given a choice of music to listen to and taught to focus on the melody, style or emotional tone, different instruments and lyrics. Their analyses focused on the degree of tension the patients experienced during the dressing change and the number of intrusive and catastrophic thoughts they had during and after the procedures. The distraction procedure resulted in fewer intrusive thoughts and less tension during the procedure than the emotion-focusing procedure. However, patients who did not focus on the tasks assigned, but tried to ignore the sensations without this focus, experienced the most intrusive thoughts and tension during the dressing change. It seems that having a focused concentration on something other than the pain is beneficial – but unfocused attempts simply to ignore it are less so.

Catastrophic thoughts
Automatic thoughts that exaggerate the negative aspects of any situation.

Relaxation. A second relatively simple approach that can be taught to patients is the use of relaxation. This involves teaching people to relax the muscles throughout their body, particularly those close to the site of the pain (see Chapter 13). This has a number of advantages. First, it can be used to reduce any muscular tension that can contribute to the experience of pain. Second, because relaxation instructions may explicitly involve thinking about pleasant images or at least images inconsistent with the painful situation, it may act as a form of distraction. The concentration involved in relaxing may also distract from pain sensations. Finally, there is evidence that relaxation promotes endorphin release and thus has a direct impact on the pain experience. There is ample evidence that relaxation procedures can help reduce levels of pain and distress associated with post-operative pain. Renzi *et al.* (2000), for example, reported that patients undergoing major bowel surgery who used relaxation experienced less pain, less distress and better sleep following surgery than a control group receiving 'standard care'. Similarly, Friesner *et al.* (2007) found that relaxation combined with the use of opiate drugs was superior to opiate drugs alone during a short but painful surgical procedure involving removal of a tube inserted into the chest during coronary artery bypass surgery. The evidence in support of relaxation is so consistent that the American National Institutes of Health consensus panel (National Institutes of Health Technology Assessment Panel 1996) concluded that relaxation procedures should be adopted for general use.

Hypnosis

Hypnosis is a procedure during which a health professional suggests that a patient experience changes in sensations, perceptions, thoughts or behaviour. The hypnotic context is generally established by an induction procedure. Although there are many different hypnotic inductions, most include suggestions for relaxation, calmness and wellbeing. Instructions to imagine or think about pleasant experiences are also commonly included in hypnotic inductions. It has been shown to have a reliable and significant effect on acute pain. Lang *et al.* (2006), for example, found self-hypnosis to reduce both pain and anxiety associated with having a needle breast biopsy. Not only can hypnosis reduce pain, but it may also aid patients' physical recovery. Ginandes *et al.* (2003) examined the effects of hypnosis on pain and wound healing following breast surgery. They allocated women to three interventions following surgery: usual care (normal analgesia); sessions with a counsellor providing unstructured support; and hypnosis, in which they focused on relaxation and 'accelerated wound healing' as part of the instructions ('Imagine your wound healing well'). They measured the women's pain and level of wound healing one week and seven weeks following the interventions and found that the wounds of the women in the hypnosis condition healed significantly more quickly than those in the others. They also experienced less pain over the course of their recovery. The benefits of self-hypnosis need not be restricted to adults: Liossi *et al.* (2006) found self-hypnosis combined with local anaesthetic to be more effective than anaesthetic alone in young people aged between 6 and 16 years receiving a lumbar puncture. Of note also was that the benefits of hypnosis varied according to the hypnotisability of individual participants.

Treating chronic pain

Transcutaneous electrical nerve stimulation (TENS)

Before examining psychological interventions to reduce pain, we first consider a popular method of pain control, based on the electrical stimulation of A beta fibres in order to compete with the pain signals of pain-related nerves (see discussion earlier in the chapter) and stimulate C fibres to result in endorphin release. Transcutaneous electrical nerve stimulation (TENS) involves the use of a small electrical device, about the size of a personal stereo, that is connected by wires to electrodes, placed on the skin in the area of the pain. This allows a small, low-intensity electric charge to be passed across the area. Such stimulation devices are typically used for between fifteen to twenty minutes, several times a day, and are controlled by the user. Search the internet using the acronym TENS, and you will find a multiplicity of websites selling TENS machines, many of which claim it to be an effective form of treatment. A Canadian review (Reeve *et al.* 1996) in which the authors surveyed TENS use across Canada, was broadly supportive of this use. They surveyed 50 hospitals with 200 or more beds, and estimated that over 450,000 uses of TENS take place in Canadian hospitals each year with widespread use in the treatment of acute pain (used by 93 percent of hospitals), pain associated with labour and delivery (43 percent), and chronic pain (96 percent).

Unfortunately, a series of subsequent reviews and empirical studies suggest this use is largely inappropriate. Khadilkar *et al.* (2005), for example, in conducting a Cochrane review of the area found only two studies that were of sufficient methodological rigour to provide a meaningful test of the approach's effectiveness. One study (Cheing and Hui-Chan 1999) found some short-term benefits compared to placebo; another (Deyo *et al.* 1990) found no such benefit. In a review of studies of post-operative pain, Carroll *et al.* (1996b) concluded that TENS was no better than placebo in 15 out of 17 of them. Other reviews have come to similar conclusions. Unfortunately, studies into the effectiveness of TENS are frequently small or uncontrolled. Al-Smadi *et al.* (2003) found, for example, that TENS was no better than TENS placebo in the treatment of low back pain in people with multiple sclerosis. However, they randomly allocated only 5 people to each treatment group – making any statistically significant treatment effect almost impossible to find. With this lack of high quality of evidence in mind, *Bandolier* (www.jr2.ox.ac.uk/bandolier/band37/b37-3.html) argued that better evidence in still needed, but in the meantime 'those of you who see full-page adverts in the national newspapers full of happy souls extolling the virtues of TENS might like to refer the Advertising Standards Authority to these reviews.'

Behavioural interventions

The first modern psychological intervention for pain involved behavioural interventions, based on operant conditioning processes. The treatment model, initially developed by Fordyce (1976), is based on the premise that we cannot truly understand the pain experience of others; all we can do is observe 'pain behaviour'. Fordyce argued that this behaviour should, therefore, form the target of any intervention, not the unobservable inner experience. Operant theory states that pain behaviour may be established and controlled not only by the experience of pain but also by how others respond to expressions of pain. Pain behaviour may be as subtle as gentle winces or as obvious as lying down unable to move as a result of apparently unbearable pain. It may be reinforced by expressions of sympathy, being 'let off' tasks about the home, given analgesia, and so on (see Bokan *et al.* 1981, earlier in the chapter).

The aim of behavioural interventions is to reduce disability by changing the environmental contingencies that influence pain behaviour – to remove the individual from any reinforcement of their pain behaviour. Instead, non-pain-related, adaptive behaviour is reinforced. The methods used include:

- reinforcement of adaptive behaviour such as appropriate levels of exercise;
- withdrawal of attention or other rewards that were previous responses to pain behaviour;
- providing analgesic medication at set times rather than in response to behaviour.

In this way, new forms of behaviour are encouraged through appropriate reinforcement, and older maladaptive behaviour is extinguished through non-reinforcement. The approach may involve both health professionals and others with whom the patient interacts, including their partner or even friends.

Depending on the nature of the presenting problem, these processes may be added to by other interventions. In the case of lower back pain, for example, where disuse may have resulted in a weakening of the back muscles, patients may take part in exercise programmes. In these, patients will typically engage in a number of exercise trials to identify their tolerance for various lifting activities and movements. The programme will then advance them through a series of progressively more difficult steps towards full mobility and strength. Success at each stage of the intervention is positively rewarded by the health-care professionals involved in the treatment programme.

Early studies of this approach were often case histories, as the approaches used to treat individual cases were necessarily quite different. Fordyce (1976), for example, reported a case in which they moved a hospital patient who was engaging in excessive pain behaviour into a single room, the door of which could be closed if necessary. This prevented the patient trying to attract the attention of nurses in the ward. Rewards for non-pain behaviour and 'punishments' for pain-related behaviour were achieved by entering and leaving the room if the patient inappropriately demanded pain medication or staying for social chat if they did not do so. These various case reports indicated the potential for this type of treatment. More recently, the development of standardised behavioural programmes in the treatment of a variety of disorders, including back pain, has meant that their effectiveness can be assessed using group designs.

Back pain is frequently treated using behavioural methods, possibly because it is a common disorder that often has no obvious pathology but which can cause significant impairment. They are also very effective in treating the disorder. Van Tulder *et al.* (2003), for example, reported a meta-analysis of the effects of behavioural programmes on lower back pain, and concluded that there was strong evidence that behavioural treatments were of significant benefit on measures of reported pain, improvements in mobility and lifting capacity, and on behaviour away from the clinic.

Cognitive-behavioural interventions

Behavioural interventions clearly work by changing behaviour, but these changes may also influence other parts of the pain experience. Active engagement in activities may distract patients from negative cognitive and emotional responses to pain. Re-engaging in activities previously stopped may increase self-efficacy beliefs and optimism ('Wow – I didn't think I was going to be able to do that. Perhaps I can do some other things I've stopped doing'). That is, behavioural programmes may *indirectly* change pain-related cognitions, and these changes may contribute to any improvements that patients make. Cognitive-behavioural approaches tackle these issues more directly. They focus on the cognitions mediating our emotional and behavioural responses to pain. Cognitions are seen as central to our experience of pain, and our reactions to it. As such, the model does not contradict the model of pain provided by the gate control model – it focuses on one group of variables that influence the gate. The goals of cognitive-behavioural therapy for pain are threefold:

1. To help patients alter their beliefs that their problems are unmanageable. To help them to become 'resourceful problem solvers' and move away from feeling unable to cope with their pain.
2. To help patients identify the relationship between their thoughts, emotions and behaviour, and in particular how catastrophic or other negatively biased thoughts can lead to increased perceptions of pain, emotional distress and psychosocial difficulties.
3. To provide patients with strategies to manage their pain, emotional distress and psychosocial difficulties, and in particular to help them to develop effective and adaptive ways of thinking, feeling and behaving.

Cognitive-behavioural interventions can take the form of both individual and group interventions. Cognitive change is brought about in a number of stages. In these, patients are helped to identify any maladaptive thoughts that are increasing their experience of pain or their disability. This can be achieved by discussion in therapy sessions in which patients reflect back on periods of pain or when they have been frightened to engage in particular behaviour. Any thoughts that occurred at such times are identified and discussed. Patients may also be asked to monitor their thoughts during their day-to-day activities by completing a diary in which they record their level of pain, accompanying thoughts and mood.

Once patients have begun to identify how their thoughts influence the level of pain they experience, their behaviour and their mood, they are taught to change the nature of their thoughts to more adaptive ones. This may involve two types of cognitive intervention. The first is known as self-instruction training. In this, patients are taught to change the commentary in their head at times of worry or concern about their pain or activities to a more positive commentary. This can be pre-rehearsed and thought through with the therapist. Such thoughts include reassuring commentaries, such as *'I've had pain like this before and it didn't do me any harm in the long run'* or *'The pain only means I'm extending myself, not doing myself any damage'*. Other thoughts may involve reminders to use other strategies to help to control the pain: *'OK! When the pain starts, remember to relax so I don't add to it with tension'*, and so on.

A more complex cognitive process involves trying to identify the thoughts that are driving any emotional distress or inhibiting behaviour and challenging them. This involves treating them not as truths but as hypotheses, and challenging the hypotheses by looking for contrary evidence. In practice, these types of challenge may not be that different to the self-instructions, but they may be more targeted at particular worries or concerns:

> *Oh no! My back's beginning to hurt again. I know that means I'm going to be in pain for hours – I'd better stop now and take it easy. Hang on! Remember the last time this happened; I didn't feel that bad, particularly after relaxing and slowing down a bit. So take it easy – keep going . . . I'll feel better in myself for trying.*

These cognitive interventions are often accompanied by a programme of gradually increasing exercise. This may have a number of advantages. First, and most obviously, it will increase fitness and minimise restriction of activities. In addition, it allows patients to learn from their own experience that they will not be harmed by exercising – and therefore confirm some of the new beliefs that the cognitive therapy is trying to instil.

Other interventions may also be provided. One frequently used intervention involves teaching people to relax their muscles throughout their body and, particularly, close to the site of the pain (see above in the case of acute pain). Hanson and Gerber (1990) summarised a number of strategies for coping with periods of particularly intense pain that can be taught in a cognitive-behavioural programme, including:

- stop and ask myself if I can identify the pain trigger or learn anything from this pain;
- begin slow, deep breathing and remind myself to keep calm; review my alternatives;
- identify some distracting activities – a conversation with my partner about anything but the pain, a crossword puzzle, baking biscuits, etc.;
- take a long, hot shower;
- listen to relaxation or self-hypnosis tape;
- use positive self-talk – *'The pain won't last. I can handle this on my own'*;
- use pain-modification imagery – *'Imagine a block of ice resting on my back, see my endorphins working to counter the pain'*, and so on.

Cognitive-behavioural interventions have proved very effective in the treatment of chronic pain. Morley and Williams (1999), for example, found twenty-five trials suitable for meta-analysis that examined their effectiveness in the treatment of pain resulting from medical conditions, including back problems, arthritis and musculo-skeletal problems but excluding headaches. Overall, cognitive-behavioural treatments proved more effective than no treatment on measures of reported pain, mood, cognitive coping and appraisals, behavioural activity and social engagement. They proved more effective than pharmacological, educational and occupational therapy interventions on measures of reported pain, cognitive coping and appraisal, and in reducing the frequency of pain-related behaviour. Perhaps surprisingly, however, cognitive-behavioural interventions were no more effective than the others in reducing negative, fearful or catastrophic thoughts. Nor were they more effective in changing mood. This may be because the most important therapeutic process in these interventions was that patients engaged in higher levels of activity than they previously had. As we suggested earlier in the chapter, this may change their beliefs about their ability to exercise, to control their pain while doing so, and their mood.

Whatever the cause, there is mounting evidence that cognitive change is an important mediator of change in therapy. In a relatively early study of this phenomenon, Burns *et al.* (2003) found that the cognitive changes patients made in the early stages of a cognitive-behavioural programme were strongly predictive of pain outcomes later in therapy. They took measures of catastrophising and pain at the beginning, end and middle of a four-week cognitive-behavioural pain management programme. Early changes on the measure of catastrophising were predictive of pain measures taken at the end of therapy. By contrast, early changes in pain did not predict changes in catastrophising. Turner *et al.* (2007) came to similar conclusions using data from patients with **temporomandibular disorder pain**. In this group, changes in pain beliefs (control over pain, disability and pain signals harm), catastrophising and self-efficacy for managing pain mediated the effects of CBT on pain, activity interference and jaw use limitations at one year.

Temporomandibular disorder pain
A variety of conditions that cause tenderness and pain in the temporomandibular joint (hinge joint of the jaw).

One of the difficulties many patients who are referred for cognitive-behavioural therapy experience is that it presents a very different model of pain and its treatment to that which they are used to. Often because patients are frequently offered cognitive-behavioural therapy at the end of a long chain of medical or surgical treatments – most of which have failed – but which have emphasised the medical rather than psychological aspects of their condition:

> *I [Mr Brown] came to this clinic [for cognitive-behavioural therapy] after years of looking for a treatment for my back pain. The doc sends you here, there, everywhere looking for the answer. I've had pain killers, TENS, physiotherapy, manipulation . . . and then surgery. Every time you go to the next treatment, you have that little ray of hope that this will provide the cure! I've even gone to the alternative people in the hope that they would help. The weirdest thing I have had was something called cranial manipulation . . . supposed to relieve the nerves or something. But every one you hope the pain will go . . . even if you don't believe it quite as strongly with different treatments! But this has been different. Rather than trying to take the pain away, the course has focused on helping me cope with the pain. That was the first shock on the course – and it was disappointing. I expected that you could get rid of it, not keep it . . . and let me cope better! I was quite depressed for a few days when I learned this . . . but I guess I had to stick it out. I don't have much choice. But I must admit, as the course has gone on, it has helped. The relaxation really helps me. I can take myself away from the pain for a while if I imagine stuff. And at least I know I can cope with the pain, and won't let it stop me doing things like I used to . . .*

Relaxation and biofeedback

Relaxation can be used to relax the whole body or to relax specific muscle groups such as those on the forehead or back, which contribute to headaches and back pain, respectively. The latter may be of particular benefit in some patients. Turk (1986), for example, noted that many patients taught general relaxation for the treatment of back pain generally reported reductions in pain. However, one small subgroup of individuals reported either no benefit or even an increase in pain following the intervention. Closer assessment revealed that while many people in this group had been able to relax most of their muscles, they had been unable to relax the particular muscles in their back that were contributing to their pain. To do this, they needed guidance on relaxing these specific muscles. This can be achieved through the use of **biofeedback** techniques, including electromyographic biofeedback, galvanic skin response and thermal biofeedback:

Biofeedback
Technique of using monitoring devices to provide information regarding an autonomic bodily function, such as heart rate or blood pressure. Used in an attempt to gain some voluntary control over that function.

- *Electromyographic (EMG) biofeedback*: measures the small amount of electrical current in the muscles. The voltage equates with muscle tension: higher voltage = higher tension. Uses electrodes stuck to the skin over specific muscles that contribute to pain.

- *Galvanic skin response (GSR)*: measures general tension in the body by measuring subtle changes in the moisture (sweat) typically of the hand. Increased sweat relates to increased general muscle tension – although the relationship is far from one to one.
- *Thermal biofeedback*: based on a theory that warming the skin can reduce the pain of headaches. Skin temperature is measured by a thermistor, often placed on the back of the fingers to avoid sweat and to provide a more accurate gauge of body temperature.

Whatever the mode of measurement, biofeedback helps patients to make changes (relax, increase finger temperature) guided by auditory or visual feedback of any physiological changes they produce. In the case of auditory feedback, for example, a tone may become lower as the person relaxes their muscles. Visual feedback may involve moving an indicator along a scale as they do the same. In this way, changes in physiology that the patient may not recognise are made apparent and the patient can learn how to change their muscle tension.

One area in which biofeedback has been used with some success is in the treatment of chronic headaches. Rains *et al.* (2005), for example, reported that biofeedback interventions resulted in between 35 percent and 55 percent improvements in migraine and tension-type headaches. These improvements are about three times as large as any gains following some form of placebo intervention, and the equivalent to gains achieved by medication (Andrasik 2007). However, while biofeedback may be an effective intervention in other forms of pain, it is generally no more effective than relaxation alone. As relaxation is both simpler and cheaper to implement, this should perhaps be the first-line treatment rather than biofeedback.

If relaxation techniques are to be augmented, it may be better to do so using strategies that address other aspects of the pain experience than the physiological ones. More complex cognitive-behavioural interventions, for example, may add to the benefits of relaxation in the treatment of tension headaches, particularly where an individual is facing significant stresses in their lives which add to their overall stress or inhibit their use of simple relaxation strategies.

While relaxation can be beneficial in managing chronic pain, antidepressants have also proven efficacious. No research thus far has been able to fully explain why antidepressant medication helps to reduce pain, nevertheless it has consistently been shown to do so. One study, by Jackson et al., (2010) found that tricyclic antidepressants reduced pain in patients with migraine and tension headaches. In another study, Patetsos and Horjales-Araujo (2016) reviewed 36 studies investigating the link between antidepressants and chronic pain. A total of 1898 patients were included in their analysis with chronic pain conditions including fibromyalgia, lower back pain, tension type headache or migraine, diabetic painful neuropathy, noncardiac chest pain and musculoskeletal pain. They established that more than 70% of the studies they reviewed found that Selective Serotonin Reuptake Inhibitors (SSRIs), a type of antidepressant, effectively treated chronic pain.

Many individuals presenting with chronic pain experience comorbid mental health conditions such as depression (Holmes, Christelis & Arnold, 2012). Thus, an alternative strategy for the treatment of chronic pain has been to combine relaxation with antidepressant medication. These treatment methods are best delivered as part of a collaborative, multidisciplinary team of pain management experts. In support of the effectiveness of combined pharmacological and therapeutic treatment of chronic pain, is research by Holroyd et al. (2001). They compared treatment with antidepressant medication, training in relaxation techniques, a combination of the two, and a placebo drug therapy. The results were encouraging for both interventions. Both antidepressant and cognitive-behavioural techniques proved to be more effective than the placebo on measures including the frequency of headaches, analgesic medication use and restrictions in activity as a result of the headache. Although both single active interventions were equally effective, patients who received the pharmacological medication experienced these changes more quickly than those in the cognitive-behavioural intervention. Despite these gains, the combined therapy proved the most effective. This resulted in clinically significant reductions on a combined index of headache severity in 64 percent of participants with this condition. This compared with

Table 12.1 Outline of a typical pain management programme, in this case run at the Gloucester Royal Hospital in the UK

WEEK 1	Welcome, introduction and housekeeping Pain management philosophy What is chronic pain? – questions answered Introduction to exercise – sitting and standing Pacing everyday activities The stress response and introduction to diaphragmatic breathing
WEEK 2	Recap pacing Goal setting and action plans Introduction to exercise – lying Sitting and chairs Introduction to stretch and relax Video patients doing exercises for comparison at end of group
WEEK 3	How pain works: the gate control theory of pain How pain works: pain pathways Thoughts and feelings about pain Exercises Stretch and relax Action plans
WEEK 4	Recommended use of medication for chronic pain Communication and relationships Pain management graduate perspective talk Exercises Introduction to relaxing your mind Action plans
WEEK 5	Lifting and bending Managing everyday activities Sexual relationships The benefits of exercise Exercise Relaxing your mind Action plans
WEEK 6	Introduction to fitness and fitness equipment Doctor's talk: medication, treatments and surgery for chronic pain, sleeping and beds/positions to ease pain Action plans Relaxation
WEEK 7	Flare-ups and setbacks Helpful sleep habits Video exercises and compare with the beginning of the course Introduction to brief relaxation techniques Reviewing progress, and setting goals for the follow-up sessions

38 percent of those in the antidepressant condition, 35 percent of those receiving stress management, and 29 percent of those in the placebo condition.

Pain management clinics

So far, we have considered treatments for pain in isolation, without considering who provides the treatment or where patients may go for treatment. Nowadays, many hospitals provide services specifically for people with chronic pain – of whatever origin. These services will involve a number of people. Doctors, usually anaesthetists, provide expertise in the pharmacological and even surgical treatment of pain. Physiotherapists work with patients to develop exercise programmes that they can realistically expect to be able to engage in. Occupational therapists may work with patients to consider how they can improve their day-to-day activities around the home if their mobility is restricted. Specialist nurses may work with patients to develop pain management plans for individuals or groups of individuals. Psychologists may also contribute to and develop such programmes. Table 12.1 shows the outline of a typical outpatient pain management programme – conducted at the Gloucester Royal Hospital in the UK.

[A]Morrison, V., & Bennett, P. (2009). Pain. In V. Morrison & P. Bennett (Eds.), *An introduction to health psychology* (2nd ed., pp. 479–510). Harlow, Essex: Pearson Education.

Summary

Pain is a widely prevalent phenomenon. Over 20 percent of the general population are experiencing chronic pain at any one time, and the personal and social consequences of chronic pain are significant. Various types of pain have been identified:

- *acute*: lasting up to between three and six months;
- *chronic*: lasting more than three to six months; can be further categorised as chronic benign and chronic progressive pain.

Pain can also be defined in terms of its nature: its type, severity and pattern.

The experience of pain is moderated by a variety of physical and psychological factors, including:

- the degree of attention paid to the pain;
- the mood of the individual;
- the person's beliefs about the nature of the pain, including its cause and controllability.

Early specificity and pattern theories that did not take account of these psychological factors proved to be unsuccessful in explaining the various ways in which pain can be experienced. A more complex model developed by Melzack and Wall, known as the gate theory of pain, has superseded these models of pain. This suggests that pain is the outcome of a number of complementary or competing processes. Any model of pain has to take into account how psychological factors affect the perception of pain. The gate theory of pain suggests that:

- Afferent nerves carry pain messages up to the substantia gelatinosa and then through the spinal gate mechanism to the brain.
- At the same time, psychological processes influence the activity of nerves leading from the brain to the spinal gate.
- Activation of both systems results in a variety of chemicals being produced within the gate (substantia gelatinosa), some of which 'open' the pain gate, some of which 'close' it. The main chemicals involved in reducing pain sensations in the substantia gelatinosa are endorphins.

Melzack has developed a more complex neurological model of pain, known as the neuromatrix, which accounts for phenomena previously difficult to account for by the gate theory (including phantom limb pain).

TENS is a physiological intervention based on the gate control theory of pain. Unfortunately, consistent evidence of its effectiveness is lacking.

Both behavioural and cognitive-behavioural interventions have proved to be effective in the treatment of both acute and more chronic pain. Cognitive changes appear to mediate changes in the experience of pain.

Biofeedback interventions can help to reduce pain, but their overall effectiveness is no greater than more general relaxation procedures. They may be best used when there are individual muscle groups contributing to the pain that are not relaxed following more general relaxation instructions, or for the treatment of headaches.

Psychological interventions may be combined (at least in some cases) with antidepressant medication to provide maximal benefit.[A]

Review questions

A. Fill in the missing words to complete the following statements.

1. The various types of pain which include ______ pain, ________ pain, ____________ pain, ________________________ pain.

2. The simplest theory of pain, known as the ____________________ indicated that 'pain receptors' in the skin and body transmit information from the brain to provide a sensory experience of pain.

B. Please select one statement that best answers each of the following questions.

3. Which of the following best describes chronic benign pain?
   a) pain which last < 3 to 6 months, usually involving some from of injury, may only occur once, and generally the pain disappears once the damaged tissue has healed
   b) pain that becomes progressively worse over time as a result of disease progression such as rheumatoid arthritis
   c) long-term pain that is experienced over time such as lower back pain
   d) none of the above

4. Earlier theories of pain were critiqued as they:
   a) could not explain the phenomenon of pain experienced in the absence of pain receptors
   b) could not explain the influence of psychological factors on the experience of pain
   c) could not explain how some 'pain receptors' do not actually transmit pain messages
   d) all the above

5. Which of the following statement/s are TRUE in regards to pain?
   a) there is evidence of a reciprocal relationship between pain and mood
   b) the use of distraction techniques can reduce pain while increasing attention to pain can result in increased reporting of pain
   c) Young people don't experience debilitating pain
   d) both a and b

6. Which of the following statements are FALSE in regards the experience of pain?
   a) our thoughts influence our pain experience
   b) the placebo effect does not work
   c) our beliefs regarding our ability to tolerate pain does not influence our pain experience
   d) People who feel able to tolerate their main are less likely to be restricted by their pain

7. Which of the following statements are TRUE in regards to the gate control theory of pain developed by Melzack and Wall (1965):
   a) it is considered to be one of the most influential theories of pain
   b) it recognised the importance of both the mind and brain in pain perception
   c) when the "gates" close, pain messages are prevented from reaching the brain and may not be experienced at all
   d) all of the above

8. True or False: The **Substantia Gelatinosa** in the dorsal horn controls whether the "gate" is open or closed. An "open gate" means that the transmission cells (i.e., t-cells) can carry signals to the brain where pain is perceived; a "closed gate" stops the t-cells from firing and no pain signal is sent to brain.

9. As health practitioners, measuring pain can at times be challenging given the objective nature of pain. Which of the following methods are correct measures of pain?
   a) exploring the type of pain, the emotional response to the pain, the intensity of the pain, the timing of the pain
   b) exploring the type of pain, the cognitions surrounding the pain, the intensity of the pain, the timing of the pain
   c) exploring verbal vocalisations, motor behaviour, exploring treatment attitudes to the pain
   d) none of the above

10. Galvanic skin response (GSR) is a biofeedback technique that measures:
   a) small electrical currents in the muscles to detect muscle tension
   b) subtle changes in moisture (sweat) in the body to detect muscle tension
   c) skin temperature through the use of a thermistor to gauge the body temperature
   d) all of the above

C. Read the following questions and answer with some examples to illustrate your understanding.

11. There are various treatments to manage chronic pain. Some of these approaches to pain management include:

____

____

CHAPTER 13

Emotions

The content in this section has been compiled from:
Robbins, Chapter 6

Robbins, S. P., Judge. T. A., Millet, B., & Jones, M. (2010). Emotions and moods. In S. P. Robbins, T. A. Judge, B. Millet, & M. Jones (Eds.), *OB: The essentials* (pp. 154–160), Frenchs Forest, NSW: Pearson Australia.

Lilienfeld, Chapter 11

Lilienfeld, S. O., Lynn, S. J., Namy, L. L., Woolf, N. J., Jamieson, G., Marks, A., & Slaughter, V. (2015). Emotion and motivation. In S. O. Lilienfeld, S. J. Lynn, L. L. Namy, N. J. Woolf, G. Jamieson, A. Marks, & V. Slaughter (Eds.), *Psychology: From inquiry to understanding* (2nd ed., pp. 449–460). Melbourne, VIC: Pearson Australia.

CHAPTER 13

Emotions

Emotion is a complex phenomenon and thus difficult to define, though it comprises universal responses involving: physical arousal, expressive behaviour and conscious involvement. To understand emotion, we will explore different theories that try to explain the function and purpose of emotion. Additionally, non-verbal expressions of emotion (e.g. body language) are explored. Consideration and knowledge of nonverbal expression of emotion of facilitates positive interactions between clients and/or patients and health care professionals.

After studying this chapter you should be able to:

- Describe how moods differ from emotions
- Describe fundamental aspects of emotions
- Describe theories of emotion:
  - James–Lange theory of emotion
  - Somatic marker theory (Damasio, 1994)
  - Cannon-Bard theory of emotion
  - Two-factor theory of emotion (Schachter & Singer, 1962)
- Describe non-verbal expressions of emotions.

What are emotions and moods?

How do moods differ from emotions?

Although we don't want to obsess over definitions, before we can proceed with our analysis we need to clarify three terms that are closely intertwined: *affect*, *emotions* and *moods*.

Affect is a generic term that covers a broad range of feelings that people experience. It is an umbrella concept that encompasses both emotions and moods (George, 1996). **Emotions** are intense feelings that are directed at someone or something (Frijda, 1993). **Moods** are feelings that tend to be less intense than emotions and that often (though not always) lack a contextual stimulus (Weiss & Cropanzano, 1996).

Affect
A broad range of feelings that people experience.

Emotions
Intense feelings that are directed at someone or something.

Moods
Feelings that tend to be less intense than emotions and that lack a contextual stimulus.

Most experts believe that emotions are more fleeting than moods (Ekman & Davidson, 1994). For example, if someone is rude to you, you will feel angry. That intense feeling of anger probably comes and goes fairly quickly, maybe even in a matter of seconds. When you are in a bad mood, though, you can feel bad for several hours.

Emotions are reactions to a person (seeing a good friend at work may make you feel glad) or an event (dealing with a rude client may make you feel angry). You show your emotions when you are 'happy about something, angry at someone, afraid of something' (Frijda, 1993). Moods, in contrast, aren't usually directed at a person or event. But emotions can turn into moods when you lose focus on the event or object that started the feeling. And, by the same token, good or bad moods can make you more emotional in response to an event. So, when a colleague criticises how you spoke to a client, you might become angry at him. That is, you show emotion (anger) towards a specific object (your colleague). But as the specific emotion dissipates, you might just feel generally dispirited. You can't attribute this feeling to any single event; you are just not your normal self. You might then overreact to other events. This affect state describes a mood. Figure 13.1 shows the relationships among affect, emotions and moods.

First, as the figure shows, *affect* is a broad term that encompasses emotions and moods. Second, there are differences between emotions and moods. Some of these differences—that emotions are more likely to be caused by a specific event, and emotions are more fleeting than moods—as just discussed. Other differences are more subtle. For example, unlike moods, emotions tend to be more clearly revealed with facial expressions (anger, disgust).

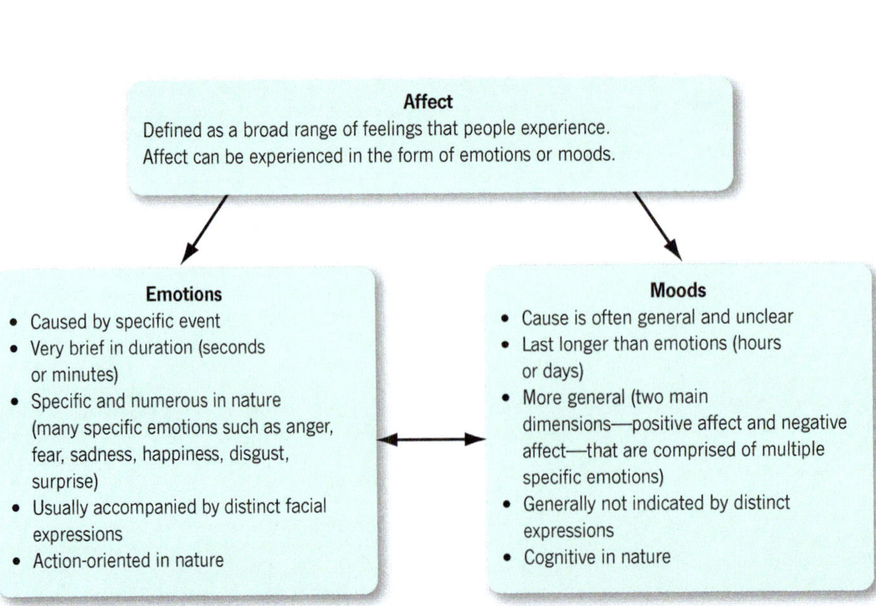

Figure 13.1 Affect, emotions and moods

Also, some researchers speculate that emotions may be more action-oriented—they may lead us to some immediate action—while moods may be more cognitive, meaning they may cause us to think or brood for a while (Ekman & Davidson, 1994).

Finally, the figure shows that emotions and moods can mutually influence each other. For example, an emotion, if it is strong and deep enough, can turn into a mood: getting your dream job may generate the emotion of joy, but it also can put you in a good mood for several days. Similarly, if you are in a good or bad mood, it might make you experience a more intense positive or negative emotion than would otherwise be the case. For example, if you are in a bad mood, you might 'blow up' in response to a fellow employee's comment when normally it would have just generated a mild reaction. Because emotions and moods can mutually influence each other, there will be many points throughout the chapter where emotions and moods will be closely connected. Although affect, emotions and moods are separable in theory, in practice the distinction isn't always crystal clear. In fact, in some areas, researchers have studied mostly moods, and in other areas, mainly emotions. So, when we review the topics on emotions and moods, you may see more information on emotions in one area and moods in another. This is reflecting the current state of the research.

Also, the terminology can be confusing. For example, the two main mood dimensions are positive affect and negative affect, yet we have defined affect more broadly than mood. So, although the topic can be fairly dense in places, hang in there.

A basic set of emotions

How many emotions are there? In what ways do they vary? There are dozens of emotions. They include anger, contempt, enthusiasm, envy, fear, frustration, joy, love, disappointment, embarrassment, disgust, happiness, hate, hope, jealousy, pride, surprise and sadness. There have been numerous research efforts to limit and define the dozens of emotions into a fundamental or basic set of emotions (Shaver, Schwartz, Kirson & O' Connor, 1987; Ekman, 1992; Izard, 1992 & Plutchik , 1994). But some researchers argue that it makes no sense to think of basic emotions, because even emotions we rarely experience, such as shock, can have a powerful effect on us (Solomon, 2002). Other researchers, even philosophers, argue that there are universal emotions common to all of us. René Descartes, often called the founder of modern philosophy, identified six 'simple and primitive passions'—wonder, love, hatred, desire, joy and sadness—and argued that 'all the others are composed of some of these six or are species of them' (Descartes, 1649). Other philosophers (such as Hume, Hobbes and Spinoza) identified categories of emotions. Though these philosophers were helpful, the burden to provide conclusive evidence for the existence of a basic set of emotions still rests with contemporary researchers.

In contemporary research, psychologists have tried to identify basic emotions by studying facial expressions (Ekman, 2003). One problem with this approach is that some emotions are too complex to be easily represented on our faces. Take love, for example. Many think of love as the most universal of all emotions (Shaver, Morgan & Wu, 1996), yet it isn't easy to express a loving emotion with one's face only. Also, cultures have norms that govern emotional expression, so how we *experience* an emotion isn't always the same as how we *show* it. Showing pleasure through facial expressions at the cards dealt to a poker player would definitely be a disadvantage to winning. Further, many companies today offer anger-management programs to teach people how to contain or even hide their inner feelings (Solomon, 2002).

It is unlikely that psychologists or philosophers will ever completely agree on a set of basic emotions, or even whether it makes sense to think of basic emotions. Still, enough researchers have agreed on six essentially universal emotions—anger, fear, sadness, happiness, disgust and surprise—with most other emotions subsumed under one of these six categories (Weiss & Cropanzano, 1996). Some researchers even plot these six emotions along a continuum: ranging from happiness at one end through to surprise to fear to sadness to anger and finally to disgust at the other end (Woodworth, 1938). The closer any two emotions are to each other on this continuum, the more likely it is that people will confuse them. For instance, we sometimes mistake happiness for surprise, but rarely do we confuse happiness and disgust. In addition, as we will see later, cultural factors can also influence interpretations.

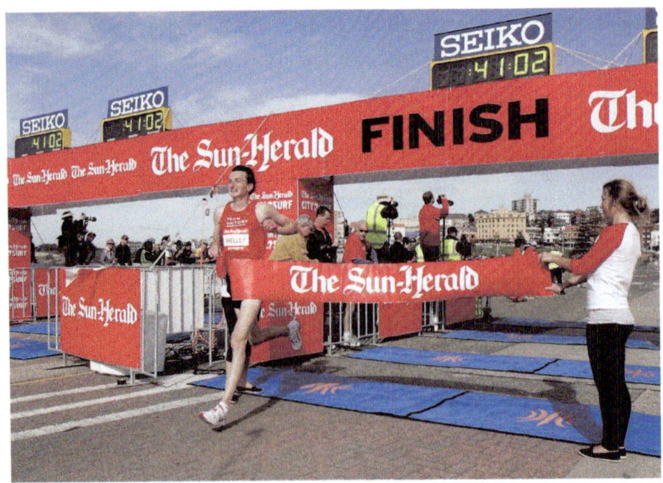

After running for 41 minutes, Martin Shelley crossed the finish line ahead of 75 000 other competitors to win the 14-kilometre Sydney City to Surf fun run in 2009. Shelley celebrated his win with a tear-filled embrace with his father. This expression of joy is one of the dozens of basic emotions that originate in our brain's limbic system to help us interpret events. As a positive emotion, joy expresses a favourable evaluation of feeling. (**Source:** Sasha Woolley/FairfaxPhotos.com)

Some aspects of emotions

There are some other fundamental aspects of emotions that we need to consider. These aspects include the biology of emotions, their intensity, as well as their frequency and duration, the relationship between rationality and emotions, and the functions of emotions. Let's deal with each of these aspects in turn.

Biology

All emotions originate in the brain's limbic system, which is about the size of a walnut and near our brain stem at the base of the skull (Nolte, 2002). People tend to be happiest (report more positive than negative emotions) when their limbic system is relatively inactive. When the limbic system 'heats up', negative emotions such as anger and guilt dominate over positive ones such as joy and happiness. Overall, the limbic system provides a lens through which you interpret events. When it is active, you see things in a negative light. When it is inactive, you interpret information more positively.

Not everyone's limbic system is the same. Moderately depressed people have more active limbic systems, particularly when they encounter negative information (Tucker, Luu, Frishkoff, Quiring & Poulsen, 2003). And women tend to have more active limbic systems than men, which, some argue, explains why women are more susceptible to depression than men and are more likely to emotionally bond with children (Gur, Gunning-Dixon, Bilker & Gur, 2002). Of course, as always, these are average differences—women are more likely to be depressed than men, but naturally that doesn't mean that all depressed people are women, or that men are incapable of bonding with their kids.

Intensity

People give different responses to identical emotion-provoking stimuli. In some cases, personality is responsible for the difference. Other times, it is a result of the job requirements.

People vary in their inherent ability to express emotional intensity. You may know people who almost never show their feelings. They rarely get angry. They never show rage. In contrast, you probably also know people who seem to be on an emotional roller-coaster. When they are happy, they are ecstatic. When they are sad, they are deeply depressed. We will explore the impact that personality has on an individual's emotions in more detail later in the chapter.

Jobs make different demands on our emotions. For instance, air traffic controllers, surgeons and trial judges are expected to be calm and controlled, even in stressful situations. Conversely, the effectiveness of television evangelists, announcers at sporting events and lawyers in court situations can depend on their ability to alter their emotional intensity as the need arises.

Frequency and duration

Sean Wolfson is basically a quiet and reserved person. He loves his job as a financial planner. The part of his job that he dislikes involves giving speeches, but these are necessary as they increase his visibility and promote his programs. 'If I had to speak to large audiences every day, I'd quit this business,' he says. 'I think this works for me because I can fake excitement and enthusiasm for an hour, a couple of times a month.' Whether an employee can successfully meet the emotional demands of a given job depends not only on what emotions need to be displayed and their intensity, but also on how frequently and for how long they need to make the effort.

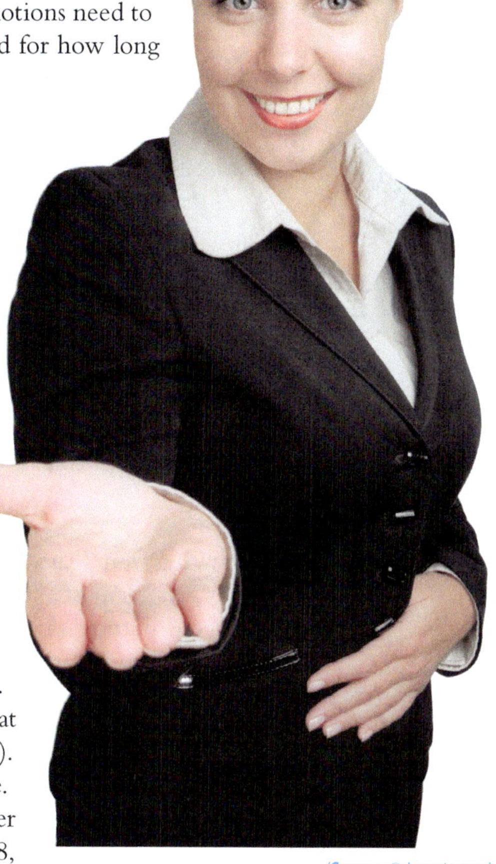

(**Source:** © Jumpingsack/ Dreamstime.com)

Do emotions make us irrational?

How often have you heard someone say, 'Oh, you're just being emotional'? You might have been offended. The famous astronomer Carl Sagan once wrote, 'Where we have strong emotions, we're liable to fool ourselves.' These observations suggest that rationality and emotion are in conflict with one another and that if you exhibit emotion, you are likely to act irrationally. One team of authors argues that displaying an emotion such as sadness to the point of crying is so toxic to a career that we should leave the room rather than allow others to witness our emotional display (Poverney and Picascia, 2011). The famous author Lois Frankel advises that women should avoid being emotional at work because it will undermine how others rate their competence (Frankel, 2004). These perspectives suggest that the demonstration, or even experience, of emotions is likely to make us seem weak, brittle or irrational. However, the research disagrees and is increasingly showing that emotions are actually critical to rational thinking (Damasio, 1994). In fact, there has been ample evidence of such a link for a long time.

Take the example of Phineas Gage. Gage was a railroad worker in Vermont, in the United States. One September day in 1848, while setting an explosive charge at work, an iron bar a metre in length flew into Gage's lower left jaw and out through the top of his skull, almost like an arrow. Remarkably, Gage survived his injury. He was still able to read and speak, and he performed well above average on cognitive ability tests. However, it became clear that Gage had lost his ability to experience emotion. He was emotionless at even the saddest misfortunes or happiest occasions. Gage's inability to express emotion eventually took away his ability to reason. He started making irrational choices about his life, often behaving erratically and against his self-interests. Despite being an intelligent man whose intellectual abilities were unharmed by the accident, Gage drifted from job to job, eventually taking up with a circus. In commenting on Gage's condition, one expert noted: 'Reason may not be as pure as most of us think it is or wish it were … emotions and feelings may not be intruders in the bastion of reason at all: they may be enmeshed in its networks, for worse and for better' (Damasio, 1994).

The example of Phineas Gage and of many other brain injury studies shows us that emotions are critical to rational thinking. In other words, to be rational, we must have the ability to experience emotions. Why? Because our emotions provide important information about how we understand the world around us. Although we might think of a computer as intellectually superior, a human so void of emotion would be unable to function. The whole theme of Isaac Asimov's story *I Robot* (made into a movie of the same name starring Will Smith) was based

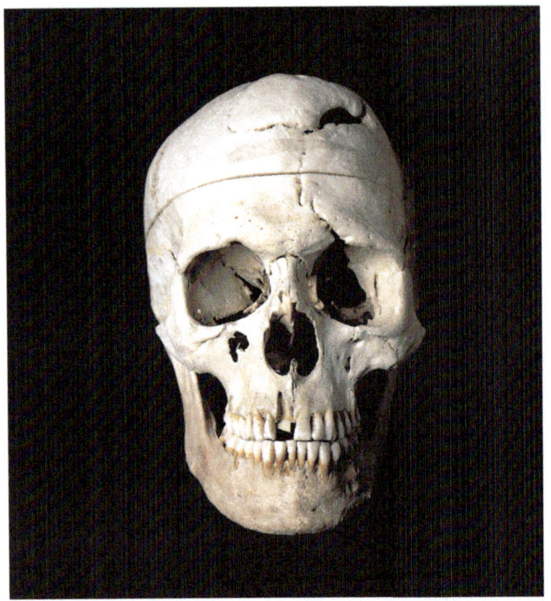
By studying the skull of Phineas Gage, shown here, and other brain injuries, researchers discovered an important link between emotions and rational thinking. They found that losing the ability to emote led to the loss of the ability to reason. From this discovery, researchers learned that our emotions provide us with valuable information that helps our thinking process.

on the question of what would happen if computer-driven robots gained the ability to feel emotion. Think about a manager making a decision to fire an employee. Would you really want the manager to make the decision without regarding either her or the employee's emotions? The key to good decision making is to employ both thinking and feeling wisely in one's decisions.

What functions do emotions serve?

Why do we have emotions? What role do they serve? We just discussed one function—that we need them to think rationally. Charles Darwin, however, took a broader approach. In *The Expression of the Emotions in Man and Animals*, Darwin argued that emotions developed over time to help humans solve problems. Emotions are useful, he said, because they motivate people to engage in actions important for survival—actions such as foraging for food, seeking shelter, choosing mates, guarding against predators and predicting others' behaviours. For example, disgust (an emotion) motivates us to avoid dangerous or harmful things (such as rotten foods). Excitement (also an emotion) motivates us to take on situations in which we require energy and initiative (for example, tackling a new career).

Evolutionary psychology
An area of inquiry that argues that we must experience the emotions that we do because they serve a purpose.

Drawing from Darwin are researchers who focus on **evolutionary psychology**. This field of study says we must experience emotions—whether they are positive or negative—because they serve a purpose (Cosmides & Tooby, 2000). For example, you would probably consider jealousy to be a negative emotion. Evolutionary psychologists would argue that it exists in people because it has a useful purpose. Males may feel jealousy to increase the chance that their genes, rather than a rival's genes, are passed on to the next generation (Buss, 2001). Although we tend to think of anger as being 'bad', it actually can help us protect our rights when we feel they are being violated. For example, a person showing anger when she's double-crossed by a colleague is serving a warning for others not to repeat the same behaviour. Consider another example. Rena Weeks was a secretary at a prominent law firm. Her boss wouldn't stop touching and grabbing her. His treatment made her angry. So, she did more than just quit—she sued, and won a multimillion-dollar case for sexual harassment in the workplace (Hundley, 2004). It isn't that anger is always good. But as with all other emotions, it exists because it serves a useful purpose. Positive emotions also serve a purpose. For example, a service employee who feels empathy for a customer may provide better customer service.

But some researchers aren't firm believers in evolutionary psychology. Why? Think about fear (an emotion). It is just as easy to think of the harmful effects of fear as it is the beneficial effects. For example, running in fear from a predator increases the likelihood of survival. But what benefit does freezing in fear serve? Evolutionary psychology provides an interesting perspective on the functions of emotions, but it isn't clear whether this perspective is always valid (Laland & Brown, 2002).

Mood as positive and negative affect

One way to classify emotions is by whether they are positive or negative (Watson, Clark & Tellegen, 1988). Positive emotions—such as joy and gratitude—express a favourable evaluation or feeling. Negative emotions—such as anger or guilt—express the opposite. Keep in mind that emotions can't be neutral. Being neutral is being non-emotional (Ben-Ze'ev, 2000).

When we group emotions into positive and negative categories, they become mood states because we are now looking at them more generally instead of isolating one particular emotion. In Figure 13.2, *excited* is a specific emotion that is a pure marker of high positive affect, while *boredom* is a pure marker of low positive affect. Similarly, *nervous* is a pure marker of high negative affect, while *relaxed* is a pure marker of low negative affect. Finally, some emotions—such as *contentment* (a mixture of high positive affect and low negative affect) or *sadness* (a mixture of low positive affect and high negative affect)—are in between. You will notice that this model doesn't include all emotions. There are two reasons why. First, we can fit other emotions such as enthusiasm or depression into the model, but we are short on space. Second, some emotions, such as surprise, don't fit well because they aren't as clearly positive or negative.

So, we can think of **positive affect** as a mood dimension consisting of positive emotions such as excitement, self-assurance and cheerfulness at the high end, and boredom, sluggishness and tiredness at the low end. **Negative affect** is a mood dimension consisting of nervousness, stress and anxiety at the high end, and relaxation, tranquillity and poise at the low end. (Note that positive and negative affect are moods. We are using these labels, rather than positive and negative *mood*, because that's how researchers label them.)

Positive affect
A mood dimension consisting of specific positive emotions such as excitement, self-assurance and cheerfulness at the high end, and boredom, sluggishness and tiredness at the low end.

Negative affect
A mood dimension consisting of nervousness, stress and anxiety at the high end, and relaxation, tranquillity and poise at the low end.

Positive affect and negative affect play out at work (and beyond work, of course) in that they colour our perceptions, and these perceptions can become their own reality. For example, a flight attendant posted an anonymous blog on the Web that said: 'I work in a pressurised aluminium tube and the environment outside my "office" cannot sustain human life. That being said, the human life inside is not worth sustaining sometimes … in fact, the passengers can be jerks, and idiots. I am often treated with no respect, nobody listens to me … until I threaten to kick them off the plane …' (Flight attendant war stories, 2011) Clearly, if a flight attendant is in a bad mood, it is going to influence his or her perceptions of passengers, which will influence his or her behaviour in turn.

Importantly, negative emotions are more likely to translate into negative moods. People think about events that created strong negative emotions five times as long as they do about events that created strong positive ones (Ben-Ze'ev, 2000). So, we should expect people to recall negative experiences more readily than positive ones. Perhaps one of the reasons is that,

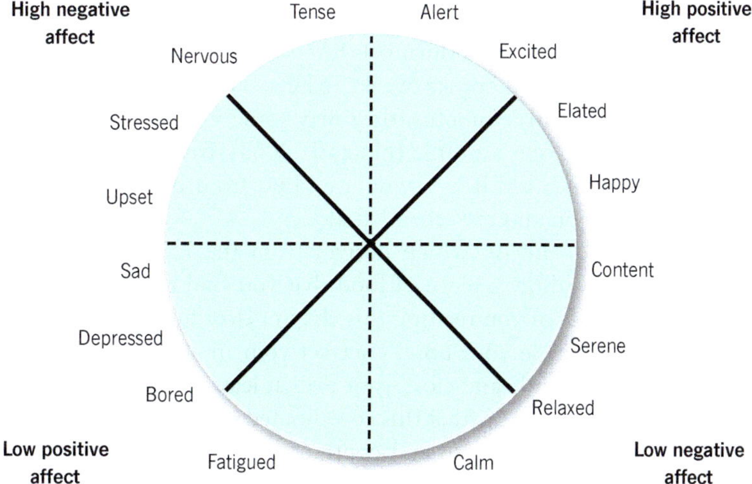

Figure 13.2 The structure of mood

Positivity offset
Tendency of most individuals to experience a mildly positive mood at zero input (when nothing in particular is going on).

for most of us, they are also more unusual. Indeed, research shows that there is a **positivity offset**, meaning that at zero input (when nothing in particular is going on), most individuals experience a mildly positive mood (Cacioppo & Gardner, 1999). So, for most people, positive moods are somewhat more common than negative moods. The positivity offset also appears to operate at work. For example, one study of customer service representatives in a British call centre (probably a job where it is pretty hard to feel positive) revealed that people reported experiencing positive moods 58 percent of the time (Holman, 2005).[A]

Theories of emotion: what causes our feelings?

Almost all of us experience emotions. Yet psychologists do not have a firm definition of emotion, nor do they agree fully on what causes our emotions, or even on what distinguishes emotions from thoughts. One definition of emotion is: a relatively brief response state involving synchronised physiological, subjective and behavioural elements. This is a rather dry definition for this rich dimension of our psychological lives, but, as we will see, emotion is a complex phenomenon that is difficult to capture meaningfully in a single definition. To understand emotion, the best approach is to explore the different theories that try to explain it.

Discrete emotions theory: emotions as evolved expressions

Discrete emotions theory
Theory that humans experience a small number of distinct emotions.

According to **discrete emotions theory**, humans experience a small number of distinct emotions, even if they combine in complex ways (Ekman & Friesen, 1971; Griffiths, 1997; Izard, 1971; 1994; Tomkins, 1962). Advocates of this theory further propose that emotions have distinct biological roots and serve evolutionary functions. Each emotion, they suggest, is associated with a distinct 'motor program': a set of genetically influenced physiological responses that are essentially the same in all people.

Support for an evolutionary basis of emotions

The fact that some emotional expressions emerge even without direct reinforcement suggests that they may be by-products of innate motor programs (Freedman, 1964; Panksepp, 2007). Newborn infants smile spontaneously during REM sleep, the sleep stage during which most vivid dreaming occurs. At about six weeks, babies start to smile whenever they see a favourite face, and at about three months, they may smile when they are learning to do something new, even when no one is around (Plutchik, 2003). Irenäus Eibl-Eibesfeldt (1973) showed that even three-month-old babies who are blind from birth smile in response to playing and tickling and frown and cry when left alone.

Consider the emotion of *disgust*, which derives from the Latin term for 'bad taste'. Imagine we asked you to swallow a piece of food that you find repulsive, like a dried-up cockroach (apologies to those of you reading this chapter over lunch or dinner). The odds are high that you would wrinkle your nose, contract your mouth, stick out your tongue, turn your head slightly to one side and close your eyes at least partly (Phillips et al., 1997). Discrete emotions theorists would say that this coordinated set of reactions is evolutionarily adaptive. When you wrinkle your nose and contract your mouth, you are reducing the

---

[A]From Robbins, S.P., Judge. T.A., Millet, B., & Jones, M. (2010). Emotions and moods, In *OB: The essentials* (pp. 154-160), Frenchs Forest, NSW:Pearson Australia.

chances you will ingest this substance; by sticking out your tongue, you are increasing the chances you will expel it; by turning your head, you are doing your best to avoid it; and by closing your eyes, you are limiting the damage it can do to your visual system. Other emotions similarly prepare us for biologically important actions (Frijda, 1986). When we are angry, our teeth and fists often become clenched, readying us to bite and fight. And when we are afraid, our eyes open wide, allowing us to better spot potential dangers, like predators, lurking in our environment. Charles Darwin (1872) was among the first to point out the similarities between the emotional expressions of humans and many non-human animals. He noted that the angry snarl of dogs, marked by the baring of their fangs, is reminiscent of the dismissive sneer of humans. Eugene Morton (1977; 1982) showed deep-seated similarities in communication across most animal species, especially mammals and birds, further suggesting that the emotions of humans and non-human animals share the same evolutionary heritage. For example, across the animal kingdom, high-pitched sounds are associated with friendly interactions; low-pitched sounds, with hostile interactions. Jaak Panksepp (2005) discovered that rats emit a high-pitched chirp, perhaps similar to human laughter, when tickled. The high-pitched panting of dogs during play also seems similar in many ways to human laughter, as does the chuckling of chimpanzees (Provine, 2012). Of course, the mere fact that two things are superficially similar doesn't prove that they share evolutionary roots. In the case of emotions, however, we know that all mammals share an evolutionary ancestor. The fact that many mammals display similar emotional reactions during similar social behaviours, such as tickling and play, lends itself to a parsimonious hypothesis: perhaps these reactions share the same evolutionary origins.

Culture and emotion

Another way of evaluating claims that discrete emotions are products of evolution is to examine the *universality* of emotional expressions. If we humans evolved to express emotions a certain way, we would expect expressions to communicate the same meaning across cultures. We would also expect people across the world to recognise emotions similarly.

RECOGNITION OF EMOTIONS ACROSS CULTURES. One telling piece of evidence for discrete emotions theory derives from research showing that people recognise and generate the same emotional expressions across cultures (Izard, 1971). Nevertheless, this research is vulnerable to a rival explanation: because these people have all been exposed to Western culture, the similarities may be due to shared experiences rather than a shared evolutionary heritage.

To rule out this explanation, in the late 1960s American psychologist Paul Ekman travelled to southeastern New Guinea to study a group of people who had never been exposed to people or things from modern Western cultures. With the aid of a translator, Ekman read them a brief story (for example, 'His mother has died, and he feels very sad'), along with a display of photographs of Americans depicting various emotions, like happiness, sadness and anger. Then, Ekman asked them to select the photograph that matched the story. He later went further, asking American university students to guess which emotions the New Guineans were displaying (Ekman & Friesen, 1971).

Ekman (1994; 1999) and his colleagues (Ekman & Friesen, 1986) concluded that a small number of **primary emotions**—perhaps seven—are cross-culturally universal. Specifically, they found that the facial expressions associated with these emotions are recognised across most, if not all, cultures. Discrete emotions theorists call these emotions 'primary' because they are presumably the biologically based emotions from which other emotions arise:

- Happiness
- Sadness
- Surprise
- Anger
- Disgust
- Fear
- Contempt

Primary emotions
Small number (perhaps seven) of emotions believed by some theorists to be cross-culturally universal.

Recent research suggests that pride may be the eighth cross-culturally universal emotion, as it, too, is recognised across diverse cultures, from the United States to Italy to remote tribal villages in West Africa (Tracy & Robins, 2008).

Ekman and his colleagues found that certain primary emotions are easier to detect than others. Happiness tends to be the most easily recognised emotion (Elfenbein & Ambady, 2002); their New Guinea participants correctly recognised happiness in Americans more than 90 percent of the time (Ekman, 1994). In contrast, negative emotions tend to be more difficult to recognise; many participants confuse disgust with anger, anger with fear, and fear with surprise (Elfenbein & Ambady, 2002; Tomkins & McCarter, 1964). Although people across widely different cultures do not always agree on which facial expressions go with which emotions (Russell, 1994), they agree often enough to provide some support for discrete emotions theory.

Secondary emotions

Primary emotions do not tell the whole story of our feelings. Just as talented painters create a magnificently complex palette of secondary paint colours, like various shades of green and purple, from a few primary paint colours, like blue and yellow, many theorists believe that our brains 'create' an enormous array of *secondary emotions* from a small number of primary emotions. For example, the secondary emotion of 'alarm' may be a mixture of fear and surprise, whereas the secondary emotion of 'hatred' may be a mixture of anger and disgust (Plutchik, 2000).

Moreover, some of these complex emotion blends possess names in other languages, but have no equivalent in English. Take *schadenfreude*, a German term that refers to the glee we experience at witnessing the misfortune of others, especially those we see as arrogant (Ortony, Clore & Collins, 1988). It appears to be a hybrid of several emotions, such as happiness, anger and pride. We experience *schadenfreude* when we feel secretly happy when a classmate who brags about getting high distinctions on all of his assignments unexpectedly fails an exam.

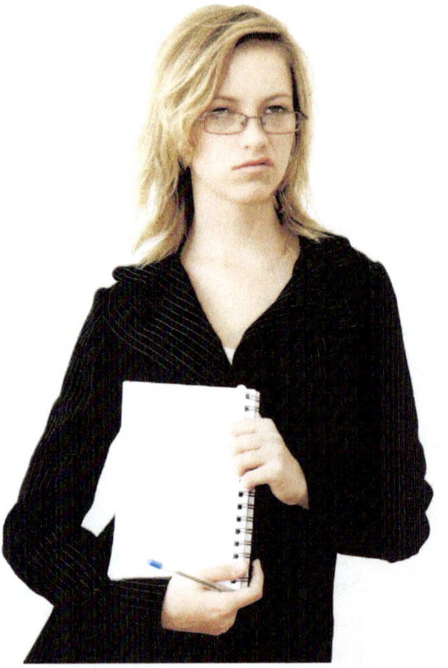

The facial reaction of contempt is frequently marked by an asymmetrical turning upward of the lips. (**Source:** Kelliem/Dreamstime.)

Accompaniments of emotional expressions

According to discrete emotions theorists, each primary emotion is associated with a distinctive constellation of facial expressions. For example, in anger our lips consistently narrow and our eyebrows move downwards. In contempt, we frequently lift and tighten our lips on one side of our face, generating a smirk (Matsumoto & Ekman, 2004), or roll our eyes upwards, in effect communicating 'I'm above (superior to) you'. Interestingly, John Gottman and his colleagues have found that contempt, and the facial expressions that go along with it, are among the best predictors of divorce in married couples (Gladwell, 2005; Gottman & Levenson, 1999).

EMOTIONS AND PHYSIOLOGY. We can also differentiate at least some primary emotions by their patterns of physiological responding (Ax, 1953; Rainville et al., 2006). The mere act of making a face associated with a specific emotion alters our bodily reactions in characteristic ways (Ekman, Levenson & Friesen,

1983). Our heart rates tend to increase more when we make angry and fearful facial expressions than when we make happy or surprised facial expressions (Cacioppo et al., 1997), probably because the first two emotions are more closely linked to the emergency reactions we experience when threatened. The heart kicks into high gear when we are in danger, mobilising us for action (Frijda, 1986). Yet even fear and anger differ physiologically. When we are afraid, our digestive system tends to slow down. In contrast, when we are angry, our digestive system tends to speed up, which explains why our 'stomach churns' when we are furious (Carlson & Hatfield, 1992).

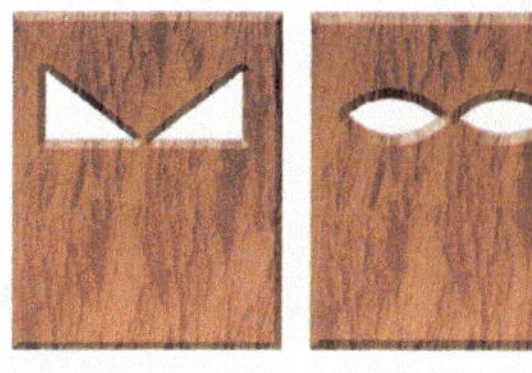

Pair 1

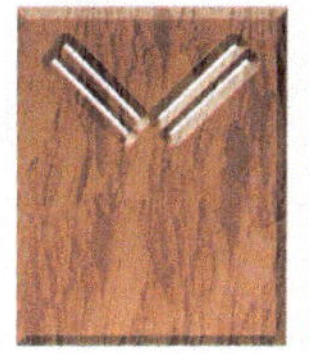

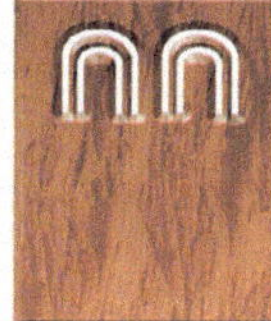

Pair 2

Figure 13.3 Which mask conveys a threat?

In hunter–gatherer societies, people often construct masks to convey threat, especially anger. These two pairs of shapes are based on wooden masks worn in these societies. In both cases, the shape on the left communicates more threat. Even American university students can distinguish the threatening from non-threatening mask at higher-than-chance levels.

(**Source:** Aronoff, Barclay & Stevenson, 1988.)

Brain imaging data also provide at least some evidence for discrete emotions. Fear, disgust and anger tend to show different patterns of brain activation (Murphy, Nimmo-Smith & Lawrence, 2003). Fear seems to be relatively specific to the amygdala, disgust to the *insula*, a region within the limbic system, and anger to a region of the frontal cortex behind our eyes (see Figure 13.3).

Yet in many other cases we cannot distinguish different emotions by means of their physiology (Cacioppo, Tassinary & Berntson, 2000; Feldman Barrett, 2006; Feldman Barrett et al., 2007). Surprisingly, happiness and sadness are not terribly different in their patterns of brain activation (Murphy, Nimmo-Smith & Lawrence, 2003). Moreover, there is almost certainly no single 'fear processor', 'disgust processor' and so on, in the brain, because multiple brain regions participate in all emotions (Schienle et al., 2002).

REAL VERSUS FAKE EMOTIONS. We can use certain facial expressions to help us distinguish real from fake emotions. In genuine happiness, we see an upward turning of the corners of the mouth, along with a drooping of the eyelids and a crinkling of the corners of the eyes (Ekman, Davidson & Friesen, 1990). Emotion theorists distinguish this genuine emotional expression, called the *Duchenne smile* after the neurologist who discovered it, from the fake or *Pan Am smile*, which is marked by a movement of the mouth but not the eyes. The term 'Pan Am smile' derives from a 1970s American television commercial featuring the now-defunct airline Pan Am, in which all of the flight attendants flashed obviously fake smiles. If you flick through your family albums, you will probably find an abundance of Pan Am smiles, especially in posed photographs. If you happen to be in a good mood when viewing these photos, you will be more likely to accept the fake smiles as being real, according to researchers from the University of New South Wales (Forgas & East, 2008).

In line with the facial feedback hypothesis describe below, some research indicates that simply putting on a happy facial expression will generate feelings of happiness in the smiler (Levenson, Ekman & Friesen, 1990). Interestingly, though, among participants asked to produce facial expressions, only Duchenne smiles are associated with increased activity of the front region of the left hemisphere, which is the brain region that appears to be specialised for positive emotions (Ekman, Davidson & Friesen, 1990).

Motivation-structural rules

Indirect evidence for discrete emotions theory comes from research on animal communication. According to Eugene Morton's (1977; 1982) **motivation-structural rules**, there are deep-seated similarities in communication across most animal species, especially mammals and birds. These rules suggest that certain crucial aspects of emotional expression are products of natural selection, as discrete emotions theorists claim.

Motivation-structural rules Deep-seated similarities in communication across most animal species.

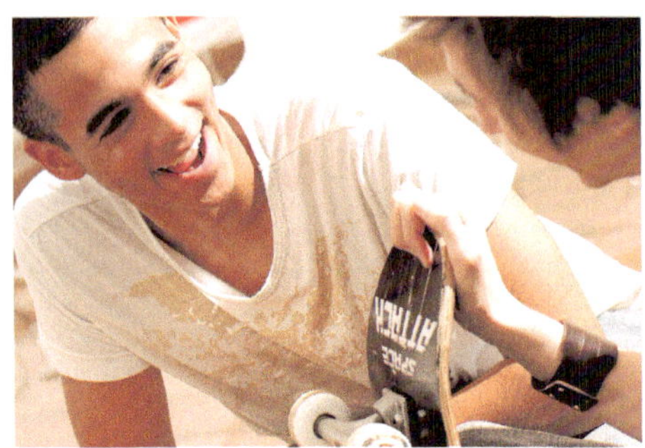

The Duchenne (genuine) smile is marked by a turning upward of the corners of the mouth and changes in the eyelids and corners of the eye.
(**Source:** Steve Shott/Pearson Education Ltd.)

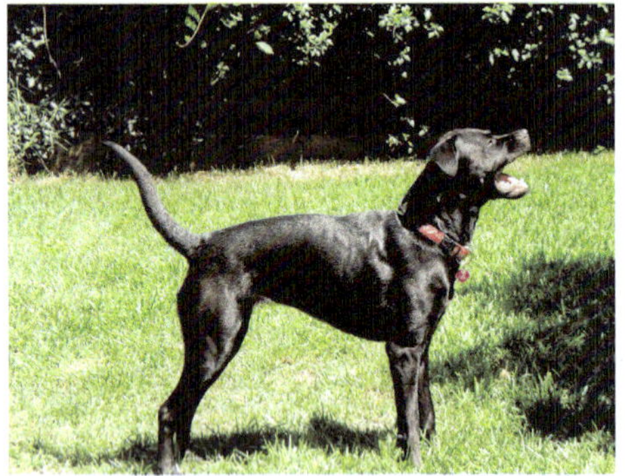

Dog barks conform to motivation-structural rules. Dogs tend to let out high-pitched barks when they are giving chase, begging for food or preparing to go for a walk. In contrast, they let out low-pitched barks when they are angry or confronting a stranger (Pongracz et al., 2005).

Cultural differences in emotional expression: display rule

The finding that certain emotions exist across most or all cultures does not mean that cultures are identical in their emotional expressions. In part, that is because cultures differ in **display rules**, their societal guidelines for how and when to express emotions (Ekman & Friesen, 1975; Matsumoto et al., 2005). In Western culture, parents teach most boys not to cry, whereas they typically teach girls that crying is acceptable (Plutchik, 2003). Australians are typically taught to be restrained in expressing affection in public, and so can be taken aback when a visitor from South America, the Middle East or some European countries, like Russia, greets them with a warm hug and a gooey kiss on the cheek.

Cognitive theories of emotion: think first, feel later

As we have seen, discrete emotions theorists emphasise the biological underpinnings of emotion. For them, emotions are largely innate physiological and motor programs triggered by certain stimuli. Advocates of **cognitive theories of emotion** disagree. For them, emotions are products of thinking. What we feel in response to a situation is determined by how we interpret it (Scherer, 1988). The way we appraise situations influences whether we find them stressful (Lazarus & Folkman, 1984). If we see an upcoming job interview as a potential catastrophe, we will be hopelessly stressed; if we see it as a healthy challenge, we will be appropriately geared up for it. Moreover, for cognitive theorists, there are no discrete emotions, because the boundaries across emotions are fuzzy (Barrett & Russell, 1999; Ortony & Turner, 1990). They believe that there are as many different kinds of emotions as there are kinds of thoughts.

James-Lange theory of emotion
Theory proposing that emotions result from our interpretations of our bodily reactions to stimuli.

Display rules
Cross-cultural guidelines for how and when to express emotions.

Cognitive theories of emotion
Theories proposing that emotions are products of thinking.

James-Lange theory of emotion

Perhaps the oldest cognitive theory of emotion, and still one of the most influential, owes its origins to American psychologist William James (1890). Because Danish researcher Carl Lange (1885) advanced a similar version of this theory around the same time, psychologists refer to it as the **James-Lange theory of emotion**. According to the James–Lange theory, emotions result from our interpretations of our bodily reactions to stimuli.

To take James's famous example, imagine that while walking through the bush we come upon a snake. What happens next? Common wisdom tells us that we first become scared and then run away. Yet, as James recognised, the link between our fear and running away is only a correlation; this link does not demonstrate that our fear *causes* us to run away. Indeed, James and Lange argued that the causal arrow is reversed: *we are afraid because we run away.* That is, we observe our physiological and behavioural reactions to a stimulus, in this case our heart pounding, our palms sweating and our feet running, and then conclude that we must have been scared (see Figure 13.4).

In support of this theory, a researcher examined five groups of patients with injuries in different regions of their spinal cord (Hohmann, 1966). Patients with injuries high in their spinal cord had lost almost all of their bodily sensation, and those with lower injuries had lost only part of their bodily sensation. Just as James and Lange would have predicted, patients with higher spinal cord damage reported less emotion—fear and anger—than those with lower spinal cord damage. Presumably, patients with lower injuries could feel more of their bodies, which allowed them a greater range of emotional reactions. Still, some researchers have criticised these findings because of a possible experimenter expectancy effect: the researcher knew which spinal cord patients were which when he assessed their emotions, and this knowledge could have biased the results (Prinz, 2004).

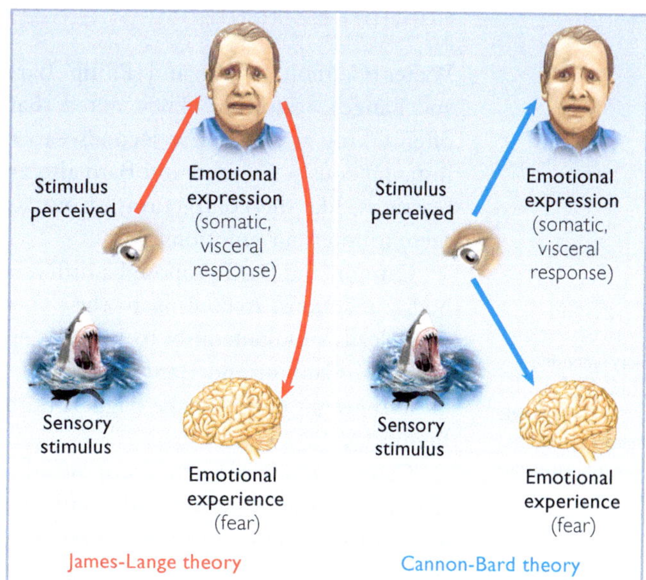

Figure 13.4 What triggers emotions? The James–Lange and Cannon–Bard theories differ in their views of how emotions are generated.
(**Source:** Adapted from Cardoso.)

Somatic marker theory

Few scientists today are strict believers in the James–Lange theory, but it continues to influence modern-day thinking about emotion. Antonio Damasio's (1994) **somatic marker theory** (*somatic* means 'physical') proposes that we use our 'gut reactions'—especially our autonomic responses, like our heart rate and sweating—to gauge how we should act. Damasio contends that this process occurs almost instantaneously, so we are typically unaware of it. According to Damasio, if we feel our heart pounding during a first date, we use that information as a 'marker' or signal to help us decide what to do next, like ask that person out for a second date. People with damage to the frontal cortex may make irrational decisions because the frontal cortex is the input station for information from the brain's sensory regions. In turn, the individual may have lost access to somatic markers of emotion (Damasio, 1994).

Somatic marker theory
Theory proposing that we use our 'gut reactions' to help us determine how we should act.

Still, it is not clear that we need to use somatic markers as guideposts for all of our decisions. There is evidence that people can make decisions solely on the basis of external knowledge and without any bodily feedback (Maia & McClelland, 2004). One team of investigators examined a group of patients who suffered from a rare condition called *pure autonomic failure* (PAF), which is marked by a deterioration of autonomic nervous system neurons beginning in middle age (Heims et al., 2004). These patients do not experience increases in autonomic activity, such as heart rate or sweating, in response to emotional stimuli. Yet the researchers found that these patients had no difficulty on a gambling task that required them to make decisions about monetary risks. These findings do not completely refute the somatic marker theory, as it is possible that somatic markers are helpful to us when making decisions. But they suggest that somatic markers are not *necessary* for wise choices, even if they sometimes give us a bit of extra guidance.

Cannon-Bard theory of emotion

Walter Cannon (1929) and Philip Bard (1942) pointed out several flaws with James's and Lange's reasoning. They noted that most physiological changes occur too slowly—often taking at least a few seconds—to trigger emotional reactions, which happen almost instantaneously. Cannon and Bard also argued that we are not aware of many of our bodily reactions, like the contractions of our stomach or liver. As a consequence, we cannot use them to infer our emotions.

Cannon and Bard proposed a different model for the correlation between emotions and bodily reactions. According to the **Cannon-Bard theory of emotion**, an emotion-provoking event leads simultaneously to both an emotion and bodily reactions. To return to James's example, Cannon and Bard would say that when we see a snake while walking in the bush, the sight of that snake triggers both fear and running at the same time (again refer to Figure 13.4).

Cannon-Bard theory of emotion Theory proposing that an emotion-provoking event leads simultaneously to an emotion and to bodily reactions.

Cannon and Bard further proposed that the *thalamus*, which is a relay station for the senses, triggers both an emotion and bodily reactions. Cannon and Bard were probably wrong about this, because later researchers showed that numerous regions of the limbic system, including the hypothalamus and the amygdala, also play key roles in emotion (Carlson & Hatfield, 1992; Plutchik & Kellerman, 1986). Still, their model of emotion has encouraged investigators to explore the bases of emotion in the brain.

Two-factor theory of emotion

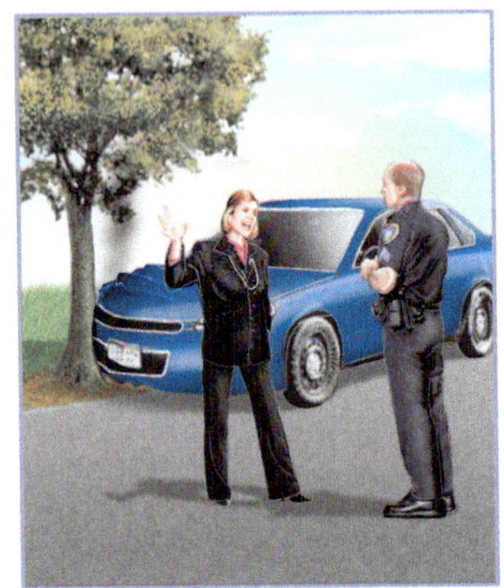

According to Schachter and Singer's two-factor theory of emotion, we first experience arousal after an emotion-provoking event, like a car accident, and then seek to interpret the cause of that arousal. The resulting label we attach to our arousal is the emotion.

Stanley Schachter and Jerome Singer (1962) argued that both the James–Lange model and the Cannon–Bard model of emotion were too simple. They agreed with James and Lange that our cognitive interpretations of our bodily reactions play a crucial role in emotions, but they disagreed with James and Lange that these bodily reactions are sufficient for emotion. According to their **two-factor theory of emotion** (Schachter & Singer, 1962), two psychological events are required to produce an emotion:

1. After encountering an emotion-provoking event, we experience an underdifferentiated state of arousal-that is, alertness. By 'undifferentiated', Schachter and Singer meant that this arousal is the same across emotions.
2. We try to explain the source of this autonomic arousal. Once we attribute the arousal to an occurrence, either an occurrence within us or an occurrence in the external environment, we experience an emotion. Once we figure out what is making us aroused, we 'label' that arousal with an emotion. This labelling process, Schachter and Singer proposed, typically occurs so rapidly that we are not even aware of it. According to this view, emotions are the explanations we attach to our arousal.

Two-factor theory of emotion Theory proposing that emotions are produced by an undifferentiated state of arousal along with an attribution (explanation) of that arousal.

To illustrate, imagine we are walking in the bush yet again and, sure enough, we come upon a snake. According to Schachter and Singer, we first become physiologically aroused; evolution assures that we do so that we are ready to fight—probably not an especially smart idea in this case—or flee. Then, we try to figure out the source of that arousal. You need not have a PhD in psychology to infer that our arousal probably has something to do with the snake. So we label this arousal as fear, and that is the emotion we experience.

It sounds plausible, but do our emotions really work this way? In a classic study, Schachter and Singer (1962) decided to find out. As a 'cover story', they informed participants that they were testing the effectiveness of a new vitamin supplement—'Suproxin'—on vision. But in reality, they were testing the effects of *adrenaline*, a chemical that produces physiological arousal. Schachter and Singer randomly assigned some participants to receive an injection of Suproxin (again, actually adrenaline) and others an injection of placebo.

While the adrenaline was entering their systems, Schachter and Singer randomly assigned participants to two additional conditions: one in which a confederate (an undercover research assistant) acted in a happy fashion while completing questionnaires, and second in which a confederate acted in an angry fashion while completing questionnaires. The confederate was blind as to whether participants had received an injection of adrenaline or the placebo. Finally, Schachter and Singer asked participants to describe how strongly they were experiencing different emotions.

Schachter and Singer's results dovetailed with two-factor theory. The emotions of the participants who had received the placebo were not influenced by the behaviour of the confederate, but the emotions of the participants who received adrenaline were. Participants exposed to the happy confederate reported feeling happier, and those exposed to the angry confederate reported feeling angrier—but in both cases only if they had received adrenaline. Emotion, Schachter and Singer concluded, requires *both* physiological arousal *and* an attribution of that arousal to an emotion- inducing event.

The award for the most creative test of the two-factor theory probably goes to two researchers Dutton & Aron (1974), who asked an attractive female confederate to approach male undergraduates on the University of British Columbia campus. She asked them for help with a survey and gave them her phone number in case they had any questions. Half of the time, she approached them on a sturdy bridge that did not move, and half of the time she approached them on a swaying suspension bridge high above a river. Although only 30 percent of males in the first condition called her, 60 percent of males in the second condition did. The wobbly bridge in the second condition presumably increased male students' arousal, leading them to feel more intense romantic emotions. In a related study of 'love at first fright', investigators approached participants either immediately before or after a roller-coaster ride and showed them a photograph of an attractive member of the opposite sex. Participants who had just got off the roller-coaster rated the person in the photograph as more attractive—and indicated more of an interest in dating him or her—than did participants who were just about to get on the roller-coaster (Meston & Frohlich, 2003).

Still, the support for two-factor theory has been mixed. Not all researchers have replicated Schachter and Singer's (1962) results (Marshall & Zimbardo, 1979; Maslach, 1979). Moreover, research suggests that, although arousal often intensifies emotions, emotions can occur in the absence of arousal (Reisenzein, 1983). Contrary to what Schachter and Singer claimed, arousal is not necessary for emotional experience.

Putting it all together

So which of these theories should we believe? As is so often the case in psychology, there is probably a kernel of truth in several explanations. Discrete emotions theory is probably correct that our emotional reactions are shaped in part by natural selection and that these reactions serve crucial adaptive functions. Nevertheless, discrete emotions theory does not exclude the possibility that our thinking influences our emotions in significant ways, as

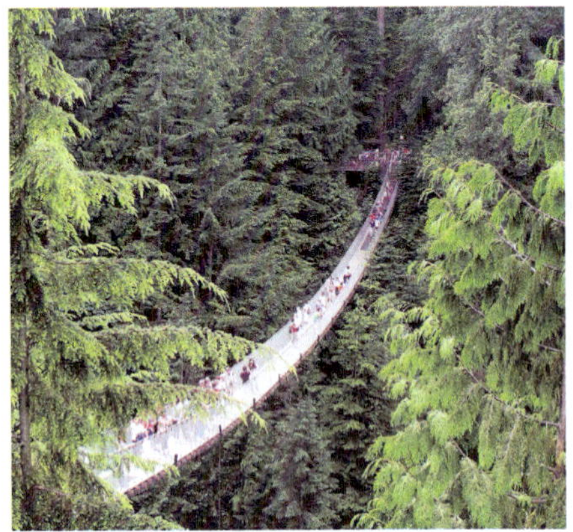

This swaying suspension bridge on the University of British Columbia campus allowed psychologists to test Schachter and Singer's two-factor theory of emotion. (**Source:** Samuel Strickler/Dreamstime.)

cognitive theorists propose. Indeed, the James–Lange and somatic marker theories are probably correct in assuming that our inferences concerning our bodily reactions can influence our emotional states. Finally, two-factor theory may also be right that physiological arousal plays a key role in the intensity of our emotional experiences, although it is unlikely that all emotions require such arousal.

Unconscious influences on emotion

In recent decades, researchers have become especially interested in *unconscious influences on emotion*: factors outside our awareness that can affect our feelings. One piece of evidence for unconscious influences on emotion comes from research on *automatic behaviours*.

Automatic generation of emotion

As we discussed earlier, research suggests that a good deal of our behaviour is produced automatically—that is, with no voluntary influence on our part (Bargh & Ferguson, 2000). Yet we often perceive such behaviour as intentional (Kirsch & Lynn, 1999; Wegner, 2002). The same may hold for our emotional reactions; many may be generated more or less automatically, like the knee-jerk reflex that the doctor elicits when she taps on your knees with a hammer.

For example, two investigators visually presented some participants with a set of words describing positive stimuli (such as 'friends' and 'music') and others describing negative stimuli (such as 'cancer' and 'cockroach'). These stimuli appeared so quickly that they were *subliminal*—that is, below the threshold for awareness. Even though participants could not identify what they saw at better-than-chance levels, those exposed to positive stimuli reported being in a better mood than those exposed to negative stimuli (Bargh & Chartrand, 1999).

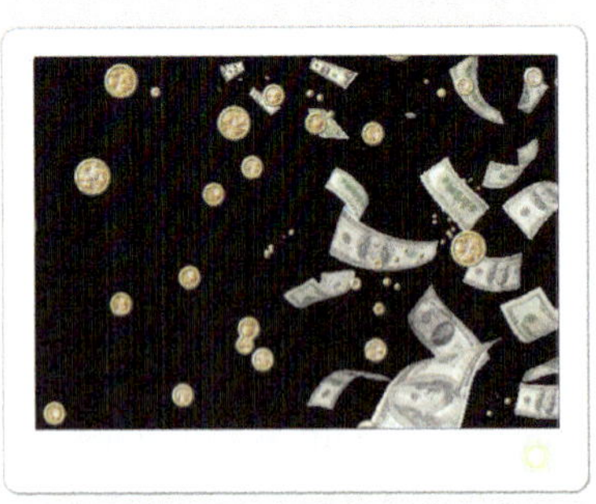

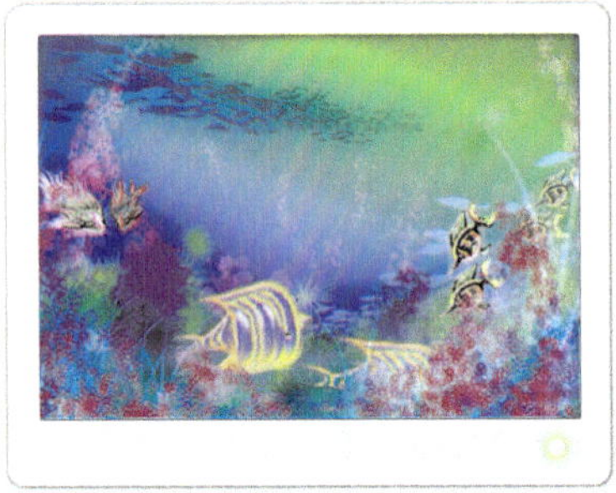

Stimuli can influence our emotional behaviour even when we do not recognise them as the culprits. In an American study, participants subtly reminded of money by watching a computer screensaver of floating currency (*top*) later put more physical distance between themselves and a stranger than did participants who watched a screensaver of floating fish (*bottom*), presumably because thinking of money makes people more self-centred (Vohs, Mead & Goode, 2006).

Mere exposure effect

- *Psychology: From Inquiry to Understanding*
- *Psychology: From Inquiry to Understanding*
- *Psychology: From Inquiry to Understanding*
- *Psychology: From Inquiry to Understanding*

After reading the four lines above, how do you feel about our textbook? Do you like it better than you did before?

Popular wisdom would say no. It tells us that 'familiarity breeds contempt': the more often we have seen or heard something, the more we come to dislike it. There is surely some truth to this notion, as most of us have had the experience of hearing a jingle on the radio that grates on our nerves increasingly with each passing repetition. Yet research by Robert Zajonc and others on the **mere exposure effect** suggests that the opposite is actually more common: that is, familiarity breeds *comfort* (Zajonc, 1968). The mere exposure effect refers to the fact that repeated exposure to a stimulus makes us more likely to feel favourably towards it (Bornstein, 1989; Kunst-Wilson & Zajonc, 1980).

Mere exposure effect
Phenomenon in which repeated exposure to a stimulus makes us more likely to feel favourably towards it.

Of course, the finding that we like things we have seen many times before is not itself terribly surprising. This correlation could be due to the fact that we repeatedly seek out things we like. If we love ice-cream, we are likely to spend more time seeing ice-cream than are people who hate ice-cream. So to find out whether mere exposure actually exerts an effect on preferences, we need to turn from correlational studies to experiments.

Some of the best evidence for the mere exposure effect derives from experiments using meaningless material, for which individuals are unlikely to have any prior feelings. Experiments show that repeated exposure to various stimuli, such as nonsense syllables (like 'zab' and 'gar'), Chinese letters (to non-Chinese participants) and polygons of various shapes, results in greater liking towards these stimuli compared with little or no exposure (see Figure 13.5). These effects have been replicated by multiple investigators using quite different stimuli, attesting to their generality. The mere exposure effect even extends to faces. We tend to prefer an image of ourselves as we appear in the mirror to an image of ourselves as we appear in a photograph (Mita, Dermer & Knight, 1977), probably because we see our reflection in the mirror just about every day. Our friends, in contrast, generally prefer the photographic image. Of course, advertisers are well aware of the mere exposure effect and capitalise on it mercilessly (Baker, 1999; Fang, Singh & AhluWalia, 2007; Pechman & Stewart, 1989). Repetitions of an advertisement tend to increase our liking for the product, especially if we are positively inclined towards it to begin with.

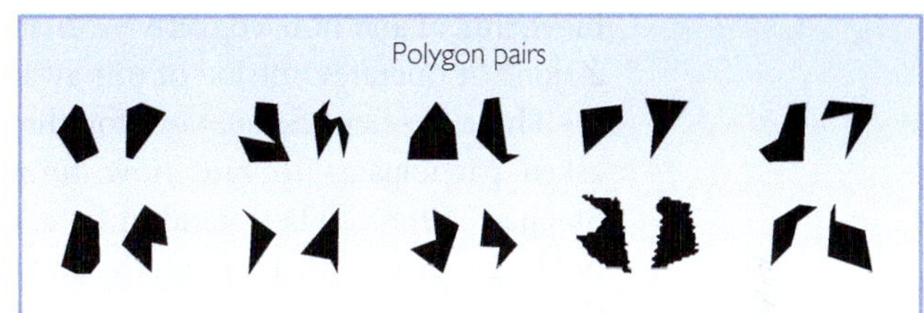

Figure 13.5 Which polygon pair do you prefer?

Pairs of polygons used in the mere exposure research of Robert Zajonc and his colleagues. Participants exposed repeatedly to only one polygon within the pair prefer that polygon, even if they do not recall having seen it.
(**Source:** Epley, 2006.)

There is evidence that the mere exposure effect can operate unconsciously, because it emerges even when experimenters present meaningless stimuli subliminally, below the threshold of awareness (Bornstein, 1989; Zajonc, 2001). Even when people aren't aware of having seen a stimulus, like a specific polygon, they report liking it better than stimuli, like slightly different polygons, they have never seen. Mere exposure effects may be even larger for subliminally than for *supraliminally* (consciously) presented stimuli (Bornstein, 1989). Still, there is controversy about just how enduring the mere exposure effect is. It seems to influence short-term, but not long-term, preferences (Lazarus, 1984).

No one knows why mere exposure effects occur. They may be an example of *habituation*, a primitive form of learning we examined earlier. The more frequently we encounter a stimulus without anything bad happening, the more comfortable we feel in its presence. Alternatively, we may prefer things we find easier to process (Harmon-Jones & Allen, 2001; Mandler, Nakamura & Van Zandt, 1987). The more often we experience something, the less effort it typically takes to comprehend it. Recall that we are *cognitive misers*: we prefer less mental work to more. So all other things being equal, you will like this paragraph better after having read it a few times than after you read it the first time!

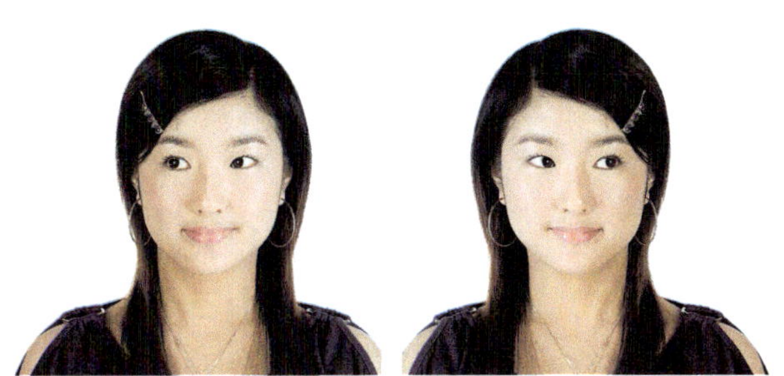

Most people prefer their mirror image to their image as taken by a photographer. In this case, this person is more likely to prefer the photograph on the left, presumably because she is more accustomed to this view of herself.
(**Source:** Nigel Riches/imagesource.com.)

Facial feedback hypothesis

If no one is near you, and you are not afraid of looking foolish, make a big smile and hold it for a while, maybe 15 seconds. How do you feel (other than silly)? Next, make a big frown, and again hold it for a while. How do you feel now?

Facial feedback hypothesis Theory that blood vessels in the face feed back temperature information to the brain, altering our experience of emotions.

According to the **facial feedback hypothesis**, you are likely to feel emotions that correspond to your facial features—first happy, and then sad or angry (Adelmann & Zajonc, 1989; Niedenthal, 2007; Zajonc, Murphy & Inglehart, 1989). This hypothesis originated with none other than Charles Darwin (1872), although Robert Zajonc revived it in the 1980s. Zajonc went beyond Darwin by proposing that changes in the blood vessels of the face 'feed back' temperature information to the brain, altering our emotions in predictable ways. Like James and Lange, Zajonc argued that our emotions typically arise from our behaviours and physiological reactions. But unlike James and Lange, Zajonc viewed this process as purely biochemical and non-cognitive—that is, as involving no thinking. Moreover, according to Zajonc, it operates outside of our awareness.

There is scientific support for the facial feedback hypothesis. In one study, researchers asked participants to rate how funny they found various cartoons (Strack, Martin & Stepper, 1988). They randomly assigned some participants to watch cartoons while holding a pen with their teeth, and others to watch cartoons while holding a pen with their lips. If you have a pen around, try doing both. You will discover that when you hold a pen with your teeth, you tend to smile; when you hold a pen with your lips, you tend to frown. Sure enough, the investigators found that participants who held a pen with their teeth rated the cartoons as funnier than did other participants.

Still, it is not clear that these effects work by means of facial feedback to the brain, as Zajonc claimed. An alternative hypothesis for these effects is classical conditioning. Over the course of our lives, we have experienced countless conditioning 'trials' in which we smile while feeling happy and frown while feeling unhappy. Eventually, smiles become conditioned stimuli for happiness, frowns for unhappiness.

Assess your knowledge FACT or FICTION?

1. Psychological research demonstrates that emotion and reason are direct opposites of each other. **(True/False)**
2. Some emotions, such as happiness, appear to be recognised by a substantial majority of people in all cultures. **(True/False)**
3. According to the James–Lange theory, emotions follow from our bodily reactions. **(True/False)**
4. Two-factor theory proposes that arousal is necessary for emotion. **(True/False)**
5. The mere exposure effect refers to the finding that repeated presentations of a stimulus lead to less liking of that stimulus. **(True/False)**

Answers: (1) F; (2) T; (3) T; (4) T; (5) F

Nonverbal expression of emotion: the eyes, bodies and cultures have it

Much of our emotional expression is nonverbal. Not only do our facial expressions frequently change when we experience a strong emotion, but so do our gestures and postures. What is more, our nonverbal behaviours are often more valid indicators of our emotions than our words, largely because we are better at disguising our verbal language than our gestures and tone of voice (DePaulo, 1992). **Nonverbal leakage**—an unconscious spillover of emotions into nonverbal behaviour—is often a powerful cue that we're trying to hide an emotion. In sharp contrast to our verbal behaviours, we're frequently unaware of our nonverbal behaviours. So when we ever so subtly roll our eyes while agreeing to our boss's unreasonable request to house-sit her dogs over the weekend ('Sure, I'd be happy to do it'), we can be confident that the 'eyes have it'.

Nonverbal leakage
Unconscious spillover of emotions into nonverbal behaviour.

We often take for granted how important nonverbal behaviour is to our everyday communication—until we do not have access to it. Without nonverbal cues to our emotions, embarrassing miscommunications sometimes arise. Many of us have experienced this effect through email, when a person to whom we send an innocuous or humorous message misinterprets it as hostile. Without being able to hear our vocal inflections or see our facial emotions, recipients of our email messages may misinterpret what we meant to say. This problem is exacerbated by the fact that we overestimate how easily others can figure out the intended meanings of our email messages (Kruger et al., 2005). More broadly, psychologists refer to this problem as the *curse of knowledge*: when we know something, in this case what we intend to say, we often make the mistake of thinking others know it, too (Birch & Bloom, 2003).

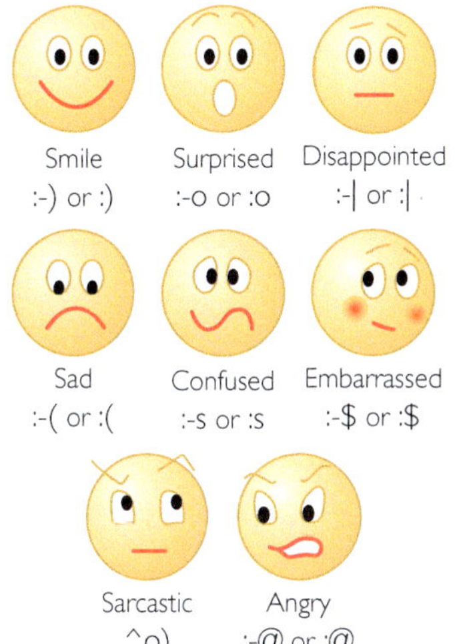

Figure 13.6 Emoticons. Because email messages are devoid of nonverbal cues, people have developed a variety of 'emoticons' to convey various emotions that might not be obvious over email and instant messaging.
(**Source:** Microsoft Corporation.)

Body language and gestures

Our postures can convey a lot about our emotional states. Slumped posture can convey sadness, and upright posture can convey happiness or excitement, although an upright posture involving a lot of body tension may also convey anger (Duclos et al, 1989). When interpreting the emotional states of others, we typically take both facial and body information into account. Research on embodied cognition even shows that our postures affect our readiness to engage in certain behaviours. When participants are insulted, they are more likely to display brain responses typical of anger (activation of the left frontal lobes) when sitting straight up than when reclining (Harmon-Jones & Peterson, 2009). That is probably because we are more prepared to strike others when we are upright than lying down. And when experimenters ask participants to adopt 'high power' poses, which are marked by having one's body and arms spread open wide, participants are more likely to feel powerful and to gamble on money than participants who adopt 'low power' poses (Carney, Cuddy & Yap, 2010). So if you want to feel powerful, look powerful.

Gestures

Gestures come in a seemingly endless variety of forms. When talking, we often use *illustrators* (Ekman, 2001), gestures that highlight or accentuate speech. For example, while making a particularly important point, we may forcefully move our hands forward. When stressed, we may engage in *manipulators*, gestures in which one body part strokes, presses, bites or otherwise touches another body part. For example, while revising for an exam, we may twirl our hair or bite our fingernails.

We are all familiar with *emblems* (Ekman, 2001), gestures that convey conventional meanings that are recognised by members of a culture, such as the hand wave, the OK sign and the nodding of the head. Some emblems are surprisingly consistent across cultures, such as crossing one's fingers as a sign of hoping for good luck (Plutchik, 2003). Yet others differ across cultures, which should serve as a word of warning to unwary foreign travellers

(Archer, 1997). For example, the 'thumbs up' is a sign of approval among Westerners, but an insult in much of the Muslim world. Many overseas students from the Middle East find it challenging to adjust their emotional responses to this emblem.

Personal space

Have you ever walked into a virtually empty movie theatre and taken a seat, only to find that someone sits right next to you? Or have you approached someone to whom you were attracted, only to find them taking a step away from you? These are among the phenomena addressed by **proxemics**—the study of personal space.

Proxemics
Study of personal space.

Anthropologist Edward Hall (1966), who coined the term *proxemics*, observed that personal distance is correlated positively with emotional distance. That is, the further we stand from a person, the less emotionally close we usually feel to him or her, and vice versa. But there are exceptions. When we are trying to intimidate people, we typically get closer to them. For example, lawyers tend to stand closer to witnesses they are challenging (Brodsky et al., 1999).

According to Hall, there are four levels of personal space. Nevertheless, like most distinctions in psychology, the separations between these levels are not clear-cut:

1. *Public distance* (3 metres or more): typically used for public speaking, such as lecturing.
2. *Social distance* (1–3 metres): typically used for conversations among strangers and casual acquaintances.
3. *Personal distance* (0.5–1 metre): typically used for conversations among close friends or romantic partners.
4. *Intimate distance* (0–0.5 metres): typically used for kissing, hugging, whispering 'sweet nothings' and affectionate touching.

When these implicit rules are violated, we usually feel uncomfortable, as when a stranger gets 'in our face' to ask us for a favour.

Hall (1976) argued that cultures differ in personal space. In many Latin and Middle Eastern countries, personal space is relatively close, whereas in many Scandinavian and Asian countries, personal space is more distant. Nevertheless, data suggest that although these cultural differences are real and often important in their implications for everyday interaction, they are not as large as Hall believed (Hayduk, 1983; Jones, 1979). There are also sex differences in personal space, with women tending to prefer closer space than men (Vrugt & Kerkstra, 1984). Personal space also increases from childhood to early adulthood (Hayduk, 1983), largely because the young have not yet developed clear interpersonal boundaries.[B]

[B] Lilienfeld, S. O., Lynn, S. J., Namy, L. L., Woolf, N. J., Jamieson, G., Marks, A., & Slaughter, V. (2015). Emotion and motivation. In S. O. Lilienfeld, S. J. Lynn, L. L. Namy, N. J. Woolf, G. Jamieson, A. Marks, & V. Slaughter (Eds.), *Psychology: From inquiry to understanding* (2nd ed., pp. 449–460). Melbourne, VIC: Pearson Australia.

Summary

- Emotions are more fleeting than moods.
- Moods are not usually directed at a person or event.
- The time of day and day of the week, stressful events, social activities and sleep patterns are all factors that influence emotions and moods.
- Emotions and moods are driven by a number of personal and environmental influences. These include personality, the moment in time, the weather, stress, the social situation, sleep, exercise, age and gender.
- According to discrete emotions theory, humans experience a small number of distinct emotions.
- Ekman and his colleagues concluded that there are about seven primary emotions, and these are cross-culturally universal.
- The James-Lange theory of emotion proposes that emotions result from our interpretations of our bodily reactions to stimuli.
- Antonio Damasio's (1994) somatic marker theory proposes that we use our 'gut reactions' to help us determine how we should act.
- The Cannon-Bard theory of emotion proposes that an emotion-provoking event leads simultaneously to an emotion and to bodily reactions.
- The two-factor theory of emotion proposes that emotions are produced by an undifferentiated state of arousal along with an attribution (explanation) of that arousal.
- Much of our emotional expression is nonverbal. Not only do our facial expressions frequently change when we experience a strong emotion, but so do our gestures and postures.

Review questions

A. Fill in the missing words to complete the following statements.

1. __________ is a term that describes a range of feelings experienced. __________ are intense feelings that are derived from a person, situation or experience, are an outward expression of behaviour that is action-oriented in nature. __________ are feelings that are often less intense than __________ and are cognitive in nature.
2. Affect is a broad term that can be experienced in the form of emotions or moods. Is this statement true or false? ___________
3. Cannon-Bard's theory of emotion was developed in response to the James-Lang theory of emotion. In contrast, Cannon-Bard argues that we experience emotions and physiological arousal _________________.
4. The two-factor theory of emotion states that emotion is based on two components being _________________ and _________________.
5. _________________________ (1885) is one of the most influential and longest standing theories of emotion. The theory states that emotions result from our interpretation of physiological reactions to stimuli. For example, I see a bear. My heart starts racing and my muscles tense. I feel scared and run away.

B. Please select one statement that best answers each of the following questions.

6. Evolutionary psychology argues that emotions are essential daily life experiences as:
   - **a)** emotions are the product of cultures and societies
   - **b)** different individuals will respond to the same event with different emotions, or the same individual may at different times respond differently to the same stimulus
   - **c)** the experience of both positive and negative emotions serve a functional purpose
   - **d)** all of the above
7. Low positive affect includes which of the following moods?
   - **a)** sadness, depression, boredom and stress
   - **b)** sadness, depression, stress, fatigue
   - **c)** sadness, depression, boredom, fatigue
   - **d)** sadness, depression, nervousness, fatigue
8. Which of the following best describe a secondary emotion?
   - **a)** emotions we experience in relation to other emotional reactions
   - **b)** feeling fear, anger, sadness or happiness
   - **c)** a person may feel guilty as a result of becoming sad or depressed
   - **d)** both a) and c)
9. Which of the following statements best describes Antonia Damasio's (1994) somatic marker theory?
   - **a)** the emotions we experience are a result of our thinking
   - **b)** our 'gut reactions' such as our autonomic responses are unreliable in guiding how we should respond to a situation or event
   - **c)** our 'gut reactions' such as our autonomic responses guide how we should respond to a situation or event
   - **d)** none of the above

10. Which of the following describes a non-verbal expression of emotions?

a) gestures

b) nonverbal leakage

c) proxemics

d) all of the above

CHAPTER 14

Stress

The content in this section has been compiled from:

Lilienfeld, Chapter 12

Lilienfeld, S. O., Lynn, S. J., Namy, L. L., Woolf, N. J., Jamieson, G., Marks, A., & Slaughter, V. (2015). Stress, coping and health. In S. O. Lilienfeld, S. J. Lynn, L. L. Namy, N. J. Woolf, G. Jamieson, A. Marks, & V. Slaughter (Eds.), *Psychology: From inquiry to understanding* (2nd ed., pp. 503–510, 510–521). Melbourne, VIC: Pearson Australia.

Smith, Chapter 5

Smith, J. (1993). The transactional matrix. In J. Smith (Ed.), *Understanding stress and coping* (pp. 69–89). New York, NY: Macmillan.

Donatelle, Chapter 3

Donatelle, R. J. (2015). Managing stress and coping with life's challenges. In R. J. Donatelle (Ed.), *Health: The basics* (11th ed., pp. 75–83). Upper Saddle River, NJ: Pearson Education.

Smith, Chapter 8

Smith, J. (1993). The transactional matrix. In J. Smith (Ed.), *Understanding stress and coping* (pp. 133–146). New York, NY: Macmillan.

CHAPTER 14

Stress

Stress is a type of response, which can consist of tension, discomfort and physical symptoms that arise when a situation (i.e. a stressor – a type of stimulus) strains our ability to cope effectively. In the health care setting, it is essential to understand the client and/or patient as a whole. As members of a health care team, it is important to be able to recognise if or when an individual is encountering stressful stimuli, and identify if they have the coping resources to manage the process and meaning of the stressful stimuli. This chapter examines key theories of stress to explain both the physiological and psychosocial components of stress to foster your 'stress-literacy' – (i.e. provide you with powerful knowledge for helping and supporting others as well as yourself)!

After studying this chapter you should be able to:

- Explain how stress is defined
- Identify different approaches to measuring stress:
  - Social Readjustment Rating Scale
  - Hassles Scale
- Describe how people adapt to stress: Selye's general adaptation syndrome (GAS)
- Describe the Transactional model of coping and appraisal: Lazarus and Folkman (1984)
- Describe the biopsychosocial effects of stress
- Describe how stress can impact health
- Describe the role of social support and different types of control in coping with stress.

What is stress?

Before we proceed further, it is important to distinguish two terms—*stress* and *trauma*— that are commonly confused. **Stress**—a type of response—consists of the tension, discomfort or physical symptoms that arise when a situation, called a *stressor*—a type of stimulus—strains our ability to cope effectively. A *traumatic* event is a stressor that is so severe that it can produce long-term psychological or health consequences.

The field's thinking about stress has evolved over the years (Cooper & Drewe, 2004). Before the 1940s, scientists rarely used the term 'stress' outside of the engineering profession (Hayward, 1960, p. 185), where it referred to stresses on materials and building structures. A building was said to withstand stress if it did not collapse under intense pressure. It was not until 1944 that the term *stress* found its way into the psychological literature (Jones & Bright, 2001). This engineering analogy highlights the notion that 'if the body were like a machine and machines are subject to wear and tear then so too would be the body' (Doublet, 2000, p. 48). But, just as two buildings can withstand differing amounts of stress before weakening and collapsing, people differ widely in their personal resources, the meaning and significance they attach to stressful events, and their ability to grapple with them.

Stress in the eye of the beholder: three approaches

Researchers have approached the study of stress in three different, yet interrelated, ways (Kessler, Price & Wortman, 1985). Each approach has yielded valuable insights, illuminating the big and small events that generate distress and the ways we perceive and respond to stressful situations.

Stressors as stimuli

The stressors-as-stimuli approach focuses on identifying different types of stressful events. This approach has succeeded in pinpointing categories of events that most people find dangerous and unpredictable, as well as the people who are most susceptible to stress following different events (Collins et al., 2003; Costa & McCrae, 1990). For example, first-year university students show a greater response to such negative life events as the break-up of a relationship, than older men or women (Jackson & Finney, 2002). When people are retired, the combination of low income and physical disability can make matters worse, suggesting that stressful situations can produce cumulative effects (Smith et al., 2005).

Victims of natural disasters sometimes suffer from collective trauma that damages the bonds among them. In the aftermath of the Black Saturday bushfires in Victoria, survivors and state government officials argued over whether or not enough had been done to alert community members to the severity and threat of the fires. But disasters can also unify communities and bring out the best in us, exemplified in Victoria in the numerous stories of people risking their lives to warn others of the approaching fires. Indeed, stressful circumstances that touch the lives of an entire community can increase social awareness, cement interpersonal bonds, and enhance a variety of positive personal characteristics (Peterson & Seligman, 2003).

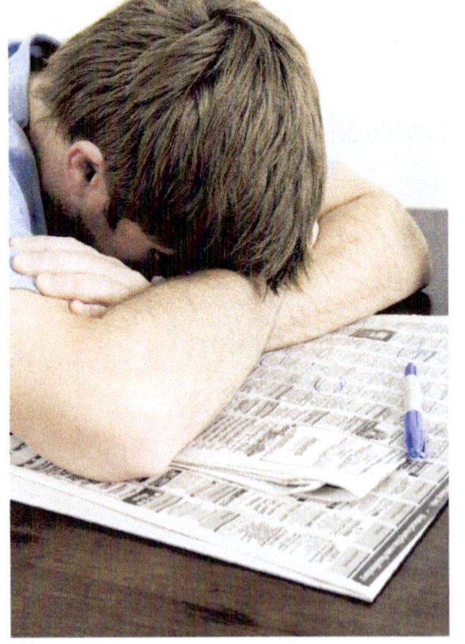

The stress of unemployment includes not only the frustration and despair of looking for a new job, but the economic hardship of living on a sharply reduced income.
(**Source:** Stephanie Swartz/Dreamstime.)

Stress as a response

Stress researchers also study stress as a response—that is, they assess people's psychological and physical reactions to stressful circumstances. Typically, scientists expose participants to independent variables such as stress-producing stimuli; in other cases, they study people who have encountered real-life stressors. Then they measure a host of dependent variables: stress-related feelings such as depression, hopelessness and hostility; and physiological responses such as heart rate, blood pressure and the release of stress hormones called **corticosteroids**. These hormones activate the body and prepare us for stressful circumstances. But measuring the size and impact of stressors on mental and physical functioning can be challenging.

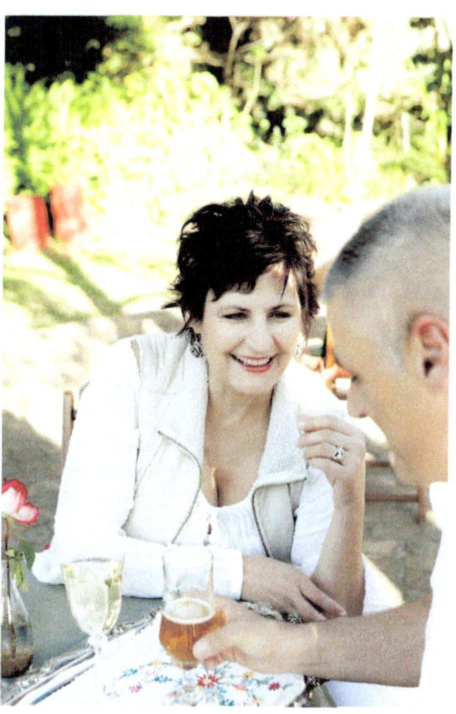

Emotion-focused coping may encourage people who have divorced to begin dating again.
(**Source:** Luba V Nel/Dreamstime.)

Stress as a transaction

Stress is a subjective experience. Some people are devastated by the break-up of a meaningful relationship, whereas others are optimistic about the opportunity to start afresh. People's varied reactions to the same event suggest that we can view stress as a transaction between people and their environments (Coyne & Holroyd, 1982; Lazarus, 1999; Lazarus & Folkman, 1984). Researchers who study stress as a transaction examine how people interpret and cope with stressful events. Richard Lazarus and his colleagues contended that a critical factor determining whether we experience an event as stressful is our appraisal—that is, our evaluation—of the event. When we encounter a potentially threatening event, we initially engage in **primary appraisal**—that is, we first decide whether the event is harmful and then make a **secondary appraisal** about how well we can cope with it (Lazarus & Folkman, 1984).

When we believe we cannot cope, we are more likely to experience a full-blown stress reaction than when we believe we can (Lazarus, 1999). When we are optimistic and think we can achieve our goals, we are more likely to engage in **problem-focused coping**, a coping strategy in which we tackle life's challenges head-on (Carver & Scheier, 1999; Lazarus & Folkman, 1984). When situations arise that we cannot avoid or control, we are more likely to adopt **emotion-focused coping**, a coping strategy in which we try to place a positive spin on our feelings or predicaments and engage in behaviours to reduce painful emotions (Carver, Scheier & Weintraub, 1989; Lazarus & Folkman, 1984). After the break-up of a relationship, we may remind ourselves that we were unhappy months before it occurred and look forward to meeting someone new.

Corticosteroids
Stress hormones that activate the body and prepare us to respond to stressful circumstances.

Primary appraisal
Initial decision regarding whether an event is harmful.

Secondary appraisal.
Perceptions regarding our ability to cope with an event that follow primary appraisal.

Problem-focused coping
Coping strategy by which we tackle life's challenges head-on.

Emotion-focused coping
Coping strategy that features a positive outlook on feelings or situations accompanied by behaviours that reduce painful emotions.

No two stresses are created equal: measuring stress

Measuring stress is a tricky business, largely because what is exceedingly stressful for one person, like an argument with a boss, may be a mere annoyance for another. Two scales—the Social Readjustment Rating Scale and the Hassles Scale—endeavour to gauge the nature and impact of differing stressful events.

Major life events

Adopting the view that stressors are stimuli, David Holmes and his colleagues developed the Social Readjustment Rating Scale (SRRS), the first of many efforts to measure life events systematically. The SRRS is based on 43 life events such as 'jail term' and 'personal injury or illness', ranked in terms of their stressfulness as rated by participants (Holmes & Rahe, 1967; Miller & Rahe, 1997) (see Figure 14.1). Studies using the SRRS and related measures

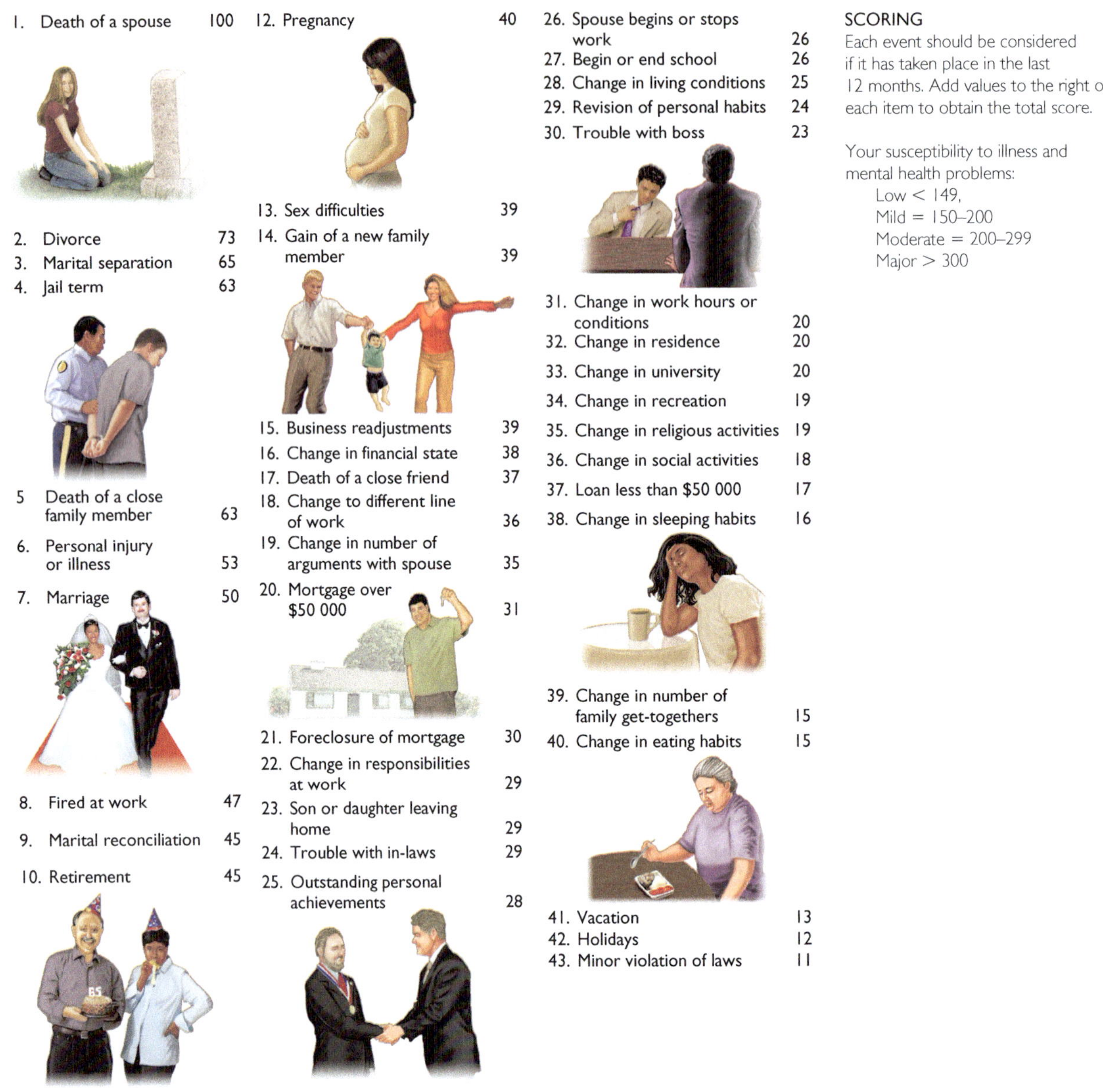

Figure 14.1 Social readjustment rating scale.
(**Source:** Holmes & Rahe, 1967.)

indicate that the number of stressful events people report over the previous year or so is associated with a variety of physical disorders (Dohrenwend & Dohrenwend, 1974; Holmes & Masuda, 1974) and psychological disorders like depression (Coyne, 1992; Holahan & Moos, 1991; Schmidt et al., 2004).

Nevertheless, the sheer number of stressful life events is far from a perfect predictor of who will become physically or psychologically ill (Coyne & Racioppo, 2000). That is because this approach to measuring stressors doesn't consider other crucial factors, including people's interpretation of events, coping behaviours and resources, and difficulty recalling events accurately (Coyne & Racioppo, 2000; Lazarus, 1999). In addition, it neglects to take into account some of the more 'chronic', or ongoing, stressors that many individuals experience.

Even subtle forms of discrimination or differential treatment based on race, gender, sexual orientation or religion, for example, can be a significant source of stress even though they rarely are prompted by or lead to a single stressful event we can check off a list. This approach also neglects the fact that some stressful life events, such as divorce and troubles with the boss, can be *consequences* rather than *causes* of people's psychological problems (Depue & Monroe, 1986). That is because people's psychological difficulties, such as severe depression and anxiety, can create a host of interpersonal problems, such as difficult interactions with loved ones and co-workers.

Hassles: don't sweat the small stuff

We have all had days when just about everything goes wrong and everybody seems to get on our nerves. Our daily lives are often loaded with **hassles**, minor annoyances or nuisances that strain our ability to cope. But can a lot of hassles add up to be as taxing as the monumental events that shake the foundations of our world?

Hassles
Minor annoyances or nuisances that strain our ability to cope.

Researchers (DeLongis, Folkman & Lazarus, 1988; Kanner et al., 1981) developed the Hassles Scale to measure how stressful events, ranging from small annoyances to major daily pressures, impact our adjustment. Both major life events and hassles are associated with poor general health. Nevertheless, the frequency and perceived severity of hassles are better predictors of physical health, depression and anxiety than are major life events (Fernandez & Sheffield, 1996; Kanner et al., 1981).

Still, it is possible that major stressful events are the real culprits, because they set us off when we already feel hassled, or create hassles with which we then need to cope. To test this alternative hypothesis, researchers have used statistical procedures to show that even when the influence of major life events is subtracted from the mix, hassles still predict psychological adjustment (Forshaw, 2002; Kanner et al., 1981).

Yet questions about the measurement of hassles remain. Some of the items on the scale, such as difficulties with relaxing and insomnia, may reflect symptoms of psychological disorders, such as depression or anxiety, rather than hassles (Monroe, 1983). However, when the scale developers (DeLongis, Folkman & Lazarus, 1988) revised the scale by removing all words related to symptoms, they found that hassles were still associated with health outcomes.

To recap, it is important to assess not only events that require major life adaptations but everyday hassles as well. Information about how people appraise stressful situations (Peacock & Wong, 1990), their coping abilities and strategies in specific situations (Carver, 1997), and their goals and available social support (Billings & Moos, 1984) can also help us predict who will and will not thrive in the face of potentially stressful circumstances (Brown & Harris, 1978; 1986).

Assess your knowledge — FACT or FICTION?

1. Most people at one time or another will experience an extremely stressful event. **(True/False)**
2. The effects of stressors can be cumulative. **(True/False)**
3. Natural disasters may sometimes result in stronger community bonds. **(True/False)**
4. According to the stress as a transaction viewpoint, almost all people respond to stressful events in the same way. **(True/False)**
5. Major life events have a greater effect on adjustment than do everyday hassles. **(True/False)**

Answers: (1) T; (2) T; (3) T; (4) F; (5) F

How we adapt to stress: change and challenge

As anyone who has had to confront a harrowing event, such as a car accident or a high-pressure interview for a big job, knows, adapting to stress is not easy. Yet natural selection has endowed us with a set of responses for coping with anxiety-provoking circumstances.

The mechanics of stress: Selye's general adaptation syndrome

In 1956, Canadian doctor Hans Selye ignited the field of modern-day stress research by publishing *The Stress of Life*, a landmark book that unveiled his decades of study on the effects of prolonged stress on the body. Selye's search for a new sex hormone in rats led him to discover that animals reacted with similar physical symptoms to a variety of injections. Ironically, Selye never discovered a new sex hormone. However, his genius was to recognise a connection between his injections and symptoms of stress in the animals, including stomach ulcers and increases in the size of the adrenal gland, which produces stress hormones. Selye further connected this stress response in animals with his observations of ill patients, who showed a consistent pattern of stress-related responses.

Dovetailing with the engineering analogy we have already discussed, Selye believed that too much stress leads to breakdowns. He argued that we are equipped with a sensitive physiology that responds to stressful circumstances by kicking us into high gear. He called the pattern of responding to stress the **general adaptation syndrome (GAS)**. According to Selye, all prolonged stressors take us through three stages of adaptation: *alarm, resistance* and *exhaustion* (see Figure 14.2).

General adaptation syndrome (GAS) Stress-response pattern proposed by Hans Selye that consists of three stages: alarm, resistance and exhaustion.

To illustrate key aspects of the GAS, and the extent to which our appraisals determine our reactions to stress, consider the experience of a participant in a treatment study for acrophobia (fear of heights) run by University of Queensland researchers (Coelho et al., 2008). We will call the participant Mark, and home in on what he experienced during the third treatment session. As Mark stood on an eighth floor balcony of a downtown hotel, his cold, clammy hands clutched the railing. His mouth was dry. His heart pounded. His breathing was rapid and shallow. He felt light-headed and dizzy. Images of bodies falling from buildings that he had seen on television popped uncontrollably into his mind. On some level he knew he was safe, but that did not help.

Mark knows he is safe because he is not actually on a hotel balcony; he is in a virtual environment, created by sophisticated, computer-controlled equipment that simulates the experience. The head-mounted display that Mark wears provides him with visual input specifying being up very high, and when he moves, the world below appears to shift as if he were looking at it from on high. Altogether, the effect is so convincing that much of the time he forgets he is in a laboratory.

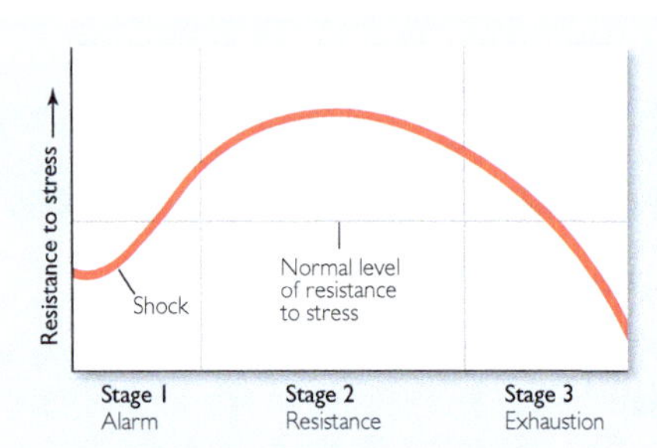

Figure 14.2 Selye's general adaptation syndrome. According to Selye's general adaptation syndrome, our level of resistance to stress drops during the alarm phase, increases during the resistance phase, and drops again during the exhaustion phase.
(**Source:** Adapted from Selye, 1956.)

Over the course of three sessions, Mark successfully confronted and tamed his fear of heights. In treatment, he learned anxiety management techniques, including deep breathing, and learned to recognise that his uncomfortable physical reactions are responses to his negative thoughts about being up high. He was 'virtually' exposed to higher and higher balconies and encouraged to walk back and forth across them. Research shows that 70 percent of participants who complete virtual exposure therapy like this become less afraid (Rothbaum et al, 2006). We can examine Mark's experiences in terms of the GAS.

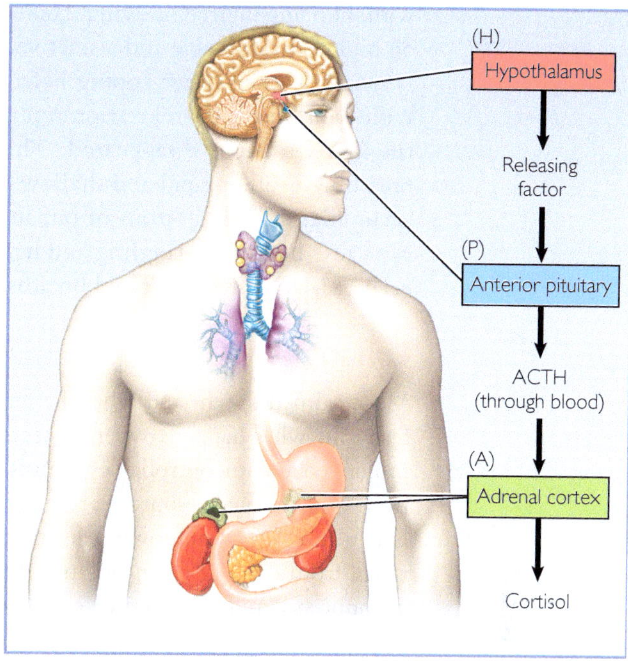

Figure 14.3 The hypothalamus-pituitary-adrenal (HPA) axis.

The alarm reaction

Selye's first stage, the *alarm reaction*, involves excitation of the autonomic nervous system, the discharge of the stress hormone adrenaline, and physical symptoms of anxiety. Joseph LeDoux (1996) and others have identified the seat of anxiety within a region of the midbrain—dubbed the *emotional brain*—that consists of the amygdala, hypothalamus and hippocampus. Mark's swift emotional reaction to his perception of falling is tripped largely by the amygdala, where vital emotional memories are stored and create gut feelings of a possible fall.

The hypothalamus sits atop a mind–body link known as the *hypothalamus-pituitary-adrenal* (HPA) axis, shown in Figure 14.3. When the hypothalamus (H) receives signals of fear, it hooks up with the pituitary gland (P), which releases hormones, including adrenaline, that trigger anxiety. Blood pressure rises as adrenaline (A) readies Mark for the **fight-or-flight response**, which Walter Cannon first described in 1915. This response is a set of physiological or psychological reactions that mobilise us to either confront or leave a threatening situation. Cannon noted that when people or animals face a threat, they have two options: *fight* (actively attack the threat or cope in the immediate situation) or *flee* (escape). Of course, Mark can take flight from the balcony and go inside the virtual hotel room, but given that he has agreed to complete the virtual reality (VR) treatment, he is 'stuck' confronting the source of his anxiety. So his fear escalates, with his hippocampus retrieving terrifying images in the news of people falling from great heights.

Fight-or-flight response
Physical and psychological reaction that mobilises people and animals to either defend themselves (fight) or escape (flee) a threatening situation.

Resistance

After the initial rush of adrenaline, Mark enters Selye's second stage of the GAS: *resistance*. He adapts to the stressor and finds ways to cope with it. The instant Mark's hippocampus detected danger from the first apparent view of the city below, it opened up a gateway to portions of his cerebral cortex, which LeDoux (1996) called the 'thinking brain'. Confronted with a stressful situation, we examine each new development as it unfolds, consider alternative solutions and direct our efforts towards constructing a coping plan.

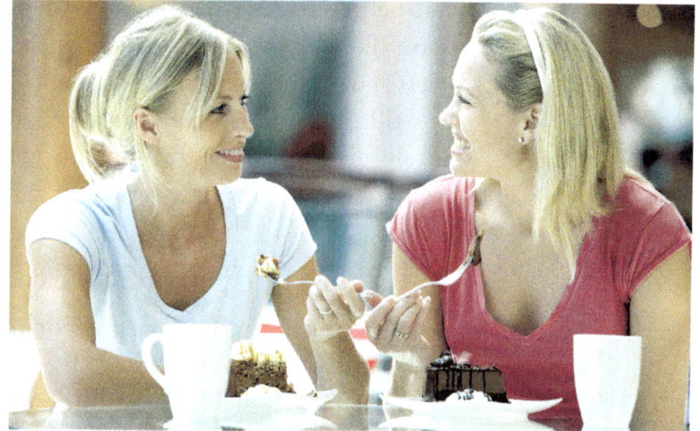

In stressful times, women often rely on friendships for support and comfort, a pattern that psychologist Shelley Taylor has called 'tend and befriend'. **(Source:** Monkey Business Images/Dreamstime.)

At one point, Mark experienced a sudden impulse to tear off the VR headset, but his basal ganglia, linked to the frontal cortex of his thinking brain, wisely led him to think better of it. Mark slowly but surely got a handle on his fears. He reminded himself that people live in tall apartment buildings all over the world, without being injured or dying. He recalled that most people consider views of the city from on high to be desirable and attractive.

Mark learned other coping behaviours. He reminded himself to breathe slowly, and with each breath his relaxation replaced tension. He no longer felt light-headed, and his tingling sensations disappeared. This exercise helps because when we are anxious our breathing is often rapid and shallow. When we do not exhale sufficiently, carbon dioxide accumulates at the bottom of our lungs, and even tiny increases in carbon dioxide level can cause numbness, tingling and light-headedness. Excess oxygen that accumulated with each of Mark's shallow, rapid breaths made his heart beat strongly and rapidly.

Exhaustion

Mark calmed down, and when he left the simulated balcony he felt more in control of his fear. But what happens when a stressor, such as wartime combat lasting months, is more prolonged and uncontrollable? This is when the third stage of Selye's GAS—*exhaustion*—sets in. If our personal resources are limited and we lack good coping measures, our resistance may ultimately break down, causing our levels of activation to bottom out. The results can range from damage to an organ system, to depression and anxiety, to a breakdown in the immune system (which we discuss later in the chapter).

The diversity of stress responses

Not all of us react to stressors with a fight-or-flight response. Our reactions vary from one stressor to another, and these reactions may be shaped by gender.

Fight or flight, or tend and befriend?

Tend and befriend
Reaction that mobilises people to nurture (tend) or seek social support (befriend) under stress.

Shelley Taylor and her colleagues coined the catchy phrase **tend and befriend** to describe a common pattern of reacting to stress among women (Taylor et al., 2000), although some men display it, too. Taylor observed that in times of stress, women generally rely on their social contacts and nurturing abilities—they *tend* to those around them and to themselves—more than men do. When stressed out, women typically *befriend*, or turn to others for support.

That is not to say that women lack a self-preservation instinct. They do not shirk from defending themselves and their children or from attempting to escape when physically threatened. However, compared with men, women generally have more to lose—especially when they are pregnant, nursing or caring for children—if they are injured or killed fighting or fleeing. Therefore, over the course of evolutionary history, they have developed a tend-and-befriend rather than a fight-or-flight pattern of reacting to stressful circumstances to boost the odds of their and their offspring's survival. The hormone *oxytocin* further counters stress and promotes the tend-and-befriend response (Kosfeld et al., 2005; Taylor et al., 2000).

Still, men and women are more alike than different in how they respond to stressors. Surely many men are invested in close relationships and caring for children, and many women react with a fight-or-flight response when endangered.

Long-lasting stress reactions

Bad things happen to all of us. For most of us, life goes on. But others experience long-lasting psychological repercussions, including posttraumatic stress disorder (Meichenbaum, 1994; Yehuda et al., 1993). On the morning of 26 December 2004, 20-year-old Sumithra was preparing to leave her village home on the west coast of Sri Lanka after a short holiday from university, to return to the city to prepare for final exams. After saying her temporary goodbyes, she set off for the bus station. On the way, she heard people shouting that the sea was approaching. She climbed onto the roof of a nearby building and watched as the first wave of the 2004 Boxing Day tsunami rushed by, taking people and debris with it. Afterwards, she ran home to find her house and family gone. She was taken to safety by neighbours before the second and third waves came. Over the next week, Sumithra found her siblings and parents in different camps around the area. She returned with them to rebuild their home, but she suffered constant fear of a new wave coming. She could not sleep and would not return to university for fear of being separated from those she loved (Hettiarachchi, 2007).

Sumithra displays some of the hallmark symptoms of *posttraumatic stress disorder* (PTSD), a condition that sometimes follows extremely stressful life events. Its telltale symptoms include vivid memories, feelings and images of traumatic experiences, known commonly as *flashbacks*. Other symptoms of PTSD include efforts to avoid reminders of the trauma, feeling detached or estranged from others, and symptoms of increased arousal, such as difficulty sleeping and

Research and Applications

Almost All People are Traumatised by Highly Aversive Events

A widespread view in popular psychology is that most people exposed to trauma develop PTSD or other serious psychological disorders. Immediately following the Victorian bushfires, for example, many mental health professionals were concerned that there would be an epidemic of PTSD cases across Australia. But the data suggest otherwise. For instance, Parslow, Jorm and Christensen (2006) surveyed victims of the 2003 Canberra bushfires and found that three months after the tragedy, only 5 percent of respondents met the criteria for PTSD. Although this rate is higher than the Australian PTSD prevalence of 1.5 percent (Rosenman, 2002) and indicates that there are individuals who require psychological help following these sorts of traumatic events, it is striking that the vast majority of respondents were psychologically healthy. So when it comes to responses to trauma, resilience is the rule rather than the exception.

People who cope well in the aftermath of a serious stressor tend to display relatively high levels of functioning before the event (Bonanno et al., 2005). Yet resilience is not limited to a few particularly well-adjusted, brave or tough-minded people, or to a single type or class of events. Instead, it is actually the most common response to traumatic events. Most people who take care of a dying partner, suffer the death of a spouse, or survive a physical or sexual assault report few long-term psychological symptoms (Bonanno, 2004). Table 14.1 (below) presents the rates of PTSD and acute stress disorder (a disorder similar to, although briefer in duration than, PTSD) associated with a number of other disturbing events. As can be seen, only a minority of people who contend with such events develop PTSD or acute stress disorder. Furthermore, these data are from a Western culture. In many non-Western cultural groups, life stressors such as illness and death are regarded as natural and inevitable aspects of life, rather than as traumas to be avoided. In these groups, PTSD and acute stress disorder are rarely diagnosed at all (Summerfield, 2001).

Table 14.1 Percentages of people who develop posttraumatic conditions as a function of the event

Percentage of people who develop PTSD	
Natural disaster	4–5%
Bombing	34%
Plane crash into hotel	29%
Mass shooting	28%
Percentage of people who develop acute stress disorder	
Cyclone	7%
Industrial accident	6%
Mass shooting	33%
Violent assault	19%
Vehicle accident	14%
Assault, severe burns	13%

(**Source:** Bryant, 2000, National Center for PTSD, US.)

startling easily. The lifetime prevalence of PTSD varies across the globe (Atwoli, 2013; Ferry et al., 2011; Kawakami, Tsuchiya, Umeda, Koenen & Kessler, 2014), with the highest rates generally found in countries with a history of civil conflict or natural disasters (Atwoli, Stein, Koenen & McLaughin, 2015). People who have experienced extreme and long-lasting stressors that result in displacement from their home, as is the case with many asylum seekers attempting to come to Australia, are at an especially high risk for PTSD (Murray, Davidson & Schweitzer, 2008). Findings from the 2007 National Survey of Mental Health and Wellbeing indicate that the lifetime prevalence of PTSD in Australia is 7.2% (McEvoy, Grove & Slade, 2011).

Assess your knowledge | FACT or FICTION?

1. People's first reaction to an extreme stressor involves activation of the autonomic nervous system. (True/False)
2. Physical illness can be a reaction to a prolonged stressor. (True/False)
3. Men and women are equally likely to exhibit a 'tend-and-befriend' response. (True/False)
4. The likelihood of developing PTSD is unrelated to the severity or duration of the stressor. (True/False)
5. Few people are resilient in the face of extreme stress. (True/False)

Answers: (1) T; (2) T; (3) F; (4) F; (5) F

A

Transactional approaches

As discussed earlier, the theories we have described are "cold" (Lazarus & Folkman, 1984) in that they simply describe how arousal, or appraisal, happens. The very same processes, whether they are those described by James and Lange, Cannon, or Schachter and Singer, can occur for nonstressful emotion. Parallel to these theories, a different set of approaches developed in experimental psychology. These can be described as "hot" and place central importance on motivational factors or valued wants that energise and direct our actions.

The transactional model of coping and appraisal

As discussed earlier in the chapter, stress is a subjective experience. Lazarus and Folkman's (1984) transactional model of coping and appraisal states that we are under stress when something we need or want is threatened and there is not much we think we can do about the situation. Notice that this view of stress always involves some type of transaction concerning needs and wants. Stressful transactions are not unlike life's many other transactions, such as the give-and-take of dealing with problems, negotiating a complex path, bargaining, and debating. This perspective also emphasises the complexity of a stressful encounter and the ongoing interrelationship among variables.

We can now present a formal definition of the transactional model of stress (Lazarus & Folkman, 1984, p. 19): *"A particular relationship between the person and the environment that is appraised by the person as taxing or exceeding his or her resources and endangering his or her well-being,"* [italics added]. Note that this definition sees stress in terms of cognitive appraisal and coping. Cognitive appraisal is the continuous "categorising of an encounter, and its various facets, with respect to its significance for well-being" (Lazarus & Folkman, 1984, p. 31). There are two types of appraisal: *primary appraisal* and *secondary appraisal*. Primary appraisal concerns the stakes a person has in a stressful encounter. He asks, "What do I want?" and "Given my

[A] Lilienfeld, S. O., Lynn, S. J., Namy, L. L., Woolf, N. J., Jamieson, G., Marks, A., & Slaughter, V. (2015). Stress, coping and health. In S. O. Lilienfeld, S. J. Lynn, L. L. Namy, N. J. Woolf, G. Jamieson, A. Marks, & V. Slaughter (Eds.), *Psychology: From inquiry to understanding* (2nd ed., pp. 503–510). Melbourne, VIC: Pearson Australia.

wants, am I in trouble or being benefited, now or in the future, and in what way?" There are four types of primary appraisal: benefit, harm/loss, threat, and challenge. An appraisal of benefit means that a person's wants are being met, limiting the possibility for stress. Harm/loss is a perception that some damage has already occurred, such as an injury, illness, or harm to social or self steem. An appraised threat is a harm or loss that is anticipated but has not yet taken place. Appraised challenge is similar to threat, except there is a possibility for growth or gain.

Secondary appraisal concerns the options and prospects for coping with a stressful situation. The key question of secondary appraisal is, "What, if anything, could be done about it?" At this point, it is appropriate to note Bandura's (1977, 1982) two components of *self-efficacy: efficacy expectancy,* or the perceived ability or intention (Kirsch, 1985, 1990) to perform a behaviour, and *outcome expectancy,* or the belief that a particular behaviour will produce a desired outcome. Outcome expectancies can include *stimulus expectancies,* or beliefs about the occurrence of external events (reinforcements such as money, grades, and social approval), and *response expectancies,* or beliefs about potentially rewarding or aversive internal reactions to events (such as joy, pleasure, pain, or fear).

A few examples can clarify these types of appraisal. Consider a student who is very anxious about an upcoming exam. Her primary appraisal may be that the exam threatens the grade point average she wants. Stress may increase if she lacks efficacy expectancy, and believes she does not have the ability to complete the exam or does not intend even to make the effort to complete it. If she believes that clearly written answers, no matter how good, will not help her exam grade, she has low stimulus outcome expectancy (the stimulus being the grade). If she believes that she will remain anxious no matter how well she does, she has low response (anxiety) outcome expectancy.

A different pattern can be illustrated by a boy dealing with the possible pain of dental surgery. His dentist has informed him that the pain will be minimal (response outcome expectancy = low pain). Furthermore, his mother has promised that they will have a special dinner the day after surgery (stimulus outcome expectancy = dinner). Just before surgery; the dentist instructs his patient in a simple pain-reduction coping strategy: "Divert your attention and think about your favorite TV show." As a result, our patient believes he is able to tolerate surgery and intends to go through with it (efficacy expectation = ability and intention to have surgery).

"I'M A FAILURE! EVERYONE EISE IS SO SMART!"

" TAKE ONE QUESTION AT A TIME. I KNOW I'VE GOT WHAT IT TAKES."

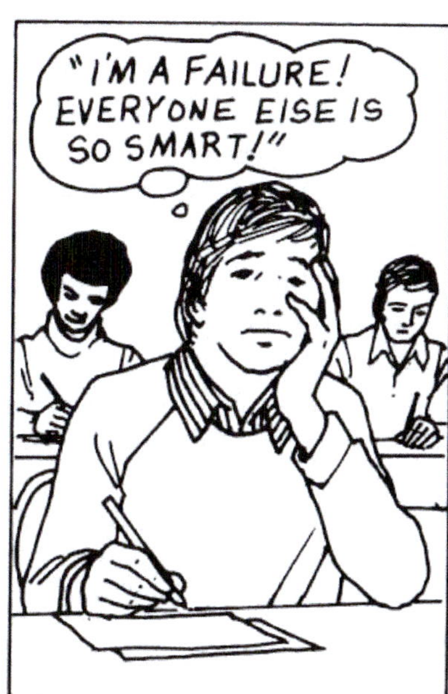

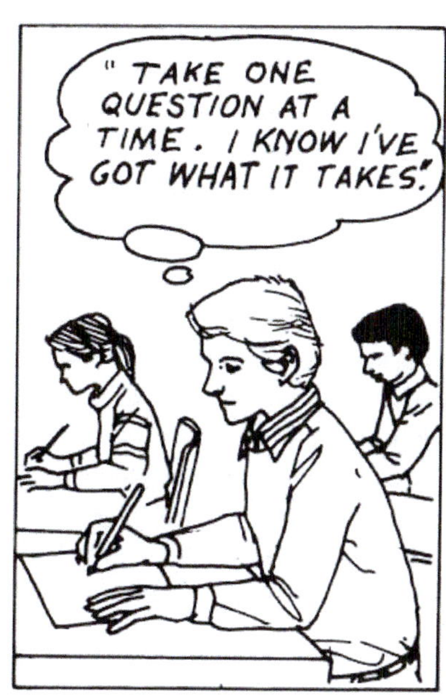

With appraisal a person determines the stakes of a stressful encounter as well as the prospects of coping with it. With coping, a person acts. *Problem-focused coping* involves planful actions to change a stressful situation by acting on the environment or oneself. Examples include the use of active coping, planning, confrontive coping, self-control, and instrumental social support. *Emotion-focused coping* involves attempting to reduce the upset or discomfort associated with a stressful situation without actively trying to change the situation itself. Some emotion-focused strategies involve changing how attention is deployed. Attention can be diverted from distress through strategies involving distancing, avoidance, or escape. Attention can also be directed toward a stressful situation by accepting reality and responsibility, and by positively reinterpreting the situation.

Some of the most important recent work on coping has focused on specific coping processes applied in specific situations. Three lists of coping strategies are frequendy cited in the literature: Moos (1974); Folkman, Lazarus, Dunkel-Schetter, DeLongis, and Gruen (1986); and Carver, Scheier, and Weintraub (1989). No researcher claims his or her listing to be complete; they frequendy cite the need for more comprehensive lists or for lists that are tailored to certain situations. Table 14.2 presents one way of cataloging ways of coping.

It is important to recognise that any form of coping can be either problem- or emotion-focused depending on the situation. For example, planning (listed as problem-focused in Table 14.2) can reduce stressful emotion. An individual might spend the hour preceding a stressful exam planning how to approach possible questions. Even though such late-minute planning may have no effect on exam performance, it does serve to reduce anxiety. Similarly, denial listed as emotion-focused in Table 14.2) can at times be an effective part of changing a stressful situation. A cancer patient who might be demoralised by accepting the full implications of her diagnosis may deny the severity of her disorder and optimistically make important and healthy changes in life style.

Finally, the appraisal process is constantly changing with no clear beginning or ending. A person's perception of threat may be reduced or increased depending on the coping options identified. *Reappraisal* is simply a changed appraisal brought about by new information.

One key feature of the transactional approach is that it considers many interacting variables and prompts us to look at specific stress encounters as well as their antecedents and consequences. This distinguishes the transactional approach from those that preceded it. We can see the difference in an example:

> *Terry is in the study hall studying for her midterm exam. It is the night before the test. She worries about how the exam might affect her academic standing and her prospects for receiving a student loan. Although she first feels helpless and overwhelmed, Terry soon decides that such worries are getting her nowhere and that she is quite capable of coming up with a sensible study strategy. She takes a few deep breaths to clear her mind. She then organises her review for the evening and confronts the challenge of studying for the exam. After taking action, she feels more in control and is more confident that she will pass the exam.*

Knowing Terry's primary appraisal (worries about her academic standing and student loan), secondary appraisal (helplessness followed by the decision that she is capable of developing a study plan), coping (deep breaths, organising her review, and studying), and reappraisal (feeling more in control and confident) give us a very rich understanding of her problem. In contrast, earlier stimulus-based, arousal-based, and cognitive approaches to defining stress and emotion would give a less complete portrait:

Stimulus-based account: Terry faces an exam tomorrow. Her instructor assigned the exam a month ago. Terry needs to pass this exam to pass the course. Compared with other life events, such an exam earns about 15 life-change units, not enough to contribute to subsequent illness.

TABLE 14.2 Coping strategies

Problem-focused coping: Attempting to alter a stressful situation through strategies such as the following (Folkman & Lazarus, 1985):

Active coping: Actively attempting to remove or circumvent a stressful situation, or ameliorate its effects. Techniques include taking direct action, increasing effort, and executing a coping plan in reasonable steps.

Planning: Thinking through how one will cope. This involves generating strategies, and selecting and deciding how to implement steps.

Confrontational coping: Standing one's ground, assertively seeking to meet one's needs and wishes, and actively attempting to change the behaviour of others.

Suppression of competing activities: Putting other projects aside, trying to avoid becoming distracted by other events, even letting other things slide, if necessary, in order to deal with the stressor. Generally, this involves suppressing involvement in competing activities or thoughts.

Self-control: Trying to keep one's feelings to oneself.

Restraint coping: Waiting until an appropriate opportunity to act presents itself, holding oneself back, and not acting prematurely.

Search for social support for instrumental reasons: Seeking advice, assistance, or information for help in coping with a stressor.

Emotion-focused coping: Attempting to reduce the upset or discomfort associated with a stressful situation without actively trying to change the situation itself.

Some forms of emotion-focused coping involve retaining a more or less accurate appraisal of the facts of a situation, but changing other aspects of the appraisal. Such *reality-based reappraisals* include:

Acceptance of reality: Accepting and living with the fact that a stressful event has occurred, is real, and can't be changed.

Acceptance of responsibility (Folkman & Lazarus, 1985): Assuming that one has brought the problem on oneself.

Positive reinterpretation and growth (termed "positive reappraisal" by Folkman & Lazarus, 1985): Reappraising a stressful situation in positive terms by seeing how it might contribute to learning and growth.

Distancing (Folkman & Lazarus, 1985): Acknowledging a troubling situation but failing to deal with its emotional significance.

Other forms of emotion-focused coping involve taking action to achieve a *substitute satisfaction or tension release*. Strategies include:

Search for social support for emotional reasons: Seeking moral support, sympathy or understanding.

Search for alternative rewards (Moos, 1974): Changing one's activities to obtain satisfactions not available in a stressful encounter.

Reliance on religion: Praying as well as seeking and trusting in a higher spiritual power.

Focus on and venting of emotions: Concentrating on and expressing one's feelings of upset.

Tension reduction: Disengaging from a stressful situation through relaxation or exercise.

Humour: Laughing at and joking about a stressful situation (see also distancing).

Still other forms of emotion-focused coping involve some *distortion or withdrawal* from the facts of a stressful situation:

Wishful thinking (Folkman & Lazarus, 1985): Simply wishing or hoping that a stressful situation will change or go away.

Denial: Refusing to believe that a stressor exists, or acting as though it is not real or hasn't happened. The opposite of the acceptance of reality.

Behavioural disengagenment: Physically giving up or withdrawing effort from attempts to attain the goal with which the stressor is interfering.

Mental disengagement: Psychologically giving up a threatened goal. This often involves engaging in attempts at obtaining substitute satisfaction through such activities as watching TV, daydreaming, sleeping, or self-distraction.

Self-isolation (Folkman & Lazarus, 1985): Avoiding people in general and keeping others from knowing how bad things are.

Alcohol or drug use: Disengaging from a stressor through alcohol or other drugs.

Source: Loosely based on lists presented in Billings and Moos (1984); Carver, Scheier, and Weintraub (1989);Cohen, Reese, Kaplan, and Riggio (1986); Folkman, Lazarus, Dunkel-Schetter, DeLongis, and Gruen (1986); and Moos (1974).

Arousal-based account: Terry faces an exam tomorrow. She is perspiring and has a slight stomach ache caused by the excessive secretion of digestive fluids. If this gastric response were to continue, one might worry that Terry is at risk of developing an ulcer.

Neutral cognitive account (Schachter & Singer, 1962): Terry faces an exam tomorrow. She is sitting in the study hall with other students, who are worried about the exam, and begins perspiring and experiencing stomach discomfort. As others express their concerns and fears, Terry thinks, "Gosh, I'm anxious about this exam." Apparently, being in a room with other worried students gave Terry a ready label for her physical symptoms.

The transactional matrix

Lazarus and Folkman (1984) present a broader perspective that looks at appraisal and coping as well as a wide range of additional variables with which stress and coping interact I have taken the liberty of modifying and expanding their views into a general classification system. The *transactional matrix* identifies three classes of variables involved in stress and coping: situational, personal, and external.

The understanding of stress begins with the identification of a concrete and specific stress situation, for example, the final exam, the interview, the first date, or the argument with the spouse. With respect to such an encounter, we have already considered four *situational variables* that must be examined:

Primary appraisal
Needs or wants
Harm/loss, threat, challenge, benefit
Secondary appraisal
Appraised coping potential
Self-efficacy
Outcome efficacy
Coping
Problem-focused
Emotion-focused
Reappraisal

A wide range of additional variables might also influence our understanding of a stress encounter. Those that contribute or potentially contribute to coping are *resources;* those that interfere or potentially interfere with coping are *deficits*. Some resources and deficits are *personal variables* that exist within the individual, such as:*

Emotion (negative, such as fear, anger and sadness: and positive, such as joy)
Physical abilities (physical strength, flexibility, stamina, agility, etc.)
Physiological functioning level of arousal, physical illness, etc.)
Cognitive abilities, skills, knowledge
Cognitive functioning (fatigue, mental inflexibility, distracting thoughts, narrowed attention, etc.)
Social skills (assertiveness, aggressiveness, passivity, etc.)
Beliefs, values, commitments (thoughts concerning what is real, important, and worthy of action)

Other resources and deficits are *external variables,* such as:

Objective characteristics of the situation (undesirability, unpredictability, uncontrollability,event magnitude, time clustering)
Social networks
Finances
Housing
Transportation
Work
Society (politics, social upheaval, discrimination, war, etc.)
Environment (noise, crowding, pollution, etc.)

---

*Stress research occasionally considers the effects of automatic patterns of processing information. Such behaviours are usually referred to as *cognitive styles*. However, since cognitive styles can mediate reactions to successful situations, they are worth noting. *Field dependence-independence* (or global-analytic style) is perhaps the most widely researched (Witkin, Goodenough, & Oilman, 1979). Field-dependent global individuals rely heavily on external cues when making judgements about the environment. Indeed, such people have difficulty separating a figure from the background or field. When placed in a darkened room and shown a tilted luminous frame surrounding a movable rod, they have problems adjusting the rod to a true upright on the basis of bodily cues. In other words, they are so distracted by the tilted frame that it becomes their incorrect point of reference. In contrast, field-independent analytic individuals can see the rod as being separate from the frame and adjust it correctly. They have been more recently viewed as possessing an analogous "disembedding," or differentiating, ability in a variety of intellectual activities, including coping with stress. When placed in ambiguous stressful situations, field· independent fanalytic subjects appear better able to analyse and restructure a field when certainty increases. In other words, they are not bound by previous appraisals of uncertainty and appear able to reappraise when conditions are appropriate (Gaines, Smith, & Skolnick, 1977).

Additional cognitive styles include *levelling* (the tendency to view stimuli in terms of characteristics they have in common) and *sharpening* (the tendency to see stimuli in terms of their differences) as well as *focusing scanning, flexible-constructed control, equivalence range,* and *tolerance for unrealistic experiences* (Gardner, Holzman, Klein, Linton & Spence, 1959).

Such personal and external variables are too complex to be discussed in full here; indeed, they form the basis of much of the rest of this book.

Situational, personal, and external variables can be viewed on two temporal dimensions: (1) *timing,* or whether the variable is concurrent with, preceding, or following a stressful encounter; and (2) *duration,* or whether the variable is immediate and short-lived, or distant and enduring. These define five general categories of stress variables:

1. *Long-term antecedent variables:* All that exist prior to the stressful situation and have endured for a relatively long time. Examples include such situational antecedents as enduring patterns of appraisal and coping with specific and concrete stress situations similar to the one under consideration; such personal variables as personality traits and dispositions, physical health, abilities, and handicaps; and such external variables as long-term friendships, financial stability, and home life.
2. *Immediate antecedent variables:* All moods, states, and transitory events and conditions that are present just before a stress encounter.
3. *Stress event variables:* All variables present during the stressful encounter.
4. *Immediate consequence variables:* All moods, states, and transitory events and conditions that are present just after a stress encounter.
5. *Long-term consequence variables:* Long-term and lasting changes that can be identified after an encounter.

To illustrate, let us examine one personal variable, the emotion *anger,* and one external variable, *tangible social support.* Both can appear at various times and for various durations. As a long-term antecedent, anger is a continuing trait, a part of an individuals personality. As an immediate antecedent, it is the mood a person experiences just before a stressful situation ('Just before the exam, I was really angry."). As a part of a stress event, it is a mood a person feels during a stressful situation; as an immediate consequence, it is what a person feels after. Finally, as a long-term consequence, anger is again a continuing trait or an aspect of a person's personality.

The external variable, tangible social support (the nunber of friends who can supply money, physical assistance, etc.), can also exist as a long-term or immediate antecedent as well as a resource during a stressful event. An individual may have helpful friends for a long time before, just before, during, right after, and for a long time after a stressful encounter.

Finally, situational stress variables, that is, appraisal and coping, are primarily defined in terms of a stressful event. A person might appraise an exam as a threat to her overall grade, but possess the coping skills of planning and accepting responsibility. A person can display these same appraisals and coping skills immediately before ("The exam is coming up. It's a threat, but I accept responsibility for planning."), or after ("The exam is over. It's still a threat, and I still accept responsibility for planning."). These variables can exist as long-term antecedents ("All my life I have seen exams as a threat, but have accepted responsibility for planning.") and consequences ("The exam may be over, but for a long time I continued to see exams as threats and accepted responsibility for planning.").

Several principles characterise this matrix. Any single variable can be a long-term antecedent or consequence, a transitory or immediate antecedent or consequence, or part of the actual stressful encounter. Examples of situational, personal, and external variables are presented in Table 14.3.

Looking at stress through the transactional lens

The transactional matrix can be conceptualised as a lens through which a person perceives a stressful situation. The lens can focus narrowly on situational variables specific to a stressful encounter. Table 14.4 presents a narrowly focused description of a student taking an exam. However, the lens has a vertical and horizontal focus that can be broad or narrow. A broad

TABLE 14.3 Examples of variables for taking an exam on the transactional matrix

Variable	Long-Term Antecedents	Immediate Antecedents	Stressful Event	Immediate Consequences	Long-Term Consequences
Personal	-				
Emotion (depression)	Depressed personality	Depressed mood	Depressed mood	Depressed mood	Less depressed personality
Physical abilities (physically fit)	History of being physically fit	Has stopped exercise routine before event; level of fitness lower than usual	Not physically fit	Not physically fit	Joins fitness program; increases fitness
Physiological functioning (arousal)	Chronic high blood pressure	Normal blood pressure	High blood pressure	High blood pressure	Lower chronic blood pressure
Cognitive abilities, skills, knowledge (verbal and writing skills)	Good verbal and writing skills	At peak writing ability	At peak writing ability	Less verbal	Good verbal skills
Cognitive functioning (cognitively fatigued)	History of cognitive fatigue	Not fatigued	Not fatigued	Fatigued	Generally less fatigued during stressful events
Social skills (shy)	History of being shy in most social encounters	Very sociable	Not sociable	More sociable	Still sociable during stressful events
Belief, values commitments (belief in God)	Enduring belief in God	Had not considered belief in God	Did not consider belief in God	Did not consider belief in God	Not interested in religion
Situational					
Primary appraisal ("I want success; this is threatened.")	Generally driven to seek success, generally fearful it is threatened.	Not particularly concerned about success	Concerned about success	Less concerned about success	More concerned about living life, less concerned about success
Secondary appraisal ("I'm not prepared.")	Generally believes "I'm not prepared to deal with stress."	Feels "I'm not prepared."	Feels "I'm not prepared."	Feels "I'm not prepared about success."	Feels better prepared to deal with stress
Coping ("Plan one step at a time.")	Generally plans life activities	Has no plan	Has no plan	Has no plan	Faces stressful events with a plan
Reappraisal (fear of failure)	Generally has plan and does not fear failure	Fears failure because has no plan	Fears failure because has no plan	Still fears failure because has no plan	Learns to approach problems with plan; fears failure less
External					
Objective characteristics of situation (controllable)	Generally had little control over tests and exams	Had little control over available study time	Has control over how to take the exam	Has little control over grading of exam	Has control over taking of future exams
Social networks (many acquaintances, few friends)	Generally has had many acquaintances, few friends	Is with friends	Is with several friends	Is alone	Still maintains several good friends
Finances (little money on hand)	Generally has had considerable money	No financial problems	No financial problems	No financial problems	No financial problems
Housing, food (have place to stay and food)	Generally has had housing and food	No housing or food problems	No housing or food problems	No housing or food problems	No housing or food problems

TABLE 14.4 A narrow focus for taking an exam

Variable	Long-Term Antecedents	Immediate Antecedents	Stressful Event	Immediate Consequences	Long-Term Consequences
Personal					
Situational			"I wanted to get an *A* but, when I saw the exam, I realised it covered matter I hadn't studied. [appraisal of want and threat], and I didn't know what to do [appraisal of coping]. I pushed on, just answered the easy questions, and prayed for the best [actual coping].		
External					

TABLE 14.5 A broad vertical focus for taking an exam

Variable	Long-Term Antecedents	Immediate Antecedents	Stressful Event	Immediate Consequences	Long-Term Consequences
Personal			While taking this exam, I was tired and angry. This kept me awake and enabled me to keep on going.		
Situational			I wanted to get an A but, when I saw the exam I realise it covered matter I hadn't studied [appraisal of coping]. I pushed on, just answered the easy questions, and prayed for the best [actual coping].		
External			While taking this exam, my girlfriend was at home waiting for me. This helped me keep going.		

vertical focus includes personal and external variables that accompany the stressful event, as Table 14.5 shows. A broad horizontal focus, such as that depicted in Table 14.6, includes situational variables that come before and after the event. Finally, a broad vertical and horizontal focus includes all variables. This is portrayed in Table 14.7.

TABLE 14.6 A broad horizontal focus for taking an exam

Variable	Long-Term Antecedents	Immediate Antecedents	Stressful Event	Immediate Consequences	Long-Term Consequences
Personal					
Situational	I'm the kind of person who has always wanted to get an *A* on exams, but I find that exams cover material I haven't studied. I just answer the easy questions and hope for the best.	Right before the exam I really wanted to get an *A*. I was afraid that it might cover material I hadn't studied and that I might not know what to do. Well, I decided to answer just the easy questions and pray for the best.	I wanted to get an *A* but, when, I saw the exam I realise it covered matter I hadn't studied [appraisal of want and threat], and I didn't know what to do [appraisal of coping]. I pushed on, just answered the easy questions and prayed for the best [actual coping].	The exam is over and I hope I got an *A*. It was really clear to me that it covered material I hadn't studied and I didn't know what to do. I pray for the best.	On subsequent exams, I continued to seek *A*s and hope for the best. However, after exams I continued to realised that the exam covered material I hadn't studied for.
External					

TABLE 14.7 A broad vertical and horizontal focus for taking an exam

Variable	Long-Term Antecedents	Immediate Antecedents	Stressful Event	Immediate Consequences	Long-Term Consequences
Personal	People describe me as hot-headed and angry. I guess that describes part of me.	Right before this exam, I was tired and angry.	While taking this exam, I was tired and angry. This kept me awake and enabled me to keep on going.	Just after the exam, I was no longer angry. I felt a bit let down, since the worst was over.	The exam didn't change much in my life. I'm still basically an angry person.
Situational	I'm the kind of person who has always wanted to get an *A* on exams, but I find that exams cover material I haven't studied. I just answer the easy questions and hope for the best.	Right before the exam I really wanted to get an *A*. I was afraid that it might cover material I hadn't studied and that I might not know what to do. Well, I decided to answer just the easy questions and pray for the best.	I wanted to get an *A* but, when I saw the exam, I realised it covered matter I hadn't studied [appraisal of want and threat], and I didn't know what to do [appraisal of coping]. I pushed on, just answered the easy questions and prayed for the best [actual coping].	The exam is over and I hope I got an *A*. It was really clear to me that it covered material I hadn't studied and I didn't know what to do. I prayed for the best.	On subsequent exams, I continued to seek *A*s and hope for the best. However, after exams I continued to realise that the exam covered material I had not studied for.
External	For some time before the exam, I have been living with my girlfriend. She is always around when I need her.	Just before the exam, I realised my girlfriend was at home waiting for me.	While taking this exam, my girlfriend was at home waiting for me. This helped me keep going.	Just after the exam, I realised my girlfriend was at home.	For quite some time after the exam, I continued living with my girlfriend.

The transactional story and the process of stress

As noted, the transactional perspective derives its name from what is perhaps its most important feature. Stress is not static; it is a continuous, unfolding process. Different features of this process can interrelate as a transaction. Any transaction involves back-and-forth movement. In a financial transaction, a customer may inquire about a price, then bargain, and finally pay for a desired item. In a transaction between roommates, one may ask for help in cleaning the room, the other may respond that she is too busy with homework, and both may argue until some sort of compromise is, or is not, reached. In this sense, stress is also a transaction: appraisals of resources influence how we actually cope; the emotions we experience in one encounter influence how we cope in others; illness can be both a long-term consequence of stress, and a continuing, long-term antecedent.

The transactional matrix and lens can provide something of a "snapshot" of stress, a rich but static portrait of a wide array of variables. However, we would need many snapshots to see how an event unfolds and how the variables interrelate. Such repeated glimpses of a stressful event provide something of a transactional story, complete with central and peripheral characters and interweaving plots. Of course, to study the full story of a stressful event is difficult, and requires repeated testing and complex statistics. However, as we shall see, this is one direction that stress research is taking.

Research applications of the transactional matrix

Early studies that looked only at the accumulation of life events (long-term and immediate antecedents), stress-related illness (long-term consequence), or stress arousal (stressful event) had a severely restricted focus. Research is beginning to examine more elements of the transactional matrix. To illustrate, in a classic study Folkman and Lazarus (1985) examined three critical moments of a university midterm examination: anticipation, when students prepare for an exam not knowing exactly what it will be like; waiting, when the exam had been given and grades have yet to be announced; and outcome, when students deal with learning how they have done. Separate studies were conducted for each phase.

The results of the study reveal something of a changing microscopic portrait of what happens before, during, and after an exam. First, emotions change. As might be expected, threat and challenge emotions are high before and just after an exam, while harm and benefit emotions rise once the exam is taken. During the waiting period just before receiving grades), there is considerable ambiguity, and all emotions are high, both positive and negative. How did the students cope? One surprising finding is that people cope in very complex ways. On the average, nearly seven different coping strategies were used by each student. In addition, students used both problem- and emotion-focused coping, often in combination. Before the exam, students relied on problem-focused coping (studying and seeking informational social support) as well as the emotion-focused technique of emphasising the positive. After the exam, the use of problem-focused coping declined, and distancing and searching for emotional social support increased. Apparently, distancing is applied when waiting for an outcome.

Evaluating coping strategies

Which forms of coping were most useful? Generally, this question is hard to answer. Students who received poorer grades did report using more emotion-focused coping, probably to manage their disappointment However, at times emotion-focused coping can reduce interfering emotion and thereby facilitate problem-focused coping. Perhaps this is the reason problem-focused coping correlated highly with emphasising the positive and seeking social support. Generally, people use a wide variety of coping strategies, which change as a stressful situation unfolds (see Table 14.8).

We have described one study in detail because it represents an important direction in which stress research is progressing. Instead of examining global consequences or

TABLE 14.8 The transactional matrix applied to exam research

Variable	Long-Term Antecedents	Immediate Antecedents	Stressful Event	Immediate Consequences	Long-Term Consequences
Personal		Threat and challenge emotions.		Threat and challenge emotions, harm and benefit emotions. All emotions are high just before receiving grade.	
Situational		Problem-focused coping (studying and seeking informational social support) as well as emphasising the positive.		Problem-focused coping declined, and distancing and searching for emotional social support increased. Students who received poorer grades reported using more emotion-focused coping, probably to manage their disappointment.	
External					

antecedents, the emphasis is on a microanalysis of process and what people actually do in stressful situations; put simply, the aim is to discover important stress stories. The potential of this line of research is considerable. In time, we may learn which coping strategies are most appropriate for which people in which situations.

This research model is beginning to yield some tantalising results:

- Most people use nearly all forms of coping in every stressful encounter, although some may be emphasised more than others (Lazarus, 1990).
- The pattern of coping changes from one stage of a stressful encounter to another. Students coping with an examination tend to seek information before the exam, but use distancing after the exam and before grades are announced (Lazarus, 1990).
- Some forms of coping are relatively stable, whereas others are unstable. For example, problem-focused approaches tend to vary highly from one situation to another, whereas some emotion-focused strategies, such as positive reappraisal and self-control, are more stable and used in a wide variety of situations (Lazarus, 1990).
- Problem-focused and reality-based emotion-focused coping (particularly confrontive coping, acceptance of responsibility, and planning) as well as positive reappraisal predominates when people feel that something constructive can be done. In contrast, emotion-focused coping, such as distancing and disengagement from a situation, predominates when people appraise a stressor as something that cannot be changed (Folkman & Lazarus, 1980; Folkman, et al.,1986). In addition, the suppression of competing activities and search for instrumental support are also more likely to be applied in controllable situations (Carver et al., 1989).
- Unsuccessful coping appears to be more associated with confrontational and avoidant strategies as well as wishful thinking and self-blame, whereas successful coping is more associated with planful problem-solving (Folkman et al., 1986; Folton, Revenson, & Hinrichsen, 1989).
- Emotions play a complex role in stress, and can inhibit, instigate, and maintain coping behaviour. Emotion is also one important consequence of coping, and different emotions are associated with failure, success, and uncertain outcome (Folkman & Lazarus, 1991).
- Depressed people appear to feel they have more at stake in stressful encounters and use more confrontive coping and self-control (keeping feelings to themselves). They also

seek more social support, yet report more anger and hostility in their encounters. One is tempted to speculate that such strategies are counter-productive. Keeping feelings to oneself and using confrontive coping may not be conducive to the development of social support such individuals seek, thus contributing to further depression (Coyne, Aldwin, & Lazarus, 1981; Folkman & Lazarus, 1986; Folkman & Lazarus, 1988).

- Rational, planful problem-solving may be less likely to communicate hostility than confrontive coping, and may well invite the cooperation and support of others. Indeed, one study found that planful problem-solving elicited all types of support (emotional, tangible, and informational), whereas confrontive coping elicited primarily information (Dunkel-Schetter, Folkman, & Lazarus, 1987).
- Finally, causal antecedents (such as life events and personality) are poor predictors of how people actually cope during a stressful encounter as well as of the short and long-term consequences they will experience (Folkman & Lazarus, 1980; Lazarus & Folkman,1984). What a person actually does in a stressful situation is determined by a complex array of factors, including situational constraints, resources, personality, appraisals, and past coping successes and failures.

The relativity of coping: the case of denial

It should be clear that the stress research we have described does not assume that any coping strategies are either good or bad. Any particular strategy works differently for different individuals, and generalizations concerning the overall utility of coping strategies may be hard to come by. This can be seen very clearly with respect to denial, a strategy about which psychotherapists have had much to say. For example, psychodynamic therapists see denial as a sign of neurosis, and rational emotive therapists view it as irrational. However, experimental stress researchers note that people frequently engage in benign self-deceptions, such as faith in the existence (or nonexistence) of God or an afterlife, feelings of virtual immortality, and belief in unproven remedies for illness and techniques for self-improvement. Such illusions foster a sense of self-efficacy and optimism that may well be conducive to health.

In fact, there are both costs and benefits to denial. These positive and negative effects can occur in a variety of contexts, including illness, catastrophe and disaster, and developmental tasks. In general, Lazarus and Folkman (1984) and others have proposed a variety of conditions under which denial and denial-like forms of coping might have favorable or unfavorable outcomes:

- When nothing can be done to overcome a threat, denial can reduce distress without causing harm. ("I am terminally ill and that cannot be changed.")
- When certain facets of a situation can be denied, others can be attended to and managed with less disruption. ("My diabetes isn't really a serious disorder; however, I will very diligently keep up with my medications and diet")
- When a given stressful situation must be encountered again and again, denial can interfere with mastery and increase stress.
- Denial may be valuable at an early stage of coping if a person's resources are insufficient for managing a problem, such as the beginning of a crisis, a sudden illness, incapacitation, or loss of a loved one. Such denial may provide the breathing room needed to develop coping resources.
- Some kinds of denial may be more or less dangerous or helpful than others. Weisman (1972) has suggested that it may be more dangerous to deny fact (that a person has cancer) than implication (that cancer can lead to death). In addition, it may be more dangerous to deny what is clear and unambiguous (that a person is overweight, has heart disease, and should go on a diet) than what cannot be known for certain (working hard may contribute to stress).

- When an uncontrollable situation is changing and may become controllable,denial can be risky and prevent timely action.

Lazarus and Folkman (1984) have also suggested that denial that is "partial, tentative or minimal" should be less destructive and potentially more useful. Such derual is closer to a "working fiction," a sense of "as if" that is often difficult to challenge empirically (p. 137). This can serve to maintain morale and even motivate a person to cope. There comes a point when minimal denial ceases to be denial and instead becomes an accurate reappraisal, a shift of emphasis. An individual may well first view his situation as a threat and thus experience considerable stress. However, it can be just as realistic but much more adaptive to view the same situation as a challenge.

Clinical and experimental approaches to stress

Coping research in general and the example of denial in particular shows how complex stress can be. A wide range of variables may determine when any particular strategy is constructive or destructive. One overall lesson of coping research is the *importance of assessing the costs and payoffs of any coping strategies that an individual may apply.* This is the core of contemporary clinical approaches to stress management.

In addition, coping research may help the clinical process of experimenting with a wide range of coping strategies in a search for those that work. This becomes obvious when we phrase empirical questions as personal concerns:

- "An exam is coming up. How do successful students cope with their anxiety? I tend to be shy and over anxious. Are there coping strategies that would apply well to my situation?"
- "Next week I have surgery. I want to do everything possible to hasten my recovery. I know that a certain amount of fear is normal, but how can I learn to keep my fear in check? I'm the kind of person who likes to know all the details about what is going on. Are there coping strategies that are better for me?"
- "I play on the school basketball team and have to deal with many types of pressure. Sometimes I have to worry about the crowd (and my date) watching me. Sometimes it is an important game, and I think about not making the one mistake that loses the game. Sometimes we are just practicing. Are different strategies for dealing with pressure better for different situations or for my type of personality?"
- "My job is really tense. I want to do my best, but this is impossible given the enormous amount of work I must do. My concern is that heart disease runs in my family, and I don't want work stress to increase my chances of becoming ill. Should I learn to relax? Should I lower my standards? Should I just learn to accept what can't be changed? It would be helpful to know what works for other people in my situation."

The transactional matrix represents a step closer to behavioural approaches to clinical stress assessment. Typically, the clinician identifies the specifics of a problem situation, and then examines the consequences to determine problem behaviours, their seriousness, client motivation to change, and so on. An examination of antecedents helps determine coping resources that have been applied in similar situations, difficulties a client may have in learning and applying new skills, and the probability of change. In other words, clinical stress assessment begins with a narrow focus and then expands to apply a broad horizontal focus in exploring the vast array of variables suggested by the transactional matrix. Why do stress clinicians initially tend to pay less attention to personal and external antecedents and consequences? From the research examined, it appears that such variables may not provide as much predictive power as do the concrete and specific situational variables (although they can enrichen our understanding of a situation). For example, to understand how John may fare on his next interview, the first task would be to ask how he fared on previous interviews rather than to explore his overall situation, personality, and so on.

In sum, just as clinical approaches to stress have become more experimental, experimental models have ecome more clinical. The transactional matrix represents something of a meeting of the two worlds of research.

Other aspects of stress

So far we have reviewed current research and thinking on the basics of stress. Much of this work can be organised in terms of the transactional matrix. You may find it interesting to complete Application Box 14.1 which follows in relation to a stressful situation you have experienced to see how much you understand the concept of the transactional matrix.

We continue our journey with a topic that has received considerably urgent attention: stress and health. People's personalities consist of enduring patterns of behaviours, including how they habitually cope and defend themselves, and their ongoing reactions to patterns of coping failures and successes. Is there an illness-prone or health-prone personality? How do specific patterns of stress contribute to specific illnesses ? And what is the link between stress, illness, and risk behaviours such as lack of exercise, poor eating habits, smoking, alcoholism, and substance abuse?

After probing these questions, we shall step back and discuss more general contexts that have attracted considerable research: disasters, catastrophes, and crises; development and the family; work stress; and environment and the society. We shall conclude by examining the major approaches to stress management used in clinics.

Application box 14.1

Analysing stress with the transactional lens

Think of a recent stress situation. Try to recall all of the specifics. When did it happen? What did you think, do, and say? Where were you? Now try to identify examples of primary appraisal, secondary appraisal, and coping in your example. Describe these below:

Primary appraisal ____

____

Secondary appraisal ____

____

Coping ____

____

Now, let's see if we can understand your stress situation more deeply. What are all the elements in the "stress story" of this situation ? Below is an empty transactional matrix. Try to identify what came before and after the stress situation. What were your personal and external resources and deficits? What were the short and long-term costs and payoffs?

Variables	*Long-term Antecedents*	*Immediate Antecedents*	*Stress Event*	*Immediate Consequences*	*Long-term Consequences*
Personal	_______	_______	_______	_______	_______
	_______	_______	_______	_______	_______
Situational	_______	_______	_______	_______	_______
	_______	_______	_______	_______	_______
External	_______	_______	_______	_______	_______
	_______	_______	_______	_______	_______[B]

Lifetime effects of stress

Stress is often described as a "disease of prolonged arousal" that leads to a cascade of negative health effects. The longer you are chronically stressed, the more likely there will be negative health effects. Look at the stress symptoms shown in Figure 14.4.

Tension headaches, migraine, dizziness
Oily skin, skin blemishes, rashes, blushing
Dry mouth, jaw pain, grinding teeth
Backache, neck stiffness, muscle cramps, fatigue
Tightness in chest, hyperventilation, heart pounding, palpitations
Stomach ache, acid stomach, burping, nausea, indigestion, stomach "butterflies"
Diarrhea, gassiness, constipation, increased urge to urinate
Cold hands, sweaty hands and feet, hand tremor

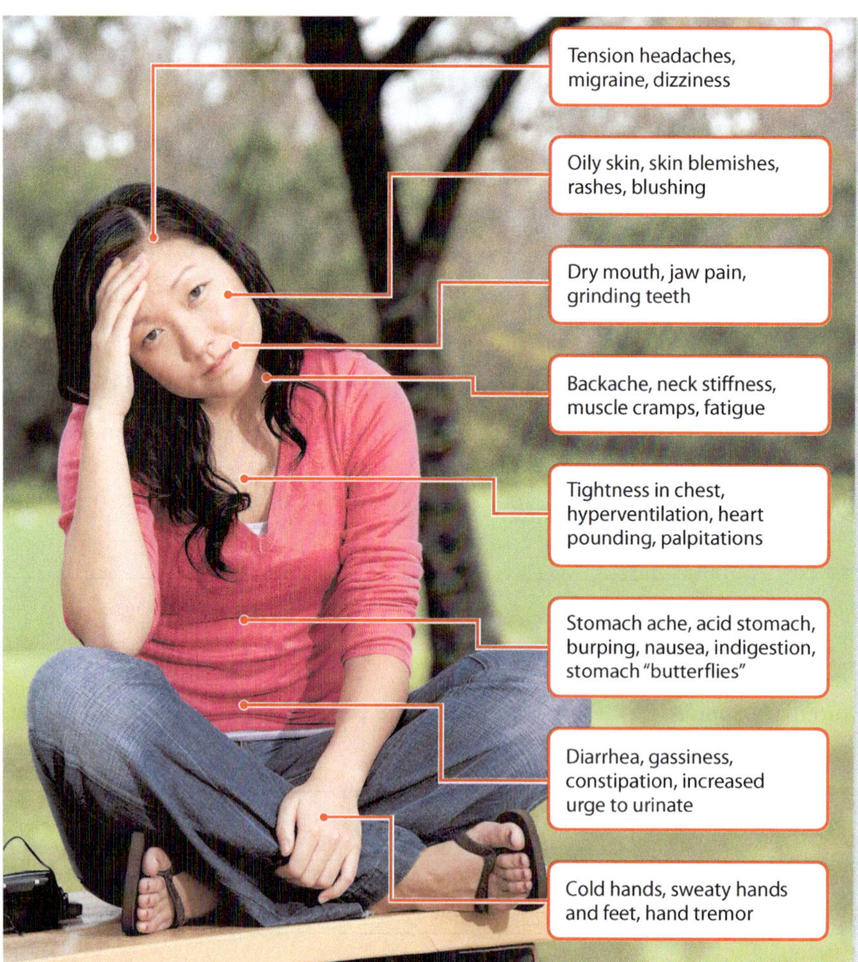

Figure 14.4 Common physical symptoms of stress

Sometimes you may not even notice how stressed you are until your body starts sending you signals. Do you frequently experience any of these physical symptoms of stress? (**Source:** Michael Krinke/nycshooter/iStockphoto.)

[B]Smith, J. (1993). The transactional matrix. In J. Smith (Ed.), *Understanding stress and coping* (pp. 69–89). New York, NY: Macmillan.

Physical effects of stress

The higher the levels of stress you experience and the longer that stress continues, the greater the likelihood of damage to your physical health (Thoits, 2010). In addition to the physical disease threats we've discussed, increases in rates of suicide, homicide, hate crimes, alcohol and drug abuse, and domestic violence are symptoms of a nation that is chronically stressed.

Stress and cardiovascular disease

Perhaps the most studied and documented health consequence of unresolved stress is cardiovascular disease (CVD). Research on CVD demonstrates the impact of chronic stress on heart rate, blood pressure, heart attack, and stroke (Backe et al, 2011; Steptoe, Rosengren & Hjemdahl, 2012).

Historically, the increased risk of CVD from chronic stress has been linked to increased arterial plaque buildup due to elevated cholesterol, hardening of the arteries, increases in inflammatory responses in the body, alterations in heart rhythm, increased and fluctuating blood pressures, and difficulties in cardiovascular responsiveness due to all of the above (Richardson et al., 2012; Marshall, 2011). In the past two decades, research into the relationship between stress and CVD contributors has shown direct links between the incidence and progression of CVD and stressors such as job strain, caregiving, bereavement, and natural disasters (Kivimaki et al, 2012; Mostofsky et al., 2012).

Stress and weight gain

Are you a "*stress*" or "*emotional eater*"? Do you run for the refrigerator when you are under pressure or feeling anxious or down? If you think that when you are extremely stressed, you tend to eat more and gain weight, you didn't imagine it. We comfort ourselves with things we love; hence that bag of chips or ice cream sundae may be just the thing to distract us. But there is more to stress eating than soothing our emotions.

Higher stress levels may drive us toward food because they may increase cortisol levels in the bloodstream. Because cortisol contributes to increased hunger and seems to activate fat-storing enzymes, people who are stressed may get a double whammy of risks from higher-circulating cortisol levels. High cortisol may also increase cravings for salty and sweet foods. Animal and human studies, including those in which subjects suffer from post-traumatic stress, seem to support the theory that cortisol plays a role in laying down extra belly fat and increasing eating behaviours (Scott, Melhorn & Sakai, 2012; Vincennati, 2011; Pagota et al', 2012).

Stress and alcohol dependence

New research has found that a specific stress hormone, the *corticotropin-releasing factor (CRF)*, is key to the development and maintenance of alcohol dependence in animals. CRF is a natural substance involved in the body's stress response, stimulating the secretion of various stress hormones. If proven to be true in humans, options for dealing with stress and alcohol may increase dramatically (Ribertim et al, 2010).

Stress and hair loss

Too much stress can lead to thinning hair, and even baldness, in men and women. The most common type of stress-induced hair loss is *telogen effluvium*. Often seen in individuals who have lost a loved one or experienced severe weight loss or other trauma, this condition pushes colonies of hair into a resting phase. Over time, hair begins to fall out. A similar stress-related condition known as *alopecia areata* occurs when stress triggers white blood cells to attack and destroy hair follicles, usually in patches (Hall-Flavin, 2012).

"Why Should I Care?"

Compelling evidence links stress and immune system functioning. Exposure to academic stressors and self-reported stress are associated with increased upper respiratory tract infection among students. Take time to de-stress, and you might avoid that bad cold.

(**Source:** Yuri Arcurs/Age Fotostock.)

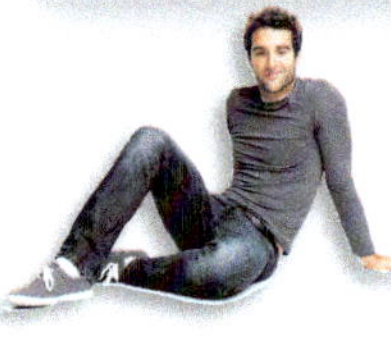

Stress and diabetes

Controlling stress levels is critical for preventing weight gain and other risk factors for type 2 diabetes, as well as for successful short- and long-term diabetes management (American Diabetes Association, 2011). People under lots of stress often don't get enough sleep, don't eat well, and may drink or take other drugs to help them get through a stressful time. All of these behaviours can alter blood sugar levels and promote development of diabetes.

Stress and digestive problems

Digestive disorders are physical conditions for which the causes are often unknown. It is widely assumed that an underlying illness, pathogen, injury, or inflammation is already present when stress triggers nausea, vomiting, stomach cramps and gut pain, or diarrhea. Although stress doesn't directly cause these symptoms, it is clearly related and may actually make your risk of having symptoms worse (National Digestive Diseases Information Clearinghouse (NDDIC), 2012). For example, people with depression or anxiety, or who feel tense, angry, or overwhelmed, are more susceptible to dehydration, inflammation, and other digestive problems. Irritable bowel syndrome may be more likely, in part, because stress stimulates colon spasms by means of the nervous system. Some relaxation techniques and mindfulness training may be helpful in coping with stressors that irritate your digestive system. These relaxation techniques reduce the activity of the sympathetic nervous system, leading to decreases in heart rate, blood pressure, and other stress responses. They also appear to reduce gastrointestinal reactivity and decrease your risks of gastrointestinal tract flare-ups (Herlong, 2013; Fang et al., 2010).

Psychoneuroimmunology (PNI)
The study of the interrelationship between mind and body, and on immune system functioning.

Stress and impaired immunity

A growing area of scientific investigation known as **psychoneuroimmunology (PNI)** analyses the intricate relationship between the mind's response to stress and the immune system's ability to function effectively. Several recent reviews of research linking stress to adverse health consequences suggest that too much stress over a long period can negatively affect various aspects of the cellular immune response. This increases risks for upper respiratory infections and certain chronic conditions, increases adverse fetal development and birth outcomes, and exacerbates problems for children and adults suffering from post-traumatic stress (Marshall, 2011; Christian, 2012). More prolonged stressors, such as the loss of a loved one, caregiving, living with a handicap, and unemployment, also have been shown to impair the natural immune response among various populations over time (Kondo, 2011; Gouln & Kiecolt-Glaser, 2011).

Intellectual effects of stress

In a recent national survey of university students, more than half of the respondents said that they had felt overwhelmed by all that they had to do within the past 2 weeks, 48.3 percent reported being exhausted, and 19.2 percent felt overwhelmed by anxiety in the same time period. About 37 percent of students felt they had been under more-than-average stress in the past 12 months, whereas over 10 percent reported being under tremendous stress during that same time period. Not surprisingly, these same students rated stress as their number one impediment to academic performance, followed by lack of sleep and anxiety (American College Health Association, 2012). Stress can play a huge role in whether students stay in school, get good grades, and succeed on their career path. It can also wreak havoc on students' ability to concentrate, affect memory, and decrease ability to understand and retain information.

Stress, memory, and concentration

Although the exact reasons stress can affect grades and job performance are complex, new research has provided possible clues. Animal studies have provided compelling indicators of how glucocorticoids—stress hormones released from the adrenal cortex—are believed to affect memory. In humans, acute stress has been shown to impair short-term memory, particularly verbal memory (Marin et al., 2011; Schwabe, Wolf & Oitzi, 2009). Recent laboratory studies with rats have linked prolonged exposure to cortisol (a key stress hormone) to actual shrinking of the hippocampus, the brain's major memory center (Dias-Ferreira, 2009; Quervan et al., 2009).

Psychological effects of stress

Stress may be one of the single greatest contributors to mental disability and emotional dysfunction in industrialised nations. Studies have shown that the rates of mental disorders, particularly depression and anxiety, are associated with various environmental stressors (Fox et al., 2010; Scottet et al, 2011). University students not only face pressure to get good grades, they also face additional new stressors stemming from housing searches, becoming financially independent, career choices and employment (or the lack thereof), relationships, interactions with family and peers, and perceived environmental threats. Coping skills and social support from family, friends, and community services can buffer the negative effects of stress overload (Hunt & Eisenbe, 2010; Segrin & Passalacqua, 2010 & Chao, 2012).

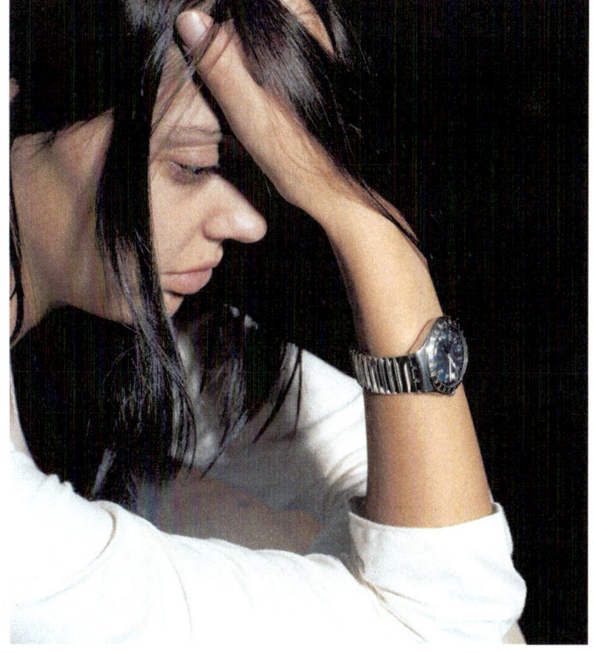

Stress and depression have complicated interconnections based on emotional, physiological, and biochemical processes. Prolonged stress can trigger depression in susceptible people, and prior periods of depression can leave individuals more susceptible to stress.
(**Source:** David De Lossy/Photodisc/Getty Images.)

What causes stress?

On any given day, we all experience eustress and distress, usually from a wide range of sources. One of the most comprehensive studies examining sources of stress among various populations is conducted annually by the Australian Psychological Association (Figure 14.5). The 2014 survey found that personal finance issues and family issues were the largest contributors to stress amongst Australians (Casey & Liang, 2014). Other commonly reported causes of stress include: personal health issues, issues with trying to maintain a healthy lifestyle, issues with the health of those close, issues in the workplace, relationship issues and issues concerning the economy (Casey & Liang, 2014). Similarly, surveys conducted by the American Psychological Association in 2012 found that concerns over money, work, the economy, and relationships were the biggest reported causes of stress for Americans (American Psychological Association, 2012). Students, in particular, face stressors that come from internal sources, as well as external pressures to succeed in a competitive environment. Awareness of the sources of stress can do much to help you develop a plan to avoid, prevent, or control the things that cause you stress.

Psychosocial stressors

Psychosocial stressors refer to the factors in our daily routines and in our social and physical environments that cause us to experience stress. Key psychosocial stressors include adjustment to change, hassles, interpersonal relationships, academic and career pressures, frustrations and conflicts, overload, and stressful environments.

39% Maintaining a Healthy Lifestyle
49% Money
32% Work
54% Family responsibilities
31% Relationships
42% Personal health concerns
36% Health problems affecting my family

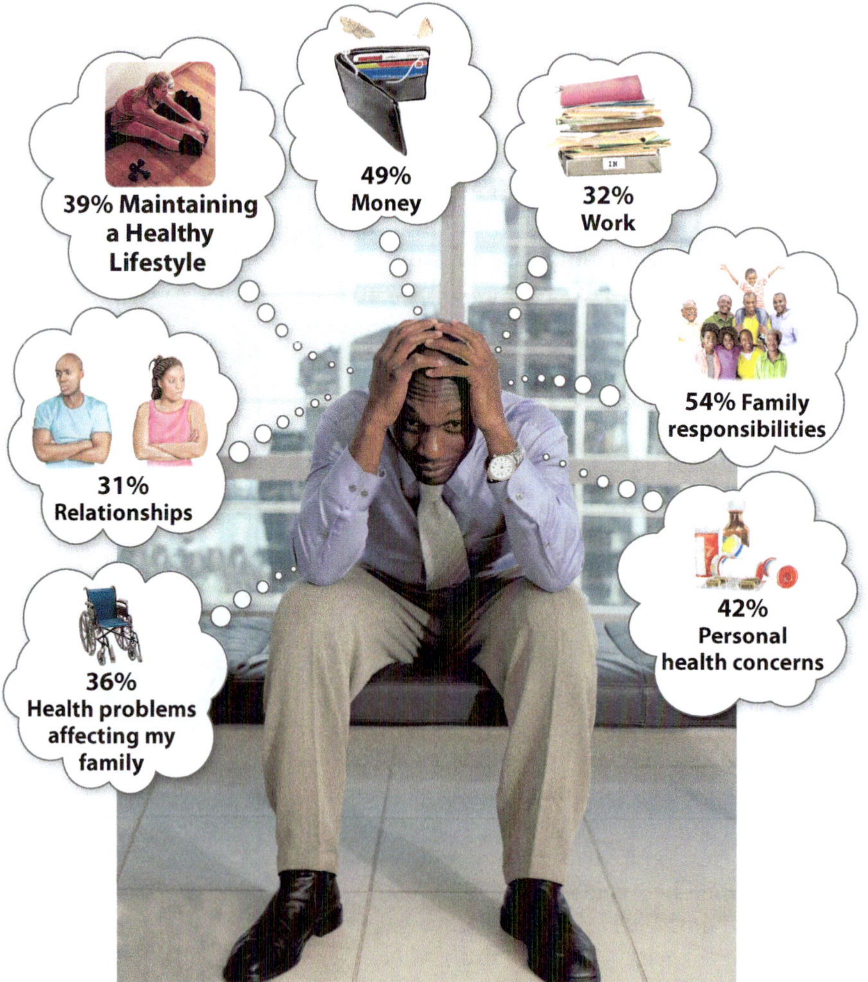

Figure 14.5 What do we say stresses us?

Over the past few years, the annual *Stress and wellbeing in Australia* survey has indicated that Australian adults are increasingly experiencing concerns finance, family, health, lifestyle, the health of others and work.

Source: Data from Australian Psychological Association, *Stress and wellbeing in Australia survey 2014*, 2013, http://www.psychology.org.au **(Source:** Thinkstock Images/ Comstock/Thinkstock.)

Adjustment to change

Anytime change, whether good or bad, occurs in your normal routine, you experience stress. The more changes you experience and the more adjustments you must make, the greater the chances are that stress will have an impact on your health. Unfortunately, although your first days on campus can be exciting, they can also be among the most stressful you will face in your life. Moving away from home, trying to fit in and make new friends from diverse backgrounds, adjusting to a new schedule, and learning to live with strangers in housing that is often lacking in the comforts of home can all cause sleeplessness and anxiety and keep your body in a continual fight-or-flight mode.

Hassles: little things that bug you

Some psychologists have proposed that the little stressors, frustrations, and petty annoyances, known collectively as *hassles,* can add up and be just as stressful as major life changes (Lazarus, 1985). Put another way, cumulative hassles add up. They tax the physiological systems of the body and cause stress-related wear and tear, known as an *allostatic load,* on the body. Listening to others monopolise class time, not finding parking on campus, continual drops on your cell phone connections, and a host of other irritants can push your buttons and trigger an acute fight-or-flight response (Hellhammer, 2010). For many people, electronic devices that are supposed to be fun can cause anxiety and sap time. See the Tech & Health box for more on technostress.

The toll of relationships

Let's face it, relationships can trigger some of the biggest fight-or-flight reactions of all time. Although romantic relationships are the ones we often think of first—the wild, exhilarating feeling of new love and the excruciating pain of breakups—relationships with friends, family, and coworkers can be sources of struggles, just as they can be sources of support. These relationships can make us strive to be the best that we can be and give us hope for the future, or they can diminish our self-esteem and leave us reeling from destructive interactions. A recent comparison of nearly 80 studies of stress and work provides strong evidence that work situations with high demands, little control, and coworkers who are difficult to get along with increase the likelihood of employee complaints about gastrointestinal ailments and sleep difficulties. Competition for rewards and systems that favor certain classes of employees or pit workers against one another are among the most stressful job situations (Nixon et al., 2011).

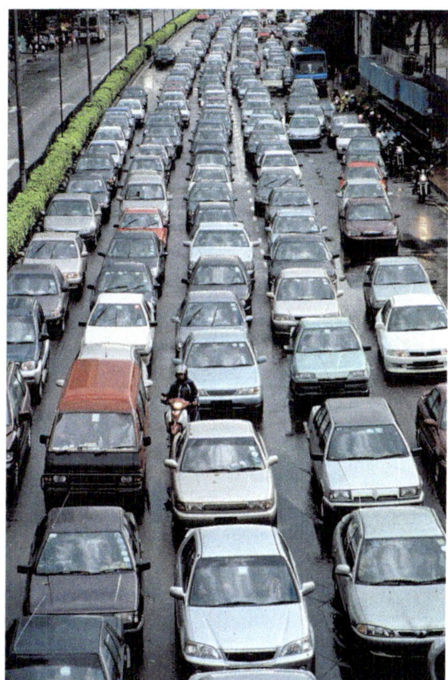

Traffic jams and noise pollution are examples of daily hassles that can add up and jeopardise our health. **(Source:** Steve Lovegrove/slovegrove/iStockphoto.)

Academic and financial pressure

It isn't surprising that today's university students face mind-boggling amounts of pressure while competing for grades, internships, athletic positions, and jobs. Challenging classes can be tough enough, but many students must juggle studies with work to pay the bills, and an economic downturn can make student dreams seem unobtainable. Increasing reports of mental health problems on university campuses may be one result of too much stress and no clear way of finding relief.

Frustrations and conflicts

Whenever there is a disparity between our goals (what we hope to obtain in life) and our behaviours (actions that may or may not lead to these goals), frustration can occur. For example, you realise that you must get good grades in university to enter graduate school, which is your ultimate goal. If your social life is cutting into your studying time, you may find your goals slipping away, leading to increased stress.

Conflicts occur when we are forced to decide among competing motives, impulses, desires, and behaviours (for example, go out partying or study) or when we are forced to face pressures or demands that are incompatible with our own values and sense of importance (for example, get good grades or play on an all-star sports team). University students who are away from their families for the first time may face a variety of conflicts among parental values, their own beliefs, and the beliefs of others who are very different from themselves.

Overload

Overload A condition in which a person feels overextended and overly pressured by demands.

Background distressors Environmental stressors of which people are often unaware.

We've all experienced times in our lives when the demands of work, responsibilities, deadlines, and relationships all seem to be pulling us underwater. **Overload** occurs when we are overextended and, try as we might, there are not enough hours in the day to do what we must get done. Students suffering from overload may experience depression, sleeplessness, mood swings, frustration, anxiety, or a host of other symptoms. Binge drinking, high consumption of junk food, lack of money, and arguments can all add fuel to the overload fire. Unrelenting stress and overload can lead to a state of physical and mental exhaustion known as *burnout.*

Stressful environments

For many students, where they live and the environment around them cause significant levels of stress. Perhaps you cannot afford quality housing, a bad roommate is producing major environmental stress, or loud neighbors are keeping you up at night. Maybe it isn't safe to walk to your car after dark on campus, or you have to leave your bicycle in a prime "rip-off" location during classes. Seemingly unending inconveniences and minor threats can wear you down.

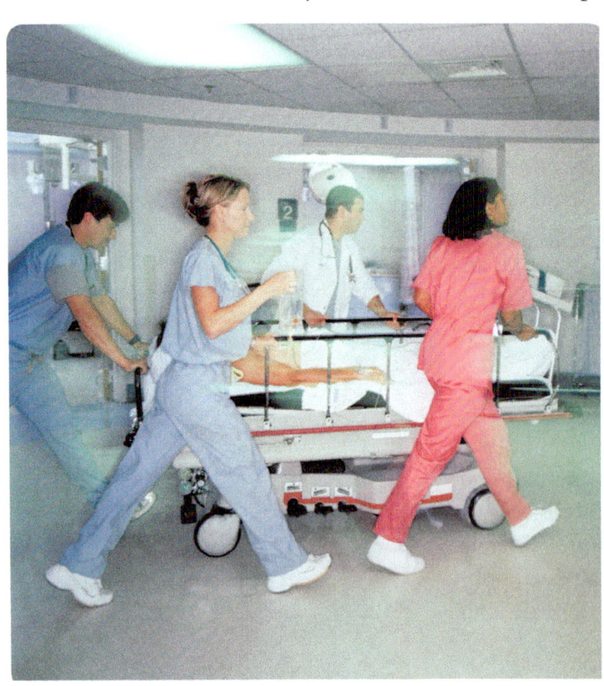

Who is most prone to stress?

Some people have careers or life circumstances that impose external pressures on them. Doctors and nurses face long work hours and a high-stakes work environment that make them especially prone to stress, overload, and burnout. (**Source:** Ryan McVay/Digital Vision/Getty Images.)

Unexpected natural disasters that affect you or others can cause great emotional upset. Superstorm Sandy and Hurricane Katrina; the Sumatra, Japan, and Haiti earthquakes; killer tornadoes in Oklahoma, Iowa, and Kansas; as well as human disasters such as the Gulf oil spill have threatened millions with mayhem and death, disrupted lives, and damaged ecosystems for the foreseeable future. Even after the initial images of suffering pass and the crisis has subsided, shortages of vital resources such as gasoline, clean water, food, housing, health care, sewage disposal, and other necessities, as well as electricity outages and transportation problems, can wreak havoc in local communities and on campuses. Although not as newsworthy as major disasters, **background distressors** in the environment, such as noise, air, and water pollution; allergy-aggravating pollen and dust; unsafe food; or environmental tobacco smoke can also be incredibly stressful. Campus violence, shootings, and highly charged political clashes on campus can also be sources of anxiety as students worry about safety.

Bias and discrimination

Racial and ethnic diversity of students, faculty members, and staff enriches everyone's educational experiences. It also challenges us to examine our personal attitudes, beliefs, and biases. As campuses become more internationalised, a diverse cultural base of vastly different life experiences, languages, and customs is emerging. Often, those perceived as dissimilar may become victims of subtle and not-so-subtle forms of bigotry, insensitivity, harassment, or hostility, or they may simply be ignored. Race, ethnicity, religious affiliation, age, sexual orientation, gender, or other differences may hang like a dark cloud over these students (Schwartz et al, 2012; Pieterse, 2010; McAleavey, Castonguay & Locke, 2011).

Evidence of the health effects of excessive stress in minority groups abounds. For example, African Americans suffer higher rates of hypertension, CVD, and most cancers than do whites (Iwamoto, Kenji & Ming, 2010). Poverty and socioeconomic status have been blamed for much of the spike in hypertension rates for African Americans and other marginalised groups. Instead, chronic, physically debilitating stress among these groups may reflect the real and perceived effects of institutional racism. More research is necessary to show direct associations between racism, stress, and hypertension. It is important to realise that all types of "isms" may influence stress-related hypertension and make it more difficult for those affected to engage in healthy lifestyle behaviours (Brondolo, 2011; Fuchs, 2011).

Appraisal
The interpretation and evaluation of information provided to the brain by the senses.

Suicidal ideation
A desire to die and thoughts about suicide.

Self-efficacy
Belief in one's ability to achieve goals and influence events in life.

Appraisal and stress

Throughout life, we encounter many different types of demands and potential stressors. It is our appraisal of these demands, not the demands themselves, that results in our experiencing stress. **Appraisal** is defined as the interpretation and evaluation of information provided to the brain by the senses. Typically, it isn't a conscious activity, but rather a natural process whereby the brain sizes up a situation. Appraisal helps us recognise stressors, evaluate them on the basis of past experiences and emotions, and decide how to cope with them.

Self-esteem and self-efficacy

Self-esteem refers to how you feel about yourself. Self-esteem can and does continually change (Karren et al., 2010). When you feel good about yourself, you are less likely to view an event as stressful and more likely to be able to cope (Seaward, 2012). Of particular concern, research with high school and university students has found that low self-esteem and stressful life events significantly predict **suicidal ideation,** a desire to die and thoughts about suicide. On a more positive note, research has also indicated that it is possible to increase an individual's ability to cope with stress by increasing self-esteem (Brown, 2011; Gomez, Miranda & Polanco, 2011).

Self-efficacy, or confidence in one's skills and ability to cope with life's challenges, appears to be a key buffer in preventing negative stress effects. Research has shown that people with high levels of self-efficacy tend to have a greater sense or feeling of being in control of stressful situations and, as such, report fewer stress effects (Glanz, Rimmer & Levis, 2008). Self-efficacy is considered one of the most important personality traits that influences psychological and physiological stress responses (Abraham, 2012). Developing self-efficacy is also vital to coping with and overcoming academic pressures and worries (Bragard, 2010). For example, by learning to handle anxiety around testing situations, you will feel more capable of handling

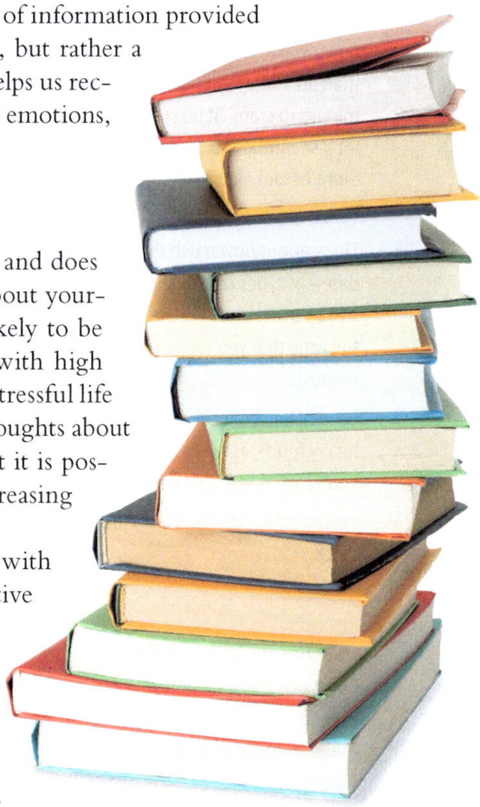

How daunting that pile of books and homework is depends on your appraisal of it.
(**Source:** kate_sept2004/E+/Getty Images.)

Hostility
The cognitive, affective, and behavioural tendencies toward anger, distrust, and cynicism.

them and your sense of academic self-efficacy will grow. For tips on how to deal with test-taking anxiety, see the Skills for behaviour Change box below.

Type A and type B personalities

It should come as no surprise to you that personality can have an impact on whether you are happy and socially well-adjusted or sad and socially isolated. However, your personality may affect more than just your social interactions: It may be a critical factor in your stress levels.

In 1974, physicians Meyer Friedman and Ray Rosenman published a book indicating that Type A individuals had a greatly increased risk of heart disease (Friedman & Rosenman, 1974). *Type A* personalities are defined as hard-driving, competitive, time-driven perfectionists. In contrast, *Type B* personalities are described as being relaxed, noncompetitive, and more tolerant of others.

Today, most researchers recognise that none of us will be wholly Type A or Type B all of the time, and we may exhibit either type in selected situations. In addition, recent research indicates that not all Type A people experience negative health consequences; in fact, some Type A individuals thrive on their supercharged lifestyles. Often Type A's who exhibit a "toxic core," that is, who have disproportionate amounts of anger; are distrustful of others; and have a cynical, glass-half-empty approach to life—a set of characteristics referred to as **hostility**—are at increased risk for heart disease (Whooley & Wong, 2011; Newman et al., 2011; Smith et al., 2012).

Skills for behaviour Change

Overcoming Test-Taking Anxiety

Testing well is a skill needed at university and beyond. Try these tips on your next exam.

BEFORE THE EXAM

- Manage your study time. Keep up with reading during the term. Make sure your preparation for the test is a review rather than an initial reading of material. Don't wait until the last minute to cram. At least 1 week before your test, start studying for a set amount of time each day. Do a limited review the night before, get a good night's sleep, and arrive for the exam early.
- Think about how much time you might need to answer different types of test questions. If you know how much time will be available for the test, make a general strategy for using the time that you can and quickly refine at the beginning of the test.
- Eat a balanced meal before the exam. Avoid sugar and rich or heavy foods, as well as foods that might upset your stomach. You want to feel your best.
- Wear a watch to class on the day of the test, in case there is no clock.

DURING THE EXAM

- Manage your time during the test. Look at how many questions there are and what each is worth. Prioritise the high-point questions, allow a certain amount of time for each, and make sure that you leave some time for the rest. Hold to this schedule.
- Slow down and pay attention. Focus on one question at a time. Check off each part of multipart questions to make sure your answers are complete.

Type C and type D personalities

In addition to CVD, personality types have often been linked to increased risk for a variety of other illnesses, ranging from asthma to cancer, even though much of this research remains in question. A type commonly discussed today is the *Type C* personality, characterised as stoic, with a tendency to stuff feelings down and conform to the wishes of others (or be "pleasers"). Preliminary research suggests that Type C individuals may be more susceptible to illnesses such as asthma, multiple sclerosis, autoimmune disorders, and cancer; however, more research is necessary to support this relationship (Mate, 2011).

A more recently identified personality type is *Type D* (distressed), which is characterised by a tendency toward excessive negative worry, irritability, gloom, and inability to express these feelings due to social inhibition. Several recent studies have indicated that Type D people may be up to eight times more likely to die of a heart attack or sudden death (Versteed, Spek & Petersen, 2011; Mols & Denollet, 2010).

Are internal stressors inescapable?

For most people most of the time, enough exposure to stressors will evoke the stress response. With the long list of stressors we've just reviewed, especially for people prone to Type A behaviour, it might seem like stress is a given. But two factors seem to break the cycle and offer some protection from stress: psychological hardiness and the shift-and-persist strategy.

Psychological hardiness

According to psychologist Susanne Kobasa, **psychological hardiness** may negate self-imposed stress associated with Type A behaviour. Psychologically hardy people are characterised by *control, commitment,* and willingness to embrace *challenge* (Kobasa, 1979). People with a sense of control are able to accept responsibility for their behaviours and change those that they discover are debilitating. People with a sense of commitment have good self-esteem and understand their purpose in life. Those who embrace challenge see change as an opportunity for growth.

The concept of hardiness has evolved to include a person's ability to cope with stress and adversity (Schetter & Dolbier, 2011). In recent years, it has become common for people to think of this general hardiness concept in terms of **psychological resilience**. Essentially, resilience refers to our capacity to maintain or regain psychological well-being in the face of challenge.[37] Resilient individuals are often able to do well in the face of adversity because of "protective factors" such as strong support networks of family, friends, and healthy communities and their own coping skills. Resilience has been studied extensively and appears to be a key indicator of good psychological and social development (Ryff et al., 2012).

Psychological hardiness
A personality trait characterised by control, commitment, and the embrace of challenge.

Psychological resilience
The capacity to maintain or regain psychological well-being in the face of adversity, trauma, tragedy, threats, or significant sources of stress.

Shift and persist
A strategy of reframing appraisals of current stressors and focusing on a meaningful future that protects a person from the negative effects of too much stress.

Shift and persist

Even though they face extreme poverty, abuse, and unspeakable living conditions as they grow up, some youth seem to thrive when their conditions are bleak. Why? An exciting, emerging body of sociological research proposes that in the midst of extreme, persistent adversity, youth—often with the help of positive role models in their lives—are able to reframe appraisals of current stressors more positively (*shifting*), while *persisting* in focusing on a future that has something to offer them. These youth are able to endure the present by adapting, holding on to meaningful things in their lives, and staying optimistic and positive. These **"shift and persist"** strategies are among the most recently identified factors that protect against the negative effects of too much stress in our lives (Chen et al., 2012).[C]

How stress impacts our health

In 1962, two Japanese doctors, Y. Ikemi and S. Nakagawa, conducted a study demonstrating the intimate connection between brain and body. Their study, which researchers today might

[C]Donatelle, R. J. (2015). Managing stress and coping with life's challenges. In R. J. Donatelle (Ed.), *Health: The basics* (11th ed., pp. 75–83). Upper Saddle River, NJ: Pearson Education.

find difficult to carry out for ethical reasons, showed how hypnotic and direct suggestions from a respected authority figure can produce dramatic skin reactions. The researchers selected 13 boys who contracted a red, itchy skin reaction when touched with the leaves of a tree similar to poison ivy. Five boys received a hypnotic induction with suggestions for relaxation and drowsiness, and another group of eight boys received no prior hypnotic induction—just suggestions administered while they were awake and alert.

In the first phase of the study, all of the boys sat with their eyes closed while a respected physician told them he was touching them with the leaves of a plant similar to poison ivy. In fact, he was touching them with leaves from a harmless plant. The reactions were remarkable. All of the boys—the hypnotic participants and the suggestion-alone participants—showed significant skin disturbance after believing they had been touched by the poison ivy–type leaves. As is so often the case in psychology, beliefs can create reality, in this case a *nocebo effect*.

In the second phase of the study, the researchers reversed the conditions: They rubbed the boys' arms with the poison ivy–type leaves, but told them the leaves were harmless. Four of the five hypnotic participants and seven of the eight suggestion-alone participants didn't show any skin reactions to the leaves. Interestingly, all had developed skin reactions to the leaves *prior* to the study (Ikemi & Nakagawa, 1962).

This study demonstrates how psychological factors, in this case the stressful idea of contracting an itchy rash, can influence physical processes. Indeed, much of what we call a 'psychological' response to events manifests itself in physiological reactions. By now you will realise that stress can spill over into multiple domains of life, creating physical difficulties that disrupt our sleep and sexual functioning. But can stress seep into our cells and weaken our body's defences against infections? A number of fascinating studies tell us that the answer is yes.

The immune system

Immune system
The body's defence system against invading bacteria, viruses and other potentially illness-producing organisms and substances.

Ordinarily (and thankfully!), we never have to think about the billions of viruses, fungi, protozoa and bacteria that share our environment or inhabit our body. That is because our **immune system** neutralises or destroys them. The immune system is our body's defence against invading bacteria, viruses and other potentially illness-producing organisms and substances. Our first shield from these foreign invaders, called *antigens*, is the skin, which blocks the entry of many disease-producing organisms, called *pathogens*. When we cough or sneeze, the lungs expel harmful bacteria and viruses. Saliva, urine, tears, perspiration and stomach acid also rid our body of pathogens.

Some viruses or bacteria penetrate these defences, but the immune system is wily, and has other means of safeguarding us. *Phagocytes* and *lymphocytes* are two types of specialised white blood cells produced in the marrow of the bones. One type of phagocyte, called a *neutrophil*, is abundant and is first at the scene of an infection to engulf an invader. Longer-lived *macrophages* also travel through the body as scavengers, sticking to and destroying remaining antigens and dead tissue. Two types of lymphocytes, *T cells* and *B cells*, are also stalwart soldiers in the night-and-day battle to keep us healthy. Killer T cells, as they are called, move through the body and attach to proteins on the surface of virus- and cancer-infected cells, popping them like balloons. Memory T cells recognise the invading cells after an initial infection and promote an efficient response upon reinfection. B cells produce proteins called *antibodies*, which stick to the surface of the invader, slow its progress and attract other proteins that destroy the foreign organism.

Under ordinary circumstances, the immune system is remarkably effective. But it is not a perfect barrier against infection. For example, some cancer cells can suppress an effective immune response, multiply and wreak havoc in the body. Serious disorders of the immune system, such as **acquired immune deficiency syndrome (AIDS)**, are life-threatening. AIDS is an incurable yet often treatable condition in which the human immunodeficiency virus (HIV) attacks and damages the immune system. When the immune system is overactive, it can launch an attack on various organs of the body, causing *autoimmune diseases* such as arthritis, in which the immune system causes swelling and pain at the joints, and multiple sclerosis, in which the immune system attacks the protective myelin sheath surrounding neurons.

Acquired immune deficiency syndrome (AIDS)
A life-threatening, incurable, yet treatable condition in which the human immunodeficiency virus (HIV) attacks and damages the immune system.

Psychoneuroimmunology
Study of the relationship between the immune system and the central nervous system.

Psychoneuroimmunology: our body, our environment and our health

The study of the relationship between the immune system and the central nervous system—the seat of our emotions and reactions to the environment—goes by the name **psychoneuroimmunology** (Cohen & Herbert, 1996). When evaluating psychoneuroimmunology, we must be careful not to fall prey to exaggerated claims. Illnesses are not the result of negative thinking, nor can positive thinking reverse serious illnesses. Nevertheless, researchers using rigorous designs have discovered at least some fascinating links between our life circumstances and our ability to fend off illnesses.

Stress and colds

Many people believe they are more likely to get a cold when they are really stressed—and they are right. Sheldon Cohen and his associates placed cold viruses into volunteers' nasal passages (Cohen, Tyrell & Smith, 1991). Other volunteers, in a placebo condition, did not receive the virus, but instead received nasal drops with a saline solution. Stressful life events in the year preceding the study predicted the number of colds people developed when exposed to the virus. Exposure to the virus was also important. People in the placebo condition did not develop as many colds, even when they experienced stressful events in the year before the study. The researchers (Cohen et al., 1998) later discovered that significant stressors, such as unemployment and interpersonal difficulties lasting at least a month, were the best predictors of who developed a cold. But a network of friends and relatives, and close ties to the community, afforded protection against colds (Cohen et al., 1997; Cohen et al., 2003).

It is possible that stress affects health-related behaviours but has no direct impact on the immune system. For instance, our susceptibility to a cold may increase because when we are under stress we tend to sleep poorly, eat non-nutritious foods, and smoke and drink alcohol excessively, all of which depress the immune system. Yet Cohen and his colleagues found that even when they controlled for these influences, the relationship between stress and colds remained.

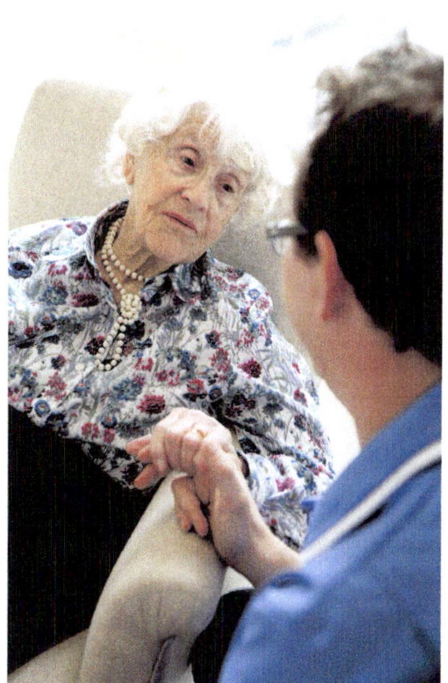

Carers of people with Alzheimer's disease experience high levels of stress, are at heightened risk of developing depression, and even show decreases in their blood's ability to clot (associated with having a stroke) in response to stressful life events (von Känel et al., 2003).
(**Source:** Lord and Leverett/Pearson Education Ltd.)

Stress and immune function: beyond the common cold

Janice Kiecolt-Glaser and her associates are pioneers in the study of the connection between stressors and the immune system. Caring for a family member with Alzheimer's disease, a form of dementia, can be exceedingly stressful and cause long-term deregulation of the immune system. Kiecolt-Glaser demonstrated that a small wound

Psychophysiological Description of illnesses such as asthma and ulcers in which emotions and stress contribute to, maintain or aggravate the physical condition.

Biopsychosocial perspective The view that an illness or a medical condition is the product of the interplay of biological, psychological and social factors.

Coronary heart disease (CHD) Damage to the heart from the complete or partial blockage of the arteries that provide oxygen to the heart.

(standardised for size) took 24 percent longer to heal in Alzheimer's caregivers compared with a group of people who were not taking care of a relative with Alzheimer's (Kiecolt-Glaser et al., 1995).

All of the following stressors can lead to disruptions in the immune system (Kiecolt-Glaser et al., 2002):

- taking an important test
- the death of a spouse
- unemployment
- marital conflict
- living near a damaged nuclear reactor
- natural disasters.

The good news is that positive emotions and social support, which we consider later in the chapter, can fortify our immune system (Esterling, Kiecolt-Glaser & Glaser, 1996; Kennedy, Kiecolt-Glaser & Glaser, 1990).

Stress-related illnesses: a biopsychosocial view

Not long ago a common myth of popular psychology was that beliefs and mental states were the root causes of many physical ailments. Certain illnesses or disorders were once called *psychosomatic*, because psychologists believed that psychological conflicts and emotional reactions were the culprits. Today, psychologists use the term **psychophysiological** to describe illnesses like asthma and ulcers in which emotions and stress contribute to, maintain or aggravate physical conditions.

Today, psychologists widely acknowledge that emotions and stress are associated with physical disorders, including coronary heart disease and AIDS. Most scientists have adopted a **biopsychosocial perspective**, which proposes that most medical conditions are neither all physical nor all psychological. Numerous physical illnesses depend on the interplay of genes, lifestyle, immunity, social support, everyday stressors and self-perceptions (Markus & Kitayama, 1991; Turk, 1996).

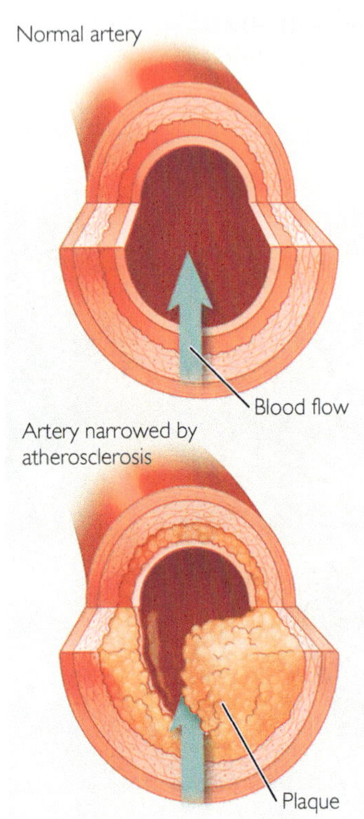

Figure 14.6 Atherosclerosis. Cholesterol deposits in the large arteries form plaque, restricting the flow of blood. This condition, called atherosclerosis, can result in stroke, heart attack and serious chest pain.

Coronary heart disease

Scientists have learned that psychological factors, including stress and personality traits, are key risk factors for **coronary heart disease (CHD)**. CHD is the complete or partial blockage of the arteries that provide oxygen to the heart. It kills more Australians than any other single disease, accounting for 17 percent of all deaths annually (Australian Institute of Health & Welfare, 2008a). Before age 65, men are more likely than women to die from CHD. But after 65, the statistics even out: one in three men and women die of CHD. CHD develops when deposits of *cholesterol*—a waxy, fatty substance that travels in the bloodstream—collects in the walls of arteries, narrowing and blocking the coronary arteries. This creates a condition called *atherosclerosis*. When atherosclerosis worsens, it can lead to chest pain and the deterioration and death of heart tissue, otherwise known as a heart attack (see Figure 14.6).

The role of stress in CHD. Many risk factors are associated with CHD, including a history of smoking, high cholesterol and high blood pressure (Clarke et al., 2009). A family history of CHD, diabetes and low levels of vitamin D—the 'sunshine vitamin'—can also boost the risk of heart disease (Wang et al., 2008).

Stress deserves a prominent place on the list of CHD risk factors. Stressful life events predict recurrences of heart attacks, high blood pressure, and enlargement of the heart (Repetti, Taylor & Seeman, 2002; Schnall et al., 1990; Troxel et al., 2003). Although only correlational, these data are consistent with this hypothesis that stressors may sometimes produce negative physiological effects. Moreover, high levels of stress hormones triggered by extreme stress can lead to disruptions in normal heart rhythm and even sudden death, as well as to atherosclerosis in people who are highly reactive to everyday stressors (Carney, Freedland & Veith, 2005; Sarafino, 2006). People with CHD also show signs of a hyped-up autonomic nervous system, with elevated heart rates and extreme responses to physical stressors (Carney, Freedland & Veith, 2005).As well as exerting a direct effect on CHD, stress is also associated with behavioural risk factors for CHD, including poor diet and inadequate exercise (Chandola et al., 2008). So at least some of the effects of stress on CHD may actually be due to the overlap between stress and these risk factors.

THE ROLE OF PERSONALITY IN CHD. In addition to stress, researchers have suggested that long-standing behaviour patterns contribute to risk for CHD. Two cardiologists, Meyer Friedman and Ray Rosenman (1959), coined the term **Type A personality**, now widely popularised in the media, to describe a curious behaviour pattern they observed among CHD patients. They noticed that the chairs in their hospital waiting room were rapidly becoming worn out around the edges. Many of their CHD patients were literally sitting and bouncing on the edge of their seats because of restlessness. Later, Friedman and Rosenman (1974) identified additional characteristics that clustered under the Type A description: perfectionistic, prone to hostility, stubborn, opinionated, cynical, controlling, and concerned with deadlines. Although early studies revealed high rates of CHD among extreme Type A individuals, later studies yielded many negative results (Gatchel & Oordt, 2003). Accordingly, scientists began to wonder whether certain Type A traits are more associated with heightened risk than other traits.

Type A personality
Personality type that describes people who are competitive, driven, hostile and ambitious.

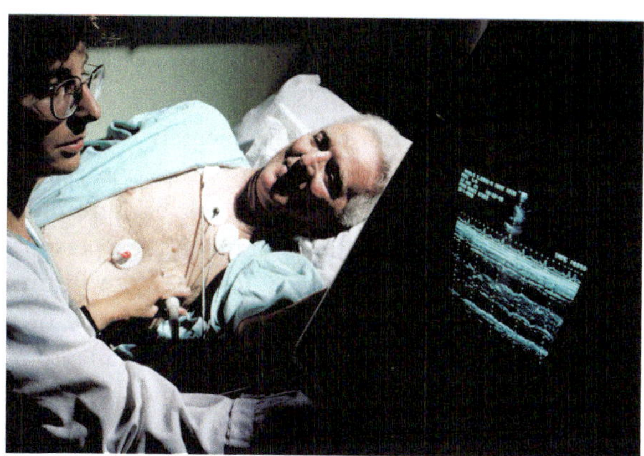

The classic Framingham Study, which began in 1948, continues to examine the health of more than 5000 American men and women in Framingham, Massachusetts. This longitudinal study has provided a treasure trove of data on risk factors for CHD.
(Source: Nathan Benn/Corbis.)

Of all Type A traits researchers have studied, hostility turned out to be most predictive of heart disease (Matthews et al., 2004; Myrtek, 2001; Nabi et al., 2008; Smith & Gallo, 2001). In a study of healthy young-to-middle-aged Australian men, angry reactions to being criticised were linked to high levels of fat and cholesterol in the blood, the greatest physical risk factor for CHD (Richards, Hof & Alvarenga, 2000). Hostility is associated with other well-documented risk factors for CHD, such as alcohol consumption, smoking and weight gain (Bunde & Suls, 2006), so an alternative hypothesis is that its effects on CHD are indirect. Nevertheless, in a study of older white men, hostility surpassed these traditional risk factors in predicting CHD (Niaura et al., 2002).

But there is a silver lining to this grey cloud: reducing anger and hostility helps. When researchers taught CHD patients techniques to curtail their anger, they found a 37 percent decrease in deaths from heart attacks compared with other patients (Dusseldorp et al., 1999; Friedman et al., 1987).

CHD, everyday experiences and socioeconomic factors

Hostility and other negative emotions do not always arise from enduring personality traits. These negative emotions can stem from the many pressures and demands we confront in our fast-paced, competitive society. Consider three sources of support for the claim that everyday experiences set the stage for many physical problems, including heart disease. First, people who experience even one significant drop in their income over a five-year period face a 30 percent increase in their risk of dying from any cause. Two such drops in income jack iflate the risk to a whopping 70 percent (Duncan, 1996). Second, the INTERHEART study of more than 11 000 people from Europe, the Middle East, Australasia and the Americas showed that CHD was associated with psychosocial factors including work stress, financial stress and other major life events. Third, CHD is associated with substantial job stress and dissatisfaction (Quick et al., 1997). Although job stress is correlated with CHD, it may not cause it in all circumstances. An interesting possibility that has yet to be fully explored is that the causal arrow is reversed: perhaps CHD causes job stress in some people.

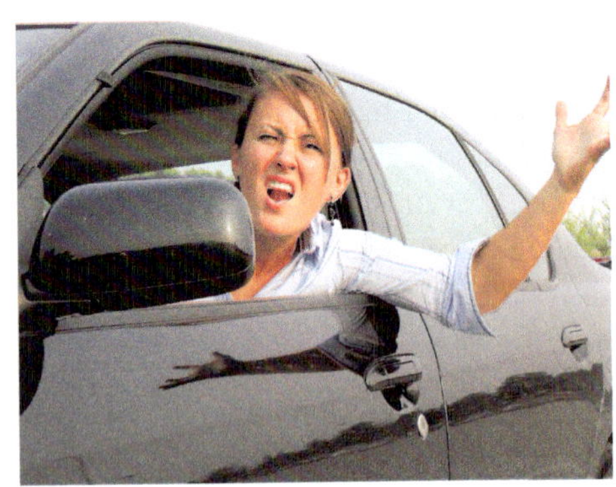

Can chronic anger be bad for our health? Research indicates that the anger component of the Type A personality can be deadly, increasing our risk for coronary heart disease. (**Source:** Kirk Johnson/Dreamstime.)

Still, these findings, along with the others we have examined, point to another possibility that has been well supported by research: the burden of most health problems is shared disproportionately by the poor. Researchers have established a strong correlation between poverty and poor health (Antonovsky, 1967; Repetti, Taylor & Seeman, 2002), but we still need to ask: 'What is responsible for this association?'

Linda Gallo and Karen Matthews (2003) addressed this question. They noted that life can prove immensely challenging for people who have little education, struggle in a bad job with a nasty supervisor and barely make enough money to pay the bills. People from low socioeconomic backgrounds who regularly encounter these circumstances experience a significant drain on their personal and interpersonal resources. This state of affairs decreases their ability to cope with future stressors, including depression, hopelessness and hostility, which can increase the risk of poor health and CHD. To make matters worse, negative thoughts and feelings can promote unhealthy habits like smoking, drinking and lack of exercise, which further increase the risk of physical problems (Gallo & Matthews, 2003).

Illness can create stress

We have seen that stress can contribute to physical disorders, such as CHD. But, of course, physical disorders can also create stress. Being diagnosed with a potentially fatal illness that has an uncertain outcome, like cancer, can be unimaginably stressful and pose innumerable challenges. The spectre of death and feelings of hopelessness, along with side-effects of treatment, including profound fatigue and embarrassing hair loss, frequently compound the distress of cancer. People who suffer from cancer often endure chronic pain and wonder whether even a slight increase in pain signals a downward, perhaps fatal, turn in the progression of their illness. Irritability, anger and frustration can also be by-products of prolonged periods of pain-related sleeplessness and the fatigue that results from it (Moffitt et al., 1991).

Asthma
medical condition in which breathing becomes difficult when the bronchial tubes in the lungs become inflamed, spasm and are clogged with mucus.

ASTHMA: CHRONIC ILLNESS AND STRESS. **Asthma** provides another example of how an illness can contribute to stress and hamper people's ability to cope with life's challenges. The prevalence of asthma in Australia is among the highest in the world, with up to 12 percent of adults suffering from the disease (Australian Institute of Health & Welfare, 2008c). Asthma sufferers find it difficult to breathe because the bronchial tubes in their lungs become inflamed, spasm and become clogged with mucus (see Figure 14.7,). People with asthma

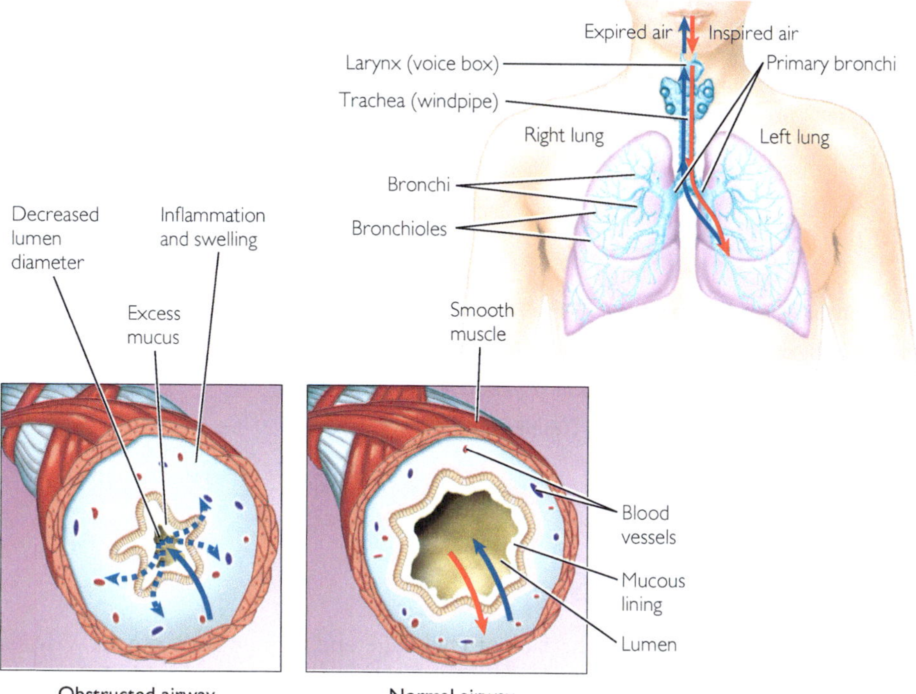

Figure 14.7 Anatomy of an asthma attack. (**Source:** Encyclopaedia Britannica, 2001.)

feel tightness in their chest, and cough and wheeze because of their lung condition. The narrowing of the bronchial tube can become so severe that it is life-threatening (Gatchel & Oordt, 2003).

When asthmatics react to an attack with fear and agitation, their symptoms can intensify to the point of being disabling. Asthma sufferers often must deal with sleep loss, absences from school and work, loss of income and restriction of everyday activities (Labott, 2004; Mailick, Holden & Walther, 1994). Understandably, asthma is associated with anxiety (Vila et al., 2000) and depression (Chaney et al., 1999). Emotions by themselves do not cause most asthma attacks, but physical responses to stress or emotional responses (such as crying, laughter and coughing) can trigger attacks and/or exacerbate attacks in some asthma patients.

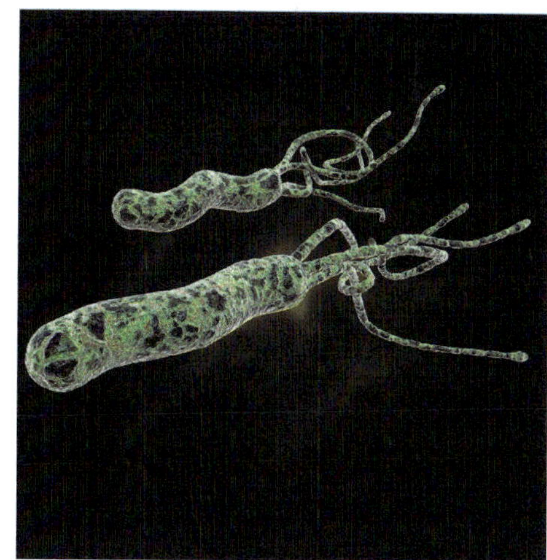

Contrary to popular belief, stress is not the major cause of ulcers. Instead, the bacterium *Helicobacter pylori* is the prime culprit. (**Source:** Pseudolongino/Dreamstime.)

ULCERS: CHANGING VIEWS OF PSYCHOPHYSIOLOGICAL DISORDERS. In the case of some psychophysiological disorders, such as ulcers, psychologists are still uncovering the role of stress.

A popular myth is that stomach ulcers—an inflamed area in the gastrointestinal tract that can cause pain, nausea, and loss of appetite—result from overindulging in spicy foods like salsas or hot chicken wings, which create excess stomach acid. Just 30 years ago, many scientists accepted this idea. However, in 1984 Australian medical scientist Barry Marshall proved that the bacteria *Helicobacter pylori* (*H. pylori*) thrives in stomach acid. He famously accomplished this by drinking a petri dish full of the stuff. His demonstration led medical researchers to realise that *H. pylori* is the cause of as many as 90 percent of stomach ulcers, and these can be effectively treated with antibiotics. But the great majority of people infected with *H. pylori* do not develop ulcers. So other influences are clearly at work, too. Research shows that the widespread belief that stress by itself causes ulcers is wrong. Yet stress probably plays some role, because higher rates of ulcers and a poor response to ulcer treatment (Levenstein, Kaplan & Smith, 1997; Overmier & Murison, 1997) are associated with earthquakes, being a prisoner of war, economic crises and other anxiety-provoking events (Levenstein et al., 1999). So stress, together with *H. pylori*, may trigger some cases of ulcers.

Assess your knowledge — FACT or FICTION?

1. Overactivity of the immune system sometimes leads to disease. **(True/False)**
2. The number one cause of death in Australia is coronary heart disease. **(True/False)**
3. Social and economic factors are largely or entirely unrelated to risk for physical diseases. **(True/False)**
4. One major cause of ulcers is eating hot spicy foods late at night. **(True/False)**

Answers: (1) T; (2) T; (3) F; (4) F

Coping with stress

Clearly, some of us adapt better in the face of challenge and change than others. Why is this so, and what can we do to reduce stress, manage our lives and stay healthy? We now take stock of how we can use social support and coping strategies to surmount stressful circumstances.

Social support

Social support
Relationships with people and groups that can provide us with emotional comfort and personal and financial resources.

Imagine that you survived the Boxing Day tsunami of 2004. What would be helpful? When we ask our students this question, many say the support of family, friends, neighbours, teachers, colleagues and clergy would be invaluable. **Social support** encompasses social relationships with people, groups and the larger community. Social support can provide us with emotional comfort, financial assistance and information to make decisions, solve problems and contend with stressful situations (Schaefer, Coyne & Lazarus, 1981; Stroebe, 2000; Wills & Fegan, 2001).

Lisa Berkman and Leonard Syme (1979) conducted a landmark study of the hypothesis that social support buffers us against the adverse effects of stress on health. They analysed data from nearly 5000 men and women in Alameda County, California, over a nine-year period. They homed in on four kinds of social ties: marriage, contact with friends, church membership, and formal and informal group associations. They then created a social network index reflecting the number of social connections and social supports available to each person.

Berkman and Syme found a strong relationship between the number of social connections, across every age group, and the probability of dying during the nine-year period. But do these findings mean that isolation increases our chances of dying? A rival hypothesis is that poor health results in few social bonds, rather than the other way around. To rule out this possibility, the researchers surveyed participants when they started the study. People with high and low levels of support reported a comparable illness history, suggesting that poor initial health cannot explain why people with the least social support are later more likely to die. Nevertheless, people are not necessarily accurate when they judge their health.

To address this concern, James House, Cynthia Robbins and Helen Metzner (1982) ensured that their 2700 participants received a medical examination *before* their study got under way. This exam provided a more objective assessment of health status. The researchers replicated Berkman and Syme's (1979) findings: even when they took initial health status into account, people with less social support had higher mortality rates.

Fortunately, the positive influence of social support is not limited to health outcomes. Supportive and caring relationships can help us cope with short-term crises and life transitions. A happy marriage, for example, is protective against depression, even when people encounter major stressors (Alloway & Bebbington, 1987; Gotlib & Hammen, 1992). But the break-up of close relationships through separation, divorce, discrimination or bereavement ranks among the most stressful events we can experience (Gardner, Gabriel & Diekman, 2000).

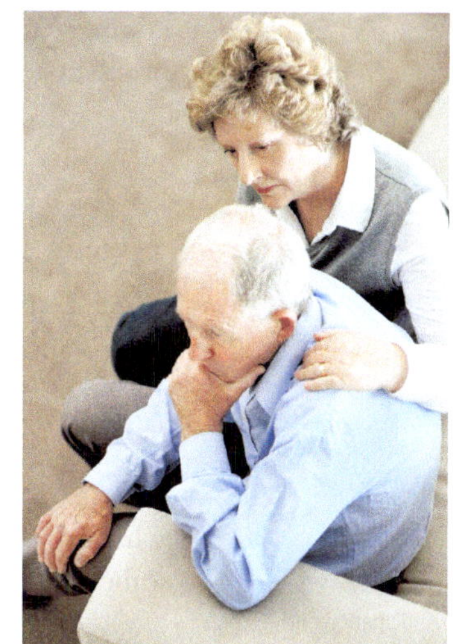

Support and comfort from others can buffer the effects of highly aversive situations. **(Source:** Yuri Arcurs/Dreamstime.)

With advancements in technology, recent research has established that online social support groups through social media sites such as Facebook can foster positive outcomes and empower those experiencing difficult circumstances (Chung, 2014; Idriss, Kvedar & Watson, 2009). For example, one study found that patients diagnosed with breast cancer, arthritis, or fibromyalgia, who participated in online support groups, described feelings of empowerment as a result of the online support they recieved (van Uden-Kraan, 2008). In particular, patients reported increased confidence in their relationship with their medical practitioner, improved acceptance of their illness and more confident regarding their treatment (van Uden-Kraan, 2008). Research in this area highlights the importance of having a support network, irrespective of whether that support is face-to-face, or not.

Gaining control

As mentioned earlier, we can also relieve stress by acquiring control of situations. Next, we discuss five types of control we can use in different situations (Bonanno, 2004; Cohen et al., 1986; Higgins & Endler, 1995; Lazarus & Folkman, 1984; Sarafino, 2006).

Behavioural control

Behavioural control is the ability to step up and do something to reduce the impact of a stressful situation. As you may recall, this type of active coping is called *problem-focused* and is generally more effective in relieving stress than *avoidance-oriented coping*—that is, avoiding action to solve our problems or giving up hope (Lazarus & Folkman, 1984; Roth & Cohen, 1986). Research shows that the more university students use problem-focused coping techniques, the less likely they are to use alcohol (Feil & Hasking, 2008).

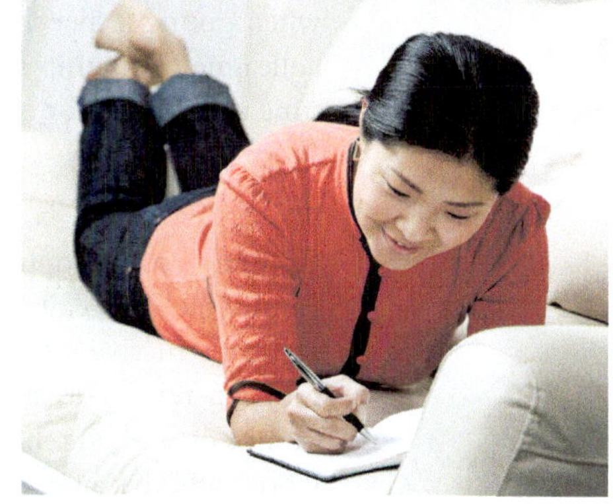

The work of James Pennebaker suggests that writing about our stressors can ward off physical illness, although this effect is only modest. **(Source:** Jonathan Ross/Dreamstime.)

Cognitive control

Cognitive control is the ability to *cognitively restructure or think differently about* negative emotions that arise in response to stress-provoking events (Higgins & Endler, 1995; Lazarus & Folkman, 1984; Skinner et al., 2003). This type of control includes *emotion-focused coping*, which we introduced earlier, a strategy that comes in handy when we are adjusting to uncertain situations or aversive events we cannot control or change. In one study (Strentz & Auerbach, 1988), experimenters exposed participants to a simulated abduction and four days of captivity. During captivity, participants who received instructions to use emotion-focused coping strategies reported less distress than did those who received instructions to use problem-focused coping.

Decisional control

Decisional control is the ability to choose among alternative courses of action (Sarafino, 2006). For instance, we can consult with trusted friends about which classes to take and which lecturers to avoid, and make decisions about which surgeon to consult to perform a high-stakes operation.

Informational control

Informational control is the ability to acquire information about a stressful event. Knowing what types of questions are on the final exam can help us prepare for them, as can knowing something about the person we will be working for when we start a new job. We engage in **proactive coping** when we anticipate stressful situations and take steps to prevent or minimise difficulties before they arise (Greenglass, 2002; Karasek & Theorell, 1990; Schwarzer & Taubert, 2002). People who engage in proactive coping tend to perceive stressful circumstances as opportunities for growth (Greenglass, 2002).

Proactive coping Anticipation and preparation for problems and stressful situations that promotes effective coping.

Emotional control

Emotional control is the ability to suppress and express emotions. Communication can strengthen social bonds, enhance problem-solving and regulate emotions (Bonanno, 2004; Ekman & Davidson, 1993). James Pennebaker and his colleagues (Pennebaker, Kiecolt-Glaser & Glaser, 1988) asked one group of uni students to write for 4 consecutive days for 20 minutes a day about their deepest thoughts and feelings about past traumas. They asked another group of students to write about superficial topics. Six weeks after the study, students who 'opened up' about their traumatic experiences made fewer visits to the health centre and showed signs of improved immune functioning compared with the students who wrote about trivial topics. Replications in laboratories around the world have confirmed that writing about traumatic events can influence a variety of academic, social and cognitive variables, and improve the health and well-being of people, ranging from arthritis sufferers to maximum-security prisoners (Campbell & Pennebaker, 2003; Pennebaker & Graybeal, 2001; Smyth et al., 1999), although scientific debate regarding the size of these effects continues (Frisina, Borod & Lepore, 2004).

Still, there are times when it is best to conceal our emotions, such as cloaking our fears when giving a speech and suppressing our anger when trying to resolve a problem with a colleague (Bonanno et al., 2004; Gross & Muñoz, 1995). As the old saying goes: 'There's a time and a place for everything.'

Is catharsis a good thing?

Contrary to the popular notion that expressing what we feel is always beneficial, disclosing painful feelings, called *catharsis*, is a double-edged sword. When it involves problem-solving and constructive efforts to make troubling situations 'right', it can be beneficial. But when catharsis reinforces a sense of helplessness, as when we stew endlessly about something we cannot or will not change, catharsis can actually be harmful (Littrell, 1998). This finding is worrisome, because a slew of popular psychotherapies rely on catharsis, encouraging clients to 'get it out of your system' or 'get things off your chest'. Some of these therapies instruct clients to yell, punch pillows or throw balls against walls when they become upset (Lewis & Bucher, 1992; Lohr et al., 2007). Yet research shows that these activities rarely reduce our long-term stress, although they may make us feel slightly better for a few moments. In other cases, they actually seem to heighten our anger or anxiety in the long run (Tavris, 1989), perhaps because emotional upset often generates a vicious cycle: we can become distressed about the fact that we are distressed.

Does psychological debriefing help?

Around the world some therapists, often those employed by fire, police or other emergency services, administer a popular treatment called *psychological debriefing*, *crisis debriefing* or *critical incidence stress debriefing*, which is designed to ward off PTSD among people exposed to trauma. For instance, after the 2001 terrorist attacks on the World Trade Center in America, several thousand debriefers travelled to New York City in a well-meaning effort to help traumatised witnesses of the attacks. Crisis debriefing is a single-session procedure, typically conducted in groups, that usually lasts three to four hours. Most often, therapists conduct this procedure within a few days of a traumatic event, such as a terrible accident. It proceeds according to standardised steps, including strongly encouraging group members to discuss and 'process' their negative emotions, listing the Post-traumatic symptoms that group members are likely to experience, and discouraging group members from discontinuing participation once the session has started.

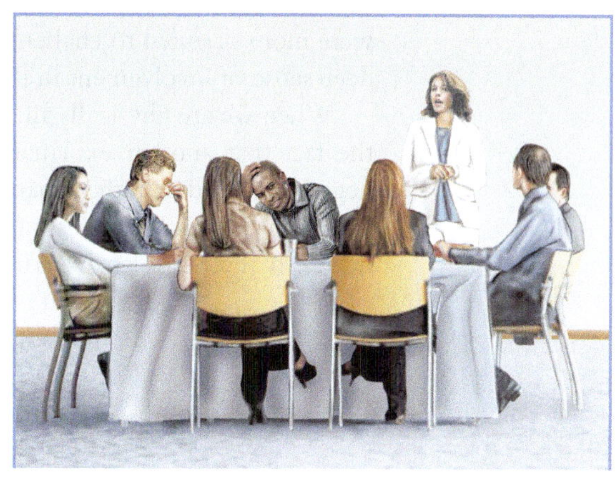

Psychological debriefing sessions, in which people discuss their reactions to a traumatic event in a group, may actually increase PTSD risk.

Recent studies indicate that psychological debriefing is not effective for trauma reactions. What is worse, several studies suggest that it may actually increase the risk of PTSD among people exposed to trauma, perhaps because it gets in the way of people's natural coping strategies (Lilienfeld, 2007; Litz et al., 2002; McNally, Bryant & Ehlers, 2003). Based on these findings, in the aftermath of the Black Saturday bushfires, the Australian Centre for Posttraumatic Mental Health did not employ psychological debriefers, but instead developed a three-tiered approach for working with survivors that included a range of immediate and longer-term psychological treatments (Forbes et al., 2010).

Indeed, there is not much evidence that merely talking about our problems when we are upset is helpful. A meta-analysis of 61 studies (Meads & Nouwen, 2005) revealed no overall benefits for emotional disclosure (compared with non-disclosure) on a variety of measures of physical and psychological health. None of this implies that we should never discuss our feelings with others when we are upset. But it does mean that doing so is most likely to be beneficial when it allows us to think about and work through our problems in a more constructive way.

Attitudes, beliefs, and personality

Some people survive almost unimaginably horrific circumstances with few or no visible psychological scars, whereas others view the world through the dark lens of pessimism and crumble when the little things in life do not go their way. Our attitudes, personality and socialisation shape our reactions—for better and worse—to potential stressors.

Hardiness
Set of attitudes marked by a sense of control over events, commitment to life and work, and courage and motivation to confront stressful events.

Spirituality
Search for the sacred, which may or may not extend to belief in God.

Hardiness: challenge, commitment and control

Over three decades ago, Salvatore Maddi and his colleagues (Kobasa, Hilker & Maddi, 1979) initiated a study of the qualities of stress-resistant people. They determined that resilient people possess a set of attitudes they called **hardiness**. Hardy people view change as a challenge rather than as a threat, are committed to their life and work, and believe they can control events. Hardy individuals have the courage and motivation to confront stressors and engage in problem-solving to contend with them (Maddi, 2004).

Suzanne Kobasa and Salvatore Maddi asked 670 managers at a large company to report their stressful experiences on a checklist. Then they selected executives who scored high on both stress and illness, and another group who scored equally high on stress but reported below-average levels of illness. Managers who showed high stress but low levels of illness were more oriented to challenge and higher in their sense of control over events, and felt a deep sense of involvement in their work and social lives.

When we are physically ill, we do not usually feel especially hardy. So we can appreciate the fact that another explanation for Kobasa and Maddi's findings is that illness creates negative attitudes, rather than the other way around. To address the question of causal direction, Maddi and Kobasa (1984) conducted a longitudinal study that examined changes in health and attitudes over time. At the end of two years, people whose attitudes towards life reflected high levels of control, commitment and challenge remained healthier than those whose attitudes did not. Hardiness also can boost stress resistance among nurses in hospice settings, immigrants adjusting to life in a new country, and military personnel who survive life-threatening stressors (Bartone, 1999; Maddi, 2002). In short, hardiness can transform stressors from potential disasters into valuable growth opportunities.

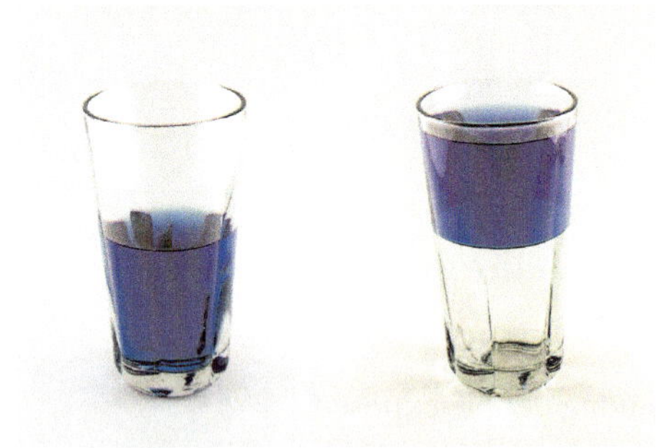

Optimists—who proverbially see the glass as 'half full' rather than 'half empty'—are more likely than pessimists to view change as a challenge.
(Source: Chad Heap/Dreamstime.)

Optimism

We know them when we meet them. Optimistic people have a rosy outlook and do not dwell on the dark side of life. Even on a cloudy day, we can bask in their sunshine. There are some distinct advantages to being optimistic. Optimistic people are more productive, focused, persistent and better at handling frustration than are pessimists (Peterson, 2000; Seligman, 1990). Optimism is also associated with a lower mortality rate (Stern, Dhanda & Hazuda, 2001), a more vigorous immune response (Segerstrom et al., 1998), lower distress in infertile women trying to have a child (Abbey, Halman & Andrews, 1992), better surgical outcomes (Scheier et al., 1989) and fewer physical complaints (Scheier & Carver, 1992).

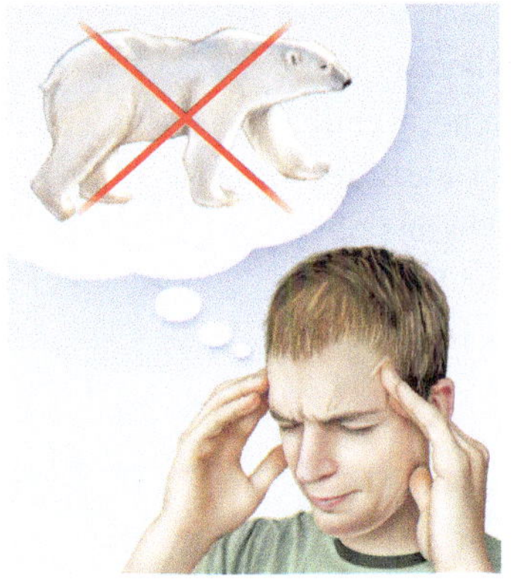

Research suggests that instructing someone *not* to think of something, like a white bear, often results in increases in the very thought the person is trying to suppress (Wegner, 1989).

Spirituality and religious involvement

Spirituality is a search for the sacred, which may or may not extend to belief in God. Spiritual and religious beliefs play vital roles in many of our lives. According to a Nielsen poll, 68 percent of Australians believe in a God or Universal Spirit (*Sydney Morning Herald*, 19 December 2009). Compared with non-religious people, religious people have lower mortality rates, improved immune system functioning, lower blood pressure and a greater ability to recover from illnesses (Koenig, McCullough & Larson, 2001; Levin, 2001; Matthews, Larson & Barry, 1993). One explanation for these findings is that religious involvements activate a healing energy that scientists cannot measure (Ellison & Levin, 1998). This is an intriguing hypothesis. Nevertheless, explanations that depend on an undetectable force or energy cannot be empirically tested and therefore lie outside the boundaries of science.

The correlation between religiosity and physical health is not easy to interpret. Some authors have measured religiosity by counting how often people attend church or other religious services, and found that such attendance is associated with better physical health. But this correlation is potentially attributable to other variables. For example people who are sick are less likely to attend religious services, so the causal arrow may be reversed (Sloan, Bagiella & Powell, 1999).

Research on the links between spirituality and religious involvement, and health, on the other, is limited. But until more definitive evidence is available, we can consider several potential reasons why spirituality and religious involvements may be a boon to many people.

1. Many religions prohibit behaviours that are actually risky to health, including consuming alcohol, taking drugs and following unsafe sexual practices.
2. Religious engagement, such as attendance at services, often boosts social support.
3. A sense of meaning and purpose, control over life, positive emotions and positive appraisals of stressful situations associated with prayer and religious activities may enhance coping (Potts, 2004).

Flexible coping

The ability to adjust coping strategies as the situation demands is critical to contending with many stressful situations (Bonanno & Kaltman, 2001; Cheng, 2003; Westphal & Bonanno, 2004). George Bonanno and his colleagues (Bonanno et al., 2004) studied students who had just started university in New York City when terrorists destroyed the World Trade Center in 2001. The researchers predicted that students who had difficulties with managing their emotions would find the transition to university life particularly difficult. Participants completed a checklist of psychological symptoms at the start of the study and then again two years later. Participants who were better at flexibly controlling their emotions by suppressing or expressing them on demand, on a laboratory task, reported less distress two years later.

Expending a great deal of effort to suppress and avoid emotions can distract us from problem-solving and lead to an unintended consequence: the emotions may return in full or with greater force. In fact, the attempt to suppress negative emotions and thoughts associated with aversive events tends to backfire and increase the very negative experiences we were struggling so hard to avoid (Beck et al., 2006; Richards, Butler & Gross, 2003; Wegner, 2005). Accepting circumstances and feelings we cannot change, and finding positive ways of thinking about our problems, can be a potent means of contending with stressful situations (Skinner et al., 2003).

Rumination: recycling the mental garbage

So far we have considered adaptive ways of coping with taxing circumstances without becoming unhinged. But some ways of reacting to stressful situations are clearly counterproductive. Susan Nolen-Hoeksema (1987) suggested that recycling negative events in our minds can lead us to become depressed. More specifically, some of us spend a great deal of time *ruminating*—focusing on how bad we feel and endlessly analysing the causes and consequences of our problems.

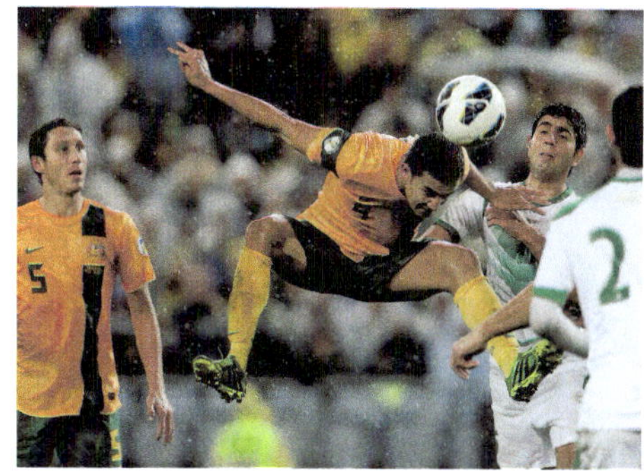

Men may be more likely than women to play sport, which often decreases the tendency to ruminate when stressed. (**Source:** Toby Zerna/Newspix/© News Ltd.)

Nolen-Hoeksema (2000; 2003) contended that women have much higher rates and more frequent bouts of depression than men because they tend to ruminate more than men. In contrast, when stressed, men are more likely to focus on pleasurable or distracting activities, such as work, watching football games or drinking copious amounts of alcohol (which we do not recommend). They also adopt a more direct approach to solving their problems than do women (Nolen-Hoeksema, 2002; 2003). Early socialisation may in part pave the way for these differing reactions (Nolen-Hoeksema & Girgus, 1994). Although parents encourage girls to analyse and talk about their problems, they often actively discourage boys from expressing their feelings and instead encourage them to take action or tough it out. Still, men and women alike can benefit from cutting down on rumination and confronting their problems head-on.[D]

Assess your knowledge — FACT or FICTION?

1. During a nine-year study, researchers found a strong connection between social support and people's chance of dying. **(True/False)**
2. Optimistic people are especially skilled at tolerating frustration. **(True/False)**
3. Participation in religious activities can increase social support. **(True/False)**
4. One general coping strategy tends to work for all situations. **(True/False)**
5. Rumination is usually an adaptive strategy for dealing with anxiety and depression. **(True/False)**

Answers: (1) T; (2) T; (3) T; (4) F; (5) F

Stress, risk behaviours, and health

There are many ways in which people injure their health. Belloc and Breslow (1972), after surveying nearly 7,000 individuals, identified seven behaviours related to the maintenance of personal health:

1. Sleeping seven to eight hours daily.
2. Eating breakfast almost every day.
3. Never or rarely eating between meals.
4. Being at or near prescribed height-adjusted weight.
5. Never smoking cigarettes.
6. Moderate or no use of alcohol.
7. Regular physical activity.

Any of these, if not maintained, can become a *risk behaviour* that contributes to illness and death. We shall see that many of these same behaviours are closely tied to stress. We will focus on three that have received the most research attention: fitness and exercise, eating and nutrition, and addiction and substance abuse.

Fitness and exercise

Many people believe that exercise helps to manage stress. Often such notions are either downplayed or overemphasised in stress clinics. But what are the facts? *Are* athletes better

[D]Lilienfeld, S. O., Lynn, S. J., Namy, L. L., Woolf, N. J., Jamieson, G., Marks, A., & Slaughter, V. (2015). Stress, coping and health. In S. O. Lilienfeld, S. J. Lynn, L. L. Namy, N. J. Woolf, G. Jamieson, A. Marks, & V. Slaughter (Eds.), *Psychology: From inquiry to understanding* (2nd ed., pp. 510–521). Melbourne, VIC: Pearson Australia.

prepared to manage stress? Can daily exercise aid in stress management at work and home? Before exploring these questions, it is important to review some basic concepts concerning fitness.

Physical fitness is defined in terms of several variables. *Muscular strength* is the maximmn force a muscle can generate; *muscular endurance* is the ability of a muscle to sustain continuous work; *cardiorespiratory endurance* is the ability of the heart, lungs, and blood vessels to sustain continuous work by supplying oxygen and nutrients and removing waste *products; flexibility* is the ability to exercise and move joints fully; *body composition* is the proportion of lean body mass (bone and muscle) to fat; and *agility* is the ability to work with speed and balance. *Aerobic fitness* is related to endurance and involves the efficiency with which one uses oxygen; aerobically fit individuals, compared with those who are unfit, use up a greater percentage of the oxygen they breathe.

To achieve fitness, a person must engage in some form of regular physical activity, including exercise. Most exercises can be classified as *isotonic, isometric,* or *isokinetic.* In addition, exercises vary the extent to which they are *aerobic.* Isotonic exercises (weight lifting, push-ups, and many calisthenics) involve moving a heavy object (including a person's own body weight) in one direction, contributing to strength and endurance. Isometric exercises involve exerting force against an immovable object, such as a wall, and are better for building strength than endurance. Isokinetic exercises involve exerting effort in more than one direction, for example, by pushing and pulling a heavy object. This type of exercise builds strength and endurance. Finally, aerobic exercises are vigorous activities that require high levels of oxygen consumption. Heart and breathing rates increase, contributing to endurance and aerobic fitness.

Exercise, particularly aerobic, has several general benefits that can indirectly help reduce the possible costs of stress on health. Exercise burns calories, which can lead to sustained weight loss. Increased metabolism that results from exercise suppresses appetite. Aerobic exercise strengthens the heart, enhances muscle tone, strength, and elasticity, and has desirable effects on blood pressure, heart pumping efficiency, and cholesterol (Brownell, 1980). Partly because of these effects, aerobic exercise decreases the risk of many diseases that can be aggravated by stress, including coronary disease, diabetes, and hypertension.

People who exercise report less anxiety, depression, and tension (Folkins & Sime, 1981). Exercise improves sleep (Folkins, Lynch, & Gardner, 1972) as well as self-concept (Hughes, 1974). Such findings, although common, leave unanswered the question of causality. Does

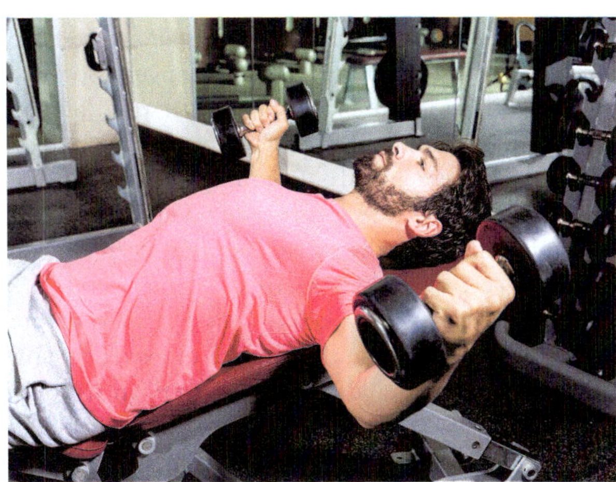

Weight lifting is a form of isotonic exercise.
(Soruce: Tono Balaguer.123rf.com)

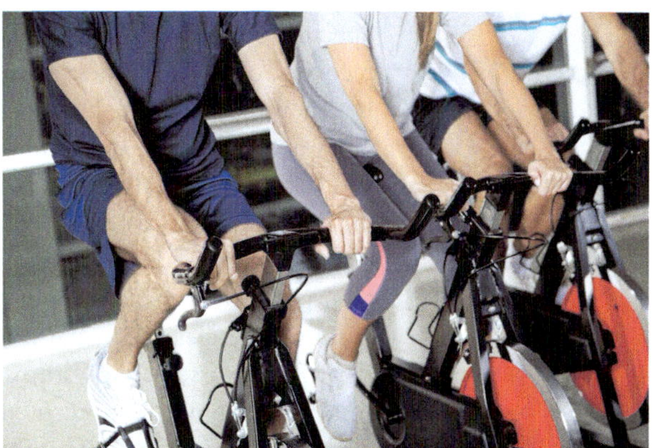

Working out on exercise bikes is a good form of aerobic exercise.
(Soruce: Tyler Olson.Shutterstock.com)

exercise contribute to reduced stress, do people with lower stress have more time and energy to exercise, or does some third variable contribute to both? In one experiment, Goldwater and Collis (1985) randomly assigned male subjects to a six-week vigorous (five days a week) aerobic exercise program and a moderate (two days a week) aerobic exercise program. The vigorous exercise increased the subject's fitness and reduced their anxiety.

In addition, those who exercise or are fit show less cardiovascular reactivity to stress and are less likely to be hypertensive (Crews & Landers, 1987). Again, questions can be asked about causal links. Research clarifies the situation. Both retrospective (Kobasa, Maddi, & Puccetti, 1982) and prospective (Roth & Holmes, 1985) studies show that people experiencing high levels of stress are much less likely to report and experience illness if they exercise. Brown (1991) found that aerobic fitness had a clear buffering effect. For unfit subjects, high life stress was strongly related to illness (measured by visits to a health center); however, for fit subjects, life stress had little ill effect.

Six mechanisms have been proposed to explain the impact of fitness and exercise on stress:

1. Exercise may *change cognitive appraisals* of a person's self image and the world. Improved physical appearance resulting from exercise can increase self-esteem (Folkins & Sime, 1981). Observable improvements in strength, flexibility, and endurance can contribute to feelings of self-efficacy and mastery (Rodin, 1986). However, Folkins and Sime (1981) suggest that participants in an exercise program feel more confident and able, even though changes in aerobic fitness may be unrelated to confidence and ability ratings. A variety of factors can contribute to such perceptions, including social support, increased feelings of control and mastery, expectations of improvement, and satisfaction with personal improvement (King, Taylor, Haskell & DeBusk, 1989).
2. Exercise may *reduce affective states,* such as anger and hostility, implicated in stress disorders (Czajkowski et al., 1990).
3. Physical fitness may *divert attention* from stressful situations and cognitions (Bahrke & Morgan, 1978). Simply taking time off from a hectic day removes one source of potentially stressful stimulation. And becoming absorbed in a vigorous sport leaves less attention for stressful worry.
4. Exercise *increases the flow of blood and oxygen to the brain,* possibly contributing to feelings of greater energy and alertness (Kostrubala, 1977).
5. Exercise (especially aerobic) may *enhance the production of certain neurotransmitters,* including catecholamines and endorphins, leading to a positive mood and feelings of euphoria.
6. Highly-fit people *show less physiological reactivity* to stress than those that are not fit. Specifically, they show lower arousal on some physiological dimensions and more rapid recovery on others. To explain, the cardiovascular and biochemical changes associated with aerobic fitness enable the body to respond more efficiently to physical stress (Sinyor, Schwartz, Peronnet, Brisson, & Seraganian, 1983). The long-distance runner, swimmer, and biker is physically conditioned to sustain the demands of running, swimming, and biking. Physiologically, their heart rate is lower, the volume of blood pumped with each stroke is increased, their heart rate returns more rapidly to normal after exercise, and their glucose, insulin, norepinephrine, and cortisol levels are lower.

It should be clear that many of the physical changes evoked by physical exertion are similar to those associated with psychological stress, even in the absence of exertion. This suggests that people who are fit may show less arousal and quicker recovery in response not only to the demands of running, swimming, and biking but also to the demands of psychological stress. Recent research is beginning to support this thinking. Holmes and Roth (1985) found that highly-fit women show lower elevations in heart rate in response to laboratory stress.

Eating and nutrition

Stress and eating are related in at least four ways. Poor nutrition can make a person more vulnerable to stress-related illnesses; stress can deplete the body of certain nutrients; some foods can evoke or aggravate the stress arousal response; and specific eating disorders may have a stress component.

Good nutrition

First, what is good nutrition? The United States Department of Agriculture's *food pyramid* suggests a balance of six food groups emphasising bread and grains, vegetables, and fruit, while placing less importance on meat, milk products, and fats and sweets. Perhaps the best way of avoiding stress-related nutrition problems is to maintain a responsible diet.

EATING AND ILLNESS. Poor nutrition can contribute to illnesses that have been linked with stress. For example, a diet high in saturated fats (found in red meats, whole milk, and butter) and cholesterol can increase the level of cholesterol in the blood, contributing to heart disease. Diets low in fiber (found in whole wheat grains, fruit, and vegetables) or high in saturated fat can contribute to breast, colon, and prostate cancers. Adequate levels of vitamins A and C may be needed to help prevent cancer of the larynx, esophagus, stomach, and lung. Cruciferous vegetables (such as broccoli, carrots, cauliflower, and spinach) contain fiber and beta carotene, which may also help prevent cancer. Finally, excess salt (sodium) can aggravate the risk of hypertension for those already at risk.

DEPLETION OF NUTRIENTS. Many components of the stress arousal response, such as cortisol production and the metabolism of carbohydrates and glucose, require the use of B complex vitamins (thiamine, riboflavin, niacin, pantothenic acid, and pyridoxine hydrochloride) as well as vitamin C. People who experience vitamin deficiencies can feel anxious, depressed, and weak, and suffer from insomnia and an upset stomach. In addition, when the "stress" vitamins are depleted, the body's ability to manufacture certain stress hormones and mount an effective stress response is impaired. Stress may also interfere with the absorption of important minerals, such as calcium, potassium, zinc, copper, and magnesium. Finally, an excessive ingestion of certain nutrients can aggravate the depletion of important stress-related vitamins and minerals. To metabolise sugar and processed (unenriched) flour, the body requires B complex vitamins, leaving less available for the production of stress hormones.

NUTRITION AND THE STRESS AROUSAL RESPONSE. Certain food substances called *pseudostressors,* or *sympathomimetics,* can mimic the sympathetic nervous system arousal response. Caffeine (contained in colas, coffee, tea, and chocolate) as well as theobromine and theophylline (found in tea) increase metabolism and stress hormone secretion. In addition, they increase the arousability of the nervous system, resulting in an exaggerated stress response to other stimuli. Caffeine's best documented physiological effect is its ability to increase blood pressure both at rest and under stress, particularly for those at risk for hypertension (Lovallo et al., 1991). However, caffeine may well have different effects and operate through different mechanisms than stress; for example, some studies show that caffeine produces a decreased heart *rate.* The debate over whether caffeine is actually a stimulant continues (Pincomb, Lovallo, Passey, Brackett, & Wilson, 1987; Robertson et al., 1978).

Excessive sugar intake can contribute to *hypoglycemia,* a condition of low blood sugar preceded by elevated blood sugar. Some people who experience "midmorning slump" or increased irritability after a breakfast or lunch consisting of a doughnut may be displaying the symptoms of hypoglycemia. For some, this disorder can be triggered by having a high intake of sugar in a short period or missing meals. Paradoxically, temporary high levels of blood sugar stimulate the release of insulin, which causes sugar to be removed form the blood into body tissue. The result is hypoglycemic sugar depletion. Symptoms of hypoglycemia, such as anxiety, headaches, dizziness, rapid heartbeat, and initability,can intensify the stress arousal response.

Finally, excessive salt intake may not only aggravate hypertension in some, but may well contribute to stress symptoms. The sodium in salt is important for regulating water balance, but too much sodium results in excessive fluid retention. This in turn may contribute to edema (abnormal accumulation of fluid) in the nervous system. One symptom of edema is increased nervous tension and stress reactivity.

EATING DISORDERS. Tens of millions of Americans are overweight or obese. Generally, people are classified as overweight if they are 10 to 20 percent overweight, and obese if they are more than 20 percent overweight (Suitor & Hunter, 1980). There are far too many causes of overeating to consider here, but stress may well play a role. Obese people may confuse nonhunger physiological cues with hunger cues, and eat in response to anxiety, fatigue, or tension (Hodgson & Miller, 1982). Overeating can be a form of emotion-focused coping and a way to maintain social support. And people with eating problems often experience more stressful life events, have lower self-esteem, possess more irrational beliefs, use avoidance coping, and are less likely to use cognitive and behavioural coping strategies (Mayhew & Edelmann, 1989; Soukup, Beiler & Terrell, 1990).

Some people who suffer from extreme malnutrition and weight loss simply do not consume enough food. Patients with anorexia nervosa have an abnormally intense concern about body image and seek an extremely thin appearance. Claiming to "feel fat" when they are actually thin, anorexics limit their food intake so that their body weight is at least 15 percent below their ideal. Bulimia is a related disorder that involves binge eating followed by induced vomiting. Both anorexics and bulimics experience considerable personal stress and depression.

A few researchers suspect that anorexic and bulimic eating may contribute to, or be caused by, a malfunctioning of the hypothalamus, the body's stress trigger (Halmi, Owen, Lasky & Stokes, 1983). Changes in the hypothalamus may alter the body's regulation of fat metabolism, water balance, endocrine gland, secretion and possibly dopamine production (associated with depression).

At the very least, episodes of binge eating or severe eating restraint can be brought on by anxiety, depression, and interpersonal stress (Carrol & Leon, 1981), and most bulimics feel relief from anxiety and depression as a result of eating. However, the relationship among anorexia, bulimia, and stress is complex. Both disorders are associated with poor overall adjustment Gohnson & Berndt, 1983), suggesting a general deficiency in coping skills.

Addiction and substance abuse

In Chapter 6 'Health-Risk Behaviours', we discussed in depth the multitude of health risk behaviours that exist in modern society. Here we aim to make the connection between some of these concepts (e.g., substance abuse) and stress. In considering substance abuse, it is useful to differentiate between addiction, dependence, and abuse. In *addiction,* a person can become physically or psychologically dependent on an addicting substance. In *physical dependence,* the body adapts to a substance so that larger and and larger doses are required to achieve an effect. When the substance is no longer ingested, a person experiences withdrawal, or a set of unpleasant physical and psychological symptoms, including anxiety, craving, nausea, and tremors. Substances differ considerably in their addictive potential. *Psychological dependence* occurs when a person feels driven to use a substance to produce a pleasant effect, even without physical addiction. The substance is used to help adjust to stress. Finally, *substance abuse* is the overuse of a substance. Generally, abuse is defined as at least a month of a clear pattern of pathological heavy use that is difficult to stop or reduce, and problems at work or home resulting from use of the substance.

Substance abuse is a complex process, promoted in part by social pressure and modeling, and maintained by avoidance of physical withdrawal symptoms. We are interested in the relationship between stress and addiction, and will consider substance abuse as a form of *emotion-focused coping* (Lazarus & Folkman, 1984), directed toward reducing distress rather than solving a stressful problem.

It is useful to consider the involvement of stress at three stages of the addictive process: initiation, or the start of the addictive process; continuation of addictive behaviour; and relapse, or the return to addictive behaviour after an attempt has been made to stop (Wills, 1990). Although much is understood about the general effects of drugs, such as depressants, stimulants, narcotics, opiates, psychedelics, hallucinogens, and tranquillisers, (see Table 14.9), most stress research has focused on tobacco and alcohol, and, to a lesser extent, the opiates. Psychedelics, hallucinogens, and tranquillisers, (see Table 14.9), most stress research has focused on tobacco and alcohol, and, to a lesser extent, the opiates. These are also the drugs we shall consider in detail.

Tobacco

Smoking has a wide range of negative effects on physical health. Not only does it contribute to lung and other forms of cancer, but it is a risk factor for hypertension, heart disease, lung disorders, impaired immune system functioning, impaired healing, and even premature wrinkling of the skin.

Research has focused on two major by-products of smoking: carbon monoxide and nicotine. (A third by-product, tars, or minute particles of burnt residue, have attracted less attention.) Carbon monoxide is readily absorbed in the blood and quickly affects its oxygen-carrying capacity. Too much carbon monoxide can impair performance.

Nicotine is a very powerful and addicting poison. Indeed, the amount found in a single cigarette would be a fatal dose if extracted and injected into a person. When a cigarette is smoked, nonfatal doses enter the bloodstream through the mouth, nose, and lungs, travel to the brain, and cause the release of catecholamines. As we have seen, this activates the central and sympathetic nervous systems, increasing heart rate and blood pressure. In short, the body is aroused. Also, in a way that is not completely understood, nicotine alters the absorption of certain neurotransmitter substances in the brain. Together, the physiological changes produce a smoker's "fix" or "lift." But there is a cost: nicotine reduces the lung's capacity to process air and take in oxygen. In addition, it is powerfully addicting, with such withdrawal symptoms as headache, nausea, fatigue, and difficulty concentrating.

Smoking behaviour can become closely tied to stress regulation in general. People smoke for *positive affect,* that is, pleasurable stimulation and reduced tension (Tomkins, 1968). People who show strong physiological reactions to their first attempts at smoking are more likely to continue, suggesting that greater physiological reactivity increases susceptibility to smoking and relapse (Abrams et al., 1987).

People usually begin smoking between the ages of twelve and sixteen. Most of the research on who starts smoking has been conducted on school-age children. A handful of studies, conducted on large samples of between several hundred and several thousand subjects, show a clear link between stress and smoking initiation. Recent negative events, school change, schoolwork stress (for males), concerns about appearance (for females), feelings of helplessness, Type A behaviour, and anger all emerge as predictors of smoking (Wills, 1990). If we examine their coping skills, nonsmokers use problem-solvirig, cognitive reappraisal, and a search for social support from adults; smokers are more likely to rely on aggression, distraction, and peer group activity (Wills, 1986).

TABLE 14.9 Psychoactive drugs and their effects

Classification	Drug	Effects	Tolerance	Psychological Dependence	Physiological Dependence
Depressants	Alcohol	Reduced tension and anxiety	Yes	Yes	Yes
	Barbituates	Reduced tension, sleep	Yes	Yes	Yes
	Tranquillisers		Yes	Yes	Yes
Stimulants	Nicotine	Alertness, reduced fatigue, increased endurance, euphoria	Yes	Yes	Yes
	Caffeine		Yes	Yes	Yes
	Amphetamines		Yes	Yes	No?
	Cocaine		Some	Yes	No?
Narcotics (opioids)	Opium	Pain relief, relaxation, euphoria, reduced tension	Yes	Yes	Yes
	Morphine		Yes	Yes	Yes
	Heroin		Yes	Yes	Yes
	Codeine		Yes	Yes	Yes
Psychedelics and hallucinogens	Marijuana	Distortions in perception, changes in mood and behaviour, loss of contact with reality	No	Yes	No
	Hashish		No	Yes	No
	Mescaline		No	Yes	No
	Psilocybin		No	Yes	No
	LCD		No	Yes	No
	PCP		No	Yes	No
Minor tranquillisers	Librium	Reduced tension, sleep	Yes	Yes	Yes
	Miltown		Yes	Yes	Yes
	Valium		Yes	Yes	Yes

Research on the continuation of smoking behaviour has focused primarily on adults. Heavy smokers report more job and family stress (Wills, 1990). Subjects are more likely to smoke on high-stress days than on low-stress days (Conway, Vickers, Ward & Rahe, 1981). In one study, smokers were presented with stressful social situations while they smoked or did not smoke (Gilbert & Spielberger, 1987). Those who smoked claimed they felt less anxiety and greater effectiveness in expressing their opinions.

Most of those who quit smoking experience at least one relapse. As with most forms of substance abuse, a relapse occurs in a discrete episode rather than as a slow process. Negative life events, personal conflict, and "negative affect smoking," that is, smoking done when one feels frustrated, tense, or anxious (Pomerleau, Adkins, & Pertschuck, 1978), predict the likelihood of relapse. Relapsers also have low expectation of success and low personal adjustment.

A growing body of research has examined the coping strategies of relapsers. Successful quitters combine both cognitive modification of self-statements (self-reward, positive self-statements, thought of consequences, intention to delay possible relapse) and behavioural coping (distracting activity, relaxation) to deal with relapse. A combination appears to be more effective than either strategy alone for dealing with crises situations in which relapse is imminent. Either approach of coping was more effective than no coping attempt. (Cuny &

Marlatt, 1985; Glasgow, Klesges, Mizes, & Pechacek, 1985; Shiffman, 1982, 1984a, 1984b). Indeed, virtually every subject who makes no attempt to cope with relapse continues smoking. Interestingly, relapsers appear to be deficient in relaxation skills as well as social skills specifically related to dealing with smoking-specific situations (such as resisting social pressure to smoke), rather than social skills in general.

Alcohol

Experts disagree on the definition of alcoholism and problem drinking. However, most would agree that an alcoholic is one with a serious drinking problem that impairs health and functioning at work and home.

Alcohol has a powerful impact on just about every organ in the body, including the brain. The more highly specialised the tissue, such as the brain, liver, pancreas, and endocrine glands, the greater the impact. Alcohol abuse is related to several clear organic brain syndromes, including alcohol dementia and alcohol amnesia (memory) syndromes, or Korsakoff's psychosis. Physical disorders include cirrhosis of the liver, gastritis, and even heart disorders. Most people are aware of the potentially serious consequences of alcohol abuse. Psychological dependence can also be destructive to overall life adjustment, contributing to deterioration in coping at home and work.

Just how alcohol affects stress is not entirely known. At low to moderate doses, alcohol reduces tension and anxiety, and produces euphoria. Its reinforcing quality may rise from its impact on neurotransmitters (Livezey, Balbkins, & Vogel, 1987). In addition, alcohol may reduce stress by facilitating the diversion of attention from stressful thoughts to ongoing activity (Gosepbs & Steele, 1990). Alcoholics may metabolise alcohol differently, which contributes to their dependency. At the very least, the cell metabolism of the person who has developed an alcohol dependency has adapted to alcohol and requires its continued presence to avoid withdrawal.

The pattern for the initiation of alcohol abuse is at times similar to that of smoking. Generally, alcohol immediately reduces tension and anxiety, while also increasing euphoria. This combination provides powerful pressure to continue drinking in spite of its maladaptive long-term consequences (Bandura, 1969; Levenson, Sher, Grossman, Newman, & Newlin, 1980). In addition, the amount of alcohol that drinkers consume a day is related to the amount of stress on that day. Generally, economic stress, feelings of vulnerability, job and marital stress, and poor physical condition all relate to alcohol use. Those who have little social support and who use avoidance coping strategies are more likely to use alcohol for coping (Cronkite & Moos, 1984).

Once a drinking pattern has developed, alcoholics show low stress tolerance, negative self-image, feelings of inadequacy, isolation, and depression. More severe impairment includes lack of responsibility, difficulty in controlling impulses, and a tendency toward deceitfulness and manipulation. It is often observed that serious alcoholics make frequent use of denial, rationalisation, and projection as defense mechanisms. Alcoholics who try but fail to quit show a pattern similar to that of smokers and opiate users: negative emotional states, increased stress, poorer coping skills, lower levels of assertiveness, and lower learned resourcefulness. Use of active cognitive and behavioural coping predicts the likelihood of staying off alcohol, where as relapsers use more avoidance and aggressive coping, such as taking their emotions out on others.

Opiates

Opiates are derived from the opium poppy, and include morphine and heroin. Opiates have both analgesic (pain-reducing) and positive mood effects resulting from the secretion of catecholarnines and endogenous opiates. As we have seen, the nerves of the brain and spine have special receptor sites for special neurotransmitters. Morphine and similar drugs block pain and evoke pleasure because they fit these sites.

The opiate user experiences an immediate euphoric spasm lasting about a minute, followed by a "high" in which one is lethargic, withdrawn, relaxed, and contented. This can last for four to six hours. Eventually there is a craving for more of the drug.

Opiate addictions have serious consequences. Not only are the drugs illegal, but the costs of addiction escalates. One becomes able to tolerate ever-increasing doses, requiring higher amounts of the drug. This can lead to the ruinous expense of maintaining a habit. Withdrawal symptoms can be severe and include sweating, pain, nausea, vomiting, and diarrhea. Finally, unsanitary conditions associated with opiate use, such as dirty needles, can lead to serious health consequences.

Predictors of more serious drug use are complex and include subjective stress, as well as rejection by family and school, and depression. How stress contributes to addiction is open to debate. According to the theory of *exposure orientation,* endorphins are released under stress and produce stress-induced analgesia. The use of opiates may lead to a breakdown of the body system that synthesises endorphins (Jaffee, 1985).

The addict then continues to use opiates because of the breakdown in the body's normal ability to block pain. Similarly, since withdrawal is a source of serious pain, there is additional incentive for opiate use.

In contrast, the *adaptive orientation* perspective (Alexander & Hadaway, 1982) states that addiction is not automatic; both the person and the situation must be considered. For example, drug use may increase under conditions of extreme stress, feelings of helplessness and low self-efficacy, and low support for refraining from drug use.

Much addiction research has focused on who stays in and who quits treatment programs for opiate dependence. Predictors of relapse include life events, stress, loss of social support, pain, depression, and low efficacy expectations for the ability to resist the relapse temptation (Wills, 1990). In addition, relapsers are more likely to lack coping skills for such unexpected stressors of the nondrug world as low-status work, unemployment, and the recreational drug use of nonaddict co-workers (Platt & Metzger, 1987).

Stress and substance abuse

In general, three models help explain the relationship between stress and substance abuse. The *affect regulation mode* assumes that tobacco, alcohol, or opiate use reduces pain and stress while providing pleasure. This then contributes to continued use (Wills, 1990). In addition, the physiological impact of such substances may distract attention from stressors or interfere with the processing of potentially upsetting information. Such an impact is in tum reinforced by the positive affect evoked by drugs.

The *self-control model* derives from the cognitive fatigue model of stress after effects (Cohen, 1980). Stressful tasks (especially those that are uncertain and unpredictable) call for increased vigilance and coping. This mental effort contributes to cognitive fatigue that can persist as a stress after effect. Fatigue can impair performance on a variety of tasks, including resisting the temptation to smoke, drink, or use drugs. In other words, when compromised by the debilitating effects of stress, one is more likely to resort to substance use as a coping mechanism and have fewer coping resources to resist substance use.

Marlatt's relapse model (Marlatt, 1985; Marlatt & George, 1984; Marlatt & Gordon, 1985) focuses more on the effect of stress on those who are attempting to quit substance use. According to this theory, the first episode of postcessation drug use is a "lapse," and a full return to drug use is a "relapse." A lapse is most likely when a person encounters a stressful situation involving interpersonal conflict and social pressure and experiences negative affect. Those who have effective coping responses should have greater feelings of self-efficacy and

TABLE 14.10 The transactional matrix for quitting smoking

Variable	Long-Term Antecedents	Immediate Antecedents	Stressful Event (Quitting)	Immediate Consequences	Long-Term Consequences
Personal		Physiological reactivity, concerns about appearance (women), feelings of helplessness, type A behavioural, anger, low personal adjustment, general absence of coping and relaxation skills		*Physiological*: Reduced blood oxygen levels, increased arousal	Heart disease, cancer, immune system impairment, addiction
				Emotional: Smoker's "lifts" reduced tension	
				Performance: Poorer performance	
Situational			Low expectation of success; failure to use problem-solving, cognitive reappraisal, and social support from adults; rely more on distraction, aggression, and peer support; smoking used to reduce stress ("negative affect smoking")		
External		Recent negative events, school change, schoolwork (males)			

a greater likelihood of actually changing a stressful situation. As a result, they should be less likely to resume substance use.

In contrast, those more likely to experience relapse and continue with substance use display an *abstinence violation effect,* a cognitive-affective reaction that has two components:(1) an attribution of the cause of the lapses to internal, stable, and global factors that are uncontrollable (for example, lack of will power and an addictive personality); and (2) negative emotions of self-blame and guilt. Presumably, increasing a person's repertoire of coping skills should reduce the abstinence violation effect and contribute to maintained abstinence.

However, relatively little is understood about the dynamics of stress and substance abuse, as well as the relationship among stress, eating, and exercise. Who is more likely to use one particular substance for emotion-focused coping? Under what conditions is this more likely to occur? What are the short- and long-term physiological, psychological, and environmental consequences of substance abuse? How do these consequences in turn help maintain substance abuse? Table 14.10 illustrates how the array of such variables can be considered in terms of the transactional matrix for quitting smoking. Clearly, researchers have just begun to understand the complex interactions of stress and substance abuse.[E]

[E] Smith, J. (1993). The transactional matrix. In J. Smith (Ed.), *Understanding stress and coping* (pp. 133–146). New York, NY: Macmillan.

Summary

What is stress?

- The effects of stress can be emotional, psychological, and physical. Reactions to stress are different in everyone, with some people expressing more physical signs, like fatigue or high blood pressure, and others expressing more emotion or psychological signs, like irritability or depression
- Researchers have approached the study of stress in three different, yet interrelated, ways. These include: stress-as-stimuli, stress as a response, and stress as a transaction
- Richard Lazarus and his colleagues contended that a critical factor determining whether we experience an event as stressful is our appraisal—that is, our evaluation—of the event.
- David Holmes and his colleagues developed the Social Readjustment Rating Scale (SRRS), the first of many efforts to measure life events systematically

How we adapt to stress: change and challenge

- Hans Selye called the pattern of responding to stress the General Adaptation Syndrome (GAS) According to Selye, all prolonged stressors take us through three stages of adaptation: alarm, resistance and exhaustion
- Shelley Taylor and her colleagues created the catchy phrase 'tend and befriend' to describe a common pattern of reacting to stress among women

Transactional approaches

- Lazarus and Folkman believed that the interpretation of stressful events was more important than the events themselves. For example, it is the perception of potential harm, threats and challenges, together with how confident an individual feels in dealing with these, that determines one's ability to cope with stress

Research applications of the transactional matrix

- Lazarus and Folkman suggested there are two types of coping responses emotion-focused and problem-focused

Lifetime effects of stress

- The higher the levels of stress you experience and the longer that stress continues, the greater the likelihood of damage to your physical, social and emotional health

How stress impacts our health

- Psychoneuroimmunology is the study of the relationship between the immune system and the central nervous system
- Janice Kiecolt-Glaser and her associates are pioneers in the study of the connection between stressors and the immune system

Coping with stress

- Lisa Berkman and Leonard Syme (1979) conducted a landmark study of the hypothesis that social support buffers us against the adverse effects of stress on health
- People can relieve stress by acquiring control of situations. There are five types of control we can use in different situations including: behavioural control, cognitive control, decisional control, informational control and emotional control

Stress, risk behaviours and health

- There are many behaviours related to the maintenance of personal health, and if any of these are not maintained, it can become a risk behaviour that contributes to illness and death

Review questions

A. Fill in the missing words to complete the following statements.

1. Stress is defined as a stimulus or event that is __________ or __________ an individual's resources which can negatively impact on ones' wellbeing.
2. ____ examined stress as a transaction of needs and wants and discovered two major factors that influence an individuals appraisal of a stress event as either a primary or secondary appraisal.
3. ____ is strategy employed during stressful situations. Emotion focused coping involves taking a ____________ outlook on a situation or event in order to manage difficult emotional reactions related to that event.
4. The term ____________ is a psychoanalytic principle known as an emotional release.

B. Please select one statement that best answers each of the following questions.

5. A primary appraisal of a stressful situation involves which of the following processes?
   a) a coping strategy whereby a positive outlook is encouraged
   b) deciding whether or not you can cope with the event
   c) deciding whether or not the event is harmful
   d) none of the above
6. Which of the following statements is true in regards to Selye's General Adaptation Syndrome (GAS)?
   a) our level of resistance to stress drops in the alarm stage, increases during the resistance stage and drops again during the exhaustion stage
   b) our level of resistance to stress drops in the alarm stage, decreases during the resistance stage and drops again during the exhaustion stage
   c) our level of resistance to stress increases in the alarm stage, decreases during the resistance stage and drops again during the exhaustion stage
   d) our level of resistance to stress increases in the alarm stage, increases during the resistance stage and drops again during the exhaustion stage
7. True or False? During stressful situations, women typically tend-and-befriend rather than fight-or-flight.
8. Outcome expectancy is referred to as which of the following?
   a) the belief that a specific behaviour will result in a desired outcome
   b) an individual's perceptions regarding their own abilities
   c) an individual's belief system regarding their personal reaction to various rewarding or aversive events
   d) all of the above
9. According to Lazarus and Folkman's (1984) Transactional Model of Coping and Appraisal, the term reappraisal relates to which of the following?
   a) individual factors that influence our reactions to stress such as our abilities, deficits and personal variables
   b) individual factors that influence our reactions to stress such as resources, deficits and personal variables
   c) individual factors that influence our reactions to stress such as resources, deficits, personal and external variables
   d) none of the above

10. An individual with type C personality is most likely to be described as?
    a) perfectionistic, competitive and get things done on time.
    b) calm, reflective, creative, analytical and laid back
    c) detail oriented, non-assertive and people pleasers
    d) negative outlook on life, irritable and prone to depression

11. Which of the following statements is true in terms of rumination?
    a) describes the tendency to repetitively think about the causes and consequences of our negative emotional experience
    b) during stressful circumstances, men are more likely to focus on pleasurable or distracting activities (e.g., work) whereas, women are more likely to ruminate over a situation
    c) rumination can be counterproductive and is linked to depression
    d) all of the above

Review answers

Chapter 1

A. Fill in the missing words to complete the following statements.

1. conditioned stimulus (CS); unconditioned stimulus (US)
2. learning; conditioned stimulus (CS); unconditioned stimulus (UCS); conditioned response (CR)
3. operant conditioning
4. decreases
5. variable-ratio schedule

B. Read the following sentences and answer with the most correct definition.

6. extinction
7. stimulus generalisation
8. law of effect
9. negative reinforcement

C. Please select one statement that best answers each of the following questions.

10. a) neutral stimulus is paired with an unconditioned stimuls
11. a) does not elicit and unconditioned response
12. e) extinction
13. b) stimulus discrimination
14. a) conditioned stimulus
15. b) operant conditioning

Chapter 2

A. Fill in the missing words and/or key concepts to complete the following tables.

1. Stages of lifespan development

Stage	Age period
Prenatal	Conception to birth
Infancy	Birth at full term to about 18 months
Early childhood	**About 18 months to about 6 years**
Middle childhood	**About 6 years to about 11 years**
Adolescence	About 11 years to about 20 years
Early adulthood	**About 20 years to about 40 years**
Middle adulthood	About 40 years to about 65 years
Late adulthood	**About 65 years and older**

2. Piaget's stages of cognitive development

Stages	Age	Characteristics and major accomplishments
Sensorimotor	0-2	**The child learns by doing: looking, touching, sucking. Child develops object permanence and the beginning of symbolic thought.**
Preoperational	2-7	**The child uses symbols (words and images) to represent objects. Imagination is strong, but complex abstract thought is still difficult. Child's thought is marked by egocentrism and centration.**
Concrete Operational	7–11	**The child achieves understanding of conservation, as well as cause-and-effect relationships. The child can reason with respect to concrete, physical objects.**
Formal Operations	11+	**The individual demonstrates abstract thinking, including logic, deductive reasoning and hypothetical thinking.**

3. Erikson's psychosocial stages

Approximate age	Crisis
0 – 1.5	Trust vs. mistrust
1.5 – 3	Autonomy vs. self-doubt
3 – 6	**Initiative vs. guilt**
6 – puberty	**Competence vs. inferiority**
Adolescent	Identity vs. role confusion
Early adult	Intimacy vs. isolation
Middle adult	**Generativity vs. stagnation**
Later adult	**Ego integrity vs. despair**

B. Fill in the missing words to complete the following statements.

4. Longitudinal; cross-sectional
5. puberty
6. egocentrism
7. generativity
8. I. An individual can be at only one stage at a given time.
   II. Everyone goes through the stages in a fixed order.
   III. Each stage is more comprehensive and complex than the preceding.
   IV. The same stages occur in every culture.

C. Read the following statements and answer with the most correct definition.

9. teratogen
10. foetal
11. assimilation
12. internalisation

D. Please select one statement that best answers each of the following questions.

13. a) sensorimotor, preoperational, concrete operational, formal operational
14. c) trust vs. mistrust
15. d) school age
16. b) formal operational
17. d) You feel capable of developing closeness and commitment to another vs. feeling isolated and alone
18. a) object permanence
19. c) egocentrism
20. b) industry (competence) vs. inferiority

Chapter 3

A. Fill in the missing words to complete the following statements.

1. storage; retrieval
2. Elaboration; elaborating

B. Read the following statements and answer with the most correct definition.

3. chunking
4. encoding
5. iconic

C. Please select one statement that best answers each of the following questions.

6. b) short-term memory
7. d) both a and c
8. a) anterograde amnesia
9. c) hippocampus

D. Fill in the missing words and/or key concepts to complete the following diagram.

10.

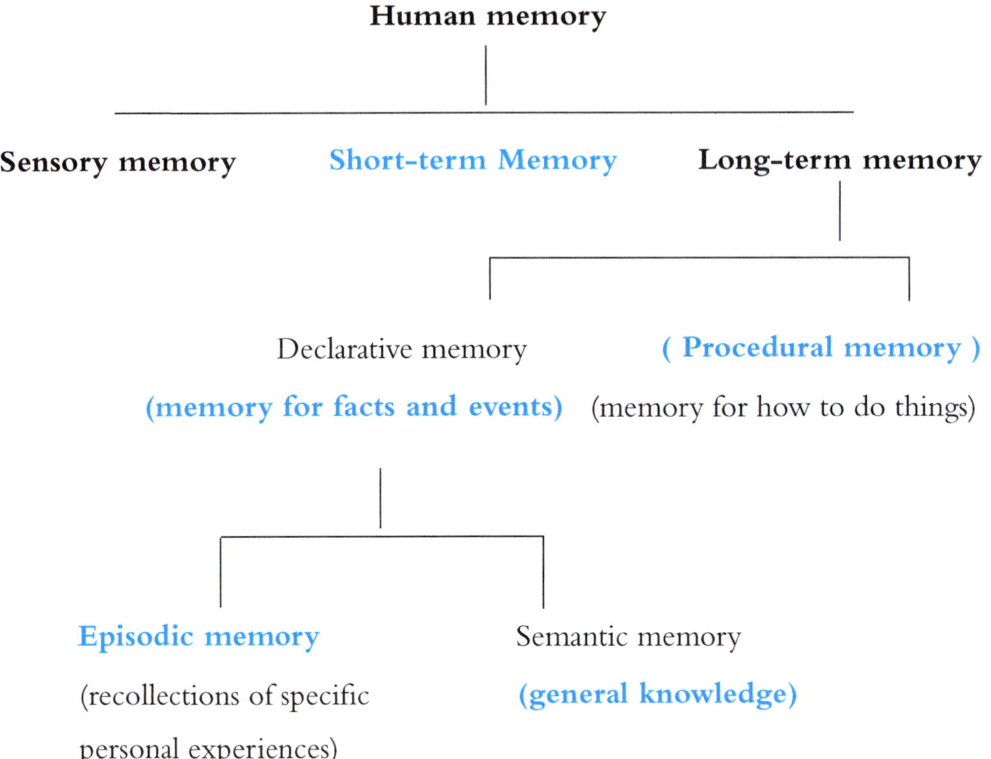

Chapter 4

A. Fill in the missing words to complete the following statements.

1. physical; physical
2. aptitude; natural intelligence
3. mental; physical
4. general knowledge; digit span; vocabulary; arithmetic; comprehension; similarities; picture completion; picture arrangement; block design; digit symbol, object assembly
5. the reliability of intelligence tests; the validity of intelligence tests; whether the usefulness of intelligence tests is over-emphasised
6. malnutrition; years in school; father's economic status; average TV viewing; selfconfidence
7. accurately perceiving emotions; using emotions to facilitate meaning; understanding emotional meanings; managing emotions

B. Read the following statements and answer with the most correct definition.

8. intellectual disability

C. Please select one statement that best answers each of the following questions.

9. a) because the Simon-Binet test did not work effectively cross-culturally
10. b) specific intelligence and general intelligence
11. d) both a and c
12. b) fluid intelligence
13. b) affects crystallised intelligence
14. b) he achieved an average IQ score compared to other people
15. d) all of the above
16. c) be aware, regulate our behaviour, and be self-motivated

Chapter 5

A. Fill in the missing words to complete the following statements.

1. culture
2. Diagnostic and Statistical Manual of Mental Disorders (DSM)
3. insomnia; significant weight loss; two; diminished interest or pleasure in everyday activities

B. Read the following statements and answer with the most correct definition.

4. comorbidity.
5. posttraumatic stress disorder (PTSD).
6. attention-deficit hyperactivity disorder (ADHD).

C. Please select one statement that best answers each of the following questions.

7. a) confusion of fantasy and reality.
8. a) dependent
9. a) dissociative identity disorder.
10. b) somatoform disorders.
11. c) greatly out of proportion to the situation.
12. a) a generalized anxiety disorder.
13. c) phobias
14. d) delusions
15. d) avoidant
16. b) somatisation disorder
17. b) amnesia
18. c) multiple personality
19. b) hallucinations
20. b) obsessive-compulsive

Chapter 6

A. Fill in the missing words to complete the following statements.

1. 'Alamenda Seven'
2. 0.05-0.07%; 0.25-0.34%
3. genetic predisposition / an individual's biological parents' substance use status; social group; positive family attitudes to alcohol
4. four or more drinks; fetal alcohol syndrome (FAS)

B. Fill in the missing words and/or key concepts to complete the following table.

5.

Class of drug	Effect on body	Example
Stimulants	**Increases nerve and brain activity**	Nicotine, caffeine, cocaine, ecstasy, ritalin
Depressants	Slows down brain and nerve activity OR (Central nervous system depressants)	**Alcohol, valium, barbiturates**
Hallucinogens	**Alters what we see and hear**	LSD, Ketamine, mushrooms
Narcotics	Blocks nerve impulses	**Heroin, morphine, codeine**

6.

Treatment modality	Aim of therapy
Cognitive Behavioural therapy	**Helps clients to identify unhelpful thoughts, feelings and behaviours to help cope with drug and alcohol difficulties**
Multidimensional family therapy	Includes the client and their family in addressing the patterns and influences of drug and alcohol abuse
Motivational interviewing	**Is a client-centered approach that enhances intrinsic motivation to change by exploring and resolving ambivalence**
Motivational incentives (contingency management)	**Encourages abstinence by employing positive reinforcement strategies**
12-Step Programs	Meetings are open to anyone at no membership cost. Work is focused on personal recovering using the 12-step approach.

C. Please select one statement that best answers each of the following questions.

7. d) both b) and c)
8. c) over 1 in 4 Australian children and adolescents are now overweight or obese, and rates are 2 times higher than for their parent's generation.
9. d) all the above
10. d) all the above

Chapter 7

A. Fill in the missing words to complete the following statements.

1. sensing a need or desire; activating and guiding the organism; reducing the sensation of need
2. achievement; affiliation; power
3. low-risk; the easily attained; achievements
4. Biological needs; Safety needs; Love, attachment, and affiliation needs; Esteem needs; Self-actualization.
5. Homeostasis

B. Read the following statements and answer with the most correct definition.

6. extrinsic motivation.
7. intrinsic motivation.

C. Fill in the missing words and/or key concepts to complete the following table.

8.

Theories of Motivation Compared

Theories	Emphasis	Examples
Intrinsic theory	Biological processes that motivate behaviour patterns specific to a species	Bird migration, fish schooling
Drive theory	Needs produce drives that motivate behaviour until drives are reduced	Hunger, thirst
Freud's theory	Motivation arises from unconscious desires; developmental changes in these urges appear as we mature	Sex, aggression
Maslow's theory	Motives result from needs, which occur in a priority order (a need hierarchy)	Esteem needs, self-actualisation
Evolutionary theory	Priority of motives determined by functional, proximal, and developmental factors	Food odor (proximal stimulus) may raise the priority of hunger drive

D. Please select one statement that best answers each of the following questions.

9. d) extrinsic/intrinsic
10. d) all of the above
11. d) both (a) and (c)
12. a) intrinsic motivation
13. c) primary need
14. a) knowing
15. a) drive reduction

Chapter 8

A. Fill in the missing words to complete the following statements.

1. barriers to change.
2. pre-contemplation; contemplation
3. preparation
4. action
5. maintenance

B. Please select statement that best answers each of the following questions.

6. d) action
7. d) none of the above
8. b) describes an individual's belief related to their ability to successfully cope with a particular task or situation.
9. d) both b) and c)
10. c) pre-contemplation, contemplation, preparation, action, maintenance and termination
11. a) address the issue, assess the client, advise the client and arrange for a follow-up
12. d) all of the above
13. b) developing discrepancy
14. c) rolling with resistance

Chapter 9

A. Fill in the missing words to complete the following statements.

1. primacy effect; recency effect
2. inferential; impression; judgments
3. heuristic; anchor; adjusts
4. Internal (or dispositional); external (or situational) influences
5. theory of correspondent inferences; underlying disposition
6. internal or personal factors; situational or external factors

B. Please select one statement that best answers each of the following questions.

7. d) both a) and b)
8. d) all of the above
9. c) schema
10. a) pre-attentive analysis, focal attention, comprehension, elaborative reasoning
11. c) both a) and b)
12. d) attribution theory
13. c) fundamental attribution error
14. c) fundamental attribution error
15. a) expertise, popularity and attractiveness, rapid speech, perceived manipulation, linguistic power and fear
16. c) tactics for requests

17. d) all of the above
18. d) agentic state

C. Fill in the missing words to complete the following table.

19.

Types of Schemas	Definition	Example
Script	Schema about events	20 years later, I remember going to the 1996 footy grand final
Person schema	Schemas about individuals or specific knowledge about someone	**My sister is very creative but a poor athlete**
Role schema	**Schemas about various occupations or roles**	**A real police officer should be dressed blue police uniform**

Chapter 10

A. Fill in the missing words to complete the following statements.

1. Touch; spatial
2. personal; interpersonal; intragroup; intergroup

B. Read the following statements and answer with the most correct definition.

3. b) intrapersonal, interpersonal, small group discussion, organisational communication
4. d) all of the above
5. b) it is an important component of verbal communication and includes, pitch, tone, speed, volume, emotional quality, stress and accent.
6. d) all of the above
7. c) conflict related to when members within a family, group or community do not agree with each other
8. a) collaboration, avoidance, accommodation, competition, compromise, and mediation
9. b) hearing client's stories and learning what their symptoms and distress mean to them by taking the clients lead, asking clarifying questions, offering reflections and validation to ensure a strong therapeutic relationship is developed and maintained.

Chapter 11

A. Fill in the missing words to complete the following statements.

1. empathic; congruence
2. somatotypes; physique; temperament
3. cardinal; central; secondary

B. Please select one statement that best answers each of the following questions.

4. b) Albert Bandura and Julian Rotter
5. d) all of the above
6. d) physiological
7. c) occurs when an individual's actual self and ideal self are congruent with each other
8. c) melancholic, phlegmatic, choleric and sanguine
9. b) big-boned with well-defined muscles
10. True
11. c) introversion versus extraversion, neuroticism versus stability and psychoticism versus socialisation
12. d) extraversion

Chapter 12

A. Fill in the missing words to complete the following statements.

1. acute; chronic; chronic benign; chronic progressive
2. specificity theory
3. c) long-term pain that is experienced over time, such as lower back pain
4. d) all the above
5. d) both a) and b)
6. c) our beliefs regarding our ability to tolerate pain does not influence our pain experience
7. d) all of the above
8. True
9. a) exploring the type of pain, the emotional response to the pain, the intensity of the pain, the timing of the pain.
10. b) subtle changes in moisture (sweat) in the body to detect muscle tension

Read the following questions and answer with some examples to illustrate your understanding.

11. Relaxation and biofeedback, transcutaneous electrical nerve stimulation and behavioural interventions, cognitive-behavioural interventions

Chapter 13

A. Fill in the missing words to complete the following statements.

1. Affect; emotions; moods; emotions
2. true
3. simultaneously
4. physiological arousal; cognitive label
5. James-Lang's theory of emotion

B. Please select one statement that best answers each of the following questions.

6. c) the experience of both positive and negative emotions serve a functional purpose
7. c) sadness, depression, boredom, fatigue
8. d) Both a) and c)
9. c) our 'gut reactions' such as our autonomic responses guide how we should respond to a situation or event.
10. d) all of the above

Chapter 14

A. Fill in the missing words to complete the following statements.

1. taxing; exceeding
2. The transactional model of coping and appraisal
3. Emotion focused coping; positive
4. catharsis

B. Please select one statement that best answers each of the following questions.

5. c) deciding whether or not the event is harmful
6. a) our level of resistance to stress drops in the alarm stage, increases during the resistance stage and drops again during the exhaustion stage.
7. True
8. a) the belief that a specific behaviour will result in a desired outcome
9. c) individual factors that influence our reactions to stress such as resources, deficits, personal and external variables
10. c) detail oriented, non-assertive and people pleasers
11. d) All of the above

References

Chapter 1

Aarons, L. (1976). Sleep-assisted instruction. *Psychological Bulletin, 83*(1), 1–40.

Akins, C. K. (2004). The role of Pavlovian conditioning in sexual behavior: a comparative analysis of human and nonhuman animals. *International Journal of Comparative Psychology, 17*(2–3), 241–262.

American Psychiatric Association. (2000). *Diagnostic and Statistical Manual of Mental Disorders: DSM-IV-TR* (4th ed.). Washington, DC: American Psychiatric Association.

Anderson, A. K., Christoff, K., Stappen, I., Panitz, D., Ghahremani, D. G., Glover, G. et al. (2003). Dissociated neural representations of intensity and valence in human olfaction. *Nature Neuroscience, 6*, 196–202.

Anderson, C. A. & Bushman, B. J. (2002a). Media violence and the American public revisited. *American Psychologist, 57*, 448–450.

Anderson, C. A. & Bushman, B. J. (2002b). The effects of media violence on society. *Science, 295*, 2377–2378.

Anderson, C. A., Gentile, D. A. & Buckley, K. E. (2007). *Violent Video Game Effects on Children and Adolescents: Theory, Research, and Public Policy*. Oxford: Oxford University Press.

Andresen, G. V., Birch, L. L. & Johnson, P. A. (1990). The scapegoat effect on food aversions after chemotherapy. *Cancer, 66*(7), 1649–1653.

Ayllon, T. & Milan, M. (2002). Token economy: guidelines for operation. In M. Hersen & W. Sledge (eds), *Encyclopedia of Psychotherapy*. New York: Academic Press, pp. 829–833.

Azar, B. (2005). How mimicry begat culture. *American Psychological Association Monitor, 36*(9). Retrieved 26 May 2008, from www.apa.org/monitor/ oct05/mirror.html.

Azrin, N. H. & Holz, W. C. (1966). Punishment. In W. K. Honig (ed.), *Operant Behavior: Areas of Research and Application*. New York: Appleton-Century- Crofts, pp. 380–447.

Bandura, A. (1965). Vicarious processes: a case of no-trial learning. In L. Berkowitz (ed.), *Advances in Experimental Social Psychology* (Vol. 2). New York: Academic Press, pp. 3–55.

Bandura, A. (1977). Self-efficacy: toward a unifying theory of behavioral change. *Psychological Review, 84*, 191–215.

Bandura, A., Ross, D. & Ross, S. A. (1961). Transmission of aggression through imitation of aggressive models. *Journal of Abnormal and Social Psychology, 63*, 575–582.

Bandura, A., Ross, D. & Ross, S. A. (1963). Imitation of film mediated aggressive models. *Journal of Abnormal and Social Psychology, 66*, 3–11.

Blodgett, H. C. (1929). The effect of the introduction of reward upon the maze performance of rats. *University of California Publications in Psychology, 4*, 113–134.

Bloom, C., Venard, J., Harden, M. & Seetharaman, S. (2007). Non-contingent positive and negative reinforcement schedules of superstitious behaviors. *Behavioural Processes, 75*, 8–13.

Bolles, R. C. (1979). *Learning Theory*. New York: Holt, Rinehart & Winston.

Bond, N. W. & Siddle, D. A. T. (1996). The preparedness account of social phobia: some data and alternative explanations. In R. M. Rapee (ed.), *Current Controversies in the Anxiety Disorders*. London: Guilford, pp. 291–316.

Bouton, M. E. (1994). Context, ambiguity, and classical conditioning. *Current Directions in Psychological Science, 3*, 1–5.

Bradbard, M. R., Martin, C. L., Endsley, R. C. & Halverson, C. E. (1986). Influence of sex stereotypes on children's exploration and memory: a competence versus performance distinction. *Developmental Psychology, 22*(4), 481–486.

Brennan, P. A. & Mednick, S. A. (1994). Learning theory approach to the deterrence of criminal recidivism. *Journal of Abnormal Psychology, 103*, 430–440.

Brewer, W. F. (1974). There is no convincing evidence for operant or classical conditioning in adult humans. In W. B. Weimer & D. S. Palemo (eds), *Cognition and the Symbolic Processes*. Hillsdale, NJ: Erlbaum, pp. 1–42.

Brown, P. L. & Jenkins, H. M. (1968). Auto-shaping of the pigeon's key-peck. *Journal of the Experimental Analysis of Behavior, 11*(1), 1–18.

Bushman, B. J. & Anderson, C. A. (2001). Media violence and the American public: scientific facts versus media misinformation. *American Psychologist, 56*, 477–489.

Carnagey, N. L., Anderson, C. A. & Bartholow, B. D. (2007). Media violence and social neuroscience: new questions and new opportunities. *Current Directions in Psychological Science, 16*(4), 178–182.

Carr, J. E., Fraizer, T. J. & Roland, J. P. (2005). Token economy. In A. M. Gross & R. S. Drabman (eds) *Encyclopedia of Behavior Modification and Cognitive Behavior Therapy—Volume 2: Child Clinical Applications.* Thousand Oaks, CA: Sage, pp. 1075–1079.

Church, R. M. (1969). Response suppression. In B. Campbell & R. Church (eds), *Punishment and Aversive Behavior.* New York: Appleton-Century-Crofts, pp. 111–156.

Collins, H. & Pinch, T. (1993). *The Golem: What You Should Know About Science.* Cambridge: Cambridge University Press.

D'Amato, E. (1998, January/February). Mystery of disgust. *Psychology Today.* Retrieved 26 May 2008 from http://psychologytoday.com/articles/pto-19980201-000032.html.

Damisch, L., Stoberock, B. & Mussweiler, T. (2010). Keep your fingers crossed! How superstition improves performance. *Psychological Science, 21(7)*, 1014–1020.

Danaher, B. C. (1974). Theoretical foundations and clinical applications of the Premack principle: review and critique. *Behavior Therapy, 5*(3), 307–324.

Dawes, R. M. (1994). *House of Cards: Psychology and Psychotherapy Built on Myth.* New York: The Free Press.

deBell, C. S. & Harless, D. K. (1992). B. F. Skinner: myth and misperception. *Teaching of Psychology, 19*(2), 68–73.

Denniston, J. C., Chang, R. & Miller, R. R. (2003). Massive extinction prevents the renewal effect. *Learning and Motivation, 34*, 68–86.

DiLalla, L. F. & Gottesman, I. I. (1991). Biological and genetic contributors to violence—Widom's untold tale. *Psychological Bulletin, 109*, 125–129.

DiNardo, P. A., Guzy, L. T. & Bak, R. M. (1988). Anxiety response patterns and etiological factors in dog-fearful and non-fearful subjects. *Behaviour and Research Therapy, 26*(3), 245–251.

Fabbri-Destro, M. & Rizzolatti, G. (2008). Mirror neurons and mirror systems in monkeys and humans. *Physiology, 23*, 171–179.

Fang, X. & Corso, P. S. (2007). Child maltreatment, youth violence, and intimate partner violence: developmental relationships. *American Journal of Preventive Medicine, 33*, 281–290.

Ferguson, C. J. (2009). Violent video games: dogma, fear, and pseudoscience. *Skeptical Inquirer, 33*(5), 38–54.

Fowles, D. C. (1980). The three arousal model: implications of Gray's two-factor learning theory for heart rate, electrodermal activity, and psychopathy. *Psychophysiology, 17*, 87–104.

Freedman, J. L. (1984). Effect of television violence on aggressiveness. *Psychological Bulletin, 96*(2), 227–246.

Freedman, J. L. (2002). *Media Violence and its Effects on Aggression: Assessing the Scientific Evidence.* Toronto: University of Toronto Press.

Gallese, V. & Goldman, A. (1998). Mirror neurons and the simulation theory of mind-reading. *Trends in Cognitive Sciences, 2*(12), 493–501.

Garcia, J. & Hankins, W. G. (1977). On the origin of food aversion paradigms. In L. M. Barker, M. R. Best & M. Domjan (eds), *Learning Mechanisms in Food Selection.* Houston, TX: Baylor University Press, pp. 3–22.

Garcia, J. & Koelling, R. A. (1966). The relation of cue to consequence in avoidance learning. *Psychonomic Science, 4*, 123–124.

García-Montes, J. M., Álvarez, M. P., Sass, L. A. & Cangas, A. J. (2008). The role of superstition in psychopathology. *Philosophy, Psychiatry, & Psychology, 15*, 227–237.

Gershoff, E. T. (2002). Corporal punishment by parents and associated child behaviors and experiences: a meta-analytic and theoretical review. *Psychological Bulletin, 128*(4), 539–579.

Gewirtz, J. C. & Davis, M. (2000). Using Pavlovian 'higher-order' conditioning paradigms to investigate the neural substrates of emotional learning and memory. *Learning and Memory, 7*, 257–266.

Gorn, G. J. (1982). The effects of music in advertising on choice behavior: a classical conditioning approach. *Journal of Marketing, 46*, 94–101.

Gould, J. L. & Gould, C. G. (1994). *The Animal Mind.* New York: Scientific American Library/Scientific American Books.

Green, G. (1996). Early behavioral intervention for autism: what does research tell us? In C. Maurice, G. Green & S. Luce (eds), *Behavioral Intervention for Young Children with Autism: A Manual for Parents and Professionals.* Austin, TX: PRO-E, pp. 29–44.

Gresham, L. G. & Shimp, T. A. (1985). Attitude toward the advertisement and brand attitudes: a classical conditioning perspective. *Journal of Advertising, 14*, 10–49.

Grings, W. W. (1973). Cognitive factors in electrodermal conditioning. *Psychological Bulletin, 79*(3), 200–210.

Haney, R. E. (1969). Classical conditioning of a plant: *Mimosa pudica. Journal of Biological Psychology, 11*, 5–12.

Herbert, J. D., Sharp, I. R. & Gaudiano, B. A. (2002). Separating fact from fiction in the etiology and treatment of autism: a scientific review of the evidence. *Scientific Review of Mental Health Practice, 1*, 25–45.

Herrnstein, R. J. (1966). Superstition: a corollary of the principles of operant conditioning. In W. K. Honig (ed.), *Operant Behavior: Areas of Research and Application.* New York: Appleton-Century-Crofts, pp. 33–51.

Hoffmann, H. (2011). Hot and bothered: classical conditioning of sexual incentives in humans. In T. R. Schachtman & S. Reilly (eds), *Associative Learning and Conditioning Theory: Human and Non-human Applications.* New York: Oxford University Press, pp. 532–550.

Huesmann, L. R., Moise-Titus, J., Podolski, C. & Eron, L. D. (2003). Longitudinal relations between children's exposure to TV violence and their aggressive and violent behavior in young adulthood: 1977–1992. *Developmental Psychology, 39*(2), 201–221.

Iacoboni, M. (2009). Imitation, empathy, and mirror neurons. *Annual Review of Psychology, 60*, 653–670.

Jones, M. C. (1924). The elimination of children's fears. *Journal of Experimental Psychology*, 7, 382–390.

Joukhador, J., Blaszczynski, A. & Maccallum, F. (2004). Superstitious beliefs in gambling among problem and non-problem gamblers: preliminary data. *Journal of Gambling Studies, 20*, 171–180.

Kazdin, A. E. (1982). The token economy: a decade later. *Journal of Applied Behavior Analysis, 15*(3), 431–445.

Kendler, K. S., Neale, M. C., Kessler, R. C., Heath, A. C. & Eaves, L. J. (1992). The genetic epidemiology of phobias in women: the interrelationship of agoraphobia, social phobia, situational phobia, and simple phobia. *Archives of General Psychiatry, 49*(4), 273–281.

Kirsch, I., Lynn, S. J., Vigorito, M. & Miller, R. R. (2004). The role of cognition in classical and operant conditioning. *Journal of Clinical Psychology, 60*, 369–392.

Knapp, T. J. (1976). Premack principle in human experimental and applied settings. *Behaviour Research and Therapy, 14*(2), 133–147.

Köhler, W. (1925). An aspect of Gestalt psychology. *Pedagogical Seminary and Journal of Genetic Psychology, 32*(4), 691–723.

Köksal, F., Domjan, M., Kurt, A., Sertel, O., Orüng, S., Bowers, R. et al. (2004). An animal model of fetishism. *Behaviour Research and Therapy, 42*(12), 1421–1434.

Krueger, R. F., Hicks, B. M. & McGue, M. (2001). Altruism and antisocial behavior: independent tendencies, unique personality correlates, distinct etiologies. *Psychological Science, 12*, 397–402.

LeDoux, J. (1996). *The Emotional Brain: The Mysterious Underpinnings of Emotional Life.* New York: Simon & Schuster.

Lovaas, O. I. (1987). Behavioral treatment and normal educational and intellectual functioning in young autistic children. *Journal of Consulting and Clinical Psychology, 55*(1), 3–9.

Lowenstein, L. F. (2002). Fetishes and their associated behavior. *Sexuality and Disability, 20*, 135–147.

Lozanov, G. (1978). *Suggestology and Outlines of Suggestopedy.* (M. Hall-Pozharlieva & K. Pashmakova, trans.). Oxford: Gordon & Breach.

Lykken, D. T., Iacono, W. G., Harioan, K., McGue, M. & Bouchard, T. J. (1988). Habituation of the skin-conductance response to strong stimuli—a twin study. *Psychophysiology, 25*(1), 4–15.

Lynch, S. K., Turkheimer, E., D'Onofrio, B. M., Mendle, J., Emery, R. E., Slutske, W. S. et al. (2006). A genetically informed study of the association between harsh punishment and offspring behavioral problems. *Journal of Family Psychology, 20*(2), 190–198.

Matson, J. L., Benavidez, D. A., Compton, L. S., Paclawskyj, T. & Baglio, C. (1996). Behavioral treatment of autistic persons: a review of research from 1980 to the present. *Research in Developmental Disabilities, 17*(6), 433–465.

McConnell, J. V. (1962). Memory transfer through cannibalism in planarianns. *Journal of Neuropsychiatry, 3* (Suppl. 1), 542–548.

McCord, J. (2006). Punishments and alternate routes to crime prevention. In A. K. Hess & I. B. Weiner (eds), *The Handbook of Forensic Psychology* (3rd ed.). Hoboken, NJ: John Wiley, pp. 701–721.

McEachin, J. J., Smith, T. & Lovaas, O. I. (1993). Long-term outcome for children with autism who received early intensive behavioral treatment. *American Journal on Mental Retardation, 97*(4), 359–372.

McNamara, H. J., Long, J. B. & Wike, E. L. (1956). Learning without response under two conditions of external cues. *Journal of Comparative and Physiological Psychology, 49*(5), 477–480.

Mineka, S. & Cook, M. (1993). Mechanisms involved in the observational conditioning of fear. *Journal of Experimental Psychology: General, 122*, 23–38.

Mischel, W. (1973). Toward a cognitive social learning reconceptualization of personality. *Psychological Review, 80*, 252–283.

Moffitt, T. E. (1983). The learning theory model of punishment: implications for delinquency deterrence. *Criminal Justice and Behavior, 10*, 131–158.

Molenberghs, P., Cunnington, R. & Mattingley, J. B. (2012). Brain regions with mirror properties: a meta-analysis of 125 human fMRI studies. *Neuroscience and Biobehavioral Reviews, 36:* 341–349.

Morokuma, S., Fukushima, K., Kawai, N., Tomonaga, M., Satoh, S. & Nakano, H. (2004). Fetal habituation correlates with functional brain development. *Behavioural Brain Research, 153*(2), 459–463.

Morse, W. H. & Skinner, B. F. (1957). A second type of superstition in the pigeon. *American Journal of Psychology, 70*(2), 308–311.

Mowrer, O. H. (1947). On the dual nature of learning—a re-interpretation of 'conditioning' and 'problem-solving.' *Harvard Educational Review, 17*, 102–148.

Ohman, A., Flykt, A. & Esteves, F. (2001). Emotion drives attention: detecting the snake in the grass. *Journal of Experimental Psychology: General, 130*, 466–478.

Ohman, A. & Mineka, S. (2001). Fears, phobias, and preparedness: toward an evolved module of fear and fear learning. *Psychological Review, 108*(3), 483–522.

Ohman, A. & Mineka, S. (2003). The malicious serpent: snakes as a prototypical stimulus for an evolved module of fear. *Current Directions in Psychological Science, 12*(1), 5–9.

Paul, G. & Lentz, R. J. (1977). *Psychosocial Treatment of Chronic Mental Patients: Milieu Versus Social-Learning Programs.* Cambridge, MA: Harvard University Press.

Pavlov, I. P. (1927). *Conditioned Reflexes.* Oxford: Oxford University Press.

Pinker, S. (1997, 1994). *How the Mind Works.* New York: Norton.

Plotkin, H. (2004). *Evolutionary Thought in Psychology: A Brief History.* Oxford: Blackwell.

Premack, D. (1965). Reinforcement theory. In D. Levine (ed.), *Nebraska Symposium on Motivation.* Lincoln, NE: University of Nebraska Press, pp. 123–180.

Purkis, H. M. & Lipp, O. V. (2008). Are snakes and spiders special? Acquisition of negative valence and modified attentional processing by non-fear-relevant animal stimuli. *Cognition & Emotion, 23*(3), 430–452.

Rachman, S. (1977). The conditioning theory of fear-acquisition: a critical examination. *Behaviour Research and Therapy, 15*, 375–387.

Rachman, S. & Hodgson, R. J. (1968). Experimentally induced 'sexual fetishism': replication and development. *Psychological Record, 18*, 25–27.

Ramachandran, V. S. (2000). Mirror neurons and imitation learning as the driving force behind 'the great leap forward' in human evolution. *Edge.* Retrieved 15 January 2006 from www.edge.org/3rd_culture/ramachandran/ramachan-dran_p1.html.

Rescorla, R. A. (1990). The role of information about the response-outcome relations in instrumental discrimination learning. *Journal of Experimental Psychology: Animal Behavior Processes, 16*, 262–270.

Rescorla, R. A. & Wagner, A. R. (1972). A theory of Pavlovian conditioning: variations in effectiveness of reinforcement and non-reinforcement. In A. H. Black & W. F. Prokasy (eds), *Classical Conditioning II: Current Research and Theory.* New York: Appleton-Century-Crofts, pp. 64–98.

Rilling, M. (1996). The mystery of the vanished citations: James McConnell's forgotten 1960s quest for planariann learning, a biochemical engram, and celebrity. *American Psychologist, 51*(1), 1039.

Rizzolatti, G., Fadiga, L., Gallese, V. & Fogassi, L. (1996). Premotor cortex and the recognition of motor actions. *Cognitive Brain Research, 3*(2), 131–141.

Robbins, T. W., Granon, S., Muir, J. L., Durantou, F., Harrison, A. & Everitt, B. J. (1998). Neural systems underlying arousal and attention: implications for drug abuse. In J. A. Harvey & Kosofsky, B. E. (eds), *Cocaine: Effects on the Developing Brain.* New York: New York Academy of Sciences, pp. 222–237.

Romanczyk, R. G., Arnstein, L., Soorya, L. V. & Gillis, J. (2003). The myriad of controversial treatments for autism: a critical evaluation of efficacy. In S. O. Lilienfeld, S. J. Lynn & J. M. Lohr (eds), *Science and Pseudoscience in Clinical Psychology.* New York: Guilford, pp. 363–395.

Rozin, P. & Fallon, A. (1987). A perspective on disgust. *Psychological Review, 94*, 23–41.

Rozin, P., Markwith, M. & Ross, B. (1990). The sympathetic magical law of similarity, nominal realism and neglect of negatives in response to negative labels. *Psychological Science, 1*(6), 383–384.

Rozin, P., Millman, L. & Nemeroff, C. (1986). Operation of the laws of sympathetic magic in disgust and other domains. *Journal of Personality and Social Psychology, 50*, 703–712.

Schopler, E., Short, A. & Mesibov, G. (1989). Relation of behavioral treatment to 'normal functioning': comment on Lovaas. *Journal of Consulting and Clinical Psychology, 57*(1), 162–164.

Seligman, M. E. (1971). Phobias and preparedness. *Behavior Therapy, 2*, 307–320.

Seligman, M. E. & Hager, J. L. (1972). Sauce-béarnaise syndrome. *Psychology Today, 6*(3), 59.

Shadish, W. R., Cook, T. D. & Campbell, D. T. (2002). *Experimental and Quasi-Experimental Designs for Generalized Causal Inference.* Boston, MA: Houghton Mifflin.

Siegelbaum, S. A., Camardo, J. S. & Kandel, E. R. (1982). Serotonin and cyclic AMP close single K^+ channels in Aplysia sensory neurons. *Nature, 299,* 413–417.

Simon, C. W. & Emmons, W. H. (1955). Learning during sleep? *Psychological Bulletin, 52*(4), 328–342.

Skinner, B. F. (1938). *The Behavior of Organisms: An Experimental Analysis.* New York: Appleton-Century-Crofts.

Skinner, B. F. (1948). Superstition in the pigeon. *Journal of Experimental Psychology, 38,* 168–172.

Skinner, B. F. (1953). *Science and Human Behavior.* New York: Macmillan.

Skinner, B. F. (1969). *Contingencies of Reinforcement.* East Norwalk, CT: Appleton-Century-Crofts.

Skinner, B. F. (1971). *Beyond Freedom and Dignity.* New York: Knopf.

Skinner, B. F. (1990). Can psychology be a science of mind? *American Psychologist, 4,* 1206–1210.

Smalheiser, N. R., Manev, H. & Costa, E. (2001). RNAi and memory: was McConnell on the right track after all? *Trends in Neuroscience, 24,* 216–218.

Smith, R. A. (2001). *Challenging Your Preconceptions: Thinking Critically About Psychology.* Pacific Grove, CA: Wadsworth.

Staddon, J. E. R. (2003). Humanism and Skinner's radical behaviorism. In K. A. Lattal & P. N. Chase (eds), *Behavior Theory and Philosophy.* New York: Kluwer Academic/Plenum, pp. 129–146.

Staddon, J. E. R. & Simmelhag, V. L. (1971). Superstition experiment—a re-examination of its implications for principles of adaptive behavior. *Psychological Review, 78*(1), 3.

Straus, M. A. & McCord, J. (1998). Do physically punished children become violent adults? In S. Nolen-Hoeksema (ed.), *Clashing Views on Abnormal Psychology: A Taking Sides Custom Reader.* Guilford, CT: Dushkin/McGraw-Hill, pp. 130–155.

Straus, M. A., Sugarman, D. B. & Giles-Sims, J. (1997). Spanking by parents and subsequent antisocial behavior of children. *Archives of Pediatrics and Adolescent Medicine, 151*(8), 761–767.

Stuart, E. W., Shimp, T. A. & Engle, R. W. (1987). Classical conditioning of consumer attitudes: four experiments in an advertising context. *Journal of Consumer Research, 14,* 334–349.

Tear, M. J. & Nielsen, M. (2013). Failure to demonstrate that playing violent video games diminishes prosocial behavior. *PLoS One, 8,* e68382.

Thompson, R. & McConnell, J. (1955). Classical conditioning in the planariann, *Dugesia dorotocephala. Journal of Comparative and Physiological Psychology, 48*(1), 65–68.

Thorndike, E. L. (1898). *Animal Intelligence: An Experimental Study of the Associative Processes in Animals.* New York: Macmillan.

Thorndike, E. L. (1911). *Animal Intelligence: Experimental Studies.* New York: Macmillan.

Tice, D. M. & Baumeister, R. F. (1997). Longitudinal study of procrastination, performance, stress, and health: the costs and benefits of dawdling. *Psychological Science, 8*(6), 454–458.

Tolman, E. C. (1932). *Purposive Behavior in Animals and Men.* Oxford: Appleton-Century.

Tolman, E. C. (1948). Cognitive maps in rats and men. *Psychological Review, 55,* 189–208.

Tolman, E. C. & Honzik, C. H. (1930). Introduction and removal of reward, and maze performance in rats. *University of California Publications in Psychology, 4,* 257–275.

Tomarken, A. J., Mineka, S. & Cook, M. (1989). Fear-relevant selective associations and covariation bias. *Journal of Abnormal Psychology, 98*(4), 381–394.

Tomarken, A. J., Sutton, S. K. & Mineka, S. (1995). Fear-relevant illusory correlations: what types of associations promote judgmental bias? *Journal of Abnormal Psychology, 104*(2), 312–326.

Tsang, E. W. K. (2004). Toward a scientific inquiry into superstitious business decision-making. *Organization Studies, 25,* 923–946.

Vaitl, D. & Lipp, O. V. (1997). Latent inhibition and autonomic responses: a psychophysiological approach. *Behavioral Brain Research, 88*(1), 85–93.

Veit, R., Flor, H., Erb, M., Hermann, C., Lotze, M., Grodd, W. et al. (2002). Brain circuits involved in emotional learning in antisocial behavior and social phobia in humans. *Neuroscience Letters, 328*(3), 233–236.

Vyse, S. A. (1997). *Believing in Magic.* New York: Oxford University Press.

Wakefield, J. C. (2006). Is behaviorism becoming a pseudo-science? Power versus scientific rationality in the eclipse of token economies by biological psychiatry in the treatment of schizophrenia. *Behavior and Social Issues, 15,* 202–221.

Watanabe, S., Sakamoto, J. & Wakita, M. (1995). Pigeons' discrimination of paintings by Monet and Picasso. *Journal of the Experimental Analysis of Behavior, 63,* 65–174.

Watson, J. B. & Rayner, R. (1920). Conditioned emotional reactions. *Journal of Experimental Psychology, 3*, 1–14.

Weinberg, M. S., Williams, C. J. & Calhan, C. (1995). If the shoe fits . . . Exploring male homosexual foot fetishism. *Journal of Sex Research, 31*(1), 17–27.

Williams, T. M. (1986). *The Impact of Television: A Naturalistic Study in Three Communities.* Orlando, FL: Academic Press.

Wilson, J. Q. & Herrnstein, R. J. (1985). *Crime and Human Nature: The Definitive Study of the Causes of Crime.* New York: Simon & Schuster.

Winerman, L. (2005, October). The mind's mirror. *American Psychological Association Monitor, 36*(9). Retrieved 26 May 2008 from www.apa.org/monitor/oct05/ mirror.html.

Wolpe, J. (1990). *The Practice of Behavior Therapy* (4th ed.). Elmsford, NY: Pergamon.

Wood, W., Wong, F. Y. & Chachere, J. G. (1991). Effects of media violence on viewers' aggression in unconstrained social interaction. *Psychological Bulletin, 109*, 371–383.

Woodworth, R. S. (1929). *Psychology* (rev. ed.). Oxford: Holt.

Wyatt, W. J. (2001). Some myths about behaviorism that are undone by B. F. Skinner's 'The Design of Cultures'. *Behavior and Social Issues, 11*(1), 28–30.

Chapter 2

Adams, R.E. & Laursen, B. (2007). The correlates of conflict: Disagreement is not necessarily detrimental. *Journal of Family Psychology, 21*, 445–458.

Ainsworth, M.D.S., Blehar, M., Waters, E. & Wall, S. (1978). *Patterns of attachment*. Hillsdale, NJ: Erlbaum.

Allen, J.P. & Land, D. (1999). Attachment in adolescence. In J. Cassidy & P. R. Shaver (Eds.), *Handbook of attachment: Theory, research, and clinical applications*. New York: Guilford Press.

Allen, J.P., Porter, M.R. & McFarland, F.C. (2006). Leaders and followers in adolescent close relationships: Susceptibility to peer influence as a predictor of risky behavior, friendship instability, and depression. *Development and Psychopathology, 18*, 155–172.

Amato, P.R. & Hohmann-Marriott, B. (2007). A comparison of high- and low-distress marriages that end in divorce. *Journal of Marriage and Family, 69*, 621–638.

Arnett, J.J. (1999). Adolescent storm and stress reconsidered. *American Psychologist, 54*, 317–326.

Australian Bureau of Statistics (2013). *Australian Social Trends* (cat. no. 4102.0). Canberra, Australia: Australian Bureau of Statistics. Retrieved from http://www.abs.gov.au/AUSSTATS/abs@.nsf/Lookup/4102.0Main+Features10July+2013" \l "number" www.abs.gov.au/AUSSTATS/abs@.nsf/Lookup/4102.0Main+Features10July+2013#number

Australian Bureau of Statistics (2014). *Marriages and Divorces, Australia* (cat. no. 3310.0). Canberra, Australia: Australian Bureau of Statistics. Retrieved from http://www.abs.gov.au/AUSSTATS/abs@.nsf/DetailsPage/3310.02014?OpenDocument" www.abs.gov.au/AUSSTATS/abs@.nsf/DetailsPage/3310.02014?OpenDocument

Australian Institute of Health and Welfare (2007). Child Protection Australia 2005–06. Child welfare series no. 40. cat. no. CWS 28. Canberra: AIHW.

Australian Institute of Health and Welfare. (2012). *Dementia in Australia* (cat. no. AGE 70). Canberra, Australia, Australian Institute of Health and Welfare. Retrieved from <http://www.aihw.gov.au/WorkArea/DownloadAsset.aspx?id=10737422943>

Bahrick, H.P., Bahrick, P.O. & Wittlinger, R.P. (1975). Fifty years of memory for names and faces: A cross-sectional approach. *Journal of Experimental Psychology: General, 104*, 54–75.

Bailey, B.A. & Sokol, R.J. (2008). Pregnancy and alcohol use: Evidence and recommendations for prenatal care. *Clinical Obstetrics and Gynecology, 51*, 436–444.

Balsam, K.F., Beauchaine, T.P., Rothblum, E.D. & Solomon, S.E. (2008). Three-year follow-up of same-sex couples who had civil unions in Vermont, same-sex couples not in civil unions, and heterosexual married couples. *Developmental Psychology, 44*, 102–116.

Baltes, P.B. (1993). The aging mind: Potential and limits. *The Gerontologist, 33*, 580–594.

Baltes, P.B. & Kunzmann, U. (2003). Wisdom. *Psychologist, 16*, 131–133.

Baltes, P.B. & Staudinger, U.M. (1993). The search for a psychology of wisdom. *Current Directions in Psychological Science, 2*, 75–80.

Baltes, P.B. & Staudinger, U.M. (2000). Wisdom: A metaheuristic (pragmatic) to orchestrate mind and virtue toward excellence. *American Psychologist, 55*, 122–136.

Baltes, P.B., Smith, J. & Staudinger, U.M. (1992). Wisdom and successful aging. In T.B. Sonderegger (Ed.), *The Nebraska Symposium on Motivation: Vol. 39. The psychology of aging* (pp. 123–167). Lincoln: University of Nebraska Press.

Bauminger, N., Finzi-Dottan, R., Chason, S. & Har-Even, D. (2008). Intimacy in adolescent friendship: The roles of attachment, coherence, and self-disclosure. *Journal of Social and Personal Relationships, 25*, 409–428.

Bayley, N. (1956). Individual patterns of development. *Child Development, 27*, 45–74.

Belsky, J., Vandell, D.L., Burchinal, M., Clarke-Stewart, K.A., McCartney, K., Owen, M.T. & The NICHD Early Child Care Research Network. (2007). Are there longterm effects of early child care? *Child Development, 78*, 681–701.

Benedict, R. (1938). Continuities and discontinuities in cultural conditioning. *Psychiatry, 1*, 161–167.

Benenson, J.F. & Heath, A. (2006). Boys withdraw from one-on-one interactions, whereas girls withdraw more in groups. *Developmental Psychology, 42*, 272–282.

Benenson, J.F., Apostoleris, N.H. & Parnass, J. (1997). Age and sex differences in dyadic and group interaction. *Developmental Psychology, 33*, 538–543.

Bennett, D.S., Bendersky, M. & Lewis, M. (2008). Children's cognitive ability from 4 to 9 years old as a function of prenatal cocaine exposure, environmental risk, and maternal verbal intelligence. *Developmental Psychology, 44*, 919–928.

Bielak, A.A.M., Hughes, T.F., Small, B.J. & Dixon, R.A. (2007). It's never too late to engage in lifestyle activities: Significant concurrent but not change relationships between lifestyle activities and cognitive speed. *Journal of Gerontology: Psychological Sciences, 62B*, 331–339.

Blos, P. (1965). *On adolescence: A psychoanalytic interpretation*. New York: The Free Press.

Boekee, K. & Brown, T. (2015). Gender stereotypes of children's toys: Investigating the perspectives of adults who have and do not have children. *Journal of Occupational Therapy, Schools, & Early Intervention*, 8, 97–107. Taylor & Francis Group, LLC. doi: 10.1080/19411243.2015

Bohlin, G., Hagekull, B. & Rydell, A.-M. (2000). Attachment and social functioning: A longitudinal study from infancy to middle childhood. *Social Development, 9*, 24–39.

Boldizar, J.P., Perry, D.G. & Perry, L.C. (1989). Outcome Values and Aggression. *Child Development, 60*(3), 571–579.

Bolhuis, J.J. & Honey, R.C. (1998). Imprinting, learning and development: From behaviour to brain and back. *Trends in Neurosciences, 21*, 306–311.

Bowlby, J. (1969). *Attachment and loss, Vol. 1. Attachment*. New York: Basic Books.

Bowlby, J. (1973). *Attachment and loss, Vol. 2. Separation, Anxiety, and Anger*. London: Penguin Books.

Brainerd, C.J. (1996). Piaget: A centennial celebration. *Psychological Science, 7*, 191–195.

Branje, S.J.T., Frijns, T., Finkenaer, C., Engels, R. & Meeus, W. (2007). You are my best friend: Commitment and stability in adolescents' same-sex friendships. *Personal Relationships, 14*, 587–603.

Bretherton, I. (1996). Internal working models of attachment relationships as related to resilient coping. In G.G. Noam & K.W. Fischer (Eds.), *Development and vulnerability in close relationships* (pp. 3–27). Mahwah, NJ: Erlbaum.

Bronfenbrenner, U. (Ed.) (2004). *Making human beings human: Bioecological perspectives on human development*. Thousand Oaks, CA: Sage Publications.

Brown, F.B. & Klute, C. (2003). Friendships, cliques, and crowds. In G.R. Adams & M.D. Berzonsky (Eds.), *Blackwell handbooks of developmental psychology* (pp. 330–348). Malden, MA: Blackwell Publishing.

Buchler, N.E.G. & Reder, L.M. (2007). Modeling age-related memory deficits: A two-parameter solution. *Psychology and Aging, 22*, 104–121.

Cabeza, R. (2002). Hemispheric asymmetry reduction in older adults: The HAROLD model. *Psychology and Aging, 17*, 85–100.

Cabeza, R., Daselaar, S.M., Dolcos, F., Prince, S.E., Budde, M. & Nyberg, L. (2004). Task-independent and task-specific age effects on brain activity during working memory, visual attention and episodic retrieval. *Cerebral Cortex, 14*, 364–375.

Cahill, L., Uncapher, M., Kilpatrick, L., Alkire, M.T. & Turner, J. (2004). Sex-related hemispheric lateralization of amygdale function in emotionally influenced memory: An fMRI investigation. *Learning & Memory, 11*, 261–266.

Campos, J.J., Bertenthal, B.I. & Kermoian, R. (1992). Early experience and emotional development: The emergence of wariness of heights. *Psychological Science, 3*, 61–64.

Canli, T., Desmond, J.E., Zhao, Z. & Gabrieli, J.D.E. (2002). Sex differences in the neural basis of emotional memories. *Proceedings of the National Academy of Sciences, 99*, 10789–10794.

Carstensen, L.L. (1991). Selectivity theory: Social activity in life-span context. In K.W. Schaie (Ed.), *Annual review of geriatrics and gerontology* (11). New York: Springer.

Carstensen, L.L. (1998). A life-span approach to social motivation. In J. Heckhausen & C.S. Dweck (Eds.), *Motivation and self-regulation across the life span* (pp. 341–364). New York: Cambridge University Press.

Carstensen, L.L. & Freund, A.M. (1994). The resilience of the aging self. *Developmental Review, 14*, 81–92.

Carter, J.H. (1982). The effects of aging on selected visual functions: Color vision, glare sensitivity, field of vision, and accommodation. In R. Sekuler, D. Kline & K. Dismukes (Eds.), *Aging and human visual function* (pp. 121–130). New York: Liss.

Casey, B.J., Getz, S. & Galvan, A. (2008). The adolescent brain. *Developmental Review, 28*, 62–77.

Champoux, M., Boyce, W.T. & Suomi, S.J. (1995). Biobehavioral comparisons between adopted and nonadopted rhesus monkey infants. *Journal of Developmental and Behavioral Pediatrics, 16*, 6–13.

Chomsky, N. (1965). *Aspects of a theory of syntax*. Cambridge, MA: MIT Press.

Chomsky, N. (1975). *Reflections on language*. New York: Pantheon Books.

Cicchetti, D. & Carlson, V. (Ed.) (1989). *Child Maltreatment: Theory and Research on the Causes and Consequences of Child Abuse and Neglect*. Boston: Cambridge University Press.

Clark, A. E., Diener, E., Georgellis, Y. & Lucas, R. E. (2008). Lags and leads in life satisfaction: A test of the baseline hypothesis. *The Economic Journal, 118* (529), 222–243.

Clarke-Stewart, K.A. (1993). *Daycare*. Cambridge, MA: Harvard University Press.

Clarke-Stewart, A. & Alhusen, V.D. (2005). *What we know about childcare*. Cambridge, MA: Harvard University Press.

Clopton, N.A. & Sorell, G.T. (1993). Gender differences in moral reasoning: Stable or situational? *Psychology of Women Quarterly, 17*, 85–101.

Cohn, D., Passel, J. S., Wang, W. & Livingston, G. (2011). *Barely Half of U.S. Adults Are Married – A Record Low*. Retrieved from http://www.pewsocialtrends.org/2011/12/14/barely-half-of-u-s-adults-are-married-a-record-low/

Collins, W.A., Maccoby, E.E., Steinberg, L., Hetherington, E.M. & Bornstein, M.H. (2000). Contemporary research on parenting: The case for nature and nurture. *American Psychologist, 55*, 218–232.

Corso, J.F. (1977). Auditory perception and communication. In J.E. Birren & K.W. Schaie (Eds.), *Handbook of the psychology of aging* (pp. 535–553). New York: Van Nostrand Reinhold.

Cowan, C.P. & Cowan, P. (2000). *When partners become parents: The big life change for couples*. Mahwah, NJ: Erlbaum.

Cowan, C.P., Cowan, P.A., Heming, G., Garrett, E., Coysh, W.S., Curtis-Boles, H. & Boles, A.J., III. (1985). Transitions to parenthood: His, hers, and theirs. *Journal of Family Issues, 6*, 451–481.

Cowan, W.M. (1979, September). The development of the brain. *Scientific American, 241*, 106–117.

Darling, N. & Steinberg, L. (1993). Parenting style as context: An integrative model. *Psychological Bulletin, 113*, 487–496.

De Santis, M., Cavaliere, A.F., Straface, G. & Caruso, A. (2006). Rubella infection in pregnancy. *Reproductive Toxicology, 21*, 390–398.

DeCasper, A.J. & Prescott, P.A. (1984). Human newborns' perception of male voices: Preference, discrimination, and reinforcing value. *Developmental Psychology, 17*, 481–491.

Dejin-Karlsson, E., Hsonson, B.S., Oestergren, P.-O., Sjoeberg, O. & Karel, M. (1998). Does passive smoking in early pregnancy increase the risk of small-for-gestational age infants? *American Journal of Public Health, 88*, 1523–1527.

DeLamater, J.D. & Sill, M. (2005). Sexual desire in later life. *The Journal of Sex Research, 42*, 138–149.

Dennerstein, L., Dudley, E. & Guthrie, J. (2003). Empty nest or revolving door? A prospective study of women's quality of life in midlife during the phase of children leaving and re-entering the home. *Psychological Medicine, 32*, 545–550.

DiPietro, J.A., Hodgson, D.M., Costigan, K.A. & Johnson, T.R.B. (1996). Fetal antecedents of infant temperament. *Child Development, 67*, 2568–2583.

Dixon, R.A. (1999). Concepts and mechanisms of gains in cognitive aging. In D.C. Park & N. Schwarz (Eds.), *Cognitive aging: A primer* (pp. 23–41). Philadelphia: Psychology Press.

Dixon, R.A. (2003). Themes in the aging of intelligence: Robust decline with intriguing possibilities. In R.J. Sternberg, J. Lautrey & T.I. Lubart (Eds.), *Models of intelligence: International perspectives* (pp. 151–167). Washington, DC: American Psychological Association.

Dixon, R.A. & de Frias, C.M. (2004). The Victoria longitudinal study: From characterizing cognitive aging to illustrating changes in memory compensation. *Aging Neuropsychology and Cognition, 11*, 346–376.

Donleavy, G. D. (2008). No man's land: Exploring the space between Gilligan and Kohlberg. *Journal of Business Ethics*, 80, 807-822. doi:10.1007/s10551-007-9470-9

Donovan, W., Leavitt, L., Taylor, N. & Broder, J. (2007). Maternal sensitivity, mother-infant 9-month interaction, infant attachment status: Predictors of mother-toddler interaction at 24 months. *Infant Behavior & Development, 30*, 336–352.

Erikson, E. (1963). *Childhood and society.* New York: Norton.

Fantz, R.L. (1963). Pattern vision in newborn infants. *Science, 140*(3564), 296–297.

Federal Interagency Forum on Aging-Related Statistics. (2008). *Older Americans 2008: Key indicators of well-being.* Washington, DC: US Government Printing Office. Retrieved from <http://agingstats.gov/agingstatsdotnet/Main_Site/Data/Data_2008.asp>.

Feldman, D.H. (2004). Piaget's stages: The unfinished symphony of cognitive development. *New Ideas in Psychology, 22*, 175–231.

Fingerman, K. (2000). We had a nice little chat: Age and generational differences in mothers' and daughters' descriptions of enjoyable visits. *The Journals of Gerontology, 55* (2), 95-106.

Flavell, J.H. (1985). *Cognitive development* (2nd ed.). Englewood Cliffs, NJ: Prentice Hall.

Flavell, J.H. (1996). Piaget's legacy. *Psychological Science, 7*, 200–203.

Friesdorf, R., Conway, P. & Gawronski, B. (2015). Gender differences in responses to moral dilemmas: A process dissociation analysis. *Personality and Social Psychology Bulletin, 41*(5), 696-713.

Freud, A. (1946). *The ego and the mechanisms of defense.* New York: International Universities Press.

Freud, A. (1958). Adolescence. *Psychoanalytic Study of the Child, 13*, 255–278.

Freund, A.M. & Baltes, P.B. (1998). Selection, optimization, and compensation as strategies of life management: Correlations with subjective indicators of successful aging. *Psychology and Aging, 13*, 531–543.

Gardner, M. & Steinberg, L. (2005). Peer influence on risk taking, risk preference, and risky decision making in adolescence and adulthood: An experimental study. *Developmental Psychology, 41*, 625–635.

Gauvain, M., Perez, S. M., & Beebe, H. (2013). Authoritative Parenting and Parental Support for Children's Cognitive Development. In A. S. Morris, R. E. Larzelere, & A. Harrist (Eds.), *Authoritative parenting: Synthesizing nurturance and discipline for optimal child development*, (pp. 211-233). Washington, DC: American Psychological Association.

Gelman, S.A. (2003). *Origins of essentialism in everyday thought.* London: Oxford University Press.

Gelman, S.A. & Raman, L. (2002). Folk biology as a window into cognitive development. *Human Development, 45*, 61–68.

Gelman, S.A. & Wellman, H.M. (1991). Insides and essences: Early understandings of the non-obvious. *Cognition, 38*, 213–244.

Gibbs, J.C., Basinger, K.S., Grime, R.L. & Snarey, J.R. (2007). Moral judgment development across culture: Revisiting Kohlberg's universality claims. *Developmental Review, 27*, 443–500.

Gibson, E.J. & Walk, R.D. (1960). The ëvisual cliff', *Scientific American, 202*, 67–71.

Gilligan, C. (1982). *In a different voice: Psychological theory and women's development.* Cambridge, MA: Harvard University Press.

Goldberg, A.E. & Perry-Jenkins, M. (2007). The division of labor and perceptions of parental roles: Lesbian couples across the transition to parenthood. *Journal of Social and Personal Relationships, 24*, 297–318.

Goldberg, A.E. & Sayer, A. (2006). Lesbian couples' relationship quality across the transition to parenthood. *Journal of Marriage and Family, 68*, 87–100.

Goldstein, J.M., Seidman, L.J., Horton, N.J., Makris, N., Kennedy, D.N., Caviness, V.S., Jr., Faraone, S.V. & Tsuang, M.T. (2001). Normal sexual dimorphism of the human brain assessed by in vivo magnetic resonance imaging. *Cerebral Cortex, 11*, 490–497.

Golombok, S., Rust, J., Zervoulis, K., Croudace, T., Golding, J. & Hines, M. (2008). Developmental trajectories of sex-typed behavior in boys and girls: A longitudinal general population study of children aged 2.5–8 years. *Child Development, 79*, 1583–1593.

Golombok, S., Rust, J., Visualizer, K., Golding, J. & Hines, M. (2012). Continuity in sex-typed behavior from preschool to adolescence: a longitudinal population study of boys and girls aged 3-13 years. Archives of Sexual Behavior, 41(3), 591-7. doi: 10.1007/s10508-011-9784-7

Grady, C.L., McIntosh, A.R. & Craik, F.I.M. (2005). Task-related activity in prefrontal cortex and its relation to recognition memory performance in young and old adults. *Neuropsychologia, 43*, 1466–1481.

Grady, C.L., Springer, M.V., Hongwanishkul, D., McIntosh, A.R. & Winocur, G. (2006). Age-related changes in brain activity across the adult lifespan. *Journal of Cognitive Neuroscience, 18*, 227–241.

Gray, M.R. & Steinberg, L. (1999). Unpacking authoritative parenting: Reassessing a multidimensional construct. *Journal of Marriage and the Family, 61*, 574–587.

Green, C.S. & Bavelier, D. (2008). Exercising your brain: A review of human brain plasticity and training-induced learning. *Psychology & Aging, 23*(4), 692–701.

Gur, R.C., Gunning-Dixon, F., Bilker, W.B. & Gur, R.E. (2002). Sex differences in temporo-limbic and frontal brain volumes of healthy adults. *Cerebral Cortex, 12*, 998–1003.

Haas, S.M. & Stafford, L. (2005). Maintenance behaviors in same-sex and marital relationships: A matched sample comparison. *Journal of Family Communication, 5*, 43–60

Haidt, J. (2007). The new synthesis in moral psychology. *Science, 316*, 998–1002.

Hall, G.S. (1904). *Adolescence: Its psychology and its relations to physiology, anthropology, sociology, sex, crime, religion and education* (Vols. 1 and 2). New York: D. Appleton.

Hamlin, J.K., Hallinan, E.V. & Woodward, A.L. (2008). Do as I do: 7-month-old infants selectively reproduce other's goals. *Developmental Science, 11*, 487–494.

Harlow, H.F. & Zimmerman, R.R. (1958). The development of affectional responses in infant monkeys. *Proceedings of the American Philosophical Society, 102*, 501–509.

Herek, G.M. (2006). Legal recognition of same-sex relationships in the United States: A social science perspective. *American Psychologist, 61*, 607–621.

Hess, T.M. (2005). Memory and aging in context. *Psychological Bulletin, 131*, 383–406.

Hess, T.M. & Hinson, J.T. (2006). Age-related variation in the influences of aging stereotypes on memory in adulthood. *Psychology and Aging, 21*, 621–625.

Holmbeck, G.N. & O'Donnell, D. (1991). Discrepancies between perceptions of decision making and behavioral autonomy. In R.L. Paikoff (Ed.), *Shared views in the family during adolescence* (pp. 51–69). San Francisco: Jossey-Bass.

Hultsch, D.F., Hertzog, C., Dixon, R.A. & Small, B.J. (1998). *Memory change in the aged.* Cambridge, UK: Cambridge University Press.

Huston, A.C. (2005). The effects of welfare reform and poverty policies on children and families. In D.B. Pillemer & S.H. White (Eds.), *Developmental psychology and social change: Research, history, and policy* (pp. 83–103). New York: Cambridge University Press.

Jaffee, S. & Hyde, J.S. (2000). Gender differences in moral orientation: A meta-analysis. *Psychological Bulletin, 126*, 703–726.

Jensen, L.A. (2008). Through two lenses: A cultural-developmental approach to moral psychology. *Developmental Review, 28*, 289–315.

Joh, A.S. & Adolph, K.E (2006). Learning from falling. *Child Development, 77*, 89–102.

Kagan, J. & Snidman, N. (1991). Infant predictors of inhibited and uninhibited profiles. *Psychological Science, 2*, 40–44.

Kagan, J. & Snidman, N. (2004). *The long shadow of temperament.* Cambridge, MA: Belknap Press.

Karavasilis, L., Doyle, A.B. & Markiewicz, D. (2003). Associations between parenting style and attachment to mother in middle childhood and adolescence. *International Journal of Behavioral Development, 27*, 153–164.

Kesebir, P. & Diener, E. (2008). In pursuit of happiness: Empirical answers to philosophical questions. *Perspectives on Psychological Science, 3*, 117–125.

Kimura, D. (1999). *Sex and cognition.* Cambridge, MA: MIT Press.

Kisilevsky, B.S. & Low, J.A. (1998). Human fetal behavior: 100 years of study. *Developmental Review, 18*, 1–29.

Kisilevsky, B.S., Hains, S.M.J., Lee, K., Xie, X., Huang, H., Ye, H.H., Zhang, K. & Wang, Z. (2003). Effects of experience on fetal voice recognition. *Psychological Science, 14*, 220–224.

Knickmeyer, R., Baron-Cohen, S., Raggatt, P. & Taylor, K. (2005). Foetal testosterone, social relationships, and restricted interests in children. *Journal of Child Psychology and Psychiatry, 46*, 198–210.

Kohen, D.E., Leventhal, T., Dahinten, V.S. & McIntosh, C.N. (2008). Neighborhood disadvantage: Pathways of effects for young children. *Child Development, 79*, 156–169.

Kohlberg, L. (1964). Development of moral character and moral ideology. In M.L. Hoffman & L.W. Hoffman (Eds.), *Review of child development research* (Vol. 1). New York: Russell Sage Foundation.

Kohlberg, L. (1981). *The philosophy of moral development.* New York: Harper & Row.

Kolb, B. (1989). Development, plasticity, and behavior. *American Psychologist, 44*, 1203–1212.

Krebs, D.L. (2008). Morality: An evolutionary account. *Perspectives on Psychological Science, 3*, 149–172.

Kujawski, J.H. & Bower, T.G.R. (1993). Same-sex preferential looking during infancy as a function of abstract representation. *British Journal of Developmental Psychology, 11*, 201–209.

Lachman, M.E. (2004). Development in midlife. *Annual Review of Psychology, 55*, 305–331.

Lawrence, E., Nylen, K. & Cobb, R.J. (2007). Prenatal expectations and marital satisfaction over the transition to parenthood. *Journal of Family Psychology, 21*, 155–164.

Lenroot, R.K., Gogtay, N., Greenstein, D.K., Wells, E. M., Gregory L., Wallace, G.L., Clasen, L.V., Blumenthal, J.D., Lerch, J., Zijdenbos, A.P., Evans, A.C., Thompson, P.M. & Giedda, J.N. (2007). Sexual dimorphism of brain developmental trajectories during childhood and adolescence. *NeuroImage, 36*, 1065–1073.

Levenson, R.W., Carstensen, L.L. & Gottman, J.M. (1993). Long-term marriage: Age, gender, and satisfaction. *Psychology and Aging, 8*, 301–313.

Lindau, S.T., Schumm, L.P., Laumann, E.O., Levinson, W., O'Muircheartaigh, C.A. & Waite, L.J. (2007). A study of sexuality and health among older adults in the United States. *The New England Journal of Medicine, 357*, 762–775.

LoBue, V. & DeLoache, J. S. (2011). Pretty in pink: The early development of gender-stereotyped colour preferences. *British Journal of Developmental Psychology, 29*(3), 656-667.

Lourenço, O. & Machado, A. (1996). In defense of Piaget's theory: A reply to 10 common criticisms. *Psychological Review, 103*, 143–164.

Lyons, N. (1983). Two perspectives: On self, relationships, and morality. *Harvard Educational Review, 53*, 125–146.

Macchi Cassia, V., Turati, C. & Simion, F. (2004). Can a nonspecific bias toward top-heavy patterns explain newborns' face preference? *Psychological Science, 15*, 379–383.

Maccoby, E.E. (2002). Gender and group processes: A developmental perspective. *Current Directions in Psychological Science, 11*, 54–58.

Maccoby, E.E. & Martin, J.A. (1983). Socialization in the context of the family: Parent–child interaction. In E.M. Hetherington (Ed.), *Handbook of child psychology: Vol. 4. Socialization, personality, and social development* (pp. 1–101). New York: Wiley.

Martin, C.L. & Ruble, D. (2004). Children's search for gender cues: Cognitive perspectives on gender development. *Current Directions in Psychological Science, 13*, 67–70.

Martin, C.L., Ruble, D.N. & Szkrybalo, J. (2002). Cognitive theories of early gender development. *Psychological Bulletin, 128*, 903–933.

Martin, C. L., Kornienko, O., Schaefer, D., Hanish, L. D., Fabes, R. A. & Goble, P. (2013). The role of peers and gender-typed activities in young children' peer affiliative networks: A longitudinal analysis of selection and influence. *Child Development,* 84, 921-937.

Maslow, A.H. (1968). *Toward a psychology of being* (2nd ed.). Princeton, NJ: Van Nostrand.

Maslow, A.H. (1970). *Motivation and personality* (rev. edn). New York: Harper & Row.

McAdams, D.P. & de St. Aubin, E. (1992). A theory of generativity and its assessment through self-report, behavioral acts, and narrative themes in autobiography. *Journal of Personality and Social Psychology, 62*, 1003–1015.

McGue, M., Elkins, I., Walden, B. & Iacono, W.G. (2005). Perceptions of the parent-adolescent relationship: A longitudinal investigation. *Developmental Psychology, 41*, 971–984.

McHale, S.M., Crouter, A.C. & Whiteman, S.D. (2003). The family contexts of gender development in childhood and adolescence. *Social Development, 12*, 125–148.

Mead, M. (1928). *Coming of age in Samoa.* New York: Morrow. Mead, M. (1939). *From the South Seas: Studies of adolescence and sex in primitive societies.* New York: Morrow.

Milburn, N.G., Rotheram-Borus, M.J., Rice, E., Mallett, S. & Rosenthal, D. (2006). Cross-national variations in behavioural profiles among homeless youth. *American Journal of Community Psychology, 37*(1–2), 63–76.

Miller, J.G., Bersoff, D.M. & Harwood, R.L. (1990). Perceptions of social responsibilities in India and in the United States: Moral imperatives or personal decisions? *Journal of Personality and Social Psychology, 58*, 33–47.

Miller, K.A., Fisher, P.A., Fetrow, B. & Jordan, K. (2006). Trouble on the journey home: Reunification failures in foster care. *Children and Youth Services Review, 28*, 260–274.

Morris, J.A., Jordan, C.L. & Breedlove, S.M. (2004). Sexual differentiation of the vertebrate nervous system. *Nature Neuroscience*, 7, 1034–1039.

Myrskylä, M. & Margolis, R. (2014). Happiness: before and after the kids. Demography, 51(5), 1843-1866.

Mulvey, K. L., & Killen, M. (2015). Challenging gender stereotypes: Resistance and exclusion. *Child Development, 86*, 681–694. doi:HYPERLINK "http://dx.doi.org/10.1111/cdev.12317" 10.1111/cdev.12317

Neilsen, M. A. (2015). *Same-sex marriage: Issues for the 44th Parliament.* Canberra, Australia: Parliament of Australia. ISSN: 2203-5249

Niccols, A. (2007). Fetal alcohol syndrome and the developing socio-emotional brain. *Brain and Cognition, 65*, 135–142.

NICHD National Institute of Child Health and Human Development, Early Child Care Research Network. (1997). The effects of infant child care on infant-mother attachment security: Results of the NICHD Study of Early Child Care. *Child Development, 68*, 860–879.

NICHD National Institute of Child Health and Human Development, Early Child Care Research Network. (2002). Early child care and children's development prior to school entry. Results from the NICHD Study of Early Child Care. *American Educational Research Journal, 39,* 133–164. doi:10.3102/00028312039001133

NICHD National Institute of Child Health and Human Development, Early Child Care Research Network. (2006). Infant-mother attachment classification: Risk and protection in relation to changing maternal caregiving quality. *Developmental Psychology, 42*, 38–58.

Orbuch, T.L., Veroff, J., Hassan, H. & Horrocks, J. (2002). Who will divorce: A 14-year longitudinal study of black couples and white couples. *Journal of Social and Personal Relationships, 19*, 179–202.

Parr, W.V. & Siegert, R. (1993). Adults' conceptions of everyday memory failures in others: Factors that mediate the effects of target age. *Psychology and Aging, 8*, 599–605.

Patterson, C.J. (2002). Lesbian and gay parenthood. In M. H. Bornstein (Ed.), *Handbook of parenting: Vol. 3. Being and becoming a parent* (2nd edn, pp. 317–338). Mahwah, NJ: Erlbaum.

Paus, T. (2005). Mapping brain maturation and cognitive development during adolescence. *Trends in Cognitive Sciences, 9*, 60–68.

Pederson, D.R. & Moran, G. (1996). Expressions of the attachment relationship outside of the strange situation. *Child Development, 67*, 915–927.

Pfeifer, M., Goldsmith, H.H., Davidson, R.J. & Rickman, M. (2002). Continuity and change in inhibited and uninhibited children. *Child Development, 73*, 1474–1485.

Piaget, J. (1929). *The child's conception of the world.* New York: Harcourt, Brace.

Piaget, J. (1954). *The construction of reality in the child.* New York: Basic Books.

Piaget, J. (1965). *The moral judgment of the child* (M. Gabain, Trans.). New York: Macmillan.

Piaget, J. (1977). *The development of thought: Equilibrium of cognitive structures.* New York: Viking Press.

Pitts, D.G. (1982). The effects of aging on selected visual functions: Dark adaptation, visual acuity, stereopsis, and brightness contrast. In R. Sekuler, D. Kline & K. Dismukes (Eds.), *Aging and human visual function* (pp. 131–159). New York: Liss.

Posada, R. & Wainryb, C. (2008). Moral development in a violent society: Columbian children's judgments in the context of survival and revenge. *Child Development, 79*, 882–898.

Prior, M., Smart, D., Sanson, A. & Oberklaid, F. (2000). Does shy-inhibited temperament in childhood lead to anxiety problems in adolescence? *Journal of the American Academy of Child and Adolescent Psychiatry, 39*(4), 461–468.

Rogoff, B. (1990). *Apprenticeship in thinking: Cognitive development in social context.* New York: Oxford University Press.

Rogoff, B. (2003). *The cultural nature of human development.* London: Oxford University Press.

Rogoff, B. & Chavajay, P. (1995). What's become of research on the cultural basis of cognitive development? *American Psychologist, 50*, 859–877.

Roisman, G.I., Clausell, E., Holland, A., Fortuna, K. & Elieff, C. (2008). Adult romantic relationships as contexts of human development: A multimethod comparison among same-sex couples with opposite-sex dating, engaged, and married dyads. *Developmental Psychology, 44*, 91–101.

Rose, A.J. & Rudolph, K.D. (2006). A review of sex-differences in peer relationship processes: Potential trade-offs for the emotional and behavioral development of girls and boys. *Psychological Bulletin, 132*, 98–131.

Rothbart, M.K. (2007). Temperament, development, and personality. *Current Directions in Psychological Science, 16*, 207–212.

Rural Health Education Foundation (RHEF) (2005, 30 September). *Growing Healthy Aboriginal Kids—The Early Years 1–5.* Television Broadcast on the Rural Health Education Foundation Satellite Network. Retrieved from <www.rhef.com.au/programs/509b/509b.html>.

Russell, A., Hart, C., Robinson, C. & Olsen, S. (2003). Children's sociable and aggressive behaviour with peers: A comparison of the US and Australia, and contributions of temperament and parenting styles. *International Journal of Behavioral Development, 27*(1), 74–86.

Ryff, C.D. (1989). In the eye of the beholder: Views of psychological well-being among middle-aged and older adults. *Psychology and Aging, 4*, 195–210.

Salihu, H.M. & Wilson, R.E. (2007). Epidemiology of prenatal smoking and perinatal outcomes. *Early Human Development, 83*, 713–720.

Salthouse, T.A. (1996). The processing-speed theory of adult age differences in cognition. *Psychological Review, 103*, 403–428.

Salthouse, T.A. (2006). Mental exercise and mental aging: Evaluating the validity of the 'use it or lose it' hypothesis. *Perspectives on Psychological Science, 1*, 68–87.

Savage, J., Brodosky, N.L., Malmud, E., Giannetta, J.M. & Hurt, H. (2005). Attentional Functioning and Impulse Control in Cocaine-Exposed and Control Children at Age Ten Years. *Journal of Developmental & Behavioural Pediatrics, 26*(1), 42–47.

Scaramella, L.V., Neppl, T. K., Ontai, L.L. & Conger, R.D. (2008). Consequences of socioeconomic disadvantage across three generations: Parenting behavior and child externalizing problems. *Journal of Family Psychology, 22*, 725–733.

Schaie, K.W. (2005). *Developmental influences on adult intelligence: The Seattle longitudinal study*. New York: Oxford University Press.

Schick, B., Marschark, M. & Spencer, P.E. (Eds.) (2006). *Advances in the sign language development of deaf children*. New York: Oxford University Press.

Scholnick, E.K., Nelson, K., Gelman, S.A. & Miller, P.H. (1999). *Conceptual development: Piaget's legacy*. Mahwah, NJ: Erlbaum.

Schweinhart, L.J. (2004). *The High/Scope Perry preschool study through age 40: Summary, conclusions, and frequently asked questions*. Retrieved from <www.highscope.org/Research/PerryProject/PerryAge40SumWeb.pdf>.

Serpell, R. (2000). Intelligence and culture. In R.J. Sternberg (Ed.), *Handbook of intelligence* (pp. 549–577). Cambridge, UK: Cambridge University Press.

Serpell, R. & Boykin, A.W. (1994). Cultural dimensions of cognition: A multiplex, dynamic system of constraints and possibilities. In R.J. Sternberg (Ed.), *Handbook of perception and cognition: Vol. 2. Thinking and problem solving* (pp. 369–408). Orlando, FL: Academic Press.

Sheppard, L.D. & Vernon, P.A. (2008). Intelligence and speed of information-processing: A review of 50 years of research. *Personality and Individual Differences, 44*, 535–551.

Shmueli-Goetz, Y., Target, M., Fonagy, P. & Datta, A. (2008). The child attachment interview: A psychometric study of reliability and discriminant validity. *Developmental Psychology, 44*, 939–956.

Shuwairi, S.M., Albert, M.K. & Johnson, S.P. (2007). Discrimination of possible and impossible objects in infancy. *Psychological Science, 18*, 303–307.

Silverman, A.B., Reinherz, H.Z. & Giaconia, R.M. (1996). The long-term sequelae of child and adolescent abuse: A longitudinal community study. *Child Abuse & Neglect, 20*, 709–723.

Singer, L.T., Arendt, R., Minnes, S., Farkas, K., Salvator, A., Kirchner, H.L. & Kliegman, R. (2002). Cognitive and motor outcomes of cocaine-exposed infants. *Journal of the American Medical Association, 287*, 1952–1960.

Singer, T., Verhaegen, P., Ghisletta, P., Lindenberger, U. & Baltes, P.B. (2003). The fate of cognition in very old age: Six-year longitudinal findings in the Berlin Aging Study (BASE). *Psychology & Aging, 18*, 318–331.

Sireteanu, R. (1999). Switching on the infant brain. *Science, 286*, 59–61.

Smetana, J.G., Campione-Barr, N. & Metzger, A. (2006). Adolescent development in interpersonal and societal contexts. *Annual Review of Psychology, 57*, 255–284.

Smith, J. & Baltes, P.B. (1990). Wisdom-related knowledge: Age/cohort differences in response to life-planning problems. *Developmental Psychology, 26*, 494–505.

Sommerville, J.A., Woodward, A.L. & Needham, A. (2005). Action experience alters 3-month-old infants' perception of others' actions. *Cognition, 96*, B1–B11.

Soska, K.C. & Johnson, S.P. (2008). Development of three-dimensional object completion in infancy. *Child Development, 79*, 1230–1236.

Spence, M.J. & DeCasper, A.J. (1987). Prenatal experience with low-frequency maternal-voice sounds influences neonatal perception of maternal voice samples. *Infant Behavior and Development, 10*, 133–142.

Spence, M.J. & Freeman, M.S. (1996). Newborn infants prefer the maternal low-pass filtered voice, but not the maternal whispered voice. *Infant Behavior and Development, 19*, 199–212.

Spitz, R.A. & Wolf, K. (1946). Anaclitic depression. *Psychoanalytic Study of Children, 2*, 313–342.

Springer, M.V., McIntosh, A., Wincour, G. & Grady, C.L. (2005). The relation between brain activity during memory tasks and years of education in young and older adults. *Neuropsychology, 19*, 181–192.

Steinberg, L. (2008). A social neuroscience perspective on adolescent risk-taking. *Developmental Review, 28*, 78–106.

Story, L.B. & Bradbury, T.N. (2004). Understanding marriage and stress: Essential questions and challenges. *Clinical Psychology Review, 23*, 1139–1162.

Suomi, S.J. (1999). Developmental trajectories, early experiences, and community consequences: Lessons from studies with rhesus monkeys. In D.P. Keating & C. Hertzman (Eds.), *Developmental health and the wealth of nations: Social, biological, and educational dynamics* (pp. 185–200). New York: Guilford Press.

Thomas, A. & Chess, S. (1977). *Temperament and development.* New York: Brunner/Mazel.

Tranter, L.J. & Koustaal, W. (2008). Age and flexible thinking: An experimental demonstration of the beneficial effects of increased cognitively stimulating activity on fluid intelligence in healthy older adults. *Aging, Neuropsychology, and Cognition, 15,* 184–207.

Trautner, H.M., Ruble, D.N., Cyphers, L., Kirsten, B., Behrendt, R. & Hartmann, P. (2005). Rigidity and flexibility of gender stereotypes in childhood: Developmental or differential? *Infant and Child Development, 14,* 365–381.

Twenge, J.M., Campbell, W.K. & Foster, C.A. (2003). Parenthood and marital satisfaction: A meta-analytic review. *Journal of Marriage and Family, 65,* 574–583.

United States Census Bureau (2008a). *2007 American community survey.* Retrieved from <www.census.gov/acs/www/index.html>.

United States Census Bureau (2008b). *Families and living arrangements: 2007.* Retrieved from <www.census.gov/population/www/socdemo/hh-fam.html>.

United States Department of Health and Human Services. (2005a). *Child maltreatment 2003.* Washington, DC: U.S. Government Printing Office. Retrieved from <www.acf.hhs.gov/programs/cb/pubs/cm03/index.htm>.

United States Department of Health and Human Services. (2005b). The AFCARS Report. Retrieved from <www.acf.hhs.gov/programs/cb/stats_research/afcars/tar/report13.htm>.

Urban, J., Carlson, E., Egeland, B. & Stroufe, L.A. (1991). Patterns of individual adaptation across childhood. *Development and Psychopathology, 3,* 445–460.

Vaillant, G.E. (1977). *Adaptation to life.* Boston: Little, Brown. Valkenburg, P.M., Schouten, A.P. & Peter, J. (2005). Adolescents' identity experiments on the internet. *New Media & Society,* 7, 383–402.

Van IJzendoorn, M.H. & Kroonenberg, P.M. (1988). Cross-cultural patterns of attachment: A meta-analysis of the Strange Situation. *Child Development, 59,* 147–156.

Van Zeijl, J., Mesman, J., Van IJzendoorn, M.H., Bakermans-Kranenburg, M.J., Juffer, F., Stolk, M.N., Koot, H.M. & Alink, L.R.A. (2006). Attachment-based intervention for enhancing sensitive discipline in mothers of 1- to 3-year-old children at risk for externalizing behavior problems: A randomized controlled trial. *Journal of Consulting and Clinical Psychology, 74,* 994–1005.

Wang, S., Baillargeon, R. & Brueckner, L. (2004). Young infants' reasoning about hidden objects: Evidence from violation-of-expectation tasks with test trials only. *Cognition, 93,* 167–198.

Ward, C.D. & Cooper, R.P. (1999). A lack of evidence in 4-month-old human infants for paternal voice preference. *Developmental Psychobiology, 35,* 49–59.

Weinfield, N.S., Ogawa, J.R. & Sroufe, L.A. (1997). Early attachment as a pathway to adolescent peer competence. *Journal of Research on Adolescence,* 7(24), 1–265.

Wellman, H.M. & Inagaki, K. (1997). *The emergence of core domains of thought.* San Francisco: Jossey-Bass.

Werker, J.F. & Tees, R.C. (1999). Influences on infant speech processing: Toward a new synthesis. *Annual Review of Psychology, 50,* 509–535.

White, L. & Edwards, J.N. (1990). Emptying the nest and parental well-being: An analysis of national panel data. *American Sociological Review, 55,* 235–242.

Wismer Fries, A.B., Ziegler, T.E., Kurian, J.R., Jacoris, S. & Pollak, S.D. (2005). Early experience in humans is associated with changes in neuropeptides critical for regulating social behavior. *Proceedings of the National Academy of Sciences, 102,* 17237–17240.

Witherington, D.C., Campos, J.J., Anderson, D.I., Lejeune, L. & Seah, E. (2005). Avoidance of heights on the visual cliff in newly walking infants. *Infancy,* 7, 285–298.

Wood, E., Desmarais, S. & Gugula, S. (2002). The impact of parenting experience of gender stereotyped toy play of children. *Sex Roles, 47,* 39–49.

Yeo, S.S. (2003). Bonding and attachment of Australian Aboriginal children. *Child Abuse Review, 12*(5), 292–304.

Zeanah, C.H., Smyke, A.T., Koga, S.F. & Carlson, E. (2005). Attachment in institutionalized and community children in Romania. *Child Development, 76,* 1015–1028.

Zelazo, P.D., Helwig, C.C. & Lau, A. (1996). Intention, act, and outcome in behavioral prediction and moral judgment. *Child Development, 67,* 2478–2492.

Zelinski, E.M., Gilewski, M.J. & Schaie, K.W. (1993). Individual differences in cross-sectional and 3-year longitudinal memory performance across the adult life span. *Psychology and Aging, 8,* 176–186.

Zosuls, K., Miller, C., Ruble, D., Martin, C. & Fabes, R. (2011). Gender development research in sex roles: Historical trends and future directions. *Sex Roles, 64*(11), 826–842. doi:10.1007/s11199-010-9902-3

Chapter 3

Anderson, J.R. (1987). Skill acquisition: Compilation of weak-method problem-solutions. *Psychological Review, 94*, 192–210.

Anderson, J.R. (1996). ACT: A simple theory of complex cognition. *American Psychologist, 51*, 355–365.

Anderson, V.L., Levinson, E.M., Barker, W. & Kiewra, K.R. (1999). The effects of meditation on teacher perceived occupational stress, state and trait anxiety, and burnout. *School Psychology Quarterly, 14*, 3–25.

Australian Institute of Health and Welfare. (2012). *Dementia in Australia* (cat. no. AGE 70). Canberra, Australia, Australian Institute of Health and Welfare. Retrieved from http://www.aihw.gov.au/WorkArea/DownloadAsset.aspx?id=10737422943

Baddeley, A.D. (1986). *Working memory.* New York: Oxford University Press.

Baddeley, A.D. (1992). Working memory. *Science, 255*, 556–559.

Baddeley, A.D. (1994). The magical number seven: Still magic after all these years? *Psychological Review, 101*, 353–356.

Baddeley, A.D. & Andrade, J. (2000). Working memory and the vividness of imagery. *Journal of Experimental Psychology: General, 129*, 126–145.

Ball, L. J., Shoker, J., & Miles, J. N. V. (2010). Odour-based context reinstatement effects with indirect measures of memory: The curious case of rosemary. *British Journal of Psychology,* 101, 655-678.

Bartlett, F.C. (1932). *Remembering: A study in experimental and social psychology.* Cambridge, UK: Cambridge University Press.

Becker, M.W., Pashler, H. & Anstis, S.M. (2000). The role of iconic memory in change-detection tasks. *Perception, 29*, 273–286.

Benjamin, A.S. (2005). Response speeding mediates the contributions of cue familiarity and target retrievability to metamnemonic judgments. *Psychonomic Bulletin & Review, 12*, 874–879.

Bergman, E.T. & Roediger, H.L., III. (1999). Can Bartlett's repeated reproduction experiments be replicated? *Memory & Cognition, 27*, 937–947.

Bohannon, J.N. III, Gratz, S. & Cross, V.S. (2007). The effects of affect and input source on flashbulb memories. *Applied Cognitive Psychology, 21*, 1023–1036.

Bond, C.F., Pitre, U., Van Leeuwen, M.D. (1991). Encoding operations and the next-in-line effect. *Personality and Social Psychology Bulletin.* 17(4), 435–441.

Bowers, J.S. & Marsolek, C.J. (Eds.). (2003). *Rethinking implicit memory.* London: Oxford University Press.

Braun, K.A., Ellis, R. & Loftus, E.F. (2002). Make my memory: How advertising can change our memories of the past. *Psychology & Marketing, 19*, 1–23.

Brown, R. & Kulik, J. (1977). Flashbulb memories. *Cognition, 5*, 73–99.

Buchner, A. & Wippich, W. (2000). On the reliability of implicit and explicit memory measures. *Cognitive Psychology, 40*, 227–259.

Burnett, R.C., Medin, D.L., Ross, N.O. & Blok, S.V. (2005). Ideal is typical. *Canadian Journal of Experimental Psychology, 59*, 3–10.

Carter, S.J. & Cassaday, H.J. (1998). State-dependent retrieval and chlorpheniramine. *Human Psychopharmacology, 13*, 513–523.

Chase, W.G. & Ericsson, K.A. (1981). Skilled memory. In J.R. Anderson (Ed.), *Cognitive skills and their acquisition.* Hillsdale, NJ: Erlbaum.

Conway, A.R., Kane, M.J., Bunting, M.F., Hambrick, D.Z., Wilhelm, O. & Engle, R.W. (2005). Working memory span tasks: A methodological review and user's guide. *Psychonomic Bulletin & Review, 12*, 769–786.

Cowan, N. (2001). The magical number 4 in short-term memory: A reconsideration of mental storage capacity. *Behavioral and Brain Sciences, 24*, 87–185.

Craik, F.I.M. & Lockhart, R.S. (1972). Levels of processing: A framework for memory research. *Journal of Verbal Learning and Verbal Behavior, 11*, 671–684.

Crowder, R.G. (1992). Eidetic imagery. In L.R. Squire (Ed.), *Encyclopedia of learning and memory* (pp. 154–156). New York: Macmillan.

Curci, A. & Luminet, O. (2006). Follow-up of a cross-national comparison on flashbulb and event memory for the September 11th attacks. *Memory, 14*, 329–344.

Daneman, M. & Carpenter, P.A. (1980). Individual differences in working memory and reading. *Journal of Verbal Learning and Verbal Behavior, 19*, 450–466.

Daselaar, S.M., Rice, H.J., Greenberg, D.L., Cabeza, R., LaBar, K.S. & Rubin, D.C. (2008). The spatial dynamics of autobiographical memory: Neural correlates of recall, emotional intensity, and reliving. *Cerebral Cortex, 18*, 217–229.

Ericsson, K.A. & Chase, W.G. (1982). Exceptional memory. *American Scientist, 70*, 607–615.

Esler, W.P. & Wolfe, M.S. (2001). A portrait of Alzheimer secretases—new features and familiar faces. *Science, 293*, 1449–1454.

Fuster, J. M. (2009). Cortex and memory: emergence of a new paradigm. *Journal of Cognitive Neuroscience, 21*(11), 2047-2072.

Gallace, A., Tan, H.Z., Haggard, P. & Spence, C. (2008). Short term memory for tactile stimuli. *Brain Research, 1190*, 132–142.

Gooden, D.R. & Baddeley, A.D. (1975). Context-dependent memory in two natural environments: On land and under water. *British Journal of Psychology, 66*, 325–331.

Habib, R., Nyberg, L. & Tulving, E. (2003). Hemispheric asymmetries of memory: the HERA model revisited. *TRENDS in Cognitive Sciences, 7*, 241–245.

Hamilton, M. & Rajaram, S. (2001). The concreteness effect in implicit and explicit memory tests. *Journal of Memory and Language, 44*, 96–117.

Hardy, J. & Selkoe, D.J. (2002). The amyloid hypothesis of Alzheimer's disease: Progress and problems on the road to therapeutics. *Science, 297*, 353–356.

Hart, J.T. (1965). Memory and the feeling-of-knowing experience. *Journal of Educational Psychology, 56*, 208–216.

Hasson, U., Furman, O., Clark, D., Dudai, Y. & Davachi, L. (2008). Enhanced intersubject correlations during movie viewing correlate with successful episodic encoding. *Neuron, 57*, 452–462.

Helmuth, L. (2002). Long-awaited technique spots Alzheimer's toxin. *Science, 297*, 752–753.

Holen, M.C. & Oaster, T.R. (1976). Serial position and isolation effects in a classroom lecture simulation. *Journal of Educational Psychology. 68*(3), 293–296.

Hope, L., Ost, J., Gabbert, F., Healey, S. & Lenton, E. (2008). 'With a little help from my friends . . .': The role of co-witness relationship in susceptibility to misinformation. *Acta Psychologia, 127*, 476–484.

Jahnke, J.C. (1965). Primacy and recency effects in serial-position curves of immediate recall. *Journal of Experimental Psychology, 70*, 130–132.

Jensen, A.R. (1962). Spelling errors and the serial position effect. *Journal of Educational Psychology, 53*, 105–109.

Kane, M.J., Brown, L.H., McVay, J.C., Silvia, P. J., Myin-Germeys, I. & Kwapil, T.R. (2007). For whom the mind wanders, and when: An experience-sampling study of working memory and executive control in daily life. *Psychological Science, 18*, 614–621.

Kearins, J. (1976) Skills of desert Aboriginal children. In G.E. Kearney & D.W. McElwain (Eds.), *Aboriginal cognition, retrospect and prospect.* Canberra: Australian Institute of Aboriginal Studies.

Kearins, J.M. (1981, July). Visual spatial memory in Australian Aboriginal children of desert regions. *Cognitive Psychology. 13*(3), 434–460.

Kelemen, W. L. & Creeley, C. E. (2003). State-dependent memory effects using caffeine and placebo do Not extend to metamemory. *The Journal of General Psychology, 130*(1), 70-86.

Klekamp, J., Riedel, A., Harper, C. & Kretschmann, H.J. (1989). Morphometric study on the growth of non-cortical brain regions in Australian Aborigines and Caucasians. *Brain Research, 485*, 79–88.

Klich, L.Z. & Davidson, G.R. (1983) A cultural difference in visual memory: On le voit, on ne le voit plus. *International Journal of Psychology. 18*(3–4), 189–201.

Koriat, A. & Fischoff, B. (1974). What day is today? An inquiry into the process of time orientation. *Memory & Cognition, 2*, 201–205.

Koriat, A. & Levy-Sadot, R. (2001). The combined contributions of cue-familiarity and accessibility heuristics to feelings of knowing. *Journal of Experimental Psychology: Learning, Memory, and Cognition, 27*, 34–53.

Lampinen, J.M., Copeland, S.M. & Neuschatz, J.S. (2001). Recollections of things schematic: Room schemas revisited. *Journal of Experimental Psychology: Learning, Memory, and Cognition, 27*, 1211–1222.

Lashley, K.S. (1929). *Brain mechanisms and intelligence.* Chicago: University of Chicago Press.

Lashley, K.S. (1950). In search of the engram. In *Physiological mechanisms in animal behavior: Symposium of the Society for Experimental Biology* (pp. 454–482). New York: Academic Press.

Lockhart, R.S. & Craik, F.I.M. (1990). Levels of processing: A retrospective commentary on a framework for memory research. *Canadian Journal of Psychology, 44*, 87–122.

Loftus, E.F. (1979). *Eyewitness testimony.* Cambridge, MA: Harvard University Press.

Loftus, E.F. (2005). Planting misinformation in the human mind: A 30-year investigation of the malleability of memory. *Learning & Memory, 12*, 361–366.

Loftus, E.F. & Palmer, J.C. (1974). Reconstruction of automobile destruction: An example of the interaction between language and memory. *Journal of Verbal Learning and Verbal Behavior, 13*, 585–589.

Loftus, E.F., Miller, D.G. & Burns, H.J. (1978). Semantic integration of verbal information into a visual memory. *Journal of Experimental Psychology: Human Learning and Memory, 4*, 19–31.

Marian, V. & Kaushanskaya, M. (2007). Language contexts guides memory content. *Psychonomic Bulletin & Review, 14*, 925–933.

Markowitsch, H.J. (2000). Neuroanatomy of memory. In E. Tulving & F.I.M. Craik (Eds.), *The Oxford handbook of memory* (pp. 465–484). Oxford, UK: Oxford University Press.

Marx, J. (2001). New leads on the 'how' of Alzheimer's. *Science, 293*, 2192–2194.

Metcalfe, J. (2000). Metamemory: Theory and data. In E. Tulving & F.I.M. Craik (Eds.), *The Oxford handbook of memory* (pp. 197–211). Oxford, UK: Oxford University Press.

Miller, G.A. (1956). The magic number seven plus or minus two: Some limits in our capacity for processing information. *Psychological Review, 63*, 81–97.

Mishra, J. & Backlin, W. (2007). The effects of altering environmental and instrumental context on the performance of memorized music. *Psychology of Music, 35*, 1–20.

Mitchell, K.J. & Johnson, M.K. (2000). Source monitoring: Attributing mental experiences. In E. Tulving & F.I.M. Craik (Eds.), *The Oxford handbook of memory* (pp. 179–195). London: Oxford University Press.

Modirrousta, M. & Fellows, L.K. (2008). Medial prefrontal cortex plays a critical and selective role in 'feeling of knowing' meta-memory judgments. *Neuropsychologia, 46*, 2958–2965.

Murphy, G.L. (2002). *The big book of concepts.* Cambridge, MA: MIT Press.

Murphy, K.J., Troyer, A.K., Levine, B. & Moscovitch, M. (2008). Episodic, but not semantic, autobiographical memory is reduced in amnestic mild cognitive impairment. *Neuropsychologia, 46*, 3116–3123.

National Institute on Aging. (2005). *Alzheimer's Disease fact sheet.* Retrieved from <www.nia.nih.gov/Alzheimers/Publications/adfact.htm>.

Neath, I. & Crowder, R.G. (1990). Schedules of presentation and temporal distinctiveness in human memory. *Journal of Experimental Psychology: Learning, Memory, and Cognition, 16*, 316–327.

Neath, I. & Surprenant, A.M. (2003). *Human memory: An introduction to research, data, and theory* (2nd edn). Belmont, CA: Wadsworth.

Neath, I., Brown, G.D.A., McCormack, T., Chater, N. & Freeman, R. (2006). Distinctiveness models of memory and absolute identification: Evidence for local, not global, effects. *Quarterly Journal of Experimental Psychology, 59*, 121–135.

Neisser, U. (1967). *Cognitive psychology.* New York: Appleton-Century-Crofts.

Nosofsky, R.M. & Stanton, R.D. (2005). Speeded classification in a probabilistic category structure: Contrasting exemplar-retrieval, decision-boundary, and prototype models. *Journal of Experimental Psychology: Human Perception and Performance, 31*, 608–629.

Nyberg, L. & Cabeza, R. (2000). Brain imaging of memory. In E. Tulving & F.I.M. Craik (Eds.), *The Oxford handbook of memory* (pp. 501–519). Oxford, UK: Oxford University Press.

O'Connor, M.G. & Lafleche, G. (2005). Amnesic syndromes. In P.J. Snyder, P.D. Nussbaun & D.L. Robins (Eds.), *Clinical neuropsychology: A pocket handbook for assessment* (2nd edn) (pp. 463–488). Washington, DC: American Psychology Association.

Ono, K. & Yamada, M. (2011). Low-n oligomers as therapeutic targets of Alzheimer's disease. *Journal of Neurochemistry, 117*, 19–28.

Paivio, A. (1995). Imagery and memory. In M.S. Gazzaniga (Ed.), *The cognitive neurosciences* (pp. 977–986). Cambridge, MA: MIT Press.

Parker, A., Ngu, H. & Cassaday, H.J. (2001). Odour and Proustian memory: Reduction of context-dependent forgetting and multiple forms of memory. *Applied Cognitive Psychology, 15*, 159–171.

Peterson, L.R. & Peterson, M.J. (1959). Short-term retention of individual verbal items. *Journal of Experimental Psychology, 58*, 193–198.

Radvansky, G.A. (2006). *Human memory.* Boston: Allyn & Bacon.

Rajaram, S. & Roediger, H.L., III (1993). Direct comparison of four implicit memory tests. *Journal of Experimental Psychology: Learning, Memory, and Cognition, 19*, 765–776.

Roediger, H.L. III, Gallo, D.A. & Geraci, L. (2002). Processing approaches to cognition: The impetus from the levels-of-processing framework. *Memory, 10*, 319–332.

Rolls, E.T. (2000). Memory systems in the brain. *Annual Review of Psychology, 51*, 599–630.

Rosch, E.H. (1973). Natural categories. *Cognitive Psychology, 4*, 328–350.

Rosch, E.H. (1978). Principles of categorization. In E. Rosch & B.B. Lloyd (Eds.), *Cognition and categorization* (pp. 27–48). Hillsdale, NJ: Erlbaum.

Rosch, E.H. & Mervis, C.B. (1975). Family resemblances: Studies in the internal structure of categories. *Cognitive Psychology, 7*, 573–605.

Rosch, E.H., Mervis, C.B., Gray, W.D., Johnson, D.M. & Boyes-Braem, P. (1976). Basic objects in natural categories. *Cognitive Psychology, 8*, 382–439.

Roth, J. K., Serences, J. T., & Courtney, S. M. (2006). Neural system for controlling the contents of object working memory in humans. *Cerebral Cortex, 16*(11), 1595-1603.

Rubin, D.C. & Kontis, T.C. (1983). A schema for common cents. *Memory & Cognition, 11*, 335–341.

Seamon, J.G., Philbin, M.M. & Harrison, L.G. (2006). Do you remember proposing marriage to the Pepsi machine? False recollections from a campus walk. *Psychonomic Bulletin & Review, 13*, 752–756.

Shiffrin, R.M. (2003). Modeling memory and perception. *Cognitive Science, 27*, 341–378.

Sloman, S.A., Hayman, C.A.G., Ohta, N., Law, J. & Tulving, E. (1988). Forgetting in primed fragment completion. *Journal of Experimental Psychology: Learning, Memory, and Cognition, 14*, 223–239.

Sperling, G. (1960). The information available in brief visual presentations. *Psychological Monographs, 74*, 1–29.

Sperling, G. (1963). A model for visual memory tasks. *Human Factors, 5*, 19–31.

Talarico, J.M. & Rubin, D.C. (2003). Confidence, not consistency, characterizes flashbulb memories. *Psychological Science, 14*, 455–461.

Talarico, J.M. & Rubin, D.C. (2007). Flashbulb memories are special after all; in phenomenology, not accuracy. *Applied Cognitive Psychology, 21*, 527–578.

Tijus, C.A. & Reeves, A. (2004). Rapid iconic erasure without masking. *Spatial Vision, 17*, 483–495.

Travis, J. (2005). Saving the mind faces high hurdles. *Science, 309*, 731–734.

Tulving, E. (1972). Episodic and semantic memory. In E. Tulving & W. Donaldson (Eds.), *Organization of memory*. New York: Academic Press.

Tulving, E. & Thomson, D.M. (1973). Encoding specificity and retrieval processes in episodic memory. *Psychological Review, 80*, 352–373.

Underwood, B.J. (1948). Retroactive and proactive inhibition after five and forty-eight hours. *Journal of Experimental Psychology, 38*, 28–38.

Underwood, B.J. (1949). Proactive inhibition as a function of time and degree of prior learning. *Journal of Experimental Psychology, 39*, 24–34.

Verfaelli, M., Martin, E., Page, K., Parks, E. & Keane, M.M. (2006). Implicit memory for novel conceptual associations in amnesia. *Cognitive, Affective, and Behavioral Neuroscience, 6*, 91–101.

Voorspoels, W., Vanpaemel, W. & Storms, G. (2008). Exemplars and prototypes in natural language concepts: A typicality-based evaluation. *Psychonomic Bulletin & Review, 15*, 630–637.

Weissenborn, R. & Duka, T. (2000). State-dependent effects of alcohol on explicit memory: The role of semantic associations. *Psychopharmacology, 149*, 98–106.

Wells, G.L. & Loftus, E.F. (2003). Eyewitness memory for people and events. In A.M. Goldstein (Ed.), *Handbook of psychology: Forensic psychology* (Vol. 11, pp. 149–160). New York: Wiley.

Chapter 4

Amabile, T.M. (1983). *The social psychology of creativity*. New York: Springer-Verlag.

American Association on Mental Retardation. (1992). *Mental retardation: Definition, classification, and systems of supports* (9th edn). Washington, DC: American Association on Mental Retardation.

American Association on Mental Retardation. (2002). *Mental retardation: Definition, classification, and systems of supports* (10th edn). Washington, DC: American Association on Mental Retardation.

Anderson, N. and Shackleton, V. (1993). *Successful selection interviewing*. Blackwell: Oxford.

Austin, E. J., Farrelly, D., Black, C. and Moore, H. (2007). Emotional intelligence, Machiavellianism and emotional manipulation: Does EI have a dark side? *Personality and Individual Differences, 43*, 179–189.

Baghurst, P. A., McMichael, A. J., Wigg, N. R. *et al.* (1992). Environmental exposure to lead and children's intelligence at the age of seven years: The Port Pirie cohort study. *New England Journal of Medicine, 327*, 1279–1284.

Bailey, B. N., Delaney-Black, V., Covington, C. Y. *et al.* (2004). Prenatal exposure to binge drinking and cognitive and behavioral outcomes at age 7 years. *American Journal of Obstetrics and Gynecology, 191*, 1037–1043.

Baker, L. D. and Daniels, D. (1990). Nonshared environmental influences and personality differences in adult twins. *Journal of Personality and Social Psychology, 58*, 103–110.

Banks, W.C. (1990). *In Discovering Psychology, Program 16* [PBS video series]. Washington, DC: Annenberg/CPB Program.

Bar-On, R. (1997). *The Emotional Quotient Inventory (EQ-i): A test of emotional intelligence*. Toronto, Canada: Multi-Health Systems, Inc. Bar-On, R. (2005). The Bar-On model of emotional-social intelligence.

In P. Fernández-Berrocal and N. Extremera (guest eds), Special Issue on Emotional Intelligence. *Psicothema, 17.*

Barrick, M. R. and Mount, M. K. (1991). The big Five personality dimensions and job performance: A meta-analysis. *Personnel Psychology, 44*, 1–26.

Batty G.D., Wennerstad K.M., Davey Smith G. *et al.* (2009). IQ in late adolescence/early adulthood and mortality by middle age: cohort study of one million Swedish men. *Epidemiology, 20*, 100–9.

Batty, G. D., Deary, I. J. and Gottfredson, L. S. (2007). Premorbid (early life) IQ and later mortality risk: Systematic review. *Annals of Epidemiology, 17*, 278–288.

Beiser, M. & Gotowiec, A. (2000). Accounting for native/non-native differences in IQ scores. *Psychology in the Schools, 37*, 237–252.

Belmont, L. and Marolla, F. A. (1973). Birth order, family size, and intelligence. *Science, 182*, 1096–1101.

Bennett, D.S., Bendersky, M. & Lewis, M. (2008). Children's cognitive ability from 4 to 9 years old as a function of prenatal cocaine exposure, environmental risk, and maternal verbal intelligence. *Developmental Psychology, 44*, 919–928.

Benson, E. (2003). Intelligent intelligence testing. *APA Monitor on Psychology, 34.*

Benton, D. and Roberts, G. (1988). Effect of vitamin and mineral supplementation on intelligence of a sample of schoolchildren. *Lancet, i*, 140–144.

Bertua, C., Anderson, N. and Salgado, J. F. (2005). The predictive validity of cognitive ability tests: A UK meta-analysis. *Journal of Occupational and Organizational Psychology, 78*, 387–409.

Binet, A. (1916). New methods for the diagnosis of the intellectual level of subnormals. In E. S. Kite (trans.), *The development of intelligence in children.* Vineland, NJ: Publications of the Training School at Vineland. (Originally published 1905 in *L'Année Psychologique, 12*, 191–244.)

Binet, A. and Simon, T. (1911). *La mesure du développement de l'intelligence chez les jeunes enfants.* Paris: A. Coneslant.

Binet, A. and Simon, T. (1916). *The development of intelligence in children.* Baltimore, MD: Williams & Wilkins. (Reprinted 1973, New York: Arno Press; reprinted 1983, Salem, NH: Ayer.) The 1973 volume includes reprints of many of Binet's articles on testing.

Blake, J. (1981). Family size and the quality of children. *Demography, 18*, 421–442.

Bouchard, T. J. (1993). The genetic architecture of intelligence. In P. A. Vernon (ed.), *Biological approaches to the study of human intelligence.* Norwood, NJ: Ablex.

Bouchard, T. J. (1994). Genes, environment, and personality. *Science, 264*, 1700–1701.

Bouchard, T. J. and McGue, M. (1981). Family studies of intelligence: A review. *Science, 212*, 1055–1059.

Bouchard, T. J. and Segal, N. L. (1985). Environment and IQ. In B. B. Wolman (ed.), *Handbook of intelligence: Theories, measurements, and applications* (pp. 391–464). New York: Wiley.

Bouchard, T. J. Jr and Loehlin, J. C. (2001). Genes, personality, and evolution. *Behavioural Genetics, 31*, 243–273.

Bowden, E.M. & Beeman, M.J. (2003). Normative data for 144 compound remote associates problem. *Behavior Research Methods, Instruments, and Computers, 35*, 634–639.

Boyatzis, R. E. (1994). Stimulating self-directed learning through the Managerial Assessment and Development Course. *Journal of Management Education, 18*, 304–323.

Boyatzis, R. E. and Van Oosten, E. (2002). Developing emotionally intelligent organizations. In R. Millar (ed.), *International executive development programmes* (7th edn). London: Kogan Page.

Boyatzis, R. E., Cowen, S. S. and Kolb, D. A. (1995). *Innovations in professional education: Steps on a journey from teaching to learning.* San Francisco: Jossey-Bass.

Bratko, D., Chamorro-Premuzic, T. and Saks, Z. (2006). Personality and school performance: Incremental validity of self- and peer ratings over intelligence. *Personality and Individual Differences, 41*, 131–142.

Braungart, J. M., Plomin, R., DeFries, J. C. and Fulker, D. W. (1992a). Genetic influence on tester-rated infant temperament as assessed by Bayley's Infant Behavior Record: Nonadoptive and adoptive siblings and twins. *Developmental Psychology, 28*, 40–47.

Broman, S.H., Nichols, P.I. & Kennedy, W.A. (1975). *Preschool IQ: Prenatal and early developmental correlates.* Hillsdale, NJ: Erlbaum.

Cahan, S. and Cohen, N. (1989). Age versus schooling effects on intelligence development. *Child Development, 60*, 1239–1249.

Calvin, C. M., Batty, G. D. and Deary, I. J. (2011). Cognitive epidemiology: Concepts, evidence and future directions. In T. Chamorro-Premuzic, S. von Stumm and A. A, Furnham, Th*e Wiley-Blackwell handboook of individual differences.* Chichester: Wiley/Blackwell.

Cannon, W. B. (1929). *Bodily changes in pain, hunger, fear and rage: An account of recent research into the function of emotional excitement* (2nd edn). New York: Appleton-Century-Cross.

Carroll, J. B. (1982). The measurement of intelligence. In R. J. Sternberg (ed.), *Handbook of human intelligence* (pp. 29–120). Cambridge: Cambridge University Press.

Carroll, J. B. (1992). Cognitive abilities: The state of the art. *Psychological Science, 3*, 266–270.

Carroll, J. B. (1993). *Human cognitive abilities: A survey of factoranalytic studies*. New York: Press Syndicate of the University of Cambridge.

Carroll, J. B. (1997a). Psychometrics, intelligence, and public perception. *Intelligence, 24*, 25–52.

Carroll, J. B. (1997b). Three three-stratum theory of cognitivenabilities. In D. P. Flanagan, J. L. Gensha_ and P. L. Harrison (eds), *Contemporary intellectual assessment: Theories, tests, and issues* (pp. 122–130). New York: Guilford.

Cattell, R. B. (1950). *Personality: A systematic, theoretical, and factual study*. New York: McGraw-Hill.

Cattell, R. B. (1957). *Personality and motivation: Structure and measurement*. New York: Harcourt, Brace & World.

Cattell, R. B. (1965). *The scientific analysis of personality*. Baltimore, MD: Penguin.

Cattell, R. B. (1971). *Abilities, their structure, growth, and action*. New York: Houghton Mifflin.

Cattell, R. B. (1973). *Personality and mood by questionnaire*. New York: Jossey-Bass.

Cattell, R. B. (1979). *Personality and learning theory* (Vol. 1: *A systems theory of maturation and structured learning*). New York: Springer.

Cattell, R. B. (1980). *Personality and learning theory* (Vol. 2: *A systems theory of maturation and structured learning*). New York: Springer.

Cattell, R. B. (1982). *The inheritance of personality and ability*. New York: Academic Press.

Cattell, R. B. and Child, D. (1975). *Motivation and dynamic structure*. New York: Wiley.

Cattell, R. B. and Kline, P. (1977). *The scientific analysis of personality and motivation*. New York: Academic Press.

Cattell, R. B., Eber, H. W. and Tatsuoka, M. M. (1970). *Handbook for the Sixteen-Personality Factor questionnaire*. Champaign, IL: Institute for Personality and Ability Testing.

Ceci, S. J. (1990). *On intelligence . . . more or less*. Englewood Cli_s, NJ: Prentice Hall.

Ceci, S. J. (1991). How much does schooling influence general intelligence and its cognitive components? A reassessment of the evidence. *Developmental Psychology, 24*, 703–722.

Ceci, S.J. (1999). Schooling and intelligence. In S.J. Ceci & W.M. Williams (Eds.), *The nature-nurture debate: The essential readings* (pp. 168–175). Oxford, UK: Blackwell.

Chamoro-Premuzic, T., Bennett, E. and Furnham, A. (2007). Th happy personality: Mediational role of trait emotional intelligence. *Personality and Individual Differences, 42*, 1633–1639.

Chamorro-Premuzic, T., Harlaar, N., Greven, C. U. and Plomin, R. (2010). More than just IQ: A longitudinal examination of selfperceived abilities as predictors of academic performance in a large sample of UK twins. *Intelligence, 38*, 385–392.

Chapman, P.D. (1988). *Schools as sorters: Lewis M. Terman, applied psychology, and the intelligence testing movement, 1890–1930*. New York: New York University Press.

Charbonneau, D. and Nicol, A. A. M. (2002). Emotional intelligence and leadership in adolescents. *Personality and Individual Differences, 33*, 1101–1113.

Chipeur, H., Rovine, M. and Plomin, R. (1990). LISREL modelling: Genetic and environmental influences on IQ revisited. *Intelligence, 14*, 11–29.

Clark, B. (1992). *Growing up gifted*, 5th edn. New Jersey: Prentice Hall.

Costa, P. T. Jr and McCrae, R. R. (1980). Influence of extraversion and neuroticism on subjective well-being: happy and unhappy people. *Journal of Personality and Social Psychology, 38*, 668–678.

Costa, P. T. Jr and McCrae, R. R. (1985). *The NEO Personality Inventory manual*. Odessa, FL: Psychological Assessment Resources.

Costa, P. T. Jr and McCrae, R. R. (1989). Personality continuity and the changes in adult life. In M. Storandt and G. R. Vanden Bos (eds), *The adult years: Continuity and change* (pp. 45–77). Washington, DC: American Psychological Association.

Costa, P. T. Jr and McCrae, R. R. (1992). *Revised NEO Personality Inventory (NEO-PI-R) and NEO Five-Factor Inventory (NEOFFI) professional manual*. Odessa, FL: Psychological Assessment Resources.

Costa, P. T. Jr and McCrae, R. R. (1997). Stability and change in personality assessment: The revised NEO Personality Inventory in the year 2000. *Journal of Personality and Assessment, 68*, 86–94.

Cote, S. and Miners, C. T. H. (2006). Emotional intelligence, cognitive intelligence and job performance. *Administrative Science Quarterly, 51*, 1–28.

Davis O. S., Haworth, C. M. and Plomin, R. (2009). Dramatic increase in heritability of cognitive development from early to middle childhood: an 8-year longitudinal study of 8700 pairs of twins. *Psychological Science, 20*, 1301–1308.

Day, A. L. and Carroll, S. A. (2004). Using an ability-based measure of emotional intelligence to predict individual performance, group performance, and group citizenship behaviours. *Personality and Individual Differences, 36*, 1443–1458.

De Corte, W., Lievens, F. & Sackett, P.R. (2007). Combining predictors to achieve optimal trade-offs between selection quality and adverse impact. *Journal of Applied Psychology, 92*, 1380–1393.

Deary, I. J, Yang, J., Davies, G. *et al.* (2012). Genetic contributions to stability and change in intelligence from childhood to old age. *Nature, 482*, 212–215.

Deary, I. J. (2012). Intelligence. *Annual Review of Psychology, 63*, 453–482.Deary I. J. and Der G. (2005). Reaction time explains IQ's association with death. *Psychological Science, 16*, 64–69.

Deary, I. J., Strand, S., Smith, P. and Fernandes, C. (2007). Intelligence and educational achievement. *Intelligence, 35*, 13–21.

Deary, I. J., Thorpe, G., Wilson, V., Starr, J. M. and Whalley, L. J. (2003). Population sex differences in IQ at age 11: the Scottish mental survey 1932. *Intelligence, 31*, 533–542.

Deary, I. J., Whalley, L. J., Lemmon, H., Crawford, H. and Starr, J. M. (2000). The stability of individual differences in mental ability from childhood to old age: Follow-up of the 1932 Scottish Mental Survey. *Intelligence, 28*, 49–55.

Deary, I. J., Whiteman, M. C., Starr, J. M., Whalley, L. J. and Fox, H. C. (2004). The impact of childhood intelligence on later life: Following up the Scottish Mental Surveys of 1932 and 1947. *Journal of Personality and Social Psychology, 86*, 130–147.

Deaux, K., Bikmen, N., Gilkes, A., Ventuneac, A., Joseph, Y., Payne, Y.A. & Steele, C.A. (2007). Becoming American: Stereotype threat effects in Afro-Caribbean immigrant groups. *Social Psychology Quarterly, 70*, 384–404.

Department of Immigration and Citizenship. (2009). Fact sheet 8: Abolition of the 'White Australia' policy. Canberra: Commonwealth of Australia. Retrieved from <www.immi.gov.au/media/fact-sheets/08abolition.htm>.

Devlin, B., Daniels, M. and Roeder, K. (1997). Heritability of IQ. *Nature, 388*, 468–471.

Dickens, W.T. & Flynn, J.R. (2006). Black Americans reduce the racial IQ gap: Evidence from standardization samples. *Psychological Science, 17*, 913–920.

Dollinger, S. J. and Orf, L. A. (1991). Personality and performance in 'personality': Conscientiousness and openness. *Journal of Research in Personality, 25*, 276–284.

Downey, D. B. (2001). Number of siblings and intellectual development: The resource dilution explanation. *American Psychologist, 56*, 497–504.

Downey, G., Feldman, S. and Ayduk, O. (2000). Rejection sensitivity and male violence in romantic relationships. *Personal Relationships, 7*, 45–61.

Downey, L. A., Mountstephen, J., Lloyd, J., Hansen, K. and Stough, C. (2008). Emotional intelligence and scholastic achievement in Australian adolescents. *Australian Journal of Psychology, 60*, 10–17.

Drinkwater, B.A. (1976). Verbal thinking and learning skills of Australian Aboriginal children. *Topics in Culture Learning, 4*, 10–12.

Dumitrashku, T. A. (1996). Family structure and children's cognitive development. *Voprosy Psikhologii, 2*, 104–111.

Emmerling, R. J. and Goleman, D. (2003). *Emotional intelligence: Issues and common misunderstandings*. Consortium for Research on Emotional Intelligence in Organizations. Available online at www.eiconsortium.org/research/ei_issues_and_common_misunderstandings_caruso_comment.htm; accessed 27 December 2005.

Evans, M. & Farley, A. (1998). Institutional characteristics and the relationship between students' first year university and final year secondary school academic performance. Working Paper, 18, Department of Econometrics and Business Statistics, Monash University, p. 3.

Eysenck, H. J. (1990b). Genetic and environmental contributions to individual differences: The three major dimensions of personality. *Journal of Personality, 58*, 245–261.

Fletcher, R. (1991). *Science, ideology and the media: Cyril Burt scandal.* New Brunswick, NJ: Transaction Books.

Furnham, A. (1985). Just world beliefs in an unjust society: A cross-cultural comparison. *European Journal of Social Psychology, 15*, 363–366.

Furnham, A. (2000). Parents' estimations of their own and children's multiple intelligences. *British Journal of Developmental Psychology, 18*, 583–594.

Furnham, A. (2001). Self-estimates of intelligence: Culture and gender difference in self and other estimates of both general (g) and multiple intelligences. *Personality and Individual Differences, 31*, 1381–1405.

Furnham, A. and Bunclark, K. (2006). Sex differences in parents' estimations of their own and their children's intelligence. *Intelligence, 34*, 1–14.

Furnham, A. and Heaven, P. (1999). *Personality and social behaviour.* New York: Oxford University Press.

Furnham, A. and Petrides, K. V. (2004) Parental estimates of five types of intelligence. *Australian Journal of Psychology, 56*, 1017.

Furnham, A. and Proctor, E. (1989). Belief in a just world: Review and critique of the individual difference literature. *British Journal of Social Psychology, 28*, 365–384.

Furnham, A., Chamorro-Premuzic, T. and McDougall, F. (2003). Personality, cognitive ability, and beliefs about intelligence as predictors of academic performance. *Learning and Individual Differences, 14*, 49–66.

Furnham, A., Hosoe, T. and Tang, T. (2002). Male hubris and female humility? A cross-cultural study of ratings of self, parental and sibling multiple intelligence in America, Britain and Japan. *Intelligence, 30*, 101–115.

Galton, F. (1865). Hereditary talent and character. *Macmillan's Magazine, 12*, 157–166, 318–327.

Galton, F. (1869). *Hereditary genius: An inquiry into its laws and consequences.* London: Macmillan.

Galton, F. (1874). *English men of science: their nature and nurture.* New York: Appleton.

Galton, F. (1875). The history of twins, as a criterion of the relative powers of nature and nurture. *Fraser's Magazine, 92*, 566–576

Galton, F. (1884). Measurement of character. *Fortnightly Review, 36*, 179–185.

Gardner, H. (1993). *Multiple intelligences: The theory in practice.* New York: Basic Books.

Gardner, H. (1995). Cracking open the IQ box. *The American Prospect, 20*, 71–80.

Gassió, R., Artuch, R., Vilaseca, M.A., Fusté, E., Boix, C., Sans, A. & Campistol, J. (2005). Cognitive functions in classic phenylketonuria and mild hyperphenylalaninaemia: Experience in a paediatric population. *Developmental Medicine & Child Neurology, 47*, 443–448.

Goleman, D. and Boyatzis, R. (2005). *Emotional Competence Inventory (ECI).* Boston: Hay Resources Direct.

Goleman, D. P. (1995). *Emotional intelligence: Why it can matter more than IQ for character, health and lifelong achievement.* New York: Bantam.

Goleman, D. P. (1998). *Working with emotional intelligence.* London: Bloomsbury.

Goleman, D. P. (2001). An EI-based theory of performance. In C. Cherniss and D. Goleman, (eds), *The emotionally intelligent workplace* (pp. 27–44). New York: Jossey-Bass.

Goleman, D., Boyatzis, R. E. and McKee, A. (2002). *Primal leadership: Realizing the power of emotional intelligence.* Boston: Harvard Business School Press.

Grigorenko, E.L. (2000). Heritability and intelligence. In R.J. Sternberg (Ed.), *Handbook of intelligence* (pp. 53–91). Cambridge, UK: Cambridge University Press.

Grigorenko, E.L., Meier, E., Kipka, J., Mohatt, G., Yanez, E. & Sternberg, R.J. (2004). Academic and practical intelligence: A case study of the Yup'ik in Alaska. *Learning and Individual Differences, 14*, 183–207.

Guilford, J. P. (1950). Creativity. *American Psychologist, 5*, 444–454.

Guilford, J. P. (1959). Three faces of intellect. *American Psychologist, 14*, 469–479.

Guilford, J. P. (1967). *The nature of human intelligence.* New York: McGraw-Hill.

Guilford, J. P. (1977). *Way beyond the IQ: Guide to improving intelligence and creativity.* Buffalo, NY: Creative Education Foundation.

Guilford, J. P. (1982). Cognitive psychology's ambiguities: Some suggested remedies. *Psychological Review, 89*, 48–59.

Guilford, J. P. and Hoepfner, R. (1967, 1971). *The nature of human intelligence.* New York: McGraw-Hill.

Guilford, J. P. and Hoepfner, R. (1971). *The analysis of intelligence.* New York: McGraw-Hill.

Haier, R.J., Jung, R.E., Yeo, R.A., Head, K. & Alkire, M.T. (2004). Structural variation and general intelligence. *NeuroImage, 23*, 425–433.

Harris, J. R. (1995). Where is the child's environment? A group socialization theory of development. *Psychological Review, 102*, 458–489.

Hauser, R. M. (2007). Will practitioners benefit from metaanalysis? *Academy of Management Perspectives, 21*, 24–28.

Hauser, R. M. (2010). Causes and consequences of cognitive functioning across the life course. *Educational Researcher, 39*, 95–109.

Helms, J.E. (2006). Fairness is not validity or cultural bias in racial-group assessment: A quantitative perspective. *American Psychologist, 61*, 845–859.

Hernnstein, R.J. & Murray, C. (1994). *The bell curve.* New York: The Free Press.

Hoekstra, R.A., Bartels, M. & Boomsma, D.I. (2007). Longitudinal genetic study of verbal and nonverbal IQ from early childhood to young adulthood. *Learning and Individual Differences, 17*, 97–114.

Holahan, C.K. & Sears, R.R. (1995). The gifted group in later maturity. Stanford, CA: Stanford University Press.

Horn, J. L. (1965). A rationale and test for the number of factors in factor analysis. *Psychometrika, 30*, 179–185.

Horn, J. L. and Cattell, R. B. (1967). Age differences in fluid and crystallized intelligence. *Acta Psychologica, 26*, 107–129.

Hough, L. M. (1992). The 'Big Five' personality variables–construct confusion: Descriptive versus predictive. *Human Performance, 5*, 139–155.

Hough, L. M. (1997). The millennium for personality psychology: New horizons or good old daze. *Applied Psychology International Review, 47*, 233–261.

Hough, L. M. (1998). Personality at work: Issues and evidence. In M. Hakel (ed.), *Beyond multiple choice: Evaluating alternatives and traditional testing for selection* (pp. 131–159). Hillsdale, NJ: Erlbaum.

Hough, L. M. and Oswald, F. L. (2000). Personal selection: Looking toward the future – remembering the past. *Annual Review of Psychology, 51*, 631–664.

Huizink, A.C. & Mulder, E.J.H. (2006). Maternal smoking, drinking or cannabis use during pregnancy and neurobehavioral and cognitive functioning in human offspring. *Neuroscience and Biobehavioral Reviews, 30*, 24–41.

Hunt, E. & Carlson, J. (2007). Considerations relating to the study of group differences in intelligence. *Perspectives on Psychological Science, 2*, 194–213.

Hunter, J. E. and Hunter, R. F. (1984). Validity and utility of alternative predictors of job performance. *Psychological Bulletin, 96*, 72–98.

Jacobson, S. W., Jacobson, J. L., Sokol, R. J., Chiodo, L. M. and Corobana, R. (2004). Maternal age, alcohol abuse history, and quality of parenting as moderators of the e_ects of prenatal alcohol exposure on 7.5-year intellectual function. *Alcoholism: Clinical and Experimental Research, 28*, 1732–1745.

Jarvis, P. (1995). *Adult and continuing education: Theory and practice* (2nd edn). London: Routledge.

Jones, H. E. and Bayley, N. (1941). The Berkeley Growth Study. *Child Development, 12*, 167–173.

Joynson, R. B. (1989). *The Burt affair.* New York: Routledge.

Kamin, L. J. and Goldberger, A. S. (2002). Twin studies in behavioural research: A skeptical view. *Theoretical Population Biology, 61*, 83–95.

Kantrowitz, B. & McGinn, D. (2000, 19 June). When teachers are cheaters. *Newsweek*, pp. 48–49.

Kassebaum, N.L. (1994). Head Start: Only the best for America's children. *American Psychologist, 49*, 1123–1126.

Kaufman, A. S. (1984). K-ABC and giftedness. *Roeper Review, 7*, 83–88.

Kaufman, A. S. (1990). *Assessing adolescent and adult intelligence.* Boston: Allyn & Bacon.

Kaufman, A. S. and Kaufman, N. L. (2001). *Specific learning disabilities and difficulties in children and adolescents: Psychological assessment and evaluation.* Cambridge: Cambridge University Press.

Kaufman, A. S. and Lichtenberger, E. O. (2005). *Assessing adolescent and adult intelligence* (3rd edn). Boston: Allyn & Bacon.

Kodituwakku, P. W., Handmaker, N. S., Cutler, S. K., Weathersby, E. K. and Handmaker, S. D. (1995). Specific impairments in self-regulation in children exposed to alcohol prenatally. *Alcoholism: Clinical and Experimental Research, 19*, 1558–1564.

Kolb, D. A. (1981). *The learning style inventory.* Boston: McBer.

Kolb, D. A. (1984). *Experiential learning: Experience as the source of learning and development.* Englewood Cliffs, NJ: Prentice Hall.

Kolb, D. A. and Fry, R. (1975). Toward an applied theory of experiential learning. In C. Cooper (ed.), *Theories of group process.* London: Wiley.

Landy, F. J. (2005). Some historical and scientific issues related to research on emotional intelligence. *Journal of Organizational Behavior, 26*, 411–424.

Lecci, L. & Myers, B. (2008). Individual differences in attitudes relevant to juror decision making: Development and validation of the Pretrial Juror Attitude Questionnaire (PJAQ). *Journal of Applied Social Psychology, 38*, 2010–2038.

Lennon, R.T. (1985). Group tests of intelligence. In B.B. Wolman (Ed.), *Handbook of intelligence* (pp. 825–847). New York: Wiley.

Leung, A.K.-Y., Maddux, W.W., Galinsky, A.D. & Chiu, C.-Y. (2008). Multicultural experience enhances creativity: The when and how. *American Psychologist, 63*, 169–181.

Locurta, C. (1991). *Sense and nonsense about IQ: The case for uniqueness.* New York: Praeger.

Loehlin, J. C. (1989). Partitioning environmental and genetic contributions to behavioral development. *American Psychologist, 44,* 1285–1292.

Loehlin, J. C. (1992). *Genes and environment in personality development.* Newberry Park, CA: Sage. Loehlin, J. C. and Martin, N. G. (2001). Age changes in personality traits and their heritabilities during the adult years: Evidence from Australian Twin Registry samples. *Personality and Individual Differences, 30,* 1147–1160.

Loehlin, J. C., Willerman, L. and Horn, J. M. (1985). Personality resemblances in adoptive families when the children are late-adolescent or adult. *Journal of Personality and Social Psychology, 48,* 376–392.

Maccoby, E. E. (2000). Parenting and its effects on children: On reading and misreading behavior genetics. *Annual Review of Psychology, 51,* 1–27.

Maccoby, E. E. and Jacklin, C. N. (1974). *_e psychology of sex differences.* Stanford, CA: Stanford University Press.

Mackintosh, N. J. (1998). *IQ and human intelligence.* Oxford: Oxford University Press.

Mackintosh, N. J. (2000). *IQ and human intelligence.* Oxford: Oxford University Press.

Mascie-Taylor, C. G. N. (1984). Biosocial correlates of IQ. In C. J. Turner and H. B. Miles (eds), *The biology of human intelligence.* London: Proceedings of the 20th Annual Symposium of the Eugenics Society.

Matthews, G., Zeidner, M. and Roberts, R. D. (2004). *Emotional intelligence: Science and myth.* London: MIT Press.

Mattson, S. N. and Riley, E. P. (1998). A review of the neurobehavioral deficits in children with fetal alcohol syndrome or prenatal exposure to alcohol. *Alcoholism: Clinical and Experimental Research, 22,* 279–294.

Mattson, S. N., Riley, E. P., Delis, D. C., Stern, C. and Jones, K. L. (1996). Verbal learning and memory in children with fetal alcohol syndrome. *Alcoholism: Clinical and Experimental Research, 20,* 810–816.

Mayer, J. D. (1995). A framework of the classification of personality components. *Journal of Personality, 63,* 819–877.

Mayer, J. D. (1998). A systems framework for the field of personality psychology. *Psychological Inquiry, 9,* 118–144.

Mayer, J. D. (2005a). A tale of two visions: Can a new view of personality help integrate psychology? *American Psychologist, 60,* 294–307.

Mayer, J. D. (2005b). *Personality psychology: A systems approach* (3rd edn). Boston: Pearson Custom.

Mayer, J. D. and Salovey, P. (1997). What is emotional intelligence? In P. Salovey and D. Sluyter (eds), *Emotional development and emotional intelligence: Implications for educators* (pp. 3–31). New York: Basic Books.

Mayer, J. D., Salovey, P. and Caruso, D. R. (2000). Models of emotional intelligence. In R. J. Sternberg (ed.), *Handbook of intelligence* (pp. 396–420). Cambridge: Cambridge University Press.

Mayer, J. D., Salovey, P. and Caruso, D. R. (2002). *Mayer-Salovey- Caruso Emotional Intelligence Test (MSCEIT).* Toronto, Canada: Multi-Health Systems.

Mayer, J. D., Salovey, P., Caruso, D. R. and Sitarenios, G. (2003). Measuring emotional intelligence with the MSCEIT V2.0. *Emotion, 3,* 97–105.McMichael, A. J., Vimpani, G. V., Robertson, E. F., Baghurst, P. A. and Clark, P. D. (1986). The Port Pirie cohort study: Maternal blood lead and pregnancy outcome. *Journal of Epidemiology and Community Health, 40,* 18–25.

Mayer, J.D., Roberts, R.D. & Barsade, S.G. (2008a). Human abilities: Emotional intelligence. *Annual Review of Psychology, 59,* 507–536.

Mayer, J.D., Salovey, P. & Caruso, D.R. (2008b). Emotional intelligence: New ability or eclectic traits. *American Psychologist, 63,* 503–517.

McPherson, K.S. (1985). On intelligence testing and immigration legislation. *American Psychologist, 40,* 242–243.

Mortensen, E. L., Michaelsen, K. F., Sanders, S. A. and Reinisch, J. M. (2005). A dose-response relationship between maternal smoking during late pregnancy and adult intelligence in male offspring. *Paediatric & Perinatal Epidemiology, 19,* 4.

Neisser, U. (1998a). (ed.), *The rising curve: Long-term gains in IQ and related measures.* Washington, DC: American Psychological Association.

Neisser, U. (1998b). Introduction: rising test scores and what they mean. In U. Neisser (ed.), *The rising curve: Long-term gains in IQ and related measures.* (pp. 3–24). Washington, DC:American Psychological Association.

Neisser, U., Boodoo, O., Bouchard, T. J. *et al.* (1996). Intelligence: Knowns and unknowns. *American Psychologist, 51,* 77–101.

O'Connor, M. C. and Paunonen, S. V. (2007). Big Five personality predictors of post-secondary academic performance. *Personality and Individual Di_erences*, *43*, 971–99.

Oddy, W. H., Sherriff, J. L., de Klerk, N. H. *et al.* (2004). The relation of breastfeeding and body mass index to asthma and atopy in children: A prospective cohort study to age 6 years. *American Journal of Public Health*, *94*, 1531–1537.

Olszewski-Kubilius, P. & Lee, S.Y. (2004). The role of participation in in-school and outside-of-school activities in the talent development of gifted students. *Journal of Secondary Gifted Education*, *15*, 107–123.

Plomin, R. & Petrill, S.A. (1997). Genetics and intelligence: What's new? *Intelligence*, *24*, 53–77.

Plomin, R. & Spinath, F.M. (2004). Intelligence: Genetics, genes, and genomics. *Journal of Personality and Social Psychology*, *86*, 112–129.

Plomin, R. (1986). Behavioral genetic methods. *Journal of Personality*, *54*, 226–261.

Plomin, R. (2004). *Nature and nurture: An introduction to human behavioral genetics*. London: Wadsworth.

Plomin, R. and Daniels, D. (1987). Why are children in the same family so different from one another? *Behavioral Brain Sciences*, *10*, 1–16.

Plomin, R. and Rowe, D. C. (1979). Genetic and environmental etiology of social behavior in infancy. *Developmental Psychology*, *15*, 62–72.

Plomin, R., Chipuer, H. M. and Loehlin, J. C. (1990). Behavioral genetics and personality. In L. A. Pervin (ed.), *Handbook of personality:Theory and research* (pp. 225–243). New York: Guilford.

Plomin, R., DeFries, J. C., McClearn, G. E. and McGu_n, P. (2000). *Behavioral genetics: A primer*. London: Freeman.

Poropat, A. E. (2009). A meta-analysis of the Five-Factor Model of personality and academic performance. *Psychological Bulletin*, *135*, 322–338.

Posthuma, D., de Geus, E.J.C. and Boomsma, D.I. (2001). Perceptual speed and IQ are associated through common genetic factors. *Behavioural Genetics, 31*, 593–602.

Preckel, F., Holling, H. & Wiese, M. (2006). Relationship of intelligence and creativity in gifted and non-gifted students: An investigation of threshold theory. *Personality and Individual Differences*, *40*, 159–170.

Raven, J. C. (1962). *Standard Progressive Matrices*. London: Lewis.

Raven, J. C. (2004). *Standard Progressive Matrices*. San Antonio, TX: Harcourt Assessment

Reiss, D. (1997). Mechanisms linking genetic and social influences in adolescent development: Beginning a collaborative search. *Current Directions in Psychological Science*, *6*, 100–105.

Renzulli, J.S. (2005). The three-ring conception of giftedness: A developmental model for promoting creative productivity. In R.J. Sternberg & J.E. Davidson (Eds.), *Conceptions of giftedness* (2nd edn) (pp. 246–279). New York: Cambridge University Press.

Reynolds, A.J., Temple, J.A., Robertson, D.L. & Mann, E.A. (2001). Long-term effects of an early childhood intervention on educational achievement and juvenile arrest: A 15-year follow up of low-income children in public schools. *Journal of the American Medical Association*, *285*, 2339–2346.

Ridley, M. (1999). *Genome: The autobiography of a species in 23 chapters*. London: Fourth Estate.

Robertson, I. T. (2001). Undue diligence. *People Management*, 7 (22 November), 42–43.

Rode, J.C., Mooney, C.H., Arthaud-Day, M.L., Near, J.P., Baldwin, T.T., Rubin, R.S. & Bommer, W.H. (2007). Emotional intelligence and individual performance: Evidence of direct and moderated effects. *Journal of Organizational Behavior*, *28*, 399–421.

Rodgers, J. L., Cleveland, H. H., van den Oord, E. and Rowe, D. C. (2000). Resolving the debate over birth order, family size, and intelligence. *American Psychologist*, *55*, 599–612.

Roid, G. (2003). *Stanford-Binet intelligence scale* (5th edn). Itasca, IL: Riverside Publishing.

Ruch, R. (1937). *Psychology and life*. Glenview, IL: Scott, Foresman.

Rushton, J. P. (1994). Victim of scientific hoax (Cyril Burt and the genetic IQ controversy). *Society*, *31*, 40.

Sak, U. (2004). A synthesis of research on psychological types of gifted adolescents. *Journal of Secondary Gifted Education*, *15*, 70–79.

Salgado, J. F. (2003). Predicting job performance using FFM and non-FFM personality measures. *Journal of Occupational and Organizational Psychology*, *76*, 323–346.

Salovey, P. and Mayer, J. D. (1990). Emotional intelligence. *Imagination,Cognition, and Personality*, *9*, 185–211.

Schalock, R.L., Luckasson, R.A. & Shogren, K.A. (2007). The renaming of *Mental Retardation*: Understanding the change to the term *Intellectual Disability*. *Intellectual and Developmental Disabilities*, *45*, 116–124.

Schulte, M. J., Ree, M. J. and Carretta, T. R. (2004). Emotional intelligence: Not much more than *g* and personality. *Personality and Individual Differences*, *37*, 1059–1068.

Schweinhart, L.J. (2004). *The High/Scope Perry preschool study through age 40: Summary, conclusions, and frequently asked questions.* Retrieved from <www.highscope.org/Research/PerryProject/PerryAge40SumWeb.pdf>

Serpell, R. (2001). Intelligence and culture. In R. J. Sternberg (ed.), *Handbook of intelligence* (pp. 549–577). Cambridge: Cambridge University Press

Smith, D. M. and Kolb, D. A. (1986).*The user's guide for the Learning Style Inventory: A manual for teachers and trainers.* Boston: McBer & Company Spearman, C. E. (1904a). 'General intelligence', objectively determined and measured. *American Journal of Psychology, 15,* 201–293.

Smith, M., Durkin, M. S., Hinton, V., Bellinger, D. and Kuhn, L. (2003). Influence of breastfeeding on cognitive outcomes at age 6–8 years: Follow-up of very low birth weight infants. *American Journal of Epidemiology, 158,* 1075–1082.

Spearman, C. E. (1904b). Proof and measurement of association between two things. *American Journal of Psychology, 15,* 72–101.

Spearman, C. E. (1927). *The abilities of man: Their nature and measurement.* New York: Macmillan.

Spearman, C. E. and Jones, L. W. (1951). *Human abilities.* London: Macmillan

Sternberg, R. J. (1985b). Implicit theories of intelligence, creativity, and wisdom. *Journal of Personality and Social Psychology, 49,* 607–627.

Sternberg, R. J. (1988). *The triarchic mind: A new theory of human intelligence.* New York: Cambridge University Press.

Stevenson, H.W., Chen, C. & Lee, S.Y. (1993). Mathematics achievement of Chinese, Japanese, and American children: Ten years later. *Science, 259,* 53–58.

Tennant, M. (1997). *Psychology and adult learning* (2nd edn). London: Routledge.

Terman, L. M. (1916). *The measurement of intelligence.* Boston: Houghton Mifflin.

Terman, L. M. (1921). Intelligence and its measurement: A symposium (II). *Journal of Educational Psychology, 12,* 127–133.

Terman, L. M. (1925). *Genetic studies of genius* (Vol. 1: *Mental and physical traits of a thousand gifted children).* Stanford, CA: Stanford University Press.

Terman, L. M. and Oden, M. H. (1947). *Genetic studies of genius* (Vol. 4: *The gifted child grows up).* Stanford, CA: Stanford University Press.

Terman, L. M. and Oden, M. H. (1959). *Genetic studies of genius* (Vol. 5: *The gifted group at mid-life).* Stanford, CA: Stanford University Press.

Thorndike, R.L., Hagen, E.P. & Sattler, J.M. (1986). *Stanford-Binet intelligence scale* (4th edn). Chicago: Riverside.

Thurstone, L. L. (1953). *Examiner Manual for Thurstone Temperament Schedule.* Chicago: Science Research Associates.

Triandis, H.C. (1990). Cross-cultural studies of individualism and collectivism. In J. Berman (Ed.), *Nebraska Symposium on Motivation, 1989* (pp. 41–133). Lincoln: University of Nebraska Press.

Uecker, A. and Nadel, L. (1996). Spatial locations gone awry:Object and spatial memory deficits in children with fetal alcohol syndrome. *Neuropsychologia, 34,* 209–223.

van der Zee, K., Schakel, L. and _ijs, M. (2002). The relationship of emotional intelligence with academic intelligence and the big Five. *European Journal of Personality, 16,* 103–125.

Vernon, P. E. (1950). *The structure of human abilities.* London: Methuen.

Wahlsten, D. (1997). The malleability of intelligence is not constrained by heritability. In B. Devlin, S. E. Fienberg and K. Roeder (eds), *Intelligence, genes, and success: Scientists respond to* The Bell Curve (pp. 71–87). New York: Springer.

Wiggins, J.S. (1973). *Personality and prediction: Principles of personality assessment.* Reading, MA: Addison-Wesley.

Williamson, P., McLeskey, J., Hoppey, D. & Rentz, T. (2006). Educating students with mental retardation in general education classrooms. *Exceptional Children, 72,* 347–361.

Winner, E. (2000). The origins and ends of giftedness. *American Psychologist, 55,* 159–169.

Winship, C. and Korenman, S. (1997). Does staying in school make you smarter? The effect of education on IQ in *The Bell Curve.* In B. Devlin, S. E. Fienberg and K. Roeder (eds), *Intelligence, genes, and success: Scientists respond to* The Bell Curve (pp. 215–234). New York: Springer.

Zafra, E. L., Jimenez, M. I. and Espartal, N. R. (2008). Emotional intelligence and academic performance: An overview. *International Journal of Psychology, 3–4,* 793.

Zajonc, R. B. (1976). Family con_guration and intelligence: Variations in scholastic aptitude scores parallel trends in family size and the spacing of children. *Science, 192,* 227–236.

Zajonc, R. B. and Markus, H. (1975). Birth order and intellectual development. *Psychological Review, 82*, 74–88

Chapter 5

Abramson, L., Seligman, Y. & Teasdale, M. (1978). Learned helplessness in humans: critique and reformulation. *Journal of Abnormal Psychology, 87*, 49–74.

Acocella, J. (1999). *Creating Hysteria: Women and Multiple Personality Disorder.* San Francisco: Jossey-Bass.

Afifi, T. O., Asmundson, G. J., Taylor, S. & Jang, K. L. (2010). The role of genes and environment on trauma exposure and posttraumatic stress disorder symptoms: a review of twin studies. *Clinical Psychology Review, 30*, 101–112.

Akiskal, H. S. & McKinney, W. T. (1973). Depressive disorders: toward a unified hypothesis. *Science, 182*, 20–29.

Alda, M. (1997). Bipolar disorder: from families to genes. *Canadian Journal of Psychiatry, 42*(4), 378–387.

Allen, J. J. B. & Movius, H. L. (2000). The objective assessment of amnesia in dissociative identity disorder using event-related potentials. *International Journal of Psychophysiology, 38*, 21–41.

Alloy, L. B. & Abramson, L. Y. (1979). Judgment of contingency in depressed and non-depressed students: sadder but wiser? *Journal of Experimental Psychology: General, 108*, 441–485.

Alloy, L. B. & Abramson, L. Y. (1988). Depressive realism: four theoretical perspectives. In L. B. Alloy (ed.), *Cognitive Process in Depression*. New York: Guilford, pp. 223–265.

American Psychiatric Association (APA). (2000). *Diagnostic and Statistical Manual of Mental Disorders: DSM-IV-TR* (4th ed.). Washington, DC: American Psychiatric Association.

American Psychiatric Association (APA). (2013). *Diagnostic and Statistical Manual of Mental Disorders* (5th ed.). Washington, DC: American Psychiatric Association.

Anderson, K. W., Taylor, S. & McLean, P. (1996). Panic disorder associated with blood-injury-reactivity: the necessity of establishing functional relationships among maladaptive behaviors. *Behavior Therapy, 27*, 463–472.

Andreasen, N. C., Arndt, S., Alliger, R., Miller, D. & Flaum, M. (1995). Symptoms of schizophrenia: methods, meanings, and mechanisms. *Archives of General Psychiatry, 52*, 341–351.

Andreasen, N. C., Rezai, K., Alliger, R., Swayze, V. W. II, Flaum, M., Kirchner, P. et al. (1992). Hypofrontality in neuroleptic-naive patients and in patients with chronic schizophrenia: assessment with xenon 133 single-photon emission computed tomography and the Tower of London. *Archives of General Psychiatry, 49*, 943–958.

Andrews, G., Hobbs, M. J., Borkovec, T. D., Beesdo, K., Craske, M. G., Heimberg, R. G. et al. (2010). Generalized worry disorder: a review of DSM-IV generalized anxiety disorder and options for DSM-V. *Depression and Anxiety, 27*(2), 134–147.

Andrews-McClymont, J., Lilienfeld, S. O. & Duke, M. P. (2013). Evaluating an animal model of compulsive hoarding in humans. *Review of General Psychology, 17*, 399–419.

Angold, A. (1999). Comorbidity. *Journal of Child Psychology and Psychiatry, 40*, 57–87.

Angst, J., Cui, L., Swendsen, J. J., Rothen, S., Cravchik, A., Kessler, R. et al. (2010). Major depressive disorder with sub-threshold bipolarity in the National Comorbidity Survey Replication. *The American Journal of Psychiatry, 167*(10), 1194.

Arieti, S. (1959). Manic-depressive psychosis. In S. Arieti (ed.), *American Handbook of Psychiatry*. New York: Basic Books.

Arseneault, L., Cannon, M., Poulton, R., Murray, R., Caspi, A. & Moffitt, T. E. (2002). Cannabis use in adolescence and risk for adult psychosis: longitudinal prospective study. *British Medical Journal, 325*, 1212–1213.

Australian Bureau of Statistics (ABS). (2007). *National Survey of Mental Health and Wellbeing: Summary of Results*. ABS Cat. no. 4326.0. Canberra: ABS.

Australian Bureau of Statistics (2016). *Causes of Death, Australia, 2015* (cat. no. 3303.0). Canberra, Australia: Australian Bureau of Statistics. Retrieved from http://www.abs.gov.au/AUSSTATS/abs@.nsf/DetailsPage/3303.02015?OpenDocument

Australian Bureau of Statistics (2016). *Causes of Death, Australia, 2015* (cat. no. 3303.0). Canberra, Australia: Australian Bureau of Statistics. Retrieved from http://www.abs.gov.au/AUSSTATS/abs@.nsf/DetailsPage/3303.02015?OpenDocument

Babiak, P. & Hare, R. D. (2006). *Snakes in Suits: When Psychopaths Go To Work.* New York: Regan Books.

Bahnson, C. B. & Smith, K. (1975). Autonomic changes in a multiple personality. *Psychosomatic Medicine, 37*, 85–86.

Barkley, R. A. (1997). *ADHD and the Nature of Self-control.* New York: Guilford.

Barkley, R. A. (2006). *Attention-deficit-hyperactivity Disorder: A Handbook for Diagnosis and Treatment.* New York: Guilford.

Barlow, D. H. (2000). Unraveling the mysteries of anxiety and its disorders from the perspective of emotion theory. *American Psychologist, 55,* 1247–1263.

Barlow, D. H. (2002). *Anxiety and its Disorders: The Nature and Treatment of Anxiety and Panic.* New York: Guilford.

Barlow, D. H., Chorpita, B. F. & Turovsky, J. (1996). Fear, panic, anxiety, and disorders of emotion. In D. A. Hope (ed.), *Perspectives on Anxiety, Panic, and Fear* (The 43rd Annual Nebraska Symposium on Motivation). Lincoln, NE: University of Nebraska Press, pp. 251–328.

Barrett, P. M., Rapee, R. M., Dadds, M. M. & Ryan, S. M. (1996). Family enhancement of cognitive style in anxious and aggressive children. *Journal of Abnormal Child Psychology, 24,* 187–203.

Barta, P. E., Pearlson, G. D., Powers, R. E., Richards S. S. & Tune, L. E. (1990). Auditory hallucinations and smaller superior temporal gyral volume in schizophrenia. *American Journal of Psychiatry, 147,* 1457–1462.

Baum, A., Cohen, L. & Hall, M. (1993). Control and intrusive memories as possible determinants of chronic stress. *Psychosomatic Medicine, 55,* 274–286.

Bayer, R. (1981). *Homosexuality and American Psychiatry: The Politics of Diagnosis.* Princeton, NJ: Princeton University Press.

Bayne, T. & Levy, N. (2005). Amputees by choice: body integrity identity disorder and the ethics of amputation. *Journal of Applied Philosophy, 22,* 75–86.

Beck, A. T. (1964). Thinking and depression. *Archives of General Psychiatry, 9,* 324–333.

Beck, A. T. (1976). *Cognitive Therapy and the Emotional Disorders.* New York: International Universities Press.

Beck, A. T. (1987) Cognitive models of depression. *Journal of Cognitive Psychotherapy, 1,* 5–37.

Beck, J. (1995). *Cognitive Therapy: Basics and Beyond.* New York: Guilford.

Belli, R. F., Winkielman, P., Read, J. D., Schwarz, N. & Lynn, S. J. (1998). Recalling more childhood events leads to judgments of poorer memory: implications for the recovered/false memory debate. *Psychonomic Bulletin and Review, 5,* 318–323.

Bentall, R. P. (2000). Hallucinatory experiences. In E. Cardena, S. J. Lynn & S. Krippner (eds), *Varieties of Anomalous Experience: Examining the Scientific Evidence.* Washington, DC: American Psychological Association, pp. 85–120.

Bergner, R. M. (1997). What is psychopathology? And so what? *Clinical Psychology: Science and Practice, 4,* 235–248.

Bird, H. R. (2002). The diagnostic classification, epidemiology, and cross-cultural validity of ADHD. In P. S. Jensen & J. R. Cooper (eds) *Attention Deficit Hyperactivity Disorder: State of the Science, Best Practices.* Kingston, NJ: Civil Research Institute, pp. 212–216.

Blanchette, I. & Richards, A. (2003). Anxiety and the interpretation of ambiguous stimuli: beyond the emotion-congruent effect. *Journal of Experimental Psychology: General, 13,* 294–309.

Blaney, P. H. (1975). Implications of the medical model and its alternatives. *American. Journal of Psychiatry, 132,* 911–914.

Blashfield, R. K. & Intoccia, V. (2000). Growth of the literature on the topic of personality disorders. *American Journal of Psychiatry, 157,* 472–473.

Blatt, S. J. (1974). Levels of object representation in anaclitic and introjective depression. *Psychoanalytic Studies of the Child, 29,* 107–157.

Boos, H. B. M., Aleman, A., Pol, H. H., Cahn, W. & Kahn, R. (2007). Brain volumes in relatives of patients with schizophrenia: a meta-analysis. *Schizophrenia Bulletin, 33,* 329.

Brende, J. O. (1984). The psychophysiologic manifestations of dissociation: electrodermal responses in a multiple personality patient. *Psychiatry Clinics of North America, 7,* 41–50.

Brody, J. (2007, 17 April). When a brain forgets where memory is. *New York Times.* Retrieved from http://www.nytimes.com/2007/04/17/health/ psychology/17brody.html.

Brown, A. S., Begg, M. D., Gravenstein, S., Schaefer, C. A., Wyatt, W. J., Bresnahan, M., et al. (2004). Serologic evidence for prenatal influenza in the etiology of schizophrenia. *Archives of General Psychiatry, 61,* 774–780.

Brown, G. W., Monck, E. M., Carstairs, G. M. & Wing, J. K. (1962). Influence of family life on the course of schizophrenic illness. *British Journal of Preventive and Social Medicine, 16,* 55–68.

Brugha, T. S. (ed.). (1995). *Social Support and Psychiatric Disorder Research Findings and Guidelines for Clinical Practice.* Cambridge: Cambridge University Press.

Burns, A. B., Brown, J. S., Plant, A., Sachs-Ericsson, N. & Joiner, T. E. (2006). On the specific depressotypic nature of excessive reassurance-seeking. *Personality and Individual Differences, 40*, 135–145.

Busatto, G. F., Pilowsky, L. S., Costa, D. C., Ell, P. J., Verhoeff, N. P. & Kerwin, R. W. (1995). Dopamine D_2 receptor blockade in vivo with the novel antipsychotics risperidone and remoxipride: an 123I–IBZM single photon emission tomography (SPET) study. *Psychopharmacology, 117*(1), 55–61.

Butler, B. (2006). NGRI revisited: venirepersons' attitudes toward the insanity defense. *Journal of Applied Social Psychology, 36*, 1833–1847.

Butzlaff, R. L. & Hooley, J. M. (1998). Expressed emotion and psychiatric relapse: a meta-analysis. *Archives of General Psychiatry*, 55, 547–552.

Caldwell, M. F. (2011). Treatment-related changes in behavioral outcomes of psychopathy facets in adolescent offenders. *Law and Human Behavior, 35*, 275–287.

Cannon, T. D., Mednick, S. A. & Parnas, J. (1989). Genetic and perinatal determinants of structural brain deficits in schizophrenia. *Archives of General Psychiatry, 46*, 883–889.

Carlsson, A. (1995). Towards a new understanding of dopamine receptors. Symposium: dopamine receptor subtypes in neurological and psychiatric diseases. *Clinical Neuropharmacology, 18*(Suppl.), 65–135.

Carpenter, R. W., Tomko, R. L., Trull, T. J. & Boomsma, D. I. (2013). Gene- environment studies and borderline personality disorder: a review. *Current Psychiatry Reports, 15*, 1–7.

Caspi, A., Sugden, K., Moffitt, T. E., Taylor, A., Craig, I., Harrington, H. L. et al. (2003). Influence of life stress on depression: moderation by a polymorphism in the 5-HTT gene. *Science, 301*, 386–389.

Cechnicki, A., Bielaska, A., Hanuszkiewicz, I. & Daren, A. (2012). The predictive validity of Expressed Emotions (EE) in schizophrenia: a 20-year prospective study. *Journal of Psychiatric Research, 47*, 208–214.

Centers for Disease Control and Prevention (2013). *Autism Spectrum Disorders: Data and Statistics*. Retrieved from http://www.cdc.gov/ncbddd/autism/data. html.

Chang, K., Adleman, N. E., Dienes, K., Simeonova, D. I., Menon, V. & Reiss, A. (2004). Anomalous prefrontal-subcortical activation in familial pediatric bipolar disorder—a functional magnetic resonance imaging investigation. *Archives of General Psychiatry, 61*(8), 781–792.

Chapman, L. J., Chapman J. P. & Raulin M. L. (1978). Body-image aberration in schizophrenia. *Journal of Abnormal Psychology, 87*, 399–407.

Chentsova-Dutton, Y. E. & Tsai, J. L. (2006). Cultural factors influence the expression of psychopathology. In S. O. Lilienfeld & W. O'Donoghue (eds), *The Great Ideas of Clinical Science: The 17 Concepts that Every Mental Health Practitioner and Researcher Should Understand*. New York: Brunner-Taylor.

Chodoff, P. (1976). The case for involuntary hospitalization of the mentally ill. *American Journal of Psychiatry, 133*, 396–501.

Cima, M., Tonnaer, F. & Hauser, M. D. (2010). Psychopaths know right from wrong but don't care. *Social Cognitive and Affective Neuroscience, 5*, 59–67. Retrieved from http:// dx.doi.org/10.1093/scan/nsp051.

Clark, D. M. (1986). A cognitive approach to panic. *Behaviour Research and Therapy, 24*, 156–163.

Cleckley, H. (1941/1988). *The Mask of Sanity*. St Louis, MO: Mosby.

Compton, M. T., Kelley, M. E., Ramsay, C. E., Pringle, M., Goulding, S. M., Esterberg, M. L. et al. (2009). Association of pre-onset cannabis, alcohol, and tobacco use with age at onset of prodrome and age at onset of psychosis in first-episode patients. *American Journal of Psychiatry, 166*, 1251–1257.

Coons, P. M., Bowman, E. S. & Milstein, V. (1988). Multiple personality disorder: a clinical investigation of 50 cases. *Journal of Nervous and Mental Disease, 176*, 519–527.

Cornblatt, B. A., Green, M. F. & Walker, E. F. (1999). Schizophrenia: etiology and neurocognition. In T. Millon, P. H. Blaney & R. D. Davis (eds), *Oxford Textbook of Psychopathology*. New York: Oxford University Press, pp. 227–310.

Cornblatt, B. A. & Keilp, J. G. (1994). Impaired attention, genetics, and the pathophysiology of schizophrenia. *Schizophrenia Bulletin, 20*, 31–46.

Coryell, W., Scheftner, W., Keller, M., Endicott, J., Maser, J. & Klerman, G. L. (1993). The enduring psychosocial consequences of mania and depression. *American Journal of Psychiatry, 150*(5), 720–727.

Coryell, W., Solomon, S., Leon, A., Fiedorowicz, J. G., Schettler, P., Judd, L. et al. (2009). Does major depressive disorder change with age? *Psychological Medicine, 39*, 1689–1695.

Cox, B. J. & Taylor, S. (1998). Anxiety disorders: panic and phobias. In T. Millon, P. H. Blaney & R. D. Davis (eds), *Oxford Textbook of Psychopathology*. New York: Oxford University Press, pp. 81–113.

Coyne, J. C. (1976). Depression and the response of others. *Journal of Abnormal Psychology, 85*, 186–193.

Craddock, N., O'Donovan, M. C. & Owen, M. J. (2005). The genetics of schizophrenia and bipolar disorder: dissecting psychosis. *Journal of Medical Genetics, 42*, 193–204.

Cramer, A. O., Waldorp, L. J., van der Maas, H. L. & Borsboom, D. (2010). Comorbidity: a network perspective. *Behavioral and Brain Sciences, 33*(2-3), 137–150.

Craske, M. G., Rapee, R. M., Jackel, L. & Barlow, D. H. (1989). Qualitative dimensions of worry in DSM-III-R generalized anxiety disorder subjects and nonanxious controls. *Behaviour Research and Therapy, 27*, 397–402.

Crowell, S. E., Beauchaine, T. P. & Linehan, M. M. (2009). A biosocial developmental model of borderline personality disorder: elaborating and extending Linehan's theory. *Psychological Bulletin, 135*, 495–510.

Dalenberg, C. J., Brand, B. L., Gleaves, D. H., Dorahy, M. J., Loewenstein, R. J., Cardeña, E. et al. (2012). Evaluation of the evidence for the trauma and fantasy models of dissociation. *Psychological Bulletin, 138*, 550–588.

Davies, G., Welham, J., Chant, D. Torrey, E. F. & McGrath, J. (2003). A systematic review and meta-analysis of northern hemisphere season of birth in schizophrenia. *Schizophrenia Research, 29*, 587–593.

Davis, K. L., Kahn, R. S., Ko, G. & Davidson, M. (1991). Dopamine in schizophrenia: review and reconceptualization. *American Journal of Psychiatry, 148*, 1474–1486.

Degenhardt, L. & Hall, W. (2006). Is cannabis a contributory cause of psychosis? *Canadian Journal of Psychiatry*, 51, 556–565.

Degenhardt, L., Hall, W. D., Lynskey, M., McGrath, J. M., McLaren, J., Calabria, B. et al. (2009). Should burden of disease estimates include cannabis use as a risk factor for psychosis? *PLoS Medicine, 6*. e1000133. Retrieved from doi:10.1371/journal.pmed.1000133.

De Leo, D., Dudley, M. J., Aebersold, C. J., Mendoza, J. A., Barnes, M. A., Harrison, J. E. et al. (2010). Achieving standardised reporting of suicide in Australia: rationale and program for change. *Medical Journal of Australia, 192*, 452–456.

Depue, R. & Iacono, W. (1989). Neurobehavioral aspects of affective disorders. *Annual Review of Psychology, 40*, 457–492.

Dickey, M. (1994). *Anxiety Disorders*. National Institute of Mental Health. Washington: US Government Printing Office.

Dimidjian, S., Hollon, S. D., Dobson, K. S., Schmaling, K. B., Kohlenberg, R. J., Addis, M. E. et al. (2006). Randomized trial of behavioral activation, cognitive therapy and antidepressant medication in the acute treatment of adults with mild depression. *Journal of Consulting and Clinical Psychology, 74*, 658–670.

Disner, S. G., Beevers, C. G., Haigh, E. A. & Beck, A. T. (2011). Neural mechanisms of the cognitive model of depression. *Nature Reviews Neuroscience, 12*(8), 467–477.

Doessel, D. P., Scheurer, R. W., Chant, D. C. & Whiteford, H. A. (2005). Australia's National Mental Health Strategy and deinstitutionalization: some empirical results. *Australian and New Zealand Journal of Psychiatry, 39*, 989–994.

Dolan, A. (2006). The obsessive disorder that haunts my life. *Mail Online*. Retrieved from http://www.dailymail.co.uk/tvshowbiz/article-381802/The-obsessivedisorder-haunts-life.html.

Dolnick, E. (1998). *Madness on the Couch: Blaming the Victim in the Heyday of Psychoanalysis*. New York: Simon & Schuster.

Douglas, K. S., Guy, L. S. & Hart, S. D. (2009). Psychosis as a risk factor for violence to others: a meta-analysis. *Psychological Bulletin, 135*, 679–706.

Durães, D., Martins, J., Borralho, R. & Paiva, A. (2015). Postpartum onset obsessive-compulsive disorder – an overlooked condition. *European Psychiatry, 30*(1), 1504.

Dutton, K. (2012). *The Wisdom of Psychopaths: What Saints, Spies, and Serial Killers Can Teach Us About Success*. New York: Scientific American/Farrar, Straus & Giroux.

Ellis, A. (1962). *Reason and Emotion in Psychotherapy*. Secaucus, NJ: Citadel.

Ellis, A. & Dryden, W. (1997). *The Practice of Rational-Emotive Behavior Therapy*. New York: Springer.

Elzinga, B. M., van Dyck, R. & Spinhoven, P. (1998). Three controversies about dissociative identity disorder. *Clinical Psychology and Psychotherapy, 5*, 13–23.

Fawcett, J. (1997). The detection and consequences of anxiety in clinical depression. *Journal of Clinical Psychiatry, 58*, 35–40.

Feldman, E. (1991). Identifying the genes for diabetes and schizophrenia. *British Medical Journal, 303*, 124.

Fieve, R. (1976). *Moodswing: The Third Revolution in Psychiatry*. New York: Bantam.

Fincham, F. D., Diener, C. I. & Hokoda, A. (2011). Attributional style and learned helplessness: relationship to the use of causal schemata and depressive symptoms in children. *British Journal of Social Psychology, 26(1)*, 1–7.

Finlay-Jones, R. A. & Brown, G. W. (1981). Types of stressful life event and the onset of anxiety and depressive disorder. *Psychological Medicine, 11*, 803–815.

Fisher, L., Marikar, S. & Shaw, A. (2013). Leana Dunham and 9 more stars with OCD. *ABC News*. Retrieved from http://abcnews.go.com/Entertainment/lenadunham-stars-obsessive-compulsive-disorder/story?id=18513623#3.

Foa, E. B. & Kozak, M. J. (1986). Emotional processing of fear: exposure to corrective information. *Psychological Bulletin, 99*, 20–35.

Foa, E. B. & Rothbaum, B. O. (1998). *Treating the Trauma of Rape: Cognitive Behavioural Therapy for PTSD.* New York: Guilford.

Foley, H. A., Carlton, C. O. & Howell, R. J. (1996). The relationship of attention deficit hyperactivity disorder and conduct disorder to juvenile delinquency: legal implications. *Bulletin of the American Academy of Psychiatry and the Law, 24*, 333–345.

Folsom, D. & Jeste, D. V. (2008). Schizophrenia in homeless persons: a systematic review of the literature. *Acta Psychiatrica Scandinavica, 105*, 404–413.

Forbes, E. E., Shaw, D. S. & Dahl, R. E. (2007). Alterations in reward-related decision making in boys with recent and future depression. *Biological Psychiatry, 61*, 633–639.

Fowler, K. A., O'Donohue, W. T. & Lilienfeld, S. O. (2007). Personality disorders in perspective. In W. T. O'Donohue, K. A. Fowler & S. O. Lilienfeld (eds), *Personality Disorders: Toward the DSM–V.* Los Angeles, CA: Sage, pp. 1–19.

Fowles, D. C. & Dindo, L. (2009). Temperament and psychopathy: a dual-pathway model. *Current Directions in Psychological Science, 18*, 179–183.

Frances, A. (2012, 3 December). DSM-5 is a guide, not a bible: simply ignore its 10 worst changes. *Huffington Post.* Retrieved from http://www.huffingtonpost. com/allen-frances/dsm-5_b_2227626.html.

Frances, A. J. & Widiger, T. (2012). Psychiatric diagnosis: lessons from the DSM-IV past and cautions for the DSM-5 future. *Annual Review of Clinical Psychology, 8*, 109–130.

Franklin, M. E. & Foa, E. B. (2008). Obsessive compulsive disorder. In D. Barlow (ed.), *Clinical Handbook of Psychological Disorders: A Step-By-Step Treatment Manual.* New York: Guilford, pp. 164–215.

Freedman, R., Lewis, D. A., Michels, R., Pine, D. S., Schultz, S. K., Tamminga, C. A. et al. (2013). The initial field trials of DSM-5: new blooms and old thorns. *American Journal of Psychiatry, 170*(1), 1–5.

Freud, S. (1917/1953). 'Mourning and melancholia' in *The Standard Edition of the Complete Psychological Works of Sigmund Freud* (Vol. 14). (James Strachey, trans. and ed.). London: Hogarth Press.

Friedman, R. A. (2006). Mental illness and violence: how strong is the link? *New England Journal of Medicine, 355*, 2064–2066.

Frisher M., Crome, I., Martino, O. & Croft, P. (2009). Assessing the impact of cannabis use on trends in diagnosed schizophrenia in thc United Kingdom from 1996 to 2005. *Schizophrenia Research, 113*, 123–128.

Frith, C. D. (1992). *The Cognitive Neuropsychology of Schizophrenia.* Hillsdale, NJ: Lawrence Erlbaum.

Frost, R., Steketee, G., Tolin, D. & Brown, T. (2006). Diagnostic issues in compulsive hoarding. Paris: Paper presented at the European Association of Behavioural and Cognitive Therapies.

Frost, R. O. & Gross, R. C. (1993). The hoarding of possessions. *Behavioural Research and Therapy, 31*(4), 367–381.

Fullana, M. A., Mataix-Cols, D., Caspi, A., Harrington, H., Grisham, J. R., Moffitt, T. E. et al. (2009). Obsessions and compulsions in the community: prevalence, interference, help seeking, developmental stability, and co-occurring psychiatric conditions. *The American Journal of Psychiatry, 166*, 329–336.

Fuller, R. L., Luck, S. J., Braun, E. L., Robinson, B. M., McMahon, R. P. & Gold, J. M. (2006). Impaired control of visual attention in schizophrenia. *Journal of Abnormal Psychology, 115*, 266–275.

Garb, H. N. (1998). *Studying the Clinician: Judgment, Research, and Psychological Assessment.* Washington, DC: American Psychological Association.

Gause, C., Morris, C., Vernekar, S., Pardo-Villamizar, C., Grados, M. A. & Singer, H. S. (2009). Antineuronal antibodies in OCD: comparisons in children with OCD-only, OCD+chronic tics and OCD+PANDAS. *Journal of Neuroimmunology, 214*, 118–124.

Geller, B., Zimmerman, B., Williams, M., DelBello, M. P., Bolhofner, K., Craney, J. L. et al. (2002). DSM-IV mania symptoms in a prepubertal and early adolescent bipolar disorder phenotype compared to attention deficit hyperactive and normal controls. *Journal of the American Academy of Child and Adolescent Psychopharmacology, 12*, 11–25.

Gernsbacher, M. A., Dawson, M. & Goldsmith, H. H. (2005). Three reasons not to believe in an autism epidemic. *Current Directions in Psychological Science, 14*, 55–58.

Gibb, B. E. & Alloy, L. B. (2006). A prospective test of the hopelessness theory of depression in children. *Journal of Clinical Child and Adolescent Psychology, 35*, 264–274.

Giesbrecht, T., Lynn, S. J., Lilienfeld, S. O. & Merckelbach, H. (2008). Cognitive processes in dissociation: an analysis of core theoretical assumptions. *Psychological Bulletin, 134*, 617–647.

Gleaves, D. H. (1996). The sociocognitive model of dissociative identity disorder: a reexamination of the evidence. *Psychological Bulletin, 120*, 42–59.

Gleaves, D. H., May, M. C. & Cardeña, E. (2001). An examination of the diagnostic validity of dissociative identity disorder. *Clinical Psychology Review, 21*, 577–608.

Goldenberg, J. N., Brown, S. B. & Weiner, W. J. (2004). Coprolalia in younger patients with Gilles de la Tourette syndrome. *Movement Disorders, 9*, 622–625.

Golin, S., Terrell, T. & Johnson, B. (1977). Depression and the illusion of control. *Journal of Abnormal Psychology, 86*, 440–442.

Goodwin F. K. & Jamison K. R. (1990). *Manic-Depressive Illness.* New York: Oxford University Press.

Gorenstein, E. E. (1984). Debating mental illness: implications for science, medicine, and social policy. *American Psychologist, 39*, 50–56.

Gottesman, I. I. (1991). *Schizophrenia Genesis: The Origins of Madness.* New York: W. H. Freeman.

Gottesman, I. I. & Shields, J. (1972). *Schizophrenia and Genetics: A Twin Study Vantage Point.* New York: Academic Press.

Grace, A. A. (1991). The cortical regulation of dopamine system responsivity—a hypothesis regarding its role in the etiology of schizophrenia. *Schizophrenia Research, 4*(3), 345.

Granello, D. H. & Beamish, P. M. (1998). Reconceptualizing codependency in women: a sense of connectedness, not pathology. *Journal of Mental Health Counseling, 20*, 344–358.

Grant, B. F., Hansin, D. S., Stinson, F. S., Dawson D. A., June Ruan, W., Goldstein, R. B. et al. (2005). Prevalence, correlates, co-morbidity, and comparative disability of DSM-IV generalized anxiety disorder in the USA: results from the National Epidemiologic Survey on alcohol and related conditions. *Psychological Medicine, 35*, 1747–1759.

Grinker, R. R. (2007). *Unstrange Minds: Remapping the World of Autism.* New York: Basic Books.

Grinker, R. R. & Werble, B. (1977). *The Borderline Patient.* New York: Aronson.

Grinnell, R. (2008). Word salad. In J. M. Grohol, *Encyclopedia of Psychology.* Retrieved from http://psychcentral.com/encyclopedia.

Grob, G. N. (1997). Deinstitutionalization: the illusion of policy. *Journal of Policy History, 9*, 48–73.

Gunderson, J. G., Stout, R. L., McGlashan, T. H., Shea, M. T., Morey, L. C., Grilo, C. M. et al. (2011). Ten-year course of borderline personality disorder: psychopathology and function from the Collaborative Longitudinal Personality Disorders Study. *Archives of General Psychiatry, 68*, 827–837.

Gusow, W. (1963). A preliminary report of kayak-angst among the Eskimo of West Greenland: a study in sensory deprivation. *International Journal of Social Psychiatry, 9*, 18–26.

Haack, L. J., Metalsky, G. I., Dykman, B. M. & Abramson, L. Y. (1996). Use of current situational information and causal inference: do dysphoric individuals make 'unwarranted' causal inferences? *Cognitive Therapy and Research, 20*(4), 309–331.

Haaga, D. A., Dyck, M. J. & Ernst, D. (1991). Empirical status of cognitive theory of depression. *Psychological Bulletin, 110*, 215–236.

Hall, J. R. & Benning, S. D. (2006). The 'successful' psychopath: adaptive and sub-clinical manifestations of psychopathy in the general population. In C. J. Patrick (ed.), *Handbook of Psychopathy.* New York: Guilford, pp. 459–478.

Hallmayer, J., Cleveland, S., Torres, A., Phillips, J., Cohen, B., Torigoe, T., et al. (2011). Genetic heritability and shared environmental factors among twin pairs with autism. *Archives of General Psychiatry, 68*, 1095.

Halweg, K., Goldstein, M. J., Neuchterlein, K. H., Magana, A. B., Mintz, J., Doane, J. A. et al. (1989). Expressed emotion and patient-relative interaction in families of recent onset schizophrenics. *Journal of Consulting and Clinical Psychology, 57*, 11–18.

Hames, J. L., Hagan, C. R. & Joiner, T. E. (2013). Interpersonal processes in depression. *Annual Review of Clinical Psychology, 9*(1), 355–377.

Hammen, C. (1991). Generation of stress in the course of unipolar depression. *Journal of Abnormal Psychology, 100*, 555–561.

Hanson, D. R. & Gottesman, I. I. (2005). Theories of schizophrenia: a genetic-inflammatory-vascular synthesis. *Biomed Central Medical Genetics, 6.* Published online 11 February. Doi: 10.1186/1471-2350-6-7.

Hare, E. H. (1962). Masturbatory insanity: the history of an idea. *Journal of Mental Science, 108*, 2–25.

Hare, R. D. (1978). Electrodermal and cardiovascular correlates of psychopathy. In R. D. Hare & D. Schalling (eds), *Psychopathic Behavior: Approaches to Research.* Chichester: John Wiley, pp. 107–144.

Hare, R. D. (1993). *Without Conscience: The Disturbing World of the Psychopaths Among Us*. New York: Simon & Schuster.

Hare, R. D. (2003). *The Hare Psychopathy Checklist—Revised.* Toronto: Multi-Health Systems.

Hariri, A. R., Mattay, V. S., Tessitore, A., Kolachana, B., Fera, F., Goldman, D. et al. (2002). Serotonin transporter genetic variation and the response of the human amygdala. *Science, 297*, 400–403.

Harkness, A. R. (2007). Personality traits are essential for a complete clinical science. In S. O. Lilienfeld and W. O'Donohue (eds), *The Great Ideas of Clinical Science: 17 Concepts That Every Mental Health Professional Should Understand.* New York: Routledge, pp. 263–290.

Harkness, A. R. & Lilienfeld, S. O. (1997). Individual differences science for treatment planning: personality traits. *Psychological Assessment, 9*, 349–360. Retrieved from http://dx.doi.org/10.1037/1040-3590.9.4.349.

Harkness, K. L. & Luther, J. (2001). Clinical risk factors for the generation of life events in major depression. *Journal of Abnormal Psychology, 110*, 564–572.

Harris, E. C. & Barraclough, B. (1997). Suicide as an outcome for mental disorders—a meta-analysis. *British Journal of Psychiatry, 170*, 205–228.

Harrow, M., Grossman, L. S., Jobe, T. H. & Herbener, E. S. (2005). Do patients with schizophrenia ever show periods of recovery? A 15-year multi-follow-up study. *Schizophrenia Bulletin, 31*, 723–734.

Harvey, J. H. & Weary, G. (1984). Current issues in attribution theory and research. *Annual Review of Psychology, 35*, 427–460.

Harvey, P. D., Reichenberg, A. & Bowie, C. R. (2006). Cognition and aging in psychopathology: focus on schizophrenia and depression. In S. Nolen-Hoeksema, T. D. Cannon & T. Widiger (eds), *Annual Review of Clinical Psychology* (Vol. 2). Palo Alto, CA: Annual Reviews, pp. 389–409.

Haslam, N., Holland, E. & Kuppens, P. (2012). Categories versus dimensions in personality and psychopathology: a quantitative review of taxometric research. *Psychological Medicine, 1(1)*, 1–18.

Haslam, N., Williams, B., Prior, M., Haslam, R., Graetz, B. & Sawyer, M. (2006). Testing the latent structure of ADHD: a taxometric analysis. *Australian and New Zealand Journal of Psychiatry, 40*, 639–647.

Hawton, K., Casanas, I., Comabella, C., Haw, C. & Saunders, K. (2013). Risk factors for suicide in individuals with depression: a systematic review. *Journal of Affective Disorders, 147*(3), 17-28.

Hazlett-Stevens, H., Pruitt, L. D. & Collins, A. (2008). Phenomenology of generalized anxiety disorder. In M. M. Anthony & M. B. Stein (eds), *Oxford Handbook of Anxiety and Related Disorders*. New York: Oxford University Press, pp. 47–64.

Heimberg, R. G. & Juster, H. R. (1995). Cognitive-behavioral treatments: literature review. In R. G. Heimberg, M. R. Liebowitz, D. A. Hope & F. R. Schneier (eds), *Social Phobia: Diagnosis, Assessment, and Treatment.* New York: Guilford.

Hempel, A., Hempel, E., Schönknecht, P., Stippich, C. & Schröder, J. (2003). Impairment in basal limbic function in schizophrenia during affect recognition. *Psychiatry Research, 122*, 115–124.

Henriques, G., Wenzel, A., Brown, G. K. & Beck, A. T. (2005). Suicide attempters' reaction to survival as a risk factor for eventual suicide. *American Journal of Psychiatry, 162*, 2180–2182.

Herbert, J. D., Sharp, I. R. & Gaudiano, B. A. (2002). Separating fact from fiction in the etiology and treatment of autism: a scientific review of the evidence. *Scientific Review of Mental Health Practice, 1*, 25–45.

Hinshaw, S. P. (2002). Is ADHD an impairing condition in childhood and adolescence? In P. S. Jensen & J. R. Cooper (eds), *Attention Deficit Hyperactivity Disorder: State of the Science—Best Practices*. Kingston, NJ: Civic Research Institute, pp. 515–521.

Hollander, E., Zohar, J., Sirovatka, M. S. & Regier, D. A. (2011). *Obsessive-compulsive Spectrum Disorders: Refining the Research Agenda for DSM-V.* Washington, DC: American Psychiatric Publishing.

Honda, H., Shimizu, Y. & Rutter, M. (2005). No effect of MMR withdrawal on the incidence of autism: a total population study. *Journal of Child Psychology and Psychiatry, 46*, 572–579.

Howes, O. D. & Salkovskis, P. M. (1998). Health anxiety in medical students. *Lancet, 351*, 1332.

Howland, R. H. & Thase, M. E. (1998). Cyclothymic disorder. In T. A. Widiger (ed.), *DSM-IV Sourcebook*. Washington, DC: American Psychiatric Association.

Hoyer, E. H., Licht, R. & Mortensen, P. B. (2009). Risk factors of suicide in inpatients and recently discharged patients with affective disorders. A case-control study. European Psychiatry, 24 (5), 317-321.

Hoza, B. (2007). Peer functioning in children with ADHD. *Journal of Pediatric Psychology, 32*, 665–663.

Hunter, R. A. & Macalpine, I. (1963). *Three Hundred Years of Psychiatry: 1535–1860.* London: Oxford University Press.

Huntjens, R. J., Verschuere, B. & McNally, R. J. (2012). Inter-identity autobiographical amnesia in patients with dissociative identity disorder. *PLoS One*, 7(7), e40580.

Iacono, W. G. (1985). Psychophysiologic markers of psychopathology: a review. *Canadian Psychology, 26*, 96–112.

Ilardi, S. S. & Feldman, D. (2001). The cognitive neuroscience paradigm: a unifying meta-theoretical framework for the science and practice of clinical psychology. *Journal of Clinical Psychology, 57*, 1067–1088.

Ingram, R. (2003). Origins of cognitive vulnerability to depression. *Cognitive Therapy and Research, 27*, 77–88.

Jardri, R., Pouchet, A., Pins, D. & Thomas, P. (2011). Cortical activations during auditory verbal hallucinations in schizophrenia: a coordinate-based meta-analysis. *The American Journal of Psychiatry, 168*, 73–81.

Jensvold, M. F. & Turner, S. M. (1988). The woman who hadn't been out of her house in 25 years. In J. A. Talbott & A. Z. A. Manevitz (eds), *Psychiatric House Calls*. Washington, DC: American Psychiatric Association Press, pp. 161–167.

Jerome, L. (2000). Central auditory processing disorder and ADHD. *Journal of the American Academy of Child & Adolescent Psychiatry, 39*, 399–400.

Job, D., Whalley, H. C., Johnstone, E. C. & Lawrie, S. M. (2005). Grey matter changes over time in high risk subjects developing schizophrenia. *NeuroImage, 25*, 1023–1030.

Johnson, S. L., Cueller, A. K., Ruggero, C., Winett-Perlman, C., Goodnick, P. & White, R. (2008). Life events as predictors of mania and depression in bipolar 1 disorder. *Journal of Abnormal Psychology, 117*, 268–277.

Johnson, S. L. & Miller, I. (1997). Negative life events and time to recovery from episodes of bipolar disorder. *Journal of Abnormal Psychology, 106*, 449–457.

Johnson, S. L., Sandrow, D., Meyer, B., Winters, R., Miller, I., Solomon D. et al. (2000). Increases in manic symptoms after life events involving goal attainment. *Journal of Abnormal Psychology, 109*, 721–727.

Joiner, T. E. & Coyne, J. C. (1999). *The Interactional Nature of Depression: Advances in Interpersonal Approaches*. Washington, DC: American Psychological Association.

Jones, J. C. & Barlow, D. H. (1990). The etiology of posttraumatic stress disorder. *Clinical Psychology Review, 10*, 299–328.

Judd, F., Komiti, A. & Jackson, H. J. (2008). How does being female assist help-seeking for mental health problems? *Australian and New Zealand Journal of Psychiatry, 42*, 24–29.

Karg, K., Burmeister, M., Shedden, K. & Sen, S. (2011). The serotonin transporter promoter variant (5-HTTLPR), stress, and depression meta-analysis revisited: evidence of genetic moderation. *Archives of General Psychiatry, 68*(5), 444–454.

Karlin, R. A. & Orne, M. T. (1996). Commentary on *Borawick v. Shay:* hypnosis, social influence, incestuous child abuse, and satanic ritual abuse: the iatrogenic creation of horrific memories for the remote past. *Cultic Studies Journal, 13*(1), 42–94.

Keefe, R. & Henry, P. S. (1994). *Understanding Schizophrenia: A Guide to the New Research on Causes and Treatment*. New York: Free Press.

Keefe, R. S., Silverman, J. M., Mohs, R. C., Siever, L. J., Harvery, P. D., Friedman, L. et al. (1997). Eye tracking, attention, and schizotypal symptoms in nonpsychotic relatives of patients with schizophrenia. *Archives of General Psychiatry, 54*, 169–176.

Keith, S. J., Gunderson, J. G., Reifman, A., Buchsbaum, S. & Mosher, L. R. (1976). Special report: schizophrenia, 1976. *Schizophrenia Bulletin, 2*, 510–565.

Kelly, E. (2009). *Encyclopedia of Attention Deficit Hyperactivity Disorder.* New York: Greenwood.

Kendell, R. E. (1975). The concept of disease and its implications for psychiatry. *British Journal of Psychiatry, 127*, 305–315.

Kendler, K. S. & Diehl, S. R. (1993). The genetics of schizophrenia: a current, genetic-epidemiologic perspective. *Schizophrenia Bulletin, 19*, 261–285.

Kendler, K. S., Gardner, C. O. & Prescott, C. A. (2003). Personality and the experience of environmental adversity. *Psychological Medicine, 33*, 1193–1202.

Kendler, K. S. & Karkowski-Shuman, L. (1997). Stressful life events and genetic liability to major depression: genetic control of exposure to the environment? *Psychological Medicine, 27*, 539–547.

Kendler, K. S., Neale, M. C., Kessler, R. C., Heath, A. C. & Eaves, L. J. (1993). A test of the equal-environment assumption in twin studies of psychiatric illness. *Behavior Genetics, 23*, 21–27.

Kernberg, O. (1967). Borderline personality organization. *Journal of American Psychoanalytical Association, 15*, 641–685.

Kernberg, O. (1975). *Borderline Conditions and Pathological Narcissism*. New York: Jason Aronson.

Kessler, R. C., Angermeyer, M., Anthony, J. C., de Graff, R. O. N., Demyttenaere, K., Gasquet, I. et al. (2007). Lifetime prevalence and age-of-onset distributions of mental disorders in the World Health Organization's World Mental Health Survey Initiative. *World Psychiatry, 6*, 168–176.

Kessler, R. C., Berglund, P., Demler, O., Jin, R. & Walters, E. E. (2005). Lifetime prevalence and age-of-onset distributions of DSM-IV disorders in the National Comorbidity Survey Replication. *Archives of General Psychiatry, 62*, 593–602.

Kessler, R. C., Coccaro, E. F., Fava, M., Jaeger, S., Jin, R. & Walters, E. (2006). The prevalence and correlates of DSM-IV intermittent explosive disorder in the National Comorbidity Survey Replication. *Archives of General Psychiatry, 63*(6), 669–678.

Kessler, R. C., McGonagale, K. A., Zhao, S., Nelson, C. B., Hughes, M., Eshleman, S. et al. (1994). Lifetime and 12-month prevalence of DSM-III-R psychiatric disorders in the United States: results from the National Comorbidity Survey. *Archives of General Psychiatry, 51*, 8–19.

Kihlstrom, J. F. (2005). Dissociative disorders. In S. Nolen-Hoeksema, T. D. Cannon & T. Widiger (eds), *Annual Review of Clinical Psychology, 1*, 227–254.

Kim, E. Y. & Miklowitz, D. J. (2002). Childhood mania, attention deficit hyperactivity disorder and conduct disorder: a critical review of diagnostic dilemmas. *Bipolar Disorders, 4*, 215–225.

King, B. (ed.). (1997). *Lustmord: The Writings and Artifacts of Murderers*. Burbank, CA: Bloat.

King, J. (2000). Treatment of schizophrenia. What in fact is schizophrenia? *British Medical Journal, 320*(7237), 800.

Kippes, C. & Garrison, C. B. (2006). Are we in the midst of an autism epidemic? A review of prevalence data. *Missouri Medicine, 103*(1), 65–68.

Kirk, S. A. & Kutchins, H. (1992). *The Selling of DSM: The Rhetoric of Science in Psychiatry*. Hawthorne, NY: Aldine de Gruyter.

Kirmayer, L. J. & Young, A. (1999). Culture and context in the evolutionary concept of mental disorder. *Journal of Abnormal Psychology, 108*, 446–452.

Kistner, J. A., David-Ferdon, C. F., Repper, K. K. & Joiner, T. E. Jr (2006). Bias and accuracy of children's perceptions of peer acceptance: prospective associations with depressive symptoms. *Journal of Abnormal Child Psychology, 34*, 349–361.

Kleinknecht, R. A., Dinnel, D. L., Tanouye-Wilson, S. & Lonner, W J. (1994). Cultural variation in social anxiety and phobia: a study of Taijin Kyofusho. *The Behavior Therapist, 17*(8), 175–178.

Kleinman, A. (1988). *Rethinking Psychiatry: From Cultural Category to Personal Experience*. New York: Free Press.

Klerman, G. L. (1986). The National Institute of Mental Health—Epidemiologic Catchment Area (NIMH-ECA) Program—background, preliminary findings and implications. *Social Psychiatry, 21*(4), 159–166.

Klonsky, E. D., Kotov, R., Bakst, S., Rabinowitz, J. & Bromet, E. J. (2012). Hopelessness as a predictor of attempted suicide among first admission patients with psychosis: A 10-year cohort study. *Suicide and Life-Threating Behaviour, 42*(1), 1-10.

Kluft, R. P. (1984). Multiple personality in childhood. *Psychiatric Clinics of North America, 7*, 121–134.

Knyazeva, M. G., Jalili, M., Meuli, R., Hasler, M., DeFeo, O. & Do, K. Q. (2008). Alpha rhythm and hypofrontality in schizophrenia. *Acta Psychiatrica Scandinavica, 118*, 188–199.

Kollman, D. M., Brown, T. A., Liverant, G. I. & Hofmann, S. G. (2006). A taxometric investigation of the latent structure of social anxiety disorder in outpatients with anxiety and mood disorders. *Depression and Anxiety, 23*, 190–199.

Koran, L. M., Faber, R. J., Aboujaoude, E., Large, M. D. & Serpe, R. T. (2006). Estimated prevalence of compulsive buying behavior in the United States. *American Journal of Psychiatry, 163*(10), 1806–1812.

Kramer, G. M., Wolbransky, M. & Heilbrun, K. (2007). Plea bargaining recommendations by criminal defense attorneys: evidence strength, potential sentence, and defendant preference. *Behavioral Sciences & the Law, 25*, 573–585.

Krueger, R. & Piasecki, T. M. (2002). Toward a dimensional and psychometrically informed approach to conceptualizing psychopathology. *Behaviour Research and Therapy, 40*, 485–499.

Krueger, R. F., Skodol, A. E., Livesley, W. J., Shrout, P. E. & Huang, Y. (2007). Synthesizing dimensional and categorical approaches to personality disorders: refining the research agenda for DSM-V Axis II. *International Journal of Methods in Psychiatric Research, 16*, S65–S73.

Kruger, S., Seminowicz, D., Goldapple, K., Kennedy, S. H. & Mayberg, H. S. (2003). State and trait influences on mood regulation in bipolar disorder: blood flow differences with an acute mood challenge. *Biological Psychiatry, 54*(11), 1274–1283.

Kuipers, L. (2011). Expressed emotion: a review. *British Journal of Social and Clinical Psychology, 18*, 237–243.

Kuperberg, G. R., Sitnikova, T., Goff, D. & Holcomb, P. J. (2006). Making sense of sentences in schizophrenia: electrophysiological evidence for abnormal interactions between semantic and syntactic processing. *Journal of Abnormal Psychology, 115*, 251–265.

Kurlan, R. & Kaplan, E. L. (2004). The pediatric autoimmune neuropsychiatric disorders associated with streptococcal infection (PANDAS) etiology for tics and obsessive-compulsive symptoms: hypothesis or entity. Practical considerations for the clinician. *Pediatrics, 112*, 884–886.

Lamb, H. R. & Bachrach, L. L. (2001). Some perspectives on deinstitutionalization. *Psychiatric Services, 52*, 1039–1045.

Langdon, R., Ward, P. B. & Coltheart, M. (2010). Reasoning anomalies associated with delusions in schizophrenia. *Schizophrenia Bulletin, 36*, 321–330.

Lawrence, D., Johnson, S., Hafekost, J., Boterhoven de Haan, K., Sawyer, M., Ainley, J. & Zubrick, S. R. (2015). *The Mental Health of Children and Adolescents. Report on the second Australian Child and Adolescent Survey of Mental Health and Wellbeing.* Canberra, Australia: Department of Health.

Leeper, P. (1988). Having a place to live is vital to good health. *News Report, 38*, 5–8.

LeFever, G. B., Arcona, A. P. & Antonuccio, D. O. (2004). ADHD among American schoolchildren: evidence of overdiagnosis and overuse of medication. *Scientific Review of Mental Health Practice, 2*(1), 49–60.

Leichsenring, F., Leibing, E., Kruse, J., New, A. S. & Leweke, F. (2011). Borderline personality disorder. *Lancet, 377*(9759), 74–84.

Leistico, A. M. R., Salekin, R. T., DeCoster, J. & Rogers, R. (2008). A large-scale meta-analysis relating the Hare measures of psychopathy to antisocial conduct. *Law and Human Behavior, 32*, 28–45.

Lenzenweger, M. F., McLachlan, G. & Rubin, D. B. (2007). Resolving the latent structure of schizophrenia endophenotypes using expectation-maximization-based finite mixture modeling. *Journal of Abnormal Psychology, 116*, 16–29.

Leonard, B. E. (1997). The role of noradrenaline in depression: a review. *Journal of Psychopharmacology, 11*, S39–S47.

Levy-Reiner, S. (1996). The decade of the brain: library and NIMH hold symposia on mental illness. *Library of Congress Information Bulletin, 55*, 326–327.

Lewinsohn, P. M. (1974). A behavioral approach to depression. In R. J. Friedman & M. M. Katz (eds), *Psychology of Depression: Contemporary Theory and Research.* Oxford: John Wiley, pp. 157–158.

Lewinsohn, P. M., Holm-Denoma, J. M., Small, J. W., Seeley, J. R. & Joiner, T. E. (2008). Separation in childhood as a risk factor for future mental illness. *Journal of the American Academy for Child and Adolescent Psychiatry, 47*(5), 548–555.

Lichtenstein, P., Yip, B. H., Björk, C., Pawitan, Y., Cannon, T. D., Sullivan, P. F. et al. (2009). Common genetic determinants of schizophrenia and bipolar disorder in Swedish families: a population-based study. *Lancet, 373*(9659), 234–239.

Lidz, C. W., Mulvey, E. P. & Gardner, W. (1993). The accuracy of predictions of violence to others. *Journal of the American Medical Association, 269*, 1007–1111.

Lidz, T. (1973). *The Origin and Treatment of Schizophrenic Disorders.* New York: Basic Books.

Lieberman, J. A. & Koreen, A. R. (1993). Neurochemistry and neuroendocrinology of schizophrenia: a selective review. *Schizophrenia Bulletin, 2*, 371–428.

Lilienfeld, S. O. (1994). Conceptual problems in the assessment of psychopathy. *Clinical Psychology Review, 14*, 17–38.

Lilienfeld, S. O. (1997). The relation of anxiety sensitivity to higher and lower order personality dimensions: implications for the etiology of panic attacks. *Journal of Abnormal Psychology, 106*(4), 539–544.

Lilienfeld, S. O. & Arkowitz, H. (2007). Autism: an epidemic? *Scientific American Mind, 18*(2), 82–83.

Lilienfeld, S. O. & Landfield, K. (2008). Issues in diagnosis. In E. Craighead, D. J. Miklowitz & L. W. Craighead (eds), *Psychopathology: History, Diagnosis, and Empirical Foundations.* New York: Wiley.

Lilienfeld, S. O. & Lynn, S. J. (2003). Dissociative identity disorder: multiple personality, multiple controversies. In S. O. Lilienfeld, S. J. Lynn & J. M. Lohr (eds), *Science and Pseudoscience in Psychology.* New York: Guilford.

Lilienfeld, S. O., Lynn, S. J., Kirsch, I., Chaves, J. F., Sarbin, T. R., Ganaway, G. K. et al. (1999). Dissociative identity disorder and the sociocognitive model: recalling the lessons of the past. *Psychological Bulletin, 125*, 507–523.

Lilienfeld, S. O. & Marino, L. (1995). Mental disorder as a Roschian concept: a critique of Wakefield's 'harmful dysfunction' analysis. *Journal of Abnormal Psychology, 104*, 411–420.

Lilienfeld, S. O. & Waldman, I. D. (2004). Comorbidity and Chairman Mao. *World Psychiatry, 3*, 26–27.

Lilienfeld, S. O., Waldman, I. D. & Israel, A. C. (1994). A critical examination of the use of the term 'comorbidity' in psychopathology research. *Clinical Psychology: Science and Practice, 1*, 71–83.

Linehan, M. M. (1993). *Cognitive Behavioral Treatment of Borderline Personality Disorder.* New York: Guilford.

Lorber, M. F. (2004). Autonomic psychophysiology of aggression, psychopathy, and conduct problems: a meta-analysis. *Psychological Bulletin, 130*, 531–552.

Luchins, D. J., Weinberger, D. R. & Wyatt, R. J. (1982). Schizophrenia and cerebral asymmetry detected by computed tomography. *American Journal of Psychiatry, 139*, 753–757.

Ludwig, A. M., Brandsma, J. M., Wilbur, C. B., Bendfeldt, F. & Jameson, D. H. (1972). The objective study of a multiple personality: or, are four heads better than one? *Archives of General Psychiatry, 26*, 298–310.

Lundström, S., Haworth, C., Carlström, E., Gillberg, C., Mill, J., Råstam, M. et al. (2010). Trajectories leading to autism spectrum disorders are affected by paternal age: findings from two nationally representative twin studies. *Journal of Child Psychology and Psychiatry, 51*, 850–856.

Lykken, D. T. (1957). A study of anxiety in the sociopathic personality. *Journal of Abnormal and Social Psychology, 55*, 6–10.

Lykken, D. T. (1982). If a man be mad. *The Sciences, 22*, 11–13.

Lykken, D. T. (1995). *The Antisocial Personalities*. Mahwah, NJ: Lawrence Erlbaum.

Macrae, C. N. & Bodenhausen, G. V. (2000). Social cognition: thinking categorically about others. *Annual Review of Psychology, 51*, 93–120.

Madsen K. M., Hviid, A., Vestergaard, M., Schendel, D., Wohlfart, J., Thorsen, P. et al. (2002). A population-based study of measles, mumps and rubella vaccination and autism. *New England Journal of Medicine, 347*, 1477–1482.

Magee, W. J., Eaton, W. W., Wittchen, H. U., McGonagle, K. A. & Kessler, R. C. (1996). Agoraphobia, simple phobia, and social phobia in the National Comorbidity Survey. *Archives of General Psychiatry, 53*, 159–168.

Mangeot, S. D., Miller, L. J., McIntosh, D. N., McGrath-Clarke, J., Simon, J., Hagerman, R. J. et al. (2001). Sensory modulation dysfunction in children with attention-deficit-hyperactivity disorder. *Developmental Medicine & Child Neurology, 43*, 399–406.

Marder, S., Cohen, A., Hamilton, A., Saks, E., Glynn, S., Hollan, D. et al. (2008). Characteristics of high-functioning people with schizophrenia. *Schizophrenia Research, 102*, 232–232.

Martinelli, L. R., Binney, J. S. & Kaye, R. (2014). Separating myth from fact: unlinking mental illness and violence and implications for gun control legislation and public policy. *New England Journal on Criminal & Civil Confinement, 40* (2), 359-377.

Martinot, M.-L., Bragulat, V., Artiges, E., Dolle, F., Hinnen, F., Jouvent, R. et al. (2001). Decreased presynaptic dopamine function in the left caudate of depressed patients with affective flattening and psychomotor retardation. *American Journal of Psychiatry, 158*, 314–316.

Matarazzo, J. D. (1983). The reliability of psychiatric and psychological diagnosis. *Clinical Psychology Review, 3*, 103–145.

Mathews, A., Richards, A. & Eysenck, M. W. (1989). Interpretation of homophones related to threat in anxiety states. *Journal of Abnormal Psychology, 98*, 31–34.

Matthews, A. & MacLeod, C. (2005). Cognitive vulnerability to emotional disorders. In S. Nolen-Hoeksema, T. D. Cannon & T. Widiger (eds), *Annual Review of Clinical Psychology* (Vol. 1). Palo Alto, CA: Annual Reviews, pp. 167–196.

Mazure, C. M. (1998). Life stressors as risk factors in depression. *Clinical Psychology: Science and Practice, 5*, 291–313.

McCann, J. T., Shindler, K. L. & Hammond, T. R. (2003). The science and pseudo-science of expert testimony. In S. O. Lilienfeld, S. J. Lynn & J. M. Lohr (eds), *Science and Pseudoscience in Clinical Psychology*. New York: Guilford, pp. 77–108.

McCarty, C. A., Lau, A. S., Valeri, S. M. & Weisz, J. R. (2004). Parent–child interactions proxy for behavior. *Journal of Abnormal Child Psychology, 32*, 83–93.

McClellan, J., Kowatch, R. A. & Findling, R. L. (2007). Practice parameters for the assessment and treatment of children and adolescents with bipolar disorder. *Journal of the American Academy of Child and Adolescent Psychiatry, 46*, 107–125.

McCutcheon, L. E. & McCutcheon, L. E. (1994). Not guilty by reason of insanity: getting it right or perpetuating the myths? *Psychological Reports, 74*, 764–766.

McGrath, J., Saha, S., Chant, D. & Welham, J. (2008). Schizophrenia: a concise overview of incidence, prevalence, and mortality. *Epidemiologic Reviews, 30*, 67–76.

McGrath, M. E. (1984). 1st-person account. Where did I go? *Schizophrenia Bulletin, 10*(4), 638–640.

McGuffin, P., Rijsdijk, F., Andrew, M., Sham, P., Katz, R. & Cardino, A. (2003). The heritability of bipolar affective disorder and the genetic relationship to unipolar depression. *Archives of General Psychiatry, 60*(5), 497–502.

McGuire, P. K., Shah, G. M. S. & Murray, R. M. (1993). Increased blood flow in Broca's area during auditory hallucinations. *Lancet, 342*, 703–706.

McHugh, P. R. (1993). Multiple personality disorder. *Harvard Mental Health Newsletter, 10*(3), 4–6.

McKenna, K., & Harrison, J. E. (2012). *Hospital separations due to injury and poisoning, Australia 2008-09. Injury research and statistics series - No. 65.* (Cat. no. INJCAT 141). Canberra, ACT: Australian Institute of Health and Welfare.

McNally, R. J. (2003). *Remembering Trauma.* Cambridge, MA: Belknap Press.

McNally, R. J. (2011). *What is Mental Illness?* Cambridge, MA: Harvard University Press.

McNally, R. M. & Eke, M. (1996). Anxiety sensitivity, suffocation fear, and breath-holding duration as predictors of response to carbon dioxide challenge. *Journal of Abnormal Psychology, 105,* 146–149.

McNiel, D. E., Eisner, J. P. & Binder, R. L. (2000). The relationship between command hallucinations and violence. *Psychiatric Services, 51,* 1288–1292.

Mednick, S. A., Machon, R. A., Huttunen, M. O. & Bonett, D. (1988). Adult schizophrenia following prenatal exposure to an influenza epidemic. *Archives of General Psychiatry, 45,* 189–192.

Meehl, P. E. (1962). Schizotaxia, schizotypy, and schizophrenia. *American Psychologist, 17,* 827–838.

Meehl, P. E. (1990). Toward an integrated theory of schizotaxia, schizotypy, and schizophrenia. *Journal of Personality Disorders, 4,* 1–99.

Meehl, P. E. & Rosen, A. (1955). Antecedent probability and the efficiency of psychometric signs, patterns, or cutting scores. *Psychological Bulletin, 52,*194–216.

Mell, L. K., Davis, R. L. & Owens, D. (2005). Association between streptococcal infection and obsessive-compulsive disorder, Tourette's syndrome, and tic disorder. *Pediatrics, 116,* 56–60.

Mellinger, D. M. & Lynn, S. J. (2003). *The Monster in the Cave: How to Face Your Fear and Anxiety and Live Your Life.* New York: Berkeley.

Melton, G. B., Petrilla, J., Poythress, N. G. & Slobogin, L. A. (1997). *Psychological Evaluations for the Courts: A Handbook for Mental Health Professionals and Lawyers* (2nd ed.). New York: Guilford.

Mendelowicz, M. V. & Stein, M. B. (2000). Quality of life in individuals with anxiety disorders. *American Journal of Psychiatry, 157,* 669–682.

Merckelbach, H., Devilly, G. & Rassin, E. (2002). Alters in dissociative identity disorder: metaphors or genuine entities? *Clinical Psychology Review, 22,* 481–497.

Merikangas, K. R., Akiskal, H. S., Angst, J., Greenberg, P. E., Hirschfeld, R., Petukhova, M. et al. (2007). Lifetime and 12-month prevalence of bipolar spectrum disorder in the National Comorbidity Survey replication. *Archives of General Psychiatry, 64*(5), 543–552.

Merskey, H. (1992). The manufacture of personalities: the production of multiple personality disorder. *British Journal of Psychiatry, 160,* 327–340.

Meyer, S. E. & Carlson, G. A. (2008). Early-onset bipolar disorder. *Focus: The Journal of Lifelong Learning in Psychiatry, 6,* 271–283.

Miklowitz, D. J. & Johnson, S. L. (2006). The psychopathology and treatment of bipolar disorder. *Annual Review of Clinical Psychology, 2,* 199–235.

Miller, S. D. (1989). Optical differences in cases of multiple personality disorder. *Journal of Nervous and Mental Disease, 177,* 480–486.

Mineka, S. & Cook, M. (1993). Mechanisms involved in the observational conditioning of fear. *Journal of Experimental Psychology: General, 122,* 23–38.

Mittal, V. A., Tesser, K. D., Trottman, H. D., Esterberg, M., Dhruv, S. H., Simenova, D. I. et al. (2007). Movement abnormalities and the progression of prodromal symptomatology in adolescents at risk for psychotic disorders. *Journal of Abnormal Psychology, 116,* 260–267.

Molina, B. & Pelham, W. (2003). Childhood predictors of adolescent substance use in a longitudinal study of children with ADHD. *Journal of Abnormal Psychology, 112,* 497–507.

Monahan, J. (1992). Mental disorder and violent behavior: perceptions and evidence. *American Psychologist, 47,* 511–521.

Monahan, J., Steadman, H. J., Appelbaum, P. S., Robbins, P. C., Mulvey, E. P., Silver, E. et al. (2000). Developing a clinically useful actuarial tool for assessing violence risk. *British Journal of Psychiatry, 176,* 312–319.

Monastra, V. J. (2008). *Unlocking the Potential of Patients with ADHD.* Washington, DC: American Psychological Association.

Moore, M. T. & Fresco, D. M. (2012). Depressive realism: a meta-analytic review. *Clinical Psychology Review, 32,* 496–509.

Moreno, C., Laje, G., Blanco, C., Jiang, H., Schmidt, A. B. & Olfson, M. (2007). National trends in the outpatient diagnosis and treatment of bipolar disorder in youth. *Archives of General Psychiatry, 64,* 1032–1039.

Morrison, J. (1997). *When Psychological Problems Mask Medical Disorders: A Guide for Psychotherapists.* New York: Guilford.

Msetfi, R. M., Murphy, R. A., Simpson, J. & Kornbrot, D. E. (2005). Depressive realism and outcome density bias in contingency judgments: the effect of the context and inter-trial interval. *Journal of Experimental Psychology: General, 134*, 10–22.

Mueser, K. T. & McGurk, S. R. (2004). Schizophrenia. *Lancet, 363*, 2063–2072.

Mullen, P. (2000). Dangerousness, risk and the prediction of probability. In M. G. Gelder, J. J. Lopez-Ibor & N. Andreasen (eds), *New Oxford Textbook of Psychiatry*. London: Oxford University Press, pp. 2066–2078.

Murphy, J. A. & Byrne, G. J. (2012). Prevalence and correlates of the proposed DSM-5 diagnosis of chronic depressive disorder. *Journal of Affective Disorders, 139*(2), 172–180.

Murphy, J. B. (1976). Psychiatric labeling in cross-cultural perspective: similar kinds of disturbed behavior appear to be labeled abnormal in diverse cultures. *Science, 191*, 1019–1028.

National Institute on Alcohol Abuse and Alcoholism (NIAAA). (2000, July). *Alcohol Alert. From Genes to Geography: The Cutting Edge of Alcohol Research*. No 48. Available at http://pubs.niaaa.nih.gov/publications/aa48.htm.

Newman, J. P. & Kosson, D. S. (1986). Passive avoidance learning in psychopathic and nonpsychopathic offenders. *Journal of Abnormal Psychology, 95*, 252–256.

Nicholson, T. R., Ferdinando, S., Krishnaiah, R. B., Anhoury, S., Lennox, B. R., Mataix-Cols, D. et al. (2012). Prevalence of anti-basal ganglia antibodies in adult obsessive-compulsive disorder: cross-sectional study. *The British Journal of Psychiatry, 200*(5), 381–386.

Nicol, S. E. & Gottesman, I. I. (1983). Clues to the genetics and neurobiology of schizophrenia. *American Scientist, 71*, 398–404.

Nolen-Hoeksema, S. (2002). Gender differences in depression. In I. H. Gotlib & C. L. Hammen (eds), *Handbook of Depression*. New York: Guilford, pp. 492–509.

Nolen-Hoeksema, S. (2003). *Women Who Think Too Much: How to Break Free of Over Thinking and Reclaim Your Life*. New York: Holt.

Novick, D. M., Swartz, H. A. & Frank, E. (2010). Suicide attempts in bipolar I and bipolar II disorder: a review and meta-analysis of the evidence. *Bipolar Disorders, 12*, 1–9.

Noyes, R. Jr. (2001). Comorbidity in generalized anxiety disorder. *Psychiatric Clinics of North America, 24*, 41–55.

O'Brien, T. (1990). *The Things They Carried*. New York: Broadway.

Offit, P. A. (2008). Vaccines and autism revisited: the Hanna Poling case. *New England Journal of Medicine, 358*, 2089–2091.

Ogden, C. A., Rich, M. E., Schork, N. J., Paulus, M. P., Geyer, M. A., Lohr, J. B. et al. (2004). Candidate genes, pathways and mechanisms for bipolar (manic-depressive) and related disorders: an expanded convergent functional genomics approach. *Molecular Psychiatry, 9*, 1007–1029.

Overmier, J. B. & Seligman, M. E. P. (1967). Effects of inescapable shock upon subsequent escape and avoidance responding. *Journal of Comparative and Physiological Psychology, 63*, 28–33.

Papolos, D. & Papolos, J. (2007). *The Bipolar Child: The Definitive and Reassuring Guide to Childhood's Most Misunderstood Disorder* (3rd ed.). New York: Broadway.

Parker, R. (2010). Australia's Aboriginal population and mental health. *Journal of Nervous and Mental Disease, 198*, 3–7.

Pasewark, R. A. & Pantle, M. L. (1979). Insanity plea: legislator's view. *American Journal of Psychiatry, 136*, 222–223.

Patrick, C. J. (ed.). (2006). *Handbook of Psychopathy*. New York: Guilford.

Paykel, E. S. (2003). Life events and affective disorders. *Acta Psychiatrica Scandinavia, 108*, 61–66.

Perry, J. C. (1992). Problems and considerations in the valid assessment of personality disorders. *American Journal of Psychiatry, 149*(12), 1645–1653.

Peterson, J. K., Skeem, J., Kennealy, P., Bray, B. & Zvonkovic, A. (2014). How often and how consistently do symptoms directly precede criminal behavior among offenders with mental illness? *Law & Human Behavior, 38* (5), 439–449.

Pertusa, A., Frost, R. O., Fullana, M. A., Samuels, J., Steketee, G., Tolin, D. et al. (2010). Refining the diagnostic boundaries of compulsive hoarding: a critical review. *Clinical Psychology Review, 30*(4), 371–386.

Phillips, K. A., Menard, W., Fay, C. & Weisberg, R. (2005). Demographic characteristics, phenomenology, comorbidity, and family history in 200 individuals with body dysmorphic disorder. *Psychosomatics, 46*, 317–325.

Phillips, M. R., Wolf, A. S. & Coons, D. J. (1988). Psychiatry and the criminal justice system: testing the myths. *American Journal of Psychiatry, 145*, 605–610.

Piccinelli, M. & Wilkinson, G. (2000). Gender differences in depression—critical review. *British Journal of Psychiatry, 177,* 486–492.

Pies, R. (2012). Bereavement, complicated grief, and the rationale for diagnosis in psychiatry. *Dialogues in Clinical Neuroscience, 14*(2), 111–113.

Piper, A. (1997). *Hoax and Reality: The Bizarre World of Multiple Personality Disorder.* Northvale, NJ: Jason Aronson.

Pittinger, C. & Duman, R. S. (2008). Stress, depression, and neuroplasticity: a convergence of mechanisms. *Neuropsychopharmacology Reviews, 33,* 88–109.

Pope, H. G. & Hudson, J. I. (1992). Is childhood sexual abuse a risk factor for bulimia nervosa? *American Journal of Psychiatry, 149,* 455–463.

Pope, H. G. Jr, Poliakoff, M. B., Parker, M. P., Boynes, M. & Hudson, J. I. (2007). Is dissociative amnesia a culture-bound syndrome? Findings from a survey of historical literature. *Psychological Medicine, 37,* 225–233.

Price, R. H. & Bouffard, D. L. (1974). Behavioral appropriateness and situational constraint as dimensions of social behavior. *Journal of Personality and Social Psychology, 30,* 579–586.

Purcell, S. M., Wray, N. R., Stone, J. L., Visscher, P. M., O'Donovan, M. C., Sullivan, P. F. et al. (2009). Common polygenic variation contributes to risk of schizophrenia and bipolar disorder. *Nature, 460*(7256), 748–752.

Rachman, S. (1977). The conditioning theory of fear-acquisition: a critical examination. *Behaviour Research and Therapy, 15,* 375–387.

Rapee, R. M. & Heimberg, R. G. (1997). A cognitive-behavioural model of anxiety in social phobia. *Behaviour Research and Therapy, 35,* 741–756.

Raulin, M. L. & Lilienfeld, S. O. (1999). Research strategies for studying psychopathology. In T. Millon, P. H. Blaney & R. D. Davis (eds), *The Oxford Textbook of Psychopathology.* New York: Oxford University Press, pp. 49–78.

Raz, S. & Raz, N. (1990). Structural brain abnormalities in the major psychoses: a quantitative review of the evidence from computerized imaging. *Psychological Bulletin, 108,* 93–108.

Reis, F. L., Masson, S., de Oliveira, A. R. & Brandao, M. L. (2004). Dopaminergic mechanisms in the conditioned and unconditioned fear as assessed by the two-way avoidance and light switch-off tests. *Pharmacology, Biochemistry and Behavior, 79,* 359–365.

Reiss, S. & McNally, R. J. (1985). The expectancy model of fear. In S. Reiss & R. R. Bootzin (eds), *Theoretical Issues in Behavior Therapy.* New York: Academic Press, pp. 107–121.

Richter, M. A., Summerfeldt, L. J., Antony, M. M. & Swinson, R. P. (2003). Obsessive-compulsive spectrum conditions in obsessive-compulsive disorder and other anxiety disorders. *Depression and Anxiety, 18,* 118–127.

Rieber, R. W. (1999). Hypnosis, false memory, and multiple personality: a trinity of affinity. *History of Psychiatry, 10,* 3–11.

Rimland, B. (2004). Association between thimerosol-containing vaccine and autism. *Journal of the American Medical Association, 291,* 180.

Risch, N., Herrell, R., Lehner, T., Liang, K. Y., Eaves, L., Hoh, J. et al. (2009). The interaction between the serotonin transporter gene (5-HTTLPR), stressful life events, and risk of depression: a meta-analysis. *Journal of the American Medical Association, 301,* 2462–2471.

Robins, E. & Guze, S. B. (1970). Establishment of diagnostic validity in psychiatric illness: its application to schizophrenia. *American Journal of Psychiatry, 126,* 983–987.

Robinson, D. G., Woerner, M. G., McMeniman, M., Mendelowitz, A. & Bilder, R. M. (2004). Systematic and functional recovery from a first episode of schizophrenia or schizoaffective disorder. *American Journal of Psychiatry, 161,* 473–479.

Robinson, D. S. (2007). The role of dopamine and norepinephrine in depression. *Primary Psychiatry, 14,* 21–23.

Rosen, G. M. (2006). DSM's cautionary guideline to rule out malingering can protect the PTSD data base. *Journal of Anxiety Disorders, 20,* 530–535.

Rosenhan, D. (1973). On being sane in insane places. *Science, 179,* 250–258.

Rosenhan, D. L. & Seligman, M. E. P. (1989). *Abnormal Psychology.* New York: Norton.

Ross, C. A. (1997). *Dissociative Identity Disorder: Diagnosis, Clinical Features, and Treatment of Multiple Personality.* New York: Wiley.

Roy, M., McNeale, M. C., Pedersen, N. L., Mathe, A. A. & Kendler, K. S. (1995). A twin study of generalized anxiety disorder and major depression. *Psychological Medicine, 25,* 1037–1049.

Rudolph, K. D., Hammen, C., Burge, D., Lindberg, N., Herzberg, D. & Daley, S. E. (2000). Toward an interpersonal life-stress model of depression: the developmental context of stress generation. *Development and Psychopathology, 12*, 215–234.

Rueve, M. E. & Welton, R. S. (2008). Violence and mental illness. *Psychiatry, 5* (5), 34-48.

Ruscio, J. (2003). Diagnoses and the behaviors they denote: a critical evaluation of the labeling theory of mental illness. *Scientific Review of Mental Health Practice, 3*, 5–22.

Rutter, M. (2000). Genetic studies of autism: from the 1970s into the millennium. *Journal of Abnormal Child Psychology, 28*, 3–14.

Rutter, M. (2009). Gene-environment interactions: biologically valid pathway or artifact. *Archives of General Psychiatry, 66*, 1287–1289.

Sadoff, R. L. (1992). In defense of the insanity defense. *Psychiatric Annals, 22*(11), 556–560.

Saha, S., Chant, D., Welham, J. & McGrath, J. (2005). A systematic review of the prevalence of schizophrenia. *PLoS Medicine, 2*, e141. Retrieved from http://dx.doi.org/10.1371/ journal.pmed.0020141.

Salekin, R. T. (2002). Psychopathy and therapeutic pessimism: clinical lore or clinical reality? *Clinical Psychology Review, 22*, 79–112.

Salsman, N. L. & Linehan, M. M. (2012). An investigation of the relationships among negative affect, difficulties in emotion regulation, and features of borderline personality disorder. *Journal of Psychopathology and Behavioral Assessment, 34*(2), 260–267.

Samuels, J. F., Grados, M. A., Planalp, E. & Bienvenu, O. J. (2011). A genetic understanding of OCD and spectrum disorders. *The Oxford Handbook of Obsessive Compulsive and Spectrum Disorders*. New York: Oxford University Press, pp. 111–127.

Sanderson, W. C. & Dublin, R. A. (2010). Panic disorder. *Corsini Encyclopedia of Psychology*. Wiley Online Library.

Sar, V., Koyuncu, A., Ozturk, E, Yargic, L., Kundakci, T., Yazici, A. et al. (2007). Dissociative disorders in the psychiatric emergency ward. *General Hospital Psychiatry, 29*, 45–50.

Satel, S. L. (1999). *Drug Treatment: The Case for Coercion*. Washington, DC: American Enterprise Institute Press.

Satyanarayana, S., Enns, M. W., Cox, B. J. & Sareen, J. (2009). Prevalence and correlates of chronic depression in the Canadian community health survey: mental health and well-being. *Canadian Journal of Psychiatry. Revue Canadienne de Psychiatrie, 54*(6), 389.

Savitz, J., Solms, M., Pietersen, E., Ramesar, R. & Flor-Henry, P. (2004). Dissociative identity disorder associated with mania and change in handedness. *Cognitive and Behavioral Neurology, 17*, 233–237.

Schaler, J. (2004). *Addiction is a Choice*. La Salle, IL: Open Court Books.

Scheff, T. J. (1984). *Being Mentally Ill: A Sociological Theory*. New York: Aldine.

Scher, C. D., Ingram, R. E. & Segal, Z. V. (2005). Cognitive reactivity and vulnerability: empirical evaluation of construct activation and cognitive diatheses in unipolar depression. *Clinical Psychology Review, 25*, 487–510.

Schneidman, E. S., Farberow, N. L. & Litman, R. E. (1970). *The Psychology of Suicide*. New York: Science House.

Schreiber, F. R. (1973). *Sybil*. New York: Warner.

Schwartz, J. M. & Bayette, B. (1996). *Brain Lock. Free Yourself from Obsessive-Compulsive Behaviour: A Four-Step Self-Treatment Method to Change Your Brain Chemistry*. New York: HarperCollins.

Sciutto, M. J. & Eisenberg, M. (2007). Evaluating the evidence for and against the overdiagnosis of ADHD. *Journal of Attention Disorders, 11*, 106–113.

Segrin, C. (2000). Social skill deficits associated with depression. *Clinical Psychology Review, 20*, 379–403.

Seidman, L. J., Pantelis, C., Keshavan, M., Faraone, S., Goldstein, J., Horton, N. J. et al. (2003). A review and new report of medial temporal lobe dysfunction as a vulnerability indicator for schizophrenia: a magnetic resonance imaging morphometric family study of the parahippocampal gyrus. *Schizophrenia Bulletin, 29*, 803–830.

Selby, E. A, Anestis, M. D., Bender, T. W. & Joiner, T. E., Jr. (2009). An exploration of the emotional cascade model in borderline personality disorder. *Journal of Abnormal Psychology, 118*, 375–387.

Selby, E. A. & Joiner, T. E., Jr. (2009). Cascades of emotion: the emergence of borderline personality disorder from emotional and behavioral dysregulation. *Review of General Psychology, 12*, 219–229.

Seligman, M. E. P. (1975). *Helplessness: On Depression, Development, and Death*. San Francisco, CA: Freeman.

Seligman, M. E. P. & Maier, S. F. (1967). Failure to escape traumatic shock. *Journal of Experimental Psychology, 74*, 1–9.

Shea, S. C. (1998). *Psychiatric Interviewing: The Art of Understanding* (2nd ed). Philadelphia: W. B. Saunders.

Sher, L. (2011). Is it Possible to Predict Suicide? *Australian and New Zealand Journal of Psychiatry, 45* (4), 341.

Shih, J. H., Eberhart, N., Hammen, C. & Brennan, P. A. (2006). Differential exposure and reactivity to interpersonal stress predict sex differences in adolescent depression. *Journal of Clinical Child and Adolescent Psychology, 35*, 103–115.

Showalter, E. (1997). *Hystories: Hysterical Epidemics and Modern Culture.* New York: Columbia University Press.

Siever, L. J. & Davis, K. L. (2004). The pathophysiology of schizophrenia disorders: perspectives from the spectrum. *American Journal of Psychiatry, 161,* 398–413.

Sibley, M. H., Swanson, J. M., Arnold, L. E., Hechtman, L. T., Owens, E. B., Stehli, A., . . . Pelham, W. E. (2016, Sept). Defining ADHD symptom persistence in adulthood: optimizing sensitivity and specificity, *Journal of Child Psychology and Psychiatry.* HYPERLINK "http://dx.doi.org/10.1111/jcpp.12620" DOI: 10.1111/jcpp.12620

Silveira, J. M. & Seeman, M. V. (1995). Shared psychotic disorder: a critical review of the literature. *Canadian Journal of Psychiatry, 40,* 389–395.

Silver, E., Cirincione, C. & Steadman, H. J. (1994). Demythologizing inaccurate perceptions of the insanity defense. *Law and Human Behavior, 18,* 63–70.

Simeon, D., Gross, S., Guralnik, O., Stein, D. J., Schmeidler, J. & Hollander, E. (1997). Feeling unreal: 30 cases of DSM-III-R depersonalization. *American Journal of Psychiatry, 154,* 1107–1113.

Simon, R. I. (2006). Imminent suicide: the illusion of short-term prediction. *Suicide and Life-Threatening Behavior, 36,* 296–301.

Simons, R. C. (2001). Introduction to culture-bound syndromes. *Psychiatric Times, 18*(11), 283–292.

Simons, R. C. & Hughes, C. C. (1986). *The Culture-Bound Syndromes: Folk Illnesses of Psychiatric and Anthropological Interest.* Boston: D. Reidel.

Skeem, J. L., Monahan, J. & Mulvey, E. P. (2002). Psychopathy, treatment involvement, and subsequent violence among civil psychiatric patients. *Law and Human Behavior, 26,* 577–603.

Skeem, J. L., Polaschek, D. L., Patrick, C. J. & Lilienfeld, S. O. (2011). Psychopathic personality bridging the gap between scientific evidence and public policy. *Psychological Science in the Public Interest, 12,* 95–162.

Slade, T. & Andrews, G. (2005). Latent structure of depression in a community sample: a taxometric analysis. *Psychological Medicine, 35,* 489–497.

Slade, T., Johnston, A., Brown, M. A. O., Andrews, G. & Whiteford, H. (2009). 2007 National Survey of Mental Health and Wellbeing: methods and key findings. *Australian and New Zealand Journal of Psychiatry, 43,* 594–605.

Slater, L. (2004). *Opening Skinner's Box: Great Psychological Experiments of the 20th Century.* New York: W. W. Norton.

Snyder, S. H. (1975). *Madness and the Brain.* New York: McGraw-Hill.

Solomon, D. A., Leon, A. C., Coryell, W. H., Endicott, J., Li, C., Fiedorowicz, J. G. et al. (2010). Longitudinal course of bipolar I disorder: duration of mood episodes. *Archives of General Psychiatry, 67,* 339–347.

Spanos, N. P. (1994). Multiple identity enactments and multiple personality disorder: a sociocognitive perspective. *Psychological Bulletin, 116,* 143–165.

Spanos, N. P. (1996). *Multiple Identities and False Memories: A Sociocognitive Perspective.* Washington, DC: American Psychological Association.

Speisman, B. B., Storch, E. A. & Abramowitz, J. S. (2011). Postpartum obsessive-compulsive disorder. *Journal of Obstetric, Gynecologic, and Neonatal nursing, 40*(6), 680-690.

Spirito, A. & Esposito-Smythers, C. (2006). Attempted and completed suicide in adolescence. *Annual Review of Clinical Psychology, 2,* 237–266.

Spitzer, R. L. (1975). On pseudoscience, science, logic in remission, and psychiatric diagnosis: a critique of Rosenhan's 'On being sane in insane places'. *Journal of Abnormal Psychology, 84,* 442–452.

Staal, W. G., Pol, H. E. H., Schnack, H. G., Mechteld, L. C., Hoogendoorn, M. S. Jellema, K. et al. (2000). Structural brain abnormalities in patients with schizophrenia and their healthy siblings. *American Journal of Psychiatry, 157,* 416–421.

Starr, L. R. & Davila, J. (2008). Excessive reassurance seeking, depression, and interpersonal rejection: a meta-analytic review. *Journal of Abnormal Psychology, 17,* 762–765.

Steadman, H. J., Mulvey, E. P., Monahan, J., Robbins, P. C., Appelbaum, P., Grisso, T. et al. (1998). Violence by people discharged from acute psychiatric inpatient facilities and by others in the same neighborhoods. *Archives of General Psychiatry, 5,* 1–9.

Stein, D. J., Phillips, K. A., Bolton, D., Fulford, K. W. M., Sadler, J. Z. & Kendler, K. S. (2010). What is a mental/psychiatric disorder? From DSM-IV to DSM-V. *Psychological Medicine, 40(11),* 1759–1765.

Stein, M. B., Jang, K. L. & Livesley, W. J. (1999). Heritability of anxiety sensitivity: a twin study. *American Journal of Psychiatry, 156,* 246–251.

Stern, A. (1938). Psychoanalytic investigation of and therapy in the borderline group of neuroses. *Psychoanalytical Quarterly, 7,* 467–489.

Stirk, W., Dierks, T., Hubl, D. & Horn, H. (2008). Hallucinations, thought disorders, and the language domain in schizophrenia. *Clinical EEG and Neuroscience, 39,* 91–94.

Stone, A. A. (1982). The insanity defense on trial. *Hospital and Community Psychiatry, 33,* 636–640.

Susser, E. S. & Lin, S. P. (1992). Schizophrenia after prenatal exposure to the Dutch Hunger Winter of 1944–1945. *Archives of General Psychiatry, 49*, 983–988.

Swanson, J. M. & Castellanos, F. X. (2002). Biological bases of ADHD—neuroanatomy, genetics, and pathophysiology. In P. S. Jensen & J. R. Cooper (eds), *Attention Deficit Hyperactivity Disorder: State of the Science—Best Practices*. Kingston, NJ: Civic Research Institute.

Swartz, M., Blazer, D., George, L. & Winfield, I. (1990). Estimating the prevalence of borderline personality disorder in the community. *Journal of Personality Disorders, 4*, 257–272.

Szasz, T. (1978). Should psychiatric patients ever be hospitalized involuntarily? Under any circumstances—no. In J. P. Brady & H. K. H. Brodie (eds), *Controversy in Psychiatry*. Philadelphia: W. B. Saunders, pp. 965–977.

Szasz, T. (1991). *Insanity*. Chichester, UK: Wiley.

Szasz, T. S. (1960). The myth of mental illness. *American Psychologist, 15*, 113–118.

Szasz, T. S. (2006). *Mental Illness as a Brain Disease: A Brief History Lesson*. Cybercenter for Liberty and Responsibility. Retrieved 22 December 2006, from www.szasz.com/freeman13.html.

Tallis, F. (2011). Primary hypothyroidism: a case for vigilance in the psychological treatment of depression. *British Journal of Clinical Psychology, 32*(3), 261–270.

Taylor, J. & Lang, A. R. (2006). Psychopathy and substance use disorders. In C. J. Patrick (ed.), *Handbook of Psychopathy*. New York: Guilford, pp. 495–511.

Teplin, L. A., McClelland, G. M., Abram, K. M. & Weiner, D. (2005). Crime victimization in adults with severe mental illness: comparison with the national crime victimization survey. *Archives of General Psychiatry, 62*, 911–921.

Thase, M. E., Jindal, R. & Howland, R. H. (2002). Biological aspects of depression. In I. H. Gotlib & C. L. Hammen (eds), *Handbook of Depression*. New York: Guilford, pp. 192–218.

Thomas, P. (1997). *The Dialectics of Schizophrenia*. Bristol: Free Association Books.

Torgersen, S., Lygren, S., Oien, P. A., Skre, I., Onstad, S., Edvardsen, J. et al. (2000). A twin study of personality disorders. *Comprehensive Psychiatry, 41*, 416–425.

Torrey, E. F. (1997). *Out of the Shadows: Confronting America's Mental Illness Crisis*. New York: John Wiley.

Torrey, E. G., Miller, J., Rawlings, R. & Yolken, R. H. (1997). Seasonality of births in schizophrenia and bipolar disorder: a review of the literature. *Schizophrenia Research, 28*, 1–38.

Trull, T. J. & Durett, C. A. (2005). Categorical and dimensional models of personality disorder. *Annual Review of Clinical Psychology, 1*, 355–380.

Van der Kloet, D., Giesbrecht, T., Lynn, S.J., Merckelbach, H. & de Zutter, A. (2012). Sleep normalization and decreases in dissociative experiences: evaluation in an inpatient sample. *Journal of Abnormal Psychology, 121*, 140–150.

Van Grootheest, D. S., Cath, D. C., Beekman, A. T. & Boomsma, D. I. (2007). Genetic and environmental influences on obsessive-compulsive symptoms in adults: a population-based twin-family study. *Psychological Medicine, 37*, 1635–1644.

Verdoux, H. (2004). Perinatal risk factors for schizophrenia: how specific are they? *Current Psychiatry Reports, 6*, 162–167.

Vicary, D. A. & Westerman, T. (2004). 'That's just the way he is': some implications of Aboriginal mental health beliefs. *Australian e-Journal for the Advancement of Mental Health, 3*(3), 1–10.

Videbech, P. & Ravnkilde, B. (2004). Hippocampal volume and depression: a meta-analysis of MRI studies. *American Journal of Psychiatry, 161*, 1957–1966.

Vita, A., Dieci, G., Giobbio, A., Caputo, L., Ghrinighelli, M., Comazzi, M. et al. (1995). Language and thought disorder in schizophrenia: brain morphological correlates. *Schizophrenia Research, 15*, 243–251.

Volgmaier, M. M., Seidman, L. J., Niznikiewicz, M. A., Dickey, C. C., Shenton, M. E. & McCarley, R. W. (2000). Verbal and nonverbal neuropsychological test performance in subjects with schizotypal personality disorder. *American Journal of Psychiatry, 157*, 787–797.

Voncken, M. J., Bogels, S. M. & deVries, K. (2003). Interpretation and judgmental biases in social phobias. *Behavior Research and Therapy, 41*, 1481–1488.

Vriends, N., Pfaltz, M. C., Novianti, P. & Hadiyono, J. (2013). Taijin Kyofusho and social anxiety and their clinical relevance in Indonesia and Switzerland. *Frontiers in Psychology, 4*. doi:10.3389/fpsyg.2013.00003.

Wahl, O. R. (1997). *Media Madness: Public Images of the Mentally Ill*. New Brunswick, NJ: Rutgers University Press.

Wakefield, A. J., Murch, S., Anthony, A., Linnell, J., Casson, D. M., Casson, M. et al. (1998). Ileal lymphoid nodular hyperplasia, non-specific colitis, and regressive developmental disorder in children. *Lancet, 351*, 637–641.

Wakefield, J. C. (1992). The concept of mental disorder: on the boundary between biological facts and social values. *American Psychologist, 47*, 373–388.

Wakefield, J. C. & First, M. B. (2012). Placing symptoms in context: the role of contextual criteria in reducing false positives in Diagnostic and Statistical Manual of Mental Disorders Diagnoses. *Comprehensive Psychiatry, 53*(2), 130–139.

Waldman, I. D., Lilienfeld, S. O. & Lahey, B. B. (1995). Toward construct validity in the childhood disruptive behavior disorders: classification and diagnosis in DSM-IV and beyond. In T. H. Ollendick & R. J. Prinz (eds), *Advances in Clinical Child Psychology* (Vol. 17). New York: Plenum, pp. 323–363.

Walker, E., Kestler, L., Bollini, A. & Hochman, K. (2004). Schizophrenia: etiology and course. *Annual Review of Psychology, 55*, 401–430.

Walker, E. & Lewine, R. J. (1990). Prediction of adult-onset schizophrenia from childhood home movies of the patients. *American Journal of Psychiatry, 147*, 1052–1056.

Walker, E. F., Baum, K. & DiForio, D. (1998). Developmental changes in the behavioral expression of vulnerability for schizophrenia. In M. Lenzenweger & B. Dworkin (eds), *Experimental Psychopathology and Pathogenesis of Schizophrenia*. Washington, DC: American Psychological Association, pp. 469–492.

Walker, E. F. & DiForio, D. (1997). Schizophrenia: a neural-diathesis stress model. *Psychological Review, 104*, 1–19.

Wallechinsky, D., Wallace, D. & Wallace, H. (1977). *The Book of Lists*. New York: Bantam.

Watson, J. B. & Rayner, R. (1920). Conditioned emotional reactions. *Journal of Experimental Psychology, 3*, 1–14.

Watters, E. (2010). *Crazy Like Us: The Globalization of the American Psyche*. New York: Free Press.

Wei, M., Mallinckrodt, B., Larson, L. M. & Zakalik, R. A. (2005). Adult attachment, depressive symptoms, and validation from self versus others. *Journal of Counseling Psychology, 52*, 368–377.

Weinberger, D. R. (1987). Implications of normal brain development for the pathogenesis of schizophrenia. *Archives of General Psychiatry, 44*, 660–669.

Westerman, T. G. (2003). Development of an inventory to assess the moderating effects of cultural resilience with Aboriginal youth at risk of depression, anxiety and suicidal behaviours. Unpublished PhD thesis, Curtin University, Perth.

Widiger, T. A. & Clark, L. A. (2000). Toward DSM-V and the classification of psychopathology. *Psychological Bulletin, 126*, 946–963.

Widom, C. S. (1977). A methodology for studying noninstitutionalized psychopaths. *Journal of Consulting and Clinical Psychology, 45*, 674—683.

Willner, P. (1995). Animal models of depression—validity and applications. *Depression and Mania, 49*, 19–41.

Wilson, C. (2005). What is autism? *New Scientist, 187*, 39.

Wilson, N. (2003). Commercializing mental health issues: entertainment, advertising, and psychological advice. In S. O. Lilienfeld, S. J. Lynn & J. M. Lohr (eds), *Science and Pseudoscience in Clinical Psychology*. New York: Guilford, pp. 425–459.

Wing, L. & Potter, D. (2002). The epidemiology of autistic spectrum disorders: is the prevalence rising? *Mental Retardation and Developmental Disabilities Research Reviews, 8*, 151–161.

Wolfsdorf, B. A., Freeman, J., D'Eramo, K., Overholser, J. & Spirito, A. (2003). Mood states: depression, anger, and anxiety. In A. Spirito & J. Overholser (eds), *Evaluating and Treating Adolescent Suicide Attempters: From Research to Practice*. New York: Academic Press, pp. 53–88.

Wolke, D., Rizzo, P. & Woods, S. (2002). Persistent infant crying and hyperactivity problems in middle childhood. *Pediatrics, 109*, 1054–1060.

Woodward, L. J., Fergusson, D. M. & Horwood, L. J. (2000). Driving outcomes of young people with attentional difficulties in adolescence. *Journal of the American Academy of Child and Adolescent Psychiatry, 39*, 627–634.

Wright, A. G., Krueger, R. F., Hobbs, M. J., Markon, K. E., Eaton, N. R. & Slade, T. (2013). The structure of psychopathology: toward an expanded quantitative empirical model. *Journal of Abnormal Psychology, 122*, 281–294.

Wymbs, B. T., Pelham, W. E., Jr., Moline, B. S. B., Gnagy, E. M., Wilson, T. K. & Greenhouse, J. B. (2008). Rate and predictors of divorce among parents of youths with ADHD. *Journal of Consulting and Clinical Psychology, 76*, 735–744.

Yamey, G. & Shaw, P. (2002). Is extreme racism a mental illness? No. *Western Journal of Medicine, 176*, 5.

Yan-Meier, L., Eberhart, N. K., Hammen, C. L., Gitlin, M., Sokolski, K. & Altshuler, L. (2011). Stressful life events predict delayed functional recovery following treatment for mania in bipolar disorder. *Psychiatry Research, 186*, 267–271.

Youngren, M. A. & Lewinsohn, P. M. (1980). The functional relationship between depressed and problematic interpersonal behavior. *Journal of Abnormal Psychology, 89*, 333–341.

Yurgelun-Todd, D. A., Gruber, S.A., Kanayama, G., Killgore, W. D., Baird, A. A. & Young, A. D. (2000). fMRI during affect discrimination in bipolar affective disorder. *Bipolar Disorder, 3*, 237–248.

Zanarini, M. C., Horwood, J., Wolke, D., Waylen, A., Fitzmaurice, G. & Grant, B. F. (2011). Prevalence of DSM-IV borderline personality disorder in two community samples: 6,330 English 11-year-olds and 34,653 American adults. *Journal of Personality Disorders, 25*, 607–619.

Zborowski, M. J. & Garske, J. P. (1993). Interpersonal deviance and consequent social impact in hypothetically schizophrenia-prone men. *Journal of Abnormal Psychology, 102*, 482–489.

Zeier, J. D., Baskin-Sommers, A. R., Hiatt Racer, K. D. & Newman, J. P. (2012). Cognitive control deficits associated with antisocial personality disorder and psychopathy. *Personality Disorders: Theory, Research, and Treatment, 3*, 283–293.

Zimmerman, M. (1994). Diagnosing personality disorders: a review of issues and research methods. *Archives of General Psychiatry, 51*, 225–245.

Zinbarg, R. E. & Barlow, D. H. (1996). The structure of anxiety and the anxiety disorders: a hierarchical model. *Journal of Abnormal Psychology, 105*, 81–193.

Zivotofsky, A. Z., Edelman, S., Green, T., Fostick, L. & Strous, R. D. (2007). Hemisphere asymmetry in schizophrenia as revealed through line bisection, line trisection, and letter cancellation. *Brain Research, 1142*, 70–79.

Zubin, J. & Spring, B. (1977). Vulnerability: a new view of schizophrenia. *Journal of Abnormal Psychology, 86*, 103–126.

Zuckerman, M. (1989). Personality in the third dimension: a psychobiological approach. *Personality and Individual Differences, 10*, 391–418.

Zuroff, D. C., Mongrain, M. & Santor, D. A. (2004). Investing in the personality vulnerability research program: current dividends and future growth. Rejoinder to Coyne, Thompson, and Whiffen. *Psychological Bulletin, 130*, 518–522.

Chapter 6

Affenito, S. G., Franko, D. L., Striegel-Moore, R. H., & Thompson, D. (2012). Behavioral determinants of obesity: research findings and policy implications. *Journal of Obesity, 2012.*

Ahern, N. R., & Sole, M. L. (2010). Drinking games and college students—Part 1: Problem description. *Journal of Psychosocial Nursing and Mental Health Services, 48*(2), 17–20. doi: 10.3928/02793695-20100108-03

Alcohol and Drug Abuse Institute, University of Washington. (2012, December). Marijuana: Science-based information for the public. Retrieved from http://adai.washington.edu

American Academy of Periodontology. (2013). Gum disease risk factors. Retrieved from www.perio.org

American Cancer Society. (2010, July). Guide to quitting smoking. Retrieved from www.cancer.org

American Cancer Society. (2013). Cancer facts & figures 2013. Retrieved from www.cancer.org

American Cancer Society. (2013, January). Questions about smoking, tobacco, and health: What about more exotic forms of smoking tobacco, such as clove cigarettes, bidis, and hookahs?" Retrieved from www.cancer.org

American College Health Association. (2013). National College Health Assessment II: Reference Group Executive Summary Fall 2012. Retrieved from www.acha-ncha.org

American Heart Association. (2013). About cholesterol. Retrieved from http://www.heart.org

American Heart Association (2013). AHA statistical update: Heart disease and stroke statistics —2013 update. *Circulation, 127*, e6–e245. Retrieved from http://circ.ahajournals.org

American Heart Association. (2011). Alcohol and cardiovascular disease. Retrieved from http://www.heart.org

American Heart Association. (2012, October). Stroke risk factors. Retrieved from www.strokeassociation.org

American Lung Association. (2011, June). General smoking facts. Retrieved from www.lung.org

American Lung Association. (2012, March). Benefits of quitting. Retrieved from www.lungusa.org

American Psychiatric Association. (2000). *Diagnostic and Statistical Manual of Mental Disorders, Text Revision (DSM-IV-TR)*. Washington, DC: Author.

Arria, A. (2013, January 19). *College student success: The impact of health concerns and substance abuse.* Lecture presented at the NASPA Alcohol and Mental Health Conference, Fort Worth, TX.

Arria, A. M., Garnier-Dykstra, L. M., Caldeira, K. M., Vincent, K. B., Winick, E. R., & O'Grady, K. E. (2013). Drug use patterns and continuous enrollment in college: Results from a longitudinal study. *Journal of Studies on Alcohol and Drugs, 74*(1), 71–83.

Arria, A. M., Garnier-Dykstra, L. M., Cook, E. T., Caldeira, K. M., Vincent, K. B., Baron, R. A., & O'Grady, K. E. (2013). Drug use patterns in young adulthood and post-college employment. *Drug and Alcohol Dependence, 127*(1), 23–30.

Arriola, L., Martinez-Camblor, P., Larrañaga, N., Basterretxea, M., Amiano, P., Moreno-Iribas, C., . . . Barricarte, A. (2010). Alcohol intake and the risk of coronary heart disease in the Spanish EPIC cohort study. *Heart, 96*(2), 124–130. doi:10.1136/hrt.2009.173419

Asbridge, M., Hayden, J. A., & Cartwright, J. L. (2012). Acute cannabis consumption and motor vehicle collision risk: systematic review of observational studies and meta-analysis. *BMJ, 344*, e536. doi: 10.1136/bmj.e536

Australian Bureau of Statistics. (2014). *Australian Health Survey: Nutrition First Results - Foods and Nutrients, 2011–12* (No. 4364.0.55.007). Canberra: Author. Retrieved from http://www.abs.gov.au/ausstats/abs@.nsf/Lookup/by%20Subject/4364.0.55.007~2011-12~Main%20Features~Non-alcoholic%20beverages~701

Australian Bureau of Statistics. (2015). *National Health Survey: First Results, 2014-15* (No. 4364.0.55.001). Canberra: Author. Retrieved from http://www.abs.gov.au/ausstats/abs@.nsf/mf/4364.0.55.001

Australian Drug Foundation. (2016, May). *GHB* [Fact sheet]. Retrieved from http://www.druginfo.adf.org.au/images/GHB-25may16.pdf

Australian Institute of Health and Welfare. (2010). *Australia's health 2010* (No. AUS 122). Canberra: Author. Retrieved from http://www.aihw.gov.au/WorkArea/DownloadAsset.aspx?id=6442452962

Australian Institute of Health and Welfare. (2011). *2010 National Drug Strategy Household Survey report* (No. PHE 145). Canberra: Author. Retrieved from http://www.aihw.gov.au/WorkArea/DownloadAsset.aspx?id=10737421139&libID=10737421138

Australian Institute of Health and Welfare. (2014a). *Australia's health 2014* (No. AUS 178). Canberra: Author. Retrieved from http://www.aihw.gov.au/WorkArea/DownloadAsset.aspx?id=60129548150

Australian Institute of Health and Welfare. (2014b). *National Drug Strategy Household Survey detailed report 2013* (No. PHE 183). Canberra: Author. Retrieved from http://www.aihw.gov.au/WorkArea/DownloadAsset.aspx?id=60129549848

Australian Institute of Health and Welfare. (2016a). *Australian Cancer Incidence and Mortality (ACIM) books: Lung cancer.* Canberra: Author. Retrieved from http://www.aihw.gov.au/acim-books/

Australian Institute of Health and Welfare. (2016b). *Leading causes of death.* Canberra: Author. Retrieved from http://www.aihw.gov.au/deaths/leading-causes-of-death/#data

Barbosa, P. C. R., Mizumoto, S., Bogenschutz, M. P., & Strassman, R. J. (2012). Health status of ayahuasca users. *Drug Testing and Analysis, 4*(7–8), 601–609.

Barclay, A. W., & Brand-Miller, J. (2011). The Australian paradox: a substantial decline in sugars intake over the same timeframe that overweight and obesity have increased. *Nutrients, 3*(4), 491–504.

Barry, A. E., & Piazza-Gardner, A. K. (2012). Drunkorexia: Understanding the co-occurrence of alcohol consumption and eating/exercise weight management behaviors. *Journal of American College Health, 60*(3), 236–243. doi:10.1080/07448481.2011.587487

Begg, S., Vos, T., Barker, B., Stevenson, C., Stanley, L., & Lopez, A. D. (2007). *The burden of disease and injury in Australia 2003* (cat. no. PHE 82). Canberra: Australian Institute of Health and Welfare. Retrieved from www.aihw.gov.au/WorkArea/DownloadAsset.aspx?id=6442459747

Berkey, C. S., Willett, W. C., Frazier, A. L., Rosner, B., Tamimi, R. M., Rockett, H. R., & Colditz, G. A. (2010). Prospective study of adolescent alcohol consumption and risk of benign breast disease in young women. *Pediatrics, 125*(5), e1081–e1087. doi: 10.1542/peds.2009-2347

Bogle, K. E., & Smith, B. H. (2009). Illicit methylphenidate use: A review of prevalence, availability, pharmacology, and consequences. *Current Drug Abuse Reviews, 2*(2), 157–176.

Burke, S. C., Cremeens, J., Vail-Smith, K., & Woolsey, C. (2010). Drunkorexia: Calorie restriction prior to alcohol consumption among college freshman. *Journal of Alcohol and Drug Education, 54*(2), 17-34.

California Department of Alcohol and Drug Programs. (2012). Frequently asked questions: General [pp. 325-326].

Cameron, J. M., Heidelberg, N., Simmons, L., Lyle, S. B., Mitra-Varma, K., & Correia, C. (2010). Drinking game participation among undergraduate students attending National Alcohol Screening Day. *Journal of American College Health, 58*(5), 499–506. doi: 10.1080/07448481003599096

Campaign for Tobacco-Free Kids. (2012, March). Tobacco company marketing to kids. Retrieved from www.tobaccofreekids.org

Campaign for Tobacco-Free Kids. (2012, December). State cigarette excise tax rates & rankings. Retrieved from www.tobaccofreekids.org

Campaign for Tobacco Free Kids. (2013, February). The toll of tobacco use in the USA. Retrieved from www.tobaccofreekids.org

Cataldo, J. K., Prochaska, J. J., & Glantz, S. A. (2010). Cigarette smoking is a risk factor for Alzheimer's Disease: An analysis controlling for tobacco industry affiliation. *Journal of Alzheimer's Disease, 19*(2), 465–480. doi: 10.3233/JAD-2010-1240

Center of Behavioral Health Statistics and Quality. (2012). Nearly half of college student treatment admissions were for primary alcohol abuse. *Data Spotlight.* Retrieved from www.samhsa.gov

Centers for Disease Control and Prevention. (2006). *The health consequences of involuntary exposure to tobacco smoke: A report of the Surgeon General.* Atlanta, GA: US Department of Health and Human Services. Retrieved from www.cdc.gov

Centers for Disease Control and Prevention. (2008a). Alcohol-Related Disease Impact (ARDI). Retrieved from http://apps.nccd.cdc.gov

Centers for Disease Control and Prevention. (2008b). Smoking-attributable mortality, years of potential life lost, and productivity losses—United States, 2000-2004. *Morbidity and Mortality Weekly Report, 57*(45), 1226-1228.

Centers for Disease Control and Prevention. (2010a). Fetal alcohol spectrum disorders (FASDs) data and statistics. Retrieved from www.cdc.gov

Centers for Disease Control and Prevention. (2010b). *How tobacco smoke causes disease: the biology and behavioral basis for smoking-attributable disease: A report of the Surgeon General.* Atlanta, GA: Author. Retrieved from www.ncbi.nlm.nih.gov

Centers for Disease Control and Prevention. (2010c). Tobacco control state highlights 2010. Retrieved from www.cdc.gov

Centers for Disease Control and Prevention. (2011). CDC health disparities and inequalities report – United States, 2011, Supplement: Cigarette smoking – United States, 1965–2008. *Morbidity and Mortality Weekly Report 60*, 109–113.

Centers for Disease Control and Prevention. (2011, June). Smoking and tobacco use: Bidis and kreteks. Retrieved from www.cdc.gov

Centers for Disease Control and Prevention. (2011, October-a). Excessive drinking costs U.S. $233.5 billion. Retrieved from www.cdc.gov

Centers for Disease Control and Prevention. (2011, October-b). Injury prevention and control: Home and recreational safety: fire deaths and injuries. Retrieved from www.cdc.gov

Centers for Disease Control and Prevention. (2011, November). Tobacco use: Smoking cessation. Retrieved from www.cdc.gov

Centers for Disease Control and Prevention. (2012, January). Health effects of cigarette smoking. Retrieved from www.cdc.gov

Centers for Disease Control and Prevention. (2012, March). Smoking and tobacco use facts: Secondhand smoke (SHS) facts. Retrieved from www.cdc.gov

Centers for Disease Control and Prevention. (2012, October-a). *Excessive alcohol use and risks to women's health: 2010* [Fact sheet]. Retrieved from www.cdc.gov

Centers for Disease Control and Prevention. (2012, October-b). Ten leading causes of death by age group. Retrieved from www.cdc.gov

Centers for Disease Control and Prevention. (2012, November-a). Pregnant? Don't smoke! Learn how and why to quit for good. Retrieved from www.cdc.gov

Centers for Disease Control and Prevention. (2012, November-b). Unintentional drowning: Get the facts. Retrieved from www.cdc.gov

Centers for Disease Control and Prevention. (2012, November-c). Youth and tobacco use, smoking and tobacco. Retrieved from www.cdc.gov

Centers for Disease Control and Prevention. (2012, November 9). Current cigarette smoking among adults — United States, 2011. *Morbidity and Mortality Weekly Report, 61*(44), 889-894.

Centers for Disease Control and Prevention. (2012, December). Adult cigarette smoking in the United States: Current estimate. Retrieved from www.cdc.gov

Centers for Disease Control and Prevention. (2013, January). Tobacco use and pregnancy. Retrieved from www.cdc.gov

Chen, W. Y., Rosner, B., Hankinson, S. E., Colditz, G. A., & Willett, W. C. (2011). Moderate alcohol consumption during adult life, drinking patterns, and breast cancer risk. *Journal of the American Medical Association, 306*(17), 1884–1890. doi: 10.1001/ jama.2011.1590

Clarke, J. M., & Lockett, T. (2014). Primary prevention of colorectal cancer. In *Cancer Forum* (Vol. 38, p. 6-10). The Cancer Council Australia.

Colditz, G. A., & Bohlke, K. (2015). Preventing breast cancer now by acting on what we already know. *NPJ Breast Cancer, 1,* 1–4.

College on Problems of Drug Dependence (CPDD). (2011, July 31). Methamphetamine abuse and Parkinson's disease. Retrieved from www.cpddblog.com

Connor, K. L., Vickers, M. H., Beltrand, J., Meaney, M. J., & Sloboda, D. M. (2012). Nature, nurture or nutrition? Impact of maternal nutrition on maternal care, offspring development and reproductive function. *The Journal of Physiology, 590*(9), 2167–2180.

Davis, K. C., Norris, J., Hessler, D. M., Zawacki, T., Morrison, D. M., & George, W. H. (2010). College women's sexual decision making: Cognitive mediation of alcohol expectancy effects. *Journal of American College Health, 58*(5), 481–490. doi: 10.1080/07448481003599112

Degenhardt, L., Larney, S., Chan, G., Dobbins, T., Weier, M., Roxburgh, A., . . . McKetin, R. (2016). Estimating the number of regular and dependent methamphetamine users in Australia, 2002–2014. *Med J Aust, 204*(4), 1.e3–1.e6.

Dietz, W., et al. (2014). Despite obesity rise, U.S. calories trending downward. *American Journal of Clinical Nutrition* (March 6, 2013). Retrieved from www.nlm.nih.gov

DiFulvio, G. T., Linowski, S. A., Mazziotti, J. S., & Puleo, E. (2012). Effectiveness of the Brief Alcohol and Screening Intervention for College Students (BASICS) program with a mandated population. *Journal of American College Health, 60*(4), 269–280. doi: 10.1080/07448481.2011.599352

Dobbin, M. (2014). Pharmaceutical drug misuse in Australia. *Australian Prescriber, 37*(3), 79–81.

Dos Santos, R. G., Grasa, E., Valle, M., Ballester, M. R., Bouso, J. C., Nomdedéu, J. F., . . . Riba, J. (2012). Pharmacology of ayahuasca administered in two repeated doses. *Psychopharmacology, 219*(4), 1039–1053.

Dunn, M., & White, V. (2011). The epidemiology of anabolic–androgenic steroid use among Australian secondary school students. *Journal of Science and Medicine in Sport, 14*(1), 10–14.

Elliott, E. J., Payne, J., Morris, A., Haan, E., & Bower, C. (2008). Fetal alcohol syndrome: A prospective national surveillance study. *Archives of Disease in Childhood, 93*(9), 732–737.

Erowid DXM (Dextromethorphan, DM) Vault. (n.d.). Retrieved from www.erowid.org

Everyday Health. (2011, May). A guide to using the nicotine patch. Retrieved from www.everydayhealth .com

Fetal Alcohol Spectrum Disorders (FASD) Center for Excellence. (2013). What Is FASD? Retrieved from www.fasdcenter.samhsa.gov

Family Smoking Prevention and Tobacco Control Act of 2009 [HR 1256], 111th Congress of the United States of America. Retrieved from www.govtrack.us

Gao, C., & Ogeil, R. (2014). *Alcohol's burden of disease in Australia.* Canberra: FARE and VicHealth in collaboration with Turning Point. Retrieved from www.turningpoint.org.au/site/DefaultSite/filesystem/documents/EMBARGO-FARE-Alcohol-Burden-of-disease-Report.pdf

Garnier-Dykstra, L. M., Caldeira, K. M., Vincent, K. B., O'Grady, K. E., & Arria, A. M. (2012). Nonmedical use of prescription stimulants during college: Four-year trends in exposure opportunity, use, motives, and sources. *Journal of American College Health, 60*(3), 226–234.

Garrard, J. (2009). *Active transport: Children and young people: An overview of recent evidence.* Melbourne: Vic Health. Retrieved from http://apo.org.au/resource/active-transport-children-and-young-people-overview-recent-evidence

Giles, S. M., Champion, H., Sutfin, E. L., McCoy, T. P., & Wagoner, K. (2009). Calorie restriction on drinking days: An examination of drinking consequences among college students. *Journal of American College Health, 57*(6), 603–610. doi: 10.3200/ JACH.57.6.603-610

Gillespie, C., Gray, K., Bailey, E., & Zivalich, J. (2012). The growing concern of poverty in the United States: An exploration of food prices and poverty on obesity rates for low-income citizens. *Undergraduate Economic Review, 8*(1), 1-38.

Grover, S., Coupal, L., Kouache, M., Lowensteyn, I., Marchand, S., & Campbell, N. (2011). Estimating the benefits of patient and physician adherence to cardiovascular prevention guidelines: the MyHealthCheckup Survey. *Canadian Journal of Cardiology, 27*(2), 159–166. doi: 10.1016/j.cjca.2011.01.007

Hallett, J., Howat, P. M., Maycock, B. R., McManus, A., Kypri, K., & Dhaliwal, S. S. (2012). Undergraduate student drinking and related harms at an Australian university: Web-based survey of a large random sample. *BMC Public Health, 12*(1), 1–8.

Harte, C. B., & Meston, C. M. (2013). Association between cigarette smoking and erectile tumescence: The mediating role of heart rate variability. *International Journal of Impotence Research, 25*(4), 155–159. doi: 10.1038/ ijir.2012.43

Harvard Health Letter. (2012, January). What is it about coffee? Retrieved from www.health.harvard.edu

Hingson, R., et al. (2009). Magnitude of alcohol-related mortality and morbidity among U.S. college students ages 18–24: Changes from 1998 to 2005. *Journal of Studies on Alcohol and Drugs*, 12–20.

Housden, C. R., Morein Zamir, S., & Sahakian, B. J. (2011). Cognitive enhancing drugs: Neuroscience and society. In J. Savulescu, R. ter Meulen, & G. Kahane (Eds.), *Enhancing human capacities* (pp. 113–126). Oxford: Blackwell Publishing Ltd.

Hughes, C. (2012). All beer and skittles?: A qualitative pilot study of the role of alcohol in university college life. *Australian Universities' Review*, *54*(2), 22–28.

Insurance Institute for Highway Safety. (2012). Fatality Facts 2010: Alcohol. Retrieved from www.iihs.org

International Agency for Research on Cancer. (2007). Smokeless tobacco and some tobacco-specific N-nitrosamines, *IARC Monographs on the Evaluation of Carcinogenic Risks to Humans* 89. World Health Organization. Retrieved from http://monographs.iarc.fr

Jackson, K. M., Rohsenow, D. J., Piasecki, T. M., Howland, J., & Richardson, A. E. (2013). Role of tobacco smoking in hangover symptoms among university students. *Journal of Studies on Alcohol and Drugs*, *74*(1), 41–49.

Jha, P., Ramasundarahettige, C., Landsman, V., Rostron, B., Thun, M., Anderson, R. N., . . . Peto, R. (2013). 21st-century hazards of smoking and benefits of cessation in the United States. *New England Journal of Medicine*, *368*(4), 341–350. doi: 10.1056/NEJMsa1211128

Johns Hopkins Health Alerts. (2012, March). Emphysema: Symptoms and remedies. Retrieved from www.johnshopkinshealthalerts.com

Johnston, L. D., O'malley, P. M., Bachman, J. G., & Schulenberg, J. E. (2011). Monitoring the Future National Survey results on drug use, 1975-2010. Volume II, college students & adults ages 19-50. *Institute for Social Research*. Retrieved from www.monitoringthefuture.org

Judd, S. E., & Tangpricha, V. (2009). Vitamin D deficiency and risk for cardiovascular disease. *The American Journal of the Medical Sciences*, *338*(1), 40-44.

Karam, E., Kypri, K., & Salamoun, M. (2007). Alcohol use among college students: An international perspective. *Current Opinion in Psychiatry*, *20*(3), 213–221.

Kendall, B. J., Wilson, L. F., Olsen, C. M., Webb, P. M., Neale, R. E., Bain, C. J., & Whiteman, D. C. (2015). Cancers in Australia in 2010 attributable to overweight and obesity. *Australian and New Zealand Journal of Public Health*, *39*(5), 452–457.

Kenney, S. R., LaBrie, J. W., Hummer, J. F., & Pham, A. T. (2012). Global sleep quality as a moderator of alcohol consumption and consequences in college students. *Addictive Behaviors*, *37*(4), 507–512. doi: 10.1016/ j.addbeh.2012.01.006

Klatsky, A. L. (2010). Alcohol and cardiovascular health. *Physiology & Behavior*, *100*(1), 76–81. doi: 10.1016/j.physbeh.2009

Kokkinos, P., Sheriff, H., & Kheirbek, R. (2011). Physical inactivity and mortality risk. *Cardiology Research and Practice*, *2011*. doi: 10.4061/2011/924945

Laslett, A.-M., Catalano, P., Chikritzhs, T., Dale, C., Doran, C., Ferris, J., . . . Mugavin, J. (2010). *The range and magnitude of alcohol's harm to others*. Fitzroy, Victoria: AER Centre for Alcohol Policy Research, Turning Point Alcohol and Drug Centre, Eastern Health. Retrieved from www.fare.org .au/wp-content/uploads/research/The-Range-and-Magnitude-of-Alcohols-Harm-to-Others.pdf

Lawyer, S., Resnick, H., Bakanic, V., Burkett, T., & Kilpatrick, D. (2010). Forcible, drug-facilitated, and incapacitated rape and sexual assault among undergraduate women. *Journal of American College Health*, *58*(5), 453–460. doi: 10.1080/07448480903540515

Lee, D., Sui, X., Church, T. S., Lavie, C. J., Jackson, A. S., & Blair, S. N. (2012). Changes in fitness and fatness on the development of cardiovascular disease risk factors: Hypertension, metabolic syndrome, and hypercholesterolemia. *Journal of the American College of Cardiology*, *59*(7), 665–672. doi: 10.1016/j. jacc.2011.11.013

Levin, A. (2012). Determining alcoholism proves complicated endeavour. *Psychiatric News*, *47*(24), 20. doi: 10.1176/appi. pn.2012.12b13

Lewis, M. A., Patrick, M. E., Lee, C. M., Kaysen, D. L., Mittman, A., & Neighbors, C. (2012). Use of protective behavioral strategies and their association to 21st birthday alcohol consumption and related negative consequences: A between-and within-person evaluation. *Psychology of Addictive Behaviors*, *26*(2), 179-186. doi: 10.1037/a0023797

Lewis, S. J., Zuccolo, L., Smith, G. D., Macleod, J., Rodriguez, S., Draper, E. S., . . . Ring, S. (2012). Fetal alcohol exposure and IQ at age 8: Evidence from a population-based birth-cohort study. *PloS One*, 7(11), e49407. Retrieved from www.plosone.org

Lopez-Quintero, C., de los Cobos, J. P., Hasin, D. S., Okuda, M., Wang, S., Grant, B. F., & Blanco, C. (2011). Probability and predictors of transition from first use to dependence on nicotine, alcohol, cannabis, and cocaine: Results of the National Epidemiologic Survey on Alcohol and Related Conditions (NESARC). *Drug and Alcohol Dependence, 115*(1), 120–130. doi: 10.1016/j.drugalcdep.2010.11.004

Manning, M., Smith, C., & Mazerolle, P. (2013). *The societal costs of alcohol misuse in Australia.* Canberra: Australian Institute of Criminology. Retrieved from www98.griffith.edu.au/dspace/bitstream/handle/10072/58981/85722_1.pdf?sequence=1

Marrone, J. A., Maddalozzo, G. F., Branscum, A. J., Hardin, K., Cialdella-Kam, L., Philbrick, K. A., . . . Iwaniec, U. T. (2012). Moderate alcohol intake lowers biochemical markers of bone turnover in postmenopausal women. *Journal of the North American Menopause Society 19*(9), 974-979.

McCabe, S. E. (2008). Misperceptions of non-medical prescription drug use: A web survey of college students. *Addictive Behaviors, 33*(5), 713–724.

Mehta, A. (2010). Management of cardiovascular risk associated with insulin resistance, diabetes, and the metabolic syndrome. *Postgraduate Medicine, 122*(3), 61–70. doi: 10.3810/pgm.2010.05.2143

Miller, T. R., Levy, D. T., Spicer, R. S., & Taylor, D. M. (2006). Societal costs of underage drinking. *Journal of Studies on Alcohol, 67*(4), 519–528.

Ministerial Council on Drug Strategy. (2011). *The National Drugs Strategy 2010-2015: A framework for action on alcohol, tobacco and other drugs.* Canberra: Commonwealth of Australia. Retrieved from www.nationaldrugstrategy.gov.au/internet/drugstrategy/Publishing.nsf/content/F978442D7B6B9415CA2577E90075956E/$File/round.pdf

Nagle, C. M., Wilson, L. F., Hughes, M. C. B., Ibiebele, T. I., Miura, K., Bain, C. J., . . . Webb, P. M. (2015). Cancers in Australia in 2010 attributable to inadequate consumption of fruit, non starchy vegetables and dietary fibre. *Australian and New Zealand Journal of Public Health, 39*(5), 422–428.

Narcotic Drug Amendment Bill 2016 - Public Information Paper, Commonwealth of Australia (2016, February10). Retrieved from https://www.health.gov.au/internet/ministers/publishing.nsf/Content/5E437BF8715C3EBACA257F540078A07A/$File/Public%20Information%20Paper.pdf

National Center on Addiction and Substance Abuse at Columbia University. (2007). *Wasting the best and the brightest: Substance abuse at America's colleges and universities.* New York: Author. Retrieved from www.casacolumbia.org

National Collegiate Athletic Association. (2014). Substance use: National Study of Substance Use Trends among NCAA College Students - Athletes. Retrieved from www.ncaapublications.com

National Diabetes Information Clearinghouse, US Department of Health and Human Services. (2008). *Diabetes Prevention Program (DPP).* NIH Publication 09-5099. Retrieved from http://diabetes.niddk.nih

National Highway Traffic Safety Administration (2012, February). Motor vehicle crashes: Overview. Retrieved from www.nhtsa.gov

National Highway Traffic Safety Administration. (2012, April). *Traffic safety facts-2010 data. Alcohol-impaired driving.* Washington, DC: Author. Retrieved from www.nhtsa .gov

National Institute on Alcohol Abuse and Alcoholism. (2007). A family history of alcoholism: Are you at risk? Retrieved from http://pubs.niaaa.nih.gov

National Institute on Alcohol Abuse and Alcoholism. (2012a). Drinking can put a chill on your summer fun . Retrieved from http://pubs.niaaa.nih.gov

National Institute on Alcohol Abuse and Alcoholism. (2012b). Drinking statistics, 2012 [p. 311]. Retrieved from www.niaaa.nih.gov

National Institute on Alcohol Abuse and Alcoholism. (2012c). Moderate and binge drinking. Retrieved from www.niaaa.nih.gov

National Institute on Alcohol Abuse and Alcoholism. (2012, June). Fall semester: A time for parents to revisit discussions about college drinking. Retrieved from www.collegedrinkingprevention.gov

National Institute on Drug Abuse. (2010). Anabolic steroids. In *NIDA for Teens.* Retrieved from http://teens.drugabuse.gov

National Institute on Drug Abuse. (2010, March). MDMA (ecstasy). In *NIDA InfoFacts.* Retrieved from www.drugabuse.gov

National Institute on Drug Abuse. (2011, March). Marijuana: Facts for teens. Retrieved from www.drugabuse.gov

National Institute on Drug Abuse. (2012). *Tobacco addiction* [NIH publication no. 12-4342]. Retrieved from www.drugabuse.gov

National Institute on Drug Abuse. (2012. July). Marijuana. In *NIDA InfoFacts*. Retrieved from http://drugabuse.gov

Neighbors, C., Atkins, D. C., Lewis, M. A., Lee, C. M., Kaysen, D., Mittmann, A., . . . Rodriguez, L. M. (2011). Event-specific drinking among college students. *Psychology of Addictive Behaviors, 25*(4), 702-707. doi: 10.1037/a0024051

Niels Rosenquist, J, et al. (2010). The spread of alcohol consumption behaviour in a large social network. *Annuals of Internal Medicine*. Vol *152*(7). doi 10.7326/0003-4819-152-7-201004060-00007.

Nielsen, S. J. et al. (2012). Calories consumption from alcoholic beverages by US adults, 2007–2010. NCHS Data Brief no. 110. www.cdc.gov

Norman, P. E., & Powell, J. T. (2014). Vitamin D and cardiovascular disease. *Circulation Research, 114*(2), 379–393.

Ogden, C. L., Carroll, M. D., Kit, B. K., & Flegal, K. M. (2012). Prevalence of obesity and trends in body mass index among US children and adolescents, 1999-2010. *Journal of the American Medical Association, 307*(5), 483–490.

O'Keeffe, L. M., Kearney, P. M., McCarthy, F. P., Khashan, A. S., Greene, R. A., North, R. A., . . . Dekker, G. A. (2015). Prevalence and predictors of alcohol use during pregnancy: Findings from international multicentre cohort studies. *BMJ Open, 5*(7), 1-11.

Oksman, O. (2016, July 29). Russian Olympic team's drug usage could have long term effects on athletes' health. *The Guardian*. Retrieved from www.theguardian.com/lifeandstyle/2016/jul/28/russian-olympic-rio-team-drug-steroids-health-effects

Olsen, C. M., Wilson, L. F., Green, A. C., Bain, C. J., Fritschi, L., Neale, R. E., & Whiteman, D. C. (2015). Cancers in Australia attributable to exposure to solar ultraviolet radiation and prevented by regular sunscreen use. *Australian and New Zealand Journal of Public Health, 39*(5), 471–476.

Onyper, S. V., Thacher, P. V., Gilbert, J. W., & Gradess, S. G. (2012). Class start times, sleep, and academic performance in college: A path analysis. *Chronobiology International, 29*(3), 318–335. doi: 10.3109/07420528.2012.655868

Papafotiou Owens, K., & Boorman, M. (2011). *Evaluating the deterrent effect of random breath testing (RBT) and random drug testing (RDT): The driver's perspective: Research findings* (monograph series no. 41). Canberra: National Drug Law Enforcement Research Fund. Retrieved from www.ndlerf.gov.au/pub/Monograph_41.pdf

Partnership for Drug-Free Kids. (2012). GHB. Retrieved from www.drugfree.org

Partridge, B., Bell, S., Lucke, J., & Hall, W. (2013). Australian university students' attitudes towards the use of prescription stimulants as cognitive enhancers: Perceived patterns of use, efficacy and safety. *Drug and Alcohol Review, 32*(3), 295–302.

Pirie, K., Peto, R., Reeves, G. K., Green, J., Beral, V., & Collaborators, M. W. S. (2013). The 21st century hazards of smoking and benefits of stopping: A prospective study of one million women in the UK. *The Lancet, 381*(9861), 133–141. doi: 10.1016/S0140- 6736(12)61720-6

Plowman, S. A., & Smith, D. L. (2011). *Exercise physiology for health, fitness, and performance* (3rd ed.). Philadelphia: Lippincott Williams & Wilkins.

Poston, L., Harthoorn, L. F., & van der Beek, E. M. (2011). Obesity in pregnancy: Implications for the mother and lifelong health of the child. A consensus statement. *Pediatric Research, 69*(2), 175–180.

Puhl, R. M., & King, K. M. (2013). Weight discrimination and bullying. *Best Practice & Research Clinical Endocrinology & Metabolism, 27*(2), 117–127. doi: 10.1016/j.beem.2012.12.002

Ridoutt, B., Baird, D., Bastiaans, K., Hendrie, G., Riley, M., Sanguansri, P., . . . Noakes, M. (2016). Changes in food intake in Australia: Comparing the 1995 and 2011 National Nutrition Survey results disaggregated into basic foods. *Foods, 5*(40), 1–13. Retrieved from www.mdpi.com/2304-8158/5/2/40

Ritter, A., Lancaster, K., Grech, K., & Reuter, P. (2011). *Monograph No. 21: An assessment of illicit drug policy in Australia (1985 to 2010): Themes and trends.* Sydney: National Drug and Alcohol Research Centre. Retrieved from https://ndarc.med.unsw.edu.au/sites/default/files/ndarc/resources/21%20An%20assessment%20of%20illicit%20drug%20policy%20in%20Australia.pdf

Rohsenow, D. J., Howland, J., Winter, M., Bliss, C. A., Littlefield, C. A., Heeren, T. C., & Calise, T. V. (2012). Hangover sensitivity after controlled alcohol administration as predictor of post-college drinking. *Journal of Abnormal Psychology, 121*(1), 270-275. doi: 10.1037/ a0024706

Rosenquist, J. N., Murabito, J., Fowler, J. H., & Christakis, N. A. (2010). The spread of alcohol consumption behavior in a large social network. *Annals of Internal Medicine, 152*(7), 426–433. doi: 10.7326/0003-4819-152- 7-201004060-00007

Rothstein, J., Heazlewood, R., & Fraser, M. (2007). Health of Aboriginal and Torres Strait Islander children in remote Far North Queensland: Findings of the paediatric outreach service. *Medical Journal of Australia, 186*(10), 519-521.

Roxburgh, A., Ritter, A., Slade, T., & Burns, L. (2013). *Trends in drug use and related harms in Australia, 2001 to 2011.* Sydney: National Drug and Alcohol Research Centre, University of New South Wales. Retrieved from https://ndarc.med.unsw.edu.au/sites/default/files/ndarc/resources/Drug%20 Trends%202001-2013.pdf

Ryder, D., Walker, N, & Salmon, A. (2006). *Drug use and drug-related harm* (Second edition). Melbourne IP Communications, Melbourne.

Sallis, J. F., Floyd, M. F., Rodríguez, D. A., & Saelens, B. E. (2012). Role of built environments in physical activity, obesity, and cardiovascular disease. *Circulation, 125*(5), 729–737.

Schafer, M. H., & Ferraro, K. F. (2011). The stigma of obesity does perceived weight discrimination affect identity and physical health? *Social Psychology Quarterly, 74*(1), 76–97. doi: 10.1177/0190272511398197

Schiller, J. S., Lucas, J. W., Ward, B. W., & Peregoy, J. A. (2012). Summary health statistics for US adults: National Health Interview Survey, 2010. *Vital and Health Statistics. Series 10, Data from The National Health Survey*, (252), 1–207. Retrieved from www.cdc.gov

Schuster, M. A., Elliott, M. N., Kanouse, D. E., Wallander, J. L., Tortolero, S. R., Ratner, J. A., . . . Banspach, S. W. (2012). Racial and ethnic health disparities among fifth-graders in three cities. *New England Journal of Medicine, 367*(8), 735–745.

Silveri, M. (2012). Adolescent Brain development and underage drinking in the United States: Identifying risks of alcohol use in college populations. *Harvard Review of Psychiatry*, vol *20*(4). doi 10.3109/10673229.2012.714642.2

Spruijt Metz, D. (2011). Etiology, treatment, and prevention of obesity in childhood and adolescence: A decade in review. *Journal of Research on Adolescence, 21*(1), 129–152. doi: 10.1111/j.1532– 7795. 2010.00719.x

Stacey, D., Bilbao, A., Maroteaux, M., Jia, T., Easton, A. C., Longueville, S., . . . Büchel, C. (2012). RASGRF2 regulates alcohol-induced reinforcement by influencing mesolimbic dopamine neuron activity and dopamine release. *Proceedings of the National Academy of Sciences, 109*(51), 21128–21133. doi: 10.1073/pnas.1211844110

Stappenbeck, C. A., & Fromme, K. (2010). A longitudinal investigation of heavy drinking and physical dating violence in men and women. *Addictive Behaviors, 35*(5), 479–485. doi: 10.1016/j.addbeh. 2009.12.027

Sterling, K., Berg, C. J., Thomas, A. N., Glantz, S. A., & Ahluwalia, J. S. (2013). Factors associated with small cigar use among college students. *American Journal of Health Behavior, 37*(3), 325–333.

Stockley, C. S. (2012). Is it merely a myth that alcoholic beverages such as red wine can be cardioprotective? *Journal of the Science of Food and Agriculture, 92*(9), 1815–1821. doi: 10.1002/jsfa.5696

Substance Abuse and Mental Health Services Administration. (2009, April). Alcohol treatment: Need, utilization, and barriers. *NSDUH Report.* Retrieved from www.samhsa.gov

Substance Abuse and Mental Health Services Administration. (2012). *Results from the 2011 National Survey on Drug Use and Health: Detailed tables* (NSDUH Series H-44, HHS publication no. (SMA) 12-4713). Rockville, MD: Author.

Substance Abuse and Mental Health Services Administration. (2012, September). Results from the 2011 National Survey on Drug Use and Health: Summary of national findings 2012. Retrieved from www.samhsa.gov

Sutfin, E. L., McCoy, T. P., Berg, C. J., Champion, H., Helme, D. W., O'Brien, M. C., & Wolfson, M. (2012). Tobacco use by college students: A comparison of daily and nondaily smokers. *American Journal of Health Behavior, 36*(2), 218–229. doi: 10.5993/AJHB.36.2.7

Terer, K., & Brown, R. (2014). *Effective drink driving prevention and enforcement strategies: Approaches to improving practice.* Canberra: Australian Institute of Criminology. Retrieved from www.aic.gov.au/ media_library/publications/tandi_pdf/tandi472.pdf

Thun, M. J., Carter, B. D., Feskanich, D., Freedman, N. D., Prentice, R., Lopez, A. D., . . . Gapstur, S. M. (2013). 50-year trends in smoking-related mortality in the United States. *New England Journal of Medicine, 368*(4), 351–364. doi: 10.1056/NEJMsa1211127

Tobacco-Free Kids. (2011). 1998 tobacco settlement: Decade of broken promises. Retrieved from www .tobaccofreekids.org

Tobacco Free Providence. (2012, January). Sweet Deceit Survey results. Retrieved from www .tobaccofreeprovidence.org

Underage Drinking Enforcement Training Center. (2011, September). Underage drinking costs. Retrieved from www.udetc.org

University of Adelaide. (2012, July 17). Marijuana use prior to pregnancy doubles risk of premature birth. Retrieved from Science Daily website: www.sciencedaily.com/releases/2012/07/120717182953.htm

US Food and Drug Administration. (2009, July). *Public Health Advisory: FDA requires new boxed warnings for the smoking cessation drugs Chantix and Zyban*. Retrieved from www.fda.gov

US Department of Health and Human Services. (2010). Marijuana: Facts for teens. Retrieved from http://teens.drugabuse.gov

US Department of Health and Human Services & National Action Alliance for Suicide Prevention. (2012, September). *2012 National Strategy for Suicide Prevention: Goals and objectives for action*. Washington, DC: Author. Retrieved from www.surgeongeneral.gov

US National Library of Medicine (2011, March). Alcoholism and alcohol abuse. In *MedlinePlus*. Retrieved from www.nlm.nih.gov

Uusitupa, M., Tuomilehto, J., & Puska, P. (2011). Are we really active in the prevention of obesity and type 2 diabetes at the community level? *Nutrition, Metabolism and Cardiovascular Diseases, 21*(5), 380–389. doi: 10.1016/j.numecd.2010.12.007

Warburton, D. E., Katzmarzyk, P. T., Rhodes, R. E., & Shephard, R. J. (2007). Evidence-informed physical activity guidelines for Canadian adults. *Canadian Journal of Public Health, 98*, S16–S68.

Wells, S., Graham, K., & Purcell, J. (2009). Policy implications of the widespread practice of "pre drinking"or "pre gaming"before going to public drinking establishments—are current prevention strategies backfiring? *Addiction, 104*(1), 4–9. doi: 10.1111/j.1360- 0443.2008.02393.x

White, A. M., Hingson, R. W., Pan, I.-J., & Yi, H. (2011). Hospitalizations for alcohol and drug overdoses in young adults ages 18–24 in the United States, 1999–2008: Results from the Nationwide Inpatient Sample. *Journal of Studies on Alcohol and Drugs, 72*(5), 774–786.

Whiteman, D. C., Webb, P. M., Green, A. C., Neale, R. E., Fritschi, L., Bain, C. J., . . . Nagle, C. M. (2015). Cancers in Australia in 2010 attributable to modifiable factors: Summary and conclusions. *Australian and New Zealand Journal of Public Health, 39*(5), 477–484.

Wicki, M., Kuntsche, E., & Gmel, G. (2010). Drinking at European universities? A review of students' alcohol use. *Addictive Behaviors, 35*(11), 913–924.

Wilson, T., & Temple, N. J. (2010). Should moderate alcohol consumption be promoted? In *Nutrition guide for physicians* (pp. 107–114). Springer. doi: 10.1007/978-1-60327-431-9_9

World Cancer Research Fund & American Institute for Cancer Research. (2009). *Policy and action for cancer prevention. Food, nutrition, and physical activity: A global perspective*. Washington, DC: American Institute for Cancer Research. Retrieved from www.dietandcancerreport.org

Zhao, J., Halfyard, B., Roebothan, B., West, R., Buehler, S., Sun, Z., . . . Wang, P. P. (2010). Tobacco smoking and colorectal cancer: A population-based case-control study in Newfoundland and Labrador. *Canadian Journal of Public Health/Revue Canadienne de Sante'e Publique*, 101(4), 281–289.

Chapter 7

Ackerman, J. M., & Bargh, J. A. (2010). The purposedriven life: Commentary on Kenrick et al. (2010). *Perspectives on Psychological Science, 5,* 323–326.

Agras, W. S., Brandt, H. A., Bulik, C. M., Dolan- Sewell, R., Fairburn, C. G., Halmi, K. A., Herzog, D. B., Jimerson, D. C., Kaplan, A. S., Kaye, W. H., le Grange, D., Lock, J., Mitchell, J., Rudorfer, M. V., Street, L. L., Striegel-Moore, R., Vitousek, K. M., Walsh, B. T., & Wilfley, D. E. (2004). Report of the National Institutes of Health workshop on overcoming barriers to treatment research in anorexia nervosa. *International Journal of Eating Disorders, 35,* 509–521.

Andrews, J. D. W. (1967). The achievement motive and advancement in two types of organization. *Journal of Personality and Social Psychology, 6,* 163–168.

Ansbacher, H. L., & Ansbacher, R. R., Eds. (1956). *The individual psychology of Alfred Adler: A systematic presentation in selections from his writings*. New York: Basic Books.

APA Presidential Task Force on Evidence-Based Practice. (2006). Evidence-based practice in psychology. *American Psychologist, 61,* 271–285.

Australian Bureau of Statistics. (2015). *National Health Survey: First Results, 2014-15* (cat. no. 4364.0.55.001). Canberra: Australian Bureau of Statistics.

Baumeister, R. F., Bratslavsky, E., Muraven, M., & Tice, D. M. (1998). Ego depletion: Is the active self a limited resource? *Journal of Personality and Social Psychology, 74,* 1252–1265.

Baumeister, R. F., Vohs, K. D., & Tice, D. M. (2007). The strength model of self-control. *Current Directions in Psychological Science, 16,* 351–355.

Bell, L. (2010, July 3). Fat chance: Scientists are working out ways to rev up the body's gut-busting machinery. *Science News, 178*(1), 18–21. doi: 10.1002/scin.5591780122.

Bogaert, A. F. (2005). Sibling sex ratio and sexual orientation in men and women: New tests in two national probability samples. *Archives of Sexual Behavior, 34,* 111–116. doi: 10.1007/s10508-005-1005-9.

Bornstein, R. F. (2001). The impending death of psychoanalysis. *Psychoanalytic Psychology, 18,* 3–20. [See also: Bruner, 1992; Erdelyi, 1992; Greenwald, 1992; Jacoby et al., 1992; Kihlstrom et al., 1992; Loftus & Klinger, 1992.]

Bower, B. (2006a, July 1). Gay males' sibling link: Men's homosexuality tied to having older brothers. *Science News, 170*(1), 3.

Byne, W. (1995). The biological evidence challenged. *Scientific American, 270*(5), 50–55.

Carver, P., Egan, S., & Perry, D. (2004). Children who question their heterosexuality. *Developmental Psychology, 40,* 43–53.

Couzin, J. (2005, May 6). A heavyweight battle over CDC's obesity forecasts. *Science, 308,* 770–771.

Covington, M. V. (2000). Intrinsic versus extrinsic motivation in schools: A reconciliation. *Current Direction in Psychology Science, 9,* 22–25.

Cynkar, A. (2007a, April). Low glucose levels compromise self-control. *Monitor on Psychology, 38*(4), 13.

Csikszentmihalyi, M. (1990). *Flow: The psychology of optimal experience.* New York: Harper & Row.

DeAngelis, T. (2002a, June). A bright future for PNI. *Monitor on Psychology,* 46–50.

DeAngelis, T. (2002b, February). New data on lesbian, gay, and bisexual mental health. *Monitor on Psychology, 33*(2), 46–47.

DeAngelis, T. (2004a, January). Family-size portions for one. *Monitor on Psychology, 35*(1), 50–51.

DeAngelis, T. (2004b, January). What's to blame for the surge in super-size Americans? *Monitor on Psychology, 35*(1), 46–49. [See also: Abelson & Kennedy, 2004; Marx, 2003; Newman, 2004; Taubes, 1998; Wickelgren, 1998c.]

Devor, H. (1993). Sexual orientation identities, attractions, and practices of female-to-male transsexuals. *Journal of Sex Research, 30,* 303–315.

Diamond, L. (2008). Female bisexuality from adolescence to adulthood: Results from a 10-year longitudinal study. *Developmental Psychology, 44,* 5–14.

Diamond, M. (2007). *Psychosexual development— male or female?* Address given at the 2007 convention of the American Psychological Association in San Francisco.

Doyle, R. (2006, February). Sizing up: Roots of obesity epidemic lie in the mid-20th century. *Scientific American, 294*(2), 32.

Eisenberger, R., & Cameron, J. (1996). Detrimental effects of reward: Reality or myth? *American Psychologist, 51,* 1153–1166.

Flier, J. S. (2006, May 12). Regulating energy balance: The substrate strikes back. *Science, 312,* 861–864.

Flier, J. S., & Maratos-Flier, E. (2007, September). What fuels fat. *Scientific American, 297*(3), 72–81. [See also: Campfield et al., 1998; Comuzzie & Allison, 1998; Gura, 1998, 2003; Hill & Peters, 1998; Levine et al., 1999; Ravussin & Danforth, 1999.]

Freeman, C. (2007). Born to run: *My story.* Australia: Puffin.

Freeman, C. & Scott, G. (2004). Cathy: *My autobiography.* Newbury: Highdown.

Friedman, J. M. (2003, February 7). A war on obesity,not the obese. *Science, 299,* 856–858.

Gambrel, P. A., & Cianci, R. (2003). Maslow's hierarchy of needs: Does it apply in a collectivist culture? *Journal of Applied Management and Entrepreneurship, 8,* 143–161. Retrieved April 4, 2008, from www3 .tjcu.edu.cn/wangshangketang/ lyxgl/yuedu/21.pdf.

Gibbs, W. W. (2005, June). Obesity: An overblown epidemic. *Scientific American, 292*(6), 70–77.

Golombok, S., & Tasker, F. (1996). Do parents influence the sexual orientation of their children? Findings from a longitudinal study of lesbian families. *Developmental Psychology, 32,* 3–11. [See also: Bailey et al., 1995; Bell et al., 1981; Isay, 1990]

Greenberg, G. (1997). Right answers, wrong reasons: Revisiting the deletion of homosexuality from the *DSM. Review of General Psychology, 1,* 256–270.

Grimm, O. (2007, April/May). Addicted to food? *Scientific American Mind, 18*(2), 36–39. [See also: Gura, 2000; Woods et al., 1998.]

Guisinger, S. (2003). Adapted to flee famine: Adding an evolutionary perspective on anorexia nervosa. *Psychological Review, 110,* 745–761.

Harris, J. A. (2004). Measured intelligence, achievement, openness to experience, and creativity. *Personality & Individual Differences, 36,* 913–929.

Hasler, G., Buysse D. J., Klaghofer R., Gamma, A., Ajdacic, V., Eich D., Rössler W., & Angst J. (2004). The association between short sleep duration and obesity in young adults: A 13-year prospective study. *Sleep, 27,* 661–666.

Hazan, C., & Diamond, L. M. (2000). The place of attachment in human mating. *Review of General Psychology, 4,* 186–204.

Hébert, R. (2005, January). The weight is over. *APS Observer, 18*(1), 20–24.

Herek, G. M. (2000). The psychology of sexual prejudice. *Current Directions in Psychological Science, 9,* 19–22.

Hill, J. O., & Peters, J. C. (1998, May 29). Environmental contributions to the obesity epidemic. *Science, 280,* 1371–1374.

Hu, F. B., Li, T. Y., Colditz, G. A., Willett, W. C., & Manson, J. E. (2003, April 9). Television watching and other sedentary behaviors in relation to risk of obesity and Type 2 diabetes mellitus in women. *Journal of the American Medical Association, 289,* 1785–1791.

Hull, C. L. (1943). *Principles of behavior: An intro duction to behavior theory.* New York: Appleton-Century-Crofts.

Hull, C. L. (1952). *A behavior system: An introduction to behavior theory concerning the individual organism.* New Haven, CT: Yale University Press.

Hyde, J. S., & Jaffe, S. (2000). Becoming a heterosexual adult: The experiences of young women. *Journal of Social Issues, 56,* 283–296.

Institute of Medicine. (2002). *Dietary reference intakes for energy, carbohydrate, fiber, fat, fatty acids, cholesterol, protein, and amino acids.* Washington, DC: National Institutes of Health.

Johnson, P. M., & Kenny, P. J. (2010, March 28). Dopamine D2 receptors in addiction-like reward dysfunction and compulsive eating in obese rats. *Nature Neuroscience, 13,* 635–641. doi:10.1038/nn.2519.

Keel, P. K., & Klump, K. L. (2003). Are eating disorders culture-bound syndromes? Implications for conceptualizing their etiology. *Psychological Bulletin, 129,* 747–769.

Kesebir, S., Graham, J., & Oishi, S. (2010). A theory of human needs should be human-centered, not animal-centered: Commentary on Kenrick et al. (2010). *Perspectives on Psychological Science, 5,* 315–319.

Koltko-Rivera, M. E. (2006). Redisovering the later version of Maslow's hierarchy of needs: Selftranscendence and opportunities for theory, research, and unification. *Review of General Psychology, 10,* 302–317.

Kurdek, L. A. (2005). What do we know about gay and lesbian couples? *Current Directions in Psychological Science, 14,* 251–254.

Lepper, M. R., Greene, D., & Nisbett, R. E. (1973). Undermining children's intrinsic interest with extrinsic reward: A test of the over-justification hypothesis. *Journal of Personality and Social Psychology, 28*(1), 129–137.

Lyubomirsky, S., & Boehm, J. K. (2010). Human motives, happiness, and the puzzle of parenthood: Commentary on Kenrick et al. (2010). *Perspectives on Psychological Science, 5,* 327–334.

Mann, T., Tomiyama, A. J., Westling, E., Lew, A., Samuels, B., & Chatman, J. (2007). Medicare's search for effective obesity treatments: Diets are not the answer. *American Psychologist, 62,* 220–233.

Markus, H. R., Uchida, Y., Omoregie, H., Townsend, S. S. M., & Kitayama, S. (2006). Going for the gold: Models of agency in Japanese and American contexts. *Psychological Science, 17,* 103–112.

McAnulty, R. D., & Burnette, M. M. (2004). *Exploring human sexuality: Making healthy decisions* (2nd ed.). Boston: Allyn & Bacon.

McClelland, D. C. (1965). Achievement and entrepreneurship: A longitudinal study. *Journal of Personality and Social Psychology, 1,* 389–392.

McClelland, D. C. (1985). *Human motivation.* New York: Scott Foresman.

McClelland, D. C. (1987a). Characteristics of successful entrepreneurs. *The Journal of Creative Behavior, 21,* 219–233.

McClelland, D. C. (1987b). *Human motivation.* New York: Cambridge University Press. [See also: Cooper, 1983; French & Thomas, 1958]

McClelland, D. C. (1993). Intelligence is not the best predictor of job performance. *Current Directions in Psychological Science, 2,* 5–6.

Mintz, L. B., & Betz, N. E. (1986). Sex differences in the nature, realism, and correlates of body image. *Sex Roles, 15,* 185–195.

Munsey, C. (2009, October). Insufficient evidence to support sexual orientation change efforts. *Monitor on Psychology, 40*(9), 29.

Newman, C. (2004, August). Why are we so fat? *National Geographic, 206,* 46–61.

Nicholson, I. (2007, Fall). Maslow: Toward a psychology of being. *The General Psychologist, 42*(2), 25–26. [See also: Baumeister & Leary, 1995; Brehm, 1992; Hatfield & Rapson, 1993; Kelley et al., 1983; Weber & Harvey, 1994a,b.]

Novotney, A. (2009, April). New solutions. *Monitor on Psychology, 40*(4), 47–51.

Park, D. C. (2007). Eating disorders: A call to arms. *American Psychologist, 62,* 158.

Parker-Pope, T. (2009, June 23). How the food makers captured our brains. *New York Times*. Retrieved from www.nytimes.com/2009/06/23/ health/23well.html

Patterson, C. J. (2006). Children of lesbian and gay parents. *Current Directions in Psychological* n*Science, 15,* 241–244.

Peterson, C., & Park, N. (2010). What happened to self-actualization? Commentary on Kenrick et al. (2010). *Perspectives on Psychological Science, 5,* 320–322.

Pillard, R., & Bailey, M. (1991). A genetic study of male sexual orientation. *Archives of General Psychiatry, 48,* 1089–1096.

Popkin, B. M. (2007, September). The world is fat. *Scientific American, 297*(3), 88–95.

Raynor, J. O. (1970). Relationships between achievement-related motives, future orientation, and academic performance. *Journal of Personality and Social Psychology, 15,* 28–33.

Savin-Williams, R. C. (2006). Who's gay? Does it matter? *Current Directions in Psychological Science, 15,* 40–44.

Schaller, M., Neuberg, S. L., Griskevicius, V., & Kenrick, D. T. (2010). Pyramid power: Response to commentaries. *Perspectives on Psychological Science, 5,* 335–337.

Schultz, D. P., & Schultz, S. E. (2006). *Psychology and work today: An introduction to industrial and organizational psychology* (9th ed.). Upper Saddle River, NJ: Prentice Hall.

Striegel-Moore, R. H., & Bulik, C. M. (2007). Risk factors for eating disorders. *American Psychologist, 62,* 181–198.

Striegel-Moore, R. H., Silberstein, L. R., & Rodin, J. (1993). The social self in bulimia nervosa: Public self-consciousness, social anxiety, and perceived fraudulence. *Journal of Abnormal Psychology, 102,* 297–303.

Triandis, H. (1990). Cross-cultural studies of individualism and collectivism. In J. Berman (Ed.), b*Nebraska Symposium on Motivation, 1989* (pp. 42–133). Lincoln: University of Nebraska Press.

Wargo, E. (2009). Resisting temptation: Psychological research brings new strength to understanding willpower. *Observer, 22*(1), 10–17

Wells, B. E., & Twenge, J. M. (2005). Changes in young people's sexual behavior and attitudes, 1943–1999: A cross-temporal meta-analysis. *Review of General Psychology, 9,* 249–261.

Zimbardo, P. G., & Montgomery, K. D. (1957). The relative strengths of consummatory responses in hunger, thirst, and exploratory drive. *Journal of Comparative and Physiological Psychology, 50,* 504–508.

Chapter 8

Abbott, J., Dodd, M., Gee, L., & Webb, K. (2001). Ways of coping with cystic fibrosis: Implications for treatment adherence. *Disability and Rehabilitation, 23*(8), 315–324.

Adams, J., & White, M. (2005). Why don't stage-based activity promotion interventions work? *Health Education Research, 20*(2), 237–243.

Baker, S. M., Marshak, H. H., Rice, G. T., & Zimmerman, G. J. (2001). Patient participation in physical therapy goal setting. *Physical Therapy, 81*(5), 1118–1126.

Bandura, A. (1977). Self-efficacy: Toward a unifying theory of behavioral change. *Psychological Review, 84*(2), 191–215.

Bandura, A. (1997). *Self-efficacy: The exercise of control.* New York, NY: W. H. Freeman.

Banerjee, S. &Varma, R. P. (2013). Factors affecting non-adherence among patients diagnosed with unipolar depression in a psychiatric department of a tertiary hospital in Kolkata, India. *Depression Research and Treatment, 201,* 1-12.

Barlow, J. H., Macey, S. J., & Struthers, G. R. (1993). Health locus of control, self-help and treatment adherence in relation to ankylosing spondylitis patients. *Patient Education & Counseling, 20*(2–3), 153–166.

Barsa del Alcazar, C. (1998). Spectrum of adherence among hemodialysis patients. *Journal of Nephrology Social Work, 18,* 53–65.

Bassett, S. F., & Prapavessis, H. (2007). Home-based physical therapy intervention with adherence-enhancing strategies versus clinic-based management for patients with ankle sprains. *Physical Therapy, 87*(9), 1132–1143.

Belza, B., Topolski, T., Kinne, S., Patrick, D. L., & Ramsey, S. D. (2002). Does adherence make a difference? Results from a community-based aquatic exercise program. *Nursing Research, 51*(5), 285–291.

Beresford, S. A., Farmer, E. M., Feingold, L., Graves, K. L., Sumner, S. K., & Baker, R. M. (1992). Evaluation of a self-help dietary intervention in a primary care setting. *American Journal of Public Health, 82,* 79–84.

Bernard, B. (1991). The case for peers. *The Peer Facilitator Quarterly, 8,* 20–27.

Bodenheimer, T., Lorig, K., Holman H., & Grumbach, K. (2002). Patient self-management of chronic disease in primary care. *Journal of the American Medical Association, 288*(19), 2469–2475.

Bogardus, S. T., Bradley, E. H., Williams, C. S., Maciejewski, P. K., Gallo, W. T., & Inouye, S. K. (2004). Achieving goals in geriatric assessment: Role of caregiver agreement and adherence to recommendations. *Journal of the American Geriatric Society, 52*(1), 99–105.

Bouglanger, K. T., Campo, S., Glanville, J. L., Lowe, J. B., & Yang, J. (2012). The development and validation of the client expectations of massage scale. *International Journal of Therapeutic Massage & Bodywork, 5*(3), 3-15.

Bradley, E., Bogardus, Jr., S., Tinetti, M., & Inouye, S. (1999). Goal-setting in clinical medicine. *Social Science and Medicine, 49,* 267–278.

Brewer, B. W. (1999). Adherence to sport injury rehabilitation regimens. In S. J. Bull, (Ed.), *Adherence issues in sport and exercise.* (pp. 145–168). New York, NY: John Wiley & Sons.

Brewer, B. W., van Raalte, J. L., & Cornelius, A. E. (2000). Psychological factors, rehabilitation adherence, and rehabilitation outcome after anterior cruciate ligament reconstruction. *Rehabilitation Psychology, 45,* 20–37.

Britt E., Hudson, S. M., & Blampied, N. M. (2004). Motivational interviewing in health settings: A review. *Patient Education and Counseling, 53*(2), 147–155.

Brock, S., & Allen, J. (2000). Working with type in health care: Same words, different meanings? *Journal of Psychological Type, 53,* 4–10.

Brodie, D. A., & Inoue, A. (2005). Motivational interviewing to promote physical activity for people with chronic heart failure. *Journal of Advanced Nursing, 50*(5), 518–527.

Brody, L. (2005). Principles of self-management and exercise instruction. In C. M. Hall & L. T. Brody (Eds.), *Therapeutic exercise: Moving toward function* (pp. 35–46). Philadelphia, PA: Lippincott Williams & Wilkins.

Burton, L. C., Shapiro, S. B., & German, P. S. (1999). Determinants of physical activity initiation and maintenance among community-dwelling older persons. *Preventive Medicine, 29,* 422–430.

Bylund, C., & Makoul, G. (2002). Empathic communication and gender in the physician–patient encounter. *Patient Education and Counseling, 48,* 207–216.

Campbell, R., Evans, M., Tucker, M., Quilty, B., Dieppe, P., & Donovan, J. L. (2001). Why don't patients do their exercises? Understanding non-compliance with physiotherapy in patients with osteoarthritis of the knee. *Journal of Epidemiology and Community Health, 55,* 132–138.

Carpenter, C. J. (2010). A meta-analysis of the effectiveness of health belief model variables in predicting behavior. *Health Communication, 25*(8), 661 669. doi:10.1080/10410236.2010. 521906

Chinman, M. J., Allende, M., Weingarten, R., Steiner, J., Tworkowski, S., & Davidson, L. (1999). On the road to collaborative treatment planning: Consumer and provider perspectives. *Journal of Behavioral Health Services and Research, 26*(2), 211–218.

Chipperfield, J. G., & Perry, R. P. (2006). Primary and secondary control-enhancing strategies in later life: Predicting hospital outcomes in men and women. *Health Psychology, 25*(2), 226–236.

Coleman, E. A., Hall-Barrow, J., Coon, S., & Stewart, C. B. (2003). Facilitating exercise adherence for patients with multiple myeloma. *Clinical Journal of Oncology Nursing, 7*(5), 529–534,540.

Colombo, R., Pisano, F., Mazzone, A., Delconte, C., Micera, S., Carrozza, M. C., . . . Minuco, G. (2007). Design strategies to improve patient motivation during robot-aided rehabilitation. *Journal of Neuroengineering and Rehabilitation, 19*(4), 3.

Conn, V. S. (1998). Older adults and exercise: Path analysis of self-efficacy related constructs. *Nursing Research, 47,* 180–189.

Constantino, M. J., Arnkoff, D. B., Glass, C. R., Amertrano, R. M., & Smith, J. Z. (2011). Expectations. *Journal of Clinical Psychology, 67*(2), 184-92. doi: 10.1002/jclp.20754.

Cott, C., & Finch, E. (1991). Goal-setting in physical therapy practice. *Physiotherapy Canada, 43*(1), 19–22.

Coughlin, A. M., Bandura, A. S., Fleischer, T. D., & Guck, T. P. (2000). Multidisciplinary treatment of chronic pain patients: Its efficacy in changing patient locus of control. *Archives of Physical Medicine and Rehabilitation, 81,* 739–740.

Coyne C. (2008). Video "games" in the clinic: PTs report early results. *PT–Magazine of Physical Therapy,, 16*(5), 22–28.

Daily Mock, K. (2001). Effective clinician–patient communication. *Physician's News Digest.* Retrieved from http://www.physiciansnews.com/law/201.html

DeSousa, A. (2008). Psychological issues in oral and maxillofacial reconstructive surgery. *British Journal of Oral and Maxillofacial Surgery, 46*(8), 661–664.

DiMatteo, M. R. (2004a). Social support and patient adherence to medical treatment: A meta-analysis. *Health Psychology, 23*(2), 207–218.

DiMatteo, M. R. (2004b). Variations in patients' adherence to medical recommendations: A quantitative review of 50 years of research. *Medical Care, 42*(3), 200–209.

Duncan, K. A., & Pozehl, B. (2002). Staying on course: The effects of an adherence facilitation intervention on home exercise participation. *Progress in Cardiovascular Nursing, 17*(2), 59–65, 71.

Engstrom, L. O., & Oberg, B. (2005). Patient adherence in an individualized rehabilitation programme: A clinical follow-up. *Scandinavian Journal of Public Health, 33*(1), 11–18.

Escolar-Reina, P., Medina-Mirapeix, F., Gascón-Cánovas, J. J., Montilla-Herrador, J., Jimeno-Serrano, F. J., de Oliveira Sousa, S. L., . . . Lomas-Vega, R. (2010). How do care-provider and home exercise program characteristics affect patient adherence in chronic neck and back pain: a qualitative study. *BMC Health Services Research, 10*(10), 1-8. doi: 10.1186/1472-6963-10-60.

Gatchel, R. J. (2004). Psychosocial factors that can influence the self-assessment of function. *Journal of Occupational Rehabilitation, 14*(3), 197–206.

Goudas, M., Minardou, K., & Kotis, J. (2000). Feedback regarding goal achievement and intrinsic motivation. *Perceptual and Motor Skills, 90,* 810–812.

Green, C. A., Polen, M. R., Janoff, S. L., Castleton, D. K., Wisdom, J. P., Vuckovic, N., . . . Oken, S. L. (2008). Understanding how clinician–patient relationships and relational continuity of care affect recovery from serious mental illness: STARS study results. *Psychiatric Rehabilitation Journal, 32*(1), 9–22.

Greenfield, B. H., Anderson, A., Cox, B., & Tanner, M. C. (2008). Meaning of caring to 7 novice physical therapists during their first year of clinical practice. *Physical Therapy, 88*(10), 1154–1166.

Guay, F., Vallerand, R. J., & Blanchard, C. (2000). On the assessment of situational intrinsic and extrinsic motivation: The Situational Motivational Scale (SIMS). *Motivation and Emotion, 24,* 175–213.

Hall, L. K. (1999). Health and disease management: Expanding the cardiac and pulmonary rehabilitation model. *Clinical Exercise Physiology, 1*(1), 42–46.

Hartigan, C., Rainville, J., Sobel, J., & Hipona, M. (2000). Long-term exercise adherence after intensive rehabilitation for chronic low back pain. *Medicine & Science in Sports & Exercise, 32*(3), 551–555.

Haynes, R. B., McKibbon, K. A., & Kanani, R. (1996). Systematic review of randomised trials of interventions to assist patients to follow prescriptions for medication. *Lancet, 348*(10), 383–386.

Heisler, M., Bouknight, R. R., Hayward, R. A., Smith, D. M., & Kerr, E. A. (2002). The relative importance of physician communication, participatory decision-making and patient understanding in diabetes self-management. *Journal of General Internal Medicine, 17*(4), 243–252.

Herborg, H., Haugbolle, L. S., Sorensen, L., Rossing, C., & Dam, P. (2008). Developing a generic, individualised adherence programme for chronic medication users. *Pharmacy Practice, 6*(3), 148–157.

Hirano, P. C., Laurent, D. D., & Lorig, K. (1994). Arthritis patient education studies, 1987–1991: A review of the literature. *Patient Education Counseling, 24,* 9–54.

Hussey, L. C., & Gilliland, K. (1989). Compliance, low literacy, and locus of control. *Nursing Clinics of North America, 24,* 605–611.

Ignacio-Garcia, J. M., & Gonzalez-Santos, P. (1995). Asthma self-management education program by home monitoring of peak expiratory flow. *American Journal of Respiratory and Critical Care Medicine, 151*(2), 353–359.

Jensen, G. M., Gwyer, J., Shepard, K. F., & Hack, L. M. (2000). Expert practice in physical therapy. *Physical Therapy, 80*(1), 28–43.

Jensen, G. M., & Lorish, C. D. (2005). Promoting patient cooperation with exercise programs: Linking research, theory, and practice. *Arthritis Care & Research, 7*(4), 181–189.

Jones, J., & Kovalcik, E. (1988). Goal-setting: A method to help clients escape the negative effects of stress. *Stress Reduction, 83*(1), 257–261.

Kauppi, K., Hatonen, H., Adams, C. E., & Valimaki, M. (2015). Perceptions of treatment adherence among people with mental health problems and health care professionals. *Journal of Advanced Nursing, 71*(4), 777-788. doi: 10.1111/jan.12567.

Kearney, M. K., Weininger, R. B., Vachon, M. L. S., Harrison, R. L., & Mount, B. M. (2009). Self-care of physicians caring for patients at the end of life. *Journal of the American Medical Association, 301*(11), 1155–1164.

King, G., Strachan, D., Tucker, M., Duwyn, B., Desserud, S., & Shillington, M. (2009). The application of a transdisciplinary model for early intervention services. *Infants & Young Children, 22*(3), 211–223.

King, M. B., Whipple, R. H., & Gruman, C. A., Judge, J. O., Schmidt, J. A., & Wolfson, L. I. (2002). The Performance Enhancement Project: Improving physical performance in older persons. *Archives of Physical Medicine and Rehabilitation, 83*, 1060–1069.

Lawler, J., Dowswell, G., Hearn, J., Forster, A., & Young, J. (1999). Recovering from stroke: A qualitative investigation of the role of goal-setting in late stroke recovery. *Journal of Advanced Nursing, 30*(2), 401–409.

Lawrence, G. (1997). *Looking at type and learning styles.* Gainesville, FL: Center for Applications of Psychological Type.

Levensky, E. R., Forcehimes, A., O'Donohue, W. T., & Beitz, K. (2007). Motivational interviewing: An evidenced-based approach to counseling helps patients follow treatment recommendations. *American Journal of Nursing, 107*(10), 50–58.

Lewin, K., Dembo, T., Festinger, L., & Sears, P. S. (1944). Level of aspiration. In J. M. Hunt (Ed.), *Personality and the behavior disorders: A handbook based on experimental and clinical research* (pp. 333–378). New York, NY: Ronald Press.

Locke, E. A., Shaw, K. N., Saari, L. M., & Latham, G. P. (1981). Goal-setting and task performance. *Psychological Bulletin, 90*(1), 125–152.

Lorish, C. D., & Gale, J. R. (1999). Facilitating behavior change: Strategies for education and practice. *Journal of Physical Therapy Education, 13*(3), 31–37.

Lorish, C. D., & Gale, J. R. (2002). Facilitating adherence to healthy lifestyle behavior changes in patients. In K. F. Shepard & G. M. Jensen (Eds.), *Handbook of teaching for physical therapists* (2nd ed., pp. 351–385). Boston, MA: Butterworth-Heinemann.

Maciejewski, P. K., Prigerson, H. G., & Mazure, C. (2000). Self-efficacy as a mediator between stressful life events and depressive symptoms. *British Journal of Psychiatry, 176*, 373–378.

Mailloux, J., Finno, M., & Rainville, J. (2006). Long-term exercise adherence in the elderly with chronic low back pain. *American Journal of Physical Medicine and Rehabilitation, 85*(2), 120–126.

Marchese, V., Rai, S., Carlson, C., Hinds, P., Spearing, E., Zhang, L., . . . Ginsberg, J. (2007). Assessing functional mobility in survivors of lower-extremity sarcoma: Reliability and validity of a new assessment tool. *Pediatric Blood Cancer, 49*(2), 183–189.

McDonald, H. P., Garg, A. X., & Haynes, R. B. (2002). Interventions to enhance patient adherence to medication prescriptions. *Journal of the American Medical Association, 288*, 2868–2879.

Meyer, T. J., & Mark, M. M. (1995). Effects of psychosocial interventions with adult cancer patients: A meta-analysis of randomized experiments. *Health Psychology, 14*, 101–108.

Miller, W. R. (1983). Motivational interviewing with problem drinkers. *Behavioural Psychotherapy, 11*, 147–172.

Miller, W. R., & Rollnick, S. (1995). What is motivational interviewing? *Behavioural and Cognitive Psychotherapy, 23*, 325–334.

Miller, W. R., & Rollnick, S. (2002). *Motivational interviewing: Preparing people for change* (2nd ed.). New York, NY: Guilford Press.

Moore, J. E., von Korff, M., Cherkin, D., Saunders, K., & Lorig, K. (2000). A randomized trial of a cognitive behavioral program for enhancing back pain self care in a primary care setting. *Pain, 88*(2), 145–153.

Mostrom, E., & Shepard, K. F. (1999). Teaching and learning about patient education in physical therapy professional preparation: Academic and clinical considerations. *Journal of Physical Therapy Education, 13*(3), 8–17.

Mulvaney, S. A. (2009). Improving patient problem-solving to reduce barriers to diabetes self-management. *Clinical Diabetes, 27*(3), 99–104.

Oberle, K. (1991). A decade of research in locus of control: What have we learned? *Journal of Advanced Nursing, 16*, 800–806.

Ott, C. D., Lindsey, A. M., Waltman, N. L., Gross, G. J., Twiss, J. J., Berg, K., . . . Henricksen, S. (2004). Facilitative strategies, psychological factors, and strength/weight training behaviors in breast cancer survivors who are at risk for osteoporosis. *Orthopedic Nursing, 23*(1), 45–52.

Pampallona, S., Bollini, P., Tibaldi, G., Kupelnick, B., & Munizza, C. (2002). Patient adherence in the treatment of depression. *British Journal of Psychiatry, 180*, 104–109.

Penza-Clyve, S. M., Mansell, C., & McQuaid, E. L. (2004). Why don't children take their asthma medications? A qualitative analysis of children's perspectives on adherence. *Journal of Asthma, 41*(2), 189–197.

Platt, F. W., Gaspar, D. L., Coulehan, J. L., Fox, L., Adler, A. J., Weston, W. W., . . . Stewart, M. (2001). "Tell me about yourself": The patient-centered interview. *Annals of Internal Medicine, 134*(11), 1079–1085.

Playford, E. D., Dawson, L., Limbert, V., Smith, M., Ward, C. D., & Wells, R. (2000). Goal-setting in rehabilitation: Report of a workshop to explore professionals' perceptions of goal-setting. *Clinical Rehabilitation, 14*(5), 491–496.

Price-Lackey, P., & Cashman, J. (1996). Jenny's story: Reinventing oneself through occupation and narrative configuration. *American Journal of Occupational Therapy, 50*(4), 306–314.

Prochaska, J. O., DiClimente, C. C. & Norcross, J. C. (1992). In search of how people change. *American Psychologist, 47,* 1102–1104.

Prochaska, J. O., Redding, C. A., & Evers, K. E. (2002). The transtheoretical model and stages of change. In K. Glanz, B. Rimer, & Lewis F. M. (Eds.), *Health behavior and health education: Theory, research, and practice* (3rd ed., pp. 99–116). San Francisco, CA: Jossey Bass.

Prochaska, J. O., & Velicer, W. F. (1997). The transtheoretical model of health behavior change. *American Journal of Health Promotion, 12*(1), 38–48.

Rand, C. S. (1993). Measuring adherence with therapy for chronic diseases: Implications for the treatment of heterozygous familial hypercholesterolemia. *American Journal of Cardiology, 72,* 68D–74D.

Randall, K. E., & McEwen, I. R. (2000). Writing patient-centered functional goals. *Physical Therapy, 80*(12), 1197–1203.

Rapport, M. J., McWilliams, R. A., & Smith, B. J. (2004). Practices across disciplines in early intervention: The research base. *Infants & Young Children, 17*(1), 32–44.

Resnick, B., Palmer, M. H., Jenkins, L. S., & Spellbring, A. M. (2000). Path analysis of efficacy expectations and exercise behavior in older adults. *Journal of Advanced Nursing, 31*(6), 1309–1315.

Resnick, B., & Spellbring, A. M. (2000). Understanding what motivates older adults to exercise. *Journal of Gerontological Nursing, 26,* 34–42.

Resnicow, K., Dilorio, C., Soet, J. E., Borelli, B., Hecht, J., & Ernst, D. (2002). Motivational interviewing in health promotion: It sounds like something is changing. *Health Psychology, 21*(5), 444–451.

Robinson-Smith, G., Johnston, M. V., & Allen, J. (2000). Self-care, self-efficacy, quality of life and depression after stroke. *Archives of Physical Medicine and Rehabilitation, 81,* 460–464.

Rollnick, S., Miller, W. R., Butler, C. C., & Aloia, M. S. (2008). Motivational interviewing in health care: Helping patients change behavior. *Journal of Chronic Obstructive Pulmonary Disease,* 5(3), 203–205.

Rone-Adams, S. A., Stern, D. F., & Walker, V. (2004). Stress and compliance with a home exercise program among caregivers of children with disabilities. *Pediatric Physical Therapy, 16,* 140–148.

Rosenstock, I. M. (1966). Why people use health services. *Milbank Memorial Fund Quarterly, 44,* 94–127.

Rotter, J. B. (1966). Generalized expectancies for internal versus external control of reinforcement. *Psychological Monographs, General and Applied, 80,* 1–28.

Schenkman, M., Hall, D., Kumar, R., & Kohrt, W. M. (2008). Endurance exercise training to improve economy of movement of people with Parkinson disease: Three case reports. *Physical Therapy, 88*(1), 63–76.

Schroeder, K., Fahey, T., & Ebrahim, S. (2004). How can we improve adherence to blood pressure-lowering medication in ambulatory care? Systematic review of randomized controlled trials. *Archives of Internal Medicine, 164,* 722–732.

Sherman, B. R., Sanders, L. M., & Yearde, J. (1998). Role-modeling healthy behavior: Peer counseling for pregnant and post-partum women in recovery. *Women's Health Issues, 8*(4), 230–238.

Shinitzky, H. E., & Kub, J. (2001). The art of motivating behavior change: The use of motivational interviewing to promote health. *Public Health Nursing, 18*(3), 178–185.

Skinner, T. C. (2004). Psychological barriers. *European Journal of Endocrinology, 151*(Suppl. 2), T13–T17.

Sluijs, E. (1991). *Patient education in physical therapy.* Utrecht, Netherlands: Nederlands Institut voor Onderzoek Van de Eerstel I jnsgezondheidszorg NIVEL.

Sluijs, E. M., Kok, G. J., & van der Zee, J. (1993). Correlates of exercise compliance in physical therapy. *Physical Therapy, 73,* 771–782.

Stelzner, D. M., Rodriguez, J. W., Krapfl, B., Jordan, S. L., & Schenkman, M. L. (2003). *Instructor's adherence protocol: Instructor's guidelines for assisting participants.* Denver: Physical Therapy Program, University of Colorado at Denver and Health Sciences Center.

Sweeney, S., Taylor, G., & Calin, A. (2002). The effect of a home based exercise intervention package on outcome in ankylosing spondylitis: A randomized controlled trial. *Journal of Rheumatology, 29,* 763–766.

Symister, P., & Friend, R. (2003). The influence of social support and problematic support on optimism and depression in chronic illness: A prospective study evaluating self-esteem as a mediator. *Journal of Health Psychology, 22*(3), 123–129.

Taylor, A. H., & May, S. (1996).Threat and coping appraisal as determinants of compliance with sports injury rehabilitation: An application of protection motivation theory. *Journal of Sports Science, 14*, 471–482.

Toomey, T. C., Mann, J. D., Abashian, S., & Thompson-Pope, S. (1991). Relationship between perceived self-control of pain, pain description, and functioning. *Pain, 45,* 129–133.

Treichler, D. G. (1967). Are you missing the boat in training aids? In *Audiovisual communications*. New York, NY: United Business Publications.

Turner, G. (1999). Peer support and young people's health. *Journal of Adolescence, 22,* 567–572.

Vanderhoff, M. (2005). Patient education and health literacy. *PT–Magazine of Physical Therapy, 13*(9), 42–46.

Veenhof, C., van Hasselt, T. J., Koke, A. J., Dekker, J., Bijlsma, J. W., & van den Ende, C. H. (2006). Active involvement and long-term goals influence long-term adherence to behavioural graded activity in patients with osteoarthritis: A qualitative study. *Australian Journal of Physiotherapy, 52*(4), 273–278.

von Korff, M., Gruman, J., Schaefer, J., Curry, S. J., & Wagner, E. H. (1997). Collaborative management of chronic illness. *Annals of Internal Medicine, 127*(12), 1097–1102.

Wallston, K. A. (1992). Hocus-pocus, the focus isn't strictly on locus: Rotter's social learning theory modified for health. *Cognitive Therapy and Research, 16*(2), 182–199.

Weingarten, S. R., Henning, J. M., Badamgarav, E., Knught, K., Hasselblad, V., Gano, Jr., A., & Ofman, J. J. (2002). Interventions used in disease management programmes for patients with chronic illness—which ones work? Meta-analysis of published reports. *British Medical Journal, 325,* 925.

West, D. S., DiLillo, V., Bursac, Z., Gore, S. A., & Greene, P. G. (2007). Motivational interviewing improves weight loss in women with type 2 diabetes. *Diabetes Care, 30*(5), 1081–1087.

White III, A. A., Hill, J. A., Mackel, A. M., Rowley, D. L., Rickards, E. P., & Jenkins, B. (2007). The relevance of culturally competent care in orthopaedics to outcomes and health care disparities. *Journal of Bone and Joint Surgery, American Volume, 89*(6), 1379–1384.

Woodard, C. M., & Berry, M. J. (2001). Enhancing adherence to prescribed exercise: Structured behavioral interventions in clinical exercise programs. *Journal of Cardiopulmonary Rehabilitation, 21,* 201–209.

Woolf, S. H. (2008). The power of prevention and what it requires. *Journal of the American Medical Association, 299*(20), 2437–2439.

Woolf, S. H. (2009). Social policy as health policy. *Journal of the American Medical Association, 301*(11), 1166–1169.

World Health Organization. (2003). Adherence to long-term therapies: Evidence for action. In *Noncommunicable diseases and mental health adherence to long-term therapies project*. Geneva, Switzerland: Author.

Wrosch, C., Heckhausen, J., & Lachman, M. E. (2000). Primary and secondary control strategies for managing health and financial stress across adulthood. *Psychology and Aging, 15*(3), 387–399.

Chapter 9

Albarracín, D., & Vargas, P. (2010). Attitudes and persuasion: *From biology to social responses to persuasive* intent. In S. T. Fiske, D. T. Gilbert, & G. Lindzey (Eds.), Handbook of social psychology (5th ed., Vol. 1, pp. 394–427). New York: Wiley. Detailed and authoritative discussion of persuasion, which also covers literature on biochemical and brain scien*ce dimensions.*

Banaji, M. R., & Heiphetz, L. (2010). Attitudes. In S. T. Fiske, D. T. Gilbert, & G. Lindzey (Eds.), Handbook of social psychology (5th ed., Vol. 1, pp. 353–393). New York: Wiley. A completely up-to-date, comprehensive and detailed discussion of attitude research, *which also covers processes of attitude change—has detailed co*verage of recent social neuroscience research.

Banaji, M. R., & Heiphetz, L. (2010). Attitudes. In S. T. Fiske, D. T. Gilbert, & G. Lindzey (Eds.), Handbook of social psychology (5th ed., Vol. 1, pp. 353–393). New York: Wiley. *A completely up-to-date, compr*ehensive and detailed discussion of attitude research.

Baron, R. S., & Kerr, N. (2003). Group process, group decision, group action (2nd ed.). Buckingham, UK: Open University Press. A general overview of *some major topics in the study of* group processes; includes discussion of social influence phenomena.

Belch, G. E., & Belch, M. A. (2012). Advertising and promotion: An integrated marketing communications perspective (9th ed.). New York: McGraw-Hill. A well-known textbook that uses a communications theory approach (source, message, receiver) to explore how consumer attitudes and behaviour can be changed. It is rich with examples and illustrations of advertisements.

Bohner, G., & Dickel, N. (2011). Attitude and attitude change. Annual Review of Psychology, 62, 391–417. Topics include recent research on evaluative conditioning and on implicit and explicit models of attitude.

Bohner, G., Moskowitz, G. B., & Chaiken, S. (1995). The interplay of heuristic and systematic processing of social information. European Review of Social Psychology, 6, 33–68. An in-depth overview of the heuristic–systematic model of social information processing, which links attitude change more broadly to social influence.

Brown, R. J. (2000). Group processes (2nd ed.). Oxford, UK: Blackwell. A very readable introduction to group processes, which also places an emphasis on social influence processes within groups, especially conformity, norms and minority influence.

Cialdini, R. B., & Trost, M. R. (1998). Social influence: Social norms, conformity, and compliance. In D. Gilbert, S. T. Fiske, & G. Lindzey (Eds.), The handbook of social psychology (4th ed., Vol. 2, pp. 151–192). New York: McGraw-Hill. A thorough overview of social influence research with a particular emphasis on norms and persuasion.

Devine, P. G., Hamilton, D. L., & Ostrom, T. M. (Eds.) (1994). Social cognition: Impact on social psychology. San Diego: Academic Press. Leading experts discuss the impact that social cognition has had on a wide range of topics in social psychology.

Dijksterhuis, A. (2010). Automaticity and the unconscious. In S. T. Fiske, D. T. Gilbert, & G. Lindzey (Eds.), Handbook of social psychology (5th ed., Vol. 1, pp. 228–267). New York: Wiley. Detailed and comprehensive coverage of perhaps the core of social cognition— automatic cognitive processes.

Eagly, A. H., & Chaiken, S. (2005). Attitude research in the 21st century: The current state of knowledge. In D. Albarracin, B. T. Johnson, & M. P. Zanna (Eds.), The handbook of attitudes (pp. 742–767). Mahwah, NJ: Erlbaum. Another excellent review from two of the leading attitude researchers.

Fiske, S. T. (2010). Interpersonal stratification: Status, power, and subordination. In S. T. Fiske, D. T. Gilbert, & G. Lindzey (Eds.), Handbook of social psychology (5th ed., Vol. 2, pp. 941–982). New York: Wiley. Detailed and up-to-date overview of research on the psychology of status, which also covers research on power.

Fiske, S. T., & Berdahl, J. (2007). Social power. In A. W. Kruglanski & E. T. Higgins (Eds), Social psychology: Handbook of basic principles (2nd ed., pp. 678–692). New York: Guilford Press. A detailed overview of the social psychology of power.

Fiske, S. T., & Taylor, S. E. (2008). Social cognition: From brains to culture. New York: McGraw-Hill. This is essentially the third edition of Fiske and Taylor's classic social cognition text—it is comprehensive, detailed and well written, and covers the recent development of social neuroscience.

Fletcher, G., & Fincham, F. D. (Eds.) (1991). Cognition in close relationships. Hillsdale, NJ: Erlbaum. A collection of leading scholars provide detailed chapters on attribution and other sociocognitive approaches to close relationships.

Forgas, J. P., & Smith, C. A. (2007). Affect and emotion. In M. A. Hogg & J. Cooper (Eds.), The SAGE handbook of social psychology: Concise student edition (pp. 146–175). London: SAGE. Comprehensive and readable overview of what we know about the social cognitive antecedents and consequences of people's feelings.

Frith, C. D., & Frith, U. (2012). Mechanisms of social cognition. Annual Review of Psychology, 63, 287–313. The neural bases of cognition are explored in both animal and human studies. Applications included are observational learning, prosocial behaviour and theory of mind.

Hamilton, D. L. (Ed.) (2004). Social cognition: Essential readings. New York: Psychology Press. An edited collection of classic publications in social cognition. The book has an introductory overview chapter and shorter introductory chapters for each section.

Hewstone, M. (1989). Causal attribution: From cognitive processes to collective beliefs. Oxford: Blackwell. A comprehensive and detailed coverage of attribution theory and research, which also includes coverage of European perspectives that locate attribution processes in the context of society and intergroup relations.

Hilton, D. J. (2007). Causal explanation: From social perception to knowledge-based causal attribution. In A. W. Kruglanski & E. T. Higgins (Eds.), Social psychology: Handbook of basic principles (2nd ed., pp. 232–253). New York: Guilford. A comprehensive coverage of research on causal attribution processes and social explanation.

Hogg, M. A. (2010). Influence and leadership. In S. T. Fiske, D. T. Gilbert, & G. Lindzey (Eds.), Handbook of social psychology (5th ed., Vol. 2, pp. 1166–1207). New York: Wiley. Up-to-date and detailed coverage of research on social influence processes, with a major section on minority influence.

Johnson, E. J., Pham, M. T., & Johar, G. V. (2007). Consumer behavior and marketing. In A. W. Kruglanski & E. T. Higgins (Eds.), Social psychology: A handbook of basic principles (2nd ed., pp. 869–887). New York: Guilford Press. This current and detailed chapter also discusses persuasion and attitude change in the area of consumer behaviour.

Keltner, D., & Lerner, J. S. (2010). Emotion. In S. T. Fiske, D. T. Gilbert, & G. Lindzey (Eds.), Handbook of social psychology (5th ed., Vol. 1, pp. 317–352). New York: Wiley. Completely up-to-date and very detailed overview of what we know about affect and emotion.

Knowles, E. S., & Linn, J. A. (Eds.) (2004). Resistance and persuasion. Mahwah, NJ: Erlbaum. A discussion of persuasion with a particular emphasis on resistance to persuasion.

Lieberman, M. D. (2010). Social cognitive neuroscience. In S. T. Fiske, D. T. Gilbert, & G. Lindzey (Eds.), Handbook of social psychology (5th ed., Vol. 1, pp. 143–193). New York: Wiley. Current and very detailed overview of social neuroscience from one of its leading researchers.

Macrae, C. N., & Quadflieg, S. (2010). Perceiving people. In S. T. Fiske, D. T. Gilbert, & G. Lindzey (Eds.), Handbook of social psychology (5th ed., Vol. 1, pp. 428–463). New York: Wiley. Comprehensive coverage of what we know about person perception—how we form and use our cognitive representations of people.

Macrae, C. N., & Quadflieg, S. (2010). Perceiving people. In S. T. Fiske, D. T. Gilbert, & G. Lindzey (Eds.), Handbook of social psychology (5th ed., Vol. 1, pp. 428–463). New York: Wiley. Comprehensive coverage of what we know about person perception—how we form and use our cognitive representations of people.

Maio, G., & Haddock, G. (2010). The science of attitudes. London: SAGE. A mid- to upper-level text dedicated to the science of attitudes—written by two leading attitude researchers.

Maio, G., & Haddock, G. (2010). The science of attitudes. London: SAGE. A mid- to upper-level text dedicated to the science of attitudes—written by two leading attitude researchers.

Maio, G. R., & Haddock, G. (2007). Attitude change. In A. W. Kruglanski & E. T. Higgins (Eds.), Social psychology: Handbook of basic principles (2nd ed., pp. 565–586). New York: Guilford. Comprehensive and up-to-date coverage of what we know about processes of attitude change.

Martin, R., & Hewstone, M (Eds.) (2010). Minority influence and innovation: Antecedents, processes and consequences. Hove, UK: Psychology Press. An edited book that has contributions on minority influence by most of the leaders in the field of minority influence research.

Martin, R., & Hewstone, M. (2007). Social influence processes of control and change: Conformity, obedience to authority, and innovation. In M. A. Hogg & J. Cooper (Eds), The SAGE handbook of social psychology: Concise student edition (pp. 312–332). London: SAGE. A current and comprehensive review of social influence research, including conformity, obedience and minority influence.

McClure, J. (1991). Explanations, accounts, and illusions: A critical analysis. Cambridge, UK: Cambridge University Press. A critical, wide-ranging and eclectic discussion of attribution as social explanation.

Moscovici, S., Mugny, G., & van Avermaet, E. (2008). Perspectives on minority influence. Cambridge, UK: Cambridge University Press. An up-to-date overview of research on minority influence by leading scholars of this notably European topic.

Moskowitz, G. B. (2005). Social cognition: Understanding self and others. New York: Guilford. A relatively recent comprehensive social cognition text that is written in a relatively accessible style as an introduction to the topic.

Moskowitz, G. B. (2005). Social cognition: Understanding self and others. New York: Guilford. A relatively recent comprehensive social cognition text that is written in a relatively accessible style as an introduction to the topic.

Oppenheim, A. N. (1992). Questionnaire design, interviewing and attitude measurement (2nd ed.). London: Pinter. A well-illustrated and comprehensive guide with easy-to-follow examples.

Robinson, J. P., Shaver, P. R., & Wrightsman, L. S. (Eds.) (1991). Measures of personality and social psychological attitudes. New York: Academic Press. A source book of scales that have been used in social psychology and the study of personality.

Rothman, A. J., & Salovey, P (2007). The reciprocal relation between principles and practice: Social psychology and health behaviour. In A. W. Kruglanski & E. T. Higgins (Eds.), Social psychology: A handbook of basic principles (2nd ed., pp. 826–849). New York: Guilford Press. Detailed overview of social psychological processes in the context of health; including coverage of heath attitudes and behaviour.

Schwarz, N. (1996). Survey research: Collecting data by asking questions. In G. R. Semin & K. Fiedler (Eds.), Applied social psychology (pp. 65–90). London: SAGE. A brief bird's eye view of questionnaire design, with examples.

Smith, E. R. (1994). Social cognition contribution*s to attribution theory and* research. In P. G. Devine, D. L. Hamilton, & T. M. Ostrom (Eds.), Social cognition: Impact on social psychology (pp. 77–108). San Diego, CA: Academic Press. A focused coverage of social cognitive dimensions of attribution processes.

Terry, D. J., & Hogg, *M. A. (Eds.) (2000). Attitudes, behavior, and* social context: The role of norms and group membership. Mahwah, NJ: Erlbaum. A collection of chapters discussing attitudes and attitude phenomena from the perspective of group norms, group membership and *social identity.*

Trope, Y., & Gaunt, R. (2007). Attribution and person perception. In M. A. Hogg & J. Cooper (Eds.), The SAGE handbook of social psychology: Concise student edition (pp. 176–194). London: SAGE. A relatively recent, comprehensive and above all readable overview of attribution research.

Turner, J. C. (1991). Social influence. Buckingham, UK: Open Universit*y Press. Scholarly discussion of social influence which takes a* critical stance from a European perspective and places particular emphasis on social identity, minority influence and the role of group membership and group norms.

Visser, P. S., & Cooper, J. *(2007). Attitude change. In M. A. Hogg & J. Cooper (Eds.), The SAGE handb*ook of social psychology: Concise student edition (pp. 197–218). London: SAGE. A comprehensive and accessible overview of theory and research on attitude change.

Weary, G., Stanley, M. A., & Harvey, J. H. (1989). *Attribution. New York: Springer*-Verlag. A discussion of applications of attribution theory and the operation of attribution processes in clinical settings and everyday life outside the laboratory.

Zimbardo, P. G*., & Leippe,* M. R. (1991). The psychology of attitude change and social influence. New York: McGraw-Hill. A detailed look at attitudes and social influences in society, with particular attention to persuasion, influence and change. Well illustrated with relevant examples.

Chapter 10

Alper, S., Tjosvold, D., & Law, K. S. (1998). Interdependence and controversy in group decision-making: Antecedents to effective self-managing teams. *Organizational Behavior and Human Decision Process, 74*(1), 33–52.

Alpers, A., & Lo, B. (1999). Avoiding family feuds: Responding to surrogate demands for life-sustaining interventions. *Journal of Law, Medicine and Ethics, 27*(1), 74–88.

Ang, M. (2002). Advanced communication skills: Conflict management and persuasion. *Academic Medicine, 77*(11), 1166.

Attewell, A. (1998). Florence Nightingale's relevance to nurses. *Journal of Holistic Nursing, 16*(2), 281–291.

Barringer, B., & Glod, C. A. (1998). Therapeutic relationship and effective communication. In C. A. Glod (Ed.), *Contemporary psychiatric-mental health nursing: The brain–behavior connection* (pp. 47–61). Philadelphia, PA: F. A. Davis.

Beach, M. C., & Inui, T. (2006). Relationship-centered care research network. Relationship-centered care. A constructive reframing. *Journal of General Internal Medicine, 21*, S3–S8.

Beckwith, F., & Frankel, R. (1984). The effect of physician behavior on the collection of data. *Annals of Internal Medicine, 101*(6), 692–696.

Bonvicini, K. A., Perlin, M. J., Bylund, C. L., Carroll, G., Rouse, R. A., & Goldstein, M. G. (2008). Impact of communication training on physician expression of empathy in patient encounters. *Patient Education and Counseling, 75*, 3–10.

Boyle, D., Dwinnell, B., & Platt, F. (2005). Invite, listen and summarize: A patient-centered communication technique. *Academic Medicine, 80*(1), 29–32.

Cann, A., Zapata, C. L., & Davis, H. B. (2009). Positive and negative styles of humor in communication: Evidence for the importance of considering both styles. *Communication Quarterly, 57(4)*, 452–468.

Carney, B. T., West, P., Neily, J., Mills, P. D., & Bagian, J. P. (2010). Differences in nurse and surgeon perceptions of teamwork: Implications for use of a briefing checklist in the OR. *Association of Perioperative Registered Nurses, 91(6)*, 722–729.

Charon, R. (2001). Narrative medicine: A model for empathy, reflection, profession, and trust. *Journal of the American Medical Association, 286*(15), 1897–1902.

Coombs, M. (2003). Power and conflict in intensive care clinical decision-making. *Intensive Critical Care Nursing, 19*(3), 125–135.

Coulehan, J. L., & Block, M. R. (2001). *The medical interview: Mastering skills for clinical practice.* Philadelphia, PA: F. A. Davis.

Coulehan, J. L., Platt, F. W., Egener, B., Frankel, R., Lin, C. T., Lown, B., & Salazar, W. (2001). "Let me see if I have this right . . ." Words that help build empathy. *Annals of Internal Medicine. 135,* 221–227.

Davidhizar, R. E., Giger, J. N., & Poole, V. (1997). When change is a must. *Health Care Supervisor, 16*(2), 193–196.

Davis, C. M. (2006). *Patient practitioner interaction: An experiential manual for developing the art of health care* (4th ed.). Thorofare, NJ: Slack.

Davis, M. A. (2009). A perspective on cultivating clinical empathy. *Complementary Therapies in Clinical Practice, 15,* 76–79.

Donnelly, W. J. (1996). Taking suffering seriously: A new role for the medical case history. *Academic Medicine, 71*(7), 730–737.

Dove, M. A. (1998). Conflict: Process and resolution. *Nursing Management, 29*(4), 430–432.

Eason, F. R., & Brown, S. T. (1999). Conflict management: Assessing educational needs. *Journal for Nurses in Staff Development, 15*(3), 92–96.

Ekman, P. (1999). Facial expressions. In T. Dalgleish & M. Power (Eds.), *Handbook of cognition and emotion* (pp. 45–60). New York, NY: John Wiley & Sons.

Epstein, R. M. (1999). Mindful practice. *Journal of the American Medical Association, 282*(9), 833–839.

Epstein, R. M., & Street, R. L. (2007). *Patient-centered communication in cancer care. Promoting healing and reducing suffering* (NIH Publication No. 07-6225). Bethesda, MD: National Cancer Institute.

Fox, F. E., Rodham, K. J., Harris, M. F., Taylor, G. J., Sutton, J., Scott, J., & Robinson, B. (2009). Experiencing "the other side." A study of empathy and empowerment in general practitioners who have been patients. *Qualitative Health Research, 19*(11), 1580–1588.

Fraser, J. J. (2001). Technical report: Alternative dispute resolution in medical malpractice. *Pediatrics, 107*(3), 602–612.

Garden, R. (2008). Expanding clinical empathy: An activist perspective. *Journal of Internal Medicine, 24*(1), 122–125.

Greenfield, B. H., Anderson, A., Cox, B., & Tanner, M. C. (2008). Meaning of caring to 7 novice physical therapists during their first year of clinical practice. *Physical Therapy, 88*(10), 1154–1166.

Haidet, P., & Paterniti, D. A. (2003). "Building" a history rather than "taking" one: A perspective on information sharing during the medical interview. *Archives of Internal Medicine, 163*(10) 1134–1140.

Halstead, L. S. (2001). The power of compassion and caring in rehabilitation healing. *Archives of Physical Medicine Rehabilitation, 82,* 149–154.

Hassed, C. (2001). How humour keeps you well. *Australian Family Physician, 1,* 25–28.

Hayes, J., & Cox, C. (1999). The experience of therapeutic touch from a nursing perspective. *British Journal of Nursing, 8*(18), 1249–1254.

Henkin, A. B., Dee, J. R., & Beatus, J. (2000). Social communication skills of physical therapist students: An initial characterization. *Journal of Physical Therapy Education, 14*(2), 32–38.

Henrikson, M. (1998). Managing through conflict. Harnessing the energy and power of change. *Association of Women's Health, Obstetric and Neonatal Nurses (AWHONN) Lifelines, 2*(4), 53–54.

Herdtner, S. (2000). Using therapeutic touch in nursing practice. *Orthopaedic Nursing, 19*(5), 77–82.

Hutchinson, T. A. (2005). Coming home to mindfulness in medicine. *Canadian Medical Association Journal, 173*(4), 391–392.

Jadad, A. R., & Delamothe, T. (2004). What next for electronic communication and health care? *British Medical Journal, 328,* 1143–1144.

James, T. & Cinelli, B. (2003). Exploring gender-based communication styles. *Journal of School Health, 73*(1), 41–42.

Jensen, G., Gwyer, J., Shepard, K., & Hack, L. (2000). Expert practice in physical therapy. *Physical Therapy, 80*(1), 28–52.

Johnson, T. M., Hardt, E. R., & Kleinman, A. (1995). Cultural factors in the medical interview. In M. Lipkin, S. M. Putnam, & S. M. A. Lazare (Eds.), *The medical interview: Clinical care, education and research* (pp. 153–162). New York, NY: Springer-Verlag.

Kabat-Zinn, J. (1994). *Wherever you go, there you are.* New York, NY: Hyperion.

Kearney, M. K., Weininger, R. B., Vachon, R. L. S., Harrison, R. L., & Mount, B. M. (2009). Self-care of physicians caring for patients at the end of life. *Journal of the American Medical Association, 302*(11), 1155–1164.

Kern, D. E., Branch, Jr., W. T., Jackson, J. L., Brady, D. W., Feldman, M. D., Levinson, W., & Lipkin, M. (2005). Teaching the psychosocial aspects of care in the clinical setting: Practical recommendations. *Academic Medicine, 80*(1), 8–20.

Kleinman, A. (1988). *The illness narratives.* New York, NY: Basic Books.

Kleinman, A., Eisenberg, L., & Good, B. (1978). Culture, illness and care. *Annals of Internal Medicine, 88,* 251–258.

Kummervold, P. E., Trondsen, M., Andreassen, H., Gammon, D., & Hjortdahl, P. (2004). Patient–physician interaction over the Internet. *Tidsskr Nor Laegeforen, 124*(20), 2633–2636.

Levinson, W., Roter, D., Mullooly, J., Dull, V., & Frankel, R. (1997). Physician–patient communication: The relationship with malpractice claims among primary care physicians and surgeons. *Journal of the American Medical Association, 277,* 533–559.

Lieberman, S. (2010). *Differences in male and female communication styles.* Retrieved from http://www.simmalieberman.com/articles/maleandfemale.html

Lipcamon, J. D., & Mainwaring, B. A. (2004). Conflict resolution in healthcare management. *Radiology Management, 26*(3), 48–51.

Lipkin, M., Frankel, R. M., Beckman H. B., Charon, R., & Fein, O. (1995). Performing the medical interview. In M. Lipkin, S. M. Putnam, & S. M. A. Lazare (Eds.), *The medical interview: Clinical care, education and research* (pp. 65–82). New York, NY: Springer-Verlag.

Loscalzo, M. (1999). In coping with cancer, gender matters. *Journal of the National Cancer Institute, 91*(20), 1712–1714.

Martin, S. T. (1999). Language shapes thought. *PT—Magazine of Physical Therapy,* 7(6), 44–45.

McCray, A. T. (2005). Promoting health literacy. *Journal of the Medical Information Association, 12,* 152–163.

Mead, N., & Bower, P. (2002). Patient-centered consultations and outcomes in primary care: A review of the literature. *Patient Education and Counseling, 48,* 51–61.

Mentgen, J. L. (2001). Healing touch. *Holistic Nursing Care, 36*(1), 143–157.

Miller, B. J. (1998). The art of managing conflict. *Journal of Christian Nursing, 15*(1), 14–17.

Misra-Hebert, A., D. (2003). Physician cultural competence: Cross-cultural communication improves care. *Cleveland Clinic Journal of Medicine, 70*(4), 289–303.

Monroe, C. K. (2009). The effects of therapeutic touch on pain. *Journal of Holistic Nursing, 27*(2), 85–92.

Moore, C. (1996). *The mediation process* (2nd ed.). San Francisco, CA: Jossey-Bass.

Nelson, H. W., & Cox, D. M. (2003). The causes and consequences of conflict and violence in nursing homes: Working toward a collaborative work culture. *Health Care Management, 22*(4), 349–360.

Nibler, R., & Harris, K. L. (2003). The effects of culture and cohesiveness on intragroup conflict and effectiveness. *Journal of Social Psychology, 143*(5), 613–631.

Northouse, L. L., & Northouse, P. G. (1998). *Health communications: Strategies for health professionals* (3rd ed.). Stamford, CT: Appleton & Lange.

O'Day, B. L., Killeen, M., & Iezzoni, L. I. (2004). Improving health care experiences of persons who are blind or have low vision: Suggestions from focus groups. *American Journal of Medical Quality, 19*(5), 193–200.

Pettrey, L. (2003, February). Who let the dogs out? Managing conflict with courage and skill. *Critical Care Nurse,* pp. S21–S24.

Pillemer, K., Hegeman, C. R., Albright, B., & Henderson, C. (1998). Building bridges between families and nursing home staff: The partners in caregiving program. *The Gerontologist, 38*(4), 499–503.

Platt, F. W., Gaspar, D. L., Coulehan, J. L., Fox, L., Adler, A. J., Weston, W. W., . . . Steward, M. (2001). "Tell me about yourself": The patient-centered interview. *Annals of Internal Medicine, 134*(11), 1079–1085.

Platt, F., & Platt, C. (2003). Two collaborating artists produce a work of art. *Archives of Internal Medicine, 163*(10), 1131–1132.

Purtilo, R., & Haddad, A. (2007). *Health professional and patient interaction* (7th ed.). Philadelphia, PA: W. B. Saunders.

Raica, D. A. (2009). Effect of action-oriented communication training on nurses' communication self-efficacy. *Medical Surgical Nursing, 18*(6), 343–360.

Rakel, D. P., Hoeft, T. J., Barrett, B. P., Chewning, B.A., Craig, B. M., & Niu, M. (2009). Practitioner empathy and the duration of the common cold. *Family Medicine, 41*(7), 494–501.

Rotarius, T., & Liberman, A. (2000). Health care alliances and alternative dispute resolution: Managing trust and conflict. *Health Care Manager, 18*(3), 25–31.

Roter, D., & Hall, J. (1992). *Doctors talking with patients: Patients talking with doctors.* Westport, CT: Auburn Books.

Routasalo, P. (1999). Physical touch in nursing studies: A literature review. *Journal of Advanced Nursing, 30*(4), 843–850.

Saha, S., Beach, M. C., & Cooper, L. A. (2008). Patient centeredness, cultural competence, and healthcare quality. *Journal of the National Medical Association, 100*(11), 1275–1285.

Schacher, C. L., Stalker, C.A., & Teram, E. (1999). Toward sensitive practice issues for physical therapists working with survivors of childhood sexual abuse. *Physical Therapy, 79*(3), 248–261.

Schmitt, N. (1990). Patients' perception of laughter in a rehabilitation hospital. *Rehabilitation Nursing, 15*(3), 143–146.

Schneider, J., Kaplan, S. H., Greenfield, S., Li, W., & Wilson, I. B. (2004). Better physician–patient relationships are associated with higher reported adherence to antiretroviral therapy in patients with HIV infection. *Journal of General Internal Medicine, 19*(11), 1096–1103.

Schon, D. (1983) *The reflective practitioner: How professionals think in action*. San Francisco, CA: Jossey Bass.

Schouten, B. C., & Meeuwesen, L. (2006). Cultural differences in medical communication: A review of the literature. *Patient Education and Counseling, 64*, 21–34.

Shepard, K. (2007). Are you waving or drowning? *Physical Therapy, 87*(11), 1543–1554.

Simon, V. & Pedersen, H. (2005). Communicating with men at work: Bridging the gap with male co-workers and employees. Retrieved from http://www.itstime.com/mar2005.htm

Smith, R. C., & Hoppe, R. B. (1991). The patient's story: Integrating the patient- and physician-centered approaches to interviewing. *Annals of Internal Medicine, 115*, 470–477.

Stacey, C. L., Henderson, S., MacArthur, K. R., & Dohan, D. (2009). Demanding patient or demanding encounter? A case study of cancer. *Social Science and Medicine, 69*, 729–737.

Stiefel, F., Barth, J., Bensing, J., Fallowfield, L., Jost, L., Razavi, D., & Kiss, A. (2010). Communication skills training in oncology: A position paper based on a consensus meeting among European experts in 2009. *Annals of Oncology, 21*, 204–207.

Studdert, D. M., Mello, M. M., Burns, J. P., Puopolo, A. L., Galper, B. Z., Truog, R. D., & Brennan, T. A. (2003). Conflict in the care of patients with prolonged stay in the ICU: Types, sources, and predictors. *Intensive Care Medicine, 29*(9), 1489–1497.

Sutcliffe, K. M., Lewton, E., & Rosenthal, M. M. (2004). Communication failures: An insidious contributor to medical mishaps. *Academic Medicine, 79*(2), 186–194.

Taylor, R. R., Wook Lee, S., Kielhofner, G., & Ketkar, M. (2009). Therapeutic use of self: A Nationwide survey of practitioners' attitudes and experiences. *The American Journal of Occupational Therapy, 63*(2), 198–207.

Teal, C. R., & Street, R. L. (2009). Critical elements of culturally competent communication in the medical encounter: A review and model. *Social Science and Medicine, 68*, 533–543.

Thomas, K., & Kilmann, R. (1974). *Thomas Kilmann conflict mode instrument*. Tuxedo, NY: Xicom.

Thompson, V. L., Cavazos-Rehg, P. A., Jupka, K., Caito, N., Gratzke, J., Tate, K. Y., . . . Kreuter, M. W. (2007). Evidential preferences: Cultural appropriateness strategies in health communication. *Health Education Research, 23*(3), 549–559.

Tongue, J. R., Epps, H. R., & Forese, L. L. (2005). Communication skills for patient-centered care: Research-based, easily learned techniques for medical interviews that benefit orthopedic surgeons and their patients. *Journal of Bone and Joint Surgery, 87*(3), 652–658.

Tripicchio, B., Bykerk, K., &Wegner, J. (2009). Increasing patient participation: The effect of training physical and occupational therapists to involve geriatric patients in the concerns-clarification and goal-setting process. *Journal of Physical Therapy Education, 23*(1), 55–61.

Umbreit, A. W. (2000). Healing touch: Applications in the acute care setting. *American Association of Critical Care Nursing Clinical Issues, 11*(1), 105–119.

Umiker, W. (1997). Collaborative conflict resolution. *Health Care Supervisor, 15*(3), 70–75.

Vanderhoff, M. (2005). Patient education and health literacy. *PT–Magazine of Physical Therapy, 13*(9), 42–46.

Wainwright, S. F., Shepard, K. F., Harman, L. B., & Stephens, J. (2010). Physical therapist clinicians: A comparison of how reflection is used to inform the clinical-decision-making process. *Physical Therapy, 90*(1), 75–88.

Wanzer, M., Booth-Butterfield, M., & Booth-Butterfield, S. (2005). If we didn't use humor, we'd cry: Humorous coping communication in health care settings. *Journal of Health Communication, 10*, 105–125.

Williams, K., Kemper, S., & Hummert, M. L. (2004). Enhancing communication with older adults: Overcoming elderspeak. *Journal of Gerontological Nursing, 30*(10), 17–25.

Woltersdorf, M. (1998). Body language. *PT–Magazine of Physical Therapy, 6*(9), 112.

Xu, Y., & Davidhizar, R. (2004). Conflict management styles of Asian and Asian American nurses: Implications for the nurse manager. *Health Care Management, 23*(1), 46–53.

Young, A., & Turner, J. (2009). Developing inter-professional training for conflict resolution—A scoping audit and training pilot. *Mental Health Review Journal, 14*(1), 4–11.

Zweibel, E. B., & Goldstein, R. (2001). Conflict resolution at the University of Ottawa faculty of medicine: The pelican and the sign of the triangle. *Academic Medicine, 76*(4), 337–344.

Chapter 11

Aalto, A. M., Uutela, A. and Aro, A. R. (1997). Health-related quality of life among insulin dependent diabetics: Disease related and psychosocial correlates. *Patient Education and Counseling, 30*, 215–225.

Allen, D. G., Weeks, K. P. and Moffat, K. R. (2005). Turnover intentions and voluntary turnover: Thee moderating roles of self monitoring, locus of control, proactive personality, and risk aversion. *Journal of Applied Psychology, 90*, 980–990.

Allen, L. L., Haririfar, M., Cohen, J. and Henderson, M. J. (2000). Quality of life and locus of control of migraineurs. *Clinical Excellence in Nurse Practitioners, 4*, 41–49.

Allport, G. W. (1921). *Personality traits: Their classification and measurement.* New York: Holt.

Allport, G. W. (1937). *Personality: A psychological interpretation.* New York: Holt.

Allport, G. W. (1961). *Pattern and growth in personality.* New York: Holt, Rinehart & Winston.

Allport, G. W. (1966). Religious context of prejudice. *Journal for the Scientific Study of Religion, 5*, 447–457.

Allport, G. W. and Odbert, H. (1936). Trait names: A psycholexical study. *Psychological Monographs, 47*, 1–171.

Allport, G. W. and Ross, M. J. (1967). Personal religious orientation and prejudice. *Journal of Personality and Social Psychology, 5*, 432–443.

Ashton, M. C. and Lee, K. (2001). A theoretical basis for the major dimensions of personality. *European Journal of Personality, 15*, 327–353.

Amir, M., Roziner, I., Knoll, A. and Neufield, M. Y. (1999). Selfefficacy and social support as mediators in the relation between disease severity and quality of life in patients with epilepsy. *Epilepsia, 40*, 41–49.

Anderman, L. H. and Midgley, C. (1997). Motivation and middle school students. In J. L. Irvin (ed.), *What current research says to the middle level practitioner* (pp. 41–48). Columbus, OH: National Middle School Association.

Bandura, A. (1977). *Social learning theory.* Englewood Cliffs, NJ: Prentice Hall.

Bandura, A. (1978). The self-system in reciprocal determinism. *American Psychologist, 33*, 344–358.

Bandura, A. (1989). Human agency in social cognition. *American Psychologist, 44*, 1175–1184.

Bandura, A. (1990). Some reflections on reflection. *Psychological Inquiry, 1*, 101–105.

Bandura, A. (1991). Self-efficacy. In R. Schwarzer and R. Wicklund (eds), *Anxiety and self-focussed attention.* New York: Harwood Academic.

Bandura, A. (1994). Self-efficacy. In V. S. Ramachandran (ed.), *Encyclopaedia of human behaviour.* New York: Academic Press.

Bandura, A. (1997). *Self-efficacy: The exercise of control.* New York:Freeman.

Bandura, A. (1998). Personal and collective efficacy in human adaptation and change. In J. G. Adair, D.

Belanger and K. L. Dion (eds), *Advances in psychological science* (Vol. 1: *Personal, social and cultural aspects*). Hove, UK: Psychology Press.

Bandura, A. (1999). Social cognitive theory of personality. In L. Pervin and O. John (eds), *Handbook of Personality* (2nd edn). New York: Guilford.

Bandura, A. (2000). Exercise of human agency through collective efficacy. *Current Directions in Psychological Science, 9*, 75–78.

Bandura, A. (2001). Social cognitive theory: An agentic perspective. *Annual Review of Psychology, 52*, 1–26.

Bandura, A. (2002). Swimming against the mainstream: The early years from chilly tributary to transformative mainstream. *Behaviour Research & Therapy, 42*, 613–630.

Bandura, A. (2004). Self-efficacy. In W. E. Craighead and C. B. Nemeroff (eds), *The concise Corsini encyclopedia of psychology and behavioral science* (3rd edn). Hoboken, NJ: Wiley.

Bandura, A. (2006). Guide for creating self-efficacy scales. In F. Pajares and T. Urdan (eds), *Self-efficacy beliefs of adolescents.* Greenwich, CT: Information Age Publishing. Also available at www.des.emory.edu/mfp/self-efficacy.html.

Bandura, A. (ed.). (1995). *Self-efficacy in changing societies.* New York: Cambridge University Press.

Bandura, A. and Walters, R. H. (1963). *Social learning and personality development.* New York: Holt, Rinehart and Winston.

Benassi, V. A., Sweeney, P. D. and Dufour, C. L. (1988). Is there a relationship between locus of control orientation and depression? *Journal of Abnormal Psychology*, *97*, 357–367.

Barton, K., Dielman, T. E. and Cattell, R. B. (1971). _e prediction of school grades from personality and IQ measures. *Personality*, *2*, 325–333.

Bender, W. N. (1995). *Learning disabilities: Characteristics, identification and teaching strategies* (2nd edn). Needham Heights, MA: Allyn & Bacon.

Block, J. H. and Block, J. (1980). The role of ego control and ego resiliency in the organisation of behaviour. In W. A. Collins (ed.), *Development of cognitive, affect and social relations: The Minnesota symposium in child psychology* (pp. 39–101). Hillsdale, NJ: Erlbaum.

Block, J., and Block, J. H. (2006). Venturing a 30-year longitudinal study. *American Psychologist, 61*, 315–327.

Boyle, G. J. (1989). Re-examination of the major personality factors in the Cattell, Comrey and Eysenck scales: Were the factor solutions by Noller *et al.* optimal? *Personality and Individual Differences*, *10*, 1289–1299.

Briggs, S. R. (1989). Shyness: Introversion or neuroticism? *Journal of Research in Personality*, *22*, 290–307.

Cattell, R. B. (1950). *Personality: A systematic, theoretical, and factual study*. New York: McGraw-Hill.

Cattell, R. B. (1957). *Personality and motivation: Structure and measurement*. New York: Harcourt, Brace & World.

Cattell, R. B. (1965). *The scientific analysis of personality*. Baltimore, MD: Penguin.

Cattell, R. B. (1971). *Abilities, their structure, growth, and action*. New York: Houghton Mifflin.

Cattell, R. B. (1973). *Personality and mood by questionnaire*. New York: Jossey-Bass.

Cattell, R. B. (1979). *Personality and learning theory* (Vol. 1: *A systems theory of maturation and structured learning*). New York: Springer.

Cattell, R. B. (1980). *Personality and learning theory* (Vol. 2: *A systems theory of maturation and structured learning*). New York: Springer.

Cattell, R. B. (1982). *The inheritance of personality and ability*. New York: Academic Press.

Cattell, R. B. and Child, D. (1975). *Motivation and dynamic structure*. New York: Wiley.

Cattell, R. B. and Kline, P. (1977). *Thee scientific analysis of personality and motivation*. New York: Academic Press.

Cattell, R. B., Eber, H. W. and Tatsuoka, M. M. (1970). *Handbook for the Sixteen-Personality Factor questionnaire*. Champaign, IL: Institute for Personality and Ability Testing.

Church, A. T. and Burke, P. J. (1994). Exploratory and confirmatory tests of the Big Five and Tellegen's three- and four-dimensional models. *Journal of Personality and Social Psychology*, *66*, 93–114.

Conn, S. R. and Rieke, M. L. (1994). *The 16PF Fifth edition technical manager*. Champaign, IL: Institute for Personality and Ability Testing.

Costa, P. T. Jr and McCrae, R. R. (1992). *Revised NEO Personality Inventory (NEO-PI-R) and NEO Five-Factor Inventory (NEOFFI) professional manual*. Odessa, FL: Psychological Assessment Resources.

Costa, P. T. Jr and McCrae, R. R. (2003).Personality in adulthood: A five factor theory. London: Guildford Press.

Cvengros, J. A., Christensen, A. J. and Lawton, W. J. (2005). Health locus of control and depression in chronic kidney disease: A dynamic perspective. *Journal of Health Psychology*, *10*, 677–687.

Csikszentmihalyi, M. (1999). If we are so rich, why aren't we happy? *American Psychologist*, *54*, 821–827.

De Mann, A., Leduc, C. and Labrèche-Gauthier, L. (1992). Parental control in child rearing and multidimensional locus of control. *Psychological Reports*, *70*, 320–322.

De Raad, B. (2000). *The Big Five personality factors: The psycholexical approach to personality*. Seattle, WA: Hogrefe and Huber.

Digman, J. M. and Takemoto-Chock, N. K. (1981). Factors in the natural language of personality: Re-analysis, comparison, and interpretation of six major studies. *Multivariate Behavioral Research*, *6*, 149–170.

Dollard, J. and Miller, N. (1941). *Social learning and imitation*. New Haven, CT: Yale University Press.

Dollard, J. and Miller, N. (1950). *Personality and psychotherapy: An analysis in terms of learning, thinking, and culture*. New York: McGraw-Hill.

Eysenck, H. (1971). *Race, intelligence and education*. London: Maurice Temple Smith.

Eysenck, H. J. (1947). *Dimensions of personality*. London: Routledge and Kegan Paul.

Eysenck, H. J. (1952). The effects of psychotherapy: An evaluation. *Journal of Consulting Psychology*, *16*, 319–324.

Eysenck, H. J. (1963). *Use and abuses of psychology*. Baltimore, MD: Penguin.

Eysenck, H. J. (1965a). The effcts of psychotherapy. *International Journal of Psychiatry*, 1, 99–142.

Eysenck, H. J. (1965b). *Fact and fiction in psychology*. Baltimore, MD: Penguin.

Eysenck, H. J. (1967). *The biological basis of personality*. Springfeld, IL: Charles C. Thomas.

Eysenck, H. J. (1970). *The structure of human personality* (3rd edn).London: Methuen.

Eysenck, H. J. (1975). The structure of social attitudes. *British Journal of Social and Clinical Psychology, 14*, 323–331.

Eysenck, H. J. (1976a). *The measurement of personality*. Lancaster: Medical and Technical Publishers.

Eysenck, H. J. (1976b). Structure of social attitudes. *Psychological Reports, 39*, 463–466.

Eysenck, H. J. (1979). *The structure and measurement of intelligence*. New York: Springer-Verlag.

Eysenck, H. J. (1982a). Development of a theory. In H. J. Eysenck (ed.), *Personality, genetics and behaviour*. New York: Praeger.

Eysenck, H. J. (1982b). Left-wing authoritarianism: Myth or reality? *Political Psychology, 3*, 234–238.

Eysenck, H. J. (1986). *Decline and fall of the Freudian empire*. London: Penguin.

Eysenck, H. J. (1990a). Biological dimensions of personality. In L. A. Pervin (ed.), *Handbook of personality: Theory and research* (pp. 244–276). New York: Guilford.

Eysenck, H. J. (1990b). Genetic and environmental contributions to individual differences: The three major dimensions of personality. *Journal of Personality, 58*, 245–261.

Eysenck, H. J. (1991). Dimensions of personality: 16, 5 or 3? Criteria for a taxonomic paradigm. *Personality and Individual Differences, 12*, 773–790.

Eysenck, H. J. (1992). The definition and measurement of psychoticism. *Personality and Individual Differences, 13*, 757–786.

Eysenck, H. J. (1993). Comment on Goldberg. *American Psychologist, 48*, 1299–1300.

Eysenck, H. J. (1994). Personality: Biological foundations. In P.A. Vernon (ed.), *The neuropsychology of individual differences*. London: Academic Press.

Eysenck, H. J. (1995). *Genius: the natural history of creativity*. New York: Cambridge University Press.

Eysenck, H. J. (2000). *Intelligence: A new look*. London: Transaction Publishers.

Eysenck, H. J. and Eysenck, M. W. (1985a). *Personality and individual differences: A natural science approach*. New York: Plenum.

Eysenck, H. J. and Eysenck, M. W. (1985b). The psychophysiology of personality. In *Personality and individual di_erences: A natural science approach* (pp. 217–236). New York: Plenum.

Eysenck, H. J. and Eysenck, S. B. G. (1975). *Manual of the Eysenck Personality Questionnaire*. London: Hodder & Stoughton.

Eysenck, H. J. and Eysenck, S. B. G. (1982). Recent advances in the cross-cultural study of personality. In C. D. Spielberger and J. N. Butcher (eds), *Advances in personality assessment*. Hillsdale, NJ: Erlbaum.

Eysenck, H. J. and Eysenck, S. B. G. (1991). *Manual for the EPQRR*. Sevenoaks, England: Hodder & Stoughton.

Eysenck, S. B. G. (1965). *Manual of the junior Eysenck personality inventory*. London: Hodder & Stoughton.

Eysenck, S. B. G., Barrett, P. T. and Barnes, G. E. (1993). A crosscultural study of personality: Canada and England. *Personality and Individual Differences, 14*, 1–10.

Eysenck, S. B. G., Makaremi, A. and Barrett, P. T. (1994). A crosscultural study of personality: Iranian and English children. *Personality and Individual Differences, 16*, 203–210.

Fiske, D. W. (1949). Consistency of the factorial structures of personality ratings from di_erent sources. *Journal of Abnormal and Social Psychology, 44*, 329–344.

Goldberg, L. R. (1981). Language and individual differences: Thee search for universals in personality lexicons. In L. Wheeler (ed.), *Review of Personality and Social Psychology* (Vol. 2, pp. 141–165). Beverley Hills, CA: Sage.

Harrington, D. M., Block, H. J. and Block, J. (1987). Testing aspects of Carl Rogers' theory of creative environments and childrearing antecedents of creative potential in young adolescents. *Journal of Personality and Social Psychology, 52*, 851–856.

Holmes, A., Christelis, N., & Arnold, C. (2012). Depression and chronic pain. *Medical Journal of Australia, 1*(4), 17-20.

Jackson, J. L., Shimeall, W., Sessums, L., J DeZee, K. J., Becher, D., Diemer, M., . . . O'Malley, P.G. (2010). Tricyclic antidepressants and headaches: systematic review and meta-analysis. *British Medical Journal, 341*, 1-13. Doi: http://dx.doi.org/10.1136/bmj.c5222

Kassin, S. M., Ellsworth, P. C. and Smith, V. L. (1989). The 'general acceptance' of psychological research on eyewitness testimony. *American Psychologist, 44*, 1089–1098.

Lipsitt, L. P. (1977). Taste in human neonates: Its effects on sucking and heart rate. In J. M. Weiffenbach (ed.), *Taste and development: The genesis of sweet preference*. Washington, DC: US Government Printing Office.

Liu, X., Tein, J., Zhao, Z. and Sandler, I. N. (2005). Suicidality and correlates among rural adolescents of China. *Journal of Adolescent Health*, *37*, 443–451.

Loftus, E. F. (1979). *Eyewitness testimony*. Cambridge, MA:Harvard University Press.

Martinez, J. C. (1994). Perceived control and feedback in judgement and memory. *Journal of Research in Personality*, *28*, 374–381.

Maslow, A. H. (1954). *Motivation and personality*. New York: Harper & Row.

Maslow, A. H. (1962). Lessons from the peak experience. *Journal of Humanistic Psychology*, *2*, 9–18.

Maslow, A. H. (1964). *Religions, values and peak experiences*. Columbus: Ohio State University Press.

Maslow, A. H. (1965). *Eupsychian management: A journal*. Homewood, IL: Irwin-Dorsey.

Maslow, A. H. (1967). The creative attitude. In R. L. Mooney and T. A. Rasik (eds), *Explorations in creativity* (pp. 43–57). New York: Harper & Row.

Maslow, A. H. (1968). *Toward a psychology of being*. Princeton, NJ: Van Nostrand.

Maslow, A. H. (1970). *Motivation and personality* (2nd edn). New York: Harper & Row.

McCrae, R. R. and Costa, P. T. (1989). Reinterpreting the Myers– Briggs Type Indicator from the perspective of the Five-factor model of personality. *Journal of Personality*, *57*, 17–40.

McCrae, R. R. and Costa, P. T. Jr (1995). Trait explanations in personality psychology. *European Journal of Personality*, *9*, 231–252.

McCrae, R. R. and Costa, P. T. Jr (1997). Personality trait structure as a human universal. *American Psychologist*, *52*, 509–516.

McCrae, R. R., Costa, P. T., del Pilar, G. H., Rolland, J. P. and Parker, W. D. (1998). Cross-cultural assessment of the fivefactor model: The Revised NEO Personality Inventory. *Journal of Cross-Cultural Psychology*, *29*, 171–188.

Norman, W. T. (1963). Towards an adequate taxonomy of personality attributes: Replicated factor structure in peer nomination personality ratings. *Journal of Abnormal and Social Psychology*, *66*, 574–583.

Patetsos, E., & Horjales-Araujo, E. (2016). Treating chronic pain with SSRIs: What do we know? *Pain Research and Management, 2016*, 1-17. DOI: http://dx.doi.org/10.1155/2016/2020915

Peabody, D. and Goldberg, L. R. (1989). Some determinant of factor structures from personality trait descriptors. *Journal of Personality and Social Psychology*, *57*, 552–567.

Perugini, M. and Di-Blas, L. (2002). The Big Five Marker Scales (BFMS) and the Italian ABC5 taxonomy: Analyses from an eticemic perspective. In B. De Raad and M. Perugini (eds), *Big Five assessment* (pp. 281–304). Seattle, WA: Hogrefe and Huber.

Powell, L. (1992). The cognitive underpinnings of coronary-prone behaviours. *Cognitive Therapy and Research*, *16*, 123–142.

Préau, M. and the APROCO study group (2005). Health-related quality of life and health locus of control beliefs among HIV infected treated patients. *Journal of Psychosomatic Research*, *59*, 407–413.

Rogers, C. (1970). *Encounter Groups*. New York: Harper & Row.

Rogers, C. R. (1931). *Measuring personality adjustment in children*. Boston: Houghton Mifflin.

Rogers, C. R. (1939). *Clinical treatment of the problem child*. Boston: Houghton Mifflin.

Rogers, C. R. (1951). *Client-centered therapy: Its current practice, implications, and theory*. Boston: Houghton Mifflin.

Rogers, C. R. (1954). The case of Mrs. Oak: A research analysis. In C. R. Rogers and R. F. Dymond (eds), *Psychotherapy and personality change*. Chicago: University of Chicago Press.

Rogers, C. R. (1956). What it means to become a person. In C. E. Moustakas (ed.), *The self: Explorations in personal growth* (pp. 195–211). New York: Harper.

Rogers, C. R. (1959). A theory of therapy, personality and interpersonal relationships, as developed in the client-centred framework. In S. Koch (ed.), *Psychology: A study of a science* (Vol. 3). New York: McGraw-Hill.

Rogers, C. R. (1961). *On becoming a person: A therapist's view of psychotherapy*. Boston: Houghton Mifflin.

Rogers, C. R. (1965). *Client-centered therapy: Its current practice, implication, and theory*. Boston: Houghton Mifflin.

Rogers, C. R. (1969). *Freedom to learn*. Columbus, OH: Merrill.

Rogers, C. R. (1977). *Carl Rogers on personal power*. New York: Delacorte Press.

Rogers, C. R. (1980). *A way of being*. Boston: Houghton Mifflin.

Rogers, C. R. (1983). *Freedom to learn for the 80s*. Columbus, OH: Merrill.

Rogers, C. R. and Dymond, R. F. (eds). (1954). *Psychotherapy and personality change*. Chicago: University of Chicago Press.

Rogers, C. R. and Freiberg, H. J. (1993). *Freedom to learn* (3rd edn). New York: Merrill.

Rogers, C. R. and Stevens, B. (1967). *Person to person: The problem of being human*. New York: Simon & Schuster.

Rotter, J. B. (1966). Generalized expectancies for internal versus external control of reinforcement. *Psychological Monographs*, *80* (whole no. 609).

Rotter, J. B. (1982). *The development and application of social learning theory: Selected papers*. New York: Praeger.

Saucier, G. and Goldberg, L. R. (2001). Lexical studies of indigenous personality factors: Premises, products and prospects. *Journal of Personality*, *69*, 847–879.

Saucier, G. and Ostendorf, F. (1999). Hierarchical sub-components of the Big Five personality factors: A cross-language replica

Stelmack, R. M. and Stalikas, A. (1991). Galen and the humour theory of temperament. *Personality and Individual Differences*, *12*, 255–263.

Swann, W. B. (1984). Quest for accuracy in person perception: A matter of pragmatics. *Psychological Review*, *91*, 457–477.

Wylie, R. (1979). *The self-concept: Theory and research on selected topics* (Vol. II; rev. edn). Lincoln: University of Nebraska Press.

Zuckerman, M. (1991). *Psychobiology of personality*. Cambridge: Cambridge University Press.

Chapter 12

Melzack, R. and Wall, P.D. (1996). *The Challenge of Pain*. Penguin.

A classic. The most up-to-date text by the originators of the gate control theory – and over £200 cheaper than the more recent *Wall and Melzack's Textbook of Pain*. Written in a non-technical way for the interested 'lay' reader.

Three papers from the pain research centre at Bath University are worth a read:

Morley, S., Eccleston, C. and Williams, A. (1999). Systematic review and meta-analysis of randomized controlled trials of cognitive-behavioural therapy and behaviour therapy for chronic pain in adults, excluding headache. *Pain*, 80: 1–13.

A relatively up-to-date review of intervention studies to treat pain.

Crombez, G., Eccleston, C., De Vlieger, P. *et al.* (2008). Is it better to have controlled and lost than never to have controlled at all? An experimental investigation of control over pain. *Pain*, 137: 631–9.

An experimental study of what happens when you first provide control over pain, and then take it away.

Vowles, K.E., McCracken, L.M. and Eccleston, C. (2007). Processes of change in treatment for chronic pain: the contributions of pain, acceptance, and cata-strophizing. *European Journal of Pain*, 11: 779–87.

Another paper examining the mediating effects of changed cognitions on the experience of pain.

Morris, D.B. (1999). Sociocultural and religious meanings of pain. In R.J. Gatchel and D.C. Turk (eds), *Psychosocial Factors in Pain*. New York: Guilford Press.

Extends the discussion from psychology to other perspectives on pain.

Meredith, P., Ownsworth, T. and Strong, J. (2008). A review of the evidence linking adult attachment theory and chronic pain: presenting a conceptual model. *Clinical Psychology Review*, 28: 407–29.

A very different model of chronic pain to those discussed here.

A number of websites may also provide useful information:

http://www.jr2.ox.ac.uk/bandolier/booth/painpag/

http://www.painrelieffoundation.org.uk/

http://www.nlm.nih.gov/medlineplus/pain.html

http://www.psychnet-ukk.com/clinical_psychology/clinical_psychology_pain_management.htm

Chapter 13

Abbey, A., Halman, L. & Andrews, F. M. (1992). Psychosocial, treatment and demographic predictors of the stress associated with infertility. *Fertility and Sterility*, *57*, 122–127.

Alloway, R. & Bebbington, P. (1987). The buffer theory of social support: a review of the literature. *Psychological Medicine*, *17*, 91–108.

Antonovsky, A. (1967). Social class life expectancy and overall mortality. *Milbank Memorial Fund Quarterly*, *45*, 31–73.

Australian Bureau of Statistics (ABS). (2006). *Tobacco Smoking in Australia: A Snapshot, 2004–2005.* ABS Cat. no. 4831.0. Canberra: ABS.

Australian Bureau of Statistics (ABS). (2012). *Australian Health Survey: First Results, 2011–12.* ABS Cat. no. 4364.0.55.001. Canberra: ABS.

Australian Institute of Health & Welfare (AIHW). (2004). *A Rising Epidemic: Obesity in Australian Children and Adolescents.* Risk Factors Data Briefing Number 2. Canberra: AIHW.

Australian Institute of Health & Welfare (AIHW). (2008a). *Australia's Health #11.* AIHW Cat. no. AUS 99. Canberra: AIHW.

Australian Institute of Health & Welfare (AIHW). (2008b). *2007 National Drug Strategy Household Survey: Detailed Findings.* AIHW Cat. no. PHE 107. Canberra: AIHW.

Australian Institute of Health and Welfare. (2008c). *Asthma in Australia 2008.* AIHW Asthma Series no. 3. Cat. no. ACM 14. Canberra: AIHW.

Bagnardi, V., Blangiardo, M., LaVecchia, C. L. & Corrado, G. (2001). *Alcohol Consumption and the Risk of Cancer: A Meta-analysis.* Bethesda, MD: National Institute on Alcohol Abuse and Alcoholism.

Barbour, K. A., Houle, T. T. & Dubbert, P. M. (2003). Physical inactivity as a risk factor for chronic disease. In L. M. Cohen, D. E. McCargie & R. L. Collins (eds), *The Health Psychology Handbook.* Thousand Oaks, CA: Sage, pp. 146–168.

Bartone, P. T. (1999). Hardiness protects against war-related stress in army reserve forces. *Consulting Psychology Journal, 51,* 72–82.

Beck, J. G., Gudmundsdottir, B. Palyo, S. A., Miller, L. M. & Grant, D. M. (2006). Rebound effects following deliberate thought suppression: does PTSD make a difference? *Behavior Therapy, 37,* 170–180.

Berkman, L. F. & Syme, S. L. (1979). Social networks, host resistance, and mortality: a nine year follow-up study of Alameda County residents. *American Journal of Epidemiology, 109,* 186–204.

Ben-Ze'ev, A. (2000). *The subtlety of emotions.* Cambridge, MA: MIT Press.

Berlant, N. E. & Pruitt, S. D. (2003). Adherence to medical recommendations. In L. M. Cohen, D. E. McChargue & F. L. Collins (eds), *The Health Psychology Handbook.* Thousand Oaks, CA: Sage, pp. 208–224.

Bigbee, J. (1990). Stressful life events and illness occurrence in rural versus urban women. *Journal of Community Health Nursing, 7,* 105–113.

Billings, A. G. & Moos, R. H. (1984). Coping, stress and social resources among adults with unipolar depression. *Journal of Personality and Social Psychology, 46,* 877–891.

Blair, S. N., Kohl, H. W., Gordon, N. F. & Paffenberger, R. S. (1992). How much physical activity is good for health? *Annual Review of Public Health, 13,* 99–126.

Bonanno, G. (2004). Loss, trauma, and human resilience: have we underestimated the human capacity to thrive after extremely aversive events? *American Psychologist, 59,* 20–28.

Bonanno, G. A. & Kaltman, S. (2001). The varieties of grief experience. *Clinical Psychology Review, 21,* 705–734.

Bonanno, G. A., Moskowitz, J. T., Papa, A. & Folkman, S. (2005). Resilience to loss in bereaved spouses, bereaved parents, and bereaved gay men. *Journal of Personality and Social Psychology, 88,* 827–843.

Bonanno, G. A., Papa, A., Lalande, K., Westphal, M. & Coifman, K. (2004). The importance of being flexible: the ability to enhance and suppress emotional expression predicts long-term adjustment. *Psychological Science, 157,* 482–487.

Bouchard, C. (1995). Genetics and the metabolic syndrome. *International Journal of Obesity, 19,* 552–559.

Bouchard, L., Drapeau, V., Provencher, V., Lemieux, S., Chagnon, Y., Rice, T. et al. (2004). Neuromedin beta: a strong candidate gene linking eating behaviors and susceptibility to obesity. *American Journal of Clinical Nutrition, 80,* 478–486.

Breslau, N., Kilbey, K. M. & Andreski, P. (1993). Nicotine dependence and major depression. *Archives of General Psychiatry, 50,* 31–35.

Brown, G. W. & Harris, T. (1978). *Social Origins of Depression: A Study of Psychiatric Disorder in Women.* London: Tavistock.

Brown, G. W. & Harris, T. (1986). Establishing causal links: the Bedford College studies of depression. In H. Katching (ed.), *Life Events and Psychiatric Disorders.* Cambridge: Cambridge University Press, pp. 87–107.

Brownell, K. D. & Rodin, J. (1994). The dieting maelstrom: is it possible and advisable to lose weight? *American Psychologist, 49,* 781–791

Bryant, R. A. (2000). Cognitive behavioral therapy of violence-related post-traumatic stress disorder. *Aggression and Violent Behavior, 5,* 79–97.

Bunde, J. & Suls, J. (2006). A quantitative analysis of the relationship between the Cook-Medley Hostility Scale and traditional coronary artery disease risk factors. *Health Psychology, 25*, 493–500.

Buss, D. M. (2001, December). Cognitive biases and emotional wisdom in the evolution of conflict between the sexes. *Current Directions in Psychological Science, 10*(6), 219–123.

Cacioppo, J. T. & Gardner, W. L. (1999). Emotion. *Annual Review of Psychology, 50*, 191–214.

Campbell, R. S. & Pennebaker, J. (2003). The secret life of pronouns: flexibility in writing style and physical health. *Psychological Science, 14*, 60–65.

Campfield, L. A., Smith, F. J. & Burn, P. (1996). The OB protein (leptin) pathway: a link between adipose tissue mass and central neural networks. *Hormone and Metabolic Research, 28*, 619–632.

Campos, P. (2004). *The Obesity Myth: Why America's Obsession with Weight is Hazardous to Your Health*. New York: Gotham Books.

Carney, R. M., Freedland, K. E. & Veith, R. C. (2005). Depression, the autonomic nervous system, and coronary heart disease. *Psychosomatic Medicine, 67*, 29–33.

Carver, C. S. (1997). You want to measure coping but your protocol's too long: consider the Brief COPE. *International Journal of Behavioral Medicine, 4*, 92–100.

Carver, C. S. & Scheier, M. F. (1999). Themes and issues in the self-regulation of behavior. In R. S. Wyer Jr (ed.), *Advances in Social Cognition* (Vol. 12). Mahwah, NJ: Erlbaum.

Carver, C. S., Scheier, M. F. & Weintraub, J. K. (1989). Assessing coping strategies: a theoretically based approach. *Journal of Personality and Social Psychology, 56*, 267–283.

Chandola, T., Britton, A., Brunner, E., Hemingway, H., Malik, M., Kumari, M. et al. (2008). Work stress and coronary heart disease: what are the mechanisms? *European Heart Journal, 29*, 640–648.

Chaney, J. M., Mullins, L. L., Uretsky, D. L., Pace, T. M., Werden, D. & Hartman, V. L. (1999). An experimental examination of learned helplessness in older adolescents and young adults with long-standing asthma. *Journal of Pediatric Psychology, 24*, 259–271.

Cheng, C. (2003). Cognitive and motivational processes underlying coping flexibility: a dual-process model. *Journal of Personality and Social Psychology, 84*, 425–438.

Ching, P. I., Willett, W. C., Rimm, E. B., Colditz, G. A., Gortmaker, S. L. & Stampfer, M. J. (1996). Activity level and risk of overweight in male health professionals. *American Journal of Public Health, 86*, 25–30.

Clarke, R., Emberson, J., Fletcher, A., Breeze, E., Marmot, M. & Shipley, M. J. (2009). Life expectancy in relation to cardiovascular risk factors: 38 year follow-up of 19,000 men in the Whitehall study. *British Medical Journal, 339*, b3513.

Coelho, C. M., Santos, J. A., Silva, C. F., Tichoon, J., Hine, T. J. & Wallis, G. (2008). The role of self-motion in acrophobia treatment. *Cyberpsychology & Behavior, 11*, 723–725.

Cohen, P. & Cohen, J. (1984). The clinician's illusion. *Archives of General Psychiatry, 41*, 1178–1182.

Cohen, S., Doyle, W. J., Skoner, D. P., Rabin, B. S. & Gwaltney, J. M. (1997). Social ties and susceptibility to the common cold. *Journal of the American Medical Association, 277*, 1940–1944.

Cohen, S., Doyle, W. J., Turner, R. B., Alper, C. M. & Skoner, D. P. (2003). Emotional style and susceptibility to the common cold. *Psychosomatic Medicine, 65*, 652–657.

Cohen, S., Evans, G. W., Stokols, D. & Krantz, D. S. (1986). *Behavior, Health, and Environmental Stress*. New York: Plenum.

Cohen, S., Frank, E., Doyle, B. J., Skoner, D. P., Rabin, B. S. & Gwaltney, J. M. (1998). Types of stressors that increase susceptibility to the common cold. *Health* Psychology, *17*, 214–223.

Cohen, S. & Herbert, T. B. (1996). Health psychology: psychological factors and physical disease from the perspective of human psychoneuroimmunology. *Annual Review of Psychology, 47*, 113–142.

Cohen, S., Tyrell, D. A. J. & Smith, A. P. (1991). Psychological stress and susceptibility to the common cold. *New England Journal of Medicine, 325*, 606–612.

Collins, F. L., Sorocco, K. H., Haala, K. R., Miller, B. I. & Lovallo, W. R. (2003). Stress and health. In L. M. Cohen, D. E. McChargue & F. L. Collins (eds), *The Health Psychology Handbook: Practical Issues for the Behavioral Medicine Specialist*. London: Sage, pp. 169–186.

Cooper, C. L. & Drewe, P. J. (2004). *Stress: A Brief History*. Oxford: Blackwell.

Corbett, T. (2006). The facts about weight loss products and programs. Federal Trade Commission, Food and Drug Administration. Retrieved from <www.attorneygeneral.gov/uploadedFiles/Consumers/weight_loss>.

Cosmides, L. & Tooby, J. (2000). Evolutionary psychology and the emotions. In M. Lewis and J. M. Haviland-Jones (Eds.), *Handbook of emotions (*2nd ed.). New York: Guilford Press.

Costa, P. T. Jr & McCrae, R. R. (1990). Personality disorders and the five-factor model of personality. *Journal of Personality Disorders, 4*, 362–371.

Coyne, J. C. (1992). Cognition in depression: a paradigm in crisis. *Psychological Inquiry, 3*, 232–235.

Coyne, J. C. & Holroyd, K. (1982). Stress, coping, and illness: a transactional perspective. In T. Millon, C. Green & R. Meachem (eds), *Handbook of Clinical Health Psychology*. New York: Plenum, pp. 103–127.

Coyne, J. C. & Racioppo, M. W. (2000). Never the twain shall meet? Closing the gap between coping research and clinical intervention research. *American Psychologist, 55*, 655–664.

Crandall, C. S. (1994). Prejudice against fat people: ideology and self-interest. *Journal of Personality and Social Psychology, 66*, 882–894.

Creamer, M. C., Burgess, P. & McFarlane, A. C. (2001). Post-traumatic stress disorder: findings from the Australian National Survey of Mental Health and Well-being. *Psychological Medicine, 31*(7):1237–1247.

Damasio, A. R. (1994). *Descartes' error: Emotion, reason, and the human brain*. New York: Quill.

Danbrot, M. (2004). *The New Cabbage Soup Diet*. New York: St Martin's Press.

DeLongis, A., Folkman, S. & Lazarus, R. (1988). The impact of daily stress on health and mood: psychological and social resources as mediators. *Journal of Personality and Social Psychology, 54*, 486–495.

Depue, R. A. & Monroe, S. M. (1986). Conceptualization and measurement of human disorder in life stress research: the problem of chronic disturbance. *Psychological Bulletin, 99*(1), 36–51.

Descartes, R. (1989). *The passions of the soul* (1649). Indianapolis: Hackett.

Dohrenwend, B. S. & Dohrenwend, B. P. (eds), (1974). *Stressful Life Events: Their Nature and Effects*. New York: Wiley, pp. 245–258.

Doublet, S. (2000). *The Stress Myth*. Freemans Reach, NSW: Ipsilon Publishing.

Duncan, G. (1996). Income dynamics and health. *International Journal of Health Services, 26*, 419–444.

Dusseldorp, E., van Elderen, T., Maes, S., Meulman, J. & Kraaij, V. (1999). A meta-analysis of psychoeducational programs for coronary heart disease patients. *Health Psychology, 18*, 506–519.

Ekblad, S. & Jaranson, J. (2004). Psychosocial rehabilitation. In J. Wilson & B. Drozdek (eds), *Broken Spirits: The Treatment of Traumatized Asylum Seekers, Refugees and War and Torture Victims*. New York: Brunner Routledge, pp. 609–636.

Ekman, P. (1992, May/July). An argument for basic emotions. *Cognition and Emotion*, 169–200.

Ekman, P. (2003). *Emotions revealed: Recognizing faces and feelings to improve communication and emotional life*. New York: Times Books/Henry Holt and Co.

Ekman, P. & Davidson, R. (1993). Voluntary smiling changes regional brain activity. *Psychological Science, 5*, 342–345.

Ekman, P., & Davidson, R. J. (Eds.) (1994). *The nature of emotions: Fundamental questions*. Oxford: Oxford University Press.

Ellison, C. G. & Levin, S. L. (1998). The religion-health connection: evidence, theory, and future directions. *Health Education and Behavior, 25*, 700–720.

Esterling, B. A., Kiecolt-Glaser, J. K. & Glaser, R. (1996). Psychosocial modulation of cytokine-induced natural killer cell activity in older adults. *Psychosomatic Medicine, 58*, 264–272.

Feil, J. & Hasking, P. (2008). The relationship between personality, coping strategies and alcohol use. *Addiction Research and Theory, 16*, 526–537.

Fernandez, E. & Sheffield, J. (1996). Relative contributions of life events versus daily hassles to the frequency and intensity of headaches. *Headache, 36*, 595–602.

Fillmore, K. M., Kerr, W. C., Stockwell, T., Chikritzhs, T. & Bostrom, A. (2006). Moderate alcohol use and reduced mortality risk: systematic error in prospective studies. *Addiction Research and Theory, 14*, 101–132.

Flight attendant war stories . . . stewardess. Retrieved from www. aboutmyjob.com/main.php3?action= displayarticle&artid =2111

Fong, G., Hammond, D., Laux, F., Zanna, M., Cummings, K., Borland, R. et al. (2004). The near-universal experience of regret among smokers in four countries: findings from the International Tobacco Control Policy Evaluation Survey. *Nicotine & Tobacco Research, 6*, S341–S351.

Forbes D., Fletcher S., Wolfgang B., Varker T., Creamer M., Brymer M. J. et al. (2010). Practitioner perceptions of skills for psychological recovery: a training programme for health practitioners in the aftermath of the Victorian bushfires. *Australian and New Zealand Journal of Psychiatry, 44*(12), 1105–1111.

Forshaw, M. (2002). *Essential Health Psychology*. New York: Oxford University Press.

Foster, A. A., Hylwa, S. A., Bury, J. E., Davis, M. D., Pittelkow, M. R. & Bostwick, J. M. (2012). Delusional infestation: clinical presentation in 147 patients seen at Mayo Clinic. *Journal of the American Academy of Dermatology, 67*(4), 673. e1–10. 10.1016/j.jaad.2011.12.012.

Frankel, L. P. (2004). *Nice girls don't get the corner office*. New York: Warner Books.

Freudenmann, R. W., Lepping, P., Huber, M., Dieckmann, S., Bauer-Dubau, K., Ignatius, R. et al. (2012). Delusional infestation and the specimen sign: a European multicentre study in 148 consecutive cases. *British Journal of Dermatology, 167*(2), 247–251.

Friedman, M., Powell, L. H., Thoreson, C. E., Ulmer, D., Price, V., Gill, J. J. et al. (1987). Effect of discontinuance of Type A behavioral counseling on Type A behavior and cardiac recurrence rate of post myocardial infarction patients. *American Heart Journal, 114*, 483–490.

Friedman, M. & Rosenman, R. H. (1959). Association of a specific overt behavior pattern with increases in blood cholesterol, blood clotting time, incidence of *arcus senilis* and clinical coronary artery disease. *Journal of the American Medical Association, 169*, 1286–1296.

Friedman, M. & Rosenman, R. H. (1974). *Type A Behavior and Your Heart*. New York: Alfred A. Knopf.

Frijda, N. H. (1993). Moods, emotion episodes and emotions. In M. Lewis & J. M. Haviland (Eds), *Handbook of emotions*. New York: Guilford Press.

Frisina, P. G., Borod, J. C. & Lepore, S. J. (2004). A meta-analysis of the effects of written disclosure on the health outcomes of clinical populations. *The Journal of Nervous and Mental Disease, 192*, 629–634.

Gallo, L. C. & Matthews, K. A. (2003). Understanding the association between socioeconomic status and physical health: do negative emotions play a role? *Psychological Bulletin, 129*, 10–51.

Gardner, C. D., Kiazand, A., Alhassan, S., Kim, S., Stafford, R. S., Balise, R. et al. (2007). Comparison of the Atkins, Zone, Ornish, and LEARN diets for change in weight and related risk factors among overweight premenopausal women. *Journal of the American Medical Association, 297*, 969–977.

Gardner, W. L., Gabriel, S. & Diekman, A. B. (2000). Interpersonal processes. In J. T. Cacioppo, L. G. Tassinary & G. G. Berntson (eds), *Handbook of Psychophysiology* (2nd ed.). New York: Cambridge University Press, pp. 643–664.

Gatchel, R. J. & Baum, A. (1983). *An Introduction to Health Psychology*. Reading, MA: Addison-Wesley.

Gatchel, R. J. & Oordt, M. S. (2003). *Clinical Psychology and Primary Health Care*. Washington, DC: American Psychological Association.

George, J. M. (1996). Trait and state affect. In K. R. Murphy (Ed.), *Individual differences and behaviour in organizations*. San Francisco: Jossey-Bass.

Gortmaker, S. L., Must, A., Perrin, J. M., Sobol, A. M. & Dietz, W. H. (1993). Social and economic consequences of overweight in adolescence and young adulthood. *New England Journal of Medicine, 329*, 1009–1012.

Gortmaker, S. L., Must, A., Sobol, A. M., Peterson, K., Colditz, G. A. & Dietz, W. H. (1996). Television viewing as a cause of increasing obesity among children in the United States, 1986–1990. *Archives of Pediatrics & Adolescent Medicine, 150*(4), 356–362.

Gotlib, I. H. & Hammen, C. L. (1992). *Psychological Aspects of Depression: Towards a Cognitive-Interpersonal Integration*. New York: Wiley.

Green, J. P. (2000). Treating women who smoke: the benefits of using hypnosis. In L. Hornyak & J. P. Green (eds), *Healing from Within: The Use of Hypnosis in Women's Health Care*. Washington, DC: American Psychological Association, pp. 91–117.

Greenglass, E. (2002). Proactive coping. In E. Frydenberg (ed.), *Beyond Coping: Meeting Goals, Vision, and Challenges*. London: Oxford University Press, pp. 37–62.

Gross, J. J. & Muñoz, R. F. (1995). Emotional regulation and mental health. *Clinical Psychology: Science & Practice, 2*, 151–164.

Gur, R.C., Gunning-Dixon, F., Bilker, W. B., & Gur, R. E. (2002, September). Sex differences in temporo-limbic and frontal brain volumes of healthy adults. *Cerebral Cortex, 12*(9), 998–1003.

Hayward, L. R. C. (1960). The subjective meaning of stress. *British Journal of Psychology, 33*, 185–194.

Herskowitz, J. (1987). *The Popcorn Diet Plus*. New Delhi: Pharos Books.

Hertwig, R., Pachur, T. & Kurzenhauser, S. (2005). Judgments of risk frequencies: tests of possible cognitive mechanisms. *Journal of Experimental Psychology: Learning, Memory, and Cognition, 31*, 621–642.

Hettiarachchi, M. (2007). Brief intervention for post traumatic stress disorder with combined use of cognitive behaviour therapy and eye movement desensitisation reprocessing. *AeJAMH: Australian e-Journal for the Advancement of Mental Health, 6*, 1–5.

Higgins, J. E. & Endler, N. (1995). Coping, life stress, and psychological and somatic distress. *European Journal of Personality, 9*, 253–270.

Hingson, R., Heeren, T. & Winter, M. R. (2006). Drinking onset and alcohol dependence: age at onset, duration, and severity. *Archives of Pediatrics and Adolescent Medicine, 160*, 739–746.

Holahan, C. & Moos, R. H. (1991). Life stressors, personal and social resources and depression: a four-year structural model. *Journal of Abnormal Psychology, 100*, 31–38.

Holman, D. (2005). Call centres. In D. Holman, T. D. Wall, C. Clegg, P. Sparrow, & A. Howard (Eds.), *The essentials of the new work place: A guide to the human impact of modern working practices*. Chichester, UK: John Wiley & Sons.

Holmes, T. H. & Masuda, M. (1974). Life change and illness susceptibility. In B. S. Dohrenwend & P. P. Dohrenwend (eds), *Stressful Life Events: Their Nature and Effects*. New York: Wiley, pp. 45–72.

Holmes, T. H. & Rahe, R. H. (1967). The social readjustment scale. *Journal of Psychosomatic Research, 11*, 213–218.

House, J. S., Robbins, C. & Metzner, H. L. (1982). The association of social relationships and activities with mortality: prospective evidence from the Tecumseh Community Health Study. *American Journal of Epidemiology, 116*, 123–140.

Hundley, K. (2004, April 25). An unspoken problem—two-thirds of female lawyers say they have experienced or seen harassment at work, but few want to talk about it. *St. Petersburg Times. Retrieved from* www.sptimes.com/2005/04/24/ Business/An_unspoken_problem.shtml

Hylwa, S. A., Bury, J. E., Davis, M. D., Pittelkow, M. & Bostwick, J. M. (2011). Delusional infestation, including delusions of parasitosis: results of histologic examination of skin biopsy and patient-provided skin specimens. *Archives of Dermatology, 147*(9), 1041.

Ikemi, Y. & Nakagawa, S. (1962). A psychosomatic study of contagious dermatitis. *Kyushu Journal of Medical Science, 13*, 335–350.

Izard, C. E. (1992, November). Basic emotions, relations among emotions, and emotion–cognition relations. *Psychological Bulletin*, 561–165.

Jackson, P. B. & Finney, M. (2002). Negative life events and psychological distress among young adults. *Social Psychology Quarterly, 65*, 186–201.

Johnson, P. (2005). Obesity: epidemic or myth? *Skeptical Inquirer, 29*, 25–29.

Jones, F. & Bright, J. (2001). *Stress: Myth, Theory, and Research*. Harlow, UK: Prentice Hall.

Kanders, B. S. & Blackburn, G. L. (1992). Reducing primary risk factors by therapeutic weight loss. In T. A. Wadden & T. B. VanItallie (eds), *Treatment of the Seriously Obese Patient*. New York: Guilford, pp. 213–230.

Kanner, A. D., Coyne, J. C., Schaefer, C. & Lazarus, R. S. (1981). Comparison of two modes of stress measurement: daily hassles and uplifts versus major life events. *Journal of Behavioral Medicine, 4*, 1–39.

Karasek, R. & Theorell, T. (1990). *Health Work: Stress, Productivity and the Reconstruction of Life*. New York: Basic Books.

Kennedy, S., Kiecolt-Glaser, J. K. & Glaser, R. (1990). Social support, stress, and the immune system. In B. R. Sarason, I. G. Sarason & G. R. Pierce (eds), *Social Support: An Interactional View*. New York: Wiley, pp. 253–266.

Kessler, R., Price, R. & Wortman, C. (1985). Social factors in psychopathology: stress, social support and coping processes. *Annual Review of Psychology, 36*, 351–372.

Kessler, R., Sonnega, A., Bromet, E., Hughes, M. & Nelson, C. (1995). Post-traumatic stress disorder in the National Comorbidity Survey. *Archives of General Psychiatry, 52*, 1048–1060.

Kiecolt-Glaser, J. K., Marucha, P. T., Malarkey, W. B., Mercado, A. M. & Glaser, R. (1995). Slowing of wound healing by psychological stress. *Lancet, 346*, 1194–1196.

Kiecolt-Glaser, J. K., McGuire, L., Robles, T. F. & Glaser, R. (2002). Psychoneuroimmunology: psychological influences on immune function and health. *Journal of Consulting and Clinical Psychology, 70*, 537–547.

Klein, S., Burke, L. E., Bray, G. A., Blair, S., Allison, D. B., Pi-Sunyer, X. et al. (2004). AHA scientific statement: clinical implications of obesity with specific focus on cardiovascular disease. *Circulation, 1110*, 2952–2967.

Kobasa, S. C., Hilker, R. R. & Maddi, S. R. (1979). Who stays healthy under stress? *Journal of Occupational Medicine, 21*, 595–598.

Koenig, H. G., McCullough, M. E. & Larson, D. B. (2001). *Handbook of Religion and Health*. New York: Oxford University Press.

Kosfeld, M., Heinrichs, M., Zaks, P., Fischbacher, U. & Fehr, E. (2005). Oxytocin increases trust in humans. *Nature, 435*, 673–676.

Kurth, T., Gaziano, J. M., Berger, K., Kase, C. S., Rexrode, K. M., Cook, N. R. et al. (2003). Body mass index and the risk of stroke in men. *Archives of Internal Medicine, 163*, 2557–2662.

Labott, S. M. (2004). COPD and other respiratory diseases. In P. Camic & S. Knight (eds), *Clinical Handbook of Health Psychology*. Cambridge, MA: Hogrefe & Huber, pp. 59–74.

Laland, K. N. & Brown, G. R. (2002). *Sense and nonsense: Evolutionary perspectives on human behaviour*. Oxford: Oxford University Press.

Landers, D. M. (1998). Exercise and mental health. *Exercise Science, 7*, 131–146.

Lazarus, R. (1999). *Stress and Emotion: A New Synthesis*. New York: Springer.

Lazarus, R. S. & Folkman, S. (1984). *Stress, Appraisal, and Coping*. New York: Springer.

LeDoux, J. (1996). *The Emotional Brain: The Mysterious Underpinnings of Emotional Life*. New York: Simon & Schuster.

Levenstein, S., Ackerman, S., Kiecolt-Glaser, J. K. & Dubois, A. (1999). Stress and peptic ulcer disease. *Journal of the American Medical Association, 281*, 10–11.

Levenstein, S., Kaplan, G. A. & Smith, M. W. (1997). Psychological predictors of peptic ulcer incidence in the Alameda County Study. *Journal of Clinical Gastroenterology, 24*, 140–146.

Levin, J. (2001). *God, Faith, and Health: Exploring the Spirituality-Healing Connection*. New York: John Wiley.

Lewis, W. A. & Bucher, A. M. (1992). Anger, catharsis, the reformulated frustration-aggression hypothesis, and health consequences. *Psychotherapy, 29*, 385–392.

Lichtenstein, S., Slovic, P., Fischhoff, B., Layman, M. & Combs, B. (1978). Judged frequency of lethal events. *Journal of Experimental Psychology: Human Learning and Memory, 4*, 551–578.

Lieber, C. M. (2003). Alcohol and health: a drink a day won't keep the doctor away. *Cleveland Clinic Journal of Medicine, 70*, 945–953.

Lilienfeld, S. O. (2007). Psychological treatments that can cause harm. *Perspectives on Psychological Science, 2*, 53–70.

Littrell, J. (1998). Is the experience of painful emotion therapeutic? *Clinical Psychology Review, 18*, 71–102.

Litz, B. T., Gray, M. J., Bryant, R. & Adler, A. B. (2002). Early intervention for trauma: current status and future directions. *Clinical Psychology: Science and Practice, 9*, 112–134.

Lohr, J. M., Olatunji, B. O., Baumeister, R. F. & Bushman, B. J. (2007). The psychology of anger venting and empirically supported alternatives that do no harm. *Scientific Review of Mental Health Practice, 5*, 53–64.

Lynn, S. J. & Kirsch, I. (2006). *Essentials of Clinical Hypnosis: An Evidence-Based Approach*. Washington, DC: American Psychological Association.

Maddi, S. R. (2002). The story of hardiness: twenty years of theorizing, research, and practice. *Consulting Psychology Journal, 54*, 173–185.

Maddi, S. R. (2004). On hardiness and other pathways to resilience. *American Psychologist, 60*, 261–262.

Maddi, S. R. & Kobasa, S. C. (1984). *The Hardy Executive: Health under Stress*. Homewood, IL: Dow Jones-Irwin.

Mailick, M. D., Holden, G. & Walther, V. N. (1994). Coping with childhood asthma. *Health and Social Work, 19*, 103–111.

Mann, T., Tomiyama, A. J., Westling, E., Lew, A., Samuels, B. & Chatman, J. (2007). Medicare's search for effective obesity treatments: diets are not the answer. *American Psychologist, 62*, 220–233.

Marks, G. (2005). Income poverty, subjective poverty and financial stress. Social Policy Research Paper #29. Canberra: Australian Government Department of Families, Community Services and Indigenous Affairs (FaCSIA).

Markus, H. & Kitayama, S. (1991). Culture and the self: implications for cognition, emotion, and motivation. *Psychological Review, 98*, 224–253.

Marlatt, G. A. & Gordon, J. R. (eds) (1985). *Relapse Prevention: Maintenance Strategies in the Treatment of Addictive Behaviors*. New York: Guilford.

Matarazzo, J. D. (1980). Behavioral health and behavioral medicine: frontiers for a new health psychology. *American Psychologist, 35*, 807–817.

Matthews, D. A., Larson, D. B. & Barry, C. P. (1993). *The Faith Factor: An Annotated Bibliography of Clinical Research on Spiritual Subjects* (Vol. 1). Rockville, MD: National Institute for Mental Healthcare Research.

Matthews, K. A., Gump, B. B., Harris, K. F., Haney, T. L. & Barefoot, J. C. (2004). Hostile behaviors predict cardiovascular mortality among men enrolled in the Multiple Risk Factor Intervention Trial. *Circulation, 109*, 66–70.

McBride, P. E. (1992). The health consequences of smoking: cardiovascular diseases. *Medical Clinics of North America, 76*, 333–353.

McNally, R. J., Bryant, R. A. & Ehlers, A. (2003). Does early psychological intervention promote recovery from posttraumatic stress? *Psychological Science in the Public Interest, 4*, 45–79.

Meads, C. & Nouwen, A. (2005). Does emotional disclosure have any effects? A systematic review of the literature with meta-analyses. *International Journal of Technology Assessment in Health Care, 21*, 153–164.

Meichenbaum, D. (1994). *A Clinical Handbook/Practical Therapist Manual for Assessing and Treating Adults with Post-Traumatic Stress Disorder (PTSD)*. Clearwater, FL: Institute Press.

Miller, M. A. & Rahe, R. H. (1997). Life changes scaling for the 1990s. *Journal of Psychosomatic Research, 43*, 279–292.

Miller, W. R. & Rollnick, S. (2002). *Motivational Interviewing: Preparing People for Change.* New York: Guilford.

Miranda, J. & Green, B. L. (1999). The need for mental health services research focusing on poor young women. *Journal of Mental Health Policy and Economics, 2*, 73–89.

Moffitt, P. F., Kalucy, E. C., Kalucy, R. S., Baum, E. E. & Cooke, R. D. (1991). Sleep difficulties, pain, and other correlates. *Journal of Internal Medicine, 230*, 245–249.

Monroe, S. M. (1983). Major and minor events as predictors of psychological distress: further issues and findings. *Journal of Behavioral Medicine, 6*, 189–205.

Mozaffarian, D., Hao, T., Rimm, E. B., Willett, W. C. & Hu, F. B. (2011). Changes in diet and lifestyle and long-term weight gain in women and men. *New England Journal of Medicine, 364*(25), 2392–2404.

Mukamal, K. J., Chung, H., Jenny, N. S., Kuller, L. H., Longstreth, W. T. Jr, Mittleman, M. A. et al. (2005). Alcohol use and risk of ischemic stroke among older adults: the cardiovascular health study. *Stroke, 36*, 1830–1834.

Mukamal, K. J., Cinigrave, K. M., Mittleman, M. A., Camargo, C. A., Stampfer, M. J., Willett, W. C. et al. (2003). Roles of drinking pattern and type of alcohol consumed in coronary heart disease in men. *New England Journal of Medicine, 348*, 109–118.

Mutrie, N. (1988). Exercise as a treatment for moderate depression in the UK health service. In *Sport, Health, Psychology and Exercise Symposium Proceedings.* London: The Sports Council and Health Education Authority, pp. 96–105.

Myrtek, M. (2001). Meta-analyses of prospective studies on coronary heart disease, type A personality, and hostility. *International Journal of Cardiology, 79*, 245–251.

Nabi, H., Kivimäki, M., Zins, M., Elovainio, M., Consoli, S. M., Cordier, S. et al. (2008). Does personality predict mortality? Results from the GAZEL French prospective cohort study. *International Journal of Epidemiology, 37*, 386–396.

National Cancer Institute. (2000, 12 December). Fact sheet: questions and answers about smoking cessation. Retrieved November 2005 from www.cancer.gov/cancertopics/factsheet/tobacco/cessation.

National Heart, Lung, and Blood Institute (USA). (1998). *Behavioral Research in Cardiovascular, Lung, and Blood Health and Disease.* Washington, DC: US Department of Health and Human Services.

Niaura, R., Todaro, J. F., Stroud, L., Spiro, A., Ward, K. D. & Weiss, S. (2002). Hostility, the metabolic syndrome, and incident coronary heart disease. *Health Psychology, 21*, 588–593.

Nolen-Hoeksema, S. (1987). Sex differences in unipolar depression: evidence and theory. *Psychological Bulletin, 101*, 259–282.

Nolen-Hoeksema, S. (2000). The role of rumination in depressive disorders and mixed anxiety/depressive symptoms. *Journal of Abnormal Psychology, 109*, 504–511.

Nolen-Hoeksema, S. (2002). Gender differences in depression. In I. H. Gotlib & C. L. Hammen (eds), *Handbook of Depression.* New York: Guilford.

Nolen-Hoeksema, S. (2003). *Women Who Think Too Much: How to Break Free of Over Thinking and Reclaim Your Life.* New York: Holt.

Nolen-Hoeksema, S. & Girgus, J. S. (1994). The emergence of gender differences in depression during adolescence. *Psychological Bulletin, 115*, 424–443.

Nolte, J. (2002). *The human brain (*5th ed.). St. Louis: Mosby.

Norcross, J. C., Ratzin, A. C. & Payne, D. (1989). Ringing in the new year: the change processes and reported outcomes of resolutions. *Addictive Behaviors, 14*, 205–212.

Norcross, J. C. & Vangarelli, D. J. (1989). The resolution solution: longitudinal examination of New Year's change attempts. *Journal of Substance Abuse, 1*, 127–134.

Overmier, J. B. & Murison, R. (1997). Animal models reveal the 'psych' in the psychosomatics of peptic ulcer. *Current Directions in Psychological Research, 6*, 180–184.

Ozer, E., Best, S. & Lipsey, T. & Weiss, D. L. (2003). Predictors of posttraumatic stress disorder symptoms in adults: a meta-analysis. *Psychological Bulletin, 129*, 52–73.

Paffenbarger, R. S., Hyde, R. T., Wing, A. L. & Hsieh, C. C. (1986). Physical activity, all-cause mortality, and longevity of college alumni. *New England Journal of Medicine, 314*, 605–613.

Palmer, L. K. (1995). Effects of a walking program on attributional style, depression, and self-esteem in women. *Perceptual and Motor Skills, 81*, 891–898.

Parslow, R. A., Jorm, A. F. & Christensen, H. (2006). Associations of pre-trauma attributes and trauma exposure with screening positive for PTSD: analysis of a community-based study of 2085 young adults. *Psychological Medicine, 36(3),* 387–396.

Pate, R. R., Pratt, M., Blair, S. N., Haskell, W. L., Macera, C. A., Bouchard, C. et al. (1995). Physical activity and public health: a recommendation from the Centers for Disease Control and the American College of Sports Medicine. *Journal of the American Medical Association, 273,* 402–407.

Peacock, E. J. & Wong, P. T. (1990). The Stress Appraisal Measure (SAM): a multidimensional approach to cognitive appraisal. *Stress Medicine, 6,* 227–236.

Pearson, M. L., Selby, J. V., Katz, K. A., Cantrell, V., Braden, C. R., Parise, M. E. et al. (2012). Clinical, epidemiologic, histopathologic and molecular features of an unexplained dermopathy. *PLoS One,* 7(1), e29908.

Pennebaker, J. W. & Graybeal, A. (2001). Patterns of natural language use: disclosure, personality, and social integration. *Current Directions, 10,* 90–93.

Pennebaker, J. W., Kiecolt-Glaser, J. & Glaser, R. (1988). Disclosure of traumas and immune function: health implications for psychotherapy. *Journal of Consulting and Clinical Psychology, 56,* 239–245.

Peterson, C. (2000). The future of optimism. *American Psychologist, 55,* 44–55.

Peterson, C. & Seligman, M. E. P. (2003). *Character Strengths and Virtues: A Handbook and Classification.* New York: Oxford University Press.

Phillips, W. T., Kiernan, M. & King, A. C. (2001). The effects of physical activity on physical and psychological health. In A. Baum, T. A. Revenson & J. E. Singer (eds), *Handbook of Health Psychology.* Mahwah, NJ: Lawrence Erlbaum, pp. 627–660.

Plutchik, R. (1994). *The psychology and biology of emotion.* New York: HarperCollins.

Polivy, J., Schueneman, A. L. & Carlson, K. (1976). Alcohol and tension reduction: cognitive and physiological effects. *Journal of Abnormal Psychology, 85,* 595–600.

Potts, R. G. (2004). Spirituality, religion, and the experience of illness. In P. Camic & S. Knight (eds), *Clinical Handbook of Health Psychology: A Practical Guide to Effective Interventions.* Cambridge, MA: Hogrefe & Huber, pp. 297–314.

Poverny, L. M. & Picascia, S. (n.d.). There is no crying in business. Retrieved from www.womensmedia .com/new/crying-at-work.shtml

Pronk, N. P. & Wing, R. R. (1994). Physical activity and long-term maintenance of weight loss. *Obesity Research, 2,* 587–599.

Purcell, K. (1963). Distinctions between subgroups of asthmatic children: children's perceptions of events associated with asthma. *Pediatrics, 31,* 486–494.

Quick, J. C., Quick, J. D., Nelson, D. L. & Hurrell, J. J. (1997). *Preventive Stress Management in Organizations.* Washington, DC: American Psychological Association.

Repetti, R., Taylor, S. & Seeman, T. (2002). Risky families: family social environments and the mental and physical health of offspring. *Psychological Bulletin 128,* 330–366.

Richards, J. C., Hof, A. & Alvarenga, M. (2000). Serum lipids and their relationships with hostility and angry affect and behaviors in men. *Health Psychology, 19,* 393–398.

Richards, J. M., Butler, E. A. & Gross, J. J. (2003). Emotion regulation in romantic relationships: the cognitive consequences of concealing feelings. *Journal of Social and Personal Relationships, 20,* 599–620.

Rind, B., Tromovitch, P. & Bauserman, R. (1998). A meta-analytic examination of assumed properties of child sexual abuse using college samples. *Psychological Bulletin, 124,* 22–53.

Roberts, R. E., Strawbridge, W. J., Deleger, S. & Kaplan, G. A. (2002). Are the fat more jolly? *Annals of Behavioral Medicine, 24,* 169–180.

Rosenman, S. (2002). Trauma and posttraumatic stress disorder in Australia: findings in the population sample of the Australian National Survey of Mental Health and Wellbeing. *Australian and New Zealand Journal of Psychiatry, 36*(4), 515–520.

Roth, S. & Cohen, L. J. (1986). Approach, avoidance, and coping with stress. *American Psychology, 41,* 813–819.

Rothbaum, B. O., Anderson, P., Zimand, E., Hodges, L., Lang, D. & Wilson, J. (2006). Virtual reality exposure therapy and standard (in vivo) exposure therapy in the treatment of fear of flying. *Behavior Therapy, 37,* 80–90.

Ruscio, J. (2000). Risky business: vividness, availability, and the media paradox. *Skeptical Inquirer, 24,* 22–26.

Sarafino, E. P. (2006). *Health Psychology: Biopsychosocial Interactions* (5th ed.). Hoboken, NJ: John Wiley.

Schaefer, C., Coyne, J. C. & Lazarus R. S. (1981). The health-related functions of social support. *Journal of Behavioral Medicine, 4*, 381–406.

Scheier, M. F. & Carver, C. S. (1992). Effects of optimism on psychological and physical well-being: theoretical overview and empirical update. *Cognitive Therapy and Research, 16*, 201–228.

Scheier, M. F., Matthews, K. A., Owens, J. F., Magovern, G. J., Lefebvre, R. C., Abbott, R. A. et al. (1989). Dispositional optimism and recovery from coronary artery bypass surgery: the beneficial effects on physical and psychological well-being. *Journal of Personality and Social Psychology, 57*(6), 1024–1040.

Schmidt, P. J., Murphy, J. H., Haq, N., Rubinow, D. R. & Danaceau, M. A. (2004). Stressful life events, personal losses, and perimenopause-related depression. *Archives of Women's Mental Health, 7*, 19–26.

Schnall, P. L., Pieper, C., Schwartz, J. E., Karasek, R. A., Schlussel, Y., Devereux, R. B. et al. (1990). The relationship between 'job strain', workplace diastolic blood pressure, and left ventricular mass index: results of a case-control study. *Journal of the American Medical Association, 263*, 1929–1935.

Schoenbaum, M. (1997). Do smokers understand the mortality effects of smoking? Evidence from the health and retirement survey. *American Journal of Public Health, 87*, 755–759.

Schwartz, M. B., Vartanian, L. R., Nosek, B. A. & Brownell, K. D. (2006). The influence of one's own body weight on implicit and explicit anti-fat bias. *Obesity, 14*, 440–447.

Schwarzer, R. & Taubert, S. (2002). Tenacious goal pursuits and striving towards personal growth: proactive coping. In E. Fydenberg (ed.), *Beyond Coping: Meeting Goals, Visions and Challenges*. London: Oxford University Press, pp. 19–35.

Scollo, M. M. & Winstanley, M. H. (2008). *Tobacco in Australia: Facts and Issues* (3rd ed.). Melbourne: Cancer Council Victoria. Available from www.tobaccoinaustralia.org.au.

Segerstrom, S. C., Taylor, S. E., Kemeny, M. E. & Fahey, J. L. (1998). Optimism is associated with mood, coping, and immune change in response to stress. *Journal of Personality and Social Psychology, 74*, 1646–1655.

Seligman, M. (1990). *Learned Optimism*. New York: Knopf.

Selye, H. (1956). *The Stress of Life*. New York: McGraw-Hill.

Shade, E. D., Ulrich, C. M., Wener, M. H., Wood, B., Yasui, Y., Lacroix, K. et al. (2004). Frequent intentional weight loss is associated with lower natural killer cell cyto-toxicity in postmenopausal women: possible long-term immune effects. *Journal of the American Dietetic Association, 104*, 903–912.

Shaver, P. R., Morgan, H. J., & Wu, S. J. (1996, March). Is love a "basic" emotion? *Personal Relationships, 3*(1), 81–96.

Shaver, P., Schwartz, J., Kirson, D., & O'Connor, C. (1987, June). Emotion knowledge: Further exploration of a prototype approach. *Journal of Personality and Social Psychology*, 1061–1086.

Simon, G., von Kopff, M., Saunders, K., Miglioretti, D. L., Crane, K., Van Belle, K. et al. (2006). Association between obesity and psychiatric disorders in the U.S. population. *Archives of General Psychiatry, 63*, 824–830.

Skinner, E., Edge, K., Altman, J. & Sherwood, H. (2003). Searching for the structure of coping: a review and critique of category systems for classifying ways of coping. *Psychological Bulletin, 129*, 216–219.

Sloan, R. P., Bagiella, E. & Powell, T. (1999). Religion, spirituality, and medicine. *Lancet, 353*, 644–647.

Smith, D. M., Langa, K. M., Kabeto, M. U. & Ubel, P. A. (2005). Health, wealth, and happiness: financial resources buffer subjective well-being after the onset of a disability. *Psychological Science, 16*, 663–666.

Smith, T. W. & Gallo, L. C. (2001). Personality traits as risk factors for physical illness. In A. Baum, T. A. Revenson & J. Singer (eds), *Handbook of Health Psychology*. Mahwah, NJ: Laurence Erlbaum, pp. 139–173.

Smyth, J. M., Stonr, A. A., Hurewitz, A. & Kaell, A. (1999). Effects of writing about stressful experiences on symptom reduction in patients with asthma or rheumatoid arthritis: a randomized trial. *Journal of the American Medical Association, 281*, 1304–1309.

Solomon, R. C. (2002, June). Back to basics: On the very idea of "basic emotions". *Journal for the Theory of Social Behavior, 32*(2), 115–144.

Sommers, C. H. & Satel, S. (2005). *One Nation Under Therapy: How the Helping Culture is Eroding Self-Reliance*. New York: St Martin's Press.

Steel, Z. & Silove, D. M. (2001). The mental health implications of detaining asylum seekers. *Medical Journal of Australia, 175*, 596–599.

Stern, S. L., Dhanda, R. & Hazuda, H. P. (2001). Hopelessness predicts mortality in older Mexican and European Americans. *Psychosomatic Medicine, 63*, 344–351.

Strentz, T. & Auerbach, S. M. (1988). Adjustment to the stress of simulated captivity: effects of emotion-focused versus problem-focused preparation on hostages differing in locus of control. *Journal of Personality and Social Psychology, 55*, 652–660.

Stroebe, W. (2000). *Social Psychology and Health* (2nd ed.). Buckingham, UK: Open University Press.

Summerfield, D. (2001). The invention of post-traumatic stress disorder and the social usefulness of a psychiatric category. *British Medical Journal, 322*, 95–8.

Tavris, C. (1989). *Anger: The Misunderstood Emotion*. New York: Touchstone.

Taylor, S. E., Klein, L. C., Lewis, B. P., Gruenewald, T. L., Gurung, R. A. R. & Updegraff, J. A. (2000). Biobehavioral responses to stress in females: tend-and-befriend, not fight-or-flight. *Psychological Review, 107*, 411–429.

Thompson, D. L. & Ahrens, M. J. (2004). The grapefruit solution: lower your cholesterol, lose weight, and achieve optimal health with nature's wonderful fruit. [Brochure.] Linx Corporation.

Thompson, J. K., Herbozo, S. M., Himes, S. M. & Yamamiya, Y. (2005) Weight-related teasing in adults. In K. D. Brownell, L., Rudd, R. M. Puhl & M. B. Schwartz (eds), *Weight Bias: Nature, Consequences and Remedies*. New York: Guilford, pp. 137–149.

Troxel, W. M., Matthews, K. A., Bromberger, J. T. & Sutton-Tyrell, K. (2003). Chronic stress burden, discrimination, and subclinical carotid artery disease in African American and Caucasian women. *Health Psychology, 22*, 300–309.

Tucker, D. M., Luu, P., Frishkoff, G., Quiring, J., & Poulsen, C. (2003, November). Frontolimbic response to negative feedback in clinical depression. *Journal of Abnormal Psychology, 112*(4), 667–678.

Turk, D. C. (1996). Psychological aspects of pain and disability. *Journal of Musculoskeletal Pain, 4*, 145–154.

Turner, R. J., Wheaton, B. & Lloyd, D. A. (1995). The epidemiology of stress. *American Sociological Review, 60*, 104–125.

Tversky, A. & Kahneman, D. (1974). Judgment under uncertainty: heuristics and biases. *Science, 185*, 1124–1131.

Tyas, S. L. (2001). Alcohol use and the risk of developing Alzheimer's disease. *Alcohol Research and Health, 25*, 299–306.

Ullman, S. E., Filipas, H. H., Townsend, S. M. & Starzynski, L. L. (2005). Trauma exposure, posttraumatic stress disorder and problem drinking in sexual assault survivors. *Journal of Studies of Alcohol, 66*, 610–619.

Vila, G., Nollet-Clemencon, C., deBlic, J., Mouren-Simeoni, M.-C. & Scheinmann, P. (2000). Prevalence of DSM-IV anxiety and affective disorders in a pediatric population of asthmatic children and adolescents. *Journal of Affective Disorders, 58*, 223–231.

Vincent, P. (1971). Factors influencing patient noncompliance: a theoretical approach. *Nursing Research, 20*, 509–516.

von Känel, R., Dimsdale, J. E., Patterson, T. L. & Grant, I. (2003). Association of negative life event stress with coagulation activity in elderly Alzheimer caregivers. *Psychosomatic Medicine, 65*(1), 145–150.

Wadden, T. A. & Stunkard, A. J. (1993). Psychosocial consequence of obesity and dieting: research and clinical findings. In A. J. Stunkard & T. A. Wadden (eds), *Obesity: Theory and Therapy*. New York: Raven, pp. 163–177.

Wang, T. J., Pencina, M. J., Booth, S. L., Jacques, P. F., Ingelsson, E., Lanier, K. et al. (2008). Vitamin D deficiency and risk of cardiovascular disease. *Circulation, 117*, 503–511.

Watson, D.,Clark, L. A., & Tellegen, A. (1988). Development and validation of brief measures of positive and negative affect: The PANAS Scales. *Journal of Personality and Social Psychology*, 1063–1070.

Wegner, D. (2005). The illusion of conscious will. *Behavioral and Brain Sciences, 27*, 649–692.

Wegner, D. M. (1989). *White Bears and Other Unwanted Thoughts: Suppression, Obsession, and the Psychology of Mental Control*. London: Guilford.

Wei, M., Kampert, J. B., Barlow, C. E., Nichaman, M. Z., Gibbons, L. W., Paffenbarger, R. S. et al. (1999). Relationship between low cardiorespiratory fitness and mortality in normal weight, overweight, and obese men. *Journal of the American Medical Association, 282*, 1547–1553.

Weiss, H. M., & Cropanzano, R. (1996). Affective events theory: A theoretical discussion of the structure, causes and consequences of affective experiences at work. In B. M. Staw & L. L. Cummings (Eds.), *Research in organizational behavior* (Vol. 18, pp. 17–19). Greenwich, CT: JAI Press.

Westphal, M. & Bonanno, G. A. (2004). Emotional self-regulation. In M. Beauregard (ed.), *Consciousness, Emotional Self-Regulation, and the Brain*. Philadelphia: Benjamins, pp. 1–34.

Wills, T. A. & Fegan, M. F. (2001). Social networks and social support. In A. Baum, T. A. Revenson & J. E. Singer (eds), *Handbook of Health Psychology*. Mahwah, NJ: Lawrence Erlbaum, pp. 209–234.

Wing, R. R. & Hill, J. O. (2001). Successful weight loss maintenance. *Annual Review of Nutrition, 21*, 323–341.

Wing, R. R. & Jeffrey, R. W. (1999). Benefit of recruiting participants with friends and increasing social support for weight loss and maintenance. *Journal of Consulting and Clinical Psychology, 67*, 132–138.

Wing, R. R. & Polley, B. A. (2001). Obesity. In A. Baum, T. A. Revenson & J. E. Singer (eds), *Handbook of Health Psychology*. Mahwah, NJ: Lawrence Erlbaum, pp. 263–279.

Woloshin, S., Schwartz, L. M. & Welch, H. G. (2002). Risk charts: putting cancer in context. *Journal of the National Cancer Institute, 94*, 799–804.

Woodworth, R. D. (1938). *Experimental Psychology*. New York: Holt.

Yehuda, R., Resnick, H., Kahana, B. & Giller, E. L. (1993). Long-lasting hormonal alterations to extreme stress in humans: normative or maladaptive? *Psychosomatic Medicine, 55*, 287–297.

Young, R. M., Oei, T. P. S. & Knight, R. G. (1990). The tension reduction hypothesis revisited: an alcohol expectancy perspective. *British Journal of Addiction, 85*, 31–40.

Yusuf, S., Hawken, S., Ounpuu, S., Dans, T., Avezum, A., Lanas, F. et al. (2004). Effect of potentially modifiable risk factors associated with myocardial infarction in 52 countries (the INTERHEART study): case-control study. *Lancet, 364*, 937–952.

Chapter 14

Abraham, S. (2012). Relationship between stress and perceived self-efficacy among nurses in India. In *International Conference on Technology and Business Management* (Vol. 26, p. 28). Retrieved from www.ictbm.org

Abrams, D. B., Monti, P. M., Pinto, R. P., Elder J. P., Brown, R. A., Jacobus, S. I. (1987). Psychosocial stress and coping in smokers who relapse or quit. *Health Psychology, 6,* 289–303.

Alexander, B. K., & Hadaway, P. F. (1982). Opiate addiction: The case for an adaptive orientation. *Psychological Bulletin, 92,* 367–381.

Alloway, R. &Bebbington, P. (1987). The buffer theory of social support: a review of the literature. *Psychological Medicine, 17*, 91–108.

American College Health Association. (2013). *American College Health Association-National College Health Assessment II: Reference Group Executive Summary Fall 2012.* Hanover, MD: Author. Retrieved from www.acha-ncha.org

American Diabetes Association. (2011). How stress affects diabetes. Retrieved from www.diabetes.org

American Psychological Association. (2012). Stress in America.

American Psychological Association (2012). What is resilience? In *The road to resilience.* Washington, DC: Author. Retrieved from www.apa.org

Antonovsky, A. (1967). Social class life expectancy and overall mortality. *Milbank Memorial Fund Quarterly, 45*, 31–73.

Atwoli, L., Stein, D. J., Koenen, K. C., & McLaughin, K. A. (2015). Epidemiology of posttraumatic stress disorder: Prevalence, correlates and consequences. *Current Opinion in Psychiatry, 28*(4), 307–311.

Atwoli, L., Stein, D. J., Williams, D. R., Mclaughlin, K. A, Petukhova, M., Kessler, R. C., & Koenen, K. C. (2013). Trauma and posttraumatic stress disorder in South Africa: Analysis from the South African Stress and health study. *BMC Psychiatry, 13*, 182.

Australian Institute of Health & Welfare (AIHW). (2008a). *Australia's Health #11.* AIHW Cat. no. AUS 99. Canberra: AIHW.

Australian Institute of Health and Welfare. (2008c). *Asthma in Australia 2008.* AIHW Asthma Series no. 3. Cat. no. ACM 14. Canberra: AIHW.

Backé, E.-M., Seidler, A., Latza, U., Rossnagel, K., & Schumann, B. (2012). The role of psychosocial stress at work for the development of cardiovascular diseases: a systematic review. *International Archives of Occupational and Environmental Health, 85*(1), 67–79.

Bahrke, M. S., & Morgan, W. P. (1978). Anxiety reduction following exercise and meditation. *Cognitive Therapy and Research, 2*, 323–333.

Bandura, A. (1969). *Principles of behavior modification.* New York: Holt, Rinehart & Winston.

Bandura, A. (1977). Self-efficacy: Toward a unifying theory of behavioral change. *Psychological Review, 84,* 191–215.

Bandura, A. (1982). Self-efficacy mechanism in human agency, *American Psychologist, 37,* 122–147.

Bartone, P. T. (1999). Hardiness protects against war-related stress in army reserve forces. *Consulting Psychology Journal, 51,* 72–82.

Beck, J. G., Gudmundsdottir, B. Palyo, S. A., Miller, L. M. & Grant, D. M. (2006). Rebound effects following deliberate thought suppression: does PTSD make a difference? *Behavior Therapy, 37,* 170–180.

Belloc, N. B., & Breslow, L. (1972). Relationship of physical health status and health practices. *Preventive Medicine, 1,* 409–421.

Berkman, L. F. &Syme, S. L. (1979). Social networks, host resistance, and mortality: a nine year follow-up study of Alameda County residents. *American Journal of Epidemiology, 109,* 186–204.

Bonanno, G. (2004). Loss, trauma, and human resilience: have we underestimated the human capacity to thrive after extremely aversive events? *American Psychologist, 59,* 20–28.\

Bonanno, G. A. & Kaltman, S. (2001). The varieties of grief experience. *Clinical Psychology Review, 21,* 705–734.

Bonanno, G. A., Moskowitz, J. T., Papa, A. & Folkman, S. (2005). Resilience to loss in bereaved spouses, bereaved parents, and bereaved gay men. *Journal of Personality and Social Psychology, 88,* 827–843.

Bragard, I., Etienne, A. M., Merckaert, I., Libert, Y., & Razavi, D. (2010). Efficacy of a communication and stress management training on medical residents' self-efficacy, stress to communicate and burnout: A randomized controlled study. *Journal of Health Psychology, 15*(7), 1075–1084.

Brondolo, E., Love, E. E., Pencille, M., Schoenthaler, A., & Ogedegbe, G. (2011). Racism and hypertension: a review of the empirical evidence and implications for clinical practice. *American Journal of Hypertension, 24*(5), 518–524.

Brown, G. W. & Harris, T. (1978). *Social Origins of Depression: A Study of Psychiatric Disorder in Women.* London: Tavistock.

Brown, J. D. (1991). Staying fit and staying well: Physical fitness as a moderator of life stress. *Journal of Personality and Social Psychology, 60,* 555–561.

Brown, K. L. (2011). *Predictors of suicide ideation and the moderating effects of suicide attitudes.* Master's thesis, University of Ohio. Retrieved from http://etd.ohiolink.edu

Brownell, K. D. (1980). Obesity: Understanding and treating a serious, prevalent, and refractory disorder. *Psychological Bulletin, 88,* 370–405.

Bunde, J. &Suls, J. (2006). A quantitative analysis of the relationship between the Cook-Medley Hostility Scale and traditional coronary artery disease risk factors. *Health Psychology, 25,* 493–500.

Carney, R. M., Freedland, K. E. &Veith, R. C. (2005). Depression, the autonomic nervous system, and coronary heart disease. *Psychosomatic Medicine, 67,* 29–33.

Carrol, K., & Leon, G. R. (1981). *The bulimia-vomiting disorder within a generalized substance abuse pattern.* Paper presented at the 15th annual convention of the Association for the Advancement of Behavior Therapy, Toronto.

Carver, C. S. (1997). You want to measure coping but your protocol's too long: consider the Brief COPE. *International Journal of Behavioral Medicine, 4,* 92–100.

Carver, C. S., Schejer, M. F., & WeintrauB, J. K. (1989). Assessing coping strategies. A theoretically based approach. *Journal of Personality and Social Psychology, 56,* 267-283.

Casey, L., & Liang, R. P-T. (2014). *Stress and wellbeing in Australia survey 2014.* Melbourne: Australian Psychological Society.

Casey, L., & Liang, R. P-T. (2014). *Stress and wellbeing in Australia survey 2014.* Melbourne: Australian Psychological Society.

Chandola, T., Britton, A., Brunner, E., Hemingway, H., Malik, M., Kumari, M. et al. (2008). Work stress and coronary heart disease: what are the mechanisms? *European Heart Journal, 29,* 640–648

Chaney, J. M., Mullins, L. L., Uretsky, D. L., Pace, T. M., Werden, D. & Hartman, V. L. (1999). An experimental examination of learned helplessness in older adolescents and young adults with long-standing asthma. *Journal of Pediatric Psychology, 24,* 259–271.

Chao, R. C.-L. (2012). Managing perceived stress among college students: The roles of social support and dysfunctional coping. *Journal of College Counseling, 15*(1), 5–21.

Chen, E., Miller, G. E., Lachman, M. E., Gruenewald, T. L., & Seeman, T. E. (2012). Protective factors for adults from low childhood socioeconomic circumstances: The benefits of shift-and-persist for allostatic load. *Psychosomatic Medicine, 74*(2), 178-186. doi:10.1097/PSY.0B013e31824206fd

Cheng, C. (2003). Cognitive and motivational processes underlying coping flexibility: a dual-process model. *Journal of Personality and Social Psychology, 84,* 425–438.

Christian, L. M. (2012). Psychoneuroimmunology in pregnancy: Immune pathways linking stress with maternal health, adverse birth outcomes, and fetal development. *Neuroscience & Biobehavioral Reviews, 36*(1), 350–361. doi: 10.1016/j.neubiorev. 2011.07.005

Chung, J. E. (2014). Social networking in online support groups for health: How online social networking benefits patients. *Journal of Health Communication, 19*(6), 639-659. doi: 10.1080/10810730.2012.757396

Coelho, C. M., Santos, J. A., Silva, C. F., Tichoon, J., Hine, T. J. & Wallis, G. (2008). The role of self-motion in acrophobia treatment. *Cyberpsychology&Behavior, 11*, 723–725.

Cohen, S. & Herbert, T. B. (1996). Health psychology: psychological factors and physical disease from the perspective of human psychoneuroimmunology. *Annual Review of Psychology, 47*, 113–142.

Cohen, S. (1980). Aftereffects of stress on human performance and social behavior: A review of research and theory. *Psychological Bulletin, 88*, 82–108.

Cohen, S., Doyle, W. J., Turner, R. B., Alper, C. M. &Skoner, D. P. (2003). Emotional style and susceptibility to the common cold. *Psychosomatic Medicine, 65*, 652–657.

Cohen, S., Evans, G. W., Stokols, D. &Krantz, D. S. (1986). *Behavior, Health, and Environmental Stress.* New York: Plenum.

Cohen, S., Tyrell, D. A. J. & Smith, A. P. (1991). Psychological stress and susceptibility to the common cold. *New England Journal of Medicine, 325*, 606–612.

Collins (eds), *The Health Psychology Handbook: Practical Issues for the Behavioral Medicine Specialist.* London: Sage, pp. 169–186.Costa, P. T. Jr & McCrae, R. R. (1990). Personality disorders and the five-factor model of personality. *Journal of Personality Disorders, 4*, 362–371.

Collins, F. L., Sorocco, K. H., Haala, K. R., Miller, B. I. &Lovallo, W. R. (2003). Stress and health. In L. M. Cohen, D. E. McChargue& F. L.

Conway, T. L., Vickers, R. R., Jr., Ward, H. W., & Rahe, R. H. (1981). Occupational stress and variation in cigarette, coffee, and alcohol consumption. *Journal of Health and Social Behavior, 22,* 155–165.

Coyne, J. C, Aldwin, C., & Lazarus, R. S. (1981). Depression and toping in stressful episodes. *Journal of Abnormal Psychology, 90,* 439–447.

Coyne, J. C. & Racioppo, M. W. (2000). Never the twain shall meet? Closing the gap between coping research and clinical intervention research. *American Psychologist, 55*, 655–664.

Coyne, J. C. (1992). Cognition in depression: a paradigm in crisis. *Psychological Inquiry, 3*, 232–235.

Crews, D. J., & Landers, D, M. (1987). A meta-analytic review of aerobic fitness and reactivity to psychosocial stressors. *Medicine and Science in Sports and Exercise, 19,* S114-S120.

Cronkite, R. C, & Moos, R. H. (1984). The role of predisposing and moderating factors in the stress-illness relationship. *Journal of Health and Social Behavior, 25,* 372–393.

Curry, S. G., & Marlatt, G. A. (1985). Unaided quitters' strategies for coping with temptations to smoke. In S. Shiffman & T. A. Wills (Eds.), *Coping and substance use* (pp. 243–265). Orlando, FL: Academic Press.

Czajkowski, S. M., Hindelang, R. D., Dembroski, T. M., Mayerson, S. E., Parks, E. B., & HOLLAND, J. C. (1990). Aerobic fitness, psychological characteristics, and cardiovascular reactivity to stress. *Health Psychology, 9,* 676–692.

DeLongis, A., Folkman, S. & Lazarus, R. (1988). The impact of daily stress on health and mood: psychological and social resources as mediators. *Journal of Personality and Social Psychology, 54*, 486–495.

Depue, R. A. & Monroe, S. M. (1986). Conceptualization and measurement of human disorder in life stress research: the problem of chronic disturbance. *Psychological Bulletin, 99*(1), 36–51.

Dias-Ferreira, E., Sousa, J. C., Melo, I., Morgado, P., Mesquita, A. R., Cerqueira, J. J., ... & Sousa, N. (2009). Chronic stress causes frontostriatal reorganization and affects decision-making. *Science, 325*(5940), 621–625.

Dohrenwend, B. S. &Dohrenwend, B. P. (eds), (1974). *Stressful Life Events: Their Nature and Effects.* New York: Wiley, pp. 245–258.

Dominique, J. F., Aerni, A., Schelling, G., & Roozendaal, B. (2009). Glucocorticoids and the regulation of memory in health and disease. *Frontiers in neuroendocrinology, 30*(3), 358-370.

Dunkel-Schetter, C., Folkman, S., & Lazarus, R. S. (1987). Correlates of social suppo receipt. *Journal of Personality and Social Psychology. 53,* 71–80.

Dusseldorp, E., van Elderen, T., Maes, S., Meulman, J. &Kraaij, V. (1999). A meta-analysis of psychoeducational programs for coronary heart disease patients. *Health Psychology, 18*, 506–519.

Esterling, B. A., Kiecolt-Glaser, J. K. & Glaser, R. (1996). Psychosocial modulation of cytokine-induced natural killer cell activity in older adults. *Psychosomatic Medicine, 58*, 264–272.

Fang, C. Y., Reibel, D. K., Longacre, M. L., Rosenzweig, S., Campbell, D. E., & Douglas, S. D. (2010). Enhanced psychosocial well-being following participation in a mindfulness-based stress reduction program is associated with increased natural killer cell activity. *The Journal of Alternative and Complementary Medicine, 16*(5), 531–536.

Feil, J. &Hasking, P. (2008). The relationship between personality, coping strategies and alcohol use. *Addiction Research and Theory, 16,* 526–537.

Fernandez, E. & Sheffield, J. (1996). Relative contributions of life events versus daily hassles to the frequency and intensity of headaches. *Headache, 36,* 595–602.

Ferry, F., Bunting, B., Murphy, S., O'Neill, S., Stein, D., & Koenen, K. (2014). Traumatic events and their relative PTSD burden in Northern Ireland: A consideration of the impact of the 'Troubles'. *Social Psychiatry and Psychiatric Epidemiology, 49*(3), 435–446. doi:10.1097/YCO.0000000000000167

Ferry, F., Bunting, B., Murphy, S., O'Neill, S., Stein, D., & Koenen, K. (2014). Traumatic events and their relative PTSD burden in Northern Ireland: A consideration of the impact of the 'Troubles'. *Social Psychiatry and Psychiatric Epidemiology, 49*(3), 435-46. doi:HYPERLINK "https://dx.doi.org/10.1097%2FYCO.0000000000000167" 10.1097/YCO.0000000000000167

Folk1ns, C H., Lynch, S., & Gardner. M. M. (1972). Psychological fitness as a function of physical fitness. *Archives of Physical Medicine and Rehabilitation, 53, 503–508.*

Folkins, C. H., & Sime, W. E. (1981). Physical fitness training and mental health. *American Psychologist, 36,* 373–389.

Folkman, S., & Lazarus, R. S. (1980). An analysis of coping in a middle-aged community sample. *Journal of Health and Social Behavior, 21,* 219–239.

Folkman, S., & Lazarus, R. S. (1985). If it changes it must be a process: Study of emotion and coping during three stages of a college examination. *Journal of Personality and Social Psychology, 48,* 150–170.

Folkman, S., & Lazarus, R. S. (1991). Coping and emotion. In A. Monat & R. S. Lazarus (Eds.), *Stress and Coping (3rd* ed., pp. 207–227): New York: Columbia University Press.

Folkman, S., Lazarus, R. S., (1988). Coping as a mediator of emotion. *Journal of Personality and Social Psychology, 54,* 466–47.5.

Folkman, S., Lazarus, R. S., Dunkel-Schetter, C., DeLongis, A., & Gruen, R. J. (1986). Dynamics of a stressful encounter: Cognitive appraisal, coping, and encounter outcomes. *Journal of Personality and Social Psychology, 50,* 992–1003

Folton, B. J., Revenson, T, A., &, HinricHSEN, G. A. (1989). Stress and coping in the explanation of psychological adjustment among chronically ill patients. *Social Science and Medicine, 18* 889–898.

Forshaw, M. (2002). *Essential Health Psychology.* New York: Oxford University Press.

Foster, A. A., Hylwa, S. A., Bury, J. E., Davis, M. D., Pittelkow, M. R. &Bostwick, J. M. (2012). Delusional infestation: clinical presentation in 147 patients seen at Mayo Clinic. *Journal of the American Academy of Dermatology, 67*(4), 673. e1–10. 10.1016/j.jaad.2011.12.012.

Fox, J. K., Halpern, L. F., Ryan, J. L., & Lowe, K. A. (2010). Stressful life events and the tripartite model: Relations to anxiety and depression in adolescent females. *Journal of Adolescence, 33*(1), 43–54.

Friedman, M., & Rosenman, R. H. (1974). *Type A behavior and your heart.* New York: Knopf.

Freudenmann, R. W., Lepping, P., Huber, M., Dieckmann, S., Bauer-Dubau, K., Ignatius, R. et al. (2012). Delusional infestation and the specimen sign: a European multicentre study in 148 consecutive cases. *British Journal of Dermatology, 167*(2), 247–251.

Friedman, M. &Rosenman, R. H. (1959). Association of a specific overt behavior pattern with increases in blood cholesterol, blood clotting time, incidence of *arcus senilis*and clinical coronary artery disease. *Journal of the American Medical Association, 169,* 1286–1296.

Friedman, M. &Rosenman, R. H. (1974). *Type A Behavior and Your Heart.* New York: Alfred A. Knopf.

Friedman, M., Powell, L. H., Thoreson, C. E., Ulmer, D., Price, V., Gill, J. J. et al. (1987). Effect of discontinuance of Type A behavioralcounseling on Type A behavior and cardiac recurrence rate of post myocardial infarction patients. *American Heart Journal, 114,* 483–490.

Frisina, P. G., Borod, J. C. &Lepore, S. J. (2004). A meta-analysis of the effects of written disclosure on the health outcomes of clinical populations. *The Journal of Nervous and Mental Disease, 192,* 629–634.

Fuchs, F. D. (2011). Why do black Americans have higher prevalence of hypertension? An enigma still unsolved. *Hypertension, 57*(3), 379–380. Retrieved from http://hyper.ahajournals.org

Gallo, L. C. & Matthews, K. A. (2003). Understanding the association between socioeconomic status and physical health: do negative emotions play a role? *Psychological Bulletin, 129,* 10–51.

Gardner, R. W., Holzman, P. S. Klein, G. S., Linton, H. B., & Spence, D. P. (1959). Cognitive control: A study of Individual consistencies in cognitive behaviour. *Psychological Issues, 1,* (4).

Gatchel, R. J. &Oordt, M. S. (2003). *Clinical Psychology and Primary Health Care.* Washington, DC: American Psychological Association.

Gilbert, D, G., & Spelberger, C. D. (1987). Effects of smoking on heart rate, anxiety, and feelings of success during social interaction. *Journal of Behavioral Medicine, 10,* 629–638.

Glanz, K., Rimer, B. K., & Viswanath, K. (Eds.). (2008). *Health behavior and health education: Theory, research, and practice* (4th ed.). San Francisco: John Wiley & Sons.

Glasgow, R. E., Klesges, R. C., Mizes, J. S., & Pechacek, T. F. (1985). Quitting smoking: Strategies used and variables associated with success in a stop-smoking contest *Journal of Consulting and Clinical Psychology, 53,* 905–912.

Goldwater, B. C., & Collis, M. L. (1985). Psychologic effects of cardiovascular conditioning: A controlled experiment. *Psychosomatic Medicine, 47,* 174–181.

Gomez, J., Miranda, R., & Polanco, L. (2011). Acculturative stress, perceived discrimination, and vulnerability to suicide attempts among emerging adults. *Journal of youth and adolescence, 40*(11), 1465-1476.

Gotlib, I. H. &Hammen, C. L. (1992). *Psychological Aspects of Depression: Towards a Cognitive-Interpersonal Integration.* New York: Wiley.

Gouin, J.-P., & Kiecolt-Glaser, J. K. (2011). The impact of psychological stress on wound healing: Methods and mechanisms. *Immunology and Allergy Clinics of North America, 31*(1), 81–93.

Greenglass, E. (2002). Proactive coping. In E. Frydenberg (ed.), *Beyond Coping: Meeting Goals, Vision, and Challenges.* London: Oxford University Press, pp. 37–62.

Hall-Flavin, D.K. (2012). Stress and hair loss: Are they related? Retrieved from www.mayoclinic.com

Halmi, K. A., Owen, W., Lasky, E., & Stokes, P. (1983). Dopaminergic regulation in anorexia nervosa. *International Journal of Eating Disorders, 22,* 129–134.

Hellhammer, D. H., Stone, A. A., Hellhammer, J., & Broderick, J. (2010). Measuring stress. In G. Koob, M. Le Moal, R. F. Thompson (Eds.), *Encyclopedia of behavioural neurosciences* 3. San Diego: Elsevier.

Herlong, H. F. (2013). Digestive disorders white paper–2013. In *Johns Hopkins Health Alerts.* Retrieved from www.johnshopkinshealthalerts.com

Hettiarachchi, M. (2007). Brief intervention for post traumatic stress disorder with combined use of cognitive behaviour therapy and eye movement desensitisation reprocessing. *AeJAMH: Australian e-Journal for the Advancement of Mental Health, 6,* 1–5.

Higgins, J. E. &Endler, N. (1995). Coping, life stress, and psychological and somatic distress. *European Journal of Personality, 9,* 253–270.

Hodgson, R., & Miller, P. (1982). *Self-watching addictions, habits, and compulsions: What to do about them.* New York; Facts on File Publications.

Holahan, C. & Moos, R. H. (1991). Life stressors, personal and social resources and depression: a four-year structural model. *Journal of Abnormal Psychology, 100,* 31–38.

Holmes, D. S., & Roth, D. L. (1985). Association of aerobic fitness with pulse rate and subjective responses to psychological stress. *Psychophysiology, 22,* 525–529.

Holmes, T. H. & Masuda, M. (1974). Life change and illness susceptibility. In B. S. Dohrenwend & P. P. Dohrenwend (eds), *Stressful Life Events: Their Nature and Effects.* New York: Wiley, pp. 45–72.

Holmes, T. H. &Rahe, R. H. (1967). The social readjustment scale. *Journal of Psychosomatic Research, 11,* 213–218.

House, J. S., Robbins, C. &Metzner, H. L. (1982). The association of social relationships and activities with mortality: prospective evidence from the Tecumseh Community Health Study. *American Journal of Epidemiology, 116,* 123–140.

Hughes, C. A., (1974). A comparison of the effects of teaching techniques of body conditioning on physical fitness and self-concept. *Dissertation Abstracts International, 34,* 3957A–3958A. (University Microfilms No. 73–31, 255)

Hunt, J., & Eisenberg, D. (2010). Mental health problems and help-seeking behavior among college students. *Journal of Adolescent Health, 46*(1), 3–10.

Hylwa, S. A., Bury, J. E., Davis, M. D., Pittelkow, M. &Bostwick, J. M. (2011). Delusional infestation, including delusions of parasitosis: results of histologic examination of skin biopsy and patient-provided skin specimens. *Archives of Dermatology, 147*(9), 1041.

Idriss, S. Z., Kvedar, J. C., & Watson, A. J. (2009). The role of online support communities: Benefits of expanded social networks to patients with psoriasis. *Archives of Dermatology, 145*(1), 46–51.

Ikemi, Y. & Nakagawa, S. (1962). A psychosomatic study of contagious dermatitis. *Kyushu Journal of Medical Science, 13,* 335–350.

Iwamoto, D. K., & Liu, W. M. (2010). The impact of racial identity, ethnic identity, Asian values, and race-related stress on Asian Americans and Asian international college students' psychological well-being. *Journal of Counseling Psychology, 57*(1), 79–91.

Jaffee, J. H. (1985). Opioid dependence. In H. I. Kaplan & B. J. Sadock (Eds.), *Comprehensive textbook of psychiatry* (4th ed., vol. 1, pp. 987–1003). Baltimore: Williams & Wilkins.

Johnson, C T., & Berndt, D. J. (1983). Preliminary investigation of bulimia and life adjustment. *American Journal of Psychiatry, 140,* 774–777.

Josephs, R. A., & Steele, C. M. (1990). The two faces of alcohol myopia: Attentional mediation of psychological stress. *Journal of Abnormal Psychology, 99,* 115–126.

Kanner, A. D., Coyne, J. C., Schaefer, C. & Lazarus, R. S. (1981). Comparison of two modes of stress measurement: daily hassles and uplifts versus major life events. *Journal of Behavioral Medicine, 4,* 1–39.

Karasek, R. & Theorell, T. (1990). *Health Work: Stress, Productivity and the Reconstruction of Life.* New York: Basic Books.

Karren, K. J., Smith, L., & Gordon, K. J. (2010). *Mind/body health: The effects of attitudes, emotions, and relationships* (4th ed.). San Francisco: Pearson Education.

Kawakami, N., Tsuchiya, M., Umeda, M., Koenen, K. C., & Kessler, R. C. (2014). Trauma and posttraumatic stress disorder in Japan: Results from the World Mental Health Japan Survey. *Journal of Psychiatric Research, 53,* 57–65.

Kennedy, S., Kiecolt-Glaser, J. K. & Glaser, R. (1990). Social support, stress, and the immune system. In B. R. Sarason, I. G. Sarason& G. R. Pierce (eds), *Social Support: An Interactional View.* New York: Wiley, pp. 253–266.

Kiecolt-Glaser, J. K., Marucha, P. T., Malarkey, W. B., Mercado, A. M. & Glaser, R. (1995). Slowing of wound healing by psychological stress. *Lancet, 346,* 1194–1196.

King, A. C., Taylor, G. B., Haskell, W. L., & Debusk, R. F. (1989). Influence of regular aerobic exercise on psychological health: A randomized, controlled trial of healthy middle-aged adults. *Health Psychology, 8,* 305–324.

Kivimäki, M., Nyberg, S. T., Batty, G. D., Fransson, E. I., Heikkilä, K., Alfredsson, L., . . . Casini, A. (2012). Job strain as a risk factor for coronary heart disease: a collaborative meta-analysis of individual participant data. *The Lancet, 380*(9852), 1491–1497.

Kobasa, S. C. (1979). Stressful life events, personality, and health: An inquiry into hardiness. *Journal of Personality and Social Psychology, 37*(1), 1–11.

Kobasa, S. C., Maddi, S. R., & Puccetti, M. C., (1982). Personality and exercise as buffers in the stress-illness relationship. *Journal of Behavioral Medicine, 5,* 391–404.

Koenig, H. G., McCullough, M. E. & Larson, D. B. (2001). *Handbook of Religion and Health.* New York: Oxford University Press.

Kondo, N. (2012). Socioeconomic disparities and health: impacts and pathways. *Journal of Epidemiology, 22*(1), 2–6.

Kosfeld, M., Heinrichs, M., Zaks, P., Fischbacher, U. & Fehr, E. (2005). Oxytocin increases trust in humans. *Nature, 435,* 673–676.

Kostrubala, T. (1977). Jogging and personality change. *Today's Jogger, 1,* 14–15.

Labott, S. M. (2004). COPD and other respiratory diseases. In P. Camic& S. Knight (eds), *Clinical Handbook of Health Psychology.* Cambridge, MA: Hogrefe& Huber, pp. 59–74.

Lazarus, R. (1985). The trivialization of distress. In J. Rosen and L. Solomon (Eds.), *Preventing health risk behaviors and promoting coping with illness.* Hanover, NH: University Press of New England.

Lazarus, R. (1999). *Stress and Emotion: A New Synthesis.* New York: Springer.

Lazarus, R. S., & Folkman, S. (1984). *Stress, appraisal, and coping.* New York: Springer.

LeDoux, J. (1996). *The Emotional Brain: The Mysterious Underpinnings of Emotional Life.* New York: Simon & Schuster.

Levenson, R W., Sher, K. J., Grossman, L. M., Newman, J., & Newlin, D. B. (1980). Alcohol and stress response dampening: Pharmacological effects, expectancy, and tension reduction. *Journal of Abnormal Psychology, 89,* 529–538.

Levenstein, S., Ackerman, S., Kiecolt-Glaser, J. K. & Dubois, A. (1999). Stress and peptic ulcer disease. *Journal of the American Medical Association, 281,* 10–11.

Levenstein, S., Kaplan, G. A. & Smith, M. W. (1997). Psychological predictors of peptic ulcer incidence in the Alameda County Study. *Journal of Clinical Gastroenterology, 24,* 140–146.

Levin, J. (2001). *God, Faith, and Health: Exploring the Spirituality-Healing Connection.* New York: John Wiley.

Lewis, W. A. & Bucher, A. M. (1992). Anger, catharsis, the reformulated frustration-aggression hypothesis, and health consequences. *Psychotherapy, 29,* 385–392.

Lilienfeld, S. O. (2007). Psychological treatments that can cause harm. *Perspectives on Psychological Science, 2,* 53–70.

Littrell, J. (1998). Is the experience of painful emotion therapeutic? *Clinical Psychology Review, 18,* 71–102.

Litz, B. T., Gray, M. J., Bryant, R. & Adler, A. B. (2002). Early intervention for trauma: current status and future directions. *Clinical Psychology: Science and Practice, 9,* 112–134.

Livezey, G. T., Balbkins, N., & Vogel, W. H. (1987). The effect of ethanol (alcohol) and stress on plasma catecholamine levels in individual female and male rats. *Neuropsychobiology, 17,* 193–198.

Lovallo, W. R., Pincomb, G. A., Sung, B. H., Everson, S. A., Passey, R B. & Wilson, M. F. (1991), Hypertension risk and caffeine's effect on cardiovascular activity during mental stress in young men. *Health Psychology, 10,* 236–243.

Maddi, S. R. &Kobasa, S. C. (1984). *The Hardy Executive: Health under Stress.* Homewood, IL: Dow Jones-Irwin.

Maddi, S. R. (2002). The story of hardiness: twenty years of theorizing, research, and practice. *Consulting Psychology Journal, 54,* 173–185.

Maddi, S. R. (2004). On hardiness and other pathways to resilience. *American Psychologist, 60,* 261–262.

Mailick, M. D., Holden, G. & Walther, V. N. (1994). Coping with childhood asthma. *Health and Social Work, 19,* 103–111.

Marin, M. F., Lord, C., Andrews, J., Juster, R. P., Sindi, S., Arsenault-Lapierre, G., ... & Lupien, S. J. (2011). Chronic stress, cognitive functioning and mental health. *Neurobiology of learning and memory, 96*(4), 583–595.

Marlatt, G, A., & George, W. H. (1984). Relapse prevention: Introduction and overview of the model. *British Journal of Addictions, 79,* 261–273.

Marlatt, G. A. (1985). Relapse prevention: Theoretical rationale and overview of the model. In G.A. Marlatt & J.R Gordon (Eds.), *Relapse prevention: Maintenance strategies in the treatment of addictive behaviors,* pp. 3–70. New York: Guilford.

Marshall, G. D. (2011). The adverse effects of psychological stress on immunoregulatory balance: applications to human inflammatory diseases. *Immunology and Allergy Clinics of North America, 31*(1), 133–140.

Marshall Jr, G. D. (2011). Stress and immune-based diseases. *Immunology and Allergy Clinics of North America, 31*(1), 1–148.

Maté, G. (2011). *When the body says no: Understanding the stress-disease connection.* Hoboken, NJ: John Wiley & Sons.

Matthews, K. A., Gump, B. B., Harris, K. F., Haney, T. L. & Barefoot, J. C. (2004). Hostile behaviors predict cardiovascular mortality among men enrolled in the Multiple Risk Factor Intervention Trial. *Circulation, 109,* 66–70.

Mayhew, R., & Edelmann, R. J. (1989), Self-esteem, irrational beliefs, and coping strategies in relation to eating problems in a non-clinical population. *Personality and Individual Differences, 10,* 581–584.

McAleavey, A. A., Castonguay, L. G., & Locke, B. D. (2011). Sexual orientation minorities in college counseling: Prevalence, distress, and symptom profiles. *Journal of College Counseling, 14*(2), 127–142.

McEvoy, P. M., Grove, R., & Slade, T. (2011). Epidemiology of anxiety disorders in the Australian general population: Findings of the 2007 Australian National Survey of Mental Health and Wellbeing. *Australia and New Zealand Journal of Psychiatry, 45,* 957–967.

McNally, R. J., Bryant, R. A. & Ehlers, A. (2003). Does early psychological intervention promote recovery from posttraumatic stress? *Psychological Science in the Public Interest, 4,* 45–79.

Meads, C. &Nouwen, A. (2005). Does emotional disclosure have any effects? A systematic review of the literature with meta-analyses. *International Journal of Technology Assessment in Health Care, 21,* 153–164.

Meichenbaum, D. (1994). *A Clinical Handbook/Practical Therapist Manual for Assessing and Treating Adults with Post-Traumatic Stress Disorder (PTSD).* Clearwater, FL: Institute Press.

Miller, M. A. &Rahe, R. H. (1997). Life changes scaling for the 1990s. *Journal of Psychosomatic Research, 43,* 279–292.

Moffitt, P. F., Kalucy, E. C., Kalucy, R. S., Baum, E. E. & Cooke, R. D. (1991). Sleep difficulties, pain, and other correlates. *Journal of Internal Medicine, 230,* 245–249.

Mols, F., & Denollet, J. (2010). Type D personality in the general population: A systematic review of health status, mechanisms of disease, and work-related problems. *Health and Quality of Life Outcomes, 8*(1), 1–10. Retrieved from www.hqlo.com

Monroe, S. M. (1983). Major and minor events as predictors of psychological distress: further issues and findings. *Journal of Behavioral Medicine, 6,* 189–205.

Mostofsky, E., Maclure, M., Sherwood, J. B., Tofler, G. H., Muller, J. E., & Mittleman, M. A. (2012). Risk of acute myocardial infarction after the death of a significant person in one's life the determinants of myocardial infarction onset study. *Circulation, 125*(3), 491–496. doi:10.1161/CIRCULATIONAHA.111.061770

Murray, K., Davidson, G., & Schweitzer, R. (2008). *Psychological wellbeing of refugees resettling in Australia: A literature review prepared for the Australian Psychological Society.* Melbourne: Australian Psychological Society.

Myrtek, M. (2001). Meta-analyses of prospective studies on coronary heart disease, type A personality, and hostility. *International Journal of Cardiology, 79,* 245–251.

Nabi, H., Kivimäki, M., Zins, M., Elovainio, M., Consoli, S. M., Cordier, S. et al. (2008). Does personality predict mortality? Results from the GAZEL French prospective cohort study. *International Journal of Epidemiology, 37*, 386–396.

National Digestive Diseases Information Clearinghouse (NDDIC). (2012, December). What I need to know about irritable bowel syndrome. Retrieved from www.digestive.niddk.nih.gov

Newman, J. D., Davidson, K. W., Shaffer, J. A., Schwartz, J. E., Chaplin, W., Kirkland, S., & Shimbo, D. (2011). Observed hostility and the risk of incident ischemic heart disease: A prospective population study from the 1995 Canadian Nova Scotia Health Survey. *Journal of the American College of Cardiology, 58*(12), 1222–1228.

Niaura, R., Todaro, J. F., Stroud, L., Spiro, A., Ward, K. D. & Weiss, S. (2002). Hostility, the metabolic syndrome, and incident coronary heart disease. *Health Psychology, 21*, 588–593.

Nixon, A. E., Mazzola, J. J., Bauer, J., Krueger, J. R., & Spector, P. E. (2011). Can work make you sick? A meta-analysis of the relationships between job stressors and physical symptoms. *Work & Stress, 25*(1), 1–22.

Nolen-Hoeksema, S. (2002). Gender differences in depression. In I. H. Gotlib& C. L. Hammen (eds), *Handbook of Depression*. New York: Guilford.

Nolen-Hoeksema, S. (2003). *Women Who Think Too Much: How to Break Free of Over Thinking and Reclaim Your Life*. New York: Holt

Overmier, J. B. &Murison, R. (1997). Animal models reveal the 'psych' in the psychosomatics of peptic ulcer. *Current Directions in Psychological Research, 6*, 180–184.

Pagoto, S. L., Schneider, K. L., Bodenlos, J. S., Appelhans, B. M., Whited, M. C., Ma, Y., & Lemon, S. C. (2012). Association of post-traumatic stress disorder and obesity in a nationally representative sample. *Obesity, 20*(1), 200-205.

Pandey, A., Tripathi, P., Pandey, R., Srivatava, R., & Goswami, S. (2011). Alternative therapies useful in the management of diabetes: A systematic review. *Journal of Pharmacy and Bioallied Sciences, 3*(4), 504-512.

Parslow, R. A., Jorm, A. F. & Christensen, H. (2006). Associations of pre-trauma attributes and trauma exposure with screening positive for PTSD: analysis of a community-based study of 2085 young adults. *Psychological Medicine, 36(3)*, 387–396.

Peacock, E. J. & Wong, P. T. (1990). The Stress Appraisal Measure (SAM): a multidimensional approach to cognitive appraisal. *Stress Medicine, 6*, 227–236.

Pearson, M. L., Selby, J. V., Katz, K. A., Cantrell, V., Braden, C. R., Parise, M. E. et al. (2012). Clinical, epidemiologic, histopathologic and molecular features of an unexplained dermopathy. *PLoS One*, 7(1), e29908.

Pedersen, A., Zachariae, R., & Bovbjerg, D. H. (2010). Influence of psychological stress on upper respiratory infection—a meta-analysis of prospective studies. *Psychosomatic medicine, 72*(8), 823–832.

Pennebaker, J. W., Kiecolt-Glaser, J. & Glaser, R. (1988). Disclosure of traumas and immune function: health implications for psychotherapy. *Journal of Consulting and Clinical Psychology, 56*, 239–245.

Peterson, C. & Seligman, M. E. P. (2003). *Character Strengths and Virtues: A Handbook and Classification*. New York: Oxford University Press.

Peterson, C. (2000). The future of optimism. *American Psychologist, 55*, 44–55.

Pieterse, A. L., Carter, R. T., Evans, S. A., & Walter, R. A. (2010). An exploratory examination of the associations among racial and ethnic discrimination, racial climate, and trauma-related symptoms in a college student population. *Journal of Counseling Psychology, 57*(3), 255–263.

Pincomb, G. A., Lovallo, W. R, Passey, R. B., Brackett, D. J., & Wilson, M.F. (1987). Caffeine enhances the physiological response to occupational stress in medical students. *Health Psychology, 6*, 101–112.

Platt, J. J., & Metzger, D. S. (1987). Cognitive interpersonal problem-solving skills and the maintenance of treatment success in heroin addicts. *Journal of Addictive Behaviors, 1*, 5–13.

Pomerleau, O. F., Adkins, D., & Pertschuck, M. (1978). Predictors of outcome and recidivism in smoking cessation treatment. *Addictive Behavior, 3*, 65–70.

Purcell, K. (1963). Distinctions between subgroups of asthmatic children: children's perceptions of events associated with asthma. *Pediatrics, 31*, 486–494.

Repetti, R., Taylor, S. &Seeman, T. (2002). Risky families: family social environments and the mental and physical health of offspring. *Psychological Bulletin 128*, 330–366.

Richards, J. C., Hof, A. &Alvarenga, M. (2000). Serum lipids and their relationships with hostility and angry affect and behaviors in men. *Health Psychology, 19*, 393–398.

Richards, J. M., Butler, E. A. & Gross, J. J. (2003). Emotion regulation in romantic relationships: the cognitive consequences of concealing feelings. *Journal of Social and Personal Relationships, 20*, 599–620.

Richardson, S., Shaffer, J. A., Falzon, L., Krupka, D., Davidson, K. W., & Edmondson, D. (2012). Meta-analysis of perceived stress and its association with incident coronary heart disease. *The American Journal of Cardiology, 110*(12), 1711–1717.

Roberto, M., Cruz, M. T., Gilpin, N. W., Sabino, V., Schweitzer, P., Bajo, M., ... & Koob, G. F. (2010). Corticotropin releasing factor–induced amygdala gamma-aminobutyric acid release plays a key role in alcohol dependence. *Biological psychiatry, 67*(9), 831–839.

Robertson, D., Frouch, J. C, Carr, R.K., Watson, J. T., Hollifield, J. W., Shand, D. G., & Oates, J. A. (1978). Effects of caffeine on plasma renin activity, catecholamines, and blood pressures. *New England Journal of Medicine, 298,* 181–186.

Rodin, J. (1986). Aging and health: Effects of the sense of control. *Science, 233,* 1271–1276.

Roth, D. L., & Holmes, D. S. (1985). Influence of physical fitness in determining the impact of stressful life events on physical and psychologic health. *Psychosomatic medicine, 47,* 164–173.

Ryff, C. D., Friedman, E. M., Morozink, J. A., & Tsenkova, V. (2012). Psychological resilience in adulthood and later life: Implications for health. *Annual Review of Gerontology and Geriatrics, 32*(1), 73–92.

Sarafino, E. P. (2006). *Health Psychology: Biopsychosocial Interactions* (5th ed.). Hoboken, NJ: John Wiley.

Selye, H. (1956). *The Stress of Life.* New York: McGraw-Hill.

Scheier, M. F. & Carver, C. S. (1992). Effects of optimism on psychological and physical well-being: theoretical overview and empirical update. *Cognitive Therapy and Research, 16,* 201–228.

Scheier, M. F., Matthews, K. A., Owens, J. F., Magovern, G. J., Lefebvre, R. C., Abbott, R. A. et al. (1989). Dispositional optimism and recovery from coronary artery bypass surgery: the beneficial effects on physical and psychological well-being. *Journal of Personality and Social Psychology, 57*(6), 1024–1040.

Schetter, C. D., & Dolbier, C. (2011). Resilience in the context of chronic stress and health in adults. *Social and Personality Psychology Compass, 5*(9), 634–652. doi: 10.1111/j.1751-9004.2011.00379.x

Schmidt, P. J., Murphy, J. H., Haq, N., Rubinow, D. R. &Danaceau, M. A. (2004). Stressful life events, personal losses, and perimenopause-related depression. *Archives of Women's Mental Health, 7,* 19–26.

Schnall, P. L., Pieper, C., Schwartz, J. E., Karasek, R. A., Schlussel, Y., Devereux, R. B. et al. (1990). The relationship between 'job strain', workplace diastolic blood pressure, and left ventricular mass index: results of a case-control study. *Journal of the American Medical Association, 263,* 1929–1935.

Schwabe, L., Wolf, O. T., & Oitzl, M. S. (2009). Memory formation under stress: quantity and quality. *Neuroscience & Biobehavioral Reviews, 34*(4), 584–591.

Schwartz, S. J., Waterman, A. S., Umaña- Taylor, A. J., Lee, R. M., Kim, S. Y., Vazsonyi, A. T., . . . & Zamboanga, B. L. (2012). Acculturation and well- being among college students from immigrant families. *Journal of Clinical Psychology, 69*(4), 298-318. doi: 10.1002/jclp21847

Scott, K., Melhorn, S., & Sakai, R. (2012). Effects of chronic social stress on obesity. *Current Obesity Reports Online First, 1*(1), 16–25. doi: 10.1007/s13679-011-0006-3

Scott, K. M., Von Korff, M., Angermeyer, M. C., Benjet, C., Bruffaerts, R., De Girolamo, G., ... & Tachimori, H. (2011). Association of childhood adversities and early-onset mental disorders with adult-onset chronic physical conditions. *Archives of General Psychiatry, 68*(8), 838–844.

Seaward, B. L. (2013). *Managing stress.* Jones & Bartlett Publishers.

Segerstrom, S. C., Taylor, S. E., Kemeny, M. E. & Fahey, J. L. (1998). Optimism is associated with mood, coping, and immune change in response to stress. *Journal of Personality and Social Psychology, 74,* 1646–1655.

Segrin, C., & Passalacqua, S. A. (2010). Functions of loneliness, social support, health behaviors, and stress in association with poor health. *Health communication, 25*(4), 312–322.

Seligman, M. (1990). *Learned Optimism.* New York: Knopf.

Shiffman, S. (1982). Relapse following smoking cessation: A situational analysis. *Journal of Consulting and Clinical Psychology, 50,* 71–86.

Shiffman, S. (1984a.) Cognitive antecedents and sequelae of smoking relapse crises. *Journal of Applied Social Psychology, 14,* 296–309.

Shiffman, S. (1984b). Coping with temptations to smoke. *Journal of Consulting and Clinical Psychology, 52,* 261–267.

Sinyor, D., Schwartz, S. G., Peronnet, F., Brisson, G., & Seraganian, P. (1983). Aerobic fitness level and reactivity to psychosocial stress: Physiological, biochemical, and subjective measures. *Psychosomatic Medicine, 45,* 205–216.

Skinner, E., Edge, K., Altman, J. & Sherwood, H. (2003). Searching for the structure of coping: a review and critique of category systems for classifying ways of coping. *Psychological Bulletin, 129,* 216–219.

Smith, D. M., Langa, K. M., Kabeto, M. U. &Ubel, P. A. (2005). Health, wealth, and happiness: financial resources buffer subjective well being after the onset of a disability. *Psychological Science, 16,* 663–666.

Smith, T. W. & Gallo, L. C. (2001). Personality traits as risk factors for physical illness. In A. Baum, T. A. Revenson & J. Singer (eds), *Handbook of Health Psychology*. Mahwah, NJ: Laurence Erlbaum, pp. 139–173.

Smith, T. W., Uchino, B. N., Berg, C. A., & Florsheim, P. (2012). Marital discord and coronary artery disease: a comparison of behaviorally defined discrete groups. *Journal of Consulting and Clinical Psychology, 80*(1), 87-92.

Soukup, V. M., Beiler, M. E., & Terrell F. (1990). Stress, coping style, and problem-solving ability among eating-disorders inpatients. *Journal of Clinical Psychology, 46,* 592–599.

Steel, Z. &Silove, D. M. (2001). The mental health implications of detaining asylum seekers. *Medical Journal of Australia, 175*, 596–599.

Steptoe, A., & Kivimäki, M. (2012). Stress and cardiovascular disease. *Nature Reviews Cardiology, 9*(6), 360–370.

Steptoe, A., Rosengren, A., & Hjemdahl, P. (2011). Introduction to cardiovascular disease, stress and adaptation. In A. Steptoe, A. Rosengren, & P. Hjemdahl (Eds.), *Stress and cardiovascular disease.* New York: Springer.

Stern, S. L., Dhanda, R. &Hazuda, H. P. (2001). Hopelessness predicts mortality in older Mexican and European Americans. *Psychosomatic Medicine, 63*, 344–351.

Strentz, T. &Auerbach, S. M. (1988). Adjustment to the stress of simulated captivity: effects of emotion-focused versus problem-focused preparation on hostages differing in locus of control. *Journal of Personality and Social Psychology, 55*, 652–660.

Suitor, C. W., & Hunter M.F. (1980). *Nutrition: Principles and application in health promotion.* Philadelphia: Lippincott.

Tavris, C. (1989). *Anger: The Misunderstood Emotion.* New York: Touchstone. Stroebe, W. (2000). *Social Psychology and Health* (2nd ed.). Buckingham, UK: Open University Press.

Taylor, S. E., Klein, L. C., Lewis, B. P., Gruenewald, T. L., Gurung, R. A. R. &Updegraff, J. A. (2000). Biobehavioral responses to stress in females: tend-and-befriend, not fight-or-flight. *Psychological Review, 107*, 411–429.

Theorell, T. (2012). Evaluating life events and chronic stressors in relation to health: Stressors and health in clinical work. *Advances in Psychosomatic Medicine, 32*, 58–71.

Thoits, P. A. (2010). Stress and health major findings and policy implications. *Journal of Health and Social Behavior, 51*(1 suppl), 554–555. doi.org/10.1177/0022146510383499

Tomkens, S. (1968). A modified model of smoking behavior. E. F. Borgatta & R. R Evans (Eds.), *Smoking, health, and behavior.* Chicago: Aldine.

Troxel, W. M., Matthews, K. A., Bromberger, J. T. & Sutton-Tyrell, K. (2003). Chronic stress burden, discrimination, and subclinical carotid artery disease in African American and Caucasian women. *Health Psychology, 22*, 300–309.

van Uden-Kraan, C. F., Drossaert, C. H., Taal, E., Shaw, B. R., Seydel, E. R., & vandeLaar, M. A. (2008). Empowering processes and outcomes of participation in online support groups for patients with breast cancer, arthritis, or fibromyalgia. *Qualitative Health Research, 18*(3), 405–417.

Versteeg, H., Spek, V., Pedersen, S. S., & Denollet, J. (2012). Type D personality and health status in cardiovascular disease populations: A meta-analysis of prospective studies. *European Journal of Preventive Cardiology, 19*(6), 1373–1380. doi: 10.1177/1741826711425338

Vicennati, V., Pasqui, F., Cavazza, C., Garelli, S., Casadio, E., di Dalmazi, G., ... & Pasquali, R. (2011). Cortisol, energy intake, and food frequency in overweight/obese women. *Nutrition, 27*(6), 677–680.

Wegner, D. (2005). The illusion of conscious will. *Behavioral and Brain Sciences, 27*, 649–692.

Westphal, M. &Bonanno, G. A. (2004). Emotional self-regulation. In M. Beauregard (ed.), *Consciousness, Emotional Self-Regulation, and the Brain.* Philadelphia: Benjamins, pp. 1–34.

Whooley, M. & Wong, J. (2011). Hostility and cardiovascular disease. *Journal of the American College of Cardiology 58*(12), 1228–1230.

Wills, T. A. &Fegan, M. F. (2001). Social networks and social support. In A. Baum, T. A. Revenson & J. E. Singer (eds), *Handbook of Health Psychology.* Mahwah, NJ: Lawrence Erlbaum, pp. 209–234.

Wills, T. A. (1986). Stress and coping in early adolescence: Relationships to smoking and alcohol use in urban school samples. *Health Psychology, 5*, 503–529.

Wills, T. A. (1990). Stress and coping factors in the epidemiology of substance use. In L. T. Kozlowski, H. M. Annis, H. D. Cappell, F. B. Glaser, M.S. Goodstadt, Y. Israel, H. Kalant, E. M. Sellers, & E. R Vingilis (Eds.), *Research advances in alcohol and drug problems* (Vol. 10, pp. 215–250). New York: Plenum.

Yehuda, R., Resnick, H., Kahana, B. &Giller, E. L. (1993). Long-lasting hormonal alterations to extreme stress in humans: normative or maladaptive? *Psychosomatic Medicine, 55*, 287–297.

Index

A

ABC model 594
ability models of emotional intelligence 200–201, 208
ability traits 615
abnormality, psychological 231
Aboriginal and Torres Strait Islanders
  child development in 47, 64
  mental illness in 223, 225
abstinence violation effect 741
abstract concepts 180
abstract thought 153
abuse
  alcohol *see* alcohol abuse
  child 67
  drug *see* drug abuse; *specific drug*
accessibility 404–405
  of attitudes 452–453, 494–495
accessibility hypothesis 115
accommodation 50–51, 552–553
acetaldehyde 306
acetate 306
achievement
  attribution 422
  cross-cultural view of 345–346
  intelligence and personality factors in 213–214
  need for 344–345
acquired immune deficiency syndrome (AIDS) 721
acquisition
  in classical conditioning 6, 9–10
  defined 6
  of fears and phobias 9–10, 23–24, 31–33
  in operant conditioning 17–18
action neuromatrix 649
action research 481
action stage 378
active development 39
active listening 538–539, 559–561
actor-observer effect 428–429
acute alcohol intoxication 311–312
acute pain 637 *see also* pain
  treatment of 650–652
adaptability scales 207
adaptation to illness 370
adaptive orientation 740
Adderall 279
addiction
  alcohol *see* alcoholism
  defined 736
  drug *see* drug abuse
  nicotine 325, 335–336, 737–739 *see also* tobacco use
additive assumption 176, 180
additive genetic variation 181
A delta fibres 646–647
adherence *see also* compliance
  barriers to 375
  defined 369
  factors affecting 371–375
  role of health care providers 375–376
  strategies to enhance 376–386
Adler, Alfred 354
admixture hypothesis 194
adolescence
  cognitive development in 53
  drug abuse in 278
  obesity in 273–274
  physical development in 47–48
  sexual orientation in 362
  social development in 67–70
adoption studies
  alcohol abuse 316–317
  of intelligence 176–177, 182, 192
adrenaline (epinephrine) 203, 677
adulthood *see also* older adults
  cognitive development in 57–59
  intelligence testing in *see* intelligence tests
  personality development in 599–600
  physical changes in 48–49
  social development in 70–74
advance directives 551
advertising
  classical conditioning and 8–9
  persuasion in 462–463, 468–469
  tobacco industry 321–322, 332
aerobic exercise 732–734
aerobic fitness 732–734
affect 414–416, 443 *see also* emotions; moods
  defined 664
  negative 668–670
  positive 668–670, 737
  transfer of 469
Affect infusion model 415
affect regulation mode 740
affiliation, need for 344–345, 351
age
  attitude change and 472
  developmental 40
  mental 141–142
ageing 82 *see also* older adults
agency 572
agentic state 499
aggression 26–27, 573
agility 733
agoraphobia 221, 236–237
agreeableness 627–628
'Aha!' reaction 13–14, 29
AIDS (acquired immune deficiency syndrome) 721
Ainsworth, Mary 63
Ajzen, Icek 445–447
alarm reaction 693
alcohol 300–320
  absorption and metabolism of 306–307
  blood alcohol concentration 307–309, 315
  chemistry and potency of 305–306
  drinking patterns 300–302
  effects of 309–314
    long-term 312–314
    short-term 309–312
  during pregnancy 43–44, 185–186, 313–314
  prescription drugs combined with 318
  social costs of 318–319
  stress and 739
alcohol abuse 315–319
  causes of 316–318, 739
  identification of 316
  treatment of 298–299, 319–320
alcohol dehydrogenase 306, 308
Alcohol e-Check Up to Go (e-Chug) 304
alcoholic hepatitis 313
Alcoholics Anonymous (AA) 299, 320
alcoholism (alcohol dependence) 315–319
  causes of 316–318, 711, 739
  identification of 316
  treatment of 298–299, 319–320
alcohol poisoning 311–312
all-cause mortality 166
allostatic load 715
Allport, Gordon 435, 439, 440, 495, 613–614
alopecia areata 711
Alpha test 142
Alzheimer's disease 59, 126, 129
American Psychological Association 142, 145, 183, 504

amnesia 128–129
anterograde 128–129
dissociative 253–254
retrograde 128–129
amphetamines 285–286
amygdala 676, 693
conditioning 23
emotional intelligence 203
memory 127–128
amyl nitrite 296
amyloid *b*-peptide (Ab) 126
anabolic steroids 297–298
analysis of variance (ANOVA) 420
anchoring and adjustment 413
Anderson, Norman 409, 443
animals *see also specific animal*
depression in 246
training of 21
anorexia nervosa 356–357, 736
ANOVA 420
anterograde amnesia 128–129
antibodies 720
antidepressants 657
antigens 720
antisocial personality disorder 221
antisocial personality disorder (ASPD) 252–253
anxiety disorders 233–242
body dysmorphic disorder 239
causes of 240–241
generalised anxiety disorder 234–235, 241
obsessive-compulsive disorder 221, 238–241
panic disorder 235
posttraumatic stress disorder 237–238
prevalence of 233–234
social anxiety disorder 225–226, 237, 240
suicide risk in 248–249
Tourette's disorder 239–240
anxiety sensitivity 241
Aplysia californicus 3–4
appearance
impressions of people based on 400, 544
memory for 406
applied behaviour analysis (ABA) 22
appraisal
cognitive 414–415
coping 451, 468
defined 717
object 442
primary 689, 696–697, 700
secondary 689, 696–697, 700
threat 451, 468
transactional model of 696–699
approach-approach conflict 569
approach-avoidance conflict 569
Aristotle 608
Army intelligence tests 142–143, 169
arousal
emotional 676–677
guilt 477
sexual 360
stress 735–736
arousal-based account 699
arousal regulation, biopsychosocial model of 415
Asch, Solomon 398–399, 402, 409, 499, 505–507
Asperger's disorder 263–264
assimilation 50–51, 121, 435
associative meaning 411
assortative mating 182, 198
asthma 724–725
asylums 224
atherosclerosis 329, 722
attachment 63–64, 66, 351
attention
focus on 427, 428
pain and 643
attention-deficit/hyperactivity disorder (ADHD) 227–228, 265–266, 279
attitudes 439–461
accessibility of 452–453, 494–495
behaviour predictions from 444–457
concepts related to 457–460
coping behaviour and 729–731
defined 439
as dynamic traits 616
formation of 457
functions of 441
history of 439–440
measurement of 460
strength 453–454, 494–495
structure of 440–441
versus values 457–458
attitude change 461
cognitive dissonance and 482–491
negative 492
persuasion *see* persuasion
attitude importance 472
attitude scales 460
attributes of the observer 573
attribution 417–439
applications of 422–425
biases in 425–430
defined 397, 522
intergroup 431–439
social influence and 515–516, 522
theories of 417–422
attributional complexity scale (ACS) 423
attributional conflict 424–425
attributional style 423–424
attributional style questionnaire (ASQ) 423
audience (receiver) 464, 470–473
auditory hallucinations 258
authoritarian style 65
authoritative style 65
authority, obedience to 499–504
autism spectrum disorders (ASD) 22–23, 263–264
autoimmune diseases 721
autokinesis 504
automatic activation 453–454
automatic behaviours 678
automatic judgements 443
autonomic nervous system 647
autonomy 61, 81, 515
availability heuristic 232, 413
avoidance 552
avoidance-avoidance conflict 569
avoidance-oriented coping 727

B

babies *see* infancy
background distressors 716
backward conditioning 6
bacterial infections 720–721
Baillargeon, Renée 54
balance theory 402, 483
Baltes, Margaret 82
Baltes, Paul 82
Bandura, Albert 26–27, 570–577, 697
barbiturates 292
Bard, Philip 676
Bar-On, Reuven 206–207, 210, 213
Bartlett, Frederic 121
base-rate information 411
basic levels 117
basic needs 586–587
B cells 720
B-cognition (being cognition) 588
B complex vitamins 735
Beck, Aaron 244
behaviour
attitudes and 444–457
causal attributions *see* attribution
health *see* health behaviour
memory for 406
risky *see* risky behaviour
behavioural control 727
behavioural decision theory 410
behavioural factors 571
behavioural genetics 173–183, 190–191, 515–517
behavioural immunogens 272
behavioural interventions, for pain 653–656
behavioural model of depression 244

behavioural pathogens 272
behavioural styles 515–517
behaviour change 368–393
collaboration 386–390
barriers to 388–389
strategies for improving 389–390
motivation and adherence 369–370
barriers to 375
factors affecting 371–375
locus of control 371, 579–580
role of health care providers 375–376
strategies to enhance 376–386
behaviourism 44, 396
radical 3, 24
S-R psychology 13
behaviour potential 578
being cognition (B-cognition) 588
being motives 583
beliefs 445–451
coping behaviour and 729–731
in a just world 430
persuasibility and 472–473
belief strength 445
belongingness 31, 585
Bem, Daryl 422, 490
Benedict, Ruth 68
benzodiazepines 292
Berkeley Growth Study 167–168
Beta test 142–143, 169
biases
in attribution 425–430, 438
cognitive 456–457, 473
conformity 512–513
disconfirmation 472–473
in forming impressions 399–401
outcome 419, 426, 433
social desirability 443
stress caused by 717
bidis 326
Big Five model 230, 627–629
Binet, Alfred 140, 141, 160
Binet-Simon scale 140, 141, 160
binge drinking 300–302
biofeedback 656–658
biological drive 349–350
biological influences
anxiety disorders 241
depression 246–247
emotions 666, 672–673, 693
hunger 355–356
pain 641–645
schizophrenia 260–261
sexuality 361–362
biological needs 351
biological psychology
intelligence 183–186
learning 30–33
biologisation 197
biomedical model interview 555–556
biopsychosocial model of arousal regulation 415
biopsychosocial perspective 229, 243, 722–726
bipolar disorder 221, 242, 247–248, 266
birth order
intelligence and 194–195
sexual orientation and 361–362
bisexuality 360–361
black tar heroin 290
Bleuler, Eugen 257
blood alcohol concentration (BAC) 307–309, 315
blotter acid (LSD) 293
B-love 585
blue-green studies 516, 518
B-motives 583
Bobo doll study 572
body composition 733
body dysmorphic disorder (BDD) 239
body image 357, 373
body language 539–541, 681–682
body-self matrix 649
body weight 272–274, 357–358, 711, 736
borderline personality disorder 251–252
Bowlby, John 63
brain
in Alzheimer's disease 126
in bipolar disorder 248
conditioning and 23
development of *see also* cognitive development
during adolescence 47–48, 69
sex differences 75–76
effects of alcohol on 312
emotional structures 203, 666, 676, 693
hunger mechanisms in 355
memory structures 127–132
mind-body connection 720
pain perception in 646–648
in schizophrenia 260
brain imaging 130–132
Alzheimer's disease 126
anxiety disorders 240, 241
bipolar disorder 248
emotions 673
schizophrenia 258, 260
social neuroscience 397–398, 416
breast feeding, intelligence and 184
Brehm, Jack 492
Brewer's dual-process model 409
Brief Alcohol Screening and Intervention for College Students (BASICS) 304
British Associationists 4
British National Child Development Study (NCDS) 192
bronchitis, chronic 330
bulimia nervosa 356–357, 736
buprenorphine 291
bupropion 335
burnout 716

C

Cacioppo, John 409–410, 473–474
caffeinated alcoholic beverages (CABs) 307
caffeine 104, 286, 735
cancer 276, 313, 327–329, 721
cannabinoids 287–290
Cannon, Walter 203, 676, 693
Cannon-Bard theory of emotion 676
capillaries 276
carbon monoxide 325
cardinal traits 613
cardiorespiratory endurance 733
cardiovascular disease 276, 312, 329–330, 711, 722–723
caregivers, as health determinant 374
care plans 387–388
caring for others 80
caring touch 540
Carroll, John B. 157–160
Caruso, David 208–210, 212
catastrophic thoughts 651
catastrophising 241, 648
catatonic symptoms 259
categorical model 230
categorisation 116–117
self-categorisation 511, 520–521
social 401–403, 405
category-consistent manner 405
category-incongruent manner 405
catharsis 728–729
cats, puzzle box study 13
Cattell, Raymond B. 153, 157–160, 614–620
Cattell-Horn-Carroll (CHC) theory of cognitive abilities 157–160
causal attributions *see* attribution
causal schemata 421
causal unit 427
cause-and-effect inferences 27–28
central executive 99
central nervous system (CNS) *see also* brain
effects of alcohol on 309, 312
central route processing 409–410, 474
central traits 398–399, 613

centration 52
cerebellum 127–128
cerebral cortex 127–128
cerebrospinal fluid 309
Chaiken, Shelley 410, 474–475
chaining 21
change 39
Chantix (varinicline) 335
characteristics of the model 572–573
CHC (Cattell-Horn-Carroll) theory of cognitive abilities 157–160
chewing tobacco 327
child abuse 67
child-driven effects 188
child-effects model 187
childhood *see also* infancy
  cognitive development in 51–57
  eidetic imagery in 95
  gender development in 74–78
  intelligence testing in *see* intelligence tests
  moral development in 79–80
  obesity in 273–274
  personality development in 589, 597–600
  physical development in 46–47
  psychological disorders in 263–266
  social development in 62–67
Children's Activities Inventory (CAI) 77
Children's Self-Efficacy Scale 577
chimpanzees, insight learning 29–30
chlorpromazine 224
choleric temperament 609
cholesterol 276, 312, 722
chronic bronchitis 330
chronic illness, stress caused by 724–725
chronic obstructive pulmonary disease (COPD) 330
chronic pain 637 *see also* pain
  treatment of 652–658
chunking 97–98
cigarettes 325–326 *see also* tobacco use
  electronic 334, 335
cigars 326
cirrhosis 313
classical conditioning 4–11
  anxiety disorders and 240
  applications of 8–11
  backward 6
  defined 5
  higher-order 8
  versus operant conditioning 12
  operant conditioning combined with 23–24
  Pavlov's discovery of 4–5
  phenomenon 5–6
  placebo response 645
  principles of 6–8
client-centred interview 556–557
client-centred therapy 592–607
client-practitioner relationship *see* therapeutic relationship
client-sensitive language 535–536
clinical judgement 410
cliques 69
clove cigarettes 326
club drugs 294–295
cocaine 44, 282–285
Code of Ethics (APA) 504
coercive power 497
cognition
  being 588
  deficiency 588
  defined 442
  evaluation and 442–443
  need for 471
  pain and 643–644
  social 396–398, 416–417
cognitive algebra 409, 443
cognitive appraisals 414–415
cognitive-behavioural interventions, for pain 654–656
cognitive biases 456–457, 473
cognitive conditioning 24
cognitive consistency 397, 442, 482
cognitive control 727–728
cognitive development 50–59
  adolescence 53
  adulthood 57–59
  childhood 51–57
  defined 50
  sex differences 75–76
  in social psychology 396–398
  theories of
    contemporary 53–57
    Piaget 50–53
    Vygotsky 56–57
cognitive dissonance 442, 461, 481, 482–491
cognitive distortions 245
cognitive epidemiology 165–166
cognitive maps 25–26
cognitive misers 397, 425, 679
cognitive models
  of depression 244–245
  of emotion 674–678
  of learning 24–30
cognitive psychology 24–25, 349–350
cognitive styles 700
cohort 41
cold, common 721
cold medicines 278
cold pressor test 643
collaboration 386–390
  barriers to 388–389
  as conflict strategy 553–554
  strategies for improving 389–390
collective agency 572
collectivism 345–346
college students *see* university students
colour perception task 516, 518
command hallucinations 258
commitment, involuntary 233
common cold 721
common personality traits 613
common traits 616
communication 529–564
  barriers to 543–546
  conflict *see* conflict
  defined 531
  electronic 541–542, 550–551, 681
  elements of 532–533
  humour in 542–543
  levels of 533
  mindfulness in 536–537
  nonverbal 539–541
    emotions 672–673, 680–682
  persuasive *see* persuasion
  sex differences 75
  in therapeutic relationship 531–536
    see also therapeutic relationship
  verbal 537–539
  written 541–542
communicator 463–465
community 81
community resources 373, 726–727
comorbidity 230
comparative advertising 466
comparison process 517
compensation 82
compensatory model of emotional intelligence 211
competence 25, 61
  emotional 205
competition 553
compliance 476–481 *see also* adherence
  defined 476, 495
  induced 485–486
  obedience and 495–496, 499–504
  tactics for enhancing 477–480
comprehension 403
compromise 553
compulsions 238–239
concentration, stress and 713
concepts 116–117
concrete operations stage 52–53
concurrent validity 168
conditioned response (CR) 5–6
conditioned stimulus (CS) 5–6
conditioned taste aversions 30–31

conditioning
- classical *see* classical conditioning
- cognitive 24
- defined 4
- operant *see* operant conditioning

conditions of worth 595
Condition Your Professor (game) 15
configural model 398–399, 402, 409
conflict 546–554
- attributional 424–425
- levels of 548–549
- management strategies 551–554
- post-decisional 486
- sources of 549–551
- stress caused by 715–716
- types of 569

confluence model 194
conformity 504–511
- compliance and 495–496
- defined 504, 513
- individual characteristics 507–508
- majority group pressure 505–507
- norms 504–505
- processes of 509–511
- situational factors in 508–509

conformity bias 512–513
congeners 310
conscientiousness 627–628
consensus information 420
consequences 79
- of imitating behaviour 573
- stress variables 701

conservation 52–53
consistency
- as behavioural style 515
- cognitive 397, 442, 482
- preference for 471–472
- self-consistency 479, 489

consistency information 420
conspiracy theories 435–436
constitutional traits 615
contact comfort 66
contemplation stage 378
contents 154
content-free schemas 403
content issues 549–550
content-of-thinking hypothesis 517
context-dependent memory 104
context shock 103–104
contextual distinctiveness 105–107
continuous reinforcement 18
continuum model 409
control
- habits and 456
- illusion of 245, 430
- impulse 358–359
- locus of *see* locus of control
- perceived behavioural 447
- as stress reliever 727–729

control-enhancing strategies 385–386
controllability 422
convenience sampling 144
conventional condition 106
convergent-divergent theory 519–520
conversion effect 517
conversion theory 517–519
Cook, Michael 31–32
Cooper, Joel 490–491
coping appraisal 451, 468
coping behaviour
- avoidance-oriented 727
- denial 707–708
- emotional intelligence 203–204, 210–211
- emotion-focused 689, 698–699, 727, 737
- evaluation of 705–707
- flexible 731–732
- individual differences in 729–731
- older adults 82
- pain 651–652
- proactive 728
- problem-focused 689, 698–699, 727
- self-efficacy and 372–373
- spirituality 730–731
- stress 726–732
- transactional model of *see* transactional model of stress

core conditions of counseling 602–605
coronary heart disease (CHD) 329, 722–723
corporal punishment 16
correlational designs 27
correlations, illusory 32, 264, 411–412
correspondence bias 425–428, 438
correspondent inference 418–420
corticosteroids 689
corticotropin-releasing factor (CRF) 711
cortisol 711
Cotard's syndrome 258
cough syrups 278
counseling
- community resources for 373
- core conditions of 602–605
- motivational interviewing 379–381
- Rogerian 600–605

counter-attitudinal actions 486–488
covariation 411–412
covariation model 420–421
Coyne, James 244
C polymodal fibres 646–647
crack cocaine 284
creativity 588
crisis debriefing 729
criterion performance 110
critical incidence stress debriefing 729
cross-fostering 66
cross-sectional design 41
crowds 69
crystallised intelligence 57, 153, 158
Csikszentmihalyi, Mihaly 347, 588
cue familiarity hypothesis 115
cultural influences
- achievement 345–346
- adolescence 68
- alcohol abuse 317–318
- attachment 64
- attribution 427, 437–438
- cognitive development 56–57
- communication 546, 681–682
- conformity 508
- defined 196
- eating habits 356
- emotions 671–672, 674
- gender development 74–78
- intelligence 196–197
- intelligence tests 151, 169
- moral development 80–81
- motivation 352
- pain 640
- personal space 682
- psychological disorders 225–226, 229–230, 242

cultural universality 226, 671–672
culture-bound syndromes 225–226
cumulative records 14
cupboard theory of attachment 66
curse of knowledge 681

D

Damasio, Antonio 675
Darwin, Charles 139, 173–174, 206, 668, 680
date rape drug (Rohypnol) 292
Davis, Keith 418–420
D-cognition (deficiency cognition) 588
death of loved one 73, 243
debriefing 729
deception, in research 503–504
decisional control 728
decision making
- advance directives 551
- alcohol use and 311
- attitudes and 443–444
- emotions and 667–668
- safe sex 448–449

decision rules, for psychological disorders 229
declarative memory 91
decontextualisation 196–197
deep judgments 109
defence mechanisms (Freudian) 567–568

deficiency cognition (D-cognition) 588
deficiency motives 583
dehumanisation 502
dehydration 309
deinstitutionalisation 224–225
delirium tremens (DTs) 320
delusions 257–258
demandingness 64–65
demonic model 223
denial 298, 707–708
depersonalisation disorder 253
depressants 290–293, 309, 738
depression *see* major depressive disorder
depressive realism 245
deprivation 67
depth perception 45–46
derealisation disorder 253
Descartes, René 665
designer drugs 294–295
despair 61–62, 74
detoxification 298, 320
development *see* human development
developmental age 40
developmental approach to motivation 350
developmental level of analysis 352
developmental psychology 39
deviation IQ 148–150
dextromethorphan (DXM) 278
diabetes 276, 712
diachronic studies 424
Diagnostic and Statistical Manual of Mental Disorders (DSM) 229–233
diagnostic criteria, for psychological disorders 229
diathesis-stress models 262–263
diet pills 278
differential forgetting 427
differential-influence hypothesis 518
difficult patients 370
digestive problems 712
dimensional model 230
dipping (tobacco) 327
direct access 415
direction-of-attention hypothesis 517
disability, adaptation to 370
discipline 17
disconfirmation bias 472–473
discount 420
discrepancy variables 464–465
discrete emotions theory 670–674, 677
discrimination 717
discriminative stimulus (S_d) 17
disgust reactions 10–11
disorganised speech 258–259
display rules 674
dispositional (internal) attribution 418
disruptive mood dysregulation disorder 266
dissociative amnesia 253–254
dissociative disorders 253–256
dissociative fugue 254
dissociative identity disorder (DID) 254–256
dissolution phase 424
dissonance 442, 461, 481, 482–491
distillation 305
distinctiveness information 420
distracting behaviours 541
distraction 651
distractor task 97
disuse 48, 58
divinity 81
divorce 72
Dix, Dorothea 224
D-love 585
DNA analysis, in heritability studies 179
dogs
  classical conditioning in 4–8, 12, 23
  learned helplessness in 245–246
  operant conditioning in 17–20
Dollard, John 567–570
dominant genetic variance 181
Domjan, Michael 10
door-in-the-face tactic 479–480
dopamine 247, 248
dopamine hypothesis 260–261
double approach-avoidance conflict 569
Down syndrome 171
drive for satisfaction 594
drive theory 349–350
driving
  alcohol use and 309, 315
  drug use and 288, 309
drugs *see also specific drug*
  for ADHD 265–266
  for mental disorders 224
  for pain relief 649–651, 657
  for smoking cessation 335–336
  use during pregnancy 44
drug abuse 277–300
  alcohol *see* alcohol abuse
  common drugs of abuse 282–298
  harm reduction strategies 299–300
  illicit drugs 279–282
  over-the-counter drugs 277–278
  prescription drugs 278–279, 318
  stress and 736–741
  treatment and recovery 298–299
drunkorexia 304
dual-process dependency model 496, 510–511
dual-process models of persuasion 473–475
Duchenne smile 673
Durkheim, Emile 459
dynamic lattice 616
dynamic traits 615–616
dysphoria 294

E

early-onset bipolar disorder 266
eating
  high-calorie foods 273
  motivation for 354–359
  stress and 711, 735–736
eating disorders 356–357, 736
Ebbinghaus, Hermann 110–112
echolalia 259
e-cigarettes 334, 335
ecstasy (drug) 294–295
ectomorphy 611
education *see also* university students
  emotional intelligence in 211
  humanistic theories applied to 581–582
  intelligence and 195–196, 213–214
  intelligence testing in 163, 169–170
  patient 382–383, 389
  personality factors in 213–214
  student-centred 599
efficacy expectancy 697
effort justification 483–485
egocentrism 52
ego integrity 61–62, 74
Eichmann, Adolf 499
eidetic imagery 95
Ekman, Paul 671–672
elaboration-likelihood model (ELM) 409–410, 473–474
elaborative reasoning 403
elaborative rehearsal 112–113
elderly people *see* older adults
elderspeak 536
electromyographic (EMG) biofeedback 656
electronic cigarettes 334, 335
electronic communication 541–542, 550–551, 681
elicited response 12
e-mail 542, 550–551, 681
emblems 681
embryonic stage 42
emic approach 627
emitted response 12
emoticons 681
emotions 414–416, 662–685
  basic set of 665–666
  biology of 666, 672–673, 693
  defined 664
  expressed 259–260
  versus facts 468–469, 667–668

emotions (*Continued*)
- frequency and duration of 667
- functions of 668
- intensity of 666
- *versus* moods 664–665
- negative 668–670
- nonverbal expression of 672–673, 680–682
- persuasion and 475
- positive 668–670
- primary 671–672
- secondary 672
- theories of 670–680
  - cognitive 674–678
  - discrete emotions 670–674
  - evaluation of 677–678
- unconscious influences on 678–680

emotional cascade model 251
Emotional Competence Inventory 205–206
emotional competencies 205
emotional control 728
emotional development, sex differences 75
emotional intelligence 199–214
- defined 199
- in education and workplace 211
- measurement of 201–202, 205–206, 212–214
- models of
  - Bar-On 206–207, 210, 213
  - compensatory 211
  - contexts for understanding 207–210
  - critical consideration of 213–214
  - Goleman 203–206, 208–210, 212
  - Salovey-Mayer 199–202, 208–210, 212
- sex differences 212–213
- trait 210

emotional manipulation scale 212
Emotional Quotient Inventory (EQ-i) 207, 213
emotion-focused coping 689, 698–699, 727, 737
empathic understanding 603
empathy 532, 533
emphysema 330
empiricism 50
empowerment 374, 382–383
empty nest 72
encoding
- context and 103–107
- defined 91–92
- processes 107–110
- social 403–405
- specificity 104–105

endomorphy 611
endorphins 290, 648
energy drinks 307
engrams 127
environmental factors
- alcohol abuse 316–318
- conformity 508–509
- defined 571
- *versus* genetics *see* nature-nurture debate
- intelligence *see* intelligence
- obesity 273–274, 358, 711
- personality development 625
- sexuality 362
- stress 716

environmental-mold traits 615
environmental tobacco smoke (ETS) 329, 331–332
epidemiology, cognitive 165–166
epinephrine (adrenaline) 203, 677
episodic memory 102–103
epistasis 181
epistatic genetic variance 181
EQ-i (Emotional Quotient Inventory) 207, 213
equipotentiality 31
ergs 616
Erikson's psychosocial stages 60–62, 70–71, 73
eros 350
essentialism 426–427
esteem needs 351, 586
ethanol 305
ethics, of research design 9, 503–504
ethnicity *see* cultural influences
ethnocentrism 431
ethology 348
ethyl alcohol 305
etic approach 627
evaluation 442–443, 445
evaluative advertising 468–469
evolutionary psychology
- adolescence 48
- emotional intelligence 206
- emotions 668, 670–671
- fear and phobias 31–32
- habituation 4
- intelligence 198–199
- morality 78
- motivation 350, 353
- obesity 358
- stress response 694

exam-taking anxiety 701–705, 718
exemplars 119
exemplification 477
exercise 274–277, 356, 732–734
exhaustion 694
existential philosophy 582
expectancies 447, 578, 697
- generalised 578

expectancy-value model 445–446, 460
expectations
- learning and 24–25
- of pain relief 644–645

experiential branch 200
expert power 497–498
explanatory model of care 557–558
explicit use of memory 90
exposure orientation 740
expressed emotion (EE) 259–260
The Expression of Emotion in Man and Animals (Darwin) 206, 668
expressive touch 540
external (situational) attribution 418
external validity 28
extinction 6–7, 17–18
extinction burst 18
extraversion 622, 627–628
extraverts 622
extrinsic motivation 344
eyewitness memory 124–125, 406–407
Eysenck, Hans 620–626
Eysenck, Sybil 625
Eysenck Personality Questionnaire (EPQ) 624

F

face validity 168
facial expressions
- in communication 540
- of emotions 672–673, 680–682

facial feedback hypothesis 673, 680
facilitating branch 200
factor analysis
- of intelligence 152–160
- of personality 614–620, 627–629

facts *versus* feelings 468–469, 667–668
factual advertising 468–469
fading 21
fake smile 673
fallacies
- family size and intelligence 193–194
- gambler's 20

false consensus effect 429
false perceptions 258
family environment
- adolescence and 68–69
- adult interactions within 71–72
- alcohol abuse and 316–317
- behaviour change and 387–388
- intelligence and 186–195
- schizophrenia and 259–260
- socialisation within 62

family resemblance 117
family resemblance view of mental disorders 223
family size, intelligence and 193–194

family studies, of intelligence 176–177
Fantz, Robert 45
fatty liver 312
Fazio, Russell 452, 490–491
fears
  acquisition of 9–10, 23–24, 31–33, 240–241
  irrational *see* phobias
  persuasive messages using 466–467
feedback loops 188, 383–384
feelings *see* emotions
feelings-of-knowing 114–115, 129
females *see also* gender; sex differences
  alcohol abuse 318
  body image in 357
  emotional intelligence 212–213
  gender development 74–78
  intelligence 198
  menarche in 47
  menopause in 49
  moral reasoning 80–81
  smoking by 321, 330–331
  stress response 694, 732
fermentation 305
fertilisation 42
fertility problems, smoking-related 330
Festinger, Leon 481, 482, 488, 490
fetishism 10
fibrosis 312
field dependence-independence 700
field studies 28
fight-or-flight response 203–204, 693–694
filtered cigarettes 325
Fishbein, Martin 445–447
Fiske and Neuberg's continuum model 409
five A's behavioural intervention protocol 379
five D's of pain environment 640
five-factor model of personality 213, 626–630
fixed-action patterns 348
fixed interval (FI) schedule 19–20
fixed ratio (FR) schedule 19
flashbacks 695
flashbulb memories 122–124
flexibility 733
flexible coping 731–732
flow 347
fluid intelligence 57, 153, 158
focal attention 403
focus on attention 427, 428
foetal alcohol spectrum disorders (FASD) 314
foetal alcohol syndrome (FAS) 43–44, 185, 314
foetal stage 42–43, 75–76
folie à deux 258
follow-up, with patients 383–384
food pyramid 735
foods *see also* eating
  grasshoppers as 487
  high-calorie 273
foot-in-the-door tactic 477–479
forbidden fruit labels 492
forethought 572–573
forewarning 492
Forgas, Joe 415
forgetting 110–112 *see also* amnesia
  differential 427
formal operation stage 53
formation stage 424
foundational theories 56
frame of reference 504
framing a message 469–470
freebase (cocaine alkaloid) 284
free choice 488
Freeman, Cathy 342–343
free recall 105
Freud, Anna 60, 68, 70
Freud, Sigmund 66, 243, 350, 567–570
friendships
  adolescence 69–70
  adulthood 71
frontal lobes
  during adolescence 47–48
  memory and 127–128
  sex differences 75–76
front-loading 303
frustrations 715–716
fully functioning person 599–600
functional level of analysis 352
functional magnetic resonance imaging (fMRI) 130–131, 397–398
functional programs 385
fundamental attribution error 425–428

G

g *see* general intelligence
Gage, Phineas 667
gains 39
Galen 609
Galton, Francis 139–140, 160, 173–174, 176, 612
galvanic skin response (GSR) 657
gambler's fallacy 20
gamma-hydroxybutyrate (GHB) 293
Garcia, John 31
Gardner, Howard 169
gastrointestinal disorders 712
gate control theory of pain 646–648
gender 74–78 *see also* sex differences
gender identity 76–77
gender roles 72, 76–77
gender stereotypes 76
general adaptation syndrome (GAS) 692–694
general attitudes 446
General Certificate of Secondary Education (GCSE) 163
general intelligence (g) 143–152
  compensatory model of 211
  defined 144
  hierarchical theories of 155–160
  measurement of 143–152, 160, 167–168
  multifactor theories of 152–155
generalisation gradient 7
generalised anxiety disorder (GAD) 234–235, 241
generalised expectancies 578
general mood 207
General Perceived Self-Efficacy Scale 576
General Self-Efficacy Scale 576
generativity 61, 73–74
genetic heritability
  ADHD 265
  alcohol abuse 316–318
  anxiety disorders 241
  autism 263–264
  bipolar disorder 247–248
  defined 175
  depression 246–247
  versus environmental factors *see* nature-nurture debate
  intelligence *see* intelligence
  obesity 358
  personality traits 625
  phobias 33
  schizophrenia 261–262
genetic model of social influence 515–517
genetics, behavioural 173–183, 190–191, 515–517
genetic variance 181
German measles (rubella) 43
germinal stage 42
Gestalt psychology 397, 399, 402
gestures 681–682
GHB (gamma-hydroxybutyrate) 293
ghrelin 355
Gibson, Eleanor 45–46
giftedness 172–173
Gilligan, Carol 80
girls *see* females
goal setting 381–382, 387, 389
Goleman, Daniel 199, 203–206, 208–210, 212
Gorn, Gerald 8–9
'grandma's rule' 22
grasshoppers 487

Greenwald, Tony 442–443
grossly disorganised behaviour 259
group characteristics, conformity and 507–508
group conflict 549
group discussion 533
group-enhancing bias 431
group factors 157
group identification 455
group norms 504
group pressure 502, 505–507
group-protective bias 431
group size 508–509
group socialisation theory 190–191
group therapy 607
groupthink 513–515
group unanimity 509
growth
  in childhood 46–47
  personal 582, 602–605
growth motives 583
growth spurt, pubescent 47
Guilford, J. P. 154–155
guilt 61
guilt arousal 477

H

h^2 (estimated average of genetic heritability) 175
habits
  anxious responses as 240–241
  attitudes and 450, 456
  defined 568
  learning of 568–569
habitual responses 621
habituation 3–4, 679
hair loss 711
Hall, Edward 682
Hall, G. Stanley 68
hallucinations 258
hallucinogens 293–296, 738
Halpern, Diane F. 170
hangover 310
hardiness 719, 730
Harlow, Harry 66
harm reduction 299–300
hashish 287
hassles 691, 715
Hassles Scale 691
health
  effects of stress on 719–726
  social determinants of 373–375
health behaviour 270–339
  changes in *see* behaviour change
  defined 272
  drug abuse *see* drug abuse
  obesity 272–274, 311, 357–358, 711, 736
  physical activity 274–277, 732–734
  stress and 732–741
health belief model 376–379
health care information 374, 382–383, 389, 541–542
health care providers
  client relationship *see* therapeutic relationship
  introduction by 560–561
  role in adherence 375–376
  touching style 540
health literacy 561
health outcomes
  attitudes and 450–451
  emotional intelligence and 210–211
  IQ score and 164
  self-efficacy and 372–373
  stress-related illness 722–726
hearing
  adulthood 49
  infancy 44
heart disease 276, 312, 329–330, 711, 722–723
hedonic contingency hypothesis 475
hedonic relevance 419
Heider, Fritz 417–418
helplessness, learned 245–246
Hereditary Genius (Galton) 139, 173
heritability *see* genetic heritability
heroin 290–291, 739–740
heterosexuality 71–72, 360–362
heuristic processing 415, 474
heuristics 412–413, 488
heuristic-systematic model (HSM) 410, 474–475
hierarchical theories of intelligence 155–160
hierarchies 117
hierarchy of needs 348, 351–353, 584–586
high-density lipoproteins (HDLs) 276, 312
high-distress relationships 72
higher-order conditioning 8
high functions 209–210
high memory span 99
hippocampus 127–128, 693
Hippocrates 609
Hitler, Adolf 461–462
HIV (human immunodeficiency virus) 721
hoarding behaviour 239–240
homeostasis 349, 355
home programs, functional 385
homosexuality 71–72, 360–362
Honzik, C. H. 25
hookahs 326
Horn, John Leonard 157–160
hostility 718
Hovland, Carl 462
human development 37–86
  cognitive *see* cognitive development
  physical *see* physical development
  sex differences 74–78
  study of 39–41
human immunodeficiency virus (HIV) 721
humanistic personality theories
  in education 581–582
  history and elements of 582–607
humour 542–543
hunger 354–359
Hyman, Misty 345
hypnosis 652
hypnotic drugs 292
hypochondriasis 234
hypofrontality 260
hypoglycemia 735–736
hypothalamus 355, 647, 676, 693
hypothalamus-pituitary-adrenal (HPA) axis 693

I

iconic memory 93–95
id 350
ideal category members 117
ideal self 601
identity
  gender 76–77
  versus role confusion 61, 68
  self-identity 457
  social 190–191, 408, 433, 455, 511, 520–521
ideology 458–459
IE Scale 579
Ikemi, Y. 720
illicit drugs 279–282 *see also* drug abuse; *specific drug*
illness
  adaptation to 370
  nutrition and 735
  stress-related 722–726
illusion of control 430
illusory control 245
illusory correlations 32, 264, 411–412
illustrators 681
imitating behaviour, consequences of 573
immediacy
  of authority figure 502
  of victim 502
immediate antecedent variables 701
immediate consequence variables 701
immune system 720–721
  stress and 712, 721–722
implicit personality theories 400

implicit use of memory 90, 108–110
impressions of other people 398–401, 544
imprinting 63
impulse control 358–359
incentive 573
independence 68–69
Indigenous people *see* Aboriginal and Torres Strait Islanders
individual differences 41
  attitudes 456, 729–731
  attributional styles 423–424
  conformity 507–508
  coping behaviour 729–731
  persuasibility 471–472
individualism 345–346
induced compliance 485–486
indulgent style 65
infancy
  cognitive development in 51–55
  personality development in 598
  physical development in 44–46
infections 720–721
inferences
  cause-and-effect 27–28
  correspondent 418–420
  social 409–414
inferiority 61
influence *see* social influence
influence phase 518
information
  in actor-observer effect 428–429
  in covariation model 420
  health care 374, 382–383, 389, 541–542
  social 410
informational control 728
informational influence 510, 520–521
informational power 497
information integration theory 443
information processing 89, 443
ingratiation 477
inhalants 296–297
inhibition, latent 9, 32–33
initiative 61
innovation 513
inoculation 492–494
inoculation defence 493
insanity defence 232
insight 13
insight learning 29–30
instinctoid tendencies 583
instinct theory 348–350
institutionalisation
  of children 67
  for drug abuse treatment 299, 320
  of mentally ill 224–225, 233
instrumental touch 540
instrumental values 457
intellectual disabilities 171–172
intelligence 137–218
  in adulthood 57–58
  crystallised 57, 153, 158
  emotional *see* emotional intelligence
  environmental influences 183–199
    biological variables 183–186
    culture 196–197
    education 195–196
    family environment 186–195
    framework for 198–199
    genetics and 180
    prenatal factors 185–186
  extremes of 170–173
  fluid 57, 153, 158
  general (g) 143–152
  heritability of 173–183
    assessment of 176–183
    environment and 180
    framework for 198–199
  measurement of *see* intelligence tests
  personality and 213–214
  sensorimotor 50
  sex differences in 198
  theories of 139–160
    hierarchical 155–160
    multifactor 152–155
    triarchic 169
    two-factor 144
intelligence quotient (IQ) 141
  deviation 148–150
  fluctuations in 167–168
  mortality and 165
Intelligence Task Force 168
intelligence tests *see also specific test*
  history of 139–160
  reliability of 166–168
  standardised 144–152, 161–162
  types of 160–161
  typical features of 161–162
  uses of 162–166, 169–170
  validity of 168–169
intentions 79, 445–451
interference 111–112
intergroup attribution 431–439
intergroup conflict 549
intermittent reinforcement 18
internal (dispositional) attribution 418
internalisation 56
internal reliability 166–167
internal self-regulatory processes 574
internal validity 28
internal working model 63
Internet *see* websites
interpersonal conflict 548
interpersonal (secondary) gain 639
interpersonal level of communication 533
interpersonal model of depression 244
interpersonal relationships *see* relationships
interpersonal skills 207
interval reinforcement schedules 19–20
interviewing
  client 554–561
  motivational 379–381
intimacy 61, 70–71
intimate distance 682
intimidation 477
intragroup conflict 549
intrapersonal (primary) gain 639
intrapersonal level of communication 533
intrapersonal skills 207
intrinsic motivation 344, 353
introduction, in client interview 560–561
introversion 622
introverts 622
investment 515
invite, listen, summarize strategy 559
involuntary commitment 233
involuntary smoking 329, 331–332
I/O psychology 344–345
IQ *see* intelligence quotient
isokinetic exercise 733
isolation 61, 70–71
isometric exercise 733
isotonic exercise 733

J

James, William 674–675
James-Lange theory of emotion 674–675, 678
Japan, mental illness in 225–226
Jensen, Arthur 151
job satisfaction 345
job stress 724
Johnson, M. B. 158
Joiner, Thomas 251
Jones, Mary Cover 10
Jones, Ned 418–420
Junior Eysenck Personality Questionnaire 625
justice 80
just world, belief in 430

K

Kagan, Jerome 62
Kandel, Eric 3
Kant, Immanuel 609
Kelley, Harold 420–421

Kernberg, Otto 251
ketamine 296
Kleinman, Arthur 557–558
'k:m' factor 156–157
knowledge
  curse of 681
  organised 116
knowledge compilation 91
Kohlberg's stages of moral reasoning 79–80
Köhler, Wolfgang 29–30
Kraepelin, Emil 257

L

labelling theorists 228
laboratory studies 27–28
Lange, Carl 674–675
language *see also* communication
  attribution and 428
  body language 539–541, 681–682
  client-sensitive 535–536
  as communication barrier 546
  intelligence tests and 151, 169
  paralanguage 537–538
language-dependent memory 105
language development, sex differences 75
Latané, Bibb 522
latent inhibition 9, 32–33
latent learning 25–26
laughing gas 296
laughter 542–553
law of effect 12–13
law of large numbers 410
lay theories of personality 400
Lazarus and Folkman's transactional model *see* transactional model of stress
L-data 617
leadership, power and 498
lead poisoning 185
learned behavioural tolerance 309
learned helplessness 245–246
learning 1–34
  biological influences on 30–33
  cognitive models of 24–30
  by conditioning *see* conditioning
  defined 3
  famous psychologists on 3
  insight 29–30
  latent 25–26
  mindset and 347
  observational 26–29, 570, 572
  self-directed 370
  types of 3
learning disorders 172
learning history 24
learning models of anxiety 240–241
learning styles 383
learning theory
  applied to personality 567–570
  social learning 570–577
legal issues
  eyewitness memory 124–125, 406–407
  mental illness 231–233
legitimate power 497–498
leniency contract 521–522
leptin 355
leukoplakia 329
levelling 121, 435
levels of analysis (or explanation) 432
levels-of-processing theory 107–108
Lewin, Kurt 397, 481, 504
Lewinsohn, Peter 244
lexical hypothesis 612–613, 626–627
life events
  conflict caused by 551
  depression and 243–244, 246–248
  stress caused by 689–691, 715, 724
lifelong openness hypothesis 472
life stages hypothesis 472
limbic system
  during adolescence 47–48
  conditioning 23
  emotional intelligence 203
  emotions originating in 666, 676
  pain perception 647
Linehan, Marsha 251
linguistic factors *see* language
listening, active 538–539, 559–561
Little Albert (case study) 9, 240
Little Peter (case study) 10
liver disease 312–313
Locke, John 50
locomotion 47
locus of control
  attribution and 422
  behaviour change and 371, 579–580
  defined 577
  personality and 577–580
longitudinal design 27, 40
long-term antecedent variables 701
long-term consequence variables 701
long-term memory (LTM) 100–115
  defined 101
  encoding
    context and 103–107
    process 107–110
  forgetting 110–112, 427
  improvement of 112–113
  metamemory 113–115, 129
  for people 405
  retrieval cues 101–103
  retrieval process 107–110
  structures in 116–126
Lorenz, Konrad 63
losses 39
Lovaas, Ivar 22–23
love needs 351, 585
low-ball tactic 480
low-density lipoproteins (LDLs) 276
low-distress relationships 73
low functions 209–210
low memory span 99
LSD (lysergic acid diethylamide) 293–294
lung cancer 327–329
lymphocytes 720
lysergic acid diethylamide (LSD) 293–294

M

Machiavellianism 211–212
macrophages 720
magic mushrooms 296
magnetic resonance imaging (MRI) 130–131, 397–398
mainlining (heroin) 291
mainstream smoke 331
maintenance rehearsal 96
maintenance stage 378, 424
major depressive disorder
  in chronic pain patients 639
  explanations for 243–247, 666
  prevalence of 242–243, 732
  suicide risk in 248–249
  symptoms of 243
major depressive episode 242, 247
major group factors 156–157
majority group pressure 505–507
majority influence 517, 520–522
males *see also* gender; sex differences
  emotional intelligence 212–213
  gender development 74–78
  intelligence 198
  moral reasoning 80–81
  stress response 694, 732
Malkin, Peter 499
managing branch 200
manic-depressive disorder *see* bipolar disorder
manic episode 247
manipulators 681
marijuana 260, 287–290
marketing *see* advertising
Marlatt's relapse model 740–741
marriage 71–72, 424–425
Maslow, Abraham 70, 348, 350–353, 583–592
maternal effects model 186
maturation 46–47

Mayer, John D. 199–202, 208–210, 212
Mayer-Salovey-Caruso Emotional Intelligence Test 201–202, 212
maze tests 26
McClelland, David 344–346
McGill pain questionnaire 650
McGuire, Bill 492–494
MDMA (methylene-dioxymethamphetamine) 294–295
Mead, Margaret 68
mediation 554
media violence 27–28
medical marijuana 288–289
medical model 223–224
medium, message and 469
melancholic temperament 609
membership groups 496
memory 87–136
  in adulthood 58–59, 126, 129
  attitudes as association in 452
  biological aspects of 127–132
  causal information in 427
  defined 89
  eyewitness 124–125, 406–407
  forgetting 110–112, 427 *see also* amnesia
  iconic 93–95
  improvement of 112–113
  long-term *see* long-term memory
  metamemory 113–115, 129
  for people 405–409
  processes 91–93
  reconstructive 121–126
  short-term 95–98, 405
  stress and 713
  structures 116–126
  types of 90–91
  working 98–100, 405
memory span 96, 99
men *see* gender; males; sex differences
menarche 47
menopause 49
mental abilities, multifactor theory of 152–153
mental age 141–142
mental disorder defence 232
mental illness *see* psychological disorders; *specific disorder*
mental operations 52
mental representations 92
mental retardation 171
Mental Survey Committee (Scotland) 164, 168
menthol cigarettes 326
mere exposure effect 678–679
mescaline 295–296
mesomorphy 611
message (signal) 464, 466–470
meta-analysis 164, 446
metabolic syndrome 276
metacontrast principle 511
metamemory 113–115, 129
metaneeds 586
methadone 291
methamphetamine 285–286
method of loci 113
methylene-dioxymethamphetamine (MDMA) 294–295
microdots (LSD) 293
middle functions 209–210
migraine 637
Milgram, Stanley 499–504
Miller, Neal 567–570
mind-body connection 720
mindfulness 536–537
mindlessness 480
mindset 347
mind wandering 100
Mineka, Susan 31–32
Minnesota Study of Twins Reared Apart 177
minor group factors 157
minority influence 512, 517, 520–522
mirror neurons 28–29
mistrust 60
mixed models of emotional intelligence 205, 208
MMR vaccine 264
M'Naghten rule 232
mnemonics 113
modelling, in learning 26–28, 573
moderator variables 455–457, 472
monkeys
  fear learning 31–32
  social development in 66
moods
  attitudes and 456
  defined 664
  versus emotions 664–665
  general 207
  pain and 642
  persuasion and 475
  structure of 668–670
mood-congruence effect 415
mood disorders 242–250
  bipolar disorder 221, 242, 247–248, 266
  in childhood 266
  defined 242
  depression *see* major depressive disorder
  prevalence of 242–243
moral development 78–81
morality 78
moral treatment 224
moral values 450
morphine 739–740
mortality, IQ and 165
Morton, Eugene 673
Moscovici, Serge 434–435, 459, 512–513, 515–517
motivated processing 415
motivated tactitians 397, 425
motivation 340–366
  for behaviour change *see* behaviour change
  defined 343
  extrinsic 344
  hunger 354–359
  instinct 583
  intrinsic 344, 353
  rewards and 346–347
  sexual 360
  social 354
  theories of 348–353
    comparison of 350
    drive 349–350
    Freud's 350
    instinct 348–350
    McClelland's 344–346
motivational hierarchy 352–353
motivational interviewing 304, 379–381
motivation-structural rules 673
motor development 46–47
multifactor theories of intelligence 152–155
multiple abstract variance analysis (MAVA) 615
multiple-act criterion 446
multiple requests 477–480
multiple-systems model of hunger 354–356
Murray, Henry 344
muscular endurance 733
muscular strength 733
mushrooms 296
Myers-Briggs Type Inventory 628

N

naive psychology 56, 397, 417–418
Nakagawa, S. 720
naltrexone 291
narcolepsy 278
narcotics 290–293, 738, 739–740
narrow occluder 54
National Intelligence Test 143
National Longitudinal Survey of Youth (NLSY) 193
nativist view 50
natural selection 31

nature-nurture debate
  cognitive development 50, 56–57
  gender development 74–78
  intelligence 173–174, 180, 198–199
  moral development 81
needs
  for achievement 344–345
  for affiliation 344–345, 351
  basic 586–587
  biological 349–351
  for cognition 471
  defined 349
  hierarchy of 348, 351–353, 584–586
  metaneeds 586
  for power 344
  safety 584–585
  for self-actualisation 586
negative affect 668–670
negative assortative mating 182
negative attitude change 492
negative feedback loops 188
negative punishment 15
negative reinforcement 14, 23–24, 240
negative symptoms 261
negativity 399–400
neglecting style 65
Nemeth, Charlan 519–520
neuromatrix 648–649
neurons 28–29, 203
neuroscience, social 397–398, 416
neuroticism 243, 622, 627–628
Neuroticism, Extraversion, Openness Personality Inventory (NEO-PI-R) 627
neurotransmitters, in schizophrenia 260–261
neutral cognitive account 699
neutrophils 720
newborns, physical development in 44–45
New General Self-Efficacy Scale 576
new look model of dissonance 490–491
next-in-line effect 113
Nick A. (case study) 128–129
nicotine 324–325, 335, 737–739 *see also* tobacco use
nicotine poisoning 325
nicotine replacement products 335
nicotine withdrawal 335
nitrous oxide 296
nocebo effect 720
nociceptors 646–647
nomothetic approach to personality 608
non-common effects 419
nonseminoma 289
non-shared environments 186–187
nonverbal communication 539–541
  emotions 672–673, 680–682
nonverbal leakage 681
noradrenaline (norepinephrine) 203, 247, 248
norepinephrine (noradrenaline) 203, 247, 248
normal distribution, of IQ scores 149–150
normalisation 513
normality, psychological 231
normative influence 510, 520
normative investigations 40
normative models 410
norm referencing 162
norms
  attitudes and 455
  defined 495
  formation and influence of 504–505
nucleus accumbens 23
numerical rating scales 649–650
nurture *see* nature-nurture debate
nutrition *see also* eating
  intelligence and 183–184
  stress and 735–736

O

obedience 495–496, 499–504
obesity 272–274, 311, 357–358, 711, 736
object appraisal 442
object permanence 52, 54–55
observational learning 26–29, 570, 572
observer, attributes of 573
obsessions 238
obsessive-compulsive disorder (OCD) 221, 238–241
OCEAN 627–628
older adults
  cognitive functioning in 57–58
  hearing loss in 49
  memory impairment in 58–59, 126, 129
  sexuality 49
  social development in 72–74
  successful ageing 82
one-component attitude model 440
online systems *see* websites
openness 627–628
operant 12
operant chamber 14
operant conditioning 11–23
  anxiety disorders and 240
  applications of 21–23
  versus classical conditioning 12
  classical conditioning combined with 23–24
  defined 11–12
  law of effect 12–13
  pain response and 653
  schedules of reinforcement 18–20
  terminology of 14–18
operations 154
opioids 290–293, 738, 739–740
optimisation 82
optimism 730
options 39
organic conditions, *versus* psychological disorders 229
organised knowledge 116
organism 24
organismic valuing 598
organizational communication 533
organizational conflict 549
The Origin of Species (Darwin) 139, 173
outcome 15 *see also* health outcomes
outcome bias 419, 426, 433
outcome expectancy 697
outpatient behavioural treatment 298–299, 320
outside-family factors 190–191
overjustification 346
overload 716
  sensory 543–544
over-the-counter (OTC) drugs, abuse of 277–278
overweight 272–274, 311, 357–358, 711, 736
oxytocin 694

P

pain 635–661
  defined 637
  living with 638–641
  measurement of 649–650
  nature of 638
  prevalence of 638
  theories of
    biological 641–645
    neuromatrix 648–649
    psycho-biological 646–648
  treatment of 649–658
    acute pain 650–652
    chronic pain 652–658
    expectations of 644–645
    pain management clinics 658
  types of 637–638
pain management clinics 658
pain receptors 641–642, 646–647
paired distinctiveness 411
pairings 325
Pan Am smile 673
panic attacks 235, 241
panic disorder 235
  example of 221
paralanguage 537–538

parental influence, on self-concept 597–598
Parental Self-Efficacy Scale 577
parent-effects model 189
parenthood, transition to 72
parenting practices 66
  gender roles 72, 76–77
parenting style 64–66
partial reinforcement 18
partial-report procedure 94
participant modelling 575
passive development 39
passive model 187
passive smoking 329, 331–332
pathogens 720
patient-centred therapy 592–607
patient-controlled analgesia (PCA) 650–651
patient education 382–383, 389
patient-practitioner relationship *see* therapeutic relationship
patient-sensitive language 535–536
Pavlov, Ivan 3–6 *see also* classical conditioning
PCP (phencyclidine) 295
peak experiences 588
Pearson, Karl 145
peer relationships
  adolescence 69–70
  adulthood 71
  gender socialisation 77–78
peer support groups 384–385
peg-word method 113
people-first language 535–536
perceived behavioural control 447
perceiving branch 200
perception
  in actor-observer effect 428
  depth 45–46
  false 258
  in infants 44–46
  of pain 642–645
  self-perception theory 422, 490
performance phase 570
peripheral route processing 410, 474
peripheral traits 398–399
personal agency 572
personal conflict 548
personal constructs 400
personal disposition 613
personal distance 682
personal factors 571
personal growth 582, 602–605
personalism 419
personality 565–634
  Big Five model 230, 627–629
  coping behaviour and 729–731
  development of 589, 597–600
  heart disease and 722–723
  humanistic theories of 581–582
  impressions of people and 398–401
  learning theory applied to 567–570
    social learning 570–577
  nomothetic approach to 608
  psychopathic 252–253, 622–623
personality disorders 250–256
  antisocial 252–253
  borderline 251–252
personality system framework 209–210
personality traits
  achievement and 213–214
  attributional style 423–424
  defined 609–611
  emergence of 608–611
  memory for 406
  theories of 608–611
    Allport's approach 613–614
    Cattell's approach 614–620
    development of 611–612
    evaluation of 629–630
    Eysenck's approach 620–626
    five-factor model 213, 626–630
    lexical hypothesis 612–613, 626–627
personality types 621, 718–719, 723
personal orientation inventory (POI) 591
personal space 540–541, 682
personal variables 700
person-centred therapy 592–607
person memory 405–409
person schemas 402
persuasion 461–476
  audience in 464, 470–473
  defined 462
  dual-process models of 473–475
  message in 464, 466–470
  resistance to 491–495
  source in 463–465
  Yale approach to 462–463
Petrides, Konstantin Vasily 210
Petty, Richard 409–410, 473–474
phagocytes 720
phantom limb pain 637, 641, 648
phencyclidine (PCP) 295
phenomenology 582, 593
phenotypes 181
phenylketonuria (PKU) 171
philosophies of human nature 400
phlegmatic temperament 609
phobias 235–237
  acquisition of 7, 9–10, 23–24, 32–33, 223
  agoraphobia 221, 236–237
  defined 223, 235
  preparedness 31–33
  renewal effect 7
  social 225–226, 237, 240
  specific 237
  types of 10
phonological loop 98
photographic memory 95
physical activity 274–277, 356, 732–734
physical appearance
  impressions of people based on 400, 544
  memory for 406
physical dependence 736
physical development 42–49
  adolescence 47–48
  adulthood 48–49
  childhood 46–47
  defined 42
  infancy 44–46
  prenatal *see* prenatal development
physical punishment 16
physique, types of 611
Piaget, Jean 50–53
Pinel, Phillippe 224
pipes 326
placebo response 644–645
planned behaviour 447–451
plants, conditioning in 5
platelet adhesiveness 329
political ideologies 458–459
population concepts 180
positive affect 668–670, 737
positive assortative mating 182
positive feedback loops 188, 383–384
positive manifold 144
positive punishment 15
positive reinforcement 14
positive symptoms 261
positivity 399–400
positivity offset 670
positron emission tomography (PET) 130
post-decisional conflict 486
Postman, Leo 435
post-message behaviour 494–495
postpartum obsessive-compulsive disorders 239
posttraumatic model of dissociative disorders 255
posttraumatic stress disorder (PTSD) 237–238, 694–695, 729
poverty *see* socioeconomic status
power 497–499
  need for 344
  will 358–359

Pratkanis, Anthony 442–443
pre-attentive analysis 403
pre-contemplation stage 378
predictive validity 168
preference for consistency 471–472
prefrontal cortex (PFC) 129, 248
pre-gaming 303
pregnancy, foetal development during *see* prenatal development
Premack principle 21–22
prenatal development 42–44
  sex differences 75–76
  teratogens 43–44, 185–186, 313–314, 330
preoperational stage 52
preparation stage 378
preparedness 31–33
Preschool Activities Inventory (PSAI) 77
prescription drug abuse 278–279, 318
prevalence
  defined 229
  of pain 638
  of psychological disorders 229, 234, 236, 242–243
  of smoking 321
prewired for survival 44–46
primacy effect 105, 399
primary appraisal 689, 696–697, 700
primary control-enhancing strategies 385–386
primary drives 568
primary emotions 671–672
primary (intrapersonal) gain 639
primary reinforcers 22, 568
priming 108–109, 404–405
print media 469, 541–542
proactive coping 728
proactive interference 111–112
problem-focused coping 689, 698–699, 727
procedural components of conflict 550
procedural memory 91
procedural touch 540
procrastination 21–22
products 154
Progressive Matrices (Raven) 150–153, 160, 169
proof (alcoholic drink) 305
proportional condition 106
proportion of shared variance 175
propositional model of memory 405
proprium 614
protection motivation theory 450–451, 468
prototypes 119
proxemics 540–541, 682
proximal level of analysis 352
proxy agency 572
pseudopatients 228
pseudostressors 735
psilocin 296
psilocybin 296
psychedelics 293–294, 738
psychoactive drugs 738 *see also* *specific drug*
psychoanalytic theory 567–570, 582, 593
psycho-biological theory of pain 646–648
psychodynamic theory 350
psychological debriefing 729
psychological dependence 736–737
psychological disorders 219–269 *see also* *specific disorder*
  childhood 263–266
  cultural influences 225–226, 229–230, 242
  defined 222–223
  diagnosis of 226–233
  examples of 221
  historical concepts of 223–225
  legal issues 231–233
  prevalence of 229, 234, 236, 242–243
  stress 712–713
  treatment of 224–225
    Eysenck's approach 625
    Maslow's approach 589–590
    Rogers' approach 600–605
psychological elements of conflict 550
psychological hardiness 719, 730
psychological motives 350, 356
psychological present 100
psychological resilience 719
psychological subsystems 209–210
psychology
  biological *see* biological psychology
  cognitive 24–25, 349–350
  developmental 39
  emotional intelligence in 210–212
  evolutionary *see* evolutionary psychology
  social *see* social psychology
psychoneuroimmunology (PNI) 712, 721–722
psychopathic personality 252–253, 622–623
psychopathology 221, 226, 570, 625
psychophysiological disorders 722, 725–726
psychosocial factors
  obesity 274, 358, 711, 736
  pain 642–645
  stress 714–719
psychosocial stages (Erikson) 60–62
psychosomatic disorders 722
psychotherapy 570
psychoticism 622–623
psychotic symptoms 258
puberty 47, 68
public distance 682
punishment 15–17
pure autonomic failure (PAF) 675
purpose in life test (PIL) 591
puzzle box (Thorndike) 13

Q

Q-data 617
Q-sort 605
quantification 197
questioning, during client interview 556–558

R

racial inequality 438, 717
radical behaviourism 3, 24
radio media 469, 541–542
rape 292, 311
rational-emotive behaviour therapy 594
ratio reinforcement schedules 19–20
Raven, John Carlyle 150
Raven Progressive Matrices 150–153, 160, 169
Rayner, Rosalie 3, 9, 240
reactance 491–492
reappraisal 698, 700
reasoned action, theory of 445–447
reasoning *see also* cognition; thinking
  elaborative 403
  moral 79
recall 101–102, 105–107
receiver (audience) 464, 470–473
recency effect 105, 399
reciprocal causation 571
reciprocal determinism 571
reciprocity principle 477
recognition 101–102, 205
recognition illusion 120
reconstructive memory 121–126
reductionism 416
reference groups 496
referent informational influence 510–511
referent power 497
reflexes, infant 44
regression 410–411
regulation 205, 574–575
rehearsal
  defined 96–97
  elaborative 112–113
  maintenance 96
reification 197
reinforcement
  in classical conditioning 13–15
  defined 14

depression as loss of 244
learning and 25
negative 14, 23–24, 240
in operant conditioning 22–23
partial 18
positive 14
versus punishment 15–17
schedules of 18–20
self-reinforcement 573
reinforcement value 578
Reiss' models of genetic transmission 189
relationships
in adolescence 69–70
in adulthood 71–72
attributions in 424–425
social support 373–375, 726–727
stress caused by 715
therapeutic *see* therapeutic relationship
relaxation 652, 656–658
relearning 110
reliability
of intelligence tests 166–168
of psychiatric diagnosis 227
religion 730–731
Remembering: A Study in Experimental and Social Psychology (Bartlett) 121
renewal effect 7
repetition 466
representativeness heuristic 412–413, 488
repression 567–568
reproductive function
adulthood 49, 71–72
prenatal development *see* prenatal development
research design 27–28, 40–41
action research 481
correlational 27
cross-sectional 41
ethical issues 9, 503–504
field studies 28
heritability studies 176–177, 182
laboratory studies 27–28
longitudinal 27, 40
residential treatment programs 299, 320
resilience, psychological 719
resistance 693–694
resource dilution model 194
respiratory disorders 330
respondent conditioning *see* classical conditioning
response
conditioned 5–6
elicited 12
emitted 12
S-R psychology 13, 24, 568
stress as 688–689
unconditioned 5–6
response expectancies 697
responsibility, attribution of 430
responsiveness 64–65
retention interval 101
retrieval
defined 91–92
processes 107–110
retrieval cues 101–103
retroactive interference 111–112
retrograde amnesia 128–129
reversibility 53
reward 14
depression and 247
hunger and 356
motivation and 346–347
pain 639
reward power 497
ring of truth 466
riots 437
risky behaviour
during adolescence 47–48, 69–70
alcohol use and 311
attitudes and 450–451
health-related *see* health behaviour
stress and 732–741
risky shift 515
Ritalin 279
Rogers, Carl 592–607
Rohypnol 292
roles
defined 402
gender 72, 76–77
role confusion 61, 68
role uncertainty 543
rooting reflex 44
Rotter, Julian 371, 577–580
Rousseau, Jean-Jacques 50
Rozin, Paul 10–11
rubella (German measles) 43
rumination 731–732
rumour 435

S

s (specific abilities) 144, 156–157
safe sex 448–449
safety culture 545
safety needs 351, 584–585
salience 403–404
Salovey, Peter 199–202, 208–210, 212
salt intake 736
same-sex partners 71–72
sanguine temperament 609
satisfaction, drive for 594
sauce béarnaise syndrome 30–31
scapegoat food 31
Schachter, Stanley 676–677
schadenfreude 672
schedules of reinforcement 18–20
schemas 117–119, 401–403, 421, 441
schemes 50
schizophrenia 257–263
example of 221
explanations for 259–263
symptoms of 257–259
schizotypal personality disorder 262
schools *see* education
sciatica 644
scripts 401, 402
sea slugs 3–4
secondary appraisal 689, 696–697, 700
secondary control-enhancing strategies 385–386
secondary drives 568
secondary emotions 672
secondary (interpersonal) gain 639
secondary reinforcers 22, 568
secondary traits 613
secondhand smoke 329, 331–332
second-order conditioning 8
sedative-hypnotics 292
Selby, Edward 251
selective abstraction 245
selective exposure hypothesis 482
selective optimisation with compensation 82
selective social interaction theory 73
self
ideal 601
proprium 614
Rogers' conception of 594
role in cognitive dissonance 489
self-actualisation
characteristics of 587–588
defined 585, 594
developmental role of 598–600
in hierarchy of needs 351, 353
measurement of 591
need for 586
Rogers' approach to 594–596
social factors in 594–596
self-affirmation theory 489
self-awareness 205
self-blame 430
self-categorisation 511, 520–521
self-concept 403, 595–596, 601
self-consistency 479, 489
self-control 358–359
self-control model 740
self-directed learning 370
self-doubt 61
self-efficacy
attitudes and 451
behaviour change and 371–372

self-efficacy (*Continued*)
  components of 697
  improvement of 575–576
  measurement of 576–577
  as self-regulatory process 574–575
  stress and 717–718
self-enhancing bias 429–430
self-esteem
  behaviour change and 372–373
  persuasion and 470–471
  stress and 717–718
self-handicapping 430
self-identity 457
self-perception theory 422, 490
self-promotion 477
self-protecting bias 429–430
self-regulation/management 205, 574–575
self-reinforcement 573
self-schemas 119, 403
self-serving biases 429–430
self-standards 489
self-transcendence 351
Seligman, Martin 30–32, 245–246
Selye, Hans 692–694
semantic memory 102–103
sender (source) 463–465
sensitisation 4
sensorimotor intelligence 50
sensorimotor stage 51–52
sensory memory 93–94
sensory overload 543–544
sentiments 616
serial position effect 105–107
serial recall 105
serotonin 246, 248
set point 355
sex differences 74–78 *see also* gender
  alcohol abuse 318
  alcohol effects 308
  communication 544–545
  conformity 507
  depression 242–243, 666, 732
  emotional intelligence 212–213
  intelligence 198
  limbic system 666
  moral reasoning 80–81
  persuasibility 471
  smoking 321, 330–331
  stress response 694, 732
sexual assault 292, 311
sexual decision making, alcohol use and 311
sexual dysfunction, smoking-related 330
sexuality 360
  in adolescence 362
  in adulthood 49, 71–72
  safe sex 448–449
sexual motivation 360
sexual orientation 360–362
  origins of 361–362
  social development and 71–72
shallow judgments 109
shaping 21
shared environments 186–187
sharpening 121, 435
Sheldon, William 611–612
shift and persist strategies 719
short-term memory (STM) 95–98, 405
shuttle box 245–246
sidestream smoke 331
signal (message) 464, 466–470
similarity 464
Simon, Theodore 140
Singer, Jerome 676–677
situational (external) attribution 418
situational variables 455, 699–701
Situation Motivational Scale 369
Sixteen Personality Factor (16PF) questionnaire 617–619
skin conductance response 4, 24
Skinner, B. F. 13–18, 24
Skinner box 14
sleep aids 278
sleep disorders, dissociation with 254
sleeper effect 470
small group discussion 533
smokeless tobacco 326–327
smoking
  marijuana 260, 287–290
  tobacco *see* tobacco use
'snake in the grass effect' 32
snuff 327
social anxiety disorder 225–226, 237, 240
social awareness 205
social change 512–522
social cognition 396–398, 416–417
social comparative context 504
social desirability bias 443
social development 59–74
  adolescence 67–70
  adulthood 70–74
  childhood 62–67
  defined 59
  Erikson's psychosocial stages 60–62, 70–71, 73
social disorder, depression as 244
social distance 682
social encoding 403–405
social factors
  alcohol abuse 317–318
  attitudes 455
  attributions 436–437
  conformity 508–509
  health 373–375
  pain 639–640
  self-actualisation 594–596
  sexuality 362
  stress 714–719
social identity 190–191, 408, 433, 455, 511, 520–521
social impact 522
social inference 409–414
social influence 495–499
  conformity bias 512–513
  genetic model of 515–517
  groupthink 513–515
  majority 517, 520–522
  minority 512, 517, 520–522
  norms 504–505
  power and 497–499
  processes of 509–511, 513, 517
social information gathering 410
social interest 354
socialisation 62
  gender 76–78
  group theory of 190–191
social judgeability 401, 408–410
social learning theory 570–577
social memory 405–409
social neuroscience 397–398, 416
social power 498
social psychology 394–528
  affect 414–416
  aggression 26–27
  attitude *see* attitudes
  attribution theory *see* attribution
  cognition 396–398, 416–417
  compliance *see* compliance
  conformity *see* conformity
  emotion 414–416
  emotional intelligence 206–207
  impressions of other people 398–401
  intelligence 190–191
  memory for people 405–409
  motivation 354
  obedience 495–496, 499–504
  persuasive communication *see* persuasion
  social encoding 403–405
  social inference 409–414
  social influence *see* social influence
  social schemas 401–403
Social Readjustment Rating Scale (SRRS) 689–690
social representations 434–435, |459–460
social schemas 401–403
social skills/management 205
social smoking 322–323
social support 373–375, 726–727
sociobiological model of personality disorders 251

sociocognitive model 442–443
of dissociative disorders 255–256
sociocultural theory of cognitive development 56–57
socioeconomic status
attributions and 436–437
intelligence and 191–192
obesity and 274
stress-related illness and 724
somatic marker theory 675, 678
somatic symptom disorder 234
somatotypes 611–612
S-O-R psychology 24–25
source (sender) 463–465
source credibility 464–465
source traits 616
spatial distances 540–541, 682
Spearman, Charles 143–144, 150–151, 160
special education 169–170
Special K 296
specific abilities (s) 144, 156–157
specific attitudes 446
specific phobias 237 *see also* phobias
specific responses 621
speech *see also* communication; language
disorganised 258–259
spinal cord, pain transmission in 648
spirituality 730–731
spontaneous recovery 7, 17–18
Sport Injury Rehabilitation Adherence Scale (SIRAS) 369
S-R psychology 13, 24, 568
stability 422
stagnation 61, 73–74
standard drink (alcoholic) 305–306
standardised intelligence testing 144–152, 161–162
Stanford-Binet test 141–142, 160, 167, 169
state-dependent memory 104
state of mind 347
stereotypes
attribution and 433
defined 401, 432, 441
gender 76
impact of student exchanges on 483
Stern, William 141, 150
Sternberg, Robert 169
steroids 297–298
stigma of mental illness 222, 228–229
stimulants 738
abuse of 279, 282–286
for ADHD 265–266, 279
stimulus
conditioned 5–6
discriminative 17
S-R psychology 13, 24, 568
stress as 688
unconditioned 5–6
stimulus-based account 698
stimulus discrimination 7–8, 17–18
stimulus expectancies 697
stimulus generalisation 7, 17–18
stimulus-response model of personality 568–570
stomach, hunger sensors in 355
stomach ulcers 725–726
storage 91–92
storm-and-stress conception of adolescence 68–69
Strange Situation Test 63–64
strategic branch 200
streptococcal bacteria 240
stress 686–744
approaches to 688–691
causes of 713–719
clinical and experimental approaches to 708–709
coping with 726–732
health behaviour 732–741
defined 688
depression and 243, 246–248
effects of 710–712
health 719–726
physical 711–712
psychological 712–713
measurement of 689–691
responses to 692–696
symptoms of 710
transactional model of 689, 696–705
examples of 701–705, 709–710
research applications of 705–708
transactional matrix 699–701
stress arousal response 735–736
stress event variables 701
stress hormones 689, 735
stress-management scales 207
stress response 203–204
stress-sensitive gene 246–247
striatum 127–128
stroke 330
Structure of Intellect (SI) theory 154–155
students *see* university students
subliminal stimuli 678
substance abuse *see* drug abuse
substance P 647
substantia gelatinosa 647
substantive processing 415
sucking reflex 44
sudden sniffing death syndrome 297
sufficiency threshold 474
suicidal ideation 717
suicide 248–249
sulci 260
summarizing 559
Summerhill experience 589, 599
sunk costs 480
Suomi, Stephen 66
supertraits 621, 624
supplication 477
support groups 384–385
supportive defence 493
supraliminal stimuli 679
surface traits 616
sympathomimetics 735
synesthesia 293
systematic processing 474, 476
Szasz, Thomas 222

T

tabula rasa 50
tainted fruit labels 492
Takahashi, Naoko 345
talking phase 570
tar 325
target behaviours 22
taste aversions 30–31
T cells 720
T-data 617
Teacher Self-Efficacy Scale 577
television media 469, 541–542
telogen effluvium 711
Temgesic (buprenorphine) 291
temperament 62–63 *see also* personality
temperament traits 615
temporomandibular disorder pain 656
tend and befriend 694
teratogens 43–44, 185–186, 313–314, 330
Terman, Lewis 141–142, 144, 148, 150, 160, 173
terminal values 457–458
termination stage 378
terminology 535–536, 544
terror management theory 459, 468
tertiary gain 639
testosterone 75–76
test-retest reliability 167
test-taking anxiety 701–705, 718
tetrahydrocannabinol (THC) 287
thalamus 647, 676
thanatos 350
Thematic Apperception Test (TAT) 344
Theophrastus 608
theory of mind 56
theory of reasoned action (TRA) 445–447
therapeutic adherence *see* adherence
therapeutic relationship
client interview 554–561
collaboration in 386–390

therapeutic relationship (*Continued*)
communication in 531–536
see also communication
counseling in 604–605
therapeutic touch 540
thermal biofeedback 657
thimerosol 264
thinking *see also* cognition; intelligence
depression as disorder of 244–245
third-order conditioning 8
third-person effect 463, 473
Thorazine (chlorpromazine) 224
Thorndike, E. L. 12–13
Thorndike's puzzle box 13
threat appraisal 451, 468
three-component attitude model 440–441
Three-Stratum Model of Human Cognitive Abilities 157
Thurstone, L. L. 152–153, 440
tic disorders 239–240
tobacco industry 321–322, 332
tobacco use 321–336
health hazards of 327–331
physical effects of 323–327
during pregnancy 44, 186, 330
prevalence of 321
prevention of 332–333
quitting 333–336, 738–739, 741
sex differences 321, 330–331
social issues 321–322
stress and 737–739
tobacco products 325–327
token economy 22
Tolman, Edward Chace 25
top-heavy patterns 45
total genetic variance 181
touch, in communication 540
Tourette's disorder 239–240
trait emotional intelligence 210
trait theory *see* personality traits
tranquilizers 292, 738
transactional model of stress 689, 696–705
examples of 701–705, 709–710
research applications of 705–708
transactional matrix 699–701
transcutaneous electrical nerve stimulation (TENS) 652–653
transfer-appropriate processing 108–110
transfer of affect 469
transsexualism 361
transtheoretical model for health behaviour change 377–378
transvestism 361
trauma 688
treatment plans 387–388
Trexan (naltrexone) 291
triarchic theory of intelligence 169
trigeminal neuralgia 637
triglycerides 276
trust 60
Turner, John 496, 510–511
12-step programs 299
Twins Early Development Study (UK) 179
twin studies 17
anxiety disorders 241
autism 263–264
bipolar disorder 247
depression 246
of intelligence 176–177, 182
personality traits 625
schizophrenia 261–262
sexuality 361
two-component attitude model 440
two-factor theory
of emotion 676–677
of intelligence 144
two-process theory 23–24
type 2 diabetes 276, 712
type A personality 718, 723
type B personality 718
type C personality 718–719
type D personality 718–719

U

ulcers 725–726
ultimate attribution error 426, 431
unconditional positive regard 595, 603
unconditioned response (UCR) 5–6
unconditioned stimulus (UCS) 5–6
unconscious 350, 567–568
emotion and 678–680
understanding branch 200
unique traits 616
universality, cultural 226, 671–672
university students
alcohol drinking by 300–305
drug treatment and recovery for 298–299, 319–320
drug use among 279–280
emotional intelligence in 213
exam-taking anxiety 701–705, 718
smoking by 322–324
stressors for 701–705, 715
student exchange 483
testing conditions for 105
unlabelled 567

V

vaccines, autism link with 264
Vaillant, George 73–74
validation process 517
validity
external 28
of intelligence tests 168–169
internal 28
of Maslow's theory 591
of psychiatric diagnosis 227–228
of Rogers' theory 606
values 457–458
moral 450
reinforcement 578
variable interval (VI) schedule 19–20
variable ratio (VR) schedule 19–20
varinicline 335
'v:ed' factor 156–157
ventricles 260
verbal communication 537–539
Vernon, Philip E. 156–157
vested interest 521–522
vicarious dissonance 489
vicarious experience 575
vicarious (observational) learning 26–29
violence
alcohol use and 311
media 27–28
mental illness and 231–232
rape 292, 311
viral infections 720–721
virtual reality systems 386
vision
adulthood 48–49
infancy 44–46
visual analogue scales 649–650
visual cliff 45–46
visual hallucinations 258
visual memory 94–95
visuospatial sketchpad 99
vitamin deficiencies 735
vividness 404
vocabulary 535–537, 544
voice 544
volition 447–451
Vygotsky, Lev 56–57

W

Walk, Richard 45–46
Watson, John B. 3, 9, 44, 240
websites
alcohol abuse education 305
health information 541–542
Wechsler, David 145
Wechsler tests 145–150, 153, 160–161
reliability of 167
validity of 168
Wechsler Adult Intelligence Scale (WAIS) 145, 161, 171

Wechsler-Bellevue Scale 145
Wechsler Intelligence Scale for Children (WISC) 145, 161, 169
Wechsler Preschool and Primary Scale of Intelligence (WPPSI) 161
weight problems 272–274, 311, 357–358, 711, 736
Weiner, Bernard 422
Wellbutrin (bupropion) 335
whole-report procedure 94–95
wide occluder 54
will power 358–359
windowpane (LSD) 293
wisdom 57
within-family factors 187–189
women *see* females; gender; sex differences
Woodcock, Richard W. 158
Woodcock-Johnson III Tests of Cognitive Abilities 161
Woodcock-Johnson Psychoeducational Battery 158, 160
word choice 535–536, 544
working memory 98–100, 405
working memory span 99
workplace, emotional intelligence in 211–212
written communication 541–542
Wundt, Wilhelm 396, 609

xanthines 286

Yale approach to communication 462–463
Yerkes, Robert 142–144, 160
Yerkes-Dodson law 253

Z

Zajonc, Robert 680
Zyban (bupropion) 335
zygote 42